NURSE'S ESSENTIAL DRUG GUIDE 2006

NURSE'S ESSENTIAL DRUG GUIDE 2006

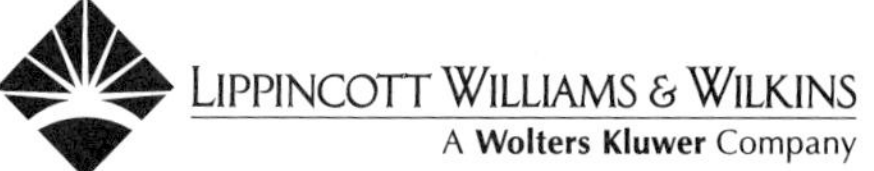

LIPPINCOTT WILLIAMS & WILKINS
A **Wolters Kluwer** Company
Philadelphia • Baltimore • New York • London
Buenos Aires • Hong Kong • Sydney • Tokyo

Staff

Executive Publisher
Judith A. Schilling McCann, RN, MSN

Editorial Director
William J. Kelly

Clinical Director
Joan M. Robinson, RN, MSN

Senior Art Director
Arlene Putterman

Art Director
Elaine Kasmer

Clinical Manager
Eileen Cassin Gallen, RN, BSN

Editorial Project Manager
Christiane L. Brownell

Clinical Editors
Christine M. Damico, RN, MSN, CRNP;
Kimberly A. Zalewski, RN, MSN

Copy Editor
Tom Wolfe

Digital Composition Services
Diane Paluba (manager),
Donald G. Knauss

Manufacturing
Patricia K. Dorshaw (director),
Beth J. Welsh

NEDG06011105-D N
07 06 05 10 9 8 7 6 5 4 3 2 1
ISBN 1-58255-974-0
ISSN 1550-8919

Contents

Contributors and consultants

At the time of publication, the contributors and consultants held the following positions.

Steven R. Abel, PharmD, FASHP
Professor and Head, Department of Pharmacy Practice
Purdue University School of Pharmacy and Pharmacy Sciences
Indianapolis, Ind.

Katrina Allen, RN, MSN, CCRN
Nursing Instructor
Faulkner State Community College
Bay Minette, Ala.

Tricia M. Berry, PharmD, BCPS
Associate Professor of Pharmacy Practice
St. Louis College of Pharmacy

Lawrence P. Carey, PharmD
Assistant Professor
Philadelphia University

Wendy Tagan Conroy, MSN, FNP-BC
Nurse Practitioner
City of Portland (Maine) Public Health Department

Jason C. Cooper, PharmD
Clinical Specialist
Medical University of South Carolina
Charleston

Melissa Devlin, PharmD
Clinical Pharmacist
Excellerx, Inc.
Philadelphia

Jennifer Faulkner, PharmD, BCPP
Clinical Pharmacy Specialist, Psychiatry
Central Texas Veterans Health Care System
Temple

Christopher A. Fausel, PharmD, BCPS, BCOP
Clinical Pharmacist, Adult Hematology and Oncology
Indiana University Hospital
Indianapolis

Dawn Feltner, PharmD
Staff Pharmacist
Acme
Burlington, N.J.

Tatyana Gurvich, PharmD
Clinical Pharmacologist
Glendale (Calif.) Adventist FPRP

Catherine Heyneman, PharmD
Assistant Professor of Pharmacy Practice
Idaho State University
Pocatello

AnhThu Hoang, PharmD
Pharmacist
North York (Ontario) General Hospital

Erin Jaynes, RN, MSN
Administrative Nurse Specialist
Medical College of Ohio
Toledo

William A. Kehoe, PharmD, MA, FCCP, BCPS
Professor of Clinical Pharmacy and Psychology
Chairman, Department of Pharmacy Practice
T.J. Long School of Pharmacy and Health Sciences
University of the Pacific
Stockton, Calif.

Mary Kate Kelly, RPh, PharmD
Publications Director
Institute for Safe Medication Practices
Huntingdon Valley, Pa.

Karla M. Killgore, PharmD
Pharmacist
University of California at San Francisco Medical Center

Thomas Lodise, PharmD
Assistant Professor
Albany (N.Y.) College of Pharmacy

Dawna Martich, RN, BSN, MSN
Clinical Trainer
American Healthways
Pittsburgh

Rickey C. Miller, RPh, PharmD, BCOP
Clinical Pharmacy Specialist
Allegheny General Hospital
Pittsburgh

Jean Nappi, PharmD, FCCP, BCPS
Professor of Pharmacy and Clinical Sciences
College of Pharmacy
Medical University of South Carolina
Charleston

William O'Hara, RPh, BS, PharmD
Clinical Team Leader
Thomas Jefferson Hospital
Philadelphia

Christine Price, PharmD
Clinical Coordinator, Department of Pharmacy
Morton Plant Mease Health Care
Clearwater, Fla.

Jeffrey B. Purcell, PharmD
Clinical Lead Pharmacist
Harborview Medical Center
Clinical Associate Professor
University of Washington School of Pharmacy
Seattle

Donna Scemons, RN, MSN, CNS, FNP-C, CWOCN
Family Nurse Practitioner
Healthcare Systems, Inc.
Castaic, Calif.

Mary Clare Schafer, RN, MS, ONC, CIC
Infection Control Coordinator, Osteoporosis Support
Rehabilitation Hospital of South Jersey
Vineland, N.J.

Mary Stahl, RN, APRN, BC, MSN, CCRN
Clinical Nurse Specialist
St. Luke's Hospital
Kansas City, Mo.

Sheryl Thomas, RN, MSN
Nursing Instructor
Wayne County Community College
Detroit

Catherine Ultrino, RN, MSN, OCN
Charge Nurse
Kindred Hospital
Tampa, Fla.

Eva M. Vasquez, PharmD, FCCP, BCPS
Associate Professor
University of Illinois at Chicago

Joanne Whitney, RPh, PharmD, PhD
Director, Drug Products Services
Associate Clinical Professor
Department of Clinical Pharmacy
University of California
San Francisco

Laurie Willhite, RPh, PharmD
Clinical Assistant Professor
University of Minnesota
Minneapolis

Margaret Wilson, RN, MSN, EdD
Nursing Professor
Cypress (Calif.) College

Guide to abbreviations

ACE	angiotensin-converting enzyme
ADH	antidiuretic hormone
AIDS	acquired immunodeficiency syndrome
ALT	alanine transaminase
AST	aspartate transaminase
AV	atrioventricular
b.i.d.	twice daily
BPH	benign prostatic hypertrophy
BSA	body surface area
BUN	blood urea nitrogen
cAMP	cyclic 3', 5' adenosine monophosphate
CBC	complete blood count
CK	creatine kinase
CMV	cytomegalovirus
CNS	central nervous system
COPD	chronic obstructive pulmonary disease
CSF	cerebrospinal fluid
CV	cardiovascular
CVA	cerebrovascular accident
D_5W	dextrose 5% in water
DIC	disseminated intravascular coagulation
dl	deciliter
DNA	deoxyribonucleic acid
ECG	electrocardiogram
EEG	electroencephalogram
EENT	eyes, ears, nose, throat
FDA	Food and Drug Administration
g	gram
G	gauge
GABA	gamma-aminobutyric acid
GFR	glomerular filtration rate
GGT	gamma-glutamyltransferase
GI	gastrointestinal
gtt	drops
GU	genitourinary
G6PD	glucose-6-phosphate dehydrogenase
H_1	histamine$_1$
H_2	histamine$_2$
HDL	high-density lipoprotein
HIV	human immunodeficiency virus
HMG-CoA	3-hydroxy-3-methylglutaryl coenzyme A
h.s.	at bedtime
I.D.	intradermal
I.M.	intramuscular
INR	International Normalized Ratio
IPPB	intermittent positive-pressure breathing
IU	international unit
I.V.	intravenous
kg	kilogram
L	liter
lb	pound
LDH	lactate dehydrogenase
LDL	low-density lipoprotein
M	molar
m^2	square meter
MAO	monoamine oxidase
mcg	microgram
mEq	milliequivalent

mg	milligram
MI	myocardial infarction
min	minute
ml	milliliter
mm^3	cubic millimeter
mo	month
msec	millisecond
NSAID	nonsteroidal anti-inflammatory drug
OTC	over-the-counter
PABA	para-aminobenzoic acid
PCA	patient-controlled analgesia
P.O.	by mouth
P.R.	by rectum
p.r.n.	as needed
PT	prothrombin time
PTT	partial thromboplastin time
PVC	premature ventricular contraction
q	every
q.i.d.	four times daily
RBC	red blood cell
RDA	recommended daily allowance
REM	rapid eye movement
RNA	ribonucleic acid
RSV	respiratory syncytial virus
SA	sinoatrial
S.C.	subcutaneous
sec	second
SIADH	syndrome of inappropriate antidiuretic hormone
S.L.	sublingual
SSRI	selective serotonin reuptake inhibitor
T_3	triiodothyronine
T_4	thyroxine
t.i.d.	three times daily
tsp	teaspoon
USP	United States Pharmacopeia
UTI	urinary tract infection
WBC	white blood cell
wk	week

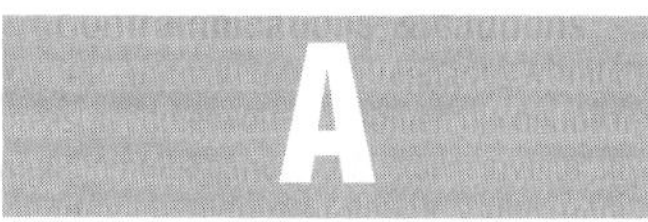

abacavir sulfate
Ziagen

Pregnancy risk category C

Indications & dosages
➲ HIV-1 infection
Adults: 300 mg P.O. b.i.d. with other antiretrovirals.
Children ages 3 months to 16 years: 8 mg/kg P.O. b.i.d., up to maximum of 300 mg P.O. b.i.d., with other antiretrovirals.

Contraindications & cautions
• Contraindicated in patients hypersensitive to drug or its components.
• Use cautiously when giving drug to patients at risk for liver disease. Lactic acidosis and severe hepatomegaly with steatosis, including fatal cases, have been reported with the use of nucleoside analogues alone or in combination, including abacavir and other antiretrovirals. Stop treatment with drug if events occur.
• Use cautiously in pregnant women because the effects of abacavir on pregnancy are unknown. Use during pregnancy only if the potential benefits outweigh the risk. Register pregnant women taking abacavir with the Antiretroviral Pregnancy Registry at 1-800-258-4263.

Adverse reactions
CNS: insomnia and sleep disorders, fever, headache.
GI: *nausea, vomiting, diarrhea, anorexia.*
Skin: rash.
Other: ***hypersensitivity reaction***.

Interactions
Drug-lifestyle. *Alcohol use:* May decrease elimination of abacavir, increasing overall exposure to drug. Monitor alcohol consumption. Discourage use together.

Nursing considerations
• Women are more likely than men to experience lactic acidosis and severe hepatomegaly with steatosis. Obesity and prolonged nucleoside exposure may be risk factors.
!!ALERT Abacavir can cause fatal hypersensitivity reactions; if patient develops signs or symptoms of hypersensitivity (such as fever, rash, fatigue, nausea, vomiting, diarrhea, or abdominal pain), stop drug and notify prescriber immediately.
!!ALERT Don't restart drug after a hypersensitivity reaction because severe signs and symptoms will recur within hours and may include life-threatening hypotension and death. To facilitate reporting of hypersensitivity reactions, register patients with the Abacavir Hypersensitivity Reaction Registry at 1-800-270-0425.
• Always give drug with other antiretrovirals, never alone.
• Because of a high rate of early virologic resistance, triple antiretroviral therapy with abacavir, lamivudine, and tenofovir shouldn't be used as new treatment regimen for naïve or pretreated patients. Monitor patients currently controlled with this combination and those who use this combination in addition to other antiretrovirals, and consider modification of therapy.
• Drug may mildly elevate glucose level.
!!ALERT Don't confuse abacavir with amprenavir.

Patient teaching
• Inform patient that abacavir can cause a life-threatening hypersensitivity reaction. Warn patient who develops signs or symptoms of hypersensitivity (such as fever, rash, severe tiredness, achiness, a generally ill feeling, nausea, vomiting, diarrhea, or stomach pain) to stop taking drug and notify prescriber immediately.
• Include information leaflet about drug with each new prescription and refill. Patient also should receive, and be instructed to carry, a warning card summarizing signs and symptoms of abacavir hypersensitivity reaction.
• Inform patient that this drug doesn't cure HIV infection. Tell patient that drug doesn't reduce the risk of transmission of HIV to others through sexual contact or blood contamination and that its long-term effects are unknown.
• Tell patient to take drug exactly as prescribed.

• Inform patient that drug can be taken with or without food.

abciximab

ReoPro

Pregnancy risk category C

Indications & dosages

➲ Adjunct to percutaneous coronary intervention (PCI) to prevent acute cardiac ischemic complications

Adults: 0.25 mg/kg as an I.V. bolus given 10 to 60 minutes before start of PCI ; then a continuous I.V. infusion of 0.125 mcg/kg/minute to a maximum of 10 mcg/minute for 12 hours.

➲ Unstable angina not responding to conventional medical therapy in patients scheduled for PCI within 24 hours

Adults: 0.25 mg/kg as an I.V. bolus; then an 18- to 24-hour infusion of 10 mcg/minute concluding 1 hour after PCI.

Contraindications & cautions

• Contraindicated in patients hypersensitive to drug, its ingredients, or murine proteins.
• Contraindicated in those with active internal bleeding, significant GI or GU bleeding within 6 weeks, CVA within past 2 years, significant residual neurologic deficit, bleeding diathesis, thrombocytopenia (platelet count under 100,000/mm^3), major surgery or trauma within 6 weeks, intracranial neoplasm, intracranial arteriovenous malformation, intracranial aneurysm, severe uncontrolled hypertension, or history of vasculitis.
• Contraindicated when oral anticoagulants have been given within past 7 days unless PT is 1.2 times control or less, or when I.V. dextran is used before or during PCI.
• Use with caution in patients at increased risk for bleeding, including those weighing less than 165 lb (75 kg) or older than age 65, those who have a history of GI disease, and those who are receiving thrombolytics. Conditions that increase patient's risk of bleeding include PCI within 12 hours of onset of symptoms for acute MI, prolonged PCI (lasting longer than 70 minutes), or failed PCI. Heparin used with drug also may contribute to the risk of bleeding.

Adverse reactions

CNS: hyperesthesia, hypoesthesia, confusion, headache, pain.
CV: *hypotension*, ***bradycardia***, peripheral edema.
EENT: abnormal vision.
GI: *nausea*, vomiting, abdominal pain.
Hematologic: ***bleeding***, ***thrombocytopenia***, anemia, leukocytosis.
Respiratory: pleural effusion, pleurisy, pneumonia.

Interactions

Drug-drug. *Antiplatelet drugs, dipyridamole, heparin, NSAIDs, other anticoagulants, thrombolytics, ticlopidine:* May increase risk of bleeding. Monitor patient closely.

Nursing considerations

• The risk of bleeding is reduced by using low-dose, weight-adjusted heparin, early sheath removal, and careful maintenance of access site immobility.
• Review and monitor other drugs patient is taking; drug is intended for use with aspirin and heparin.

!!ALERT Keep epinephrine, dopamine, theophylline, antihistamines, and corticosteroids readily available in case of anaphylaxis.

• Monitor patient closely for bleeding at the arterial access site used for cardiac catheterization and internal bleeding involving the GI or GU tract or retroperitoneal sites.
• Institute bleeding precautions. Keep patient on bed rest for 6 to 8 hours after sheath removal or end of drug infusion, whichever is later. Minimize or avoid, if possible, arterial and venous punctures, I.M. injections, urinary catheters, nasogastric tubes, automatic blood pressure cuffs, and nasotracheal intubation.
• During abciximab infusion, remove sheath only after heparin has been stopped and its effects largely reversed.
• Obtain platelet count before treatment, 2 to 4 hours after bolus dose, and 24 hours after bolus dose or before discharge, whichever is first.
• Anticipate stopping abciximab and giving platelets for severe bleeding or thrombocytopenia.

!!ALERT Don't confuse abciximab with arcitumomab.

Patient teaching

- Explain use and administration of drug to patient and family.
- Instruct patient to report adverse reactions immediately.

acamprosate calcium
Campral

Pregnancy risk category C

Indications & dosages

➲ Adjunct to management of alcohol abstinence
Adults: 666 mg P.O. t.i.d.

In patients with creatinine clearance of 30 to 50 ml/minute, give 333 mg t.i.d.

Contraindications & cautions

- Contraindicated in patients allergic to drug or its components and in those whose creatinine clearance is 30 ml/minute or less.
- Use cautiously in pregnant or breast-feeding women, elderly patients, patients with moderate renal impairment, and patients with a history of depression and suicidal thoughts or attempts.

Adverse reactions

CNS: abnormal thinking, amnesia, anxiety, asthenia, depression, dizziness, headache, insomnia, paresthesia, somnolence, ***suicidal thoughts***, syncope, tremor.
CV: hypertension, palpitations, peripheral edema, vasodilation.
EENT: abnormal vision, pharyngitis, rhinitis.
GI: abdominal pain, anorexia, constipation, *diarrhea*, dry mouth, dyspepsia, flatulence, increased appetite, nausea, taste disturbance, vomiting.
GU: impotence.
Metabolic: weight gain.
Musculoskeletal: arthralgia, back pain, chest pain, myalgia.
Respiratory: bronchitis, dyspnea, increased cough.
Skin: increased sweating, pruritus, rash.
Other: accidental injury, chills, decreased libido, flulike symptoms, infection, pain.

Interactions

None significant.

Nursing considerations

- Use only after the patient successfully becomes abstinent from drinking.
- Drug doesn't eliminate or reduce withdrawal symptoms.
- Monitor patient for development of depression or suicidal thoughts.
- Drug doesn't cause alcohol aversion or a disulfiram-like reaction if used with alcohol.

Patient teaching

- Tell patient to continue the alcohol abstinence program, including counseling and support.
- Advise patient to notify his prescriber if he develops depression, anxiety, thoughts of suicide, or severe diarrhea.
- Caution patient's family or caregiver to watch for signs of depression or suicidal ideation.
- Tell patient that drug may be taken without regard to meals, but that taking it with meals may help him remember it.
- Tell patient not to crush, break, or chew the tablets but to swallow them whole.
- Advise women to use effective contraception while taking this drug. Tell patient to contact her prescriber if she becomes pregnant or plans to become pregnant.
- Explain that this drug may impair judgment, thinking, or motor skills. Urge patient to use caution when driving or performing hazardous activities until drug's effects are known.
- Tell patient to continue taking acamprosate and to contact his prescriber if he resumes drinking alcohol.

acarbose
Prandase†, Precose

Pregnancy risk category B

Indications & dosages

➲ Adjunct to diet to lower glucose level in patients with type 2 (non–insulin-dependent) diabetes whose hyperglycemia can't be managed by diet alone or by diet and a sulfonylurea; adjunct to insulin or metformin therapy in patients with type 2 (non–insulin-dependent) diabetes whose hyperglycemia can't be managed

by diet, exercise, and insulin or metformin alone
Adults: Individualized. Initially, 25 mg P.O. t.i.d. with first bite of each main meal. Adjust dosage q 4 to 8 weeks, based on 1-hour postprandial glucose level and tolerance. Maintenance dosage is 50 to 100 mg P.O. t.i.d.

For patients weighing less than 60 kg (132 lb), don't exceed 50 mg P.O. t.i.d. For patients weighing more than 60 kg, don't exceed 100 mg P.O. t.i.d.

Contraindications & cautions

- Contraindicated in patients hypersensitive to drug and in those with diabetic ketoacidosis, cirrhosis, inflammatory bowel disease, colonic ulceration, renal impairment, partial intestinal obstruction, predisposition to intestinal obstruction, chronic intestinal disease with marked disorder of digestion or absorption, or conditions that may deteriorate because of increased intestinal gas formation.
- Contraindicated in pregnant or breastfeeding patients and those with creatinine level greater than 2 mg/dl.
- Use cautiously in patients receiving a sulfonylurea or insulin.
- Safety and efficacy of drug haven't been established in children.

Adverse reactions

GI: *abdominal pain, diarrhea, flatulence.*
Metabolic: hypocalcemia.

Interactions

Drug-drug. *Calcium channel blockers, corticosteroids, estrogens, fosphenytoin, hormonal contraceptives, isoniazid, nicotinic acid, phenothiazine, phenytoin, sympathomimetics, thiazides and other diuretics, thyroid products:* May cause hyperglycemia when used together or hypoglycemia when withdrawn. Monitor glucose level.
Digestive enzyme preparations containing carbohydrate-splitting enzymes (such as amylase, pancreatin), intestinal adsorbents (such as activated charcoal): May reduce effect of acarbose. Avoid using together.
Digoxin: May reduce digoxin level. Monitor digoxin level.

Nursing considerations

- Closely monitor patients receiving a sulfonylurea or insulin; acarbose may increase risk of hypoglycemia. If hypoglycemia occurs, treat patient with oral glucose (dextrose). Severe hypoglycemia may require I.V. glucose infusion or glucagon administration. Because dosage adjustments may be needed to prevent further hypoglycemia, report hypoglycemia and treatment required to prescriber.
- Insulin therapy may be needed during increased stress (infection, fever, surgery, or trauma). Monitor patient closely for hyperglycemia.
- Monitor patient's 1-hour postprandial glucose level to determine therapeutic effectiveness of acarbose and to identify appropriate dose. Report hyperglycemia to prescriber. Thereafter, measure glycosylated hemoglobin level every 3 months.
- Monitor transaminase level every 3 months in first year of therapy and periodically thereafter in patients receiving more than 50 mg three times a day. Report abnormalities; dosage adjustment or drug withdrawal may be needed.

Patient teaching

- Tell patient to take drug daily with first bite of each of three main meals.
- Explain that therapy relieves symptoms but doesn't cure disease.
- Stress importance of adhering to therapeutic regimen, specific diet, weight reduction, exercise, and hygiene programs. Show patient how to monitor glucose level and to recognize and treat hyperglycemia.
- Teach patient taking a sulfonylurea how to recognize hypoglycemia. Advise treating symptoms with a form of dextrose rather than with a product containing table sugar.
- Urge patient to wear or carry medical identification at all times.
- Advise patient that adverse reactions usually occur in the first few weeks of therapy and diminish over time.

acetaminophen (APAP, paracetamol)

Abenol† ◇, Acephen, Aceta ◇, Acetaminophen ◇, Actamin ◇, Aminofen ◇, Apacet ◇, Apo-Acetaminophen† ◇, Atasol† ◇, Banesin ◇, Dapa ◇, Exdol†, Feverall ◇, Genapap ◇, Genebs ◇, Liquiprin ◇, Neopap ◇, Oraphen-PD ◇, Panadol ◇, Redutemp ◇, Robigesic† ◇, Rounox† ◇, Snaplets-FR ◇, St. Joseph Aspirin-Free Fever Reducer for Children ◇, Suppap ◇, Tapanol ◇, Tempra ◇, Tylenol ◇, Valorin ◇

Pregnancy risk category B

Indications & dosages

➲ Mild pain or fever

P.O.

Adults: 325 to 650 mg P.O. q 4 to 6 hours; or 1 g P.O. t.i.d. or q.i.d., p.r.n. Or, two extended-release caplets P.O. q 8 hours. Maximum, 4 g daily. For long-term therapy, don't exceed 2.6 g daily unless prescribed and monitored closely by health care provider.

Children older than age 14: 650 mg P.O. q 4 to 6 hours, p.r.n.

Children ages 12 to 14: 640 mg P.O. q 4 to 6 hours, p.r.n.

Children age 11: 480 mg P.O. q 4 to 6 hours, p.r.n.

Children ages 9 to 10: 400 mg P.O. q 4 to 6 hours, p.r.n.

Children ages 6 to 8: 320 mg P.O. q 4 to 6 hours, p.r.n.

Children ages 4 to 5: 240 mg P.O. q 4 to 6 hours, p.r.n.

Children ages 2 to 3: 160 mg P.O. q 4 to 6 hours, p.r.n.

Children ages 12 to 23 months: 120 mg P.O. q 4 to 6 hours, p.r.n.

Children ages 4 to 11 months: 80 mg P.O. q 4 to 6 hours, p.r.n.

Children up to age 3 months: 40 mg P.O. q 4 to 6 hours, p.r.n. Or, 10 to 15 mg/kg/dose q 4 hours, p.r.n. Don't exceed five doses in 24 hours.

P.R.

Adults: 650 mg P.R. q 4 to 6 hours, p.r.n. Maximum, 4 g daily. For long-term therapy, don't exceed 2.6 g daily unless prescribed and monitored closely by health care provider.

Children ages 6 to 12: 325 mg P.R. q 4 to 6 hours, p.r.n.

Children ages 3 to 6: 120 to 125 mg P.R. q 4 to 6 hours, p.r.n.

Children ages 1 to 3: 80 mg P.R. q 4 to 6 hours, p.r.n.

Children ages 3 months to 11 months: 80 mg P.R. q 6 hours, p.r.n.

Contraindications & cautions

- Contraindicated in patients hypersensitive to drug.
- Use cautiously in patients with long-term alcohol use because therapeutic doses cause hepatotoxicity in these patients.

Adverse reactions

Hematologic: hemolytic anemia, ***neutropenia, leukopenia, pancytopenia.***
Hepatic: jaundice.
Metabolic: ***hypoglycemia.***
Skin: rash, urticaria.

Interactions

Drug-drug. *Barbiturates, carbamazepine, hydantoins, rifampin, sulfinpyrazone:* High doses or long-term use of these drugs may reduce therapeutic effects and enhance hepatotoxic effects of acetaminophen. Avoid using together.

Lamotrigine: May decrease lamotrigine level. Monitor patient for therapeutic effects.

Warfarin: May increase hypoprothrombinemic effects with long-term use with high doses of acetaminophen. Monitor INR closely.

Zidovudine: May decrease zidovudine effect. Monitor patient closely.

Drug-herb. *Watercress:* May inhibit oxidative metabolism of acetaminophen. Discourage use together.

Drug-food. *Caffeine:* May enhance analgesic effects of acetaminophen. Products may combine caffeine and acetaminophen for therapeutic advantage.

Drug-lifestyle. *Alcohol use:* May increase risk of hepatic damage. Discourage use together.

Nursing considerations

!!ALERT Many OTC and prescription products contain acetaminophen; be aware of this when calculating total daily dose.

• Use liquid form for children and patients who have difficulty swallowing.
• In children, don't exceed five doses in 24 hours.

Patient teaching

• Tell parents to consult prescriber before giving drug to children younger than age 2.
• Advise patient that drug is only for short-term use and to consult prescriber if giving to children for longer than 5 days or adults for longer than 10 days.
!!ALERT Advise patient or caregiver that many OTC products contain acetaminophen; be aware of this when calculating total daily dose.
• Tell patient not to use for marked fever (temperature higher than 103.1° F [39.5° C]), fever persisting longer than 3 days, or recurrent fever unless directed by prescriber.
!!ALERT Warn patient that high doses or unsupervised long-term use can cause liver damage. Excessive alcohol use may increase the risk of liver damage. Caution long-term alcoholics to limit acetaminophen intake to less than or equal to 2 g/day.
• Tell breast-feeding woman that acetaminophen appears in breast milk in low levels (less than 1% of dose). Drug may be used safely if therapy is short-term and doesn't exceed recommended doses.

acetylcysteine

Acetadote, Mucomyst, Mucosil-10, Mucosil-20

Pregnancy risk category B

Indications & dosages

➲ Adjunct therapy for abnormal viscid or thickened mucous secretions in patients with pneumonia, bronchitis, bronchiectasis, primary amyloidosis of the lung, tuberculosis, cystic fibrosis, emphysema, atelectasis, pulmonary complications of thoracic surgery, or CV surgery
Adults and children: 1 to 2 ml 10% or 20% solution by direct instillation into trachea as often as q hour. Or, 1 to 10 ml of 20% solution or 2 to 20 ml of 10% solution by nebulization q 2 to 6 hours, p.r.n.

➲ Acetaminophen toxicity
Adults and children: Initially, 140 mg/kg P.O.; then 70 mg/kg P.O. q 4 hours for 17 doses (total). Or, a loading dose of 150 mg/kg I.V. over 15 minutes; then I.V. maintenance dose of 50 mg/kg infused over 4 hours, followed by 100 mg/kg infused over 16 hours.

Contraindications & cautions

• Contraindicated in patients hypersensitive to drug.
• Use cautiously in elderly or debilitated patients with severe respiratory insufficiency. Use I.V. formulation cautiously in patients with asthma or a history of bronchospasm.

Adverse reactions

CNS: fever, drowsiness, abnormal thinking, gait disturbances.
CV: tachycardia, hypotension, hypertension, flushing, chest tightness.
EENT: *rhinorrhea*, ear pain, eye pain, pharyngitis, throat tightness.
GI: *stomatitis, nausea, vomiting.*
Respiratory: rhonchi, ***bronchospasm***, dyspnea, cough.
Skin: rash, clamminess, diaphoresis, pruritus, urticaria.
Other: ***angioedema***, chills, *anaphylactoid reaction.*

Interactions

Drug-drug. *Activated charcoal:* May limit acetylcysteine's effectiveness. Avoid using activated charcoal before or with acetylcysteine.

Nursing considerations

• Use plastic, glass, stainless steel, or another nonreactive metal when giving by nebulization. Hand-bulb nebulizers aren't recommended because output is too small and particle size too large.
• Drug is physically or chemically incompatible with tetracyclines, erythromycin lactobionate, amphotericin B, and ampicillin sodium. If given by aerosol inhalation, nebulize these drugs separately. Iodized oil, trypsin, and hydrogen peroxide are physically incompatible with acetylcysteine; don't add to nebulizer.
• Drug smells strongly of sulfur. Mixing oral form with juice or cola improves its taste.

• Drug delivered through nasogastric tube may be diluted with water.
• Monitor cough type and frequency.
!!ALERT Monitor patient for bronchospasm, especially if he has asthma.
• Use fresh dilutions within 1 hour. Store undiluted solutions that have been opened in the refrigerator for up to 96 hours.
• Ingestion of more than 150 mg/kg of acetaminophen may cause liver toxicity. Measure acetaminophen level 4 hours after ingestion to determine risk of liver toxicity.
!!ALERT Acetylcysteine is used to treat acetaminophen overdose within 24 hours after ingestion. Start treatment immediately as prescribed; don't wait for results of acetaminophen level. Acetadote should be given within 8 to 10 hours after acetaminophen ingestion to minimize hepatic injury.
• If you suspect acetaminophen overdose, get baseline AST, ALT, bilirubin, PT, BUN, creatinine, glucose, and electrolyte levels.
• Dilute oral doses used in treating acetaminophen overdose with cola, fruit juice, or water before giving. Dilute the 20% solution to 5% (add 3 ml of diluent to each milliliter of acetylcysteine). If patient vomits within 1 hour of receiving loading or maintenance dose, repeat dose. Use diluted solution within 1 hour.
!!ALERT Monitor patient receiving I.V. acetylcysteine for anaphylactoid reactions.
• Be aware that facial erythema may occur within 30 to 60 minutes after the start of an I.V. infusion and usually resolves without infusion interruption.
• When acetaminophen level returns to below toxic level according to nomogram, acetylcysteine therapy may be stopped.
!!ALERT Don't confuse acetylcysteine with acetylcholine.

Patient teaching

• Warn patient that drug may have a foul taste or smell that some patients find distressing.
• For maximum effect, instruct patient to clear his airway by coughing before aerosol administration.

activated charcoal

Actidose ◇, Actidose-Aqua ◇, Actidose with Sorbitol ◇, CharcoAid ◇, CharcoAid 2000 ◇, CharcoCaps ◇, Liqui-Char ◇

Pregnancy risk category C

Indications & dosages

➲ Flatulence, dyspepsia
Adults: 600 mg to 5 g P.O. as single dose or 0.975 to 3.9 g P.O. t.i.d. after meals.
➲ Poisoning
Adults and children: Initially, 1 to 2 g/kg (30 to 100 g) P.O. or 10 times the amount of poison ingested as a suspension in 120 to 240 ml (4 to 8 ounces) of water.

Contraindications & cautions

No known contraindications.

Adverse reactions

GI: *black stools*, nausea, constipation, ***intestinal obstruction***.

Interactions

Drug-drug. *Acetaminophen, barbiturates, carbamazepine, digitoxin, digoxin, furosemide, glutethimide, hydantoins, methotrexate, nizatidine, phenothiazines, phenylbutazone, propoxyphene, salicylates, sulfonamides, sulfonylureas, tetracyclines, theophyllines, tricyclic antidepressants, valproic acid:* May reduce absorption of these drugs. Give charcoal at least 2 hours before or 1 hour after other drugs.
Acetylcysteine, ipecac: May inactivate these drugs. Give charcoal after vomiting has been induced by ipecac; remove charcoal by nasogastric tube before giving acetylcysteine.
Drug-food. *Milk, ice cream, sherbet:* May decrease adsorptive capacity of charcoal. Discourage use together.

Nursing considerations

• Although there are no known contraindications, drug isn't effective for treating all acute poisonings.
!!ALERT Drug is commonly used for treating poisoning or overdose with acetaminophen, aspirin, atropine, barbiturates, dextropropoxyphene, digoxin, poisonous mushrooms, oxalic acid, parathion, phenol, phenytoin, propantheline, propoxyphene,

strychnine, or tricyclic antidepressants. Check with poison control center for use in other types of poisonings or overdoses.
- Give after emesis is complete because activated charcoal absorbs and inactivates ipecac syrup.
- For maximal effect, give within 30 minutes after poison ingestion.
- Mix powder (most effective form) with tap water to consistency of thick syrup. Adding a small amount of fruit juice or flavoring makes mix more palatable. Don't mix with ice cream, milk, or sherbet because these decrease adsorptive capacity of activated charcoal.

!! ALERT Don't aspirate or allow patient to aspirate charcoal powder; this has resulted in death.
- Give by large-bore nasogastric tube after lavage, if needed.
- If patient vomits shortly after administration, be prepared to repeat dose.
- Space doses at least 1 hour apart from other drugs if treatment is for indications other than poisoning.
- Follow treatment with stool softener or laxative to prevent constipation unless sorbitol is part of product ingredients. Preparations made with sorbitol have a laxative effect that lessens risk of severe constipation or fecal impaction.
- Don't use charcoal with sorbitol in fructose-intolerant patients or in children younger than age 1.

!! ALERT Drug is ineffective for poisoning or overdose of cyanide, mineral acids, caustic alkalis, and organic solvents; it's not very effective for overdose of ethanol, lithium, methanol, and iron salts.

!! ALERT Don't confuse Actidose with Actos.

Patient teaching

- Explain use and administration of drug to patient (if awake) and family.
- Warn patient that stools will be black until all the charcoal has passed through the body.
- Instruct patient to drink 6 to 8 glasses of liquid per day because charcoal can cause constipation.

acyclovir (systemic)
Avirax†, Zovirax

acyclovir sodium
Avirax†, Zovirax

Pregnancy risk category C

Indications & dosages

➲ First and recurrent episodes of mucocutaneous herpes simplex virus (HSV-1 and HSV-2) infections in immunocompromised patients; severe first episodes of genital herpes in patients who aren't immunocompromised

Adults and children age 12 and older: 5 mg/kg given I.V. over 1 hour q 8 hours for 7 days. Give for 5 to 7 days for severe first episode of genital herpes.

Children younger than age 12: 10 mg/kg given I.V. over 1 hour q 8 hours for 7 days.

➲ First genital herpes episode

Adults: 200 mg P.O. q 4 hours while awake, five times daily; or 400 mg P.O. q 8 hours. Continue for 7 to 10 days.

➲ Intermittent therapy for recurrent genital herpes

Adults: 200 mg P.O. q 4 hours while awake, five times daily. Continue for 5 days. Begin therapy at first sign of recurrence.

➲ Long-term suppressive therapy for recurrent genital herpes

Adults: 400 mg P.O. b.i.d. for up to 12 months. Or, 200 mg P.O. three to five times daily for up to 12 months.

➲ Varicella (chickenpox) infections in immunocompromised patients

Adults and children age 12 and older: 10 mg/kg I.V. over 1 hour q 8 hours for 7 days. Dosage for obese patients is 10 mg/kg based on ideal body weight q 8 hours for 7 days. Don't exceed maximum dosage equivalent of 20 mg/kg q 8 hours.

Children younger than age 12: 20 mg/kg I.V. over 1 hour q 8 hours for 7 days.

➲ Varicella infection in immunocompetent patients

Adults and children weighing more than 40 kg (88 lb): 800 mg P.O. q.i.d. for 5 days.

Children age 2 and older, weighing less than 40 kg: 20 mg/kg (maximum 800 mg/dose) P.O. q.i.d. for 5 days. Start therapy as soon as symptoms appear.

➲ **Acute herpes zoster infection in immunocompetent patients**
Adults and children age 12 and older: 800 mg P.O. q 4 hours five times daily for 7 to 10 days.
➲ **Herpes simplex encephalitis**
Adults and children age 12 and older: 10 mg/kg I.V. over 1 hour q 8 hours for 10 days.
Children ages 3 months to 12 years: 20 mg/kg I.V. over 1 hour q 8 hours for 10 days.
➲ **Neonatal herpes simplex virus infection**
Neonates to 3 months old: 10 mg/kg I.V. over 1 hour q 8 hours for 10 days.

For patients receiving the I.V. form, if creatinine clearance is 25 to 50 ml/minute, give 100% of dose q 12 hours; if clearance is 10 to 24 ml/minute, give 100% of dose q 24 hours; if clearance is less than 10 ml/minute, give 50% of dose q 24 hours.

For patients receiving the P.O. form, if normal dose is 200 mg q 4 hours five times daily and creatinine clearance is less than 10 ml/minute, give 200 mg P.O. q 12 hours. If normal dose is 400 mg q 12 hours and clearance is less than 10 ml/ minute, give 200 mg q 12 hours. If normal dose is 800 mg q 4 hours five times daily and clearance is 10 to 25 ml/minute, give 800 mg q 8 hours; if clearance is less than 10 ml/minute, give 800 mg q 12 hours.

Contraindications & cautions

- Contraindicated in patients hypersensitive to drug.
- Use cautiously in patients with neurologic problems, renal disease, or dehydration, and in those receiving other nephrotoxic drugs.
- Because no adequate studies have been done in pregnant women, give acyclovir during pregnancy only if potential benefits outweigh risks to fetus.

Adverse reactions

CNS: *malaise, headache,* ***encephalopathic changes***, (including lethargy, obtundation, tremor, confusion, hallucinations, agitation, ***seizures, coma***).
GI: *nausea, vomiting,* diarrhea.
GU: hematuria, ***acute renal failure***.
Hematologic: ***thrombocytopenia, leukopenia***, thrombocytosis.
Skin: rash, itching, urticaria, *inflammation or phlebitis at injection site.*

Interactions

Drug-drug. *Interferon:* May have synergistic effect. Monitor patient closely.
Probenecid: May increase acyclovir level. Monitor patient for possible toxicity.
Zidovudine: May cause drowsiness or lethargy. Use together cautiously.

Nursing considerations

!!ALERT Don't give I.M. or S.C.
- Monitor renal function if used in patients with renal disease or dehydration and in those taking other nephrotoxic drugs.
- Encephalopathic changes are more likely to occur in patients with neurologic disorders and in those who have had neurologic reactions to cytotoxic drugs.

!!ALERT Don't confuse acyclovir sodium (Zovirax) with acetazolamide sodium (Diamox) vials, which may look alike.
!!ALERT Don't confuse Zovirax with Zyvox.

Patient teaching

- Tell patient to take drug as prescribed, even after he feels better.
- Tell patient drug is effective in managing herpes infection but doesn't eliminate or cure it. Warn patient that acyclovir won't prevent spread of infection to others.
- Tell patient to avoid sexual contact while visible lesions are present.
- Teach patient about early signs and symptoms of herpes infection (such as tingling, itching, or pain).
- Tell him to notify prescriber and get a prescription for acyclovir before the infection fully develops. Early treatment is most effective.

acyclovir (topical)
Avirax†, Zovirax

Pregnancy risk category B

Indications & dosages

➲ **Initial herpes genitalis; limited, non-life-threatening mucocutaneous herpes simplex virus infections in immunocompromised patients**
Adults and children 12 years and older: Cover all lesions q 3 hours six times daily

for 7 days. Although dose varies depending on total lesion area, use about ½ -inch (1.3-cm) ribbon of ointment on each 4-inch (10-cm) square of surface area.

➲ **Recurrent herpes labialis (cold sores)**
Adults and children 12 years and older: Apply cream five times daily for 4 days. Start therapy as early as possible after signs and symptoms start.

Contraindications & cautions

- Contraindicated in patients hypersensitive to drug and patients with chemical intolerance to drug.

Adverse reactions

Skin: eczema; *mild pain, burning or stinging*; rash; dryness; pruritus; contact dermatitis; application site reactions.
Other: ***angioedema***, anaphylaxis.

Interactions

None significant.

Nursing considerations

- Start therapy as early as possible after signs or symptoms begin.
- Apply drug with a finger cot or rubber glove to prevent autoinoculation of other body sites and transmission of infection to other persons.
- All lesions must be thoroughly covered.
- Drug is for cutaneous use only; don't apply to eye.
- Drug isn't a cure for herpes, but it helps improve signs and symptoms.

Patient teaching

- Teach patient that virus transmission can occur during treatment.
- Tell patient that there may be some discomfort with application.
- Stress importance of compliance for successful therapy.
- Teach patient that therapy should begin as soon as signs and symptoms appear.
- Tell patient to notify prescriber if adverse reactions occur.
- Instruct patient to store drug in a dry place at 59° to 77° F (15° to 25° C).

adalimumab
Humira

Pregnancy risk category B

Indications & dosages

➲ **To reduce signs and symptoms and structural damage and improve physical function in patients with moderately to severely active rheumatoid arthritis and an inadequate response to one or more disease-modifying antirheumatic drugs**
Adults: 40 mg S.C. q other week. May increase to 40 mg q week if patient isn't taking methotrexate.

Contraindications & cautions

- Contraindicated in patients hypersensitive to adalimumab or its components, in immunosuppressed patients, or those with an active chronic or localized infection.
- Use cautiously in patients with a history of recurrent infection, patients with underlying conditions that predispose them to infections, or those who have lived in areas where tuberculosis and histoplasmosis are endemic.
- Use with anakinra may cause serious infections and isn't recommended.
- Use cautiously in patients with CNS-demyelinating disorders and in elderly patients because of their higher rate of infection and malignancies.
- Don't give adalimumab to pregnant women unless benefits outweigh risks. Because of the risk of serious adverse reactions, the patient should stop breast-feeding or stop using the drug.
- The drug's safety and effectiveness in children haven't been established.

Adverse reactions

CNS: headache.
CV: hypertension.
EENT: *sinusitis.*
GI: nausea, abdominal pain.
GU: urinary tract infection, hematuria.
Hematologic: ***pancytopenia, thrombocytopenia, leukopenia.***
Metabolic: hypercholesterolemia, hyperlipidemia.
Musculoskeletal: back pain.
Respiratory: *upper respiratory tract infection*, bronchitis.

Skin: *rash.*
Other: *injection site reactions (erythema, itching, hemorrhage, pain, swelling),* ***malignancy***, flulike syndrome, *accidental injury*, allergic reactions, ***anaphylaxis***.

Interactions

Drug-drug. *Live-virus vaccines:* May cause secondary transmission of infection from live-virus vaccines. Avoid using together.
Methotrexate: May decrease clearance of adalimumab. Dosage adjustment isn't necessary.

Nursing considerations

- Drug can be given alone or with methotrexate or other disease-modifying antirheumatic drugs.
- Give first dose under supervision of experienced prescriber.
- Evaluate patient for latent tuberculosis and, if present, start treatment before giving adalimumab.
- Serious infections and sepsis, including tuberculosis and invasive opportunistic fungal infections, may occur. If patient develops new infection during treatment, monitor closely.
- Drug may increase the risk for malignancy. Patients with highly active disease may be at an increased risk for lymphoma.
- Stop drug if patient develops a severe infection, anaphylaxis, other serious allergic reaction, or evidence of a lupus-like syndrome.

!!ALERT The needle cover contains latex and shouldn't be handled by those with latex sensitivity.

Patient teaching

- Tell patient to report evidence of tuberculosis or infection.
- If appropriate, teach patient or caregiver how to give drug.

!!ALERT Warn patient to seek immediate medical attention for symptoms of blood dyscrasias or infection, including fever, bruising, bleeding, and pallor.

- Tell patient to rotate injection sites and to avoid tender, bruised, red, or hard skin.
- Teach patient to dispose of used vials, needles, and syringes properly and not in the household trash or recyclables.
- Tell patient to refrigerate adalimumab in its original container before use.

adefovir dipivoxil
Hepsera

Pregnancy risk category C

Indications & dosages

➲ Chronic hepatitis B infection
Adults: 10 mg P.O. once daily.

In patients with creatinine clearance of 20 to 49 ml/minute, give 10 mg P.O. q 48 hours. In patients with clearance of 10 to 19 ml/minute, give 10 mg P.O. q 72 hours. In patients receiving hemodialysis, give 10 mg P.O. q 7 days, after dialysis session.

Contraindications & cautions

- Contraindicated in patients hypersensitive to any component of the drug.
- Use cautiously in patients with renal dysfunction, in those receiving nephrotoxic drugs, and in those with known risk factors for hepatic disease.
- Use cautiously in elderly patients because they're more likely to have decreased renal and cardiac function.
- Pregnant women exposed to drug may call the Antiretroviral Pregnancy Registry at 1-800-258-4263 to monitor fetal outcome.
- Safety and efficacy in children haven't been established.

Adverse reactions

CNS: *asthenia*, headache, fever.
EENT: pharyngitis, sinusitis.
GI: abdominal pain, diarrhea, dyspepsia, flatulence, nausea, vomiting.
GU: ***renal failure, renal insufficiency***, *hematuria*, glycosuria.
Hepatic: ***hepatomegaly with steatosis, hepatic failure***.
Metabolic: ***lactic acidosis***.
Respiratory: cough.
Skin: pruritus, rash.

Interactions

Drug-drug. *Ibuprofen:* May increase adefovir bioavailability. Monitor patient for adverse effects.
Nephrotoxic drugs (aminoglycosides, cyclosporine, NSAIDs, tacrolimus, vancomycin): May increase risk of nephrotoxicity. Use together cautiously.

Nursing considerations

- Monitor renal function, especially in patients with renal dysfunction or concurrent treatment with nephrotoxic drugs.

!!ALERT Patients may develop lactic acidosis and severe hepatomegaly with steatosis during treatment. Risk factors include female gender, obesity, and concurrent antiretroviral therapy.

- Monitor hepatic function. Notify prescriber if patient develops signs or symptoms of lactic acidosis and severe hepatomegaly with steatosis. Treatment may have to be stopped.
- Stopping adefovir may cause severe worsening of hepatitis. Monitor hepatic function closely in patients who stop anti–hepatitis B therapy.
- The optimal duration of treatment with adefovir hasn't been established.
- Offer HIV antibody testing to patients receiving adefovir. Adefovir may promote resistance to antiretrovirals in patients with unrecognized or untreated HIV infection.

Patient teaching

- Inform the patient that adefovir may be taken without regard to meals.
- Tell patient to immediately report weakness, muscle pain, trouble breathing, stomach pain with nausea and vomiting, dizziness, light-headedness, fast or irregular heartbeat, and feeling cold, especially in arms and legs.
- Warn patient not to stop taking this drug unless directed because it could cause hepatitis to become worse.
- Instruct woman to tell her prescriber if she becomes pregnant or is breast-feeding. It's unknown if drug appears in breast milk. Use cautiously in breast-feeding women.

adenosine
Adenocard

Pregnancy risk category C

Indications & dosages

➲ To convert paroxysmal supraventricular tachycardia (PSVT) to sinus rhythm
Adults and children weighing 50 kg (110 lb) or more: 6 mg I.V. by rapid bolus injection over 1 to 2 seconds. If PSVT isn't eliminated in 1 to 2 minutes, give 12 mg by rapid I.V. push and repeat, if needed.
Children weighing less than 50 kg: Initially, 0.05 to 0.1 mg/kg I.V. by rapid bolus injection followed by a saline flush. If PSVT isn't eliminated in 1 to 2 minutes, give additional bolus injections, increasing the amount given by 0.05- to 0.1-mg/kg increments, followed by a saline flush. Continue, p.r.n., until conversion or a maximum single dose of 0.3 mg/kg is given.

Contraindications & cautions

- Contraindicated in patients hypersensitive to drug.
- Contraindicated in those with second- or third-degree heart block or sinus node disease (such as sick sinus syndrome and symptomatic bradycardia), except those with a pacemaker.
- Use cautiously in patients with asthma, emphysema, or bronchitis because bronchoconstriction may occur.

Adverse reactions

CNS: dizziness, light-headedness, numbness, tingling in arms, headache.
CV: *facial flushing.*
GI: nausea.
Respiratory: chest pressure, *dyspnea, shortness of breath.*

Interactions

Drug-drug. *Carbamazepine:* May cause high-level heart block. Use together cautiously.
Digoxin, verapamil: May cause ventricular fibrillation. Monitor ECG closely.
Dipyridamole: May increase adenosine's effects. Adenosine dose may need to be reduced. Use together cautiously.
Methylxanthines (caffeine, theophylline): May decrease adenosine's effects. Adenosine dose may need to be increased or patients may not respond to adenosine therapy.
Drug-herb. *Guarana:* May decrease patient's response to drug. Monitor patient.

Nursing considerations

!!ALERT By decreasing conduction through the AV node, adenosine may produce first-, second-, or third-degree heart block. Patients who develop high-level heart block after a single dose of adenosine shouldn't receive additional doses.

!!ALERT Because new arrhythmias, including heart block and transient asystole, may develop, monitor cardiac rhythm and be prepared to give appropriate therapy.

- Crystals may form if solution is cold. If crystals are visible, gently warm solution to room temperature. Don't use solutions that aren't clear.
- Discard unused drug; adenosine lacks preservatives.

Patient teaching

- Instruct patient to report adverse reactions promptly.
- Tell patient to report discomfort at I.V. site.
- Inform patient that he may experience flushing or chest pain lasting 1 to 2 minutes.

albuterol sulfate (salbutamol sulfate)

AccuNeb, Proventil, Proventil HFA, Proventil Repetabs, Ventolin, Ventolin HFA, Volmax, VoSpire ER

Pregnancy risk category C

Indications & dosages

➲ To prevent or treat bronchospasm in patients with reversible obstructive airway disease

Capsules for inhalation

Adults and children age 4 and older: 200 mcg inhaled q 4 to 6 hours using a Rotahaler inhalation device. Some patients may need 400 mcg q 4 to 6 hours.

Extended-release tablets

Adults and children age 12 and older: 4 to 8 mg P.O. q 12 hours. Maximum, 16 mg b.i.d.

Children ages 6 to 12: 4 mg P.O. q 12 hours. Maximum, 12 mg b.i.d.

Oral tablets

Adults and children age 12 and older: 2 to 4 mg P.O. t.i.d. or q.i.d. Maximum, 8 mg q.i.d.

Children ages 6 to 12: 2 mg P.O. t.i.d. or q.i.d. Maximum, 6 mg q.i.d.

Solution for inhalation

Adults and children age 12 and older: 2.5 mg t.i.d. or q.i.d. by nebulizer. To prepare solution, use 0.5 ml of 0.5% solution diluted with 2.5 ml of normal saline solution. Or, use 3 ml of 0.083% solution.

Children ages 2 to 12: Initially, 0.1 to 0.15 mg/kg by nebulizer, with subsequent doses adjusted to response. Don't exceed 2.5 mg t.i.d. or q.i.d. by nebulization.

Syrup

Adults and children older than age 12: 2 to 4 mg (1 to 2 tsp) P.O. t.i.d. or q.i.d. Maximum, 8 mg q.i.d.

Children ages 6 to 12: 2 mg (1 tsp) P.O. t.i.d. or q.i.d. Maximum, 24 mg daily in divided doses.

Children ages 2 to 6: Initially, 0.1 mg/kg P.O. t.i.d. Starting dose shouldn't exceed 2 mg (1 tsp) t.i.d. Maximum, 4 mg (2 tsp) t.i.d.

For elderly patients and those sensitive to sympathomimetic amines, 2 mg P.O. t.i.d. or q.i.d. as oral tablets or syrup. Maximum, 8 mg t.i.d. or q.i.d.

➲ To prevent exercise-induced bronchospasm

Adults and children age 4 and older: 200-mcg capsule for inhalation inhaled using a Rotahaler inhalation device 15 minutes before exercise. Or, 2 inhalations using the metered-dose inhaler (MDI) 15 minutes before exercise.

Contraindications & cautions

- Contraindicated in patients hypersensitive to drug or its ingredients.
- Use cautiously in patients with CV disorders (including coronary insufficiency and hypertension), hyperthyroidism, or diabetes mellitus and in those who are unusually responsive to adrenergics.
- Use extended-release tablets cautiously in patients with GI narrowing.

Adverse reactions

CNS: *tremor, nervousness,* dizziness, insomnia, *headache, hyperactivity,* weakness, CNS stimulation, malaise.

CV: *tachycardia, palpitations,* hypertension.

EENT: dry and irritated nose and throat with inhaled form, nasal congestion, epistaxis, hoarseness.

GI: heartburn, *nausea, vomiting,* anorexia, altered taste, increased appetite.

Metabolic: hypokalemia.

Musculoskeletal: muscle cramps.

Respiratory: ***bronchospasm,*** cough, wheezing, dyspnea, bronchitis, increased sputum.

Other: hypersensitivity reactions.

Interactions

Drug-drug. *CNS stimulants:* May increase CNS stimulation. Avoid using together.
Digoxin: May decrease digoxin level. Monitor digoxin level closely.
MAO inhibitors, tricyclic antidepressants: May increase adverse CV effects. Monitor patient closely.
Propranolol, other beta blockers: May cause mutual antagonism. Monitor patient carefully.

Nursing considerations

- Drug may decrease sensitivity of spirometry used for diagnosis of asthma.
- When switching patient from regular to extended-release tablets, remember that a regular 2-mg tablet every 6 hours is equivalent to an extended-release 4-mg tablet every 12 hours.
- Syrup may be taken by children as young as age 2; it contains no alcohol or sugar.
- Rarely, erythema multiforme or Stevens-Johnson syndrome has been linked to use of syrup in children.
- Ventolin HFA is a newer version of the Ventolin MDI for asthma and other obstructive lung diseases. Ventolin HFA uses the propellant hydrofluoroalkane as an alternative to chlorofluorocarbons to propel the medication.

!!ALERT Patient may use tablets and aerosol together. Monitor these patients closely for signs and symptoms of toxicity.

!!ALERT Don't confuse albuterol with atenolol or Albutein, or Flomax with Volmax.

Patient teaching

- Warn patient about risk of paradoxical bronchospasm and to stop drug immediately if it occurs.
- Teach patient to perform oral inhalation correctly. Give the following instructions for using the MDI:
  - Shake the inhaler.
  - Clear nasal passages and throat.
  - Breathe out, expelling as much air from lungs as possible.
  - Place mouthpiece well into mouth, seal lips around mouthpiece, and inhale deeply as you release a dose from inhaler. Or, hold inhaler about 1 inch (two fingerwidths) from open mouth; inhale while dose is released.
  - Hold breath for several seconds, remove mouthpiece, and exhale slowly.
- If prescriber orders more than 1 inhalation, tell patient to wait at least 2 minutes before repeating procedure.
- Tell patient that use of a spacer device may improve drug delivery to lungs.
- If patient is also using a corticosteroid inhaler, instruct him to use the bronchodilator first and then to wait about 5 minutes before using the corticosteroid. This lets the bronchodilator open the air passages for maximum effectiveness of the corticosteroid.
- Tell patient to remove canister and wash inhaler with warm, soapy water at least once a week.
- Advise patient not to chew or crush extended-release tablets or mix them with food.

alefacept
Amevive

Pregnancy risk category B

Indications & dosages

➲ Moderate to severe chronic plaque psoriasis in candidates for systemic therapy or phototherapy
Adults: 15 mg I.M. once weekly for 12 weeks. Another 12-week course may be given if CD4+ T lymphocyte count is normal and at least 12 weeks have passed since the previous treatment.

Withhold dose if CD4+ T lymphocyte count is below 250 cells/mm^3. Stop drug if CD4+ count remains below 250 cells/mm^3 for 1 month.

Contraindications & cautions

- Contraindicated in patients hypersensitive to drug or its components, in breast-feeding women, and in patients with a history of systemic malignancy or clinically important infection.
- Use cautiously in patients at high risk for malignancy, patients with chronic or recurrent infections, and pregnant patients. Give drug cautiously to elderly patients because of their increased rate of infection and malignancies.
- Safety and effectiveness in children haven't been established.

Adverse reactions

CNS: dizziness.
CV: ***coronary artery disorder, MI.***
EENT: pharyngitis.
GI: nausea.
Hematologic: **LYMPHOPENIA.**
Musculoskeletal: myalgia.
Respiratory: cough.
Skin: pruritus, *injection site pain, inflammation,* bleeding, edema, or mass.
Other: ***infection***, chills, ***malignancy***, ***hypersensitivity reaction***, accidental injury, antibody formation.

Interactions

Drug-drug. *Immunosuppressants, phototherapy:* May increase risk of excessive immunosuppression. Avoid using together.

Nursing considerations

- Monitor CD4+ T lymphocyte count weekly for the 12-week course. Ensure that CD4+ T lymphocyte count is normal before starting therapy.
- Monitor patient carefully for evidence of infection or malignancy, and stop drug if it appears.
- For I.M. administration, reconstitute 15-mg vial of alefacept with 0.6 ml of supplied diluent.
- Rotate I.M. injection sites so that the new injection is given at least 1 inch away from the old site, and not in an area that is bruised, tender, or hard.
- Because effects on fetal development aren't known, give drug only if clearly needed. Enroll pregnant women receiving alefacept into the Biogen pregnancy registry by phoning 1-800-811-0104 so that drug effects can be studied.

Patient teaching

- Tell patient about potential adverse reactions.
- Urge patient to report evidence of infection immediately.
- Tell patient that blood tests will be done regularly to monitor WBC counts.
- Tell patient to notify prescriber if she is or could be pregnant within 8 weeks of receiving drug.
- Advise patient to either stop breast-feeding or stop using the drug because of the risk of serious adverse reactions in the infant.

alendronate sodium
Fosamax, Fosamax Plus D

Pregnancy risk category C

Indications & dosages

➲ **Osteoporosis in postmenopausal women; to increase bone mass in men with osteoporosis**
Adults: 10 mg P.O. daily or 70-mg tablet P.O. once weekly.
➲ **Paget's disease of bone**
Adults: 40 mg P.O. daily for 6 months.
➲ **To prevent osteoporosis in postmenopausal women**
Adults: 5 mg P.O. daily or 35-mg tablet P.O. once weekly.
➲ **Glucocorticoid-induced osteoporosis in men and women receiving glucocorticoids in a daily dose equivalent to 7.5 mg or more of prednisone and who have low bone mineral density**
Adults: 5 mg P.O. daily. For postmenopausal women not receiving estrogen, recommended dose is 10 mg P.O. daily.

Contraindications & cautions

- Contraindicated in patients hypersensitive to drug and in those with hypocalcemia, severe renal insufficiency, or abnormalities of the esophagus that delay esophageal emptying.
- Use cautiously in patients with active upper GI problems (dysphagia, symptomatic esophageal diseases, gastritis, duodenitis, ulcers) or mild to moderate renal insufficiency.

Adverse reactions

CNS: headache.
GI: abdominal pain, nausea, dyspepsia, constipation, diarrhea, flatulence, acid regurgitation, esophageal ulcer, vomiting, dysphagia, abdominal distention, gastritis, taste perversion.
Musculoskeletal: musculoskeletal pain.

Interactions

Drug-drug. *Antacids, calcium supplements, many oral drugs:* May interfere with absorption of alendronate. Instruct patient to wait at least 30 minutes after taking alendronate before taking other drug orally.

Aspirin, NSAIDs: May increase risk of upper GI adverse reactions with drug doses greater than 10 mg daily. Monitor patient closely.
Ranitidine (I.V. form): May increase availability of alendronate. Reduce dosage, as needed.
Drug-food. *Any food:* May decrease absorption of drug. Advise patient to take with full glass of water at least 30 minutes before food, beverages, or ingestion of other drugs.

Nursing considerations

- Correct hypocalcemia and other disturbances of mineral metabolism (such as vitamin D deficiency) before therapy begins.
- When used to treat osteoporosis, disease may be confirmed by findings of low bone mass on diagnostic studies or by history of osteoporotic fracture.
- The recommended daily intake of vitamin D is 400 to 800 IU. Fosamax Plus D provides 400 IU daily when taken once weekly. Patients at risk for vitamin D deficiency, such as those who are chronically ill, nursing home bound, who have a GI malabsorption syndrome, or who are older than age 70 may require additional supplementation.
- When used to treat Paget's disease, drug is indicated for patients with alkaline phosphatase level at least two times upper limit of normal, for those who are symptomatic, and for those at risk for future complications from the disease.

!!ALERT Give drug with 6 to 8 ounces of water at least 30 minutes before patient's first food or drink of the day, to facilitate delivery to the stomach. Don't allow patient to lie down for 30 minutes after taking drug.

- Monitor patient's calcium and phosphate levels throughout therapy.

!!ALERT Don't confuse Fosamax with Flomax.

Patient teaching

- Stress importance of taking tablet only with 6 to 8 ounces of water at least 30 minutes before ingesting anything else, including food, beverages, and other drugs. Tell patient that waiting longer than 30 minutes improves absorption.
- Warn patient not to lie down for at least 30 minutes after taking drug to facilitate delivery to stomach and to reduce risk of esophageal irritation.
- Advise patient to report adverse effects immediately, especially chest pain or difficulty swallowing.
- Advise patient to take supplemental calcium and vitamin D if dietary intake is inadequate.
- Tell patient about benefits of weight-bearing exercises in increasing bone mass. If applicable, explain importance of reducing or eliminating cigarette smoking and alcohol use.

alfuzosin hydrochloride
Uroxatral

Pregnancy risk category B

Indications & dosages

➲ **BPH**
Adult men: 10 mg P.O. immediately after same meal each day.

Contraindications & cautions

- Contraindicated in patients with Child-Pugh categories B and C and those hypersensitive to alfuzosin or its ingredients.
- Use cautiously in patients with severe renal insufficiency, congenital or acquired QT-interval prolongation, or symptomatic hypotension and hypotensive responses to other drugs.

Adverse reactions

CNS: dizziness, fatigue, headache, pain.
EENT: pharyngitis, sinusitis.
GI: abdominal pain, constipation, dyspepsia, nausea.
GU: impotence.
Respiratory: bronchitis, upper respiratory tract infection.

Interactions

Drug-drug. *Antihypertensives (diltiazem):* May cause hypotension. Monitor blood pressure, and use together cautiously.
Atenolol: May cause hypotension and reduce heart rate. Monitor blood pressure and heart rate for these effects.
Cimetidine: May increase alfuzosin level. Use together cautiously.
CYP3A4 inhibitors (itraconazole, ketoconazole, ritonavir): May increase alfuzosin level. Avoid using together.

Nursing considerations

- Don't use alfuzosin to treat hypertension.
- Orthostatic hypotension may develop within a few hours after patient takes alfuzosin; it may not cause symptoms.
- Symptoms of BPH and prostate cancer are similar; rule out prostate cancer before starting therapy.
- Stop alfuzosin if angina pectoris develops or worsens.

Patient teaching

- Tell patient to take alfuzosin just after same meal each day.
- At start of therapy, warn patient about possible hypotension, and explain that it may cause dizziness. Caution patient against performing hazardous activities until he knows how the drug affects him.
- Tell patient to avoid situations in which he could be injured if he became light-headed or fainted.
- Warn patient not to crush or chew the tablets.

allopurinol

Apo-Allopurinol†, Zyloprim

allopurinol sodium

Aloprim

Pregnancy risk category C

Indications & dosages

➲ Gout or hyperuricemia

Adults: Mild gout, 200 to 300 mg P.O. daily; severe gout with large tophi, 400 to 600 mg P.O. daily. Maximum 800 mg daily. Dosage varies with severity of disease; can be given as single dose or divided, but doses greater than 300 mg should be divided.

➲ Hyperuricemia caused by malignancies

Adults and children older than age 10: 200 to 400 mg/m^2 daily I.V. as a single infusion or in equally divided doses q 6, 8, or 12 hours. Maximum 600 mg daily.

Children age 10 and younger: Initially, 200 mg/m^2 daily I.V. as single infusion or in equally divided doses q 6, 8, or 12 hours. Then titrate according to uric acid levels. For children ages 6 to 10, give 300 mg P.O. daily or divided t.i.d.; for children younger than age 6, give 150 mg P.O. daily.

➲ To prevent acute gout attacks

Adults: 100 mg P.O. daily; increase at weekly intervals by 100 mg without exceeding maximum dose (800 mg) until uric acid falls to 6 mg/dl or less.

➲ To prevent uric acid nephropathy during cancer chemotherapy

Adults: 600 to 800 mg P.O. daily for 2 to 3 days, with high fluid intake.

➲ Recurrent calcium oxalate calculi

Adults: 200 to 300 mg P.O. daily in single or divided doses.

If creatinine clearance is 10 to 20 ml/minute, give 200 mg P.O. or I.V. daily; if clearance is less than 10 ml/minute, give 100 mg P.O. or I.V. daily; if clearance is less than 3 ml/minute, give 100 mg P.O. or I.V. at extended intervals.

Contraindications & cautions

- Contraindicated in patients hypersensitive to drug and in those with idiopathic hemochromatosis.

Adverse reactions

CNS: fever, drowsiness, headache, paresthesia, peripheral neuropathy, neuritis.
CV: hypersensitivity vasculitis, necrotizing angiitis.
EENT: epistaxis.
GI: nausea, vomiting, diarrhea, abdominal pain, gastritis, taste loss or perversion, dyspepsia.
GU: ***renal failure***, uremia.
Hematologic: ***agranulocytosis***, anemia, ***aplastic anemia***, ***thrombocytopenia***, ***leukopenia***, leukocytosis, eosinophilia.
Hepatic: ***hepatitis***, ***hepatic necrosis***, hepatomegaly, cholestatic jaundice.
Musculoskeletal: arthralgia, myopathy.
Skin: ***rash;*** exfoliative, urticarial, and purpuric lesions; ***erythema multiforme;*** severe furunculosis of nose; ichthyosis; alopecia; ***toxic epidermal necrolysis***.
Other: ecchymoses, chills.

Interactions

Drug-drug. *Amoxicillin, ampicillin:* May increase possibility of rash. Avoid using together.
Anticoagulants: May increase anticoagulant effect. Dosage may need to be adjusted.
Antineoplastics: May increase potential for bone marrow suppression. Monitor patient carefully.

Chlorpropamide: May increase hypoglycemic effect. Avoid using together.
Ethacrynic acid, thiazide diuretics: May increase risk of allopurinol toxicity. Reduce allopurinol dosage, and monitor renal function closely.
Uricosurics: May have additive effect. May be used to therapeutic advantage.
Urine-acidifying drugs (ammonium chloride, ascorbic acid, potassium or sodium phosphate): May increase possibility of kidney stone formation. Monitor patient carefully.
Xanthines: May increase theophylline level. Adjust dosage of theophylline, as needed.
Drug-lifestyle. *Alcohol use:* May increase uric acid level. Discourage use together.

Nursing considerations

- Monitor uric acid level to evaluate drug's effectiveness.
- Monitor fluid intake and output; daily urine output of at least 2 L and maintenance of neutral or slightly alkaline urine are desirable.
- Periodically monitor CBC and hepatic and renal function, especially at start of therapy.
- Optimal benefits may need 2 to 6 weeks of therapy. Because acute gout attacks may occur during this time, concurrent use of colchicine may be prescribed prophylactically.
- Don't restart drug in patients who have a severe reaction.

!!ALERT Don't confuse Zyloprim with ZORprin.

Patient teaching

- To minimize GI adverse reactions, tell patient to take drug with or immediately after meals.
- Encourage patient to drink plenty of fluids while taking drug unless otherwise contraindicated.
- Drug may cause drowsiness; tell patient not to drive or perform hazardous tasks requiring mental alertness until CNS effects of drug are known.
- If patient is taking allopurinol for recurrent calcium oxalate stones, advise him also to reduce his dietary intake of animal protein, sodium, refined sugars, oxalate-rich foods, and calcium.
- Tell patient to stop drug at first sign of rash, which may precede severe hypersensitivity or other adverse reactions. Rash is more common in patients taking diuretics and in those with renal disorders. Tell patient to report all adverse reactions.
- Advise patient to avoid alcohol during therapy.
- Teach patient importance of continuing drug even if asymptomatic.

almotriptan malate
Axert

Pregnancy risk category C

Indications & dosages

➲ **Acute migraine with or without aura**
Adults: 6.25-mg or 12.5-mg tablet P.O., with one additional dose after 2 hours if headache is unresolved or recurs. Maximum, two doses within 24 hours.

For patients with hepatic or renal impairment, initially 6.25 mg, with maximum daily dose of 12.5 mg.

Contraindications & cautions

- Contraindicated in patients hypersensitive to drug.
- Contraindicated in those with angina pectoris, history of MI, silent ischemia, coronary artery vasospasm, Prinzmetal's variant angina, or other CV disease; uncontrolled hypertension; and hemiplegic or basilar migraine.
- Don't give within 24 hours after treatment with other 5-$HT_{1B/1D}$ agonists or ergotamine drugs.
- Use cautiously in patients with renal or hepatic impairment and in those with cataracts because of the potential for corneal opacities.
- Use cautiously in patients with risk factors for coronary artery disease (CAD), such as obesity, diabetes, and family history of CAD.

Adverse reactions

CNS: paresthesia, headache, dizziness, somnolence.
CV: ***coronary artery vasospasm, transient myocardial ischemia, MI, ventricular tachycardia, ventricular fibrillation.***
GI: nausea, dry mouth.

Interactions

Drug-drug. *MAO inhibitors, verapamil:* May increase almotriptan level. No dose adjustment is necessary.
CYP3A4 inhibitors such as ketoconazole: May increase almotriptan level. Monitor patient for potential adverse reaction. May need to reduce dosage.
Ergot-containing drugs, serotonin 5-HT$_{1B/1D}$ agonists: May cause additive effects. Avoid using within 24 hours of almotriptan.
SSRIs: May cause additive serotonin effects, resulting in weakness, hyperreflexia, or incoordination. Monitor patient closely if given together.

Nursing considerations

- Patients with poor renal or hepatic function should receive a reduced dosage.
- Repeat dose after 2 hours, if needed, and don't give more than two doses within 24 hours.

!!ALERT Don't confuse Axert (almotriptan) with Antivert (meclizine).

Patient teaching

- Tell patient that drug can be taken with or without food.
- Advise patient to take drug only when he's having a migraine; explain that drug isn't taken on a regular schedule.
- Advise patient to use only one repeat dose within 24 hours, no sooner than 2 hours after first dose.
- Advise patient that other commonly prescribed migraine medications can interact with almotriptan.
- Advise patient to report chest or throat tightness, pain, or heaviness.
- Teach patient to avoid possible migraine triggers, such as cheese, chocolate, citrus fruits, caffeine, and alcohol.

alosetron hydrochloride
Lotronex

Pregnancy risk category B

Indications & dosages

➲ Severe diarrhea-predominant irritable bowel syndrome (IBS)
Women: 1 mg P.O. once daily with or without food. May increase dosage to 1 mg b.i.d., if necessary, after 4 weeks. If adequate control isn't reached after 4 weeks on twice-daily therapy, stop drug.

Contraindications & cautions

- Contraindicated in patients hypersensitive to drug or any of its components and in those with a history of or current chronic or severe constipation, sequelae from constipation, intestinal obstruction, stricture, toxic megacolon, GI perforation, GI adhesions, ischemic colitis, impaired intestinal circulation, thrombophlebitis, or hypercoagulable state.
- Contraindicated in patients with a history of or current Crohn's disease, ulcerative colitis, or diverticulitis and in those who are unable to understand or comply with the Patient-Physician Agreement.
- Don't use drug if predominant symptom is constipation.
- Use cautiously in patients who are pregnant, breast-feeding, or planning to become pregnant.
- Use in patients younger than age 18 hasn't been studied.

Adverse reactions

CNS: headache.
GI: CONSTIPATION, nausea, GI discomfort and pain, abdominal discomfort and pain, abdominal distention, hemorrhoids, regurgitation, reflux, ***ileus perforation, ischemic colitis, small bowel mesenteric ischemia, impaction, obstruction.***
Skin: rash.

Interactions

Drug-drug. *Hydralazine, isoniazid, and procainamide:* May cause slower metabolism of these drugs because of *N*-acetyltransferase inhibition. Monitor patient for toxicity.

Nursing considerations

- Patients appropriate for treatment should be women who experience symptoms for at least 6 months, have no anatomic or biochemical GI tract abnormalities, and haven't responded to other therapies.
- Diarrhea-predominant IBS is considered severe if one or more of the following accompanies the diarrhea:
  - frequent and severe abdominal pain or discomfort
  - frequent bowel urgency or fecal incontinence

– disability or restriction of daily activities

!!ALERT Patients taking drug have developed ischemic colitis and serious complications of constipation, resulting in death. If patient develops ischemic colitis (acute colitis, rectal bleeding, or sudden worsening of abdominal pain) while taking drug, stop therapy.

- If patient taking drug develops constipation, stop drug until symptoms subside.
- Drug is approved for use only in women with IBS. This drug isn't indicated for use in men.
- Elderly people may be at greater risk for complications of constipation.

Patient teaching

- Have patient sign a Patient-Physician Agreement before starting therapy.
- Urge patient to read the Medication Guide before starting drug and each time she refills the prescription.
- Tell patient that this drug won't cure but may alleviate some IBS symptoms.
- Inform patient that most women notice their symptoms improving after about 1 week of therapy, but some may take up to 4 weeks to get relief from abdominal pain, discomfort, and diarrhea. Let patient know that symptoms usually return within 1 week after stopping the drug.
- Advise patient that drug may be taken with or without food.
- If constipation or signs of ischemic colitis occur (rectal bleeding, bloody diarrhea, or worsened abdominal pain or cramping), tell patient to stop the drug and consult prescriber immediately. Therapy can be resumed after the situation is discussed with prescriber and constipation resolves.
- Inform patient not to share drug with other people having similar symptoms. This drug hasn't been shown to be safe or effective for men.
- Tell patient to notify the prescriber immediately if she becomes pregnant.

alprazolam

Apo-Alpraz†, Niravam, Novo-Alprazol†, Nu-Alpraz†, Xanax, Xanax XR

Pregnancy risk category D
Controlled substance schedule IV

Indications & dosages

➲ Anxiety

Adults: Usual first dose, 0.25 to 0.5 mg P.O. t.i.d. Maximum, 4 mg daily in divided doses.

Elderly patients: Usual first dose, 0.25 mg P.O. b.i.d. or t.i.d. Maximum, 4 mg daily in divided doses.

➲ Panic disorders

Adults: 0.5 mg P.O. t.i.d., increased at intervals of 3 to 4 days in increments of no more than 1 mg. Maximum, 10 mg daily in divided doses. If using extended-release tablets, start with 0.5 to 1 mg P.O. once daily. Increase by no more than 1 mg q 3 to 4 days. Maximum daily dose is 10 mg.

For debilitated patients or those with advanced hepatic disease, usual first dose is 0.25 mg P.O. b.i.d. or t.i.d. Maximum, 4 mg daily in divided doses.

Contraindications & cautions

- Contraindicated in patients hypersensitive to drug or other benzodiazepines and in those with acute angle-closure glaucoma.
- Use cautiously in patients with hepatic, renal, or pulmonary disease.

Adverse reactions

CNS: *drowsiness, light-headedness, sedation, somnolence, difficulty speaking, impaired coordination, memory impairment, fatigue, depression,* mental impairment, ataxia, paresthesia, dyskinesia, hypoesthesia, lethargy, decreased or increased libido, *confusion, anxiety,* vertigo, malaise, *headache, dizziness,* tremor, *irritability, insomnia,* nervousness, restlessness, agitation, nightmare, syncope, akathisia, mania, ***suicide***.

CV: hot flushes, palpitation, chest pain, hypotension.

EENT: sore throat, allergic rhinitis, blurred vision, nasal congestion.

GI: *dry mouth, constipation,* nausea, increased or decreased appetite, anorexia, *di-*

arrhea, vomiting, dyspepsia, abdominal pain.
GU: dysmenorrhea, sexual dysfunction, premenstrual syndrome, difficulty urinating.
Metabolic: increased or decreased weight.
Musculoskeletal: arthralgia, myalgia, arm or leg pain, back pain, muscle rigidity, muscle cramps, muscle twitch.
Respiratory: upper respiratory tract infection, dyspnea, hyperventilation.
Skin: pruritus, increased sweating, dermatitis.
Other: influenza, injury, emergence of anxiety between doses, dependence.

Interactions

Drug-drug. *Anticonvulsants, antidepressants, antihistamines, barbiturates, benzodiazepines, general anesthetics, narcotics, phenothiazines:* May increase CNS depressant effects. Avoid using together.
Azole antifungals (including fluconazole, itraconazole, ketoconazole, miconazole): May increase and prolong alprazolam level, CNS depression, and psychomotor impairment. Avoid using together.
Carbamazepine, propoxyphene: May decrease alprazolam level. Use together cautiously.
Cimetidine, fluoxetine, fluvoxamine, hormonal contraceptives, nefazodone: May increase alprazolam level. Use cautiously together, and consider alprazolam dosage reduction.
Tricyclic antidepressants: May increase levels of these drugs. Monitor patient closely.
Drug-herb. *Kava:* May increase sedation. Discourage use together.
St. John's wort: May decrease alprazolam level. Discourage use together.
Drug-food. *Grapefruit juice:* May increase alprazolam level. Discourage use together.
Drug-lifestyle. *Alcohol use:* May cause additive CNS effects. Discourage use together.
Smoking: May decrease effectiveness of benzodiazepines. Monitor patient closely.

Nursing considerations

- The optimum duration of therapy is unknown.

!!ALERT Don't withdraw drug abruptly; withdrawal symptoms, including seizures, may occur. Abuse or addiction is possible.

- Monitor hepatic, renal, and hematopoietic function periodically in patients receiving repeated or prolonged therapy.

!!ALERT Don't confuse alprazolam with alprostadil.
!!ALERT Don't confuse Xanax with Zantac or Tenex.

Patient teaching

- Warn patient to avoid hazardous activities that require alertness and good coordination until effects of drug are known.
- Tell patient to avoid alcohol while taking drug.
- Advise patient that smoking may decrease drug's effectiveness.
- Warn patient not to stop drug abruptly because withdrawal symptoms or seizures may occur.
- Tell patient to swallow extended-release tablets whole.
- Tell patient using orally disintegrating tablet to remove it from bottle using dry hands and to immediately place it on his tongue where it will dissolve and can be swallowed with saliva.
- Tell patient taking half of a scored orally disintegrating tablet to discard the unused half.
- Advise patient to discard the cotton from the bottle of orally disintegrating tablets and keep it tightly sealed to prevent moisture from dissolving the tablets.

alteplase (tissue plasminogen activator, recombinant; t-PA)

Activase, Cathflo Activase

Pregnancy risk category C

Indications & dosages

➲ Lysis of thrombi obstructing coronary arteries in acute MI
3-hour infusion
Adults: 100 mg by I.V. infusion over 3 hours, as follows: 60 mg in first hour, 6 to 10 mg of which is given as a bolus over first 1 to 2 minutes. Then 20 mg/hour infused for 2 hours. Adults weighing less than 65 kg (143 lb) should receive 1.25 mg/kg in a similar fashion (60% in first hour, 10% of which is given as a bolus; then 20% of total dose per hour for 2 hours).

Accelerated infusion
Adults weighing more than 67 kg (147 lb): 100 mg total dose. Give 15 mg I.V. bolus over 1 to 2 minutes, followed by 50 mg infused over the next 30 minutes; then 35 mg infused over the next hour.
Adults weighing 67 kg or less: 15 mg I.V. bolus over 1 to 2 minutes, followed by 0.75 mg/kg, (not to exceed 50 mg) infused over the next 30 minutes; then 0.5 mg/kg (not to exceed 35 mg) infused over the next hour.

➲ **To manage acute massive pulmonary embolism**
Adults: 100 mg by I.V. infusion over 2 hours. Heparin begun at end of infusion when PTT or thrombin time returns to twice normal or less. Don't exceed 100-mg dose. Higher doses may increase risk of intracranial bleeding.

➲ **Acute ischemic CVA**
Adults: 0.9 mg/kg by I.V. infusion over 1 hour with 10% of total dose given as an initial I.V. bolus over 1 minute. Maximum total dose is 90 mg.

➲ **To restore function to central venous access devices**
Cathflo Activase
Adults and children older than age 2: For patients weighing more than 30 kg (66 lb), instill 2 mg in 2 ml sterile water into catheter. For patients weighing 10 kg (22 lb) to 30 kg, instill 110% of the internal lumen volume of the catheter, not to exceed 2 mg in 2 ml sterile water. After 30 minutes of dwell time, assess catheter function by aspirating blood. If function is restored, aspirate 4 to 5 ml of blood to remove drug and residual clot, and gently irrigate the catheter with normal saline solution. If catheter function isn't restored after 120 minutes, instill a second dose.

➲ **Lysis of arterial occlusion in a peripheral vessel or bypass graft♦**
Adults: 0.05 to 0.1 mg/kg/hour infused intra-arterially for 1 to 8 hours.

Contraindications & cautions

- Contraindicated in patients with active internal bleeding, intracranial neoplasm, arteriovenous malformation, aneurysm, severe uncontrolled hypertension, or history or current evidence of intracranial hemorrhage, suspicion of subarachnoid hemorrhage, or seizure at onset of CVA when used for acute ischemic CVA.
- Contraindicated in patients with history of CVA, intraspinal or intracranial trauma or surgery within 2 months, or known bleeding diathesis.
- Use cautiously in patients having major surgery within 10 days (when bleeding is difficult to control because of its location); organ biopsy; trauma (including cardiopulmonary resuscitation); GI or GU bleeding; cerebrovascular disease; systolic pressure of 180 mm Hg or higher or diastolic pressure of 110 mm Hg or higher; mitral stenosis, atrial fibrillation, or other conditions that may lead to left heart thrombus; acute pericarditis or subacute bacterial endocarditis; hemostatic defects caused by hepatic or renal impairment; septic thrombophlebitis; or diabetic hemorrhagic retinopathy.
- Use cautiously in patients receiving anticoagulants, in patients age 75 and older, and during pregnancy and the first 10 days postpartum.

Adverse reactions

CNS: fever, ***cerebral hemorrhage***.
CV: hypotension, ***arrhythmias***, edema.
GI: nausea, vomiting, ***GI bleeding***, (Cathflo Activase).
Hematologic: ***spontaneous bleeding***.
Other: bleeding at puncture sites, ***cholesterol embolization***, hypersensitivity reactions, ***anaphylaxis***, ***venous thrombosis***, ***sepsis***, (Cathflo Activase).

Interactions

Drug-drug. *Aspirin, dipyridamole, drugs affecting platelet activity (abciximab), heparin, warfarin anticoagulants:* May increase risk of bleeding. Monitor patient carefully.
Nitroglycerin: May decrease alteplase antigen level. Avoid using together. If use together is unavoidable, use the lowest effective dose of nitroglycerin.

Nursing considerations

!!ALERT When used for acute ischemic CVA, give drug within 3 hours after symptoms occur and only when intracranial bleeding has been ruled out.
- Addition of 150 to 200 units/ml aprotinin to blood sample may remedy interference with coagulation and fibrinolytic test results.

- Drug may be given to menstruating women.
- To recanalize occluded coronary arteries and improve heart function, begin treatment as soon as possible after symptoms start.
- Anticoagulant and antiplatelet therapy is commonly started during or after treatment, to decrease risk of another thrombosis.
- Monitor vital signs and neurologic status carefully. Keep patient on strict bed rest.
- Have antiarrhythmics readily available, and carefully monitor ECG. Coronary thrombolysis is linked with arrhythmias caused by reperfusion of ischemic myocardium. Such arrhythmias don't differ from those commonly linked with MI.
- Avoid invasive procedures during thrombolytic therapy. Closely monitor patient for signs of internal bleeding, and frequently check all puncture sites. Bleeding is the most common adverse effect and may occur internally and at external puncture sites.
- If uncontrollable bleeding occurs, stop infusion (and heparin) and notify prescriber.

Patient teaching

- Explain use and administration of drug to patient and family.
- Tell patient to report adverse reactions promptly.

amantadine hydrochloride

Symmetrel

Pregnancy risk category C

Indications & dosages

➲ **To prevent or treat symptoms of influenza type A virus and respiratory tract illnesses**

Children age 13 or older and adults up to age 65: 200 mg P.O. daily in a single dose or 100 mg P.O. b.i.d.

Children ages 9 to 12: 100 mg P.O. b.i.d.

Children ages 1 to 8 or weighing less than 45 kg (99 lb): 4.4 to 8.8 mg/kg P.O. as a total daily dose given once daily or divided equally b.i.d. Maximum daily dose is 150 mg.

Elderly patients: 100 mg P.O. once daily in patients older than age 65 with normal renal function.

Begin treatment within 24 to 48 hours after symptoms appear and continue for 24 to 48 hours after symptoms disappear (usually 2 to 7 days). Start prophylaxis as soon as possible after exposure and continue for at least 10 days after exposure. May continue prophylactic treatment up to 90 days for repeated or suspected exposures if influenza vaccine is unavailable. If used with influenza vaccine, continue dose for 2 to 3 weeks until antibody response to vaccine has developed.

For patients with creatinine clearance of 30 to 50 ml/minute, give 200 mg the first day and 100 mg thereafter; if clearance is 15 to 29 ml/minute, give 200 mg the first day and then 100 mg on alternate days; if clearance is less than 15 ml/minute or if patient is receiving hemodialysis, give 200 mg q 7 days.

Contraindications & cautions

- Contraindicated in patients hypersensitive to drug.
- Use cautiously in elderly patients and in patients with seizure disorders, heart failure, peripheral edema, hepatic disease, mental illness, eczematoid rash, renal impairment, orthostatic hypotension, and CV disease. Monitor renal and liver function tests.

Adverse reactions

CNS: depression, fatigue, confusion, *dizziness*, hallucinations, anxiety, *irritability*, ataxia, *insomnia*, *light-headedness*, headache.

CV: peripheral edema, orthostatic hypotension, ***heart failure***.

EENT: blurred vision.

GI: anorexia, *nausea*, constipation, vomiting, dry mouth.

Skin: livedo reticularis.

Interactions

Drug-drug. *Anticholinergics:* May increase anticholinergic effects. Use together cautiously; reduce dosage of anticholinergic before starting amantadine.

CNS stimulants: May increase CNS stimulation. Use together cautiously.

Drug-herb. *Jimsonweed:* May adversely affect CV function. Discourage use together.

Drug-lifestyle. *Alcohol use:* May increase CNS effects. Discourage use together.

Nursing considerations

- Begin treatment within 24 to 48 hours after symptoms appear and continue for 24 to 48 hours after symptoms disappear (usually 2 to 7 days of therapy).
- Start prophylaxis as soon as possible after first exposure and continue for at least 10 days after exposure. For repeated or suspected exposures, if influenza vaccine is unavailable, may continue prophylaxis for up to 90 days. If used with influenza vaccine, continue dose for 2 to 3 weeks until antibody response to vaccine has developed.

!!ALERT Elderly patients are more susceptible to adverse neurologic effects. Monitor patient for mental status changes.

- Suicidal ideation and attempts have been reported in patients both with and without prior psychiatric problems.
- Drug can worsen mental problems in patients with a history of psychiatric disorders or substance abuse.

!!ALERT Don't confuse amantadine with rimantadine.

Patient teaching

- Tell patient to take drug exactly as prescribed. Taking more than prescribed can result in serious adverse reactions or death.
- If insomnia occurs, tell patient to take drug several hours before bedtime.
- If patient gets dizzy when he stands up, instruct him not to stand or change positions too quickly.
- Instruct patient to notify prescriber of adverse reactions, especially dizziness, depression, anxiety, nausea, and urine retention.
- Caution patient to avoid activities that require mental alertness until effects of drug are known.
- Advise patient to avoid alcohol while taking drug.

---

amifostine
Ethyol

Pregnancy risk category C

Indications & dosages

➲ **To reduce cumulative renal toxicity linked to repeated administration of cisplatin in patients with advanced ovarian cancer or non–small-cell lung cancer**

Adults: 910 mg/m^2 daily as a 15-minute I.V. infusion, starting 30 minutes before chemotherapy. If hypotension occurs and blood pressure doesn't return to normal within 5 minutes after stopping treatment, 740 mg/m^2 in subsequent cycles.

➲ **To reduce moderate to severe xerostomia in patients undergoing postoperative radiation treatment for head and neck cancer**

Adults: 200 mg/m^2 daily as 3-minute I.V. infusion, starting 15 to 30 minutes before standard fraction radiation therapy.

Contraindications & cautions

- Contraindicated in patients hypersensitive to aminothiol compounds or mannitol.
- Contraindicated in patients who are hypotensive, dehydrated, or receiving antihypertensives that can't be stopped 24 hours before amifostine administration.
- Drug shouldn't be used in patients receiving chemotherapy for potentially curable malignancies (including certain malignancies of germ-cell origin), except for patients involved in clinical studies.
- Use cautiously in elderly patients and in patients with ischemic heart disease, arrhythmias, heart failure, or history of CVA or transient ischemic attacks.
- Use cautiously in patients for whom common adverse effects of nausea, vomiting, and hypotension may have serious consequences.

Adverse reactions

CNS: dizziness, somnolence.
CV: *hypotension.*
GI: *nausea, vomiting.*
Metabolic: hypocalcemia.
Respiratory: hiccups, sneezing.
Other: flushing or feeling of warmth, chills or feeling of coldness, ***allergic reactions ranging from rash to rigors.***

Interactions

Drug-drug. *Antihypertensives, other drugs that could increase hypotension:* May cause profound hypotension. Monitor patient closely.

Nursing considerations

- If possible, stop antihypertensive therapy 24 hours before amifostine administration.
- Make sure patient is adequately hydrated before giving drug. Monitor patient's blood pressure before and immediately after infusion and periodically thereafter as clinically indicated.
- Give antiemetics, including dexamethasone 20 mg I.V. and a serotonin 5-HT_3-receptor antagonist, before and with amifostine. Additional antiemetics may be needed, based on chemotherapeutic drugs given.
- Monitor patient's fluid balance if drug is used with highly emetogenic chemotherapeutic drugs.
- Monitor calcium level in patients at risk for hypocalcemia, such as those with nephrotic syndrome. If needed, give calcium supplements.
- Safety and effectiveness of drug in children haven't been established.

Patient teaching

- Instruct patient to remain lying down throughout infusion.
- Advise patient not to breast-feed; it's unknown if drug appears in breast milk.

amikacin sulfate
Amikin

Pregnancy risk category D

Indications & dosages

➲ **Serious infections caused by sensitive strains of *Pseudomonas aeruginosa, Escherichia coli, Proteus, Klebsiella,* or *Staphylococcus***

Adults and children: 15 mg/kg/day I.M. or I.V. infusion, in divided doses q 8 to 12 hours.

Neonates: Initially, loading dose of 10 mg/kg I.V.; then 7.5 mg/kg q 12 hours.

➲ **Uncomplicated UTI caused by organisms not susceptible to less toxic drugs**

Adults: 250 mg I.M. or I.V. b.i.d.

➲ ***Mycobacterium avium* complex (MAC) infection ♦**

Adults: 15 mg/kg/day I.V. in divided doses q 8 to 12 hours as part of a multiple-drug regimen.

For adult patients with impaired renal function, initially, 7.5 mg/kg I.M. or I.V. Subsequent doses and frequency determined by amikacin levels and renal function studies. For adults receiving hemodialysis, give supplemental doses of 50% to 75% of initial loading dose at end of each dialysis session. Monitor drug levels and adjust dosage accordingly.

Contraindications & cautions

- Contraindicated in patients hypersensitive to drug or other aminoglycosides.
- Use cautiously in patients with impaired renal function or neuromuscular disorders, in neonates and infants, and in elderly patients.

Adverse reactions

CNS: ***neuromuscular blockade.***
EENT: *ototoxicity.*
GU: *azotemia,* ***nephrotoxicity,*** possible increase in urinary excretion of casts.
Musculoskeletal: arthralgia.
Respiratory: ***apnea.***

Interactions

Drug-drug. *Acyclovir, amphotericin B, cephalosporins, cidofovir, cisplatin, methoxyflurane, vancomycin, other aminoglycosides:* May increase nephrotoxicity. Use together cautiously, and monitor renal function test results.

Atracurium, doxacurium, mivacurium, pancuronium, rocuronium, tubocurarine, vecuronium: May increase effects of nondepolarizing muscle relaxants, including prolonged respiratory depression. Use together only when necessary, and expect to reduce dosage of nondepolarizing muscle relaxant.

Dimenhydrinate: May mask ototoxicity symptoms. Monitor patient's hearing.

General anesthetics: May increase neuromuscular blockade. Monitor patient for increased effects.

Indomethacin: May increase trough and peak amikacin levels. Monitor amikacin level.

I.V. loop diuretics (such as furosemide): May increase ototoxicity. Use together cautiously, and monitor patient's hearing.

Parenteral penicillins (such as ticarcillin): May inactivate amikacin in vitro. Don't mix.

Nursing considerations

- Obtain specimen for culture and sensitivity tests before giving first dose. Therapy may begin while awaiting results.
- Evaluate patient's hearing before and during therapy if he will be receiving drug for longer than 2 weeks. Notify prescriber if patient has tinnitus, vertigo, or hearing loss.
- Weigh patient and review renal function studies before therapy begins.
- Correct dehydration before therapy because dehydration increases risk of toxicity.
- Obtain blood for peak amikacin level 1 hour after I.M. injection and 30 minutes to 1 hour after I.V. infusion ends; for trough levels, draw blood just before next dose. Don't collect blood in a heparinized tube; heparin is incompatible with aminoglycosides.
- Peak drug levels more than 35 mcg/ml and trough levels more than 10 mcg/ml may be linked to a higher risk of toxicity.
- Monitor renal function: urine output, specific gravity, urinalysis, BUN and creatinine levels, and creatinine clearance. Report to prescriber evidence of declining renal function.
- Watch for signs and symptoms of superinfection (especially of upper respiratory tract), such as continued fever, chills, and increased pulse rate.
- Therapy usually continues for 7 to 10 days. If no response occurs after 3 to 5 days, stop therapy and obtain new specimens for culture and sensitivity testing.

!! ALERT Don't confuse Amikin with Amicar. Don't confuse amikacin (Amikin) with anakinra (Kineret).

Patient teaching

- Instruct patient to promptly report adverse reactions to prescriber.
- Encourage patient to maintain adequate fluid intake.

aminophylline (theophylline ethylenediamine)

Aminophylline, Phyllocontin†, Phyllocontin-350†, Truphylline

Pregnancy risk category C

Indications & dosages

➲ Symptomatic relief of bronchospasm (aminophylline doses)

Patients not currently receiving theophylline products who need rapid relief from symptoms: 6 mg/kg (equivalent to 4.7 mg/kg anhydrous theophylline) I.V. at 25 mg/minute or less; then begin maintenance infusion as detailed below according to age group or health status.

For otherwise healthy adult smokers: 1 mg/kg/hour I.V. for 12 hours; then 0.8 mg/kg/hour.

Nonsmoking adults and adolescents older than age 16: 0.7 mg/kg/hour I.V. for 12 hours; then 0.5 mg/kg/hour.

Children ages 9 to 16: 1 mg/kg/hour I.V. for 12 hours; then 0.8 mg/kg/hour.

Children ages 6 months to 9 years: 1.2 mg/kg/hour for 12 hours; then 1 mg/kg/hour.

For elderly patients and those with cor pulmonale, 0.6 mg/kg/hour I.V. for 12 hours; then 0.3 mg/kg/hour. For adults with heart failure or hepatic disease, 0.5 mg/kg/hour I.V. for 12 hours; then 0.1 to 0.2 mg/kg/hour.

Patients currently receiving theophylline products: Determine time, amount, route of administration, and dosage form of patient's last theophylline dose. An aminophylline infusion of 0.63 mg/kg (0.5 mg/kg anhydrous theophylline) increases theophylline level by 1 mcg/ml. Some prescribers recommend a dose of 3.1 mg/kg (2.5 mg/kg anhydrous theophylline) if no obvious signs or symptoms of theophylline toxicity develop.

➲ Chronic bronchial asthma

Adults and children: Dosage is highly individualized. The P.R. route and the P.O. route use the same dosage. Doses reflect anhydrous theophylline equivalents: 100 mg aminophylline hydrous = 78.9 mg theophylline anhydrous (tablets, suppositories, and parenteral injection); 100 mg aminophylline hydrous = 85.7 mg theophylline anhydrous.

Initially, 16 mg/kg or 400 mg (whichever is less) P.O. daily of rapidly absorbed form, in three or four divided doses q 6 to 8 hours. Increase dosage, if tolerated, by 25% daily q 2 to 3 days. Or, 12 mg/kg or 400 mg (whichever is less) P.O. daily of extended-release form, in two or three divided doses q 8 to 12 hours. Increase dosage, if tolerated, by 2 to 3 mg/kg daily q 3 days.

Regardless of dosage form, maximum doses are as follows:

Adults and children age 16 and older: 13 mg/kg daily or 900 mg/day, whichever is less.

Children ages 12 to 16: 18 mg/kg daily.

Children ages 9 to 12: 20 mg/kg daily.

Children ages 1 to 9: 24 mg/kg daily.

When maximum dosage is reached, adjust dosage based on peak theophylline level. Target theophylline level is usually 10 to 20 mcg/ml.

Contraindications & cautions

- Contraindicated in patients hypersensitive to xanthine compounds (caffeine, theobromine) and ethylenediamine and in those with active peptic ulcer disease and seizure disorders (unless they receive adequate anticonvulsant therapy).
- Rectal suppositories contraindicated in patients with irritation or infection of the rectum or lower colon.
- Use cautiously in neonates, infants, young children, and elderly patients; and in patients with heart failure, other cardiac or circulatory impairment, COPD, cor pulmonale, renal or hepatic disease, hyperthyroidism, diabetes mellitus, glaucoma, peptic ulcer, severe hypoxemia, or hypertension.

Adverse reactions

CNS: fever, *nervousness, restlessness,* headache, *insomnia,* ***seizures,*** muscle twitching, irritability, *dizziness,* confusion, psychosis.

CV: *palpitations, sinus tachycardia,* extrasystoles, flushing, marked hypotension, ***arrhythmias.***

GI: *nausea, vomiting,* diarrhea, epigastric pain, hematemesis, irritation with rectal suppositories, anorexia.

Metabolic: hyperglycemia.

Respiratory: tachypnea, ***respiratory arrest.***

Skin: urticaria.

Other: hypersensitivity reactions.

Interactions

Drug-drug. *Adenosine:* May decrease antiarrhythmic effectiveness. Higher adenosine doses may be needed.

Alkali-sensitive drugs: May reduce activity. Don't add to I.V. fluids containing aminophylline.

Barbiturates, nicotine, phenytoin, rifampin: May enhance metabolism and decrease theophylline level. Monitor patient for decreased aminophylline effect.

Calcium channel blockers, cimetidine, disulfiram, influenza virus vaccine, interferon, macrolide antibiotics (such as erythromycin), methotrexate, hormonal contraceptives, quinolone antibiotics (such as ciprofloxacin): May decrease hepatic clearance of theophylline and elevate theophylline level. Monitor theophylline level, and watch for signs and symptoms of toxicity.

Carbamazepine, isoniazid, loop diuretics: May increase or decrease theophylline level. Monitor theophylline level closely.

Carteolol, pindolol, propranolol, timolol: May act antagonistically, reducing the effects of one or both drugs. Monitor patient closely.

Ephedrine, other sympathomimetics: May produce synergistic toxicity with these drugs, predisposing patient to arrhythmias. Monitor patient closely.

Lithium: May increase lithium excretion. Monitor lithium level.

Drug-herb. *Cayenne:* May increase risk of theophylline toxicity. Advise patient to use together cautiously.

Ipriflavone: May increase risk of theophylline toxicity. Advise patient to use together cautiously.

St. John's wort: May lower theophylline level. Monitor theophylline level and discourage use together.

Drug-lifestyle. *Smoking:* May increase elimination of theophylline, increasing dosing requirements. Monitor theophylline response and level.

Nursing considerations

- Relieve GI symptoms by giving oral drug with full glass of water at meals, although food in stomach delays absorption. No evidence exists that antacids reduce adverse GI reactions. Enteric-coated tablets may delay or impair absorption.

!!ALERT Before giving loading dose, make sure patient hasn't had recent theophylline therapy.

- Suppositories are slowly and erratically absorbed. Give rectal suppository if patient can't take drug orally. Schedule dose after bowel evacuation, if possible; drug may be retained better if given before a meal. Have patient remain recumbent 15 to 20 minutes after insertion.
- Monitor vital signs; measure and record fluid intake and output. Expect improved quality of pulse and respirations.
- Aminophylline is a soluble salt of theophylline. Dosage is adjusted by monitoring response, tolerance, pulmonary function, and theophylline level. Drug levels should range from 10 to 20 mcg/ml; toxicity may occur above 20 mcg/ml.

!!ALERT Evidence of toxicity includes tachycardia, anorexia, nausea, vomiting, diarrhea, restlessness, irritability, and headache. Check theophylline level, and adjust dosage as directed.

- Patients who develop urticaria may tolerate other theophylline preparations. Urticaria may be caused by the ethylenediamine salt.

!!ALERT Don't confuse aminophylline with amitriptyline or ampicillin.

Patient teaching

- Provide dosage schedule and instructions for home use of prescribed form. Some patients may need an around-the-clock dosage schedule.
- Warn elderly patient that dizziness is common at start of therapy.
- Warn patient to check with prescriber before combining aminophylline with other drugs. Prescription or OTC remedies may contain ephedrine and theophylline salts; excessive CNS stimulation may result.
- Caution patient not to switch brands without first checking with prescriber.
- If patient smokes, tell him to notify prescriber if he quits.

amiodarone hydrochloride

Cordarone, Pacerone

Pregnancy risk category D

Indications & dosages

➲ Life-threatening recurrent ventricular fibrillation or recurrent hemodynamically unstable ventricular tachycardia unresponsive to adequate doses of other antiarrhythmics or when alternative drugs can't be tolerated

Adults: Give loading dose of 800 to 1,600 mg P.O. daily divided b.i.d. for 1 to 3 weeks until first therapeutic response occurs; then 600 to 800 mg P.O. daily for 1 month, followed by maintenance dose 200 to 600 mg P.O. daily.

Or, give loading dose of 150 mg I.V. over 10 minutes (15 mg/minute); then 360 mg I.V. over next 6 hours (1 mg/minute), followed by 540 mg I.V. over next 18 hours (0.5 mg/minute). After first 24 hours, continue with maintenance I.V. infusion of 720 mg/24 hours (0.5 mg/minute).

➲ Cardiac arrest, pulseless ventricular tachycardia, or ventricular fibrillation

Adults: 300 mg diluted in 20 to 30 ml of a compatible solution, as I.V. push.

➲ Supraventricular arrhythmias♦

Adults: Give loading dose of 600 to 800 mg P.O. daily for 1 to 4 weeks or until supraventricular tachycardia (SVT) is controlled or adverse reactions occur. Reduce gradually to maintenance dose of 100 to 400 mg P.O. daily.

➲ Ventricular and supraventricular arrhythmias♦

Children: Give loading dose of 10 to 15 mg/kg/day or 600 to 800 mg/1.73 m^2 P.O. daily for 4 to 14 days or until arrhythmia is controlled or adverse reactions occur. Reduce dosage to 5 mg/kg/day or 200 to 400 mg/1.73 m^2 for several weeks; then reduce dosage to lowest effective level.

Or, give loading dose 5 mg/kg I.V. infused over several minutes to 1 hour. Give additional 5 mg/kg doses if needed, to a maximum of 15 mg/kg/day. Or, 5 mg/kg I.V. in five divided doses of 1 mg/kg over 5 to 10 minutes to minimize exposure to diethylhexyl phthalate (DEHP).

➲ **Short-term management of atrial fibrillation♦**
Adults: 125 mg/hour I.V. for 24 hours.
➲ **Long-term management of recurrent atrial fibrillation♦**
Adults: 10 mg/kg P.O. daily for 14 days; then 300 mg P.O. daily for 4 weeks; then maintenance dose of 200 mg P.O. daily.
➲ **Heart failure (impaired left ventricular ejection fraction, impaired exercise tolerance, and ventricular arrhythmias)♦**
Adults: 200 mg P.O. daily.

Contraindications & cautions

- Contraindicated in patients hypersensitive to drug.
- Contraindicated in those with cardiogenic shock, second- or third-degree AV block, severe SA node disease resulting in bradycardia unless an artificial pacemaker is present, and in those for whom bradycardia has caused syncope.
- Use cautiously in patients receiving other antiarrhythmics.
- Use cautiously in patients with pulmonary, hepatic, or thyroid disease.

Adverse reactions

CNS: peripheral neuropathy, ataxia, paresthesia, *tremor*, insomnia, sleep disturbances, headache, *malaise*, *fatigue*.
CV: ***bradycardia***, hypotension, ***arrhythmias***, ***heart failure***, ***heart block***, ***sinus arrest***, edema.
EENT: *asymptomatic corneal microdeposits*, optic neuropathy or neuritis resulting in visual impairment, abnormal smell, *visual disturbances*.
GI: abnormal taste, anorexia, *nausea*, *vomiting*, constipation, abdominal pain.
Hematologic: ***coagulation abnormalities***.
Hepatic: hepatic dysfunction, ***hepatic failure***.
Metabolic: *hypothyroidism*, hyperthyroidism.
Respiratory: ***acute respiratory distress syndrome***, SEVERE PULMONARY TOXICITY.
Skin: *photosensitivity*, solar dermatitis, blue-gray skin.

Interactions

Drug-drug. *Antiarrhythmics:* May reduce hepatic or renal clearance of certain antiarrhythmics, especially flecainide, procainamide, and quinidine. Use of amiodarone with other antiarrhythmics, especially mexiletine, propafenone, disopyramide, and procainamide, may induce torsades de pointes. Avoid using together.
Antihypertensives: May increase hypotensive effect. Use together cautiously.
Beta blockers, calcium channel blockers: May increase cardiac depressant effects; may increase slowing of SA node and AV conduction. Use together cautiously.
Cimetidine: May increase amiodarone level. Use together cautiously.
Cyclosporine: May increase cyclosporine level, resulting in an increase in the serum creatinine level and renal toxicity. Monitor cyclosporine levels and renal function tests.
Digoxin: May increase digoxin level 70% to 100%. Monitor digoxin level closely and reduce digoxin dosage by half or stop drug completely when starting amiodarone therapy.
Fentanyl: May cause hypotension, bradycardia, and decreased cardiac output. Monitor patient closely.
Fluoroquinolones: May increase risk of arrhythmias. Avoid using together.
Methotrexate: May impair methotrexate metabolism, causing toxicity. Use together cautiously.
Phenytoin: May decrease phenytoin metabolism and amiodarone level. Monitor phenytoin level and adjust dosages of drugs if needed.
Quinidine: May increase quinidine level, causing life-threatening cardiac arrhythmias. Avoid using together, or monitor quinidine level closely if use together can't be avoided. Adjust quinidine dosage as needed.
Rifamycins: May decrease amiodarone level. Monitor patient closely.
Ritonavir: May increase amiodarone level. Avoid using together.
Theophylline: May increase theophylline level and cause toxicity. Monitor theophylline level.
Warfarin: May increase anticoagulant response with the potential for serious or fatal bleeding. Decrease warfarin dosage 33% to 50% when starting amiodarone. Monitor patient closely.
Drug-herb. *Pennyroyal:* May change rate of formation of toxic metabolites of pennyroyal. Discourage use together.
St. John's wort: May decrease amiodarone levels. Discourage use together.

Drug-lifestyle. *Sun exposure:* May cause photosensitivity reaction. Advise patient to avoid excessive sunlight exposure and to take precautions while in the sun.

Nursing considerations

- Be aware of the high risk of adverse reactions.
- Obtain baseline pulmonary, liver, and thyroid function test results and baseline chest X-ray.
- Give loading doses in a hospital setting and with continuous ECG monitoring because of the slow onset of antiarrhythmic effect and the risk of life-threatening arrhythmias.
- Divide oral loading dose into two or three equal doses and give with meals to decrease GI intolerance. Give maintenance dose once daily or divide into two doses, with meals to decrease GI intolerance.

!!ALERT Drug may pose life-threatening management problems in patients at risk for sudden death. Use only in patients with life-threatening, recurrent ventricular arrhythmias unresponsive to or intolerant of other antiarrhythmics or alternative drugs. Amiodarone can cause fatal toxicities, including hepatic and pulmonary toxicity.

!!ALERT Amiodarone is a highly toxic drug. Watch carefully for pulmonary toxicity. Risk increases in patients receiving doses over 400 mg/day.

- Watch for evidence of pneumonitis exertional dyspnea, nonproductive cough, and pleuritic chest pain. Monitor pulmonary function tests and chest X-ray.
- Monitor liver and thyroid function test results and electrolyte, particularly potassium and magnesium, levels.
- Monitor PT and INR if patient takes warfarin and digoxin level if he takes digoxin.
- Instill methylcellulose ophthalmic solution during amiodarone therapy to minimize corneal microdeposits. About 1 to 4 months after starting amiodarone, most patients develop corneal microdeposits, although 10% or less have vision disturbances. Regular ophthalmic examinations are advised.
- Monitor blood pressure and heart rate and rhythm frequently. Perform continuous ECG monitoring when starting or changing dosage. Notify prescriber of significant change in assessment results.
- Life-threatening gasping syndrome may occur in neonates given I.V. solutions containing benzyl alcohol.

!!ALERT Don't confuse amiodarone with amiloride.

Patient teaching

- Advise patient to wear sunscreen or protective clothing to prevent sensitivity reaction to the sun. Monitor patient for skin burning or tingling, followed by redness and blistering. Exposed skin may turn blue-gray.
- Tell patient to take oral drug with food if GI reactions occur.
- Inform patient that adverse effects of drug are more common at high doses and become more frequent with treatment lasting longer than 6 months but are generally reversible when drug is stopped. Resolution of adverse reactions may take up to 4 months.

amitriptyline hydrochloride
Apo-Amitriptyline†

Pregnancy risk category C

Indications & dosages

➲ Depression

Adults: Initially, 50 to 100 mg P.O. h.s., increasing to 150 mg daily. Maximum, 300 mg daily, if needed. Maintenance, 50 to 100 mg daily. Or, 20 to 30 mg I.M. q.i.d.

Elderly patients and adolescents: 10 mg P.O. t.i.d. and 20 mg h.s. daily.

Contraindications & cautions

- Contraindicated in patients hypersensitive to drug and in those who have received an MAO inhibitor within the past 14 days.
- Contraindicated during acute recovery phase of MI.
- Use cautiously in patients with history of seizures, urine retention, angle-closure glaucoma, or increased intraocular pressure; in those with hyperthyroidism, CV disease, diabetes, or impaired liver function; and in those receiving thyroid drugs.
- Use cautiously in those receiving electroconvulsive therapy.

Adverse reactions

CNS: ataxia, tremor, peripheral neuropathy, anxiety, insomnia, restlessness, drowsiness,

dizziness, weakness, fatigue, headache, extrapyramidal reactions, ***coma***, ***seizures***, ***CVA***, hallucinations, delusions, disorientation.
CV: *orthostatic hypotension*, *tachycardia*, ECG changes, hypertension, edema, ***MI***, ***arrhythmias***, ***heart block***.
EENT: blurred vision, tinnitus, mydriasis, increased intraocular pressure.
GI: *dry mouth*, nausea, vomiting, anorexia, epigastric pain, diarrhea, constipation, paralytic ileus.
GU: urine retention.
Hematologic: ***agranulocytosis***, ***thrombocytopenia***, ***leukopenia***, eosinophilia.
Metabolic: ***hypoglycemia***, hyperglycemia.
Skin: rash, urticaria, photosensitivity reactions, diaphoresis.
Other: hypersensitivity reactions.

Interactions

Drug-drug. *Barbiturates, CNS depressants:* May enhance CNS depression. Avoid using together.
Cimetidine, fluoxetine, fluvoxamine, hormonal contraceptives, paroxetine, sertraline: May increase tricyclic antidepressant level. Watch for increased antidepressant adverse effects.
Clonidine: May cause potentially life-threatening elevations in blood pressure. Avoid using together.
Epinephrine, norepinephrine: May increase hypertensive effect. Use together cautiously.
MAO inhibitors: May cause severe excitation, hyperpyrexia, or seizures, usually with high doses. Avoid using within 14 days of MAO inhibitor therapy.
Drug-herb. *Evening primrose:* May cause additive or synergistic effect, resulting in lower seizure threshold and increasing the risk of seizures. Discourage use together.
St. John's wort, SAM-e, yohimbe: May cause serotonin syndrome and decrease amitriptyline level. Discourage use together.
Drug-lifestyle. *Alcohol use:* May enhance CNS depression. Discourage use together.
Smoking: May lower drug level. Watch for lack of effect.
Sun exposure: May increase risk of photosensitivity reactions. Advise patient to avoid excessive sunlight exposure.

Nursing considerations

!!ALERT Parenteral form of drug is for I.M. administration only. Drug shouldn't be given I.V.

- Amitriptyline has strong anticholinergic effects and is one of the most sedating tricyclic antidepressants. Anticholinergic effects have rapid onset even though therapeutic effect is delayed for weeks.
- If signs or symptoms of psychosis occur or increase, expect prescriber to reduce dosage. Record mood changes. Monitor patient for suicidal tendencies and allow only minimum supply of drug.
- Because patients using tricyclic antidepressants may suffer hypertensive episodes during surgery, stop drug gradually several days before surgery.
- Monitor glucose level.
- Watch for nausea, headache, and malaise after abrupt withdrawal of long-term therapy; these symptoms don't indicate addiction.
- Don't withdraw drug abruptly.

!!ALERT Don't confuse amitriptyline with nortriptyline or aminophylline.

Patient teaching

- Whenever possible, advise patient to take full dose at bedtime, but warn him of possible morning orthostatic hypotension.
- Tell patient to avoid alcohol during drug therapy.
- Advise patient to consult prescriber before taking other drugs.
- Warn patient to avoid activities that require alertness and good psychomotor coordination until CNS effects of drug are known. Drowsiness and dizziness usually subside after a few weeks.
- Inform patient that dry mouth may be relieved with sugarless hard candy or gum. Saliva substitutes may be useful.
- To prevent photosensitivity reactions, advise patient to use a sunblock, wear protective clothing, and avoid prolonged exposure to strong sunlight.
- Warn patient not to stop drug therapy abruptly.
- Advise patient that it may take as long as 30 days to achieve full therapeutic effect.

amlodipine besylate
Norvasc

Pregnancy risk category C

Indications & dosages

➲ **Chronic stable angina, vasospastic angina (Prinzmetal's or variant angina)**
Adults: Initially, 5 to 10 mg P.O. daily. Most patients need 10 mg daily.
Elderly patients: Initially, 5 mg P.O. daily.

For patients who are small or frail or have hepatic insufficiency, initially 5 mg P.O. daily.

➲ **Hypertension**
Adults: Initially, 2.5 to 5 mg P.O. daily. Dosage adjusted according to patient response and tolerance. Maximum daily dose is 10 mg.
Elderly patients: Initially, 2.5 mg P.O. daily.

For patients who are small or frail, are taking other antihypertensives, or have hepatic insufficiency, initially 2.5 mg P.O. daily.

Contraindications & cautions

- Contraindicated in patients hypersensitive to drug.
- Use cautiously in patients receiving other peripheral vasodilators, especially those with severe aortic stenosis, and in those with heart failure. Because drug is metabolized by the liver, use cautiously and in reduced dosage in patients with severe hepatic disease.

Adverse reactions

CNS: headache, somnolence, fatigue, dizziness, light-headedness, paresthesia.
CV: *edema*, flushing, palpitations.
GI: nausea, abdominal pain.
GU: sexual difficulties.
Musculoskeletal: muscle pain.
Respiratory: dyspnea.
Skin: rash, pruritus.

Interactions

Drug-food. *Grapefruit juice:* May increase drug level and adverse reactions. Discourage use together.

Nursing considerations

!!ALERT Monitor patient carefully. Some patients, especially those with severe obstructive coronary artery disease, have developed increased frequency, duration, or severity of angina or acute MI after initiation of calcium channel blocker therapy or at time of dosage increase.
- Monitor blood pressure frequently during initiation of therapy. Because drug-induced vasodilation has a gradual onset, acute hypotension is rare.
- Notify prescriber if signs of heart failure occur, such as swelling of hands and feet or shortness of breath.

!!ALERT Don't confuse amlodipine with amiloride.

Patient teaching

- Caution patient to continue taking drug, even when feeling better.
- Tell patient S.L. nitroglycerin may be taken as needed when angina symptoms are acute. If patient continues nitrate therapy during adjustment of amlodipine dosage, urge continued compliance.

amlodipine besylate and atorvastatin calcium
Caduet

Pregnancy risk category X

Indications & dosages

➲ **Patients who need amlodipine for hypertension, chronic stable angina, or vasospastic angina and atorvastatin for heterozygous familial or nonfamilial hypercholesterolemia, mixed dyslipidemia, elevated serum triglyceride levels, primary dysbetalipoproteinemia, or homozygous familial hypercholesterolemia**
Adults: 5 to 10 mg amlodipine with 10 to 80 mg atorvastatin P.O. once daily. Determine the most effective dose for each component, and then select the most appropriate combination product.

➲ **Hypertension and heterozygous familial hypercholesterolemia in children**
Boys and postmenarchal girls age 10 and older: 5 mg amlodipine with 10 to 20 mg atorvastatin P.O. once daily. Determine the most effective dose for each component; then select the most appropriate combination product. If patient needs less than 5 mg of amlodipine, don't use the combination product.

Contraindications & cautions

- Contraindicated in pregnant women, breast-feeding women, women of childbearing potential, patients hypersensitive to any component of the product, and patients with active liver disease or an unexplained persistently elevated serum transaminase level.
- Use cautiously in patients who consume large amounts of alcohol or have a history of liver disease.
- Use cautiously in patients who take a peripheral vasodilator or have severe aortic stenosis or heart failure.

Adverse reactions

CNS: asthenia, dizziness, fatigue, *headache*, insomnia, somnolence, vertigo.
CV: chest pain, *edema*, flushing, palpitations.
EENT: pharyngitis, rhinitis, sinusitis.
GI: abdominal pain, constipation, diarrhea, dyspepsia, flatulence, nausea.
GU: urinary tract infection.
Musculoskeletal: arthralgia, arthritis, back pain, myalgia.
Respiratory: bronchitis, dyspnea.
Skin: pruritus, rash.
Other: accidental injury, ***allergic reaction***, ***anaphylaxis***, flulike syndrome, *infection*.

Interactions

Drug-drug. *Azole antifungals, cyclosporine, erythromycin, fibric acid derivatives, niacin:* May increase risk of rhabdomyolysis with acute renal failure. Assess patient for muscle pain, tenderness, or weakness.
Digoxin: May increase digoxin level. Monitor digoxin level.
Erythromycin: May increase atorvastatin level. Monitor patient.
Hormonal contraceptives: May increase hormone levels and adverse effects of hormonal contraceptive. Monitor patient.

Nursing considerations

- Monitor liver function test results before therapy starts, after 12 weeks, whenever the dosage increases, and periodically during therapy.
- Reduce dose or stop drug if AST or ALT levels increase to more than 3 times the upper limit of normal and stay elevated.
- Assess the patient for myalgias, muscle tenderness or weakness, and marked elevation in creatine (CPK) level. Stop drug if CK level exceeds 10 times the upper limit of normal or if myopathy is diagnosed or suspected.
- Stop drug if patient has evidence of myopathy or has a condition that increases the risk of renal failure secondary to rhabdomyolysis, such as a severe acute infection, hypotension, major surgery, trauma, uncontrolled seizures, or severe metabolic, endocrine, or electrolyte disorders.
- Because of risks to the fetus, drug should be given to a woman of childbearing age only if she is unable to conceive.

Patient teaching

- Advise patient to promptly report unexplained muscle pain, tenderness, or weakness, especially if accompanied by malaise or fever.
- Urge patient to continue appropriate diet, exercise, and weight loss regimens.

amoxicillin and clavulanate potassium (amoxycillin and clavulanate potassium)

Augmentin, Augmentin ES-600, Augmentin XR, Clavulin†

Pregnancy risk category B

Indications & dosages

➲ **Recurrent or persistent acute otitis media caused by *Streptococcus pneumoniae, Haemophilus influenzae,* or *Moraxella catarrhalis* in patients exposed to antibiotics within the last 3 months, who are 2 years old or younger or in day-care facilities**

Children age 3 months and older: 90 mg/kg/day Augmentin ES-600 P.O., based on amoxicillin component, q 12 hours for 10 days.

➲ **Lower respiratory tract infections, otitis media, sinusitis, skin and skin-structure infections, and UTIs caused by susceptible strains of gram-positive and gram-negative organisms**

Adults and children weighing 40 kg (88 lb) or more: 250 mg P.O., based on amoxicillin component, q 8 hours; or 500 mg q 12 hours. For more severe infections, 500 mg q 8 hours or 875 mg q 12 hours.

Children age 3 months and older and weighing less than 40 kg: 20 to 45 mg/kg P.O., based on amoxicillin component and severity of infection, daily in divided doses q 8 to 12 hours.
Children younger than age 3 months: 30 mg/kg/day P.O., based on amoxicillin component of the 125-mg/5-ml oral suspension, in divided doses q 12 hours.

Don't give the 875-mg tablet to patients with creatinine clearance less than 30 ml/minute. If clearance is 10 to 30 ml/minute, give 250 to 500 mg P.O. q 12 hours. If clearance is less than 10 ml/minute, give 250 to 500 mg P.O. q 24 hours. Give hemodialysis patients 250 to 500 mg P.O. q 24 hours with an additional dose both during and after dialysis.

➲ **Community-acquired pneumonia or acute bacterial sinusitis caused by *H. influenzae, M. catarrhalis, H. parainfluenzae, Klebsiella pneumoniae,* methicillin-susceptible *Staphylococcus aureus,* or *S. pneumoniae* with reduced susceptibility to penicillin**
Adults and children age 16 and older: 2,000 mg/125 mg Augmentin XR tablets q 12 hours for 7 to 10 days for pneumonia; 10 days for sinusitis.

In patients with creatinine clearance less than 30 ml/minute and patients receiving hemodialysis, don't use Augmentin XR.

Contraindications & cautions

- Contraindicated in patients hypersensitive to drug or other penicillins and in those with a history of amoxicillin-related cholestatic jaundice or hepatic dysfunction.
- Contraindicated in patients receiving hemodialysis and those with creatinine clearance less than 30 ml/minute.
- Use cautiously in patients with other drug allergies (especially to cephalosporins) because of possible cross-sensitivity and in those with mononucleosis because of high risk of maculopapular rash.
- Use cautiously in breast-feeding women; it's unknown if drug appears in breast milk.
- Use cautiously in hepatically impaired patients, and monitor the hepatic function of these patients.

Adverse reactions

CNS: agitation, anxiety, insomnia, confusion, behavioral changes, dizziness.
GI: nausea, vomiting, *diarrhea*, indigestion, gastritis, stomatitis, glossitis, black hairy tongue, enterocolitis, ***pseudomembranous colitis***, mucocutaneous candidiasis, abdominal pain.
GU: vaginitis, vaginal candidiasis.
Hematologic: anemia, ***thrombocytopenia***, ***thrombocytopenic purpura***, eosinophilia, ***leukopenia***, ***agranulocytosis***.
Other: hypersensitivity reactions, ***(anaphylaxis***, rash, urticaria, pruritus, ***angioedema)***, overgrowth of nonsusceptible organisms, serum sickness–like reaction.

Interactions

Drug-drug. *Allopurinol:* May increase risk of rash. Monitor patient for rash.
Hormonal contraceptives: May decrease hormonal contraceptive effectiveness. Advise use of additional form of contraception during penicillin therapy.
Probenecid: May increase levels of amoxicillin and other penicillins. Probenecid may be used for this purpose.
Drug-herb. *Khat:* May decrease antimicrobial effect of certain penicillins. Discourage khat chewing, or tell patient to take amoxicillin 2 hours after khat chewing.

Nursing considerations

- Before giving drug, ask patient about allergic reactions to penicillin. However, a negative history of penicillin allergy is no guarantee against an allergic reaction.
- Obtain specimen for culture and sensitivity tests before giving first dose. Therapy may begin pending results.
- Give drug at least 1 hour before a bacteriostatic antibiotic.
- Each Augmentin XR tablet contains 29.3 mg (1.27 mEq) of sodium.
- Augmentin XR isn't indicated for treating infections caused by *S. pneumoniae* with penicillin minimum inhibitory concentration (commonly known as MIC) 4 mcg/ml or greater.
- If large doses are given or therapy is prolonged, bacterial or fungal superinfection may occur, especially in elderly, debilitated, or immunosuppressed patients.

!!ALERT Don't interchange the oral suspensions because of varying clavulanic acid contents.

- Augmentin ES-600 is intended only for pediatric patients ages 3 months to 12 years with persistent or recurrent acute otitis media.

- Avoid use of 250-mg tablet in children weighing less than 40 kg (88 lb). Use chewable form instead.

!!ALERT Both 250- and 500-mg film-coated tablets contain the same amount of clavulanic acid (125 mg). Therefore, two 250-mg tablets aren't equivalent to one 500-mg tablet. Regular tablets aren't equivalent to Augmentin XR.

- This drug combination is particularly useful in clinical settings with a high prevalence of amoxicillin-resistant organisms.
- After reconstitution, refrigerate the oral suspension; discard after 10 days.

!!ALERT Don't confuse amoxicillin with amoxapine.

Patient teaching

- Tell patient to take entire quantity of drug exactly as prescribed, even after feeling better.
- Instruct patient to take drug with food to prevent GI upset. If he's taking the oral suspension, tell him to keep drug refrigerated, to shake it well before taking it, and to discard remaining drug after 10 days.
- Tell patient to call prescriber if a rash occurs because rash is a sign of an allergic reaction.

amoxicillin trihydrate (amoxycillin trihydrate)

Amoxil, Apo-Amoxi†, DisperMox, Novamoxin†, Nu-Amoxi†, Trimox

Pregnancy risk category B

Indications & dosages

➲ Mild to moderate infections of the ear, nose, and throat; skin and skin structure; or genitourinary tract

Adults and children weighing 40 kg (88 lb) or more: 500 mg P.O. q 12 hours or 250 mg P.O. q 8 hours.

Children older than age 3 months weighing less than 40 kg: 25 mg/kg/day P.O. divided q 12 hours or 20 mg/kg/day P.O. divided q 8 hours.

Neonates and infants up to age 3 months: Up to 30 mg/kg/day P.O. divided q 12 hours.

➲ Mild to severe infections of the lower respiratory tract and severe infections of the ear, nose, and throat; skin and skin structure; or genitourinary tract

Adults and children weighing 40 kg or more: 875 mg P.O. q 12 hours or 500 mg P.O. q 8 hours.

Children older than age 3 months weighing less than 40 kg: 45 mg/kg/day P.O. divided q 12 hours or 40 mg/kg/day P.O. divided q 8 hours.

➲ Uncomplicated gonorrhea

Adults and children weighing more than 45 kg (99 lb): 3 g P.O. with 1 g probenecid given as a single dose.

Children age 2 and older weighing less than 45 kg: 50 mg/kg to a maximum of 3 g P.O. with 25 mg/kg, to a maximum of 1 g of probenecid as a single dose. Don't give probenecid to children younger than age 2.

➲ To prevent endocarditis in patients having dental, oral, or respiratory tract procedures; in moderate-risk patients undergoing GI and GU procedures♦

Adults: 2 g P.O. 1 hour before procedure.

Children: 50 mg/kg P.O. 1 hour before procedure.

➲ To prevent penicillin-susceptible anthrax after exposure♦

Adults and children older than age 9: 500 mg P.O. t.i.d. for 60 days.

Children younger than age 9: 80 mg/kg daily P.O., divided t.i.d. for 60 days.

Contraindications & cautions

- Contraindicated in patients hypersensitive to drug or other penicillins.
- Use cautiously in patients with other drug allergies (especially to cephalosporins) because of possible cross-sensitivity.
- Use cautiously in those with mononucleosis because of high risk of maculopapular rash.

Adverse reactions

CNS: lethargy, hallucinations, ***seizures***, anxiety, confusion, agitation, depression, dizziness, fatigue.

GI: *nausea*, vomiting, *diarrhea*, glossitis, stomatitis, gastritis, enterocolitis, abdominal pain, ***pseudomembranous colitis***, black hairy tongue.

GU: interstitial nephritis, nephropathy, vaginitis.

Hematologic: anemia, ***thrombocytopenia***, ***thrombocytopenic purpura***, eosinophilia, ***leukopenia***, hemolytic anemia, ***agranulocytosis***.
Other: hypersensitivity reactions, ***anaphylaxis***, overgrowth of nonsusceptible organisms.

Interactions

Drug-drug. *Allopurinol:* May increase risk of rash. Monitor patient for rash.
Hormonal contraceptives: May decrease hormonal contraceptive effectiveness. Advise use of additional form of contraception during penicillin therapy.
Probenecid: May increase levels of amoxicillin and other penicillins. Probenecid may be used for this purpose.
Drug-herb. *Khat:* May decrease antimicrobial effect of certain penicillins. Discourage khat chewing, or tell patient to take amoxicillin 2 hours after khat chewing.

Nursing considerations

- Obtain specimen for culture and sensitivity tests before giving first dose. Therapy may begin pending results.
- Before giving, ask patient about allergic reactions to penicillin. A negative history of penicillin allergy is no guarantee against allergic reaction.
- If large doses are given or if therapy is prolonged, bacterial or fungal superinfection may occur, especially in elderly, debilitated, or immunosuppressed patients.
- Store Trimox oral suspension in refrigerator, if possible. It also may be stored at room temperature for up to 2 weeks. Make sure to check individual product labels for storage information.
- Amoxicillin usually causes fewer cases of diarrhea than does ampicillin.

!!ALERT Don't confuse amoxicillin with amoxapine.

Patient teaching

- Tell patient to take entire quantity of drug exactly as prescribed, even after he feels better.
- Instruct patient to take drug with or without food.
- Tell patient to notify prescriber if rash, fever, or chills develop. A rash is the most common allergic reaction, especially if allopurinol is also being taken.
- Tell parent to place pediatric drops directly on child's tongue for swallowing or add to formula, milk, fruit juice, water, ginger ale, or a cold drink; patient should take immediately and consume entirely.
- If patient takes DisperMox, instruct parent to mix 1 tablet in about 10 ml of water, drink the resulting solution, rinse container with a small amount of water, and drink again to ensure the whole dose is taken. Parent should mix tablet only in water. Caution against chewing tablets, swallowing them whole, or letting them dissolve in mouth.

amphotericin B cholesteryl sulfate complex

Amphotec

Pregnancy risk category B

Indications & dosages

➲ **Invasive aspergillosis in patients whose renal impairment or unacceptable toxicity precludes use of effective doses of amphotericin B deoxycholate or whose previous amphotericin B deoxycholate therapy has failed**
Adults and children: 3 to 4 mg/kg/day I.V. Dilute in D_5W and give by continuous infusion at 1 mg/kg/hour. Give a test dose before beginning new course of treatment; infuse 10 ml of final preparation containing 1.6 to 8.3 mg of drug over 15 to 30 minutes, and monitor patient for next 30 minutes. May shorten infusion time to 2 hours or lengthen infusion time based on patient's tolerance.
➲ ***Candida*** **or** ***Cryptococcus*** **infections in patients who can't tolerate or who failed to respond to conventional amphotericin B♦**
Adults: 3 to 6 mg/kg/day I.V. Dosages up to 7.5 mg/kg/day I.V. have been used for invasive fungal infections in bone marrow transplant patients.

Contraindications & cautions

- Contraindicated in patients hypersensitive to drug or its components, unless the benefits outweigh the risks.
- It's unknown if drug appears in breast milk; if it does, breast-fed infants are at risk

for serious adverse reactions. Patient should either stop breast-feeding or stop drug.

Adverse reactions

CNS: *fever*, abnormal thinking, anxiety, agitation, confusion, depression, dizziness, hallucinations, headache, hypertonia, neuropathy, nervousness, paresthesia, psychosis, ***seizures***, somnolence, speech disorder, stupor, asthenia, syncope.
CV: ***arrhythmias***, atrial fibrillation, ***bradycardia, cardiac arrest, heart failure, hemorrhage***, hypertension, hypotension, phlebitis, chest pain, orthostatic hypotension, ***shock, supraventricular tachycardia***, *tachycardia*, vasodilation, ***ventricular extrasystoles***, edema.
EENT: amblyopia, deafness, epistaxis, eye hemorrhage, pharyngitis, tinnitus, rhinitis, sinusitis.
GI: abdominal pain, anorexia; diarrhea; dry mouth; ***GI hemorrhage***; gingivitis; glossitis; hematemesis; melena; mouth ulceration; *nausea*; oral candidiasis; stomatitis; *vomiting*.
GU: albuminuria, dysuria, glycosuria, hematuria, oliguria, urinary incontinence or urine retention, ***renal failure***.
Hematologic: anemia, coagulation disorders, ecchymosis, hypochromic anemia, leukocytosis, ***leukopenia***, petechiae, ***thrombocytopenia***.
Hepatic: *hyperbilirubinemia*, jaundice, ***hepatic failure***.
Metabolic: weight changes, acidosis, dehydration, *hypokalemia*, hypocalcemia, ***hypoglycemia***, hypoproteinemia, hyperglycemia, hypervolemia, hypophosphatemia, hyponatremia, ***hyperkalemia***, hyperlipemia, hypernatremia, hypomagnesemia.
Musculoskeletal: arthralgia, myalgia, neck or back pain.
Respiratory: ***apnea***, asthma, dyspnea, hemoptysis, hyperventilation, hypoxia, increased cough, lung or respiratory tract disorders, pleural effusion, pulmonary edema.
Skin: acne, alopecia, pruritus, rash, sweating, skin discoloration, nodules, ulcers, urticaria, pain or reaction at injection site.
Other: allergic reaction, ***anaphylaxis***, *chills*, peripheral or facial edema, infection, mucous membrane disorder, ***sepsis***.

Interactions

Drug-drug. *Antineoplastics:* May enhance renal toxicity, bronchospasm, and hypotension. Use together cautiously.
Cardiac glycosides: May enhance potassium excretion and increase digitalis toxicity. Monitor potassium level closely.
Corticosteroids: May enhance potassium depletion, which may increase risk of cardiac dysfunction. Monitor electrolyte levels.
Cyclosporine, tacrolimus: May increase creatinine level. Monitor renal function.
Flucytosine: May increase toxicity by amphotericin. Use together cautiously.
Imidazoles (clotrimazole, fluconazole, ketoconazole, miconazole): May antagonize effects of amphotericin. Monitor patient closely.
Leukocyte transfusions: May increase risk of pulmonary reactions, such as acute dyspnea, tachypnea, hypoxemia, hemoptysis, and interstitial infiltrates. Use together cautiously; separate doses as much as possible, and monitor pulmonary function.
Nephrotoxic drugs (such as aminoglycosides, pentamidine): May enhance renal toxicity. Monitor renal function closely.
Skeletal muscle relaxants: May enhance muscle relaxant effects because of amphotericin. Monitor potassium level closely.

Nursing considerations

!!ALERT Dosages of different amphotericin B preparations will vary because the preparations aren't interchangeable. Confusing the preparations may cause permanent damage or death.
!!ALERT Monitor vital signs every 30 minutes during initial therapy. Acute infusion-related reactions include fever, chills, hypotension, nausea, and tachycardia, usually occur 1 to 3 hours after the I.V. infusion starts, and are usually more severe after first dose, usually diminishing with subsequent doses. If severe respiratory distress occurs, stop infusion immediately and don't treat further with drug.

- Reduce acute infusion-related reactions by pretreating with antihistamines, antipyretics, and corticosteroids; reducing infusion rate; and maintaining sodium balance.
- Reduce risk of nephrotoxicity by hydrating patient before infusion.
- Monitor intake and output; report changes in urine appearance or volume.

- Monitor renal and hepatic function test results, electrolyte levels (especially potassium, magnesium, and calcium), CBC, and PT.

Patient teaching

- Instruct patient to immediately report symptoms of hypersensitivity.
- Warn patient of possible discomfort at I.V. site.
- Advise patient of potential adverse reactions, such as fever, chills, nausea, and vomiting. Tell patient that these can be severe with first dose but usually subside with repeated doses.

amphotericin B desoxycholate
Amphocin, Amphotericin B for Injection, Fungizone

Pregnancy risk category B

Indications & dosages

➲ **Systemic fungal infection (histoplasmosis, coccidioidomycosis, blastomycosis, cryptococcosis, disseminated candidiasis, aspergillosis, phycomycosis, zygomycosis) or meningitis**

Adults: Initially, test dose of 1 mg in 20 ml of D_5W infused I.V. over 20 to 30 minutes. If that dosage is tolerated, start daily dose at 0.25 to 0.3 mg/kg by slow I.V. infusion (0.1 mg/ml) over 2 to 6 hours. Daily dose is gradually increased to maximum of 1.5 mg/kg in patients with potentially fatal infections. If drug is stopped for 1 week or longer, resume with initial dose and increase gradually.

➲ **To prevent fungal infection in bone marrow transplant patients♦**

Adults: 0.1 mg/kg/day as I.V. infusion.

Contraindications & cautions

- Contraindicated in patients hypersensitive to drug.
- Use cautiously in patients with impaired renal function.

Adverse reactions

CNS: *headache, fever,* peripheral neuropathy, transient vertigo, *malaise,* ***seizures.***
CV: hypotension, ***arrhythmias, asystole,*** hypertension, tachycardia, flushing, *phlebitis, thrombophlebitis.*
EENT: hearing loss, tinnitus, blurred vision, diplopia.
GI: *anorexia, nausea, vomiting, dyspepsia, diarrhea, epigastric pain, cramping,* melena, steatorrhea, ***hemorrhagic gastroenteritis.***
GU: *abnormal renal function with azotemia, hyposthenuria, renal tubular acidosis, nephrocalcinosis,* ***permanent renal impairment,*** anuria, oliguria.
Hematologic: *normochromic anemia, normocytic anemia,* ***thrombocytopenia, leukopenia, agranulocytosis,*** eosinophilia, leukocytosis.
Hepatic: ***hepatitis,*** jaundice, ***acute liver failure.***
Metabolic: *weight loss, hypokalemia,* ***hypoglycemia,*** hyperglycemia, hyperuricemia, hypomagnesemia.
Musculoskeletal: arthralgia, myalgia.
Respiratory: dyspnea, tachypnea, ***bronchospasm,*** wheezing.
Skin: *maculopapular rash,* pruritus, tissue damage with extravasation, *pain at injection site.*
Other: *chills, generalized pain,* ***anaphylactoid reaction.***

Interactions

Drug-drug. *Antineoplastics (such as mechlorethamine):* May cause renal toxicity, bronchospasm, and hypotension. Use together cautiously.
Cardiac glycosides: May increase risk of digitalis toxicity in potassium-depleted patients. Monitor digoxin level closely.
Corticosteroids: May increase potassium depletion. Monitor potassium level.
Flucytosine: May have synergistic effect; may cause increased toxicity of flucytosine. Monitor patient closely for toxicity.
Leukocyte transfusions: May increase risk of pulmonary reactions, such as acute dyspnea, tachypnea, hypoxemia, hemoptysis, and interstitial infiltrates. Use together cautiously; separate doses as much as possible and monitor pulmonary function if drugs are used together.
Nephrotoxic drugs such as antibiotics, pentamidine: May cause additive renal toxicity. Use together cautiously and monitor renal function studies.
Thiazides: May intensify depletion of electrolytes, especially potassium. Monitor patient for hypokalemia.

Drug-herb. *Gossypol:* May increase risk of renal toxicity. Discourage use together.

Nursing considerations

- Because of drug's dangerous adverse effects, it's used primarily to treat patients with progressive and potentially fatal fungal infections.
- Infusion-related reactions, including fever, shaking chills, hypotension, anorexia, nausea, vomiting, headache, dyspnea, and tachypnea, may occur 1 to 3 hours after starting infusion.

!!ALERT Different amphotericin B preparations aren't interchangeable, so dosages will vary. Confusing the preparations may cause permanent damage or death.

!!ALERT To reduce severe adverse effects, patient may receive premedication with antipyretics, antihistamines, antiemetics, or small doses of corticosteroids given on an alternate-day schedule. For severe reactions, stop drug and notify prescriber.

- Infusion-related reactions occur most frequently with initial doses and usually lessen with subsequent doses.
- Monitor fluid intake and output; report change in urine appearance or volume. Monitor BUN and creatinine levels or creatinine clearance at least weekly. Kidney damage may be reversible if drug is stopped at first sign of renal dysfunction.
- Hydration before infusion may reduce risk of nephrotoxicity.
- Obtain hepatic and renal function studies weekly, if ordered. Drug may be stopped if alkaline phosphatase or bilirubin level increases. If BUN level exceeds 40 mg/100 ml or if creatinine level exceeds 3 mg/100 ml, prescriber may reduce or stop drug until renal function improves. Monitor CBC weekly.
- Monitor potassium level closely and report signs of hypokalemia. Hypokalemia occurs commonly and can be life-threatening. Potassium supplementation may be needed.
- Check calcium and magnesium levels twice weekly.
- Drug is potentially ototoxic. Report evidence of hearing loss, tinnitus, vertigo, or unsteady gait.

Patient teaching

- Warn patient of possible discomfort at I.V. site and other potential adverse reactions. Instruct patient to report signs and symptoms of hypersensitivity immediately.
- Inform patient that therapy may take several months. Stress importance of compliance and follow-up.

amphotericin B lipid complex
Abelcet

Pregnancy risk category B

Indications & dosages

➲ **Invasive fungal infections, including *Aspergillus* and *Candida* species, in patients refractory to or intolerant of conventional amphotericin B therapy**
Adults and children: 5 mg/kg daily I.V. as a single infusion given at rate of 2.5 mg/kg/hour.

Contraindications & cautions

- Contraindicated in patients hypersensitive to amphotericin B or its components.
- Use cautiously in patients with renal impairment. Base the need for dosage adjustment on overall clinical status of patient. Renal toxicity is more common at higher dosages.
- It's unknown if drug appears in breast milk. Encourage the patient to either stop breast-feeding or stop treatment.

Adverse reactions

CNS: *fever*, headache, pain.
CV: chest pain, ***cardiac arrest***, hypertension, hypotension.
GI: abdominal pain, diarrhea, ***GI hemorrhage***, nausea, vomiting.
GU: ***renal failure***.
Hematologic: anemia, ***leukopenia***, ***thrombocytopenia***.
Hepatic: bilirubinemia.
Metabolic: hypokalemia.
Respiratory: dyspnea, respiratory disorder, ***respiratory failure***.
Skin: rash.
Other: *chills*, infection, MULTIPLE ORGAN FAILURE, ***sepsis***.

Interactions

Drug-drug. *Antineoplastics:* May increase risk of renal toxicity, bronchospasm, and hypotension. Use together cautiously.

Cardiac glycosides: May increase risk of digitalis toxicity from amphotericin B–induced hypokalemia. Monitor potassium level closely.
Clotrimazole, fluconazole, itraconazole, ketoconazole, miconazole: May antagonize amphotericin B. Monitor patient closely.
Corticosteroids, corticotropin: May enhance hypokalemia, which could lead to cardiac toxicity. Monitor electrolyte levels and cardiac function.
Cyclosporine: May increase renal toxicity. Monitor renal function test results closely.
Flucytosine: May increase risk of flucytosine toxicity from increased cellular uptake or impaired renal excretion. Use together cautiously.
Leukocyte transfusions: Risk of pulmonary reactions such as acute dyspnea, tachypnea, hypoxemia, hemoptysis, and interstitial infiltrates. Use together with caution; separate doses as much as possible, and monitor pulmonary function if drugs are used together.
Nephrotoxic drugs (such as aminoglycosides, pentamidine): May increase risk of renal toxicity. Use together cautiously and monitor renal function closely.
Skeletal muscle relaxants: May enhance skeletal muscle relaxant effects of amphotericin B–induced hypokalemia. Monitor potassium level closely.
Zidovudine: May increase myelotoxicity and nephrotoxicity. Monitor renal and hematologic function.

Nursing considerations

!!ALERT Different amphotericin B preparations aren't interchangeable, so dosages will vary. Confusing the preparations may cause permanent damage or death.

- Premedicate patient with acetaminophen, antihistamines, or corticosteroids to prevent or lessen severity of infusion-related reactions such as fever, chills, nausea, and vomiting, which occur 1 to 2 hours after start of infusion.
- Hydration before infusion may reduce risk of nephrotoxicity.
- Monitor creatinine and electrolyte levels (especially magnesium and potassium), liver function, and CBC during therapy.

Patient teaching

- Inform patient that fever, chills, nausea, and vomiting may occur during infusion and that these reactions usually subside with subsequent doses.
- Instruct patient to report any redness or pain at infusion site.
- Teach patient to recognize and report to prescriber signs and symptoms of acute hypersensitivity, such as respiratory distress.
- Warn patient that therapy may take several months.
- Tell patient to expect frequent laboratory testing to monitor kidney and liver function.

amphotericin B liposomal

AmBisome

Pregnancy risk category B

Indications & dosages

➲ **Empirical therapy for presumed fungal infection in febrile, neutropenic patients**
Adults and children: 3 mg/kg I.V. infusion over 2 hours daily.

➲ **Systemic fungal infections caused by *Aspergillus* species, *Candida* species, or *Cryptococcus* species refractory to amphotericin B deoxycholate or in patients for whom renal impairment or unacceptable toxicity precludes use of amphotericin B deoxycholate**
Adults and children: 3 to 5 mg/kg I.V. infusion over 2 hours daily.

➲ **Visceral leishmaniasis in immunocompetent patients**
Adults and children: 3 mg/kg I.V. infusion over 2 hours daily on days 1 to 5, 14, and 21. A repeat course of therapy may be beneficial if initial treatment fails to clear parasites.

➲ **Visceral leishmaniasis in immunocompromised patients**
Adults and children: 4 mg/kg I.V. infusion over 2 hours daily on days 1 to 5, 10, 17, 24, 31, and 38. Refer patient for expert advice regarding further treatment if initial therapy fails or patient relapses.

➲ **Cryptococcal meningitis in patients with HIV infection**
Adults and children: 6 mg/kg/day I.V. infusion over 2 hours. Reduce infusion time to

1 hour if treatment is well tolerated, and increase infusion time if discomfort occurs.

Contraindications & cautions

- Contraindicated in patients hypersensitive to drug or its components.
- Use cautiously in patients with impaired renal function, in elderly patients, and in pregnant women.
- It's unknown if drug appears in breast milk. Because of potential for serious adverse reactions in breast-fed infants, encourage the patient to either stop breast-feeding or stop treatment, taking into account importance of drug to mother.

Adverse reactions

CNS: *fever, anxiety, confusion, headache, insomnia, asthenia, pain.*
CV: *chest pain, hypotension, tachycardia, hypertension, edema, flushing.*
EENT: *epistaxis, rhinitis.*
GI: *nausea, vomiting, abdominal pain, diarrhea,* ***GI hemorrhage****.*
GU: *hematuria,* ***renal failure****.*
Hepatic: *bilirubinemia,* ***hepatotoxicity****.*
Metabolic: *hyperglycemia,* hypernatremia, *hypocalcemia, hypokalemia, hypomagnesemia.*
Musculoskeletal: *back pain.*
Respiratory: *increased cough, dyspnea,* hypoxia, *pleural effusion, lung disorder,* hyperventilation.
Skin: *pruritus, rash, sweating.*
Other: *chills, infection,* ***anaphylaxis, sepsis****, blood product infusion reaction.*

Interactions

Drug-drug. *Antineoplastics:* May enhance potential for renal toxicity, bronchospasm, and hypotension. Use together cautiously.
Cardiac glycosides: May increase risk of digitalis toxicity caused by amphotericin B–induced hypokalemia. Monitor potassium level closely.
Clotrimazole, fluconazole, ketoconazole, miconazole: May induce fungal resistance to amphotericin B. Use together cautiously.
Corticosteroids, corticotropin: May increase potassium depletion, which could cause cardiac dysfunction. Monitor electrolyte levels and cardiac function.
Flucytosine: May increase flucytosine toxicity by increasing cellular reuptake or impairing renal excretion of flucytosine. Use together cautiously.
Leukocyte transfusions: May increase risk of pulmonary reactions, such as acute dyspnea, tachypnea, hypoxemia, hemoptysis, and interstitial infiltrates. Use together cautiously; separate doses as much as possible, and monitor pulmonary function.
Other nephrotoxic drugs, such as antibiotics and antineoplastics: May cause additive nephrotoxicity. Use together cautiously; monitor renal function closely.
Skeletal muscle relaxants: May enhance effects of skeletal muscle relaxants resulting from amphotericin B–induced hypokalemia. Monitor potassium level.

Nursing considerations

- Patients also receiving chemotherapy or bone marrow transplantation are at greater risk for additional adverse reactions, including seizures, arrhythmias, and thrombocytopenia.

!! ALERT Different amphotericin B preparations aren't interchangeable, so dosages will vary. Confusing the preparations may cause permanent damage or death.

- Premedicate patient with antipyretics, antihistamines, antiemetics, or corticosteroids.
- Hydration before infusion may reduce the risk of nephrotoxicity.
- Monitor BUN and creatinine and electrolyte levels (particularly magnesium and potassium), liver function, and CBC.
- Watch for signs and symptoms of hypokalemia (ECG changes, muscle weakness, cramping, drowsiness).
- Patients treated with amphotericin B liposomal have a lower risk of chills, elevated BUN level, hypokalemia, hypertension, and vomiting than patients treated with conventional amphotericin B.
- Therapy may take several weeks to months.
- Observe patient closely for adverse reactions during infusion. If anaphylaxis occurs, stop infusion immediately, provide supportive therapy, and notify prescriber.

Patient teaching

- Teach patient signs and symptoms of hypersensitivity, and stress importance of reporting them immediately.
- Warn patient that therapy may take several months; teach personal hygiene and

other measures to prevent spread and recurrence of lesions.
- Instruct patient to report any adverse reactions that occur while receiving drug.
- Tell patient to watch for and report signs and symptoms of low levels of potassium in the blood (muscle weakness, cramping, drowsiness).
- Advise patient that frequent laboratory testing will be needed.

ampicillin
Apo-Ampi†, Novo Ampicillin†, Nu-Ampi†

ampicillin sodium
Ampicin†, Penbritin†

ampicillin trihydrate
Penbritin†, Principen

Pregnancy risk category B

Indications & dosages

➲ Respiratory tract or skin and skin-structure infections
Adults and children weighing 40 kg (88 lb) or more: 250 to 500 mg P.O. q 6 hours.
Children weighing less than 40 kg: 25 to 50 mg/kg/day P.O. in equally divided doses q 6 hours. Pediatric dosages shouldn't exceed recommended adult dosages.

➲ GI infections or UTIs
Adults and children weighing 40 kg (88 lb) or more: 500 mg P.O. q 6 hours. For severe infections, larger doses may be needed.
Children weighing less than 40 kg: 50 to 100 mg/kg/day P.O. in equally divided doses q 6 hours.

➲ Bacterial meningitis or septicemia
Adults: 150 to 200 mg/kg/day I.V. in divided doses q 3 to 4 hours. May be given I.M. after 3 days of I.V. therapy. Maximum recommended daily dose is 14 g.
Children: 150 to 200 mg/kg I.V. daily in divided doses q 3 to 4 hours. Give I.V. for 3 days; then give I.M.

➲ Uncomplicated gonorrhea
Adults and children weighing more than 45 kg (99 lb): 3.5 g P.O. with 1 g probenecid given as a single dose.

➲ To prevent endocarditis in patients having dental, GI, and GU procedures♦
Adults: 2 g I.M. or I.V. within 30 minutes before procedure. For high-risk patients, also give 1.5 mg/kg gentamicin 30 minutes before the procedure; 6 hours later, ampicillin 1 g I.M. or I.V. or amoxicillin 1 g P.O.
Children: 50 mg/kg I.M. or I.V. within 30 minutes before procedure. For high-risk patients, also give 1.5 mg/kg gentamicin 30 minutes before the procedure; 6 hours later, ampicillin 25 mg/kg I.M. or I.V. or amoxicillin 25 mg/kg P.O.

In patients with creatinine clearance of 10 to 50 ml/minute, use same dose but increase dosing interval to 6 to 12 hours; for those with a clearance less than 10 ml/minute, increase dosing interval to 12 to 24 hours.

Contraindications & cautions
- Contraindicated in patients hypersensitive to drug or other penicillins.
- Use cautiously in patients with other drug allergies (especially to cephalosporins) because of possible cross-sensitivity, and in those with mononucleosis because of high risk of maculopapular rash.

Adverse reactions
CNS: lethargy, hallucinations, ***seizures***, anxiety, confusion, agitation, depression, dizziness, fatigue.
CV: vein irritation, thrombophlebitis.
GI: *nausea*, vomiting, *diarrhea*, glossitis, stomatitis, gastritis, abdominal pain, enterocolitis, ***pseudomembranous colitis***, black hairy tongue.
GU: interstitial nephritis, nephropathy, vaginitis.
Hematologic: anemia, ***thrombocytopenia***, ***thrombocytopenic purpura***, eosinophilia, ***leukopenia***, hemolytic anemia, ***agranulocytosis***.
Skin: pain at injection site.
Other: hypersensitivity reactions, overgrowth of nonsusceptible organisms.

Interactions
Drug-drug. *Allopurinol:* May increase risk of rash. Monitor patient for rash.
H_2 antagonists, proton pump inhibitors: May decrease ampicillin absorption and serum levels. Separate administration times. Monitor patient for continued antibiotic efficacy.

Hormonal contraceptives: May decrease hormonal contraceptive effectiveness. Advise use of additional form of contraception during penicillin therapy.
Oral anticoagulants: May increase risk of bleeding. Monitor PT and INR.
Probenecid: May increase levels of ampicillin and other penicillins. Probenecid may be used for this purpose.

Nursing considerations

- Before giving drug, ask patient about allergic reactions to penicillin. A negative history of penicillin allergy is no guarantee against a future allergic reaction.
- Obtain specimen for culture and sensitivity tests before giving first dose. Therapy may begin pending results.
- Give drug I.M. or I.V. only if prescribed and the infection is severe or if patient can't take oral dose.
- Give drug 1 to 2 hours before or 2 to 3 hours after meals. When given orally, drug may cause GI disturbances. Food may interfere with absorption.
- Monitor sodium level because each gram of ampicillin contains 2.9 mEq of sodium.
- If large doses are given or if therapy is prolonged, bacterial or fungal superinfection may occur, especially in elderly, debilitated, or immunosuppressed patients.
- Watch for signs and symptoms of hypersensitivity, such as erythematous maculopapular rash, urticaria, and anaphylaxis.
- Decrease dosage in patients with impaired renal function.
- In pediatric meningitis, ampicillin may be given with parenteral chloramphenicol for 24 hours, pending cultures.
- To prevent bacterial endocarditis in patients at high risk, give drug with gentamicin.

Patient teaching

- Tell patient to take entire quantity of drug exactly as prescribed, even after he feels better.
- Instruct patient to take oral form on an empty stomach 1 hour before or 2 hours after meals.
- Inform patient to notify prescriber if rash, fever, or chills develop. A rash is the most common allergic reaction, especially if allopurinol is also being taken.
- Advise patient to report discomfort at I.V. injection site.

ampicillin sodium and sulbactam sodium
Unasyn

Pregnancy risk category B

Indications & dosages

➲ **Intra-abdominal, gynecologic, and skin-structure infections caused by susceptible strains**
Adults: 1.5 to 3 g I.M. or I.V. q 6 hours. Maximum daily dose is 12 g.
Children age 1 or older (skin and skin-structure infections only): 300 mg/kg I.V. in divided doses q 6 hours for no longer than 14 days.

If creatinine clearance in adults is 15 to 29 ml/minute, give 1.5 to 3 g q 12 hours; if clearance is 5 to 14 ml/minute, give 1.5 to 3 g q 24 hours.

Contraindications & cautions

- Contraindicated in patients hypersensitive to drug or other penicillins.
- Use cautiously in patients with other drug allergies (especially to cephalosporins) because of possible cross-sensitivity, and in those with mononucleosis because of high risk of maculopapular rash.

Adverse reactions

CV: thrombophlebitis, vein irritation.
GI: *nausea*, vomiting, *diarrhea*, glossitis, stomatitis, gastritis, black hairy tongue, enterocolitis, ***pseudomembranous colitis***.
Hematologic: anemia, ***thrombocytopenia***, ***thrombocytopenic purpura***, eosinophilia, ***leukopenia***, ***agranulocytosis***.
Skin: *pain at injection site.*
Other: hypersensitivity reactions, ***anaphylaxis***, overgrowth of nonsusceptible organisms.

Interactions

Drug-drug. *Allopurinol:* May increase risk of rash. Monitor patient for rash.
Hormonal contraceptives: May decrease hormonal contraceptive effectiveness. Advise use of additional form of contraception during penicillin therapy.

Oral anticoagulants: May increase risk of bleeding. Monitor PT and INR.
Probenecid: May increase ampicillin level. Probenecid may be used for this purpose.

Nursing considerations

- Before giving drug, ask patient about allergic reactions to penicillin. However, a negative history of penicillin allergy is no guarantee against future allergic reaction.
- Obtain specimen for culture and sensitivity tests before giving first dose. Therapy may begin pending results.
- Dosage is expressed as total drug. Each 1.5-g vial contains 1 g ampicillin sodium and 0.5 g sulbactam sodium.
- Decrease dosage in patients with impaired renal function.
- For I.M. injection, reconstitute with sterile water for injection or 0.5% or 2% lidocaine hydrochloride injection. Add 3.2 ml to a 1.5-g vial (or 6.4 ml to a 3-g vial) to yield a concentration of 375 mg/ml. Give deep into muscle.
- Don't use I.M. route in children.
- Monitor liver function test results during therapy, especially in patients with impaired liver function.
- If large doses are given or if therapy is prolonged, bacterial or fungal superinfection may occur, especially in elderly, debilitated, or immunosuppressed patients.

Patient teaching

- Tell patient to report rash, fever, or chills. A rash is the most common allergic reaction.
- Advise patient to report discomfort at I.V. insertion site.
- Warn patient that I.M. injection may cause pain at injection site.

amprenavir

Agenerase

Pregnancy risk category C

Indications & dosages

➲ **HIV-1 infection (with other antiretrovirals)**
Adults and children ages 13 to 16, weighing 50 kg (110 lb) or more: 1,200 mg (eight 150-mg capsules) P.O. b.i.d. with other antiretrovirals.
Children ages 4 to 12, or ages 13 to 16 and weighing less than 50 kg (110 lb): For capsules, give 20 mg/kg P.O. b.i.d. or 15 mg/kg P.O. t.i.d., to maximum daily dose of 2,400 mg with other antiretrovirals.

For oral solution, give 22.5 mg/kg (1.5 ml/kg) P.O. b.i.d. or 17 mg/kg (1.1 ml/kg) P.O. t.i.d., to maximum daily dose of 2,800 mg with other antiretrovirals.

For patients with a Child-Pugh score of 5 to 8, reduce dose for capsules to 450 mg P.O. b.i.d. For patients with a Child-Pugh score of 9 to 12, reduce dose for capsules to 300 mg P.O. b.i.d.

Contraindications & cautions

- Contraindicated in patients hypersensitive to drug or its components. Contraindicated in infants, children younger than age 4, pregnant women, patients with liver or kidney failure, and patients treated with disulfiram (Antabuse) or metronidazole (Flagyl).
- Use cautiously in patients with moderate or severe hepatic impairment, diabetes mellitus, a known sulfonamide allergy, or hemophilia A or B.
- Use cautiously in pregnant women because no adequate studies exist regarding the effects of amprenavir when given during pregnancy. Use during pregnancy only if the potential benefits outweigh the risks. Register pregnant woman taking amprenavir with the Antiretroviral Pregnancy Registry by calling 1-800-258-4263.

Adverse reactions

CNS: *oral and perioral paresthesia*, depression or mood disorders.
GI: abdominal pain or discomfort, *nausea, vomiting, diarrhea or loose stools*, taste disorders.
Metabolic: *hyperglycemia, hypertriglyceridemia*, hypercholesterolemia.
Skin: *rash*, ***Stevens-Johnson syndrome***.

Interactions

Drug-drug. *Antacids:* May decrease amprenavir absorption. Separate doses by at least 1 hour.
Antiarrhythmics such as amiodarone, lidocaine (systemic), quinidine; anticoagulants such as warfarin; tricyclic antidepressants: May alter levels of these drugs. Monitor patient closely.

Dihydroergotamine, midazolam, rifampin, triazolam: May cause serious and life-threatening interactions. Avoid using together.
Efavirenz: May decrease amprenavir exposure. May need to increase dose.
Ethinyl estradiol and norethindrone: May cause loss of virologic response and possible resistance to amprenavir. Advise the use of nonhormonal contraception.
HMG-CoA reductase inhibitors, such as atorvastatin, lovastatin, simvastatin: May increase levels of these drugs; may increase risk of myopathy, including rhabdomyolysis. Avoid using together.
Indinavir, nelfinavir, ritonavir: May increase amprenavir level. Monitor patient closely for adverse reactions.
Ketoconazole: May increase levels of both drugs. Monitor patient closely for adverse reactions.
Macrolides: May increase amprenavir level. Don't adjust dosage.
Methadone: May decrease amprenavir level. Consider alternative antiretroviral or pain therapy. May need to increase methadone dosage if used together.
Psychotherapeutic drugs: May increase CNS effects. Monitor patient closely.
Rifabutin: May decrease amprenavir exposure. May increase rifabutin level by 200%. May need to decrease rifabutin dose to 150 mg daily or 300 mg two to three times a week.
Saquinavir: May decrease amprenavir exposure. Monitor patient closely.
Sildenafil: May increase sildenafil level, which may increase sildenafil effects, including hypotension, visual changes, and priapism. Don't exceed 25 mg of sildenafil in 48 hours.
Drug-herb. *St. John's wort:* May decrease amprenavir level. Discourage use together.
Drug-food. *Grapefruit juice:* May affect amprenavir level. Monitor patient closely.
High-fat meals: May decrease drug absorption. Advise patient to avoid taking drug with a high-fat meal.

Nursing considerations

!! ALERT Drug can cause severe or life-threatening rash, including Stevens-Johnson syndrome. Stop therapy if patient develops a severe or life-threatening rash or a moderate rash accompanied by systemic signs and symptoms.
!! ALERT Because amprenavir may interact with many drugs, obtain patient's complete drug history. Ask patient to show you the drugs he's taking.
- Patient shouldn't take drug with high-fat foods because they may decrease absorption of amprenavir.
- Amprenavir oral solution should only be used when the capsules or other protease inhibitor formulations aren't therapeutic options.
- Monitor patient for adverse reactions. A patient taking a protease inhibitor may experience a redistribution of body fat, including central obesity, dorsocervical fat enlargement (buffalo hump), peripheral wasting, breast enlargement, and cushingoid appearance. The mechanism and long-term consequences of these effects are unknown.
- Drug provides high daily doses of vitamin E, which may worsen coagulopathy caused by vitamin K deficiency.
- Protease inhibitors have caused spontaneous bleeding in some patients with hemophilia A or B. In some patients, additional factor VIII was needed. In many of the reported cases, treatment with protease inhibitors was continued or restarted.
- Amprenavir capsules aren't interchangeable with amprenavir oral solution on a milligram-per-milligram basis.

!! ALERT Don't confuse amprenavir with abacavir.

Patient teaching

- Advise patient that drug doesn't cure HIV infection; patient may continue to develop opportunistic infections and other complications from the disease. Also, tell patient that drug doesn't reduce risk of HIV transmission through sexual contact.
- Tell patient that although drug can be taken without regard to food, he shouldn't take it with a high-fat meal because of decreased drug absorption.
- Tell patient to report adverse reactions, especially rash.
- Advise patient to take drug daily, as prescribed, with other antiretrovirals. Dosage must not be altered or stopped without prescriber's approval.

- Inform patient to take an antacid 1 hour before or after amprenavir to prevent a decrease in amprenavir absorption.
- Advise patient receiving sildenafil of increased adverse reactions. Caution against taking more than 25 mg of sildenafil in 48 hours.
- If a dose is missed by more than 4 hours, advise patient to wait and take the next dose at the regularly scheduled time. If a dose is missed by less than 4 hours, advise him to take the dose as soon as possible and then take the next dose at the regularly scheduled time. If a dose is skipped, patient shouldn't double the dose.
- Advise patient using hormonal contraception to use another contraceptive method during drug therapy.
- Advise patient to notify prescriber if pregnancy occurs during therapy.
- Advise patient not to take supplemental vitamin E because drug contains a significant amount of the vitamin.

anakinra
Kineret

Pregnancy risk category B

Indications & dosages

➲ **To reduce signs and symptoms and slow progression of structural damage in moderately to severely active rheumatoid arthritis (RA) after one or more failures with disease-modifying antirheumatic drugs (DMARDs), alone or combined with DMARDs other than tumor necrosis factor (TNF)-blocking drugs**

Adults: 100 mg S.C. daily.

Contraindications & cautions

- Contraindicated in patients hypersensitive to *Escherichia coli*–derived proteins or any components of the product, or in patients with active infections.
- Use drug cautiously in elderly patients because they have a greater risk of infection and are more likely to have renal impairment.
- Use drug cautiously in immunosuppressed patients and in those with chronic infection.
- It's unknown whether drug appears in breast milk. Use cautiously in breast-feeding women.
- Safety and effectiveness in patients with juvenile RA haven't been established.

Adverse reactions

CNS: *headache.*
EENT: sinusitis.
GI: abdominal pain, diarrhea, nausea.
Hematologic: ***neutropenia***, eosinophilia.
Respiratory: *upper respiratory tract infection.*
Skin: *injection site reactions (erythema, ecchymosis, inflammation, pain).*
Other: *infection (cellulitis, pneumonia, bone and joint)*, flulike symptoms.

Interactions

Drug-drug. *Etanercept, other TNF-blocking drugs:* May increase risk of severe infection. Use together with caution.
Vaccines: May decrease effectiveness of vaccines or may increase risk of secondary transmission of infection with live vaccines. Avoid using together.

Nursing considerations

- Don't start treatment if patient has active infection.
- Obtain neutrophil count before treatment, monthly for the first 3 months of treatment, and then quarterly for up to 1 year.
- Inject entire contents of prefilled syringe.
- Monitor patient for infections and injection site reactions.
- Stop drug if a serious infection develops.
- Monitor patient for possible anaphylactic reaction.
- Store drug in the refrigerator at 35° to 46° F (2° to 8° C). Don't freeze or shake.
- Protect drug from light.

!! ALERT Don't confuse anakinra (Kineret) with amikacin (Amikin).

Patient teaching

- Tell patient to store drug in refrigerator and not to freeze or expose to excessive heat. Advise letting drug come to room temperature before giving dose.
- Teach patient proper dosage and administration.
- Urge patient to rotate injection sites.

- Teach proper disposal of syringes in a puncture-resistant container. Also, caution patient not to reuse needles.
- Review signs and symptoms of allergic and other adverse reactions, especially signs of serious infections. Urge patient to contact prescriber if they arise.
- Inform patient that injection site reactions are common, usually mild, and typically last 14 to 28 days.
- Tell patient to avoid live-virus vaccines while taking anakinra.

anastrozole
Arimidex

Pregnancy risk category D

Indications & dosages

➲ **First-line treatment of postmenopausal women with hormone receptor–positive or hormone receptor–unknown locally advanced or metastatic breast cancer; advanced breast cancer in postmenopausal women with disease progression after tamoxifen therapy; adjunctive treatment of postmenopausal women with hormone receptor–positive early breast cancer**

Adults: 1 mg P.O. daily.

Contraindications & cautions

- Don't use in women who are or may be pregnant.
- Use cautiously in breast-feeding women.

Adverse reactions

CNS: *headache, asthenia,* dizziness, depression, paresthesia, *pain.*
CV: chest pain, edema, ***thromboembolic disease***, peripheral edema, *hot flashes.*
EENT: pharyngitis.
GI: *nausea,* vomiting, diarrhea, constipation, abdominal pain, anorexia, dry mouth.
GU: vaginal hemorrhage, vaginal dryness, pelvic pain.
Metabolic: weight gain.
Musculoskeletal: bone pain, *back pain.*
Respiratory: dyspnea, increased cough.
Skin: alopecia, rash, sweating.

Interactions

None significant.

Nursing considerations

- Give drug under supervision of a prescriber experienced in use of anticancer drugs.
- Patients with hormone receptor–negative disease and patients who didn't respond to previous tamoxifen therapy rarely respond to anastrozole.
- For patients with advanced breast cancer, continue anastrozole until tumor progresses.

Patient teaching

- Instruct patient to report adverse reactions, especially difficulty breathing or chest pain.
- Tell patient to take medication at the same time each day.
- Stress need for follow-up care.
- Counsel woman of childbearing age about risks to pregnancy during therapy.

apomorphine hydrochloride
Apokyn

Pregnancy risk category C

Indications & dosages

➲ **Intermittent hypomobility, "off" episodes caused by advanced Parkinson's disease (given with an antiemetic)**

Adults: Initially, give a 0.2-ml S.C. test dose. Measure supine and standing blood pressure q 20 minutes for the first hour. If patient tolerates and responds to drug, start with 0.2 ml S.C. p.r.n. as outpatient. Separate doses by at least 2 hours. Increase by 0.1 ml every few days, p.r.n.

If initial 0.2-ml dose is ineffective but tolerated, give 0.4 ml at next "off" period, measuring supine and standing blood pressure q 20 minutes for the first hour. If drug is tolerated, start with 0.3 ml S.C. as outpatient. If needed, increase by 0.1 ml every few days.

If patient doesn't tolerate 0.4-ml dose, give 0.3 ml as a test dose at the next "off" period, measuring supine and standing blood pressure q 20 minutes for the first hour. If drug is tolerated, give 0.2 ml as outpatient. Increase by 0.1 ml every few days, p.r.n.; doses higher than 0.4 ml usually aren't tolerated if 0.2 ml is the starting dose.

Maximum recommended dose is usually 0.6 ml p.r.n. Most patients use drug t.i.d.

Experience is limited at more than five times daily or more than 2 ml daily.

In patients with mild to moderate renal impairment, use test and starting doses of 0.1 ml S.C.

Contraindications & cautions

- Contraindicated in patients allergic to apomorphine or its ingredients, including sulfites, and in patients who take 5-HT_3 antagonists.
- Use cautiously in patients at risk for prolonged QTc interval, such as those with hypokalemia, hypomagnesemia, bradycardia, or genetic predisposition.
- Use cautiously in patients with CV or cerebrovascular disease and in those with renal or hepatic impairment.

Adverse reactions

CNS: aggravated Parkinson's disease, anxiety, *confusion*, depression, *dizziness*, *drowsiness*, fatigue, *hallucinations*, headache, insomnia, *somnolence*, syncope, weakness.
CV: *angina*, ***cardiac arrest***, *chest pain*, *chest pressure*, *edema*, flushing, ***heart failure***, *hypotension*, *orthostatic hypotension*, ***MI***.
EENT: *rhinorrhea*.
GI: constipation, *nausea*, *vomiting*, diarrhea.
GU: UTI.
Respiratory: dyspnea, pneumonia.
Metabolic: dehydration.
Musculoskeletal: arthralgia, back pain, *dyskinesias*, limb pain.
Skin: bruising, injection site reaction, pallor, sweating.
Other: *falls*, *yawning*.

Interactions

Drug-drug. *Antihypertensives, vasodilators:* May increase risk of hypotension, MI, pneumonia, falls, and joint injury. Use together cautiously.
Dopamine antagonists, metoclopramide: May reduce apomorphine efficacy. Use together cautiously.
Drugs that prolong the QTc interval: May prolong the QTc interval. Give cautiously with other drugs that prolong QTc interval.
5-HT_3 antagonists (ondansetron, granisetron, dolasetron, palonosetron, alosetron): May cause serious hypotension and loss of consciousness. Don't use together.
Drug-lifestyle. *Alcohol use:* May increase risk of sedation and hypotension. Discourage use together.

Nursing considerations

!!ALERT Drug is for S.C. injection only. Avoid I.V. use.

- Give with an antiemetic to avoid severe nausea and vomiting. Start with trimethobenzamide 300 mg P.O. t.i.d. 3 days before starting apomorphine, and continue antiemetic at least 2 months.

!!ALERT The prescribed dose should always be specified in milliliters rather than milligrams to avoid confusion; the dosing pen is marked in milliliters.

- Give test dose in a medically supervised setting to determine tolerability and effect.
- Monitor supine and standing blood pressure every 20 minutes for the first hour after starting doses or dosage changes.
- When programming the dosing pen, it's possible to select the appropriate dose even though insufficient drug remains in the pen. To avoid insufficient dosing, track the amount of drug received at each dose, and change the cartridge before drug runs out.

!!ALERT Monitor patient for drowsiness or sleepiness, which may occur well after treatment starts. Stop drug if patient develops significant daytime sleepiness that interferes with activities of daily living.

- Watch for evidence of coronary or cerebral ischemia, and stop drug if it occurs.
- Adverse effects are more likely in elderly patients, particularly hallucinations, falls, CV events, respiratory problems, and GI effects.

Patient teaching

- Tell patient to avoid sudden position changes, especially rising too quickly from lying down. A sudden drop in blood pressure, dizziness, or fainting can occur.
- Urge patient to keep taking the prescribed antiemetic because nausea and vomiting are likely.
- Instruct patient or caregiver to document each dose to make sure enough drug remains in the cartridge to provide a full next dose.
- Tell patient or caregiver to wait at least 2 hours between doses.

!!ALERT Show patient or caregiver how to read the dosing pen, and make sure he understands that it's marked in milliliters and not milligrams.
- Tell patient or caregiver to rotate injection sites and to wash hands before each injection. Applying ice to the site before and after the injection may reduce soreness, redness, pain, itching, swelling, or bruising at the site.
- Explain that hallucinations (either visual or auditory) may occur, and urge patient or caregiver to report them immediately.
- Explain that headaches may occur and tell patient to notify prescriber if they become severe or don't go away.
- Advise patient to avoid hazardous activities that require alertness until drug effects are known.
- Caution patient to avoid consuming alcohol.

aprepitant
Emend

Pregnancy risk category B

Indications & dosages

➲ **To prevent nausea and vomiting after highly emetogenic chemotherapy (including cisplatin); given with a 5-HT_3 antagonist and a corticosteroid**

Adults: On day 1 of chemotherapy, 125 mg P.O. 1 hour before treatment; then 80 mg P.O. q morning on days 2 and 3 of chemotherapy.

Contraindications & cautions

- Contraindicated in patients hypersensitive to aprepitant or its components.
- Use cautiously in patients receiving chemotherapy drugs metabolized mainly via CYP3A4 and in those with severe hepatic disease.
- Use in pregnant women only when drug's benefit clearly outweighs its risk.
- Don't use in breast-feeding women; it's unknown if drug appears in breast milk.
- Safety and efficacy haven't been established in children.

Adverse reactions

CNS: *asthenia,* dizziness, *fatigue,* fever, headache, insomnia.
EENT: mucous membrane disorder, tinnitus.
GI: abdominal pain, *anorexia, constipation, diarrhea,* epigastric pain, gastritis, heartburn, *nausea,* vomiting.
Hematologic: ***neutropenia.***
Respiratory: *hiccups.*
Other: dehydration.

Interactions

Drug-drug. *Alprazolam, midazolam, triazolam:* May increase levels of these drugs. Watch for CNS effects, such as increased sedation. Decrease benzodiazepine dose by 50%.
Carbamazepine, phenytoin, rifampin, other CYP3A4 inducers: May decrease aprepitant level. Watch for decreased antiemetic effect.
Clarithromycin, diltiazem, erythromycin, itraconazole, ketoconazole, nefazodone, nelfinavir, ritonavir, troleandomycin, other CYP3A4 inhibitors: May increase aprepitant level and risk of toxicity. Use together cautiously.
Dexamethasone, methylprednisolone: May increase levels of these drugs and risk of toxicity. Decrease P.O. corticosteroid dose by 50%; decrease I.V. methylprednisolone dose by 25%.
Diltiazem: May increase diltiazem level. Monitor heart rate and blood pressure. Avoid using together.
Docetaxel, etoposide, ifosfamide, imatinib, irinotecan, paclitaxel, vinorelbine, vinblastine, vincristine: May increase levels and risk of toxicity of these drugs. Use together cautiously.
Hormonal contraceptives: May decrease contraceptive effectiveness. Tell women to use additional birth control method during therapy.
Paroxetine: May decrease paroxetine and aprepitant effects. Monitor patient for effectiveness.
Phenytoin: May decrease phenytoin level. Monitor level carefully, and increase phenytoin dose as needed during therapy. Avoid using together.
Pimozide: May increase pimozide level. Avoid using together.
Tolbutamide: May decrease tolbutamide effects. Monitor glucose level.

Warfarin: May decrease warfarin effectiveness. Monitor INR carefully for 2 weeks after each aprepitant treatment.
Drug-herb. *St. John's wort:* May decrease antiemetic effects by inducing CYP3A4. Discourage use together.
Drug-food. *Grapefruit juice:* May increase aprepitant level and risk of toxicity. Discourage use together.

Nursing considerations

- Avoid giving drug for more than 3 days per chemotherapy cycle.

!!ALERT Before giving drug, screen patient carefully for possible drug or herb interactions.

- Don't give drug for existing nausea or vomiting.
- Expect to give drug with other antiemetics to treat breakthrough emesis.
- Monitor CBC, liver function test results, and creatinine level periodically during therapy.

Patient teaching

- Tell patient that drug is to be taken with other antiemetics and shouldn't be taken alone.
- If nausea or vomiting occurs, instruct patient to take breakthrough antiemetics rather than more aprepitant.
- Urge patient to report use of any other prescription, nonprescription, or herbal medicines.
- Caution patient against taking drug with grapefruit juice.
- Advise woman who takes a hormonal contraceptive to use an additional form of birth control during aprepitant therapy.
- Tell patient who takes warfarin that PT and INR will be monitored closely for 2 weeks after aprepitant therapy starts.

argatroban

Pregnancy risk category B

Indications & dosages

➲ **To prevent or treat thrombosis in patients with heparin-induced thrombocytopenia**
Adults: 2 mcg/kg/minute, given as a continuous I.V. infusion; adjust dose until the steady-state activated PTT is $1\frac{1}{2}$ to 3 times the initial baseline value, not to exceed 100 seconds; maximum dose 10 mcg/kg/minute.

For patients with moderate hepatic impairment, reduce first dose to 0.5 mcg/kg/minute, given as a continuous infusion. Monitor PTT closely and adjust dosage p.r.n.

➲ **Anticoagulation in patients with or at risk for heparin-induced thrombocytopenia during percutaneous coronary intervention (PCI)**
Adults: 350 mcg/kg I.V. bolus over 3 to 5 minutes. Start a continuous I.V. infusion at 25 mcg/kg/minute. Check activated clotting time (ACT) 5 to 10 minutes after the bolus dose is completed.

Use the following table to adjust the dosage.

Activated clotting time	Additional I.V. bolus	Continuous I.V. infusion
< 300 sec	150 mcg/kg	30 mcg/kg/min*
300–450 sec	None needed	25 mcg/kg/min
> 450 sec	None needed	15 mcg/kg/min*

*Check ACT again after 5 to 10 minutes.

In case of dissection, impending abrupt closure, thrombus formation during the procedure, or inability to achieve or maintain an ACT exceeding 300 seconds, give an additional bolus of 150 mcg/kg and increase infusion rate to 40 mcg/kg/minute. Check ACT again after 5 to 10 minutes.

Contraindications & cautions

- Contraindicated in patients who have overt major bleeding who are hypersensitive to drug or any of its components.
- Use cautiously in patients with hepatic disease or conditions that increase the risk of hemorrhage, such as severe hypertension.
- Use cautiously in patients who have just had lumbar puncture, spinal anesthesia, or major surgery, especially of the brain, spinal cord, or eye; patients with hematologic conditions causing increased bleeding tendencies, such as congenital or acquired bleeding disorders; and patients with GI ulcers or other lesions.

Adverse reactions

CNS: ***cerebrovascular disorder, hemorrhage***, fever, pain.

CV: ***atrial fibrillation, cardiac arrest***, hypotension, ***ventricular tachycardia***.
GI: abdominal pain, diarrhea, ***GI bleeding***, nausea, vomiting.
GU: abnormal renal function, groin bleeding, *hematuria*, UTI.
Respiratory: cough, dyspnea, pneumonia, hemoptysis.
Other: allergic reactions, brachial bleeding, infection, ***sepsis***.

Interactions

Drug-drug. *Antiplatelet drugs, heparin, thrombolytics:* May increase risk of intracranial bleeding. Avoid using together.
Oral anticoagulants: May prolong PT and INR and may increase risk of bleeding. Monitor patient closely.

Nursing considerations

- Stop all parenteral anticoagulants before giving argatroban. Giving argatroban with antiplatelets, thrombolytics, and other anticoagulants may increase risk of bleeding.
- Get results of baseline coagulation tests, platelet count, hemoglobin level, and hematocrit before starting therapy, and report any abnormalities to the prescriber.
- Check activated PTT 2 hours after giving drug; dose adjustments may be required to get a targeted activated PTT of 1.5 to 3 times the baseline, no longer than 100 seconds. Steady state is achieved 1 to 3 hours after starting argatroban.
- Draw blood for additional ACT about every 20 to 30 minutes during prolonged PCI.
- Patients receiving argatroban can hemorrhage from any site in the body. Any unexplained decrease in hematocrit or blood pressure or any other unexplained symptoms may signify a hemorrhagic event.
- To convert to oral anticoagulant therapy, give warfarin P.O. with argatroban at up to 2 mcg/kg/minute until the INR exceeds 4 on combined therapy. After argatroban is stopped, repeat the INR in 4 to 6 hours. If the repeat INR is less than the desired therapeutic range, resume the I.V. argatroban infusion. Repeat the procedure daily until the desired therapeutic range on warfarin alone is reached.
- Use cautiously in breast-feeding women; it's unknown if drug appears in breast milk.

!!ALERT Don't confuse argatroban with Aggrastat (tirofiban).

Patient teaching

- Tell patient that this drug can cause bleeding, and ask him to report any unusual bruising or bleeding (nosebleeds, bleeding gums) or tarry stools to the prescriber immediately.
- Advise patient to avoid activities that carry a risk of injury, and to use a soft toothbrush and an electric razor while receiving argatroban.
- Instruct patient to notify prescriber if he has wheezing, trouble breathing, or skin rash.
- Instruct patient to notify prescriber if she is pregnant, has recently delivered, or is breast-feeding.
- Tell patient to notify prescriber if he has GI ulcers or liver disease, or has had recent surgery, radiation treatment, falling episodes, or injury.

aripiprazole
Abilify

Pregnancy risk category C

Indications & dosages

➲ Schizophrenia
Adults: Initially, 10 to 15 mg P.O. daily; increase to maximum daily dose of 30 mg if needed, after at least 2 weeks.

When using with CYP3A4 inhibitors such as ketoconazole or CYP2D6 inhibitors such as quinidine, fluoxetine, or paroxetine, give half the aripiprazole dose. When using with CYP3A4 inducers such as carbamazepine, double the aripiprazole dose. Return to original dosing after the concomitant drugs are stopped.

➲ Bipolar mania, including manic and mixed episodes
Adults: Initially, 30 mg P.O. once daily. May reduce dose to 15 mg daily based on patient tolerance. Safety of doses greater than 30 mg daily and treatment lasting beyond 6 weeks haven't been established.

Contraindications & cautions

- Contraindicated in patients hypersensitive to aripiprazole.

- Use cautiously in patients with CV disease, cerebrovascular disease, or conditions that could predispose the patient to hypotension, such as dehydration or hypovolemia.
- Use cautiously in patients with history of seizures or with conditions that lower the seizure threshold.
- Use cautiously in patients who engage in strenuous exercise, are exposed to extreme heat, take anticholinergic medications, or are susceptible to dehydration.
- Use cautiously in patients at risk for aspiration pneumonia, such as those with Alzheimer's disease.
- Use cautiously in pregnant and breast-feeding patients.

Adverse reactions

CNS: *headache, anxiety, insomnia, lightheadedness, somnolence, akathisia*, tremor, asthenia, depression, nervousness, hostility, ***suicidal thoughts***, manic behavior, confusion, abnormal gait, cogwheel rigidity, ***seizures***, fever, tardive dyskinesia, ***neuroleptic malignant syndrome, increased suicide risk***.
CV: peripheral edema, chest pain, hypertension, tachycardia, orthostatic hypotension, ***bradycardia***.
EENT: rhinitis, blurred vision, increased salivation, conjunctivitis, ear pain.
GI: *nausea, vomiting, constipation*, anorexia, diarrhea, abdominal pain, esophageal dysmotility.
GU: urinary incontinence.
Hematologic: ecchymosis, anemia.
Metabolic: weight gain, weight loss, hyperglycemia.
Musculoskeletal: neck pain, neck stiffness, muscle cramps.
Respiratory: dyspnea, pneumonia, cough.
Skin: rash, dry skin, pruritus, sweating, ulcer.
Other: flulike syndrome.

Interactions

Drug-drug. *Antihypertensives:* May enhance antihypertensive effects. Monitor blood pressure.
Carbamazepine and other CYP3A4 inducers: May decrease levels and effectiveness of aripiprazole. Double the usual dose of aripiprazole, and monitor the patient closely.
Ketoconazole and other CYP3A4 inhibitors: May increase risk of serious toxic effects. Start treatment with one-half the usual dose of aripiprazole, and monitor patient closely.
Potential CYP2D6 inhibitors (fluoxetine, paroxetine, quinidine): May increase levels and toxicity of aripiprazole. Give half the usual dose of aripiprazole.
Drug-food. *Grapefruit juice:* May increase aripiprazole level. Tell patient not to take drug with grapefruit juice.
Drug-lifestyle. *Alcohol use:* May increase CNS effects. Discourage use together.

Nursing considerations

!!ALERT Neuroleptic malignant syndrome may occur with aripiprazole use. Monitor patient for hyperpyrexia, muscle rigidity, altered mental status, irregular pulse or blood pressure, tachycardia, diaphoresis, and cardiac dysrhythmias.
- If signs and symptoms of neuroleptic malignant syndrome occur, immediately stop drug and notify prescriber.
- Monitor patient for signs and symptoms of tardive dyskinesia. The elderly, especially elderly women, are at highest risk of developing this adverse effect.

!!ALERT Hyperglycemia may occur. Monitor patient with diabetes regularly. Patient with risk factors for diabetes should undergo fasting blood glucose testing at baseline and periodically. Monitor all patients for symptoms of hyperglycemia including increased hunger, thirst, frequent urination, and weakness. Hyperglycemia may resolve when patient stops taking drug.
- Treat patient with the smallest dose for the shortest time and periodically reevaluated for continued treatment.
- Give prescriptions only for small quantities of drug, to reduce risk of overdose.
- Substitute the oral solution on a milligram-by-milligram basis for the 5-, 10-, 15-, or 20-mg tablets, up to 25 mg. Give patients taking 30 mg tablets 25 mg of solution.

Patient teaching

- Tell patient to use caution while driving or operating hazardous machinery because psychoactive drugs may impair judgment, thinking, or motor skills.
- Tell patient that drug may be taken without regard to meals.

• Advise patients that grapefruit juice may interact with aripiprazole and to limit or avoid its use.
• Advise patient that gradual improvement in symptoms should occur over several weeks rather than immediately.
• Tell patients to avoid alcohol use while taking drug.
• Advise patients to limit strenuous activity while taking drug, to avoid dehydration.
• Tell patient to store oral solution in refrigerator and that the solution can be used for up to 6 months after opening

asparaginase
Elspar, Kidrolase†

Pregnancy risk category C

Indications & dosages

➲ Acute lymphocytic leukemia with other drugs
Adults and children: 1,000 IU/kg I.V. daily for 10 days beginning on day 22 of regimen, injected over 30 minutes. Or, 6,000 IU/m^2 I.M. at intervals specified in protocol.

➲ Sole induction drug for acute lymphocytic leukemia
Adults and children: 200 IU/kg I.V. daily for 28 days.

Contraindications & cautions

• Contraindicated in patients hypersensitive to drug (unless desensitized) and in those with pancreatitis or history of pancreatitis.
• Use cautiously in patients with hepatic dysfunction. Drug should first be given in hospital setting under close supervision.

Adverse reactions

CNS: confusion, drowsiness, depression, hallucinations, fatigue, agitation, headache, lethargy, somnolence, fever.
GI: *vomiting, anorexia, nausea,* cramps, stomatitis, HEMORRHAGIC PANCREATITIS.
GU: *azotemia,* ***renal failure,*** glycosuria, polyuria, uric acid nephropathy.
Hematologic: *anemia,* ***hypofibrinogenemia,*** depression of clotting factor synthesis, ***leukopenia, DIC.***
Hepatic: ***hepatotoxicity.***
Metabolic: weight loss, *hyperglycemia,* hyperuricemia, hyperammonemia, hypocalcemia.
Skin: *rash, urticaria.*
Other: ANAPHYLAXIS, chills, hypersensitivity reactions.

Interactions

Drug-drug. *Methotrexate:* May decrease methotrexate effectiveness. Avoid using together, or give asparaginase after methotrexate.
Prednisone: May cause hyperglycemia. Monitor glucose level.
Vincristine: May increase neuropathy. Give asparaginase after vincristine, and monitor patient closely.

Nursing considerations

• Monitor blood and urine glucose levels before and during therapy. Watch for signs and symptoms of hyperglycemia.
• Start allopurinol before therapy begins to help prevent uric acid nephropathy.
!!ALERT Risk of hypersensitivity increases with repeated doses. Perform an intradermal skin test before first dose and when drug is given after an interval of 1 week or more between doses. Give 2 IU asparaginase as intradermal injection. Observe site for at least 1 hour for erythema or a wheal, which indicates a positive response. Patient with negative skin test may still develop allergic reaction to drug. Desensitization may be needed before first treatment dose is given and with retreatment. One IU of drug may be ordered I.V. Dose is then doubled every 10 minutes, provided no reaction has occurred, until total amount given equals patient's total dose for that day.
• Drug shouldn't be used alone to induce remission unless combination therapy is inappropriate. Drug isn't recommended for maintenance therapy.
• For I.M. injection, reconstitute with 2 ml normal saline solution to the 10,000-IU vial. Refrigerate and use within 8 hours.
• Don't give more than 2 ml I.M. at one injection site.
• Don't use cloudy solutions.
• If drug touches skin or mucous membranes, wash with a generous amount of water for at least 15 minutes.
• Keep epinephrine, diphenhydramine, and I.V. corticosteroids available for treating anaphylaxis.

- Monitor CBC and bone marrow function tests.
- Obtain amylase and lipase levels to check pancreatic status. If levels are elevated, stop asparaginase.
- Increase patient's fluid intake to help prevent tumor lysis, which can result in uric acid nephropathy.
- Drug may affect clotting factor synthesis and cause hypofibrinogenemia, leading to thrombosis or, more commonly, severe bleeding. Monitor patient and bleeding studies closely.
- Because of vomiting, give fluids parenterally for 24 hours or until oral fluids are tolerated.
- Some patients may become hypersensitive to asparaginase derived from cultures of *Escherichia coli. Erwinia asparaginase,* derived from cultures of *E. carotovora,* has been used in these patients without causing cross-sensitivity.
- Drug toxicity is more likely to occur in adults than in children.
- There are several protocols for use of this drug.

Patient teaching

- Tell patient to watch for signs of infection (fever, sore throat, fatigue) and bleeding (easy bruising, nosebleeds, bleeding gums, tarry stools). Tell patient to take temperature daily.
- Stress importance of maintaining adequate fluid intake to help prevent hyperuricemia. If adverse GI reactions prevent patient from drinking fluids, tell him to notify prescriber.
- Urge patient to immediately report severe headache, stomach pain with nausea or vomiting, or inability to move a limb.
- Advise patient to report signs of a hypersensitivity reaction, including rash, itching, chills, dizziness, chest tightness, or difficulty breathing.

aspirin (acetylsalicylic acid)

Artria S.R. ◇, ASA ◇, Aspergum ◇, Bayer Aspirin ◇, Coryphen† ◇, Easprin ◇, Ecotrin ◇, Empirin ◇, Entrophen† ◇, Halfprin, Norwich Extra-Strength ◇, Novasen† ◇, ZORprin ◇

Pregnancy risk category D

Indications & dosages

➲ Rheumatoid arthritis, osteoarthritis, or other polyarthritic or inflammatory conditions
Adults: Initially, 2.4 to 3.6 g P.O. daily in divided doses. Maintenance dosage is 3.2 to 6 g P.O. daily in divided doses.

➲ Juvenile rheumatoid arthritis
Children: 60 to 110 mg/kg daily P.O. divided q 6 to 8 hours.

➲ Mild pain or fever
Adults and children older than age 11: 325 to 650 mg P.O. or P.R. q 4 hours, p.r.n.
Children ages 2 to 11: 10 to 15 mg/kg/dose P.O. or P.R. q 4 hours up to 80 mg/kg daily.

➲ To prevent thrombosis
Adults: 1.3 g P.O. daily in two to four divided doses.

➲ To reduce risk of MI in patients with previous MI or unstable angina
Adults: 75 to 325 mg P.O. daily.

➲ Kawasaki syndrome (mucocutaneous lymph node syndrome)
Adults: 80 to 180 mg/kg P.O. daily in four divided doses during febrile phase. When fever subsides, decrease to 10 mg/kg once daily and adjust according to salicylate level.

➲ Acute rheumatic fever
Adults: 5 to 8 g P.O. daily.
Children: 100 mg/kg daily P.O. for 2 weeks; then 75 mg/kg daily P.O. for 4 to 6 weeks.

➲ To reduce risk of recurrent transient ischemic attacks and stroke or death in patients at risk
Adults: 50 to 325 mg P.O. daily.

➲ Acute ischemic stroke
Adults: 160 to 325 mg P.O. daily, started within 48 hours of stroke onset and continued for up to 2 to 4 weeks.

➲ Acute pericarditis after MI
Adults: 160 to 325 mg P.O. daily. Higher doses (650 mg P.O. q 4 to 6 hours) may be needed.

Contraindications & cautions

- Contraindicated in patients hypersensitive to drug and in those with NSAID-induced sensitivity reactions, G6PD deficiency, or bleeding disorders, such as hemophilia, von Willebrand's disease, or telangiectasia.
- Use cautiously in patients with GI lesions, impaired renal function, hypoprothrombinemia, vitamin K deficiency, thrombocytopenia, thrombotic thrombocytopenic purpura, or severe hepatic impairment.

!!ALERT Oral and rectal OTC products containing aspirin and nonaspirin salicylates shouldn't be given to children or teenagers who have or are recovering from chickenpox or flulike symptoms because of the risk of developing Reye's syndrome.

Adverse reactions

EENT: *tinnitus, hearing loss.*
GI: *nausea*, GI distress, occult bleeding, dyspepsia, ***GI bleeding***.
Hematologic: ***leukopenia***, ***thrombocytopenia***, *prolonged bleeding time.*
Hepatic: ***hepatitis***.
Skin: *rash*, bruising, urticaria.
Other: ***angioedema***, hypersensitivity reactions, ***Reye's syndrome***.

Interactions

Drug-drug. *ACE inhibitors:* May decrease antihypertensive effects. Monitor blood pressure closely.
Ammonium chloride, other urine acidifiers: May increase levels of aspirin products. Watch for aspirin toxicity.
Antacids in high doses, other urine alkalinizers: May decrease levels of aspirin products. Watch for decreased aspirin effect.
Anticoagulants: May increase risk of bleeding. Use with extreme caution if must be used together.
Beta blockers: May decrease antihypertensive effect. Avoid long-term aspirin use if patient is taking antihypertensives.
Corticosteroids: May enhance salicylate elimination and decrease drug level. Watch for decreased aspirin effect.
Heparin: May increase risk of bleeding. Monitor coagulation studies and patient closely if used together.
Methotrexate: May increase risk of methotrexate toxicity. Avoid using together.
Nizatidine: May increase risk of salicylate toxicity in patients receiving high doses of aspirin. Monitor patient closely.
NSAIDs: May decrease NSAID level and increase risk of GI bleeding. Avoid using together.
Oral antidiabetics: May increase hypoglycemic effect. Monitor patient closely.
Probenecid, sulfinpyrazone: May decrease uricosuric effect. Avoid using together.
Valproic acid: May increase valproic acid level. Avoid using together.
Drug-herb. *Dong quai, feverfew, ginkgo, horse chestnut, kelpware, red clover:* May increase risk of bleeding. Monitor patient closely for increased effects. Discourage use together.
White willow: May increase risk of adverse effects. Discourage use together.
Drug-food. *Caffeine:* May increase the absorption of aspirin. Watch for increased effects.
Drug-lifestyle. *Alcohol use:* May increase risk of GI bleeding. Discourage use together.

Nursing considerations

- For inflammatory conditions, rheumatic fever, and thrombosis, give aspirin on a schedule rather than p.r.n.
- Because enteric-coated and sustained-release tablets are slowly absorbed, they aren't suitable for rapid relief of acute pain, fever, or inflammation. They cause less GI bleeding and may be better suited for long-term therapy, such as treatment of arthritis.
- For patient with swallowing difficulties, crush nonenteric-coated aspirin and dissolve in soft food or liquid. Give liquid immediately after mixing because drug will break down rapidly.
- For patients who can't tolerate oral drugs, ask prescriber about using aspirin rectal suppositories. Watch for rectal mucosal irritation or bleeding.
- Febrile, dehydrated children can develop toxicity rapidly.
- Monitor elderly patients closely because they may be more susceptible to aspirin's toxic effects.
- Monitor salicylate level. Therapeutic salicylate level in arthritis is 150 to 300 mcg/ml. Tinnitus may occur at levels above 200 mcg/ml, but this isn't a reliable indicator of toxicity, especially in very young pa-

tients and those older than age 60. With long-term therapy, severe toxic effects may occur with levels exceeding 400 mcg/ml.

- During prolonged therapy, assess hematocrit, hemoglobin, PT, INR, and renal function periodically.
- Aspirin irreversibly inhibits platelet aggregation. Stop aspirin 5 to 7 days before elective surgery to allow time for production and release of new platelets.
- Monitor patient for hypersensitivity reactions such as anaphylaxis or asthma.

!!ALERT Don't confuse aspirin with Asendin or Afrin.

Patient teaching

- Tell patient who is allergic to tartrazine dye to avoid aspirin.
- Advise patient on a low-salt diet that 1 tablet of buffered aspirin contains 553 mg of sodium.
- Advise patient to take drug with food, milk, antacid, or large glass of water to reduce unpleasant GI reactions.
- Tell patient not to crush or chew sustained-release or enteric-coated forms but to swallow them whole.
- Instruct patient to discard aspirin tablets that have a strong vinegar-like odor.
- Tell patient to consult prescriber if giving drug to children for longer than 5 days or adults for longer than 10 days.
- Advise patient receiving prolonged treatment with large doses of aspirin to watch for small round red pinprick spots, bleeding gums, and signs of GI bleeding, and to drink plenty of fluids. Encourage use of a soft-bristled toothbrush.
- Because of many possible drug interactions involving aspirin, warn patient taking prescription drugs to check with prescriber or pharmacist before taking aspirin or OTC products containing aspirin.
- Urge pregnant woman to avoid aspirin during last trimester of pregnancy unless specifically directed by prescriber.
- Aspirin is a leading cause of poisoning in children. Caution parents to keep drug out of reach of children. Encourage use of child-resistant containers.

atazanavir sulfate

Reyataz

Pregnancy risk category B

Indications & dosages

➲ HIV-1 infection, with other antiretrovirals

Adults: Give antiretroviral-experienced patients 300 mg (as two 150-mg capsules) once daily plus 100 mg ritonavir once daily with food. Give antiretroviral-naive patients 400 mg (as two 200-mg capsules) once daily with food. When drug is given with efavirenz in antiretroviral-naive patients, give atazanavir 300 mg, ritonavir 100 mg, and efavirenz 600 mg as a single daily dose with food. Dosage recommendations for efavirenz and atazanavir in treatment-experienced patients haven't been established.

In patients with Child-Pugh class B hepatic insufficiency who haven't experienced prior virologic failure, reduce dosage to 300 mg P.O. once daily.

Contraindications & cautions

- Contraindicated in patients hypersensitive to atazanavir or its ingredients.
- Contraindicated in patients taking drugs cleared mainly by CYP3A4 or drugs that can cause serious or life-threatening reactions at high levels (dihydroergotamine, ergonovine, ergotamine, midazolam, methylergonovine, pimozide, triazolam).
- Use cautiously in patients with conduction system disease or hepatic impairment.
- Use cautiously in elderly patients because of the increased likelihood of other disease, additional drug therapy, and decreased hepatic, renal, or cardiac function.

Adverse reactions

CNS: depression, dizziness, fatigue, fever, *headache*, insomnia, peripheral neurologic symptoms.
EENT: scleral yellowing.
GI: *abdominal pain, diarrhea, nausea*, vomiting.
Hepatic: jaundice, hyperbilirubinemia.
Metabolic: lipodystrophy.
Musculoskeletal: arthralgia, back pain.
Respiratory: increased cough.
Skin: *rash*.

Other: pain.

Interactions

Drug-drug. *Amiodarone, lidocaine (systemic), quinidine, tricyclic antidepressants:* May increase levels of these drugs. Monitor drug levels.
Antacids, buffered drugs, didanosine: May decrease atazanavir level. Give atazanavir 2 hours before or 1 hour after these drugs.
Atorvastatin: May increase atorvastatin levels, increasing the risk of myopathy and rhabdomyolysis. Use together cautiously.
Clarithromycin: May increase clarithromycin level and prolong QTc interval while reducing active metabolite. Avoid using together, except to treat *Mycobacterium avium* complex infection. Decrease clarithromycin by 50% when using together.
Cyclosporine, sirolimus, tacrolimus: May increase immunosuppressant level. Monitor immunosuppressant level.
Diltiazem, felodipine, nicardipine, nifedipine, verapamil: May increase calcium channel blocker level. Use together cautiously, with close ECG monitoring. Adjust calcium channel blocker dosage as needed. Decrease diltiazem dose by 50%.
Efavirenz: May alter atazanavir level. Reduce atazanavir dosage.
Ergot derivatives, pimozide: May cause serious or life-threatening reactions. Avoid using together.
Ethinyl estradiol and norethindrone: May increase ethinyl estradiol and norethindrone levels. Use cautiously together, and give the lowest effective dose of hormonal contraceptive.
H_2-receptor antagonists: May decrease atazanavir level, reducing therapeutic effect. Separate doses by at least 12 hours.
Indinavir: May increase risk of indirect (unconjugated) hyperbilirubinemia. Avoid using together.
Irinotecan: May interfere with irinotecan metabolism and increase irinotecan toxicity. Avoid using together.
Lovastatin, simvastatin: May cause myopathy and rhabdomyolysis. Avoid using together.
Midazolam, triazolam: May cause prolonged or increased sedation or respiratory depression. Avoid using together.
Proton-pump inhibitors, rifampin: May significantly reduce atazanavir level. Avoid using together.
Rifabutin: May increase rifabutin level. Reduce rifabutin dose up to 75%.
Ritonavir: May increase atazanavir level. Decrease atazanavir dose to 300 mg.
Saquinavir (soft gelatin capsules): May increase saquinavir level. Avoid using together.
Sildenafil: May increase sildenafil level, causing hypotension, visual changes, and priapism. Tell patient to use together cautiously and reduce dose to 25 mg q 48 hours; watch for adverse events.
Tenofovir: May decrease atazanavir level, causing resistance. Give both drugs with ritonavir.
Warfarin: May increase warfarin level, which may cause life-threatening bleeding. Monitor INR.
Drug-herb. *St. John's wort:* May decrease atazanavir level, reducing therapeutic effect and causing drug resistance. Discourage use together.
Drug-food. *Any food:* May increase bioavailability of drug. Tell patient to take drug with food.

Nursing considerations

!!ALERT Atazanavir may prolong the PR interval.
- Monitor the patient for hyperglycemia and new-onset diabetes or worsened diabetes. Insulin and oral hypoglycemic dosages may need adjustment.
- Monitor a patient with hepatitis B or C for elevated liver enzymes or hepatic decompensation.
- Watch for lactic acidosis syndrome (sometimes fatal) and symptomatic hyperlactatemia, especially in women and obese patients.
- If the patient has hemophilia, watch for bleeding.
- Most patients have an asymptomatic increase in indirect bilirubin, possibly with yellowed skin or sclerae. This hyperbilirubinemia will resolve when atazanavir therapy stops.
- Although cross-resistance occurs among protease inhibitors, resistance to atazanavir doesn't preclude use of other protease inhibitors.

• Give drug to a pregnant woman only if the potential benefit justifies the risk to the fetus.
• To monitor maternal-fetal outcomes among pregnant women who receive atazanavir, an Antiretroviral Pregnancy Registry has been formed. Patients can be registered by calling 1-800-258-4263.

Patient teaching

• Urge patient to take atazanavir with food every day and to take other antiretrovirals as prescribed.
• Explain that atazanavir doesn't cure HIV infection and that the patient may develop opportunistic infections and other complications of HIV disease.
• Caution the patient that atazanavir doesn't reduce the risk of transmitting the HIV virus to others.
• Tell patient that drug may cause altered or increased body fat, central obesity, buffalo hump, peripheral wasting, facial wasting, breast enlargement, and a cushingoid appearance.
• Tell patient to report yellowed skin or sclerae, dizziness, or light-headedness.
• Caution patient not to take other prescription, OTC, or herbal remedies without first consulting his prescriber.

atenolol

Apo-Atenolol†, Tenormin

Pregnancy risk category D

Indications & dosages

➲ Hypertension
Adults: Initially, 50 mg P.O. daily alone or in combination with a diuretic as a single dose, increased to 100 mg once daily after 7 to 14 days. Dosages of more than 100 mg daily are unlikely to produce further benefit.

➲ Angina pectoris
Adults: 50 mg P.O. once daily, increased p.r.n. to 100 mg daily after 7 days for optimal effect. Maximum, 200 mg daily.

➲ Reduce risk of CV-related death and reinfarction in patients with acute MI
Adults: 5 mg I.V. over 5 minutes; then another 5 mg after 10 minutes. After another 10 minutes, give 50 mg P.O.; then give another 50 mg P.O. in 12 hours. Subsequently, give 100 mg P.O. daily (as a single dose or 50 mg b.i.d.) for at least 7 days.

If creatinine clearance is 15 to 35 ml/minute, maximum dose is 50 mg daily; if clearance is below 15 ml/minute, maximum dose is 25 mg daily. Hemodialysis patients need 25 to 50 mg after each dialysis session.

Contraindications & cautions

• Contraindicated in patients with sinus bradycardia, heart block greater than first degree, overt cardiac failure, or cardiogenic shock.
• Use cautiously in patients at risk for heart failure and in those with bronchospastic disease, diabetes, hyperthyroidism, and impaired renal or hepatic function.

Adverse reactions

CNS: *fatigue*, lethargy, vertigo, drowsiness, *dizziness*, fever.
CV: ***bradycardia***, *hypotension*, ***heart failure***, intermittent claudication.
GI: nausea, diarrhea.
Musculoskeletal: leg pain.
Respiratory: dyspnea, ***bronchospasm***.
Skin: rash.

Interactions

Drug-drug. *Amiodarone:* May increase risk of bradycardia, AV block, and myocardial depression. Monitor ECG and vital signs.
Antihypertensives: May increase hypotensive effect. Use together cautiously.
Calcium-channel blockers, hydralazine, methyldopa: May cause additive hypotensive effects. Adjust dosage as needed.
Cardiac glycosides, diltiazem: May cause excessive bradycardia and increased depressant effect on myocardium. Use together cautiously.
Dolasetron: May decrease clearance of dolasetron and increase risk of toxicity. Monitor patient for toxicity.
Insulin, oral antidiabetics: May alter dosage requirements in previously stabilized diabetic patient. Observe patient carefully.
I.V. lidocaine: May reduce hepatic metabolism of lidocaine, increasing risk of toxicity. Give bolus doses of lidocaine at a slower rate and monitor lidocaine level closely.
NSAIDs: May decrease antihypertensive effects. Monitor blood pressure.

Prazosin: May increase the risk of orthostatic hypotension in the early phases of use together. Help patient stand slowly until effects are known.
Reserpine: May cause hypotension. Use together cautiously.
Verapamil: May increase the effects of both drugs. Monitor cardiac function closely and decrease dosages as necessary.

Nursing considerations

- Check apical pulse before giving drug; if slower than 60 beats/minute, withhold drug and call prescriber.
- Monitor patient's blood pressure.
- Monitor hemodialysis patients closely because of hypotension risk.
- Beta blockers may mask tachycardia caused by hyperthyroidism. In patients with suspected thyrotoxicosis, withdraw beta blocker gradually to avoid thyroid storm.
- Drug may mask signs and symptoms of hypoglycemia in diabetic patients.
- Drug may cause changes in exercise tolerance and ECG.

!!ALERT Withdraw drug gradually over 2 weeks to avoid serious adverse reactions.
!!ALERT Don't confuse atenolol with timolol or albuterol.

Patient teaching

- Instruct patient to take drug exactly as prescribed, at the same time every day.
- Caution patient not to stop drug suddenly, but to notify prescriber if unpleasant adverse reactions occur.
- Teach patient how to take his pulse. Tell him to withhold drug and call prescriber if pulse rate is below 60 beats/minute.
- Tell woman of childbearing age to notify prescriber about planned, suspected, or known pregnancy. Drug will need to be stopped.
- Advise breast-feeding mother to contact prescriber; drug isn't recommended for breast-feeding women.

atomoxetine hydrochloride
Strattera

Pregnancy risk category C

Indications & dosages

➲ Attention-deficit hyperactivity disorder (ADHD)
Adults, children, and adolescents weighing more than 70 kg (154 lb): Initially, 40 mg P.O. daily; increase after at least 3 days to a total of 80 mg/day P.O., as a single dose in the morning or two evenly divided doses in the morning and late afternoon or early evening. After 2 to 4 weeks, total dose may be increased to a maximum of 100 mg, if needed.
Children weighing 70 kg or less: Initially, 0.5 mg/kg P.O. daily; increase after a minimum of 3 days to a target total daily dose of 1.2 mg/kg P.O. as a single dose in the morning or two evenly divided doses in the morning and late afternoon or early evening. Don't exceed 1.4 mg/kg or 100 mg daily, whichever is less.

In patients with moderate hepatic impairment, reduce to 50% of the normal dose; in those with severe hepatic impairment, reduce to 25% of the normal dose. Poor metabolizers of CYP2D6 may require a reduced dose. In children weighing less than 70 kg, adjust dosage to 0.5 mg/kg daily and increase to 1.2 mg/kg daily if symptoms don't improve after 4 weeks and if first dose is tolerated. In children and adults weighing more than 70 kg, start at 40 mg daily and increase to 80 mg daily if symptoms don't improve after 4 weeks and if first dose is tolerated.

Contraindications & cautions

- Contraindicated in patients hypersensitive to atomoxetine or to components of drug, in those who have taken an MAO inhibitor within the past 2 weeks, and in those with angle-closure glaucoma.
- Use cautiously in patients with hypertension, tachycardia, or CV or cerebrovascular disease, and in pregnant or breast-feeding patients.
- Safety and efficacy haven't been established in patients younger than age 6.

Adverse reactions

CNS: dizziness, *headache*, somnolence, crying, irritability, mood swings, pyrexia, fatigue, *insomnia*, sedation, depression, tremor, early morning awakening, paresthesia, abnormal dreams, sleep disorder.
CV: orthostatic hypotension, tachycardia, hypertension, palpitations, hot flashes.
EENT: ear infection, rhinorrhea, sore throat, nasal congestion, nasopharyngitis, sinus congestion, mydriasis, sinusitis.
GI: *abdominal pain, constipation*, dyspepsia, *nausea, vomiting, decreased appetite*, gastroenteritis, *dry mouth*, flatulence.
GU: urinary retention, urinary hesitation, ejaculatory problems, difficulty in micturition, dysmenorrhea, erectile disturbance, impotence, delayed menses, menstrual disorder, prostatitis.
Metabolic: weight loss.
Musculoskeletal: arthralgia, myalgia.
Respiratory: *cough*, upper respiratory tract infection.
Skin: *dermatitis, pruritus, increased sweating.*
Other: influenza, decreased libido, rigors.

Interactions

Drug-drug. *Albuterol:* May increase CV effects. Use together cautiously.
MAO inhibitors: May cause hyperthermia, rigidity, myoclonus, autonomic instability with possible rapid fluctuations of vital signs, and mental status changes. Avoid use within 2 weeks of MAO inhibitor.
Pressor agents: May increase blood pressure. Use together cautiously.
Strong CYP2D6 inhibitors (paroxetine, fluoxetine, quinidine): May increase atomoxetine level. Reduce first dose.

Nursing considerations

- Use drug as part of a total treatment program for ADHD, including psychological, educational, and social intervention.
- Effectiveness of treatment lasting longer than 10 weeks hasn't been evaluated. Patients taking drug for extended periods must be reevaluated periodically to determine drug's usefulness.
- Monitor growth during treatment. If growth or weight gain is unsatisfactory, consider interrupting therapy.

!!ALERT Severe liver injury may occur and progress to liver failure. Notify prescriber at any sign of liver injury—yellowing of the skin or the sclera of the eyes, pruritus, dark urine, upper right-sided tenderness or unexplained flulike syndrome.

- Monitor blood pressure and pulse at baseline, after each dose increase and periodically during treatment.
- Monitor for urinary hesitancy or retention and sexual dysfunction.
- Patient can stop taking drug without tapering off.

Patient teaching

- Tell pregnant women, women planning to become pregnant, and breast-feeding women to consult prescriber before taking atomoxetine.
- Tell patient to use caution when operating a vehicle or machinery until the effects of atomoxetine are known.

atorvastatin calcium
Lipitor

Pregnancy risk category X

Indications & dosages

➲ **Adjunct to diet to reduce LDL cholesterol, total cholesterol, apolipoprotein B, and triglyceride levels and to increase HDL cholesterol levels in patients with primary hypercholesterolemia (heterozygous familial and nonfamilial) and mixed dyslipidemia (Fredrickson types IIa and IIb); adjunct to diet to reduce triglyceride level (Fredrickson type IV); primary dysbetalipoproteinemia (Fredrickson type III) in patients who don't respond adequately to diet**
Adults: Initially, 10 or 20 mg P.O. once daily. Patients who require a large reduction in LDL cholesterol (more than 45%) may be started at 40 mg once daily. Increase dose, p.r.n., to maximum of 80 mg daily as single dose. Dosage based on lipid levels drawn within 2 to 4 weeks after starting therapy.
➲ **Alone or as an adjunct to lipid-lowering treatments such as LDL apheresis to reduce total and LDL cholesterol in patients with homozygous familial hypercholesterolemia**
Adults: 10 to 80 mg P.O. once daily.

➲ Heterozygous familial hypercholesterolemia
Children ages 10 to 17 (girls should be 1 year postmenarche): Initially, 10 mg P.O. once daily. Adjustment intervals should be at least 4 weeks. Maximum daily dose is 20 mg.
➲ Prevention of CV disease by reduction of heart attack risk in patients with normal to mildly elevated cholesterol levels and other cardiovascular risk factors
Adults: 10 mg P.O. daily.

Contraindications & cautions

- Contraindicated in patients hypersensitive to drug and in those with active liver disease or unexplained persistent elevations of transaminase levels.
- Contraindicated in pregnant and breast-feeding women and in women of childbearing age.
- Use cautiously in patients with history of liver disease or heavy alcohol use.
- Withhold or stop drug in patients at risk for renal failure caused by rhabdomyolysis resulting from trauma; in serious, acute conditions that suggest myopathy; and in major surgery, severe acute infection, hypotension, uncontrolled seizures, or severe metabolic, endocrine, or electrolyte disorders.
- Use of atorvastatin in children has been limited to those older than age 9 with homozygous familial hypercholesterolemia.

Adverse reactions

CNS: *headache,* asthenia, insomnia.
CV: peripheral edema.
EENT: rhinitis, pharyngitis, sinusitis.
GI: abdominal pain, dyspepsia, flatulence, nausea, constipation, diarrhea.
GU: urinary tract infection.
Musculoskeletal: arthritis, arthralgia, myalgia.
Respiratory: bronchitis.
Skin: rash.
Other: infection, flulike syndrome, allergic reactions.

Interactions

Drug-drug. *Antacids, colestipol:* May decrease atorvastatin level. Monitor patient.
Azole antifungals, cyclosporine, erythromycin, fibric acid derivatives, niacin: May increase risk of myopathy. Avoid using together.
Digoxin: May increase digoxin level. Monitor digoxin level and patient for evidence of toxicity.
Erythromycin: May increase atorvastatin level. Monitor patient.
Fluconazole, itraconazole, ketoconazole, voriconazole: May increase atorvastatin level and adverse effects. Avoid using together; or if unavoidable, reduce dose of atorvastatin.
Hormonal contraceptives: May increase hormone levels. Consider increased hormone levels when selecting a hormonal contraceptive.
Drug-herb. *Eucalyptus, jin bu huan, kava:* May increase risk of hepatotoxicity. Discourage use together.
Red yeast rice: May increase risk of adverse reactions because herb contains compounds similar to those of statin drugs. Discourage use together.
Drug-food. *Grapefruit juice:* May increase drug levels, increasing risk of adverse reactions. Discourage use together.

Nursing considerations

- Use only after diet and other nondrug therapies prove ineffective. Patient should follow a standard low-cholesterol diet before and during therapy.
- Before starting treatment, assess patient for underlying causes for hypercholesterolemia and obtain a baseline lipid profile. Obtain periodic liver function test results and lipid levels before starting treatment and at 6 and 12 weeks after initiation, or after an increase in dosage and periodically thereafter.
- Drug may be given as a single dose at any time of day, with or without food.
- Watch for signs of myositis.

!! ALERT Don't confuse Lipitor with Levatol.

Patient teaching

- Teach patient about proper dietary management, weight control, and exercise. Explain their importance in controlling high fat levels.
- Warn patient to avoid alcohol.
- Tell patient to inform prescriber of adverse reactions, such as muscle pain, malaise, and fever.
- Advise patient that drug can be taken at any time of day, without regard to meals.

!!ALERT Tell woman to stop drug and notify prescriber immediately if she is or may be pregnant or if she's breast-feeding.

atovaquone
Mepron

Pregnancy risk category C

Indications & dosages

➲ **Acute, mild to moderate *Pneumocystis carinii* pneumonia in patients who can't tolerate co-trimoxazole**
Adults and adolescents ages 13 to 16: 750 mg P.O. b.i.d. with food for 21 days.
➲ **To prevent *P. carinii* pneumonia in patients who are unable to tolerate co-trimoxazole**
Adults and adolescents ages 13 to 16: 1,500 mg (10 ml) P.O. daily with food.

Contraindications & cautions

- Contraindicated in patients hypersensitive to drug.
- Use cautiously in breast-feeding patients; it's unknown if drug appears in breast milk.
- Use cautiously with other highly protein-bound drugs; if used together, assess patient for toxicity.

Adverse reactions

CNS: *headache, insomnia, fever, pain,* asthenia, anxiety, dizziness.
CV: hypotension.
EENT: sinusitis, rhinitis.
GI: *nausea, diarrhea, vomiting,* constipation, *abdominal pain,* anorexia, dyspepsia, *oral candidiasis,* taste perversion.
Hematologic: anemia, ***neutropenia.***
Metabolic: ***hypoglycemia,*** hyponatremia.
Respiratory: *cough.*
Skin: *rash,* pruritus, *diaphoresis.*

Interactions

Drug-drug. *Rifabutin, rifampin:* May decrease atovaquone's steady-state level. Avoid using together.

Nursing considerations

!!ALERT Monitor patient closely during therapy because of risk of concurrent pulmonary infection.

Patient teaching

- Instruct patient to take drug with meals because food significantly enhances absorption.

atovaquone and proguanil hydrochloride
Malarone, Malarone Pediatric

Pregnancy risk category C

Indications & dosages

➲ **To prevent *Plasmodium falciparum* malaria, including where chloroquine resistance has been reported**
Adults and children weighing more than 40 kg (88 lb): 1 adult-strength (250 mg atovaquone and 100 mg proguanil hydrochloride) tablet P.O. once daily with food or milk, beginning 1 or 2 days before entering a malaria-endemic area. Continue prophylactic treatment during stay and for 7 days after return.
Children weighing 31 to 40 kg (68 to 88 lb): 3 pediatric-strength (62.5 mg atovaquone and 25 mg proguanil hydrochloride) tablets P.O. once daily with food or milk, beginning 1 or 2 days before entering endemic area. Total daily dose is 187.5 mg atovaquone and 75 mg proguanil hydrochloride. Continue prophylactic treatment during stay and for 7 days after return.
Children weighing 21 to 30 kg (46 to 66 lb): 2 pediatric-strength tablets P.O. once daily with food or milk, beginning 1 or 2 days before entering endemic area. Total daily dose is 125 mg atovaquone and 50 mg proguanil hydrochloride. Continue prophylactic treatment during stay and for 7 days after return.
Children weighing 11 to 20 kg (24 to 44 lb): 1 pediatric-strength tablet P.O. daily with food or milk, beginning 1 or 2 days before entering endemic area. Total daily dose is 62.5 mg atovaquone and 25 mg proguanil hydrochloride. Continue prophylactic treatment during stay and for 7 days after return.
➲ **Acute, uncomplicated *P. falciparum* malaria**
Adults and children weighing more than 40 kg (88 lb): 4 adult-strength tablets (total daily dose 1 g atovaquone and 400 mg pro-

guanil hydrochloride) P.O. once daily, with food or milk, for 3 consecutive days.
Children weighing 31 to 40 kg (68 to 88 lb): 3 adult-strength tablets P.O. once daily, with food or milk, for 3 consecutive days. Total daily dose is 750 mg atovaquone and 300 mg proguanil hydrochloride.
Children weighing 21 to 30 kg (46 to 66 lb): 2 adult-strength tablets P.O. once daily, with food or milk, for 3 consecutive days. Total daily dose is 500 mg atovaquone and 200 mg proguanil hydrochloride.
Children weighing 11 to 20 kg (24 to 44 lb): 1 adult-strength tablet P.O. once daily, with food or milk, for 3 consecutive days.
Children weighing 9 to 10 kg (20 to 22 lb): 3 pediatric-strength tablets P.O. once daily, with food or milk, for 3 consecutive days.
Children weighing 5 to 8 kg (11 to 18 lb): 2 pediatric-strength tablets P.O. once daily, with food or milk, for 3 consecutive days.

Contraindications & cautions

- Contraindicated in patients hypersensitive to atovaquone, proguanil hydrochloride, or any component of the formulation.
- Use cautiously in patients with severe renal impairment and in those who are vomiting.
- It isn't known if elderly patients respond differently to drug than younger patients. Use cautiously in elderly patients because they have a greater frequency of decreased renal, hepatic, and cardiac function.
- It isn't known if atovaquone appears in breast milk, but proguanil hydrochloride appears in breast milk in small amounts. Use cautiously in breast-feeding patients.
- Safety and efficacy haven't been established in children who weigh less than 11 kg.

Adverse reactions

CNS: fever, asthenia, dizziness, *headache*, dreams, insomnia.
GI: *abdominal pain*, diarrhea, anorexia, dyspepsia, gastritis, *nausea*, *vomiting*, oral ulcers.
Respiratory: cough.
Skin: pruritus.

Interactions

Drug-drug. *Metoclopramide:* May decrease atovaquone bioavailability. Consider alternative antiemetics.
Rifampin, rifabutin: May decrease atovaquone level by about 50%. Avoid using together.
Tetracycline: May decrease atovaquone level by about 40%. Monitor patient with parasitemia closely.

Nursing considerations

- Atovaquone absorption may be decreased by persistent diarrhea or vomiting. Patients with persistent diarrhea or vomiting may need a different antimalarial.
- Atovaquone and proguanil hydrochloride haven't been studied for treatment of cerebral malaria or other complicated malaria forms.
- If malaria treatment or prevention using this drug fails, use a different antimalarial.
- Give atovaquone and proguanil hydrochloride at the same time each day with food or milk.
- Store tablets at controlled room temperature of 59° to 86° F (15° to 30° C).

Patient teaching

- Tell patient to take dose at the same time each day.
- Advise patient to take drug with food or milk.
- If patient vomits within 1 hour after taking a dose, tell him to repeat dose.
- Advise patient to notify prescriber if he can't complete the course of therapy as prescribed.
- Instruct patient to supplement preventive malarial with use of protective clothing, bed nets, and insect repellents.

atracurium besylate
Tracrium

Pregnancy risk category C

Indications & dosages

➲ **Adjunct to general anesthesia to facilitate endotracheal intubation and relax skeletal muscles during surgery or mechanical ventilation**
Adults and children age 2 or older: 0.4 to 0.5 mg/kg by I.V. bolus. Give maintenance dose of 0.08 to 0.1 mg/kg within 20 to 45 minutes during prolonged surgery. Give maintenance doses q 12 to 25 minutes in patients receiving balanced anesthesia. For

prolonged procedures, use a constant infusion of 5 to 9 mcg/kg/minute.
Children ages 1 month to 2 years: First dose, 0.3 to 0.4 mg/kg I.V. for children under halothane anesthesia. Frequent maintenance doses may be needed.

Contraindications & cautions

- Contraindicated in patients hypersensitive to drug.
- Use cautiously in elderly or debilitated patients and in those with CV disease; severe electrolyte disorder; bronchogenic carcinoma; hepatic, renal, or pulmonary impairment; neuromuscular disease; or myasthenia gravis.

Adverse reactions

CV: ***bradycardia***, hypotension, tachycardia.
Respiratory: ***prolonged, dose-related apnea;*** wheezing; increased bronchial secretions; dyspnea; ***bronchospasm; laryngospasm***.
Skin: *skin flushing*, erythema, pruritus, urticaria, rash.
Other: ***anaphylaxis***.

Interactions

Drug-drug. *Amikacin, gentamicin, neomycin, streptomycin, tobramycin:* May increase the effects of nondepolarizing muscle relaxant including prolonged respiratory depression. Use together cautiously. May reduce nondepolarizing muscle relaxant dose.
Carbamazepine, phenytoin, theophylline: May reverse, or cause resistance to, neuromuscular blockade. May need to increase atracurium dose.
Clindamycin, general anesthetics (enflurane, halothane, isoflurane), kanamycin, polymyxin antibiotics (colistin, polymyxin B sulfate), procainamide, quinidine, quinine, thiazide and loop diuretics, trimethaphan, verapamil: May enhance neuromuscular blockade, increasing skeletal muscle relaxation and prolonging effect of atracurium. Use together cautiously during and after surgery.
Corticosteroids: May cause prolonged weakness. Monitor patient closely.
Edrophonium, neostigmine, pyridostigmine: May inhibit drug and reverse neuromuscular block. Monitor patient closely.
Lithium, magnesium salts, opioid analgesics: May enhance neuromuscular blockade, increasing skeletal muscle relaxation and possibly causing respiratory paralysis. Reduce atracurium dosage.
Succinylcholine: May cause quicker onset of atracurium; may increase depth of neuromuscular blockade. Monitor patient.

Nursing considerations

- Dosage depends on anesthetic used, individual needs, and response. Recommended dosages must be individually adjusted.
- Give analgesics for pain. Patient may have pain but not be able to express it.
- Don't give drug by I.M. injection.
- Once spontaneous recovery starts, be prepared to reverse atracurium-induced neuromuscular blockade with an anticholinesterase (such as neostigmine or edrophonium); usually given together with an anticholinergic such as atropine. Complete reversal of neuromuscular blockade is usually achieved within 8 to 10 minutes after using an anticholinesterase.
- Monitor respirations and vital signs closely until patient has fully recovered from neuromuscular blockade, as indicated by tests of muscle strength (hand grip, head lift, and ability to cough).
- A nerve stimulator and train-of-four monitoring are recommended to confirm antagonism of neuromuscular blockade and recovery of muscle strength. Make sure spontaneous recovery is evident before attempting reversal with neostigmine.
- Prior use of succinylcholine doesn't prolong duration of action, but quickens onset and may deepen neuromuscular blockade.

!!ALERT Careful dosage calculation is essential. Always verify dosage with another health care professional.

Patient teaching

- Explain all events and procedures to patient because he can still hear.

atropine sulfate (ophthalmic)
Atropine 1, Atropisol, Isopto Atropine

Pregnancy risk category C

Indications & dosages

➲ Acute iritis, uveitis

Adults: Instill 1 or 2 drops up to q.i.d. or apply small strip of ointment to conjunctival sac up to t.i.d.

Children: Instill 1 or 2 drops of 0.5% solution up to t.i.d. or apply small strip of ointment to conjunctival sac up to t.i.d.

➲ Cycloplegic refraction

Adults: 1 or 2 drops of 1% solution 1 hour before refraction.

Children: 1 or 2 drops of 0.5% solution in each eye b.i.d. for 1 to 3 days before eye examination and 1 hour before refraction.

Contraindications & cautions

- Contraindicated in patients hypersensitive to drug or belladonna alkaloids and in those with glaucoma or adhesions between the iris and lens. Don't use atropine in infants age 3 months or younger because of possible link between cycloplegia and development of amblyopia.
- Use cautiously in elderly patients and in others who may have increased IOP. Excessive use in children or in certain susceptible patients, including those with spastic paralysis, brain damage, or Down syndrome, may produce systemic symptoms of atropine poisoning.

Adverse reactions

CNS: confusion, somnolence, headache.
CV: tachycardia.
EENT: ocular congestion with long-term use, conjunctivitis, contact dermatitis of eye, ocular edema, *blurred vision*, eye dryness, photophobia, increased intraocular pressure (IOP), transient stinging and burning, irritation, hyperemia.
GI: dry mouth, abdominal distention in infants.
Skin: dryness.

Interactions

Drug-lifestyle. *Sun exposure:* May cause photophobia. Advise patient to wear sunglasses.

Nursing considerations

!!ALERT Treat drops and ointment as poison (not for internal use); signs of poisoning are disorientation and confusion. Antidote of choice is physostigmine salicylate I.V. or I.M.

- Watch patient for signs and symptoms of glaucoma, including increased IOP, ocular pain, headache, and progressive blurring of vision; notify prescriber if they occur.

!!ALERT Don't confuse Atropisol with Aplisol.

Patient teaching

- Teach patient how to instill atropine. Advise him to wash hands before and after instillation and to apply light finger pressure on lacrimal sac for 1 minute after instillation. Warn patient not to touch tip of dropper or tube to eye or surrounding tissue.
- Warn patient to avoid hazardous activities, such as operating machinery or driving, until temporary blurring subsides.
- Advise patient to ease photophobia by wearing dark glasses or staying out of bright light.

atropine sulfate (systemic)
Sal-Tropine

Pregnancy risk category C

Indications & dosages

➲ Symptomatic bradycardia, bradyarrhythmia (junctional or escape rhythm)

Adults: Usually 0.5 to 1 mg I.V. push, repeated q 3 to 5 minutes to maximum of 2 mg p.r.n.

Children and adolescents: 0.02 mg/kg I.V., with minimum dose of 0.1 mg and maximum single dose of 0.5 mg in children or 1 mg in adolescents. May repeat dose at 5-minute intervals to a maximum total dose of 1 mg in children or 2 mg in adolescents.

➲ Antidote for anticholinesterase insecticide poisoning

Adults: Initially, 1 to 2 mg I.V.; may repeat with 2 mg I.M. or I.V. q 5 to 60 minutes until muscarinic signs and symptoms disappear or signs of atropine toxicity appear. Severe poisoning may require up to 6 mg hourly.

Children: 0.05 mg/kg I.M. or I.V. repeated q 10 to 30 minutes until muscarinic signs and symptoms disappear (may be repeated if they reappear) or until atropine toxicity occurs.

➲ **Preoperatively to diminish secretions and block cardiac vagal reflexes**

Adults and children weighing 20 kg (44 lb) or more: 0.4 to 0.6 mg I.V., I.M. or S.C. 30 to 60 minutes before anesthesia.

Children weighing less than 20 kg: 0.01 mg/kg I.V., I.M. or S.C. up to maximum dose of 0.4 mg 30 to 60 minutes before anesthesia. May repeat q. 4 to 6 hours p.r.n.

Infants weighing more than 5 kg (11 lb): 0.03 mg/kg q 4 to 6 hours p.r.n.

Infants weighing 5 kg or less: 0.04 mg/kg q 4 to 6 hours p.r.n.

➲ **Adjunct treatment of peptic ulcer disease; functional GI disorders such as irritable bowel syndrome**

Adults: 0.4 to 0.6 mg P.O. q 4 to 6 hours.

Contraindications & cautions

- Contraindicated in patients hypersensitive to drug.
- Contraindicated in those with acute angle-closure glaucoma, obstructive uropathy, obstructive disease of GI tract, paralytic ileus, toxic megacolon, intestinal atony, unstable CV status in acute hemorrhage, tachycardia, myocardial ischemia, asthma, or myasthenia gravis.
- Use cautiously in patients with Down syndrome because they may be more sensitive to drug.

Adverse reactions

CNS: *headache, restlessness,* ataxia, disorientation, hallucinations, delirium, *insomnia, dizziness,* excitement, agitation, confusion.

CV: palpitations, ***bradycardia***, tachycardia.

EENT: photophobia, *blurred vision, mydriasis,* cycloplegia, increased intraocular pressure.

GI: *dry mouth,* thirst, *constipation,* nausea, vomiting.

GU: urine retention, impotence.

Other: ***anaphylaxis***.

Interactions

Drug-drug. *Antacids:* May decrease absorption of oral anticholinergics. Separate doses by at least 1 hour.

Anticholinergics, drugs with anticholinergic effects (amantadine, antiarrhythmics, antiparkinsonians, glutethimide, meperidine, phenothiazines, tricyclic antidepressants): May increase anticholinergic effects. Use together cautiously.

Ketoconazole, levodopa: May decrease absorption of these drugs. Separate doses by at least 2 hours, and monitor patient for clinical effect.

Potassium chloride wax-matrix tablets: May increase risk of mucosal lesions. Use together cautiously.

Drug-herb. *Jaborandi tree, pill-bearing spurge:* May decrease effectiveness of drug. Discourage use together.

Jimsonweed: May adversely affect CV function. Discourage use together.

Squaw vine: Tannic acid may decrease metabolic breakdown of drug. Monitor patient.

Nursing considerations

- Many adverse reactions (such as dry mouth and constipation) vary with the dose.
- In adults, avoid doses less than 0.5 mg because of the risk of paradoxical bradycardia.

!!ALERT Watch for tachycardia in cardiac patients because it may lead to ventricular fibrillation.

- Monitor fluid intake and urine output. Drug causes urine retention and urinary hesitancy.

Patient teaching

- Teach patient receiving oral form of drug how to handle distressing anticholinergic effects.
- Instruct patient to report serious or persistent adverse reactions promptly.
- Tell patient about potential for sensitivity of the eyes to the sun and suggest use of sunglasses.

auranofin
Ridaura

Pregnancy risk category C

Indications & dosages

➲ **Rheumatoid arthritis**

Adults: 3 mg b.i.d. or 6 mg once daily. After 6 months, may increase to 3 mg t.i.d. If response is inadequate after 3 months of 9 mg/day, stop use.

Children: Initially, 0.1 mg/kg daily. Maintenance dose is 0.15 mg/kg daily; maximum dose is 0.2 mg/kg daily.

Contraindications & cautions

- Contraindicated in patients with history of severe gold toxicity or toxicity from previous exposure to other heavy metals and in those with necrotizing enterocolitis, pulmonary fibrosis, exfoliative dermatitis, bone marrow aplasia, or severe hematologic disorders.
- Contraindicated in patients with urticaria, eczema, colitis, severe debilitation, hemorrhagic conditions, or systemic lupus erythematosus and in patients who have recently received radiation therapy.
- Manufacturer recommends avoiding use during pregnancy.
- Use cautiously with other drugs that cause blood dyscrasias.
- Use cautiously in patients with rash, history of bone marrow depression, or renal, hepatic, or inflammatory bowel disease.

Adverse reactions

CNS: confusion, hallucinations, ***seizures***.
EENT: conjunctivitis.
GI: *diarrhea, abdominal pain, nausea, stomatitis,* glossitis, anorexia, metallic taste, dyspepsia, flatulence, constipation, dysgeusia, ulcerative colitis.
GU: proteinuria, hematuria, nephrotic syndrome, glomerulonephritis, ***acute renal failure***.
Hematologic: ***thrombocytopenia***, ***aplastic anemia***, ***agranulocytosis***, ***leukopenia***, eosinophilia, anemia.
Hepatic: jaundice.
Skin: *rash, pruritus, dermatitis,* exfoliative dermatitis, urticaria, erythema, alopecia.

Interactions

Drug-drug. *Phenytoin:* May increase phenytoin blood levels. Watch for toxicity.

Nursing considerations

- Monitor patient's platelet count monthly. Stop drug if platelet count falls below 100,000/mm^3, if hemoglobin level drops suddenly, if granulocyte count is less than 1,500/mm^3, or if leukopenia (WBC count less than 4,000/mm^3) or eosinophilia of more than 5% exists.

!!ALERT Monitor patient's urinalysis results monthly. If proteinuria or hematuria is detected, stop drug because it can cause nephrotic syndrome or glomerulonephritis, and notify prescriber.

- Monitor renal and liver function test results.
- Warn women of childbearing potential about risks of drug therapy during pregnancy.

Patient teaching

- Encourage patient to take drug as prescribed.
- Tell patient to continue concomitant drug therapy if prescribed.
- Remind patient to see prescriber for monthly platelet counts.
- Suggest that patient have regular urinalysis.
- Tell patient to keep taking drug if mild diarrhea occurs but to immediately report blood in stool. Diarrhea is the most common adverse reaction.
- Advise patient to report rash or other skin problems and to stop drug until reaction subsides. Itching may precede dermatitis; consider itchy skin eruptions during drug therapy to be a reaction until proven otherwise.
- Inform patient that inflammation of the mouth may be preceded by a metallic taste; tell him to notify prescriber if this occurs. Promote careful oral hygiene during therapy.
- Advise patient to report unusual bleeding or bruising.
- Inform patient that beneficial effect may be delayed as long as 3 months. If response is inadequate and maximum dose has been reached, expect prescriber to stop drug.
- Warn patient not to give drug to others. Auranofin is prescribed only for selected patients with rheumatoid arthritis.

azacitidine
Vidaza

Pregnancy risk category D

Indications & dosages

➲ **Myelodysplastic syndrome, including refractory anemia, refractory anemia with ringed sideroblasts (if patient has neutropenia or thrombocytopenia, or needs transfusions), refractory anemia with excess blasts, refractory anemia with excess blasts in transformation, or chronic myelomonocytic leukemia**

Adults: Initially, 75 mg/m^2 S.C. daily for 7 days; repeat cycle q 4 weeks. May increase to 100 mg/m^2 if no response after two treatment cycles and nausea and vomiting are the only toxic reactions. At least four treatment cycles are recommended.

If bicarbonate level is less than 20 mEq/L, reduce next dose by 50%. If BUN or creatinine levels rise during treatment, delay the next cycle until they are normal; then give 50% of previous dose.

Adjust further during therapy based on hematologic or renal toxicities.

Contraindications & cautions

- Contraindicated in patients hypersensitive to azacitidine or mannitol and in patients with advanced malignant hepatic tumors.
- Use cautiously in patients with hepatic and renal disease.

Adverse reactions

CNS: *anxiety, depression, dizziness, fatigue, headache,* hypoesthesia, *insomnia,* lethargy, *malaise, pain,* syncope, *weakness.*
CV: *cardiac murmur, chest pain, edema,* hypotension, peripheral swelling, tachycardia.
EENT: *epistaxis,* nasal congestion, *nasopharyngitis, pharyngitis,* postnasal drip, *rhinorrhea,* sinusitis.
GI: abdominal distension, *abdominal pain and tenderness, anorexia, constipation, decreased appetite, diarrhea,* dyspepsia, dysphagia, gingival bleeding, hemorrhoids, loose stools, mouth hemorrhage, *nausea,* oral mucosal petechiae, stomatitis, tongue ulceration, *vomiting.*
GU: dysuria, UTI.
Hematologic: *anemia,* FEBRILE NEUTROPENIA, hematoma, LEUKOPENIA, NEUTROPENIA, postprocedural hemorrhage, THROMBOCYTOPENIA.
Metabolic: *decreased weight.*
Musculoskeletal: *arthralgia, back pain, limb pain,* muscle cramps, *myalgia.*
Respiratory: *atelectasis, cough, crackles, dyspnea,* pleural effusion, *rales, rhonchi, pneumonia, upper respiratory tract infection,* wheezing.
Skin: *bruising,* dry skin, granuloma, *pain,* pigmentation, pruritus at injection site, swelling at injection site, cellulitis, *contusion, ecchymosis, erythema, increased sweating, injection site reaction,* night sweats, *pallor, petechiae, pitting edema, rash, skin lesion,* skin nodules, urticaria.
Other: *rigors, pyrexia,* lymphadenopathy, herpes simplex.

Interactions

None reported.

Nursing considerations

- Dilute using aseptic and hazardous substances techniques. Reconstitute with 4 ml sterile water for injection. Invert vial two to three times and gently rotate until a uniform suspension forms. The resulting cloudy suspension will be 25 mg/ml. Draw up suspension into syringes for injection (no more than 4 ml per syringe).
- Just before giving drug, resuspend drug by inverting the syringe two to three times and gently rolling between palms for 30 seconds. Divide doses greater than 4 ml into two syringes and inject into two separate sites. Give new injections at least 1 inch from previous site, and never into tender, bruised, red, or hardened skin.
- Check liver function test results and creatinine levels before therapy starts.
- Obtain CBC before each cycle or more often.
- Monitor renal function closely in elderly patients and in renally impaired patients receiving drug because renal impairment may increase toxicity.
- Store unreconstituted vials at room temperature (59° to 86° F [15° to 30° C]).
- Reconstituted drug is stable 1 hour at room temperature and 8 hours refrigerated (36° to 46° F [2° to 8° C]). After refrigera-

tion, suspension may be allowed to warm for 30 minutes at room temperature.

Patient teaching

- Inform patient that blood counts may decrease, with febrile neutropenia, thrombocytopenia, and anemia.
- Advise men and women to use birth control during azacitidine therapy.

azelaic acid cream

Azelex, Finacea, Finevin

Pregnancy risk category B

Indications & dosages

➲ Mild to moderate inflammatory acne vulgaris

Adults: Apply thin film and gently but thoroughly massage into affected areas b.i.d., in morning and evening.

➲ Mild to moderate rosacea

Adults: Apply thin film of Finacea and gently but thoroughly massage into affected areas b.i.d., in morning and evening.

Contraindications & cautions

- Contraindicated in patients hypersensitive to drug or its components.
- Use cautiously in pregnant or breast-feeding women.

Adverse reactions

Skin: pruritus, burning, stinging, tingling, dermatitis, peeling, erythema.
Other: allergic reaction.
Finacea only
Respiratory: worsening of asthma.
Skin: pruritus, *burning, stinging, tingling,* dermatitis, scaling, erythema, irritation, edema, acne.

Interactions

None significant.

Nursing considerations

- Monitor patient for early signs and symptoms of hypopigmentation, especially patient with dark complexion.
- If sensitivity or severe irritation occurs, notify prescriber, who may stop drug and order appropriate treatment.
- Avoid using occlusive dressings.

Patient teaching

- Instruct patient to wash and pat dry affected areas before applying drug and to wash hands well after application. Warn him not to apply occlusive dressings or wrappings to affected areas.
- Warn patient that skin irritation may occur, usually at start of therapy, if drug is applied to broken or inflamed skin. Tell him to notify prescriber if irritation persists.
- Advise patient to keep drug away from mouth, eyes, and other mucous membranes. If contact occurs, tell him to rinse thoroughly with water and to notify prescriber if irritation persists.
- Advise patient to report abnormal changes in skin color.
- Urge patient to use drug for full treatment period. In most patients with inflammatory lesions, improvement occurs in 1 to 2 months.
- Warn patients with rosacea to avoid foods and beverages that may cause flushing, such as spicy foods, hot food or drinks, and alcohol.
- Instruct patient to store drug at 59° to 86° F (15° to 30° C) and protect it from freezing.

azithromycin

Zithromax

Pregnancy risk category B

Indications & dosages

➲ Acute bacterial worsening of COPD caused by *Haemophilus influenzae, Moraxella catarrhalis,* or *Streptococcus pneumoniae;* uncomplicated skin and skin-structure infections caused by *Staphylococcus aureus, Streptococcus pyogenes,* or *Streptococcus agalactiae;* second-line therapy for pharyngitis or tonsillitis caused by *Staphylococcus pyogenes*

Adults and adolescents age 16 and older: Initially, 500 mg P.O. as a single dose on day 1, followed by 250 mg daily on days 2 through 5. Total cumulative dose is 1.5 g. Or, for worsening COPD, 500 mg P.O. daily for 3 days.

➲ Community-acquired pneumonia from *Chlamydia pneumoniae, H. influenzae, Mycoplasma pneumoniae,* or *S. pneumo-*

niae; **or caused by** ***Legionella pneumophila, M. catarrhalis,*** **or** ***S. aureus***
Adults and adolescents age 16 and older: For mild infections, give 500 mg P.O. as a single dose on day 1; then 250 mg P.O. daily on days 2 through 5. Total dose is 1.5 g. For more severe infections or those caused by *S. aureus*, give 500 mg I.V. as a single daily dose for 2 days; then 500 mg P.O. as a single daily dose to complete a 7- to 10-day course of therapy. Switch from I.V. to P.O. therapy at the prescriber's discretion and based on patient's clinical response.

➲ **Community-acquired pneumonia from** ***C. pneumoniae, H. influenzae, M. pneumoniae, S. pneumoniae***
Children 6 months and older: 10 mg/kg P.O. (maximum of 500 mg) as a single dose on day 1, followed by 5 mg/kg (maximum of 250 mg) daily on days 2 through 5.

➲ **Chancroid**
Adults: 1 g P.O. as a single dose.
Infants and children♦: 20 mg/kg (maximum of 1 g) P.O. as a single dose.

➲ **Nongonococcal urethritis or cervicitis caused by** ***C. trachomatis***
Adults and adolescents age 16 and older: 1 g P.O. as a single dose.

➲ **To prevent disseminated** ***Mycobacterium avium*** **complex in patients with advanced HIV infection♦**
Adults and adolescents: 1.2 g P.O. once weekly alone or with rifabutin.
Infants and children: 20 mg/kg P.O. (maximum of 1.2 g) weekly or 5 mg/kg (maximum of 250 mg) can be given P.O. daily. Children age 6 and older may also receive rifabutin 300 mg P.O. daily.

➲ ***M. avium*** **complex in patients with advanced HIV infection**
Adults: 600 mg P.O. daily with ethambutol 15 mg/kg daily.

➲ **Urethritis and cervicitis caused by** ***Neisseria gonorrhoeae***
Adults: 2 g P.O. as a single dose.

➲ **Pelvic inflammatory disease caused by** ***C. trachomatis, N. gonorrhoeae,*** **or** ***M. hominis*** **in patients who need initial I.V. therapy**
Adults and adolescents age 16 and older: 500 mg I.V. as a single daily dose for 1 to 2 days; then 250 mg P.O. daily to complete a 7-day course of therapy. Expect to switch from I.V. to P.O. therapy, based on patient's clinical response.

➲ **Otitis media**
Children older than age 6 months: 30 mg/kg P.O. as a single dose; or, 10 mg/kg P.O. once daily for 3 days; or, 10 mg/kg P.O. on day 1 and then 5 mg/kg once daily on days 2 to 5.

➲ **Pharyngitis, tonsillitis**
Children age 2 and older: 12 mg/kg (maximum 500 mg) P.O. daily for 5 days.

➲ **To prevent bacterial endocarditis in penicillin-allergic adults at moderate to high risk♦**
Adults: 500 mg P.O. 1 hour before procedure.
Children: 15 mg/kg P.O. 1 hour before procedure. Don't exceed adult dose.

➲ **Chlamydial infections; uncomplicated gonococcal infections of the cervix, urethra, rectum, and pharynx; to prevent such infections after sexual assault♦**
Adults: 1 g P.O. as a single dose, with other drugs, as recommended by the CDC.

Contraindications & cautions

- Contraindicated in patients hypersensitive to erythromycin or other macrolides.
- Use cautiously in patients with impaired hepatic function.

Adverse reactions

CNS: dizziness, vertigo, headache, fatigue, somnolence.
CV: palpitations, chest pain.
GI: *nausea, vomiting, diarrhea, abdominal pain*, dyspepsia, flatulence, melena, ***pseudomembranous colitis***.
GU: candidiasis, vaginitis, nephritis.
Hepatic: cholestatic jaundice.
Skin: rash, photosensitivity.
Other: ***angioedema***.

Interactions

Drug-drug. *Antacids containing aluminum and magnesium:* May lower peak azithromycin level. Separate doses by at least 2 hours.
Carbamazepine, cyclosporine, phenytoin: May increase levels of these drugs. Monitor drug levels.
Digoxin: May increase digoxin level. Monitor digoxin level.
Ergotamine: May cause acute ergotamine toxicity. Monitor patient closely.

Pimozide: May prolong QT interval and cause ventricular tachycardia. Monitor patient closely.
Theophylline: May increase theophylline level. Monitor theophylline level carefully.
Triazolam: May decrease triazolam clearance. Monitor patient closely.
Warfarin: May increase INR. Monitor INR carefully.
Drug-food. *Any food:* May decrease absorption of multidose oral suspension formulation. Advise patient to take drug on empty stomach.
Drug-lifestyle. *Sun exposure:* May cause photosensitivity reactions. Advise patient to avoid excessive sunlight exposure.

Nursing considerations

- Obtain specimen for culture and sensitivity tests before giving first dose. Therapy may begin pending results.
- Give multidose oral suspension 1 hour before or 2 hours after meals; don't give with antacids. Tablets and single-dose packets for oral suspension can be taken with or without food.
- Monitor patient for superinfection. Drug may cause overgrowth of nonsusceptible bacteria or fungi.
- Reconstitute single-dose, 1-g packets for suspension with 2 ounces (60 ml) water, and give to patient. Patient should rinse glass with additional 2 ounces water and drink to ensure he has consumed entire dose. Packets aren't for pediatric use.

Patient teaching

- Tell patient that tablets or oral suspension may be taken with or without food.
- Tell patient to take drug as prescribed, even after he feels better.
- Advise patient to avoid excessive sunlight and to wear protective clothing and use sunscreen when outside.
- Tell patient to report adverse reactions promptly.

aztreonam
Azactam

Pregnancy risk category B

Indications & dosages

➲ **UTIs; septicemia; infections of lower respiratory tract, skin, and skin structures; intra-abdominal infections, surgical infections, and gynecologic infections caused by susceptible *Escherichia coli, Klebsiella pneumoniae, Proteus mirabilis, Pseudomonas aeruginosa, Enterobacter cloacae, K. oxytoca, Citrobacter* species, and *Serratia marcescens;* respiratory infections caused by *Haemophilus influenzae***
Adults: 500 mg to 2 g I.V. or I.M. q 8 to 12 hours. For severe systemic or life-threatening infections, 2 g q 6 to 8 hours. Maximum dose is 8 g daily.
Children ages 9 months to 15 years: 30 mg/kg q 6 to 8 hours I.V. Maximum dose is 120 mg/kg/day.
Neonates age 1 to 4 weeks weighing more than 2 kg (4.4 lbs): 30 mg/kg I.V. q 6 hours.
Neonates age 1 to 4 weeks weighing 2 kg or less: 30 mg/kg I.V. q 8 hours.
Neonates younger than 7 days weighing more than 2 kg: 30 mg/kg I.V. q 8 hours.
Neonates younger than 7 days weighing 2 kg or less: 30 mg/kg I.V. q 12 hours.

For adults with a creatinine clearance of 10 to 30 ml/minute, give 1 to 2 g; then give 50% of the usual dose at usual interval. If clearance is less than 10 ml/minute, give 500 mg to 2 g; then give 25% of the usual dose at usual interval. For adults with alcoholic cirrhosis, decrease dose by 20% to 25%.

Contraindications & cautions

- Contraindicated in patients hypersensitive to drug or to any component of the formulation.
- Use cautiously in elderly patients and in those with impaired renal or hepatic function. Dosage adjustment may be needed. Monitor renal function tests.

Adverse reactions

CNS: ***seizures***, headache, insomnia, confusion.
CV: hypotension, thrombophlebitis.

GI: diarrhea, nausea, vomiting, ***pseudomembranous colitis***.
Hematologic: ***neutropenia***, anemia, ***pancytopenia***, ***thrombocytopenia***, leukocytosis, thrombocytosis.
Skin: discomfort and swelling at I.M. injection site, rash.
Other: hypersensitivity reactions.

Interactions

Drug-drug. *Aminoglycosides:* May have synergistic nephrotoxic effects. Monitor renal function.
Cefoxitin, imipenem: May have antagonistic effect. Avoid using together.
Probenecid: May increase aztreonam level. Avoid using together.

Nursing considerations

- Obtain specimen for culture and sensitivity tests before giving first dose. Therapy may begin pending results.
- To prepare I.M. injection, add at least 3 ml of one of the following solutions per gram of aztreonam: sterile water for injection, bacteriostatic water for injection, normal saline solution, or bacteriostatic normal saline solution.
- Give I.M. injections deep into a large muscle, such as the upper outer quadrant of the gluteus maximus or the lateral aspect of the thigh. Give doses exceeding 1 g I.V.

!!ALERT Don't give I.M. injection to children.
- Observe patient for signs and symptoms of superinfection.

!!ALERT Because drug is ineffective against gram-positive and anaerobic organisms, anticipate combining it with other antibiotics for immediate treatment of life-threatening illnesses.

!!ALERT Patients allergic to penicillins or cephalosporins may not be allergic to aztreonam. Monitor closely those who have had an immediate hypersensitivity reaction to these antibiotics, especially to ceftazidime.

Patient teaching

- Warn patient receiving I.M. drug that pain and swelling may occur at injection site.
- Tell patient to report discomfort at I.V. insertion site.
- Instruct patient to report adverse reactions and signs and symptoms of superinfection promptly.

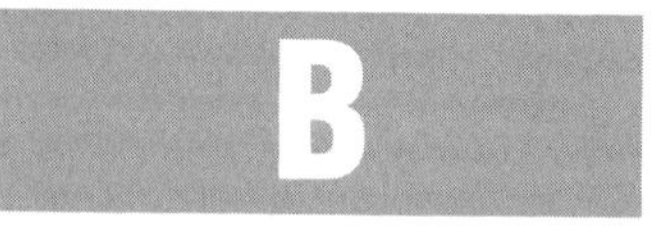

baclofen

Kemstro, Lioresal, Lioresal Intrathecal

Pregnancy risk category C

Indications & dosages

➲ Spasticity in multiple sclerosis; spinal cord injury
Adults: Initially, 5 mg P.O. t.i.d. for 3 days; then 10 mg t.i.d. for 3 days, 15 mg t.i.d. for 3 days, 20 mg t.i.d. for 3 days. Increase daily dosage, based on response, to maximum of 80 mg.

For patients with psychiatric or brain disorders and for elderly patients, increase dose gradually.

➲ To manage severe spasticity in patients who don't respond to or can't tolerate oral baclofen therapy
Adults: For screening phase, after test dose to check responsiveness, give drug via implantable infusion pump. Give test dose of 1 ml of 50-mcg/ml dilution into intrathecal space by barbotage over 1 minute or longer. Significantly decreased severity or frequency of muscle spasm or reduced muscle tone should appear within 4 to 8 hours. If response is inadequate, give second test dose of 75 mcg/1.5 ml 24 hours after the first. If response is still inadequate, give final test dose of 100 mcg/2 ml after 24 hours. Patients unresponsive to the 100-mcg dose shouldn't be considered candidates for implantable pump.
For maintenance therapy: Adjust first dose based on screening dose that elicited an adequate response. Double this effective dose and give over 24 hours. However, if screening dose efficacy was maintained for 12 hours or longer, don't double the dose. After the first 24 hours, increase dose slowly as needed and tolerated by 10% to 30% daily. During prolonged maintenance therapy, increase daily dose by 10% to 40% if needed; if patient experiences adverse effects, decrease dose by 10% to 20%. Maintenance dosages range from 12 mcg to 2,000 mcg daily, but experience with dos-

ages of more than 1,000 mcg daily is limited. Most patients need 300 to 800 mcg daily.

For patients with impaired renal function, decrease oral and intrathecal doses.

Contraindications & cautions

- Contraindicated in patients hypersensitive to drug.
- Orally disintegrating tablets contraindicated in patients hypersensitive to aspartame or other components of the drug.
- Use cautiously in patients with impaired renal function or seizure disorder or when spasticity is used to maintain motor function.

Adverse reactions

CNS: *drowsiness*, ***high fever***, *dizziness*, headache, *weakness*, *fatigue*, ***paresthesias***, hypotonia, *confusion*, insomnia, dysarthria, ***seizures with intrathecal use***.
CV: hypotension, hypertension.
EENT: blurred vision, nasal congestion, slurred speech.
GI: *nausea*, constipation, *vomiting*.
GU: urinary frequency.
Metabolic: hyperglycemia, weight gain.
Musculoskeletal: muscle rigidity or spasticity, ***rhabdomyolysis***, muscle weakness.
Respiratory: dyspnea.
Skin: rash, pruritus, excessive sweating.
Other: ***multiple organ-system failure***.

Interactions

Drug-drug. *CNS depressants:* May increase CNS depression. Avoid using together.
Drug-lifestyle. *Alcohol use:* May increase CNS depression. Discourage use together.

Nursing considerations

- Give oral form with meals or with milk to prevent GI distress.

!!ALERT Don't use oral drug to treat muscle spasm caused by rheumatic disorders, cerebral palsy, Parkinson's disease, or CVA because drug's efficacy for these indications hasn't been established. Don't give intrathecal injection by I.V., I.M., S.C., or epidural route.

- Watch for sensitivity reactions, such as fever, skin eruptions, and respiratory distress.
- Expect an increased risk of seizures in patients with seizure disorder.
- The amount of relief determines whether dosage (and drowsiness) can be reduced.
- Don't withdraw drug abruptly after long-term use unless severe adverse reactions demand it; doing so may precipitate seizures, hallucinations, or rebound spasticity.
- If patient suddenly requires a large intrathecal dose increase, check for a catheter complication such as kinking or dislodgement.
- Experience with long-term intrathecal use suggests that about 5% of patients may develop tolerance to drug. In some cases, this may be treated by hospitalizing patient and slowly withdrawing drug over a 2-week period.

!!ALERT Don't confuse baclofen with Bactroban.

Patient teaching

- Instruct patient to take oral form with meals or milk.
- Tell patients with phenylketonuria that orally disintegrating tablets contain phenylalanine (3.9 mg/10 mg tablet and 7.9 mg/20 mg tablet).
- Instruct patient to remove orally disintegrating tablet from blister pack and immediately place on the tongue to dissolve; then swallow with or without water.
- Tell patient to avoid activities that require alertness until CNS effects of drug are known. Drowsiness usually is transient.
- Tell patient to avoid alcohol and OTC antihistamines while taking drug.
- Advise patient to follow prescriber's orders regarding rest and physical therapy.

basiliximab
Simulect

Pregnancy risk category B

Indications & dosages

➲ To prevent acute organ rejection in patients receiving renal transplantation when used as part of an immunosuppressive regimen that includes cyclosporine and corticosteroids
Adults and children weighing 35 kg (77 lb) or more: 20 mg I.V. given within 2 hours before transplant surgery and 20 mg I.V. given 4 days after transplantation.

Children weighing less than 35 kg: 10 mg I.V. given within 2 hours before transplant surgery and 10 mg I.V. given 4 days after transplantation.

Contraindications & cautions

- Contraindicated in patients hypersensitive to drug or its components.
- Use cautiously and only under supervision of prescriber qualified and experienced in immunosuppressive therapy and managing organ transplantation.
- Use cautiously in elderly patients.

Adverse reactions

CNS: agitation, anxiety, asthenia, depression, dizziness, *headache*, hypoesthesia, *insomnia*, neuropathy, paresthesia, *tremor, fever*, fatigue.
CV: angina pectoris, ***arrhythmias***, atrial fibrillation, ***heart failure***, chest pain, abnormal heart sounds, aggravated hypertension, *hypertension*, hypotension, tachycardia, *leg or peripheral edema*, generalized edema.
EENT: abnormal vision, cataract, conjunctivitis, *rhinitis, pharyngitis*, sinusitis.
GI: *abdominal pain, candidiasis, constipation, diarrhea, dyspepsia*, esophagitis, enlarged abdomen, flatulence, gastroenteritis, GI disorder, ***GI hemorrhage***, gum hyperplasia, melena, *nausea*, ulcerative stomatitis, *vomiting*.
GU: abnormal renal function, albuminuria, bladder disorder, dysuria, frequent micturition, genital edema, hematuria, increased nonprotein nitrogen, oliguria, renal tubular necrosis, ureteral disorder, *UTI*, urinary retention, impotence.
Hematologic: *anemia*, hematoma, ***hemorrhage***, polycythemia, purpura, ***thrombocytopenia***, thrombosis.
Metabolic: acidosis, dehydration, diabetes mellitus, fluid overload, hypercalcemia, *hypercholesterolemia, hyperglycemia, hyperkalemia*, hyperlipemia, *hyperuricemia*, hypocalcemia, *hypokalemia*, hypomagnesemia, *hypophosphatemia*, hypoproteinemia, weight gain.
Musculoskeletal: arthralgia, arthropathy, back pain, bone fracture, cramps, hernia, leg pain, myalgia.
Respiratory: abnormal chest sounds, bronchitis, ***bronchospasm***, cough, *dyspnea*, pneumonia, pulmonary disorder, ***pulmonary edema***, *upper respiratory tract infection*.
Skin: *acne*, cyst, hypertrichosis, pruritus, rash, skin disorder or ulceration.
Other: accidental trauma, *viral infection*, infection, ***sepsis***, *surgical wound complications*, herpes zoster, herpes simplex, ***hypersensitivity reactions***.

Interactions

None significant.

Nursing considerations

- Severe acute hypersensitivity reactions can occur within 24 hours after administration. Make sure drugs for treating hypersensitivity reactions are readily available; withhold second dose if hypersensitivity reactions occur.
- Check for electrolyte imbalances and acidosis during drug therapy.
- Monitor patient's intake and output, vital signs, hemoglobin level, and hematocrit during therapy.
- Be alert for signs and symptoms of opportunistic infections during drug therapy.

Patient teaching

- Inform patient of potential benefits of and risks related to immunosuppressive therapy, including decreased risk of graft loss or acute rejection.
- Advise patient that immunosuppressive therapy increases risk of developing infection. Tell him to report signs and symptoms of infection promptly.
- Inform woman of childbearing age to use effective contraception before therapy starts and for 4 months after therapy ends.
- Instruct patient to report adverse effects immediately.
- Explain that drug is used with cyclosporine and corticosteroids.

BCG vaccine

TICE BCG

Pregnancy risk category C

Indications & dosages

➲ Tuberculosis (TB) exposure
Adults and children age 1 month and older: 0.2 to 0.3 ml (percutaneous vaccine) applied to clean skin; then apply multiple-puncture disk.

Infants younger than age 1 month: Reduce dosage by 50% by using 2 ml of sterile water without preservatives when reconstituting.

Contraindications & cautions

- Contraindicated in patients hypersensitive to vaccine and in patients with hypogammaglobulinemia, immunosuppression and a positive tuberculin reaction (when meant for use as immunoprophylactic after exposure to TB), fresh smallpox vaccinations, or burns.
- Contraindicated in patients receiving corticosteroid therapy.
- Avoid use in pregnant patients.
- Use cautiously in patients with chronic skin disease.
- Safety and effectiveness in adults and children infected with HIV haven't been determined.

Adverse reactions

Musculoskeletal: osteomyelitis.
Other: lymphadenopathy, allergic reaction, ***anaphylaxis***.

Interactions

Drug-drug. *Immunosuppressants:* May reduce response to BCG vaccine. Avoid using together.
Isoniazid, rifampin, streptomycin: May inhibit multiplication of BCG. Avoid using together.

Nursing considerations

- Don't inject vaccine I.V., S.C., or I.D.
- Inject only into healthy skin.
- Obtain history of allergies and reaction to immunization.
- Keep epinephrine 1:1,000 available to treat anaphylaxis.
- Don't shake vial after reconstitution. Use within 2 hours.
- Don't give to febrile patients unless cause is known.
- For TICE BCG, add 1 ml of sterile diluent (preservative-free saline injection) to 50-mg vial to resuspend. Leave drug and diluent in contact for 1 minute. Then mix suspension by withdrawing it into syringe and expelling it gently back into vial two or three times. Avoid producing foam; don't shake.
- Give vaccine using a multiple-puncture disc. Keep area dry for at least 24 hours after administration.
- Expect lesions in 10 to 14 days. Papules reach maximum diameter of 3 mm and then fade. Quicker results occur when the patient has tuberculosis.
- Allow at least 6 to 8 weeks between BCG and live-virus vaccines; give killed-virus vaccines 7 days before or 10 days after BCG.
- Vaccine is of no value as immunoprophylactic in patients with positive tuberculin test result.
- Tuberculin sensitivity may be rendered positive by BCG intravesical treatment. Determine patient's reactivity to tuberculin before therapy.
- Destroy live vaccine by autoclaving or treating with formaldehyde solution before disposal.

Patient teaching

- Advise patient to have tuberculin skin test 2 to 3 months after BCG vaccination.
- Tell patient to report unusual signs and symptoms after vaccination, or signs of allergic reaction, including difficulty breathing, enlarged lymph nodes, or skin ulcer or lesion at injection site.
- Urge patient to keep site dry for 24 hours and not to expose area to others because live vaccine may infect them.

---

beclomethasone dipropionate (nasal)

Beconase AQ

Pregnancy risk category C

Indications & dosages

➲ To relieve symptoms of seasonal or perennial rhinitis, to prevent nasal polyp recurrence after surgical removal

Adults and children older than age 12: 1 or 2 sprays in each nostril b.i.d., t.i.d., or q.i.d.
Children ages 6 to 12: 1 spray into each nostril t.i.d.

Contraindications & cautions

- Contraindicated in patients hypersensitive to drug and in those with untreated localized infection involving the nasal mucosa.
- Use cautiously, if at all, in patients with active or quiescent respiratory tract tuber-

culous infections or untreated fungal, bacterial, or systemic viral or ocular herpes simplex infections.
- Use cautiously in patients who have recently had nasal septal ulcers, nasal surgery, or trauma until wound healing has occurred.

Adverse reactions
CNS: headache.
EENT: nasal congestion, sneezing, dryness, epistaxis, nasopharyngeal fungal infections, *mild, transient nasal burning and stinging.*

Interactions
None significant.

Nursing considerations
- Observe patient for fungal infections.
- Drug isn't effective for acute exacerbations of rhinitis. Decongestants or antihistamines may be needed.

Patient teaching
- Advise patient to pump nasal spray three or four times before first use.
- To instill, instruct patient to blow nose to clear nasal passages, shake container, tilt head slightly forward, and insert nozzle into nostril, pointing away from septum. Tell him to hold other nostril closed and inhale gently while spraying, hold breath for a few seconds, and exhale through the mouth. Next, have him shake container and repeat in other nostril.
- Tell patient to pump nasal spray once or twice before first use each day. He should clean the cap and nosepiece of the activator in warm water every day, and then allow them to air-dry.
- Advise patient to use drug regularly, as prescribed, because its effectiveness depends on regular use.
- Explain that unlike decongestants, drug doesn't work right away. Most patients notice improvement within a few days, but some may need 2 to 3 weeks.
- Warn patient not to exceed recommended dosage because of risk of hypothalamic-pituitary-adrenal axis suppression.
- Tell patient to notify prescriber if signs and symptoms don't improve within 3 weeks or if nasal irritation persists.
- Teach patient good nasal and oral hygiene.

beclomethasone dipropionate (oral inhalation)
Qvar

Pregnancy risk category C

Indications & dosages
➲ **Chronic asthma**
Adults and children age 12 and older: Starting dose, 40 to 80 mcg b.i.d. when used with bronchodilators alone, or 40 to 160 mcg b.i.d. when used with inhaled corticosteroids. Maximum, 320 mcg b.i.d.
Children ages 5 to 12: 40 mcg b.i.d., up to 80 mcg b.i.d. when used with bronchodilators alone or with inhaled corticosteroids.

Contraindications & cautions
- Contraindicated in patients hypersensitive to drug or its ingredients and in those with status asthmaticus, nonasthmatic bronchial diseases, or asthma controlled by bronchodilators or other noncorticosteroids alone.
- Use cautiously, if at all, in patients with tuberculosis, fungal or bacterial infections, ocular herpes simplex, or systemic viral infections.
- Use cautiously in patients receiving systemic corticosteroid therapy.

Adverse reactions
EENT: *hoarseness*, fungal infection of throat, *throat irritation.*
GI: dry mouth, *fungal infection of mouth.*
Metabolic: suppression of hypothalamic-pituitary-adrenal function, adrenal insufficiency.
Respiratory: ***bronchospasm***, wheezing, cough.
Other: ***angioedema***, hypersensitivity reactions, facial edema.

Interactions
None significant.

Nursing considerations
- Check mucous membranes frequently for signs and symptoms of fungal infection.
- During times of stress (trauma, surgery, or infection), systemic corticosteroids may be needed to prevent adrenal insufficiency in previously corticosteroid-dependent patients.

- Periodic measurement of growth and development may be needed during high-dose or prolonged therapy in children.

!!ALERT Taper oral corticosteroid therapy slowly. Acute adrenal insufficiency and death have occurred in patients with asthma who changed abruptly from oral corticosteroids to beclomethasone.

Patient teaching

- Tell patient to prime the inhaler before first use, or after 10 days of not using it, by depressing canister twice into the air.
- Inform patient that drug doesn't relieve acute asthma attacks.
- Tell patient who needs a bronchodilator to use it several minutes before beclomethasone.
- Instruct patient to carry or wear medical identification indicating his need for supplemental systemic corticosteroids during stress.
- Advise patient to allow 1 minute to elapse between inhalations of drug and to hold his breath for a few seconds to enhance drug action.
- Tell patient it may take up to 4 weeks to feel the full benefit of the drug.
- Tell patient to keep inhaler clean by wiping it weekly with a dry tissue or cloth; don't get it wet.
- Advise patient to prevent oral fungal infections by gargling or rinsing his mouth with water after each use. Caution him not to swallow the water.
- Tell patient to report evidence of corticosteroid withdrawal, including fatigue, weakness, arthralgia, orthostatic hypotension, and dyspnea.
- Instruct patient to store drug at 77° F (25° C). Advise patient to ensure delivery of proper dose by gently warming canister to room temperature before using.

benazepril hydrochloride
Lotensin

Pregnancy risk category C; D in 2nd and 3rd trimesters

Indications & dosages

➲ Hypertension

Adults: For patients not receiving a diuretic, 10 mg P.O. daily initially. Adjust dosage as needed and tolerated; usually 20 to 40 mg daily in one or two divided doses. For patients receiving a diuretic, 5 mg P.O. daily initially.

If creatinine clearance is below 30 ml/minute, give 5 mg P.O. daily. Daily dose may be adjusted up to 40 mg.

Contraindications & cautions

- Contraindicated in patients hypersensitive to ACE inhibitors.
- Use cautiously in patients with impaired hepatic or renal function.

Adverse reactions

CNS: headache, dizziness, drowsiness, fatigue, somnolence.
CV: symptomatic hypotension.
GI: nausea.
GU: impotence.
Metabolic: hyperkalemia.
Musculoskeletal: arthralgia, arthritis, myalgia.
Respiratory: dry, persistent, nonproductive cough.
Skin: increased diaphoresis.
Other: hypersensitivity reactions.

Interactions

Drug-drug. *Azathioprine:* May increase risk of anemia or leukopenia. Monitor hematologic study results if used together.
Diuretics, other antihypertensives: May cause excessive hypotension. Stop diuretic or lower dosage of benazepril, as needed.
Lithium: May increase lithium level and toxicity. Use together cautiously; monitor lithium level.
Nesiritide: May increase risk of hypotension. Monitor blood pressure.
NSAIDs: May decrease antihypertensive effects. Monitor blood pressure.
Potassium-sparing diuretics, potassium supplements: May cause hyperkalemia. Monitor patient closely.
Drug-herb. *Capsaicin:* May cause cough. Discourage use together.
Ma huang: May decrease antihypertensive effects. Discourage use together.
Drug-food. *Salt substitutes containing potassium:* May cause hyperkalemia. Monitor patient closely.

Nursing considerations

- Safety and efficacy of dosages of more than 80 mg daily haven't been established.
- Monitor patient for hypotension. Excessive hypotension can occur when drug is given with diuretics. If possible, diuretic therapy should be stopped 2 to 3 days before starting benazepril to decrease potential for excessive hypotensive response. If drug doesn't adequately control blood pressure, diuretic may be cautiously reinstituted.
- Although ACE inhibitors reduce blood pressure in all races, they reduce it less in blacks taking the ACE inhibitor alone. Black patients should take drug with a thiazide diuretic for a more favorable response.
- Drug may increase risk of angioedema in black patients.
- Measure blood pressure when drug level is at peak (2 to 6 hours after administration) and at trough (just before a dose) to verify adequate blood pressure control.
- Assess renal and hepatic function before and periodically during therapy. Monitor potassium level.

!!ALERT Don't confuse benazepril with Benadryl or Lotensin with Loniten or lovastatin.

Patient teaching

- Instruct patient to avoid salt substitutes because they may contain potassium, which can cause high potassium level in patients taking drug.
- Inform patient that light-headedness can occur, especially during first few days of therapy. Tell him to rise slowly to minimize this effect and to report dizziness to prescriber. If fainting occurs, he should stop drug and call prescriber immediately.
- Warn patient to use caution in hot weather and during exercise. Inadequate fluid intake, vomiting, diarrhea, and excessive perspiration can lead to light-headedness and fainting.
- Advise patient to report signs of infection, such as fever and sore throat. Tell him to call prescriber if he develops easy bruising or bleeding; swelling of tongue, lips, face, eyes, mucous membranes, or extremities; difficulty swallowing or breathing; or hoarseness.
- Tell woman of childbearing age to notify prescriber if she becomes pregnant. Drug will need to be stopped.

benztropine mesylate

Apo-Benztropine†, Cogentin, PMS Benztropine†

Pregnancy risk category NR

Indications & dosages

➲ **Drug-induced extrapyramidal disorders (except tardive dyskinesia)**
Adults: 1 to 4 mg P.O. or I.M. once or twice daily.

➲ **Acute dystonic reaction**
Adults: 1 to 2 mg I.V. or I.M.; then 1 to 2 mg P.O. b.i.d. to prevent recurrence.

➲ **Parkinsonism**
Adults: 0.5 to 6 mg P.O. or I.M. daily. First dosage is 0.5 mg to 1 mg, increased by 0.5 mg q 5 to 6 days. Adjust dosage to meet individual requirements. Maximum, 6 mg daily.

Contraindications & cautions

- Contraindicated in patients hypersensitive to drug or its components, in those with angle-closure glaucoma, and in children younger than age 3.
- Use cautiously in hot weather, in patients with mental disorders, in elderly patients, and in children age 3 and older.
- Use cautiously in patients with prostatic hyperplasia, arrhythmias, or seizure disorders.

Adverse reactions

CNS: confusion, memory impairment, nervousness, depression, disorientation, hallucinations, toxic psychosis.
CV: tachycardia.
EENT: dilated pupils, blurred vision.
GI: *dry mouth, constipation,* nausea, vomiting, paralytic ileus.
GU: urine retention, dysuria.
Skin: decreased sweating.

Interactions

Drug-drug. *Amantadine, phenothiazines, tricyclic antidepressants:* May cause additive anticholinergic adverse reactions, such as confusion and hallucinations. Reduce dosage before giving.

Nursing considerations

- Monitor vital signs carefully. Watch closely for adverse reactions, especially in elderly

or debilitated patients. Call prescriber promptly if adverse reactions occur.
- At certain doses, drug produces atropine-like toxicity, which may aggravate tardive dyskinesia.
- Watch for intermittent constipation and abdominal distention and pain, which may indicate onset of paralytic ileus.

!! ALERT Never stop drug abruptly. Reduce dosage gradually.

!! ALERT Don't confuse benztropine with bromocriptine.

Patient teaching

- Warn patient to avoid activities that require alertness until CNS effects of drug are known.
- If patient takes a single daily dose, tell him to do so at bedtime.
- Advise patient to report signs and symptoms of urinary hesitancy or urine retention.
- Tell patient to relieve dry mouth with cool drinks, ice chips, sugarless gum, or hard candy.
- Advise patient to limit hot weather activities because drug-induced lack of sweating may cause overheating.

beractant (natural lung surfactant)

Survanta

Pregnancy risk category NR

Indications & dosages

➲ To prevent respiratory distress syndrome (RDS), also known as hyaline membrane disease, in premature neonates weighing 1,250 g (2 lb, 12 ounces) or less at birth or having symptoms consistent with surfactant deficiency

Neonates: 4 ml/kg intratracheally. Divide each dose into four quarter-doses and give each quarter-dose with infant in a different position to ensure even distribution of drug; between quarter-doses, use a hand-held resuscitation bag at 60 breaths/minute and sufficient oxygen to prevent cyanosis. Give drug as soon as possible, preferably within 15 minutes of birth. Repeat in 6 hours if respiratory distress continues. Give no more than four doses in 48 hours.

➲ Rescue treatment of RDS in premature infants

Neonates: 4 ml/kg intratracheally; before giving, increase ventilator rate to 60 breaths/minute with an inspiratory time of 0.5 second and a fraction of inspired oxygen of 1. Divide each dose into four quarter-doses and give each quarter-dose with infant in a different position to ensure even distribution of drug; between quarter-doses, continue mechanical ventilation for at least 30 seconds or until stable. Give dose as soon as RDS is confirmed by X-ray, preferably within 8 hours of birth. Repeat in 6 hours if respiratory distress continues. Give no more than four doses in 48 hours.

Contraindications & cautions

- Use of drug in infants weighing less than 600 g at birth or more than 1,750 g at birth hasn't been evaluated.

Adverse reactions

CV: TRANSIENT BRADYCARDIA, vasoconstriction, hypotension.
Hematologic: decreased oxygen saturation, hypocapnia, hypercapnia.
Respiratory: ***endotracheal tube reflux or blockage, apnea.***
Skin: pallor.

Interactions

None significant.

Nursing considerations

- Only staff experienced in caring for clinically unstable premature neonates, including neonatal intubation and airway management, should give beractant.
- Accurate weight determination is essential for proper measurement of dosage.
- Continuously monitor neonate before, during, and after giving beractant. The endotracheal tube may be suctioned before giving drug; allow neonate to stabilize before proceeding with administration.
- Refrigerate at 36° to 46° F (2° to 8° C). Warm before use by allowing drug to stand at room temperature for at least 20 minutes or by holding in hand for at least 8 minutes. Don't use artificial warming methods. Unopened vials that have been warmed to room temperature may be returned to the refrigerator within 24 hours; however, warm and return drug to the refrigerator only

once. Vials are for single use only; discard unused drug.
- Beractant doesn't need sonication or reconstitution before use. Inspect contents before giving; make sure color is off-white to light brown and that contents are uniform. If settling occurs, swirl vial gently; don't shake. Some foaming is normal.
- Use a large-bore needle (20G or larger) to draw up drug; don't use a filter. Give drug using a #5 French end-hole catheter. Premeasure and shorten catheter before use. Fill catheter with beractant and discard excess drug so that only total dose to be given remains in the syringe. Insert catheter into neonate's endotracheal tube; make sure catheter tip protrudes just beyond end of tube above neonate's carina. Don't instill drug into a mainstream bronchus.
- Even distribution of drug is important. Give each dose in four quarter-doses, with each quarter-dose being given over 2 to 3 seconds and with the patient positioned differently after each use. Between giving quarter-doses, remove the catheter and ventilate the patient. Give the first quarter-dose with the patient's head and body inclined slightly downward and the head turned to the right. Give the second quarter-dose with the head turned to the left. Then, incline the head and body slightly upward with the head turned to the right to give the third quarter-dose. Turn the head to the left for the fourth quarter-dose.
- Immediately after giving, moist breath sounds and crackles can occur. Don't suction the neonate for 1 hour unless he has other signs or symptoms of airway obstruction.
- Continuous monitoring of ECG and transcutaneous oxygen saturation are essential; frequent arterial blood pressure monitoring and frequent arterial blood gas sampling are highly desirable.
- Transient bradycardia and oxygen desaturation are common after dosing.

!!ALERT Beractant can rapidly affect oxygenation and lung compliance. Peak ventilator inspiratory pressures may need to be adjusted if chest expansion improves substantially after drug administration. Notify prescriber and adjust immediately as directed because failing to do so may cause lung overdistention and fatal pulmonary air leakage.

- Audiovisual materials that describe dosage and usage procedures are available from the manufacturer.

!!ALERT Don't confuse Survanta with Sufenta.

Patient teaching

- Inform parents of neonate's need for drug, and explain drug action and use.
- Encourage parents to ask questions, and address their concerns.

betamethasone dipropionate

Alphatrex, Diprolene, Diprolene AF, Diprosone, Maxivate, Teladar

betamethasone valerate

Betatrex, Beta-Val, Luxiq, Psorion Cream

Pregnancy risk category C

Indications & dosages

➲ Inflammation and pruritus from dermatoses responsive to corticosteroids

Adults and children older than age 12: Clean area; apply cream, ointment, lotion, aerosol spray, or gel sparingly. Give dipropionate products once daily to b.i.d.; give valerate products once daily to q.i.d. Maximum dose is 45 g/week for Diprolene cream and 50 ml/week for Diprolene lotion.

➲ Inflammation and pruritus from dermatoses of scalp responsive to corticosteroids (valerate only)

Adults: Gently massage small amounts of foam into affected scalp areas b.i.d., morning and evening, until control is achieved. If no improvement is seen in 2 weeks, reassess diagnosis.

Contraindications & cautions

- Contraindicated in patients hypersensitive to corticosteroids.

Adverse reactions

GU: glycosuria with dipropionate.
Metabolic: hyperglycemia.
Skin: burning, pruritus, irritation, dryness, erythema, folliculitis, striae, acneiform eruptions, perioral dermatitis, hypopigmentation, hypertrichosis, allergic contact dermatitis, secondary infection, maceration, atrophy, miliaria with occlusive dressings.

Other: *hypothalamic-pituitary-adrenal axis suppression*, Cushing's syndrome.

Interactions

None significant.

Nursing considerations

- Gently wash skin before applying. To prevent skin damage, rub in gently, leaving a thin coat. When treating hairy sites, part hair and apply directly to lesions.
- Avoid applying near eyes or mucous membranes or in ear canal, groin area, or axillae.
- Don't dispense foam directly into warm hands because foam will begin to melt upon contact.
- Because of alcohol content of vehicle, gel products may cause mild, transient stinging, especially when used on or near excoriated skin.
- For patients with eczematous dermatitis whose skin may be irritated by adhesive material, hold dressing in place with gauze, elastic bandages, stockings, or stockinette.

!!ALERT Don't use occlusive dressings.

- If antifungal or antibiotic combined with corticosteroid fails to provide prompt improvement, stop corticosteroid until infection is controlled.
- Systemic absorption is likely with prolonged or extensive body surface treatment. Watch for symptoms.
- Avoid using plastic pants or tight-fitting diapers on treated areas in young children. Children may absorb larger amounts of drug and be more susceptible to systemic toxicity.
- Continue drug for a few days after lesions clear.

!!ALERT Diprolene and Diprolene AF may not be replaced with generics because other products have different potencies.

Patient teaching

- Teach patient how to apply drug.
- Emphasize that drug is for external use only.
- Tell patient to wash hands after application.
- Tell patient to stop drug and report signs of systemic absorption, skin irritation or ulceration, hypersensitivity, or infection.
- Instruct patient not to use occlusive dressings.
- Discuss personal hygiene measures to reduce chance of infection.

betaxolol hydrochloride

Betoptic, Betoptic S

Pregnancy risk category C

Indications & dosages

➲ Chronic open-angle glaucoma, ocular hypertension

Adults: Instill 1 or 2 drops of 0.5% solution or 0.25% suspension b.i.d.

Contraindications & cautions

- Contraindicated in patients hypersensitive to drug and in those with sinus bradycardia, greater than first-degree AV block, cardiogenic shock, or overt heart failure.
- Use cautiously in patients with restricted pulmonary function, diabetes mellitus, hyperthyroidism, or history of heart failure.

Adverse reactions

CNS: insomnia, ***CVA***, depressive neurosis.
CV: ***arrhythmias, heart block, heart failure***, palpitations.
EENT: *eye stinging on instillation causing brief discomfort*, photophobia, erythema, itching, keratitis, occasional tearing.
Respiratory: asthma, ***bronchospasm***.

Interactions

Drug-drug. *Calcium channel blockers:* May cause AV conduction disturbances, ventricular failure, and hypotension if significant systemic absorption occurs. Monitor patient closely.
Cardiac glycosides: May cause excessive bradycardia if significant systemic absorption occurs. Patient may need ECG monitoring.
Dipivefrin, ophthalmic epinephrine: May produce mydriasis. Use together cautiously.
Inhaled hydrocarbon anesthetics: May prolong severe hypotension if significant systemic absorption occurs. Tell anesthesiologist that patient is receiving ophthalmic betaxolol.
Insulin, oral antidiabetics: May cause hypoglycemia or hyperglycemia if significant systemic absorption occurs. May need to adjust dosage of antidiabetics.
Phenothiazines: May have additive hypotensive effects; may increase risk of adverse ef-

fects if significant systemic absorption occurs. Monitor patient closely.
Prazosin: May increase risk of orthostatic hypotension in early phases of use together. Assist patient to stand slowly until effects are known.
Reserpine: May cause excessive beta blockade. Monitor patient closely.
Systemic beta blockers: May have additive effects. Monitor patient closely.
Verapamil: May increase effects of both drugs. Monitor cardiac function closely and decrease dosages as necessary.
Drug-lifestyle. *Cocaine use:* May inhibit betaxolol's effects. Tell patient about this interaction.
Sun exposure: May cause photophobia. Advise patient to wear sunglasses.

Nursing considerations

- Stabilization of intraocular pressure (IOP)–lowering response may take a few weeks. Determine IOP after 4 weeks of treatment.

Patient teaching

- Teach patient how to instill drug. Advise him to wash hands before and after instillation and to apply light finger pressure on lacrimal sac for 1 minute after instilling drug. Warn him not to touch tip of dropper to eye or surrounding tissue. Tell him to shake suspension well before instilling.
- Encourage patient to comply with b.i.d. regimen.
- Tell patient to remove contact lenses before instilling drug. Lenses may be reinserted about 15 minutes after using drops.
- Advise patient to ease sun sensitivity by wearing sunglasses.
- Tell patient to avoid using other eye products with drug.

bethanechol chloride

Duvoid, Myotonachol, Urabeth

Pregnancy risk category C

Indications & dosages

➲ **Acute postoperative and postpartum nonobstructive (functional) urine retention, neurogenic atony of urinary bladder with urine retention**
Adults: 10 to 50 mg P.O. t.i.d. to q.i.d. Or, 2.5 to 5 mg S.C. Never give I.M. or I.V.

Test dosage is 2.5 mg S.C., repeated at 15- to 30-minute intervals to total of four doses to determine the minimal effective dose; then, minimal effective dose used q 6 to 8 hours. All doses must be adjusted individually.

Contraindications & cautions

- Contraindicated in patients hypersensitive to drug or its components and in those with uncertain strength or integrity of bladder wall, mechanical obstruction of GI or urinary tract, hyperthyroidism, peptic ulceration, latent or active bronchial asthma, obstructive pulmonary disease, pronounced bradycardia or hypotension, vasomotor instability, cardiac or coronary artery disease, atrioventricular conduction defects, hypertension, seizure disorder, Parkinson's disease, spastic GI disturbances, acute inflammatory lesions of the GI tract, peritonitis, or marked vagotonia.
- Contraindicated for I.M. or I.V. use and when increased muscular activity of the GI or urinary tract is harmful.
- Use cautiously in pregnant patient.

Adverse reactions

CNS: headache, malaise.
CV: ***bradycardia***, profound hypotension with reflexive tachycardia, flushing.
EENT: lacrimation, miosis.
GI: *abdominal cramps*, *diarrhea*, excessive salivation, nausea, belching, borborygmus.
GU: urinary urgency.
Respiratory: ***bronchoconstriction***, increased bronchial secretions.
Skin: diaphoresis.

Interactions

Drug-drug. *Anticholinergics, atropine, procainamide, quinidine:* May reverse cholinergic effects. Observe patient for lack of drug effect.
Cholinesterase inhibitors, cholinergic agonists: May cause additive effects or increase toxicity. Avoid using together.
Ganglionic blockers: May cause critical drop in blood pressure, usually preceded by severe abdominal pain. Avoid using together.

Nursing considerations

- Give drug 1 hour before or 2 hours after meals because it may cause nausea and vomiting if taken soon after eating.

• Adverse effects are rare with P.O. use.
!!ALERT Never give I.M. or I.V. because of possible circulatory collapse, hypotension, severe abdominal cramping, bloody diarrhea, shock, or cardiac arrest.
• Monitor vital signs frequently, especially respirations. Always have atropine injection available, and be prepared to give 0.6 mg S.C. or by slow I.V. push. Provide respiratory support, if needed.
• Watch for toxicity, especially with S.C. administration.
• Watch closely for adverse reactions that may indicate drug toxicity.
• Oral drug absorption is poor and variable, requiring larger oral doses. Oral and S.C. doses aren't interchangeable.

Patient teaching

• Tell patient to take oral form on an empty stomach and at regular intervals.
• Inform patient that drug is usually effective 30 to 90 minutes after oral use and 5 to 15 minutes after S.C. administration.

bevacizumab
Avastin

Pregnancy risk category C

Indications & dosages

➲ First-line use with fluorouracil-based therapy for metastatic colon or rectal cancer
Adults: 5 mg/kg I.V. q 14 days until disease progresses. Infusion rate varies by patient tolerance and number of infusions.

Contraindications & cautions

• Don't use in patients with recent hemoptysis or within 28 days after major surgery.
• Use cautiously in patients hypersensitive to drug or its components, in those who need surgery, and in patients with significant CV disease.

Adverse reactions

CNS: abnormal gait, *asthenia*, confusion, *dizziness*, *headache*, pain, syncope.
CV: deep vein thrombosis, heart failure, *hypertension*, hypotension, INTRA-ABDOMINAL THROMBOSIS, ***thromboembolism***.
EENT: *epistaxis*, excess lacrimation, gum bleeding, taste disorder, voice alteration.
GI: abdominal pain, *anorexia*, colitis, *constipation*, *diarrhea*, dry mouth, *dyspepsia*, *flatulence*, ***GI hemorrhage***, nausea, *stomatitis*, *vomiting*.
GU: proteinuria, urinary urgency, ***vaginal hemorrhage***.
Hematologic: ***leukopenia***, ***neutropenia***, ***thrombocytopenia***.
Metabolic: bilirubinemia, *hypokalemia*, *weight loss*.
Musculoskeletal: *myalgia*.
Respiratory: *dyspnea*, **HEMOPTYSIS**, *upper respiratory tract infection*.
Skin: *alopecia*, *dermatitis*, *discoloration*, *dry skin*, *exfoliative dermatitis*, nail disorder, skin ulcer.
Other: decreased wound healing, hypersensitivity.

Interactions

Drug-drug. *Irinotecan:* May increase level of irinotecan metabolite. Monitor patient.

Nursing considerations

• Hypersensitivity reactions can occur during infusions.
• Stop drug in patients who have nephrotic syndrome, severe hypertension, hypertensive crisis, serious hemorrhage, GI perforation, or wound dehiscence that needs intervention.
• Stop drug before elective surgery, considering drug's half-life of about 20 days. Don't resume therapy until surgical incision is fully healed.
!!ALERT May increase risk of serious arterial thromboembolic events including MI, TIAs, CVA, and angina. Those patients at highest risk are age 65 or older, have a history of arterial thromboembolism, and have taken the drug before. If patient has an arterial thrombotic event, permanently stop drug.
• Monitor urinalysis for worsening proteinuria. Patients with 2+ or greater urine dipstick test should undergo 24-hour urine collection.
• Monitor patient's blood pressure every 2 to 3 weeks.
• It isn't known whether drug appears in breast milk. Women shouldn't breast-feed during therapy and for about 20 days after therapy stops, taking into account the drug's long half-life.

• Adverse reactions occur more often in older patients.

Patient teaching

• Inform patient about potential adverse reactions.
• Tell patient to report adverse reactions immediately, especially abdominal pain, constipation, and vomiting.
• Advise patient that blood pressure and urinalysis will be monitored during treatment.
• Caution women of childbearing potential to avoid pregnancy during treatment.
• Urge patient to alert other health care providers about treatment and to avoid elective surgery during treatment.

bimatoprost
Lumigan

Pregnancy risk category C

Indications & dosages

➲ **Increased intraocular pressure (IOP) in patients with open-angle glaucoma or ocular hypertension who can't tolerate or are unresponsive to other IOP-lowering drugs**
Adults: Instill 1 drop in conjunctival sac of affected eye once daily in the evening.

Contraindications & cautions

• Contraindicated in patients hypersensitive to bimatoprost, benzalkonium chloride, or other ingredients in product.
• Contraindicated in patients with angle-closure glaucoma or inflammatory or neovascular glaucoma.
• Use cautiously in patients with renal or hepatic impairment.
• Use cautiously in patients with active intraocular inflammation (iritis, uveitis), aphakic patients, pseudophakic patients with torn posterior lens capsule, and patients at risk for macular edema.

Adverse reactions

CNS: headache, asthenia.
EENT: *conjunctival hyperemia, growth of eyelashes, ocular pruritus,* ocular dryness, visual disturbance, ocular burning, foreign body sensation, eye pain, pigmentation of the periocular skin, blepharitis, cataract, superficial punctate keratitis, eyelid erythema, ocular irritation, eyelash darkening, eye discharge, tearing, photophobia, allergic conjunctivitis, asthenopia, increase in iris pigmentation, conjunctival edema.
Respiratory: *upper respiratory tract infection.*
Skin: hirsutism.
Other: *infection.*

Interactions

Drug-herb. *Areca, jaborandi:* May have additive IOP-lowering effects. Discourage use together.

Nursing considerations

• Temporary or permanent increased pigmentation of iris and eyelid, as well as increased pigmentation and growth of eyelashes, may occur.
• Patient should remove contact lenses before using solution. Lenses may be reinserted 15 minutes after administration.
• If more than one ophthalmic drug is being used, give drugs at least 5 minutes apart.
• Store drug in original container between 59° and 77° F (15° and 25° C).

Patient teaching

• Tell patient receiving treatment in only one eye about potential for increased brown pigmentation of iris, eyelid skin darkening, and increased length, thickness, pigmentation, or number of lashes in treated eye.
• Teach patient how to instill drops, and advise him to wash hands before and after instilling solution. Warn him not to touch tip of dropper to eye or surrounding tissue.
• If eye trauma or infection occurs or if eye surgery is needed, tell patient to seek medical advice before continuing to use multidose container.
• Advise patient to immediately report eye inflammation or lid reactions.
• Advise patient to apply light pressure on lacrimal sac for 1 minute after instillation to minimize systemic absorption of drug.
• Tell patient to remove contact lenses before using solution and that lenses may be reinserted 15 minutes after administration.
• If patient is using more than one ophthalmic drug, tell him to apply them at least 5 minutes apart.
• Stress importance of compliance with recommended therapy.

bisacodyl

Bisco-Lax ◇, Correctol, Dulcolax ◇, Feen-a-Mint, Fleet Bisacodyl ◇, Fleet Bisacodyl Enema ◇, Fleet Laxatives ◇, Laxit† ◇

Pregnancy risk category B

Indications & dosages

➲ Chronic constipation; preparation for childbirth, surgery, or rectal or bowel examination

Adults and children age 12 and older: 10 to 15 mg P.O. in evening or before breakfast. Up to 30 mg P.O., p.r.n. Or, 10 mg P.R. for evacuation before examination or surgery.
Children ages 6 to 11: 5 mg P.O. or P.R. h.s. or before breakfast. Oral dose isn't recommended if child can't swallow tablet whole.

Contraindications & cautions

- Contraindicated in patients hypersensitive to drug or its components and in those with rectal bleeding, gastroenteritis, intestinal obstruction, abdominal pain, nausea, vomiting, or other symptoms of appendicitis or acute surgical abdomen.

Adverse reactions

CNS: muscle weakness with excessive use, dizziness, faintness.
GI: *nausea, vomiting, abdominal cramps,* diarrhea with high doses, *burning sensation in rectum with suppositories,* laxative dependence with long-term or excessive use, protein-losing enteropathy with excessive use.
Metabolic: alkalosis, hypokalemia, fluid and electrolyte imbalance.
Musculoskeletal: tetany.

Interactions

Drug-drug. *Antacids:* May cause gastric irritation or dyspepsia from premature dissolution of enteric coating. Separate doses by at least 1 or 2 hours.
Drug-food. *Milk:* May cause gastric irritation or dyspepsia from premature dissolution of enteric coating. Don't use within 1 or 2 hours of drinking milk.

Nursing considerations

- Give drug at times that don't interfere with scheduled activities or sleep. Soft, formed stools are usually produced 15 to 60 minutes after rectal use.
- Before giving for constipation, determine whether patient has adequate fluid intake, exercise, and diet.
- Tablets and suppositories are used together to clean the colon before and after surgery and before barium enema.
- Insert suppository as high as possible into the rectum, and try to position suppository against the rectal wall. Avoid embedding within fecal material because doing so may delay onset of action.
- Bisco-Lax may contain tartrazine.

Patient teaching

- Advise patient to swallow enteric-coated tablet whole to avoid GI irritation. Instruct him not to take within 1 hour of milk or antacid.
- Tell patient that drug is for 1-week treatment only (stimulant laxatives are often abused). Discourage excessive use.
- Advise patient to report adverse effects to prescriber.
- Teach patient about dietary sources of bulk, including bran and other cereals, fresh fruit, and vegetables.
- Tell patient to take drug with a full glass of water or juice.

bismuth subsalicylate

Bismatrol ◇, Bismatrol Extra Strength ◇, Children's Kaopectate ◇, Extra Strength Kaopectate ◇, Kaopectate ◇, Pepto-Bismol ◇, Pepto-Bismol Maximum Strength Liquid ◇, Pink Bismuth ◇

Pregnancy risk category NR

Indications & dosages

➲ Mild, nonspecific diarrhea

Adults and children age 12 and older: 30 ml or 2 tablets P.O. q 30 minutes to 1 hour, up to maximum of eight doses and for no longer than 2 days.
Children ages 9 to 12: 15 ml or 1 tablet P.O. q 30 minutes to 1 hour, up to maximum of eight doses and for no longer than 2 days.
Children ages 6 to 9: 10 ml or 2/3 tablet P.O. q 30 minutes to 1 hour, up to maximum of eight doses and for no longer than 2 days.

Children ages 3 to 6: 5 ml or ⅓ tablet P.O. q 30 minutes to 1 hour, up to maximum of eight doses and for no longer than 2 days.

➲ Traveler's diarrhea

Adults: 2 tablets P.O. q.i.d., before meals and h.s. for up to 3 weeks when traveling in high-risk areas during instances of high risk.

Contraindications & cautions

- Contraindicated in patients hypersensitive to salicylates.
- Use cautiously in patients taking aspirin. Stop therapy if tinnitus occurs.
- Use cautiously in children and in patients with bleeding disorders or salicylate sensitivity.

Adverse reactions

GI: temporary darkening of tongue and stools.

Other: salicylism with high doses.

Interactions

Drug-drug. *Aspirin, other salicylates:* May cause salicylate toxicity. Monitor patient.

Oral anticoagulants, oral antidiabetics: May increase effects of these drugs after high doses of bismuth subsalicylate. Monitor patient closely.

Tetracycline: May decrease tetracycline absorption. Separate doses by at least 2 hours.

Nursing considerations

- Avoid use before GI radiologic procedures because bismuth is radiopaque and may interfere with X-rays.

Patient teaching

- Advise patient that bismuth subsalicylate contains salicylate. Each tablet has 102 mg salicylate. Regular-strength liquid has 130 mg/15 ml. Extra-strength liquid has 230 mg/15 ml.
- Instruct patient to shake liquid before measuring dose and to chew tablets well before swallowing.
- Tell patient to call prescriber if diarrhea lasts longer than 2 days or is accompanied by high fever.
- Advise patient to drink plenty of clear fluids to help prevent dehydration, which may accompany diarrhea.
- Urge patient to consult with prescriber before giving bismuth subsalicylate to children or teenagers during or after recovery from the flu or chickenpox.
- Inform patient that all forms of Pepto-Bismol are effective against traveler's diarrhea. Tablets and caplets may be more convenient to carry.

bivalirudin

Angiomax

Pregnancy risk category B

Indications & dosages

➲ Unstable angina in patients undergoing percutaneous transluminal coronary angioplasty (PTCA)

Adults: 1 mg/kg I.V. bolus just before PTCA; then begin 4-hour I.V. infusion at 2.5 mg/kg/hour. After first 4-hour infusion, give an additional I.V. infusion at a rate of 0.2 mg/kg/hour for up to 20 hours p.r.n. Give with 300 to 325 mg aspirin.

For patients with renal impairment, give normal bolus dose and adjust infusion dose according to creatinine clearance. For creatinine clearance of 30 to 59 ml/minute, reduce dose by 20%. For creatinine clearance of 10 to 29 ml/minute, reduce dose by 60%. For dialysis-dependent patients (off dialysis), reduce dose by 90%.

Contraindications & cautions

- Contraindicated in patients hypersensitive to drug or its components and in those with active major bleeding. Avoid using in patients with unstable angina who aren't undergoing PTCA or in patients with other acute coronary syndromes.
- Use cautiously in patients with heparin-induced thrombocytopenia or heparin-induced thrombocytopenia–thrombosis syndrome, and in patients with diseases linked to increased risk of bleeding.
- Use cautiously in breast-feeding women; it's unknown if drug appears in breast milk.

Adverse reactions

CNS: anxiety, *headache*, insomnia, nervousness, fever, *pain*.

CV: ***bradycardia***, hypertension, *hypotension*.

GI: abdominal pain, dyspepsia, *nausea*, vomiting.

GU: urine retention.

Hematologic: *severe; spontaneous bleeding (cerebral, retroperitoneal*; GU, GI).
Musculoskeletal: *back pain*, pelvic pain.
Skin: pain at injection site.

Interactions

Drug-drug. *Glycoprotein IIb/IIIa inhibitors:* Safety and effectiveness not yet established. Avoid using together.
Heparin, warfarin, other oral anticoagulants: May increase risk of bleeding. Use together cautiously. Stop heparin at least 8 hours before giving bivalirudin.

Nursing considerations

- Don't give by I.M. route.
- Hemorrhage can occur at any site in the body in patients receiving bivalirudin. Consider a hemorrhagic event if patient has unexplained decrease in hematocrit, decrease in blood pressure, or other unexplained symptom.
- Monitor coagulation test results, hemoglobin level, and hematocrit before starting therapy and periodically throughout therapy.
- Monitor venipuncture sites for bleeding, hematoma, or inflammation.
- Puncture site hemorrhage and catheterization site hematoma may occur in more patients age 65 and older than in younger patients.

Patient teaching

- Advise patient that drug can cause bleeding and tell him to report unusual bruising or bleeding (nosebleeds, bleeding gums) or tarry stools immediately.
- Counsel patient that drug is given with aspirin and caution him to avoid other aspirin-containing drugs or NSAIDs while receiving bivalirudin.
- Advise patient to avoid activities that carry a risk of injury and instruct him to use a soft toothbrush and electric razor while on drug.

bleomycin sulfate
Blenoxane

Pregnancy risk category D

Indications & dosages

➲ **Squamous cell carcinoma (head, neck, skin, penis, cervix, and vulva), non-Hodgkin's lymphoma, testicular carcinoma**
Adults: 10 to 20 units/m^2 I.V., I.M., or S.C. once or twice weekly to total of 400 units.
➲ **Hodgkin's disease**
Adults: 10 to 20 units/m^2 I.V., I.M., or S.C. one or two times weekly. After 50% response, maintenance dose is 1 unit I.V. or I.M. daily or 5 units I.V. or I.M. weekly. Total cumulative dose is 400 units.
➲ **Malignant pleural effusion**
Adults: 60 units given as single-dose bolus intrapleural injection.

Contraindications & cautions

- Contraindicated in patients hypersensitive to drug.
- Use cautiously in patients with renal or pulmonary impairment.

Adverse reactions

CNS: fever.
GI: *stomatitis, anorexia, nausea, vomiting*, diarrhea.
Metabolic: weight loss, hyperuricemia.
Respiratory: PNEUMONITIS, ***pulmonary fibrosis***.
Skin: *erythema, hyperpigmentation, acne, rash, striae, skin tenderness, pruritus, reversible alopecia*, hyperkeratosis, nail changes.
Other: *chills*, ***anaphylactoid reactions***.

Interactions

Drug-drug. *Anesthesia:* May increase oxygen requirements. Monitor patient closely.
Cardiac glycosides: May decrease digoxin level. Monitor digoxin level closely.
Fosphenytoin, phenytoin: May decrease phenytoin and fosphenytoin levels. Monitor drug levels closely.

Nursing considerations

- Obtain pulmonary function tests. Stop drug if tests show a marked decline.

!!ALERT Pulmonary toxicity appears to be dose-related, with an increase when total dose is more than 400 units. Give total doses of more than 400 units with caution.

- For intrapleural administration, dilute 60 units of drug in 50 to 100 ml normal saline solution for injection; drug is given through a thoracotomy tube.
- For I.M. use, dilute drug in 1 to 5 ml of sterile water for injection, bacteriostatic wa-

ter for injection, or normal saline solution for injection.

- Monitor injection site for irritation.

!!ALERT Adverse pulmonary reactions are more common in patients older than age 70. Pulmonary fibrosis is fatal in 1% of patients, especially when cumulative dosage exceeds 400 units. Also, pulmonary toxic adverse effects may be increased in patients receiving radiation therapy, patients with lung disease, and patients who need oxygen therapy.

- Monitor chest X-ray and listen to lungs regularly.
- Obtain pulmonary function tests and chest X-rays before each course of therapy.
- If patient's condition requires sclerosis, drug may be instilled when chest tube drainage is 100 to 300 ml/24 hours before therapy; ideally, drainage should be less than 100 ml. After instillation, thoracotomy tube is clamped and patient is moved alternately from the supine to left and right lateral positions for the next 4 hours. The clamp is then removed and suction reestablished. Amount of time chest tube is left in place after sclerosis depends on patient's condition.
- Watch for fever, which may be treated with antipyretics. Fever usually occurs within 3 to 6 hours of administration.
- Look for hypersensitivity reactions, which may be delayed for several hours, especially in patients with lymphoma. (Give test dose of 1 to 2 units before first two doses in these patients. If no reaction occurs, follow regular dosage.)
- Don't use adhesive dressings.

Patient teaching

- Warn patient that hair loss may occur but is usually reversible.
- Tell patient to report adverse reactions promptly and to take infection-control and bleeding precautions.
- For patient who is to receive anesthesia, tell him to inform anesthesiologist of previous treatment with bleomycin. High oxygen levels inhaled during surgery may enhance pulmonary toxicity of drug.

bortezomib
Velcade

Pregnancy risk category D

Indications & dosages

➲ Multiple myeloma that still progresses after at least one therapy

Adults: 1.3 mg/m^2 by I.V. bolus twice weekly for 2 weeks (days 1, 4, 8, and 11), followed by a 10-day rest period (days 12 through 21). This 3-week period is a treatment cycle. For therapy longer than 8 weeks, may adjust dosage schedule to once weekly for 4 weeks on days 1, 8, 15 and 22, followed by a rest period on days 23 through 35. Separate consecutive doses of drug by at least 72 hours.

If grade 3 nonhematologic or grade 4 hematologic toxicity (excluding neuropathy) develops, withhold drug. When toxicity has resolved, restart at a 25% reduced dose. If patient has neuropathic pain, peripheral neuropathy, or both, see the table.

Severity of neuropathy	Dosage
Grade 1 (paresthesias, loss of reflexes, or both) without pain or loss of function	No change.
Grade 1 with pain or grade 2 (function altered but not activities of daily living)	Reduce to 1 mg/m^2.
Grade 2 with pain or grade 3 (interference with activities of daily living)	Hold drug until toxicity resolves; then start at 0.7 mg/m^2 once weekly.
Grade 4 (permanent sensory loss that interferes with function)	Stop drug.

Contraindications & cautions

- Contraindicated in patients hypersensitive to bortezomib, boron, or mannitol.
- Use cautiously if patient is dehydrated, is receiving other drugs known to cause hypotension, or has a history of syncope.
- Use cautiously in patients with hepatic or renal impairment, and watch closely for evidence of toxicity.
- Safety and effectiveness haven't been established for pregnant patients. Advise

women not to become pregnant during therapy.
- Safety and effectiveness haven't been established for children.

Adverse reactions

CNS: *anxiety, asthenia, dizziness, dysesthesia, fever, headache, insomnia, paresthesia, peripheral neuropathy, rigors.*
CV: *edema, hypotension.*
EENT: *blurred vision.*
GI: *abdominal pain, constipation, decreased appetite, diarrhea, dysgeusia, dyspepsia, nausea, vomiting.*
Hematologic: *anemia,* **NEUTROPENIA, THROMBOCYTOPENIA.**
Musculoskeletal: *arthralgia, back pain, bone pain, limb pain, muscle cramps, myalgia.*
Respiratory: *cough, dyspnea, pneumonia, upper respiratory tract infection.*
Skin: rash, *pruritus.*
Other: *dehydration, herpes zoster, pyrexia.*

Interactions

Drug-drug. *Antihypertensives:* May cause hypotension. Monitor patient's blood pressure closely.
Drugs linked to peripheral neuropathy, such as amiodarone, antivirals, isoniazid, nitrofurantoin, statins: May worsen neuropathy. Use together cautiously.
Inhibitors or inducers of CYP3A4: May increase risk of toxicity or may reduce drug's effects. Monitor patient closely.
Oral antidiabetics: May cause hypoglycemia or hyperglycemia. Monitor glucose level closely.

Nursing considerations

- Watch for evidence of neuropathy, such as a burning sensation, hyperesthesia, hypoesthesia, paresthesia, discomfort, or neuropathic pain.
- The development of new or worsening peripheral neuropathy may require a change in bortezomib dose and schedule.
- Because experience with elderly patients is limited, watch carefully for adverse effects.
- Patient may need an antiemetic, antidiarrheal, or both because drug may cause nausea, vomiting, diarrhea, and constipation.
- Provide fluid and electrolyte replacement to prevent dehydration.
- Be prepared to adjust antihypertensive dosage, maintain hydration status, and give mineralocorticoids to manage orthostatic hypotension.

!!ALERT Because thrombocytopenia is common, monitor patient's CBC and platelet counts carefully during treatment, especially on day 11.

Patient teaching

- Tell patient to notify prescriber about new or worsening peripheral neuropathy.
- Urge women to use effective contraception and not to breast-feed during treatment.
- Teach patient how to avoid dehydration, and stress the need to tell prescriber about dizziness, light-headedness, or fainting spells.
- Tell patient to use caution when driving or performing other hazardous activities because drug may cause fatigue, dizziness, faintness, light-headedness, and doubled or blurred vision.

---

bosentan
Tracleer

Pregnancy risk category X

Indications & dosages

➲ Pulmonary arterial hypertension in patients with World Health Organization class III or IV symptoms, to improve exercise ability and decrease rate of clinical worsening
Adults: 62.5 mg P.O. b.i.d. in the morning and evening for 4 weeks. Increase to maintenance dosage of 125 mg P.O. b.i.d. in the morning and evening.

For patients who develop ALT and AST abnormalities, the dose may need to be decreased or the therapy stopped until ALT and AST levels return to normal. If therapy is resumed, begin with initial dose. Test levels within 3 days; then give using the table on page 90. If liver function abnormalities are accompanied by symptoms of liver injury or if bilirubin level is at least twice the upper limit of normal (ULN), stop treatment and don't restart. In patients weighing less than 40 kg, the initial and maintenance dosage is 62.5 mg b.i.d.

ALT and AST levels	Treatment and monitoring recommendations
> 3 and < 5 × upper limit of normal (ULN)	Confirm with repeat test; if confirmed, reduce dose or interrupt treatment and retest q 2 wk. Once ALT and AST levels return to pretreatment levels, continue or reintroduce treatment at starting dose.
> 5 and < 8 × ULN	Confirm with repeat test; if confirmed, stop treatment and retest at least q 2 wk. Once levels return to pretreatment levels, consider reintroduction of treatment.
> 8 × ULN	Stop treatment; don't consider restarting drug.

Contraindications & cautions

- Contraindicated in patients hypersensitive to drug, in pregnant patients, and in those taking cyclosporine A or glyburide.
- Don't use in patients with moderate to severe liver impairment or in those with elevated aminotransferase levels greater than three times the ULN.
- Use cautiously in patients with mild liver impairment.
- Drug may harm fetus. Be sure patient isn't pregnant before starting treatment.
- Because it's unknown whether drug appears in breast milk, drug isn't recommended for breast-feeding women.
- Safety and effectiveness in children haven't been established.

Adverse reactions

CNS: *headache*, fatigue.
CV: hypotension, palpitations, flushing, edema.
EENT: *nasopharyngitis*.
GI: dyspepsia.
Hematologic: *anemia*.
Hepatic: HEPATOTOXICITY.
Skin: pruritus.
Other: leg edema.

Interactions

Drug-drug. *Cyclosporine A:* May increase bosentan level and decrease cyclosporine level. Use together is contraindicated.
Glyburide: May increase risk of elevated liver function test values and decrease levels of both drugs. Use together is contraindicated.
Hormonal contraceptives: May cause contraceptive failure. Advise use of an additional method of birth control.
Ketoconazole: May increase bosentan effect. Watch for adverse effects.
Simvastatin, other statins: May decrease levels of drugs. Monitor cholesterol levels to assess need to adjust statin dose.

Nursing considerations

- Use of this drug can cause serious liver injury. AST and ALT level elevations may be dose dependent and reversible, so measure these levels before treatment and monthly thereafter, adjusting dosage accordingly. If elevations are accompanied by symptoms of liver injury (nausea, vomiting, fever, abdominal pain, jaundice, or unusual lethargy or fatigue) or bilirubin increases by greater than twice the ULN, notify prescriber immediately.
- Monitor hemoglobin after 1 and 3 months of therapy; then every 3 months.
- Gradually reduce dose before stopping drug.

Patient teaching

- Advise patient to take doses in the morning and evening, with or without food.
- Warn patient to avoid becoming pregnant while taking this drug. Hormonal contraceptives, including oral, implantable, and injectable methods, may not be effective when used together with this drug. Advise patient to use a backup method of contraception. A monthly pregnancy test must be performed.
- Advise patient to have liver function tests and blood counts performed regularly.

brimonidine tartrate
Alphagan P

Pregnancy risk category B

Indications & dosages

➲ To reduce intraocular pressure (IOP) in open-angle glaucoma or ocular hypertension
Adults: 1 drop in affected eye t.i.d., about 8 hours apart.

Contraindications & cautions

- Contraindicated in patients hypersensitive to drug or benzalkonium chloride and in those receiving MAO inhibitor therapy.
- Use cautiously in patients with CV disease, cerebral or coronary insufficiency, hepatic or renal impairment, depression, Raynaud's phenomenon, orthostatic hypotension, or thromboangiitis obliterans.

Adverse reactions

CNS: asthenia, dizziness, headache.
CV: hypertension.
EENT: *ocular hyperemia, allergic conjunctivitis,* allergic reaction, *pruritus,* burning, stinging, follicular conjunctivitis, abnormal vision, blepharitis, conjunctival edema or hemorrhage, conjunctivitis, increased tearing, dryness, pain, eyelid edema or erythema, foreign body sensation, pharyngitis, rhinitis, sinus infection, sinusitis, photophobia, superficial punctate keratopathy, visual field defect, vitreous floaters, worsened visual acuity.
GI: oral dryness, dyspepsia.
Respiratory: bronchitis, cough, dyspnea.
Skin: rash.
Other: flulike syndrome.

Interactions

Drug-drug. *Antihypertensives, beta blockers, cardiac glycosides:* May further decrease blood pressure or pulse. Monitor vital signs.
CNS depressants: May increase effects. Use cautiously together.
MAO inhibitors: May increase effects. Avoid using together.
Tricyclic antidepressants: May interfere with brimonidine's IOP-lowering effects. Use cautiously together.
Drug-lifestyle. *Alcohol use:* May increase CNS-depressant effect. Urge patient to avoid alcohol.

Nursing considerations

- Monitor IOP because drug effect may reverse after first month of therapy.

Patient teaching

- Tell patient to wait at least 15 minutes after instilling drug before wearing soft contact lenses.
- Caution patient to avoid hazardous activities because of risk of decreased mental alertness, fatigue, or drowsiness.
- Advise patient to avoid alcohol.

bromfenac
Xibrom

Pregnancy risk category C

Indications & dosages

➲ Inflammation after cataract surgery
Adults: 1 drop in affected eye(s) b.i.d., starting 24 hours after surgery and continuing for 2 weeks.

Contraindications & cautions

- Contraindicated in patients hypersensitive to drug or its ingredients. Drug contains sulfite, which may cause allergic-type reactions, including anaphylaxis and life-threatening or less-severe asthmatic episodes in patients sensitive to sulfites.
- Use cautiously in patients with bleeding tendencies, those taking anticoagulants, and those sensitive to aspirin products, phenylacetic acid derivatives, and other NSAIDs.
- Use cautiously in patients who have had complicated or repeat ocular surgeries or those with corneal denervation, corneal epithelial defects, diabetes mellitus, ocular surface diseases (such as dry-eye syndrome), or rheumatoid arthritis because of the increased risk of corneal adverse effects, which may threaten their sight.
- Use in pregnant patients only if potential benefit justifies risk.
- Avoid use late in pregnancy because NSAIDs may cause premature closure of the ductus arteriosus, a necessary structure of fetal circulation.
- Use cautiously in breast-feeding women.

Adverse reactions

CNS: headache.
EENT: abnormal sensation in the eye, burning, conjunctival hyperemia, eye irritation, eye pain, eye pruritus, eye redness, iritis, keratitis, stinging.
Other: ***anaphylaxis***, hypersensitivity reactions.

Interactions

Drug-drug. *Drugs that affect coagulation:* May further increase bleeding tendency or prolong bleeding time. Avoid using together, if possible, or monitor patient closely for bleeding.
Topical corticosteroids: May delay healing. Avoid using together, if possible, or monitor healing closely.

Nursing considerations

- Ask patient if he's sensitive to sulfites, aspirin, or other NSAIDs before treatment. Drug contains sulfite, which may cause allergic-type reactions, including anaphylaxis and life-threatening or less severe asthmatic episodes, in patients sensitive to sulfites.
- Sulfite sensitivity is more common in patients with asthma than in those without asthma. If patient has asthma, monitor closely.
- If patient takes an anticoagulant, watch closely for increased bleeding.
- Begin treatment at least 24 hours after surgery and continue for 2 weeks. Starting treatment less than 24 hours after surgery or giving for longer than 14 days increases risk of ocular adverse effects.

Patient teaching

- Advise patient not to use while wearing contact lenses.
- Teach patient how to instill the drops.
- Instruct patient to start therapy 24 hours after surgery and to continue for 14 days.
- Tell patient not to use for longer than 2 weeks after surgery or to save unused amount for other conditions.
- Tell patient the signs and symptoms of adverse effects. If bothersome or serious adverse effects occur, advise patient to stop treatment and contact prescriber.
- Tell patient to store drug at room temperature.

bromocriptine mesylate
Parlodel

Pregnancy risk category B

Indications & dosages

➲ Parkinson's disease
Adults: 1.25 mg P.O. b.i.d. with meals. Increase dosage by 2.5 mg/day q 14 to 28 days, up to 100 mg daily.
➲ Amenorrhea and galactorrhea from hyperprolactinemia; hypogonadism, infertility
Adults: 0.5 to 2.5 mg P.O. daily, increased by 2.5 mg daily at 3- to 7-day intervals until desired effect occurs. Therapeutic daily dose is 2.5 to 15 mg.
➲ Acromegaly
Adults: 1.25 to 2.5 mg P.O. with h.s. snack for 3 days. Another 1.25 to 2.5 mg may be added q 3 to 7 days until therapeutic benefit occurs. Maximum, 100 mg daily.
➲ Neuroleptic malignant syndrome♦
Adults: 2.5 to 5 mg P.O. two to six times daily.

Contraindications & cautions

- Contraindicated in patients hypersensitive to ergot derivatives and in those with uncontrolled hypertension, toxemia of pregnancy, severe ischemic heart disease, or peripheral vascular disease.
- Use cautiously in patients with impaired renal or hepatic function and in those with a history of MI with residual arrhythmias.

Adverse reactions

CNS: ***CVA***, *dizziness*, *headache*, *fatigue*, mania, light-headedness, drowsiness, delusions, nervousness, insomnia, depression, ***seizures***.
CV: *hypotension*, ***acute MI***.
EENT: nasal congestion, blurred vision.
GI: *nausea*, vomiting, *abdominal cramps*, *constipation*, diarrhea, anorexia.
GU: urine retention, urinary frequency.
Skin: coolness and pallor of fingers and toes.

Interactions

Drug-drug. *Amitriptyline, haloperidol, imipramine, loxapine, MAO inhibitors, methyldopa, metoclopramide, phenothiazines, reserpine:* May interfere with bromocriptine's

effects. Bromocriptine dosage may need to be increased.
Antihypertensives: May increase hypotensive effects. Adjust dosage of antihypertensive.
Erythromycin: May increase bromocriptine level and risk of adverse reactions. Use together cautiously.
Estrogens, hormonal contraceptives, progestins: May interfere with effects of bromocriptine. Avoid using together.
Levodopa: May have additive effects. Adjust dosage of levodopa, if needed.
Drug-lifestyle. *Alcohol use:* May cause disulfiram-like reaction. Discourage use together.

Nursing considerations

- For Parkinson's disease, bromocriptine usually is given with levodopa or levodopa and carbidopa. The levodopa and carbidopa may need to be reduced.
- Adverse reactions may be minimized if drug is given in the evening with food.

!!ALERT Monitor patient for adverse reactions, which occur in 68% of patients, particularly at start of therapy. Most reactions are mild to moderate; nausea is most common. Minimize adverse reactions by gradually adjusting dosages to effective levels. Adverse reactions are more common when drug is used for Parkinson's disease.

- Baseline and periodic evaluations of cardiac, hepatic, renal, and hematopoietic function are recommended during prolonged therapy.
- Drug may lead to early postpartum conception. After menses resumes, test for pregnancy every 4 weeks or as soon as a period is missed.

!!ALERT Don't confuse bromocriptine with benztropine or brimonidine, or Parlodel with pindolol.

Patient teaching

- Instruct patient to take drug with meals.
- Advise patient to use contraceptive methods during treatment other than oral contraceptives or subdermal implants.
- Instruct patient to avoid dizziness and fainting by rising slowly to an upright position and avoiding sudden position changes.
- Inform patient that it may take 8 weeks or longer for menses to resume and excess production of milk to slow down.
- Advise patient to avoid alcohol while taking drug.

budesonide (inhalation)
Pulmicort Respules, Pulmicort Turbuhaler

Pregnancy risk category B

Indications & dosages

➲ As a preventative in maintenance of asthma
All patients: Use lowest effective dose after stabilizing asthma.
Adults previously taking bronchodilator alone: Initially, inhaled dose of 200 to 400 mcg b.i.d. to maximum of 400 mcg b.i.d.
Adults previously taking inhaled corticosteroid: Initially, inhaled dose of 200 to 400 mcg b.i.d. to maximum of 800 mcg b.i.d.
Adults previously taking oral corticosteroid: Initially, inhaled dose of 400 to 800 mcg b.i.d. to maximum of 800 mcg b.i.d.
Children older than age 6 previously taking bronchodilator alone or inhaled corticosteroid: Initially, inhaled dose of 200 mcg b.i.d. to maximum of 400 mcg b.i.d.
Children older than age 6 previously taking oral corticosteroid: 400 mcg b.i.d., maximum.
Children ages 1 to 8: 0.25 mg Respules via jet nebulizer with compressor once daily. Increase to 0.5 mg daily or 0.25 mg b.i.d. in child not receiving systemic or inhaled corticosteroid or 1 mg daily or 0.5 mg b.i.d. in child receiving oral corticosteroid.

Contraindications & cautions

- Contraindicated in patients hypersensitive to drug and in those with status asthmaticus or other acute asthma episodes.
- Use cautiously, if at all, in patients with active or quiescent tuberculosis of the respiratory tract, ocular herpes simplex, or untreated systemic fungal, bacterial, viral, or parasitic infections.

Adverse reactions

CNS: *headache*, fever, asthenia, pain, insomnia, syncope, hypertonia.
EENT: *sinusitis*, *pharyngitis*, rhinitis, voice alteration.
GI: oral candidiasis, dyspepsia, gastroenteritis, nausea, dry mouth, taste perversion, vomiting, abdominal pain.
Metabolic: weight gain.
Musculoskeletal: back pain, fractures, myalgia.
Respiratory: *respiratory tract infections*, increased cough, ***bronchospasm***.
Skin: ecchymoses.
Other: flulike symptoms; hypersensitivity reactions.

Interactions

Drug-drug. *Ketoconazole:* May inhibit metabolism and increase level of budesonide. Monitor patient.

Nursing considerations

- When transferring from systemic corticosteroid to budesonide, use caution and gradually decrease corticosteroid dose to prevent adrenal insufficiency.
- Drug doesn't remove the need for systemic corticosteroid therapy in some situations.
- If bronchospasm occurs after using budesonide, stop therapy and treat with a bronchodilator.
- Lung function may improve within 24 hours of starting therapy, but maximum benefit may not be achieved for 1 to 2 weeks or longer.
- For Pulmicort Respules, lung function improves in 2 to 8 days, but maximum benefit may not be seen for 4 to 6 weeks.
- Watch for *Candida* infections of the mouth or pharynx.

!!ALERT Corticosteroids may increase risk of developing serious or fatal infections in patients exposed to viral illnesses, such as chickenpox or measles.

- In rare cases, inhaled corticosteroids have been linked to increased intraocular pressure and cataract development. Stop drug if local irritation occurs.

Patient teaching

- Tell patient that budesonide inhaler isn't a bronchodilator and isn't intended to treat acute episodes of asthma.
- Instruct patient to use the inhaler at regular intervals, as follows, because effectiveness depends on twice-daily use on a regular basis:
  - Tell patient to keep Pulmicort Turbuhaler upright (mouthpiece on top) during loading, to provide the correct dose.
  - Instruct patient to prime Turbuhaler when using it for the first time. To prime, hold unit upright and turn brown grip fully to the right, then fully to the left until it clicks. Repeat priming.
  - Tell patient to load first dose by holding unit upright and turning brown grip to the right and then to the left until it clicks.
  - Tell patient to turn his head away from the inhaler and breathe out.
  - During inhalation, Turbuhaler must be in the upright or horizontal position.
  - Tell patient not to shake inhaler.
  - Instruct patient to place mouthpiece between lips and to inhale forcefully and deeply.
  - Tell patient that he may not taste the drug or sense it entering his lungs, but this doesn't mean it isn't effective.
  - Tell patient not to exhale through the Turbuhaler. If more than one dose is required, repeat steps.
  - Advise patient to rinse his mouth with water and then spit out the water after each dose to decrease the risk of developing oral candidiasis.
  - When 20 doses remain in the Turbuhaler, a red mark appears in the indicator window. When red mark reaches the bottom, the unit's empty.
  - Tell patient not to use Turbuhaler with a spacer device and not to chew or bite the mouthpiece.
  - Replace mouthpiece cover after use and always keep it clean and dry.
- Tell patient that improvement in asthma control may be seen within 24 hours, although the maximum benefit may not appear for 1 to 2 weeks. If signs or symptoms worsen during this time, instruct patient to contact prescriber.
- Advise patient to avoid exposure to chickenpox or measles and to contact prescriber if exposure occurs.
- Instruct patient to carry or wear medical identification indicating need for supplementary corticosteroids during periods of stress or an asthma attack.

• Advise patient that unused Respules are good for 2 weeks after the foil envelope has been opened; however, unused Respules should be returned to the envelope to protect them from light.
• Tell patient to read and follow the patient information leaflet contained in the package.

budesonide (nasal)
Rhinocort Aqua

Pregnancy risk category C

Indications & dosages
➲ Symptoms of seasonal or perennial allergic rhinitis
Adults and children age 6 and older: 1 spray in each nostril once daily. Maximum recommended dose for adults and children 12 and older is 4 sprays per nostril once daily (256 mcg daily). Maximum recommended dose for children 6 to 12 is 2 sprays per nostril once daily (128 mcg daily).

Contraindications & cautions
• Contraindicated in patients hypersensitive to drug or its components and in those who have had recent septal ulcers, nasal surgery, or nasal trauma until total healing has occurred.
• Contraindicated in those with untreated localized nasal mucosa infections.
• Use cautiously in patients with tuberculous infections, ocular herpes simplex, or untreated fungal, bacterial, or systemic viral infections.

Adverse reactions
EENT: nasal irritation, epistaxis, pharyngitis.
Respiratory: cough, ***bronchospasm***.

Interactions
None significant.

Nursing considerations
• Systemic effects of corticosteroid therapy may occur if recommended daily dose is exceeded.

Patient teaching
• Tell patient to avoid exposure to chickenpox or measles.
• To instill drug, instruct patient to shake container before use, blow nose to clear nasal passages, and tilt head slightly forward and insert nozzle into nostril, pointing away from septum. Tell him to hold other nostril closed and inhale gently while spraying. Next, have him shake container and repeat in other nostril.
• Advise patient not to freeze, break, incinerate, or store canister in extreme heat; contents are under pressure.
• Advise patient to store canister with valve upward.
• Warn patient not to exceed prescribed dosage or use drug for long periods because of risk of hypothalamic-pituitary-adrenal axis suppression.
• Tell patient to notify prescriber if signs or symptoms don't improve or if they worsen in 3 weeks.
• Teach patient good nasal and oral hygiene.
• Tell patient to use drug within 6 months of opening the protective aluminum pouch.
• Instruct patient not to share drug because this could spread infection.

budesonide (oral)
Entocort EC

Pregnancy risk category B

Indications & dosages
➲ Mild to moderate active Crohn's disease involving the ileum, ascending colon, or both
Adults: 9 mg P.O. once daily in morning for up to 8 weeks. For recurrent episodes of active Crohn's disease, a repeat 8-week course may be given. Treatment can be tapered to 6 mg P.O. daily for 2 weeks before complete cessation.
➲ To maintain remission in mild to moderate Crohn's disease that involves the ileum or ascending colon
Adults: 6 mg P.O. daily for up to 3 months. If symptom control is maintained at 3 months, taper dose to stop therapy. Therapy for longer than 3 months doesn't have added benefit.

In patients with moderate to severe liver disease who have increased signs or symptoms of hypercorticism, reduce dose.

Contraindications & cautions

- Contraindicated in patients hypersensitive to budesonide.
- Use cautiously in patients with tuberculosis, hypertension, diabetes mellitus, osteoporosis, peptic ulcer disease, glaucoma, or cataracts; those with a family history of diabetes or glaucoma; and those with any other condition in which glucocorticosteroids may have unwanted effects.
- Glucocorticoids appear in breast milk, and infants may have adverse reactions. Use cautiously in breast-feeding women only if benefits outweigh risks.

Adverse reactions

CNS: *headache*, dizziness, asthenia, hyperkinesia, paresthesia, tremor, vertigo, fatigue, malaise, agitation, confusion, insomnia, nervousness, somnolence.
CV: chest pain, hypertension, palpitations, tachycardia, flushing.
EENT: facial edema, ear infection, eye abnormality, abnormal vision, sinusitis.
GI: *nausea, diarrhea*, dyspepsia, abdominal pain, flatulence, vomiting, anal disorder, aggravated Crohn's disease, enteritis, epigastric pain, fistula, glossitis, hemorrhoids, intestinal obstruction, tongue edema, tooth disorder, increased appetite.
GU: dysuria, micturition frequency, nocturia, intermenstrual bleeding, menstrual disorder, hematuria, pyuria.
Hematologic: leukocytosis, anemia.
Metabolic: *hypercorticism*, dependent edema, hypokalemia, increased weight.
Musculoskeletal: back pain, aggravated arthritis, cramps, arthralgia, myalgia.
Respiratory: *respiratory tract infection*, bronchitis, dyspnea.
Skin: *acne*, alopecia, dermatitis, eczema, skin disorder, increased sweating.
Other: flulike disorder, sleep disorder, candidiasis, viral infection, pain.

Interactions

Drug-drug. *CYP inhibitors (erythromycin, indinavir, itraconazole, ketoconazole, ritonavir, saquinavir):* May increase effects of budesonide. If use together is unavoidable, reduce budesonide dosage.
Drug-food. *Grapefruit juice:* May increase drug effects. Discourage use together.

Nursing considerations

- Reduced liver function affects elimination of this drug; systemic availability of drug may increase in patients with liver cirrhosis.
- Patients undergoing surgery or other stressful situations may need systemic glucocorticoid supplementation in addition to budesonide therapy.
- Carefully monitor patients transferred from systemic glucocorticoid therapy to budesonide for signs and symptoms of corticosteroid withdrawal. Watch for immunosuppression, especially in patients who haven't had diseases such as chickenpox or measles; these can be fatal in patients who are immunosuppressed or receiving glucocorticoids.
- Replacement of systemic glucocorticoids with this drug may unmask allergies, such as eczema and rhinitis, which were previously controlled by systemic drug.
- Long-term use of drug may cause hypercorticism and adrenal suppression.

Patient teaching

- Tell patient to swallow capsules whole and not to chew or break them.
- Advise patient to avoid grapefruit juice while taking drug.
- Tell patient to notify prescriber immediately if he is exposed to or develops chickenpox or measles.

bumetanide
Bumex

Pregnancy risk category C

Indications & dosages

➲ **Edema caused by heart failure or hepatic or renal disease**
Adults: 0.5 to 2 mg P.O. once daily. If diuretic response isn't adequate, a second or third dose may be given at 4- to 5-hour intervals. Maximum dose is 10 mg daily. May be given parenterally if oral route isn't feasible. Usual first dose is 0.5 to 1 mg given I.V. or I.M. If response isn't adequate, a second or third dose may be given at 2- to 3-hour intervals. Maximum, 10 mg daily.

Contraindications & cautions

- Contraindicated in patients hypersensitive to drug or sulfonamides (possible cross-sensitivity) and in patients with anuria, hepatic coma, or severe electrolyte depletion.
- Use cautiously in patients with hepatic cirrhosis and ascites, in elderly patients, and in those with depressed renal function.

Adverse reactions

CNS: *weakness*, dizziness, headache, vertigo, pain.
CV: orthostatic hypotension, ECG changes, chest pain.
EENT: transient deafness, tinnitus.
GI: nausea, vomiting, upset stomach, dry mouth, diarrhea.
GU: premature ejaculation, difficulty maintaining erection, oliguria.
Hematologic: azotemia, ***thrombocytopenia***.
Metabolic: volume depletion and dehydration, hypokalemia, hypochloremic alkalosis, hypomagnesemia, asymptomatic hyperuricemia.
Musculoskeletal: arthritic pain, muscle pain and tenderness.
Skin: rash, pruritus, diaphoresis.

Interactions

Drug-drug. *Aminoglycoside antibiotics:* May increase ototoxicity. Use together cautiously.
Antidiabetics: May decrease hypoglycemic effects. Monitor glucose level.
Antihypertensives: May increase risk of hypotension. Use together cautiously.
Cardiac glycosides: May increase risk of digoxin toxicity from bumetanide-induced hypokalemia. Monitor potassium and digoxin levels.
Chlorothiazide, chlorthalidone, hydrochlorothiazide, indapamide, metolazone: May cause excessive diuretic response, causing serious electrolyte abnormalities or dehydration. Adjust doses carefully, and monitor patient closely for signs and symptoms of excessive diuretic response.
Cisplatin: May increase risk of ototoxicity. Monitor patient closely.
Lithium: May decrease lithium clearance, increasing risk of lithium toxicity. Monitor lithium level.
Neuromuscular blockers: May prolong neuromuscular blockade. Monitor patient closely.
NSAIDs, probenecid: May inhibit diuretic response. Use together cautiously.
Other potassium-wasting drugs (such as amphotericin B, corticosteroids): May increase risk of hypokalemia. Use together cautiously.
Warfarin: May increase anticoagulant effect. Use together cautiously.
Drug-herb. *Dandelion:* May interfere with diuretic activity. Discourage use together.
Licorice: May cause unexpected rapid potassium loss. Discourage use together.

Nursing considerations

- To prevent nocturia, give drug in the morning. If second dose is needed, give in early afternoon.
- Safest and most effective dosage schedule for control of edema is intermittent dosage given on alternate days or 3 to 4 days with 1 or 2 days off between cycles.
- Monitor fluid intake and output, weight, and electrolyte, BUN, creatinine, and carbon dioxide levels frequently.
- Watch for evidence of hypokalemia, such as muscle weakness and cramps. Instruct patient to report these symptoms.
- Consult prescriber and dietitian about a high-potassium diet. Foods rich in potassium include citrus fruits, tomatoes, bananas, dates, and apricots.
- Monitor glucose level in diabetic patients.
- Monitor uric acid level, especially in patients with history of gout.
- Monitor blood pressure and pulse rate during rapid diuresis. Bumetanide can lead to profound water and electrolyte depletion.
- If oliguria or azotemia develops or increases, prescriber may stop drug.
- Bumetanide can be safely used in patients allergic to furosemide; 1 mg of bumetanide equals about 40 mg of furosemide.

!!ALERT Don't confuse Bumex with Buprenex.

Patient teaching

- Instruct patient to take drug with food to minimize GI upset.
- Advise patient to take drug in morning to avoid need to urinate at night; if patient needs second dose, have him take it in early afternoon.
- Advise patient to avoid sudden posture changes and to rise slowly to avoid dizziness upon standing quickly.

• Instruct patient to notify prescriber about muscle weakness, cramps, nausea, or dizziness.
• Instruct patient to weigh himself daily to monitor fluid status.

buprenorphine hydrochloride
Buprenex

Pregnancy risk category C
Controlled substance schedule III

Indications & dosages

➲ Moderate to severe pain
Adults and children age 13 and older: 0.3 mg I.M. or slow I.V. q 6 hours, p.r.n., or around the clock; repeat dose (up to 0.3 mg), p.r.n., 30 to 60 minutes after first dose.
Children ages 2 to 12: 2 to 6 mcg/kg I.M. or I.V. q 4 to 6 hours.
Elderly patients: Reduce dose by one-half.
In high-risk patients, such as debilitated patients, reduce dose by one-half.

➲ Postoperative pain♦
Adults: 25 to 250 mcg/hr by continuous I.V. infusion. Or, 60 mcg by epidural administration in single doses, up to a mean total dose of 180 mcg over 48 hours.

➲ Adjunct to surgical anesthesia with a local anesthetic♦
Adults: 0.3 mg by the epidural route.

➲ Severe, chronic pain in terminally ill patients♦
Adults: 0.15 to 0.3 mg by the epidural route q 6 hours, up to a mean total daily dose of 0.86 mg (range 0.15 to 7.2 mg).

➲ Adjunct to surgical anesthesia during circumcision♦
Children ages 9 months to 9 years: 3 mcg/kg I.M., followed by additional 3 mcg/kg doses postoperatively, p.r.n.

➲ To reverse fentanyl-induced anesthesia and provide analgesia after surgery♦
Adults: 0.3 to 0.8 mg I.M. or I.V. 1 to 4 hours after induction of anesthesia and 30 minutes before surgery ends.

Contraindications & cautions

• Contraindicated in patients hypersensitive to drug.
• Use cautiously in elderly or debilitated patients; in those undergoing biliary tract surgery; and in those with head injury, intracranial lesions, and increased intracranial pressure; severe respiratory, liver, or kidney impairment; CNS depression or coma; thyroid irregularities; adrenal insufficiency; and prostatic hypertrophy, urethral stricture, acute alcoholism, delirium tremens, or kyphoscoliosis.

Adverse reactions

CNS: *dizziness, sedation,* headache, confusion, nervousness, euphoria, *vertigo,* ***increased intracranial pressure,*** fatigue, weakness, depression, dreaming, psychosis, slurred speech, paresthesia.
CV: hypotension, ***bradycardia,*** tachycardia, hypertension, Wenckebach block, cyanosis, flushing.
EENT: miosis, blurred vision, diplopia, tinnitus, conjunctivitis, visual abnormalities.
GI: *nausea,* vomiting, constipation, dry mouth.
GU: urine retention.
Respiratory: ***respiratory depression,*** hypoventilation, dyspnea.
Skin: pruritus, diaphoresis, injection site reactions.
Other: chills, withdrawal syndrome.

Interactions

Drug-drug. *CNS depressants, MAO inhibitors:* May cause additive effects. Use together cautiously.
CYP3A4 inducers (carbamazepine, phenobarbital, phenytoin, rifampin): May increase clearance of buprenorphine. Monitor patient for clinical effects of drug.
CYP3A4 inhibitors (erythromycin, indinavir, ketoconazole, ritonavir, saquinavir): May decrease clearance of buprenorphine. Monitor patient for increased adverse effects.
Drug-lifestyle. *Alcohol use:* May cause additive effects. Discourage use together.

Nursing considerations

• Reassess patient's level of pain 15 and 30 minutes after parenteral administration.
• Buprenorphine 0.3 mg is equal to 10 mg of morphine and 75 mg of meperidine in analgesic potency. It has longer duration of action than morphine or meperidine.
!! ALERT Naloxone won't completely reverse the respiratory depression caused by buprenorphine overdose; an overdose may necessitate mechanical ventilation. Larger-than-

customary doses of naloxone (more than 0.4 mg) and doxapram also may be ordered.
- Treat accidental skin exposure by removing exposed clothing and rinsing skin with water.

!!**ALERT** Drug's opioid antagonist properties may cause withdrawal syndrome in opioid-dependent patients.
- If dependence occurs, withdrawal symptoms may appear up to 14 days after drug is stopped.

!!**ALERT** Don't confuse Buprenex with Bumex or bupropion.

Patient teaching
- Caution ambulatory patient about getting out of bed or walking.
- When drug is used after surgery, encourage patient to turn, cough, and breathe deeply to prevent breathing problems.

bupropion hydrochloride
Wellbutrin, Wellbutrin SR, Wellbutrin XL

Pregnancy risk category B

Indications & dosages
➲ Depression

Adults: For immediate-release, initially, 100 mg P.O. b.i.d.; increase after 3 days to 100 mg P.O. t.i.d., if needed. If patient doesn't improve after several weeks of therapy, increase dosage to 150 mg t.i.d. No single dose should exceed 150 mg. Allow at least 6 hours between successive doses. Maximum dosage is 450 mg daily. For sustained-release, initially, 150 mg P.O. q morning; increase to target dose of 150 mg P.O. b.i.d., as tolerated, as early as day 4 of dosing. Allow at least 8 hours between successive doses. Maximum dose is 400 mg daily. For extended-release, initially, 150 mg P.O. q morning; increase to target dosage of 300 mg P.O. daily, as tolerated, as early as day 4 of dosing. Allow at least 24 hours between successive doses. Maximum is 450 mg daily.

In patients with mild to moderate hepatic cirrhosis or renal impairment, reduce frequency and dose. In patients with severe hepatic cirrhosis, don't exceed 75 mg (immediate-release) P.O. daily, 100 mg (sustained-release) P.O. daily, 150 mg (sustained-release) P.O. every other day, or 150 mg (extended-release) P.O. every other day.

Contraindications & cautions
- Contraindicated in patients hypersensitive to drug, in those who have taken MAO inhibitors within previous 14 days, and in those with seizure disorders or history of bulimia or anorexia nervosa because of a higher risk of seizures.
- Don't use with Zyban or other drugs containing bupropion that are used for smoking cessation.
- Contraindicated in patients abruptly stopping use of alcohol or sedatives (including benzodiazepines).
- Use cautiously in patients with recent history of MI, unstable heart disease, or renal or hepatic impairment.

Adverse reactions
CNS: fever, *headache*, ***seizures***, anxiety, confusion, delusions, euphoria, hostility, impaired sleep quality, *insomnia*, *sedation*, *tremor*, akinesia, akathisia, *agitation*, *dizziness*, fatigue, syncope, ***suicidal behavior***.
CV: hypertension, hypotension, palpitations, *tachycardia*, ***arrhythmias***, chest pain.
EENT: *auditory disturbances*, blurred vision, epistaxis, *pharyngitis*, sinusitis.
GI: *nausea*, *vomiting*, *anorexia*, *dry mouth*, taste disturbance, increased appetite, *constipation*, dyspepsia, diarrhea, abdominal pain.
GU: impotence, menstrual complaints, urinary frequency, urine retention.
Metabolic: *weight loss*, *weight gain*.
Musculoskeletal: arthritis, myalgia, arthralgia, muscle spasm or twitch.
Respiratory: upper respiratory complaints, increase in coughing.
Skin: pruritus, rash, cutaneous temperature disturbance, *excessive diaphoresis*, urticaria.
Other: fever and chills, decreased libido, accidental injury.

Interactions
Drug-drug. *Carbamazepine:* May decrease bupropion level. Monitor patient.
Levodopa, phenothiazines, tricyclic antidepressants, recent and rapid withdrawal of benzodiazepines: May cause adverse reactions, including seizures. Monitor patient closely.

MAO inhibitors: May alter seizure threshold. Avoid using together.
Nicotine replacement agents: May cause hypertension. Monitor blood pressure.
Ritonavir: May increase bupropion level. Monitor patient closely for adverse reactions.
Drug-lifestyle. *Alcohol use:* May alter seizure threshold. Discourage use together.
Sun exposure: May increase risk of photosensitivity reactions. Advise patient to avoid excessive sunlight exposure.

Nursing considerations

- Many patients experience a period of increased restlessness, including agitation, insomnia, and anxiety, especially at start of therapy.

!!ALERT For immediate-release form, minimize risk of seizure by not exceeding 450 mg daily and by giving in three equally divided doses. Don't increase dose more than 100 mg daily in a 3-day period. For sustained-release form, minimize risk of seizure by not exceeding 400 mg daily and by giving in two equally divided doses. Don't increase doses more than 200 mg daily. For extended-release form, minimize risk of seizure by not exceeding 450 mg daily. Patients who experience seizures often have predisposing factors, including history of head trauma, seizures, or CNS tumors, or they may be taking a drug that lowers seizure threshold.

!!ALERT Patient with major depressive disorder may experience a worsening of depression and suicidal thoughts even while taking an antidepressant. Carefully monitor patient for worsening depression or suicidal thoughts, especially at the beginning of therapy and during dosage changes.

- In switching patients from regular- or sustained-release tablets to extended-release tablets, give the same total daily dose (when possible) as the once-daily dosage provided.
- Closely monitor patient with history of bipolar disorder. Antidepressants can cause manic episodes during the depressed phase of bipolar disorder. This may be less likely to occur with bupropion than with other antidepressants.

!!ALERT Don't confuse bupropion with buspirone or Wellbutrin with Wellcovorin.

Patient teaching

- Advise patient to take drug as scheduled and to take each day's dose in three divided doses (immediate-release) or two divided doses (sustained-release) to minimize risk of seizures.
- Advise patient to consult prescriber before taking other prescription or OTC drugs.
- Tell patient to avoid alcohol while taking drug because it may contribute to development of seizures.
- Advise patient to avoid hazardous activities that require alertness and good psychomotor coordination until effects of drug are known.

!!ALERT Advise patient that this drug has the same ingredients as Zyban, used to aid smoking cessation, and that the two shouldn't be used together.

- Tell patient that it may take 4 weeks to reach full therapeutic effect of drug.
- Tell patient to protect drug from light and moisture.

bupropion hydrochloride
Zyban

Pregnancy risk category B

Indications & dosages

➲ Aid to smoking cessation treatment
Adults: 150 mg P.O. daily for 3 days; increased to maximum of 300 mg P.O. daily in two divided doses at least 8 hours apart.

Contraindications & cautions

- Contraindicated in patients allergic to drug or its components, in those with seizure disorders or a current or prior diagnosis of bulimia or anorexia nervosa, and in those being treated with other drugs containing bupropion (such as Wellbutrin and Wellbutrin SR).
- Contraindicated within 2 weeks of MAO inhibitor.
- Use cautiously in patients with recent MI or unstable heart disease.
- Use cautiously in patients with history of seizures, head trauma, or other predisposition to seizures, and in those being treated with drugs that lower seizure threshold.

Adverse reactions

CNS: agitation, asthenia, depression, *dizziness*, fever, headache, *insomnia*, irritability, somnolence, tremor, thinking or dream abnormalities, disturbed concentration, anxiety, nervousness.
CV: ***complete AV block***, hypertension, hypotension, *tachycardia*, palpitations, hot flashes.
EENT: amblyopia, epistaxis, *pharyngitis*, sinusitis, tinnitus, *rhinitis, blurred vision*.
GI: *anorexia*, dyspepsia, increased appetite, abdominal pain, *nausea, constipation*, diarrhea, flatulence, *vomiting, dry mouth*, taste perversion, mouth ulcer.
GU: urinary frequency.
Musculoskeletal: arthralgia, leg cramps and twitching, myalgia, neck pain.
Respiratory: bronchitis, increased cough, dyspnea.
Skin: dry skin, pruritus, rash, urticaria, *excessive sweating*.
Other: allergic reactions, injury.

Interactions

Drug-drug. *Antidepressants, antipsychotics, systemic corticosteroids, theophylline:* May lower seizure threshold. Use together cautiously.
Carbamazepine, phenobarbital, phenytoin: May enhance metabolism of bupropion and decrease its effect. Monitor patient closely.
Cimetidine: May inhibit metabolism of bupropion and lead to increased levels. Monitor patient closely.
Levodopa: May increase risk of adverse reactions. If used together, give small first doses of bupropion and increase dosage gradually.
MAO inhibitors (phenelzine): May increase toxicity. Avoid using within 2 weeks of MAO inhibitor.
Nicotine-replacement agents: May cause hypertension. Monitor blood pressure.
Other drugs containing bupropion (Wellbutrin, Wellbutrin SR): Contains same active ingredient as bupropion. Avoid using together.
Ritonavir: May increase bupropion level. Monitor patient closely for adverse reactions.
Drug-lifestyle. *Alcohol use:* May increase risk of seizures. Discourage use together.
Sun exposure: Photosensitivity reactions may occur. Advise patient to avoid excessive sunlight exposure.

Nursing considerations

!!ALERT Excessive use of alcohol, abrupt withdrawal from alcohol or other sedatives, and addiction to cocaine, opiates, or stimulants during therapy may increase risk of seizures. Seizure risk is also increased in those using OTC stimulants, in anorectics, and in diabetic patients using oral antidiabetics or insulin.
!!ALERT Different trade names and indications exist for bupropion. Be certain the patient isn't already taking Wellbutrin.
- To reduce seizure risk, don't exceed 300 mg daily. Give 150 mg twice daily so that no single dose exceeds 150 mg.
- Therapy should stop if patient hasn't progressed toward abstinence by week 7.
- Patient can stop taking drug without tapering off.
- Therapy should begin while patient is still smoking; about 1 week is needed to achieve steady-state drug levels.

!!ALERT Don't confuse bupropion with buspirone.

Patient teaching

- Stress importance of combining drug therapy with behavioral interventions, counseling, and support services.
- Advise patient to take doses at least 8 hours apart. If insomnia occurs, tell him not to take dose at bedtime.
- Tell patient not to chew, divide, or crush tablets.
- Tell patient that it may take 1 week for effects of drug to appear, and that he should set a target date for smoking cessation during the second week of therapy.
- Tell patient that treatment usually lasts 7 to 12 weeks.
- Inform patient that tablets may have a characteristic odor.
- Advise patient to avoid alcohol while taking drug.
- Tell patient to avoid hazardous activities that require mental alertness until drug's CNS effects are known.
- Warn patient not to use drug with nicotine patches unless directed by prescriber, because this could increase blood pressure.

- Inform patient that risk of seizures increases if he has a seizure or eating disorder, exceeds the recommended dosage, or takes other drugs that either contain bupropion or lower seizure threshold.
- Advise patient to read accompanying patient information before starting drug.
- Advise patient to notify prescriber about planned, suspected, or known pregnancy.

buspirone hydrochloride

BuSpar

Pregnancy risk category B

Indications & dosages

➲ **Anxiety disorders, short-term relief of anxiety**

Adults: Initially, 10 to 15 mg daily in two or three divided doses. Increase dosage by 5-mg increments at 2- to 4-day intervals. Usual maintenance dosage is 15 to 30 mg daily in divided doses. Don't exceed 60 mg daily.

In patients also taking CYP3A4 inhibitors, initial dose is 2.5 mg P.O. once or twice daily. Increase dose based on clinical assessment.

Contraindications & cautions

- Contraindicated in patients hypersensitive to drug; also contraindicated within 14 days of MAO inhibitor therapy.
- Drug isn't recommended for patients with severe hepatic or renal impairment.

Adverse reactions

CNS: *dizziness, drowsiness,* nervousness, insomnia, *headache,* light-headedness, fatigue, numbness.
CV: tachycardia, nonspecific chest pain.
EENT: blurred vision.
GI: dry mouth, nausea, diarrhea, abdominal distress.

Interactions

Drug-drug. *CNS depressants:* May increase CNS depression. Use together cautiously.
Drugs metabolized by CYP3A4 (erythromycin, itraconazole, nefazodone): May increase buspirone level. Monitor patient; decrease buspirone dosage.
MAO inhibitors: May elevate blood pressure. Avoid using together.
Drug-food. *Grapefruit juice:* May increase buspirone level, increasing adverse effects. Give with liquid other than grapefruit juice.
Drug-lifestyle. *Alcohol use:* May increase CNS depression. Discourage use together.

Nursing considerations

- Monitor patient closely for adverse CNS reactions. Buspirone is less sedating than other anxiolytics, but CNS effects may be unpredictable.

!!ALERT Before starting buspirone therapy in a patient already receiving a benzodiazepine, don't stop the benzodiazepine abruptly because a withdrawal reaction may occur.

- Drug has shown no potential for abuse and hasn't been classified as a controlled substance.

!!ALERT Don't confuse buspirone with bupropion.

Patient teaching

- Warn patient to avoid hazardous activities that require alertness and good coordination until effects of drug are known.
- Remind patient that drug effects may not be noticeable for several weeks.
- Warn patient not to abruptly stop a benzodiazepine because of risk of withdrawal symptoms.
- Tell patient to avoid alcohol use during drug therapy.

busulfan

Busulfex, Myleran

Pregnancy risk category D

Indications & dosages

➲ **Chronic myelocytic (granulocytic) leukemia**

Adults: 4 to 8 mg P.O. daily until WBC count falls to 15,000/mm^3; stop drug until WBC count rises to 50,000/mm^3, and then resume dosage as before. Or, 4 to 8 mg P.O. daily until WBC count falls to 10,000 to 20,000/mm^3; then reduce daily dose, p.r.n., to maintain WBC count at this level. Dosage is highly variable; range is 2 mg weekly to 4 mg daily.
Children: 0.06 to 0.12 mg/kg daily or 1.8 to 4.6 mg/m^2 daily P.O.; adjust dosage to

maintain WBC count at 20,000/mm³ but never below 10,000/mm³.

➲ **Allogenic hematopoietic stem cell transplantation in patients with chronic myelogenous leukemia**

Adults: 0.8 mg/kg I.V. q 6 hours for 4 days (a total of 16 doses). Give cyclophosphamide 60 mg/kg I.V. over 1 hour daily for 2 days beginning 6 hours after the 16th dose of busulfan injection.

Children weighing more than 12 kg: 0.8 mg/kg I.V. with cyclophosphamide.

Children weighing 12 kg or less: 1.1 mg/kg I.V. with cyclophosphamide.

Contraindications & cautions

- Contraindicated in patients with chronic myelogenous leukemia resistant to drug and in those with chronic lymphocytic or acute leukemia or in the blastic crisis of chronic myelogenous leukemia.
- Use cautiously in patients recently given other myelosuppressives or radiation treatment and in those with depressed neutrophil or platelet count.
- Use cautiously in patients with history of head trauma or seizures and in those receiving other drugs that lower the seizure threshold because high-dose therapy has been linked to seizures.

Adverse reactions

CNS: *fever, headache, asthenia, pain, insomnia, anxiety, dizziness, depression,* delirium, agitation, ***encephalopathy***, *confusion,* hallucination, lethargy, somnolence, ***seizures***.

CV: *edema, chest pain, tachycardia, hypertension, hypotension,* ***thrombosis***, *vasodilation, heart rhythm abnormalities,* cardiomegaly, ECG abnormalities, ***heart failure***, ***pericardial effusion***.

EENT: *rhinitis, epistaxis, pharyngitis,* sinusitis, ear disorder, cataracts.

GI: *cheilosis (P.O.), nausea, stomatitis, mucositis, vomiting, anorexia, diarrhea, abdominal pain and enlargement, dyspepsia, constipation, dry mouth, rectal disorder,* pancreatitis.

GU: dysuria, *oliguria,* hematuria, hemorrhagic cystitis.

Hematologic: **GRANULOCYTOPENIA, THROMBOCYTOPENIA, LEUKOPENIA,** *anemia.*

Hepatic: *jaundice,* ***hepatic necrosis***, hepatomegaly.

Metabolic: *hypomagnesemia, hyperglycemia, hypokalemia, hypocalcemia, hypervolemia, weight gain, hypophosphatemia,* hyponatremia.

Musculoskeletal: *back pain, myalgia, arthralgia.*

Respiratory: *lung disorder, cough, dyspnea,* ***irreversible pulmonary fibrosis***, ***alveolar hemorrhage***, asthma, atelectasis, pleural effusion hypoxia, hemoptysis.

Skin: *inflammation at injection site, rash, pruritus, alopecia,* exfoliative dermatitis, erythema nodosum, acne, skin discoloration, *hyperpigmentation,* anhidrosis.

Other: Addison-like wasting syndrome, gynecomastia (P.O.), *chills, allergic reaction,* ***graft versus host disease***, ***infection***, *hiccup.*

Interactions

Drug-drug. *Acetaminophen, itraconazole:* May decrease busulfan clearance. Use together cautiously.

Anticoagulants, aspirin: May increase risk of bleeding. Avoid using together.

Cyclophosphamide: May increase risk of cardiac tamponade in patients with thalassemia. Monitor patient.

Myelosuppressives: May increase myelosuppression. Monitor patient.

Other cytotoxic agents causing pulmonary injury: May cause additive pulmonary toxicity. Avoid using together.

Phenytoin: May decrease busulfan level. Monitor busulfan level.

Thioguanine: May cause hepatotoxicity, esophageal varices, or portal hypertension. Use together cautiously.

Nursing considerations

- Give antiemetic before first dose of busulfan injection and then on a fixed schedule during therapy; give phenytoin to prevent seizures.
- Therapeutic effects are commonly accompanied by toxicity.
- To prevent bleeding, avoid all I.M. injections when platelet count is less than 50,000/mm³.
- Monitor patient response (increased appetite and sense of well-being, decreased total WBC count, reduced size of spleen), which usually begins in 1 to 2 weeks.
- Monitor for jaundice and liver function abnormalities in patients receiving high-dose busulfan.

• Anticipate possible blood transfusion during treatment because of cumulative anemia. Patients may receive injections of RBC colony-stimulating factor to promote RBC production and decrease the need for blood transfusions.

!! ALERT Pulmonary fibrosis may occur as late as 8 months to 10 years after treatment with busulfan. (Average duration of therapy is 4 years.)

Patient teaching

• Advise patient to watch for signs of infection (fever, sore throat, fatigue) and bleeding (easy bruising, nosebleeds, bleeding gums, tarry stools). Tell patient to take temperature daily.

• Instruct patient to report signs and symptoms of toxicity so dosage can be adjusted. Persistent cough and progressive labored breathing with liquid in the lungs, suggestive of pneumonia, may be caused by drug toxicity.

• Instruct patient to avoid OTC products containing aspirin and NSAIDs.

• Inform patient that drug may cause skin darkening.

• Advise woman of childbearing age to avoid becoming pregnant during therapy. Recommend that she consult prescriber before becoming pregnant.

• Advise patient not to breast-feed during therapy because of risk of toxicity to infant.

• Instruct patient to take drug on empty stomach to decrease nausea and vomiting.

• Because of risk of impotence and male sterility, advise man of childbearing potential about sperm banking before therapy begins.

butorphanol tartrate

Stadol, Stadol NS

Pregnancy risk category C
Controlled substance schedule IV

Indications & dosages

➲ **Moderate to severe pain**

Adults: 1 to 4 mg I.M. q 3 to 4 hours, p.r.n., or around the clock. Not to exceed 4 mg per dose. Or, 0.5 to 2 mg I.V. q 3 to 4 hours, p.r.n. or around the clock. Or, 1 mg by nasal spray q 3 to 4 hours (1 spray in one nostril); repeat in 60 to 90 minutes if pain relief is inadequate. For severe pain, 2 mg (1 spray in each nostril) q 3 to 4 hours.

Elderly patients: 1 mg I.M. or 0.5 mg I.V., allow 6 hours to elapse before repeating dose. For nasal use, 1 mg (1 spray in one nostril). May give another 1 mg in 1.5 to 2 hours. Allow 6 hours to elapse before repeating dosing sequence.

For patients with renal or hepatic impairment, increase dosage interval to 6 to 8 hours.

➲ **Labor for patients at full term and in early labor**

Adults: 1 or 2 mg I.V. or I.M.; repeat after 4 hours, p.r.n.

➲ **Preoperative anesthesia or preanesthesia**

Adults: 2 mg I.M. 60 to 90 minutes before surgery.

➲ **Adjunct to balanced anesthesia**

Adults: 2 mg I.V. shortly before induction, or 0.5 to 1 mg I.V. in increments during anesthesia.

Elderly patients: One-half usual dose at twice the interval for I.V. use.

Contraindications & cautions

• Contraindicated in patients hypersensitive to drug or to preservative, benzethonium chloride, and in those with opioid addiction; may cause withdrawal syndrome.

• Use cautiously in patients with head injury, increased intracranial pressure, acute MI, ventricular dysfunction, coronary insufficiency, respiratory disease or depression, and renal or hepatic dysfunction.

• Use cautiously in patients who have recently received repeated doses of opioid analgesic

Adverse reactions

CNS: confusion, nervousness, lethargy, headache, *somnolence, dizziness, insomnia,* asthenia, anxiety, paresthesia, euphoria, hallucinations, ***increased intracranial pressure***.

CV: flushing, palpitations, vasodilation, hypotension.

EENT: blurred vision, *nasal congestion,* tinnitus.

GI: *nausea, vomiting,* constipation, anorexia, *unpleasant taste.*

Respiratory: ***respiratory depression***.

Skin: rash, hives, clamminess, excessive diaphoresis.
Other: sensation of heat.

Interactions

Drug-drug. *CNS depressants:* May cause additive effects. Use together cautiously.
Drug-lifestyle. *Alcohol use:* May cause additive effects. Discourage use together.

Nursing considerations

- Reassess patient's level of pain 15 and 30 minutes after administration.
- Don't give by S.C. route.
- Respiratory depression apparently doesn't increase with larger dosage.
- Psychological and physical addiction may occur.
- Periodically monitor postoperative vital signs and bladder function. Because drug decreases both rate and depth of respirations, monitoring arterial oxygen saturation may help assess respiratory depression.
- Watch for nasal congestion with nasal spray use.

!!ALERT Don't confuse Stadol with sotalol.

Patient teaching

- Caution ambulatory patient about getting out of bed or walking. Warn outpatient to avoid driving and other hazardous activities that require mental alertness until it is clear how the drug affects the CNS.
- Teach patient how to give and store nasal spray, if applicable.
- Instruct patient to avoid alcohol during therapy.

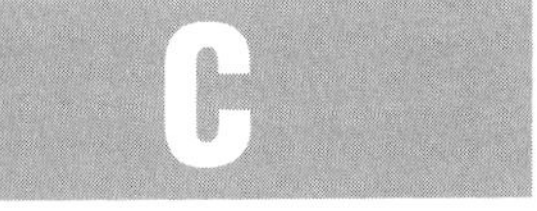

calcitonin (salmon)
Miacalcin, Salmonine

Pregnancy risk category C

Indications & dosages

➲ Paget's disease of bone (osteitis deformans)
Adults: Initially, 100 IU of calcitonin (salmon) daily I.M. or S.C. Maintenance dosage is 50 to 100 IU daily I.M. or S.C., every other day, or three times weekly.

➲ Hypercalcemia
Adults: 4 IU/kg of calcitonin (salmon) q 12 hours I.M. or S.C. If response is inadequate after 1 or 2 days, increase dosage to 8 IU/kg I.M. q 12 hours. If response remains unsatisfactory after 2 additional days, increase dosage to maximum of 8 IU/kg I.M. q 6 hours.

➲ Postmenopausal osteoporosis
Adults: 100 IU of calcitonin (salmon) daily I.M. or S.C. Or, 200 IU (one activation) of calcitonin (salmon) daily intranasally, alternating nostrils daily. Patient should receive adequate vitamin D and calcium supplements (1.5 g calcium carbonate and 400 units of vitamin D) daily.

Contraindications & cautions

- Contraindicated in patients hypersensitive to salmon calcitonin.

Adverse reactions

CNS: headache, weakness, dizziness, paresthesia.
CV: chest pressure, *facial flushing.*
EENT: eye pain, *nasal congestion, rhinitis.*
GI: *transient nausea,* unusual taste, diarrhea, anorexia, *vomiting,* epigastric discomfort, abdominal pain.
GU: *increased urinary frequency,* nocturia.
Respiratory: shortness of breath.
Skin: rash, pruritus of ear lobes, *inflammation at injection site.*
Other: hypersensitivity reactions, ***anaphylaxis***, edema of feet, chills, tender palms and soles.

Interactions

None significant.

Nursing considerations

- Skin test is usually done before starting therapy.

!!ALERT Systemic allergic reactions are possible because hormone is protein. Keep epinephrine nearby.

- Give at bedtime, when possible, to minimize nausea and vomiting.
- I.M. route is preferred if volume of dose to be given exceeds 2 ml.
- Use freshly reconstituted solution within 2 hours.

!!ALERT Observe patient for signs of hypocalcemic tetany during therapy (muscle twitching, tetanic spasms, and seizures when hypocalcemia is severe).

- Monitor calcium level closely. Watch for symptoms of hypercalcemia relapse: bone pain, renal calculi, polyuria, anorexia, nausea, vomiting, thirst, constipation, lethargy, bradycardia, muscle hypotonicity, pathologic fracture, psychosis, and coma.
- Periodic examinations of urine sediment are recommended.
- Monitor periodic alkaline phosphatase and 24-hour urine hydroxyproline levels to evaluate drug effect.
- In Paget's disease, maximum reductions of alkaline phosphatase and urinary hydroxyproline excretion may take 6 to 24 months of continuous treatment.
- In patients with good first clinical response to calcitonin who have a relapse, expect to evaluate antibody response to the hormone protein.
- If symptoms have been relieved after 6 months, treatment may be stopped until symptoms or radiologic signs recur.
- Refrigerate calcitonin (salmon) at 36° to 46° F (2° to 8° C).

!!ALERT Don't confuse calcitonin with calcifediol or calcitriol.

Patient teaching

- When drug is given for postmenopausal osteoporosis, remind patient to take adequate calcium and vitamin D supplements.
- Show home care patient and family member how to give drug. Tell them to do so at bedtime if only one dose is needed daily. If nasal spray is prescribed, tell patient to alternate nostrils daily.
- Advise patient to notify prescriber if significant nasal irritation or evidence of an allergic response occurs.
- Inform patient that facial flushing and warmth occur in 20% to 30% of patients within minutes of injection and usually last about 1 hour. Reassure patient that this is a transient effect.
- Tell patient that nausea and vomiting may occur at the onset of therapy.
- Tell patient to inform prescriber promptly if signs and symptoms of hypercalcemia occur. Inform patient that, if calcitonin loses its hypocalcemic activity, other drugs or increased dosages won't help.

calcitriol (1,25-dihydroxycholecalciferol)

Calcijex, Rocaltrol

Pregnancy risk category C

Indications & dosages

➲ **Hypocalcemia in patients undergoing long-term dialysis**

Adults: Initially, 0.25 mcg P.O. daily; may increase by 0.25 mcg daily at 4- to 8-week intervals. Maintenance dosage is 0.5 to 3 mcg daily. Or, 0.5 mcg I.V. three times weekly about every other day. If response to first dosage is inadequate, may increase by 0.25 to 0.5 mcg at 2- to 4-week intervals. Maintenance dosage is 0.5 to 3 mcg I.V. three times weekly.

➲ **Hypoparathyroidism, pseudohypoparathyroidism**

Adults and children age 6 and older: Initially, 0.25 mcg P.O. daily in the morning. Dosage may be increased at 2- to 4-week intervals. Maintenance dosage is 0.25 to 2 mcg P.O. daily.

➲ **Hypoparathyroidism**

Children ages 1 to 5: 0.25 to 0.75 mcg P.O. daily.

➲ **To manage secondary hyperparathyroidism and resulting metabolic bone disease in predialysis patients (with creatinine clearance of 15 to 55 ml/minute)**

Adults and children age 3 and older: Initially, 0.25 mcg P.O. daily. Dosage may be increased to 0.5 mcg/day if needed.

Children younger than age 3: Initially, 0.01 to 0.015 mcg/kg P.O. daily.

Contraindications & cautions

- Contraindicated in patients with hypercalcemia or vitamin D toxicity. Withhold all preparations containing vitamin D.
- Use cautiously in patients receiving cardiac glycosides and in those with sarcoidosis or hyperparathyroidism.

Adverse reactions

CNS: headache, somnolence, weakness, irritability.

CV: hypertension, ***arrhythmias***.

EENT: conjunctivitis, photophobia, rhinorrhea.

GI: nausea, vomiting, constipation, polydipsia, ***pancreatitis***, metallic taste, dry mouth, anorexia.
GU: polyuria, nocturia.
Metabolic: weight loss.
Musculoskeletal: bone and muscle pain.
Skin: pruritus.
Other: hyperthermia, nephrocalcinosis, decreased libido.

Interactions

Drug-drug. *Cardiac glycosides:* May increase risk of arrhythmias. Use together cautiously.
Cholestyramine, colestipol, excessive use of mineral oil: May decrease absorption of oral vitamin D analogues. Avoid using together.
Corticosteroids: May counteract vitamin D analogue effects. Avoid using together.
Magnesium-containing antacids: May cause hypermagnesemia, especially in patients with chronic renal failure. Avoid using together.
Phenytoin, phenobarbital: May inhibit calcitriol synthesis. Dose may need to be increased.
Thiazides: May cause hypercalcemia. Use together cautiously.

Nursing considerations

- Monitor calcium level; multiplied by phosphate level, it shouldn't exceed 70. During adjustment, determine calcium level twice weekly. Stop and notify prescriber if hypercalcemia occurs, but resume after calcium level returns to normal. Patient should receive adequate daily intake of calcium. Observe for hypocalcemia, bone pain, and weakness before and during therapy.
- Vitamin D intoxication causes various adverse effects, including headache, somnolence, weakness, irritability, hypertension, arrhythmias, conjunctivitis, photophobia, rhinorrhea, nausea, vomiting, constipation, polydipsia, pancreatitis, metallic taste, dry mouth, anorexia, nephrocalcinosis, polyuria, nocturia, weight loss, bone and muscle pain, pruritus, hyperthermia, and decreased libido.
- Protect drug from heat and light.

!!ALERT Don't confuse calcitriol with calcifediol or calcitonin.

Patient teaching

- Tell patient to immediately report early symptoms of vitamin D intoxication: weakness, nausea, vomiting, dry mouth, constipation, muscle or bone pain, or metallic taste.
- Instruct patient to adhere to diet and calcium supplementation and to avoid unapproved OTC drugs and magnesium-containing antacids.

!!ALERT Tell patient that drug mustn't be taken by anyone for whom it wasn't prescribed. It's the most potent form of vitamin D available.

---

calcium acetate
PhosLo

calcium carbonate
Apo-Cal† ◇, Cal-Carb Forte, Cal Carb-HD ◇, Calci-Chew ◇, Calciday-667 ◇, Calci-Mix ◇, Calcite 500† ◇, Calcium 600 ◇, Calglycine ◇, Cal-Plus ◇, Calsan† ◇, Caltrate 600 ◇, Chooz ◇, Dicarbosil ◇, Gencalc 600 ◇, Mallamint ◇, Nephro-Calci ◇, Nu-Cal† ◇, Os-Cal† ◇, Os-Cal 500 ◇, Os-Cal Chewable† ◇, Oysco ◇, Oysco 500 Chewable ◇, Oyst-Cal 500 ◇, Oystercal 500 ◇, Oyster Shell Calcium-500 ◇, Rolaids Calcium Rich ◇, Super Calcium 1200 ◇, Titralac ◇, Tums ◇, Tums E-X ◇

calcium chloride ◇
Calciject†

calcium citrate ◇
Citracal ◇, Citracal Liquitab† ◇

calcium glubionate
Calciquid, Calcium-Sandoz†, Neo-Calglucon

calcium gluconate

calcium lactate ◇

calcium phosphate, dibasic ◇

calcium phosphate, tribasic
Posture ◇

Pregnancy risk category C

Indications & dosages

➲ **Hypocalcemic emergency**
Adults: 7 mEq to 14 mEq calcium I.V. May give as a 10% calcium gluconate solution, 2% to 10% calcium chloride solution.
Children: 1 mEq to 7 mEq calcium I.V.
Infants: Up to 1 mEq calcium I.V.

➲ **Hypocalcemic tetany**
Adults: 4.5 mEq to 16 mEq calcium I.V. Repeat until tetany is controlled.
Children: 0.5 to 0.7 mEq/kg calcium I.V. t.i.d. to q.i.d. until tetany is controlled.
Neonates: 2.4 mEq/kg calcium I.V. daily in divided doses.

➲ **Adjunctive treatment of magnesium intoxication**
Adults: Initially, 7 mEq I.V. Base subsequent doses on patient's response.

➲ **During exchange transfusions**
Adults: 1.35 mEq I.V. with each 100 ml citrated blood.
Neonates: 0.45 mEq I.V. after each 100 ml citrated blood.

➲ **Hyperphosphatemia**
Adults: 1,334 to 2,000 mg P.O. calcium acetate or 2 to 5.2 g calcium ion t.i.d. with meals. Most dialysis patients need 3 to 4 tablets with each meal.

➲ **Dietary supplement**
Adults: 500 mg to 2 g P.O. daily.

➲ **Hyperkalemia with secondary cardiac toxicity**
Adults: 2.25 mEq to 14 mEq I.V. Repeat dose after 1 to 2 minutes if needed.

Contraindications & cautions

- Contraindicated in cancer patients with bone metastases and in patients with ventricular fibrillation, hypercalcemia, hypophosphatemia, or renal calculi.

Adverse reactions

CNS: tingling sensations, sense of oppression or heat waves with I.V. use, syncope with rapid I.V. injection.
CV: mild drop in blood pressure, vasodilation, ***bradycardia, arrhythmias, cardiac arrest with rapid I.V. injection***.
GI: irritation, *constipation*, chalky taste, hemorrhage, nausea, vomiting, thirst, abdominal pain.
GU: polyuria, renal calculi.
Metabolic: hypercalcemia.
Skin: local reactions, including burning, necrosis, tissue sloughing, cellulitis, soft-tissue calcification with I.M. use, pain, irritation at S.C. injection site.

Interactions

Drug-drug. *Atenolol, tetracyclines:* May decrease bioavailability of these drugs and calcium when oral preparations are taken together. Separate dosing times.
Calcium channel blockers: May decrease calcium effectiveness. Avoid using together.
Cardiac glycosides: May increase digoxin toxicity. Give calcium cautiously, if at all, to digitalized patients.
Ciprofloxacin, gatifloxacin, levofloxacin, lomefloxacin, moxifloxacin, norfloxacin, ofloxacin: May decrease effects of quinolone. Give calcium carbonate at least 6 hours before or 2 hours after the quinolone.
Fosphenytoin, phenytoin: Use together may decrease absorption of both drugs. Avoid using together, or monitor levels carefully.
Sodium polystyrene sulfonate: May cause metabolic acidosis in patients with renal disease. Avoid using together.
Thiazide diuretics: May cause hypercalcemia. Avoid using together.
Drug-food. *Foods containing oxalic acid (rhubarb, spinach), phytic acid (bran, whole-grain cereals), phosphorus (dairy products, milk):* May interfere with calcium absorption. Discourage use together.

Nursing considerations

- Use all calcium products with extreme caution in digitalized patients and patients with sarcoidosis and renal or cardiac disease. Use calcium chloride cautiously in patients with cor pulmonale, respiratory acidosis, or respiratory failure.
- Give I.M. injection in gluteal region in adults and in lateral thigh in infants. Use I.M. route only in emergencies when no I.V. route is available because of irritation of tissue by calcium salts.

!!ALERT Make sure prescriber specifies form of calcium to be given; crash carts may contain both calcium gluconate and calcium chloride.

• Monitor calcium levels frequently. Hypercalcemia may result after large doses in chronic renal failure. Report abnormalities.
• Signs and symptoms of severe hypercalcemia may include stupor, confusion, delirium, and coma. Signs and symptoms of mild hypercalcemia may include anorexia, nausea, and vomiting.
• To avoid constipation and bloating and to improve absorption, give calcium carbonate in divided doses.

Patient teaching

• Tell patient to take oral calcium 1 to 1½ hours after meals if GI upset occurs.
• Tell patient to take oral calcium with a full glass of water.
• Warn patient to avoid oxalic acid (in rhubarb and spinach), phytic acid (in bran and whole-grain cereals), and phosphorus (in dairy products) in the meal preceding calcium consumption; these substances may interfere with calcium absorption.
• Inform patient that some products may contain phenylalanine.

calcium carbonate

Alka-Mints ◇, Amitone ◇, Calci-Chew, Caltrate, Chooz ◇, Dicarbosil ◇, Maalox Antacid Caplets ◇, Oscal, Rolaids Calcium Rich ◇, Tums ◇, Tums E-X ◇, Tums Ultra ◇, Viactiv ◇

Pregnancy risk category C

Indications & dosages

➲ Acid indigestion, calcium supplement
Adults: 350 mg to 1.5 g P.O. or two pieces of chewing gum 1 hour after meals and h.s., p.r.n.

Contraindications & cautions

• Contraindicated in patients with ventricular fibrillation or hypercalcemia.
• Use cautiously, if at all, if patient takes a cardiac glycoside or has sarcoidosis or renal or cardiac disease.

Adverse reactions

CNS: headache, irritability, weakness.
GI: rebound hyperacidity, *nausea*, constipation, flatulence.

Interactions

Drug-drug. *Antibiotics (tetracyclines), hydantoins, iron salts, isoniazid, salicylates:* May decrease effect of these drugs because may impair absorption. Separate doses by 2 hours.
Ciprofloxacin, gatifloxacin, levofloxacin, lomefloxacin, moxifloxacin, norfloxacin, ofloxacin: May decrease quinolone effects. Give antacid at least 6 hours before or 2 hours after quinolone.
Enteric-coated drugs: May be released prematurely in stomach. Separate doses by at least 1 hour.
Drug-food. *Milk, other foods high in vitamin D:* May cause milk-alkali syndrome (headache, confusion, distaste for food, nausea, vomiting, hypercalcemia, hypercalciuria). Discourage use together.

Nursing considerations

• Record amount and consistency of stools. Manage constipation with laxatives or stool softeners.
• Monitor calcium level, especially in patients with mild renal impairment.
• Watch for evidence of hypercalcemia (nausea, vomiting, headache, confusion, and anorexia).

Patient teaching

• Advise patient not to take calcium carbonate indiscriminately or to switch antacids without prescriber's advice.
• Tell patient who takes chewable tablets to chew thoroughly before swallowing and to follow with a glass of water.
• Tell patient who uses suspension form to shake well and take with a small amount of water to facilitate passage.
• Urge patient to notify prescriber about signs and symptoms of GI bleeding, such as tarry stools or coffee-ground vomitus.

calfactant

Infasurf

Pregnancy risk category NR

Indications & dosages

➲ To prevent respiratory distress syndrome (RDS) in premature infants under 29 weeks' gestational age at high risk for RDS; to treat infants younger than 72

hours of age, who develop RDS (confirmed by clinical and radiologic findings) and need endotracheal intubation
Newborns: 3 ml/kg of body weight at birth intratracheally, given in two aliquots of 1.5 ml/kg each, q 12 hours for total of three doses.

Contraindications & cautions

None known.

Adverse reactions

CV: BRADYCARDIA.
Respiratory: AIRWAY OBSTRUCTION, APNEA, *hypoventilation, cyanosis.*
Other: ***reflux of drug into endotracheal tube***, dislodgment of endotracheal tube.

Interactions

None significant.

Nursing considerations

- Give drug under supervision of medical staff experienced in the acute care of newborn infants with respiratory failure who need intubation.
- Store drug at 36° to 46° F (2° to 8° C). It isn't necessary to warm drug before use.
- Unopened, unused vials that have warmed to room temperature can be re-refrigerated within 24 hours for future use. Avoid repeated warming to room temperature.
- Suspension settles during storage. Gentle swirling or agitation of the vial is commonly needed for redispersion. Don't shake vial. Visible flecks in the suspension and foaming at the surface are normal.

!!ALERT Drug intended only for intratracheal use; to prevent RDS, give to infant as soon as possible after birth, preferably within 30 minutes.

- Withdraw dose into a syringe from single-use vial using a 20G or larger needle; avoid excessive foaming.
- Give through a side-port adapter into the endotracheal tube. Make sure two medical staff are present while giving dose. Give dose in two aliquots of 1.5 ml/kg each. Place infant on one side after first aliquot and other side after second aliquot. Give while ventilation is continued over 20 to 30 breaths for each aliquot, with small bursts timed only during the inspiratory cycles. Evaluate respiratory status and reposition infant between each aliquot.
- Monitor patient for reflux of drug into endotracheal tube, cyanosis, bradycardia, or airway obstruction during the procedure. If these occur, stop drug and take appropriate measures to stabilize infant. After infant is stable, resume drug with appropriate monitoring.
- After giving drug, carefully monitor infant so that oxygen therapy and ventilatory support can be modified in response to improvements in oxygenation and lung compliance.
- Enter each single-use vial only once; discard unused material.

Patient teaching

- Explain to parents the function of drug in preventing and treating RDS.
- Notify parents that, although infant may improve rapidly after treatment, he may continue to need intubation and mechanical ventilation.
- Notify parents of possible adverse effects of drug, including bradycardia, reflux into endotracheal tube, airway obstruction, cyanosis, dislodgment of endotracheal tube, and hypoventilation.
- Reassure parents that infant will be carefully monitored.

candesartan cilexetil

Atacand

Pregnancy risk category C; D in 2nd and 3rd trimesters

Indications & dosages

➲ Hypertension (used alone or with other antihypertensives)
Adults: Initially, 16 mg P.O. once daily when used alone; usual range is 8 to 32 mg P.O. daily as a single dose or divided b.i.d.

➲ Heart failure
Adults: Initially, 4 mg P.O. once daily. Double the dose about every 2 weeks as tolerated, to a target dose of 32 mg once daily.

If patient takes a diuretic, consider a lower starting dose.

Contraindications & cautions

- Contraindicated in patients hypersensitive to drug or its components.
- Use cautiously in patients whose renal function depends on the renin-angiotensin-

aldosterone system (such as patients with heart failure) because of risk of oliguria and progressive azotemia with acute renal failure or death.

- Avoid use in pregnant patients, especially in the second and third trimesters.
- Use cautiously in patients who are volume- or salt-depleted because they could develop symptoms of hypotension. Start therapy with a lower dosage range and monitor blood pressure carefully.

Adverse reactions

CNS: dizziness, fatigue, headache.
CV: chest pain, peripheral edema.
EENT: pharyngitis, rhinitis, sinusitis.
GI: abdominal pain, diarrhea, nausea, vomiting.
GU: albuminuria.
Musculoskeletal: arthralgia, back pain.
Respiratory: coughing, bronchitis, upper respiratory tract infection.

Interactions

Drug-drug. *Potassium-sparing diuretics, potassium supplements:* May cause hyperkalemia. Monitor patient closely.
Drug-herb. *Ma huang:* May decrease antihypertensive effects. Discourage use together.
Drug-food. *Salt substitutes containing potassium:* May cause hyperkalemia. Monitor patient closely.

Nursing considerations

!!ALERT Drugs such as candesartan that act directly on the renin-angiotensin system can cause fetal and neonatal illness and death when given to pregnant women. These problems haven't been detected when exposure has been limited to first trimester. If pregnancy is suspected, notify prescriber because drug should be stopped.

- If hypotension occurs after a dose of candesartan, place patient in the supine position and, if needed, give an I.V. infusion of normal saline solution.
- Most of drug's antihypertensive effect is present within 2 weeks. Maximal antihypertensive effect is obtained within 4 to 6 weeks. Diuretic may be added if blood pressure isn't controlled by drug alone.
- Carefully monitor therapeutic response and the occurrence of adverse reactions in elderly patients and in those with renal disease.

Patient teaching

- Inform woman of childbearing age of the consequences of second and third trimester exposure to drug. Prescriber should be notified immediately if pregnancy is suspected.
- Advise breast-feeding woman of the risk of adverse effects on the infant and the need to stop either breast-feeding or drug.
- Instruct patient to store drug at room temperature and to keep container tightly sealed.
- Inform patient to report adverse reactions without delay.
- Tell patient that drug may be taken without regard to meals.

capecitabine
Xeloda

Pregnancy risk category D

Indications & dosages

➲ **Metastatic breast cancer resistant to both paclitaxel and an anthracycline-containing chemotherapy regimen or resistant to paclitaxel in patients for whom further anthracycline therapy isn't indicated; first-line treatment of metastatic colorectal cancer when fluoropyrimidine therapy alone is preferred; metastatic breast cancer combined with docetaxel, after failure of anthracycline-containing chemotherapy**

Adults: 2,500 mg/m^2 daily P.O., in two divided doses, about 12 hours apart and after a meal, for 2 weeks, followed by a 1-week rest period; repeat q 3 weeks.

Follow National Cancer Institute of Canada (NCIC) Common Toxicity Criteria when adjusting dosage. Toxicity criteria relate to degrees of severity of diarrhea, nausea, vomiting, stomatitis, and hand-and-foot syndrome. Refer to drug package insert for specific toxicity definitions. NCIC grade 1: Maintain dose level. NCIC grade 2: At first appearance, stop treatment until resolved to grade 0 to 1; then restart at 100% of starting dose for next cycle. At second appearance, stop treatment until resolved to grade 0 to 1 and use 75% of starting dose for next cycle. At third appearance, stop treatment until resolved to grade 0 to 1 and use 50% of starting dose for next cycle. At fourth appearance, stop treatment permanently. NCIC grade 3: At first appearance, stop treatment until resolved to grade 0 to 1 and use 75% of starting dose for next cycle. At second appearance, stop treatment until resolved to grade 0 to 1 and use 50% of starting dose for next cycle. At third appearance, stop treatment permanently. NCIC grade 4: At first appearance, stop treatment permanently or until resolved to grade 0 to 1, and use 50% of starting dose for next cycle. Reduce starting dose for patients with creatinine clearance 30 to 50 ml/minute to 75% of the starting dose.

Contraindications & cautions

- Contraindicated in patients hypersensitive to 5-FU and in those with severe renal impairment.
- Use cautiously in elderly patients and patients with history of coronary artery disease, mild to moderate hepatic dysfunction from liver metastases, hyperbilirubinemia, and renal insufficiency.
- Safety and efficacy of drug in patients age 18 or younger haven't been established.

Adverse reactions

CNS: dizziness, *fatigue*, headache, insomnia, *paresthesia*, *pyrexia*.
CV: edema, chest pain.
EENT: eye irritation, vision abnormality.
GI: *diarrhea*, *nausea*, *vomiting*, *stomatitis*, *abdominal pain*, *constipation*, *anorexia*, ***intestinal obstruction***, *dyspepsia*, taste perversion.
Hematologic: NEUTROPENIA, THROMBOCYTOPENIA, *anemia*, *lymphopenia*.
Metabolic: dehydration.
Musculoskeletal: myalgia, limb pain, back pain.
Respiratory: *dyspnea*.
Skin: *hand-and-foot syndrome*, *dermatitis*, nail disorder, alopecia.

Interactions

Drug-drug. *Antacids containing aluminum hydroxide and magnesium hydroxide:* May increase exposure to capecitabine and its metabolites. Monitor patient.
Leucovorin: May increase cytotoxic effects of 5-FU with enhanced toxicity. Monitor patient carefully.
Phenytoin: May increase toxicity or phenytoin effect. Monitor phenytoin level.
Warfarin: May decrease clearance of warfarin. Monitor PT and INR.

Nursing considerations

- Patients older than age 80 may have a greater risk of adverse GI effects.
- Assess patient for severe diarrhea, and notify prescriber if it occurs. Give fluid and electrolyte replacement if patient becomes dehydrated. Drug may need to be immediately interrupted until diarrhea resolves or becomes less intense.
- Monitor patient for hand-and-foot syndrome (numbness, paresthesia, painless or painful swelling, erythema, desquamation, blistering, and severe pain of hands or feet), hyperbilirubinemia, and severe nausea. Drug therapy must be immediately adjusted. Hand-and-foot syndrome is staged from 1 to 4; drug may be stopped if severe or recurrent episodes occur.
- Hyperbilirubinemia may require stopping drug.

!!ALERT Monitor patient carefully for toxicity, which may be managed by symptomatic treatment, dose interruptions, and dosage adjustments.

Patient teaching

- Tell patient how to take drug. Drug is usually taken for 14 days, followed by 7-day rest period (no drug), as a 21-day cycle. Prescriber determines number of treatment cycles.
- Instruct patient to take drug with water within 30 minutes after end of breakfast and dinner.
- If a combination of tablets is prescribed, teach patient importance of correctly identifying the tablets to avoid possible misdosing.
- For missed doses, instruct patient not to take the missed dose and not to double the next one. Instead, he should continue with regular dosing schedule and check with prescriber.
- Instruct patient to inform prescriber if he's taking folic acid.
- Inform patient and caregiver about expected adverse effects of drug, especially

nausea, vomiting, diarrhea, and hand-and-foot syndrome (pain, swelling or redness of hands or feet). Tell him that patient-specific dose adaptations during therapy are expected and needed.

!!ALERT Instruct patient to stop taking drug and contact prescriber immediately if he develops diarrhea (more than four bowel movements daily or diarrhea at night), vomiting (two to five episodes in 24 hours), nausea, appetite loss or decrease in amount of food eaten each day, stomatitis (pain, redness, swelling or sores in mouth), hand-and-foot syndrome, temperature of 100.5° F (38° C) or higher, or other evidence of infection.

- Tell patient that most adverse effects improve within 2 to 3 days after stopping drug. If patient doesn't improve, tell him to contact prescriber.
- Advise woman of childbearing age to avoid becoming pregnant during therapy.
- Advise breast-feeding woman to stop breast-feeding during therapy.

captopril
Capoten, Novo-Captoril†

Pregnancy risk category C; D in 2nd and 3rd trimesters

Indications & dosages

➲ Hypertension

Adults: Initially, 25 mg P.O. b.i.d. or t.i.d. If dosage doesn't control blood pressure satisfactorily in 1 or 2 weeks, increase it to 50 mg b.i.d. or t.i.d. If that dosage doesn't control blood pressure satisfactorily after another 1 or 2 weeks, expect to add a diuretic. If patient needs further blood pressure reduction, dosage may be raised to 150 mg t.i.d. while continuing diuretic. Maximum daily dose is 450 mg.

➲ Diabetic nephropathy

Adults: 25 mg P.O. t.i.d.

➲ Heart failure

Adults: Initially, 25 mg P.O. t.i.d. Patients with normal or low blood pressure who have been vigorously treated with diuretics and who may be hyponatremic or hypovolemic may start with 6.25 or 12.5 mg P.O. t.i.d.; starting dosage may be adjusted over several days. Gradually increase dosage to 50 mg P.O. t.i.d.; once patient reaches this dosage, delay further dosage increases for at least 2 weeks. Maximum dosage is 450 mg daily.

Elderly patients: Initially, 6.25 mg P.O. b.i.d. Increase gradually p.r.n.

➲ Left ventricular dysfunction after acute MI

Adults: Start therapy as early as 3 days after MI with 6.25 mg P.O. for one dose, followed by 12.5 mg P.O. t.i.d. Increase over several days to 25 mg P.O. t.i.d.; then increase to 50 mg P.O. t.i.d. over several weeks.

Contraindications & cautions

- Contraindicated in patients hypersensitive to drug or other ACE inhibitors.
- Use cautiously in patients with impaired renal function or serious autoimmune disease, especially systemic lupus erythematosus, and in those who have been exposed to other drugs that affect WBC counts or immune response.

Adverse reactions

CNS: dizziness, fainting, headache, malaise, fatigue, fever.

CV: tachycardia, hypotension, angina pectoris.

GI: abdominal pain, anorexia, constipation, diarrhea, dry mouth, dysgeusia, nausea, vomiting.

Hematologic: ***leukopenia, agranulocytosis, pancytopenia***, anemia, ***thrombocytopenia***.

Metabolic: hyperkalemia.

Respiratory: dyspnea; *dry, persistent, nonproductive cough.*

Skin: *urticarial rash, maculopapular rash,* pruritus, alopecia.

Other: ***angioedema***.

Interactions

Drug-drug. *Antacids:* May decrease captopril effect. Separate dosage times.

Digoxin: May increase digoxin level by 15% to 30%. Monitor digoxin level and observe patient for signs of digoxin toxicity.

Diuretics, other antihypertensives: May cause excessive hypotension. May need to stop diuretic or reduce captopril dosage.

Insulin, oral antidiabetics: May cause hypoglycemia when captopril therapy is started. Monitor patient closely.

Lithium: May increase lithium level and symptoms of toxicity possible. Monitor patient closely.
NSAIDs: May reduce antihypertensive effect. Monitor blood pressure.
Potassium-sparing diuretics, potassium supplements: May cause hyperkalemia. Avoid using together unless hypokalemia is confirmed.
Drug-herb. *Black catechu:* May cause additional hypotensive effect. Discourage use together.
Capsaicin: May worsen cough. Discourage use together.
Drug-food. *Salt substitutes containing potassium:* May cause hyperkalemia. Monitor patient closely.

Nursing considerations

- Monitor patient's blood pressure and pulse rate frequently.

!!ALERT Elderly patients may be more sensitive to drug's hypotensive effects.

- Assess patient for signs of angioedema.
- Drug causes the most frequent occurrence of cough, compared with other ACE inhibitors.
- In patients with impaired renal function or collagen vascular disease, monitor WBC and differential counts before starting treatment, every 2 weeks for the first 3 months of therapy, and periodically thereafter.

!!ALERT Don't confuse captopril with Capitrol.

Patient teaching

- Instruct patient to take drug 1 hour before meals; food in the GI tract may reduce absorption.
- Inform patient that light-headedness is possible, especially during first few days of therapy. Tell him to rise slowly to minimize this effect and to report occurrence to prescriber. If fainting occurs, he should stop drug and call prescriber immediately.
- Tell patient to use caution in hot weather and during exercise. Lack of fluids, vomiting, diarrhea, and excessive perspiration can lead to light-headedness and syncope.
- Advise patient to report signs and symptoms of infection, such as fever and sore throat.
- Tell women to notify prescriber if pregnancy occurs. Drug will need to be stopped.
- Urge patient to promptly report swelling of the face, lips, or mouth, or difficulty breathing.

carbachol (intraocular)
Carbastat, Miostat

carbachol (topical)
Carboptic, Isopto Carbachol

Pregnancy risk category C

Indications & dosages

➲ To produce pupillary miosis in ocular surgery
Adults: Before or after securing sutures, 0.5 ml (intraocular form) instilled gently into anterior chamber.
➲ Glaucoma
Adults: 1 or 2 drops (topical form) instilled up to t.i.d.

Contraindications & cautions

- Contraindicated in patients hypersensitive to drug and in those with conditions in which cholinergic effects, such as constriction, are undesirable (acute iritis, some forms of secondary glaucoma, pupillary block glaucoma, or acute inflammatory disease of the anterior chamber).
- Use cautiously in patients with acute heart failure, bronchial asthma, peptic ulcer, hyperthyroidism, GI spasm, Parkinson's disease, and urinary tract obstruction.

Adverse reactions

CV: syncope, ***cardiac arrhythmia***, flushing, hypotension.
EENT: spasm of eye accommodation, conjunctival vasodilation, eye and brow pain, *transient stinging and burning*, corneal clouding, bullous keratopathy, iritis, retinal detachment, ciliary and conjunctival injection, salivation.
GI: GI cramps, vomiting, diarrhea, epigastric distress.
GU: tightness in bladder, frequent urge to urinate.
Respiratory: asthma.
Other: diaphoresis.

Interactions

Drug-drug. *Pilocarpine:* May cause additive effects. Use together cautiously.

Nursing considerations

- In case of toxicity, give atropine parenterally.
- Drug is used in open-angle glaucoma, especially when patients are resistant or allergic to pilocarpine hydrochloride or nitrate.

!!ALERT Patients with hazel or brown irises may need stronger solutions or more frequent instillation because eye pigment may absorb drug.

- If tolerance to drug develops, prescriber may switch to another miotic for a short time.

Patient teaching

- Teach patient how to instill drug. Advise him to wash hands before and after instillation and to apply light finger pressure on lacrimal sac for 1 minute after drops are instilled. Warn him not to exceed recommended dosage.
- Warn patient to avoid hazardous activities, such as operating machinery or driving, until temporary blurring subsides. Reassure patient that blurred vision usually diminishes with prolonged use.
- Tell glaucoma patient that long-term use may be needed. Stress compliance. Tell him to remain under medical supervision for periodic tests of intraocular pressure.
- Warn patient to use caution during night driving and while performing other hazardous activities in reduced light.

carbamazepine

Apo-Carbamazepine†, Carbatrol, Epitol, Equetro, Novo-Carbamaz†, Tegretol, Tegretol CR†, Tegretol-XR, Teril

Pregnancy risk category D

Indications & dosages

➲ Generalized tonic-clonic and complex partial seizures, mixed seizure patterns

Adults and children older than age 12: Initially, 200 mg P.O. b.i.d. (conventional or extended-release tablets), or 100 mg P.O. q.i.d. of suspension with meals. May be increased weekly by 200 mg P.O. daily in divided doses at 12-hour intervals for extended-release tablets or 6- to 8-hour intervals for conventional tablets or suspension, adjusted to minimum effective level. Maximum, 1,000 mg daily in children ages 12 to 15, and 1,200 mg daily in patients older than age 15. Usual maintenance dosage is 800 to 1,200 mg daily.

Children ages 6 to 12: Initially, 100 mg P.O. b.i.d. (conventional or extended-release tablets) or 50 mg of suspension P.O. q.i.d. with meals, increased at weekly intervals by up to 100 mg P.O. divided in three to four doses daily (divided b.i.d. for extended-release form). Maximum, 1,000 mg daily. Usual maintenance dosage is 400 to 800 mg daily; or, 20 to 30 mg/kg in divided doses three to four times daily.

Children younger than age 6: 10 to 20 mg/kg in two to three divided doses (conventional tablets) or four divided doses (suspension). Maximum dosage is 35 mg/kg in 24 hours.

➲ Acute manic and mixed episodes associated with bipolar I disorder

Adults: Initially, 200 mg Equetro P.O. b.i.d. Increase by 200 mg daily to achieve therapeutic response. Doses higher than 1,600 mg daily haven't been studied.

➲ Trigeminal neuralgia

Adults: Initially, 100 mg P.O. b.i.d. (conventional or extended-release tablets) or 50 mg of suspension q.i.d. with meals, increased by 100 mg q 12 hours for tablets or 50 mg of suspension q.i.d. until pain is relieved. Maximum, 1,200 mg daily. Maintenance dosage is usually 200 to 400 mg P.O. b.i.d.

➲ Restless legs syndrome♦

Adults: 100 to 300 mg P.O. h.s.

➲ Non-neuritic pain syndromes (painful neuromas, phantom limb pain)♦

Adults: Initially, 100 mg P.O. b.i.d. Maintenance dose is 600 to 1,400 mg daily.

Contraindications & cautions

- Contraindicated in patients hypersensitive to carbamazepine or tricyclic antidepressants and in those with a history of previous bone marrow suppression; also contraindicated in those who have taken an MAO inhibitor within 14 days of therapy.
- Use cautiously in patients with mixed seizure disorders because they may experience an increased risk of seizures. Also, use with caution in patients with hepatic dysfunction.

Adverse reactions

CNS: *dizziness, vertigo, drowsiness*, fatigue, *ataxia*, ***worsening of seizures***, confusion, fever, headache, syncope.
CV: ***heart failure***, hypertension, hypotension, aggravation of coronary artery disease, ***arrhythmias, AV block***.
EENT: conjunctivitis, dry pharynx, blurred vision, diplopia, nystagmus.
GI: dry mouth, *nausea, vomiting*, abdominal pain, diarrhea, anorexia, stomatitis, glossitis.
GU: urinary frequency, urine retention, impotence, albuminuria, glycosuria.
Hematologic: ***aplastic anemia, agranulocytosis***, eosinophilia, leukocytosis, ***thrombocytopenia***.
Hepatic: ***hepatitis***.
Metabolic: SIADH, hyponatremia.
Respiratory: pulmonary hypersensitivity.
Skin: rash, urticaria, ***erythema multiforme, Stevens-Johnson syndrome***, excessive diaphoresis.
Other: chills.

Interactions

Drug-drug. *Atracurium, cisatracurium, doxacurium, mivacurium, pancuronium, rocuronium, tubocurarine, vecuronium:* May decrease the effects of nondepolarizing muscle relaxant, causing it to be less effective. May need to increase the dose of the nondepolarizing muscle relaxant.
Cimetidine, danazol, diltiazem, fluoxetine, fluvoxamine, isoniazid, macrolides, propoxyphene, valproic acid, verapamil: May increase carbamazepine level. Use together cautiously.
Clarithromycin, erythromycin, troleandomycin: May inhibit metabolism of carbamazepine, increasing carbamazepine level and risk of toxicity. Avoid using together.
Doxycycline, felbamate, haloperidol, hormonal contraceptives, phenytoin, theophylline, tiagabine, topiramate, valproate, warfarin: May decrease levels of these drugs. Watch for decreased effect.
Lamotrigine: May decrease lamotrigine level and increase carbamazepine level. Monitor patient for clinical effects and toxicity.
Lithium: May increase CNS toxicity of lithium. Avoid using together.
MAO inhibitors: May increase depressant and anticholinergic effects. Avoid using together.
Phenobarbital, phenytoin, primidone: May decrease carbamazepine level. Watch for decreased effect.
Drug-herb. *Plantains (psyllium seed):* May inhibit GI absorption of drug. Discourage use together.

Nursing considerations

- Watch for worsening of seizures, especially in patients with mixed seizure disorders, including atypical absence seizures.
- Obtain baseline determinations of urinalysis, BUN level, liver function, CBC, platelet and reticulocyte counts, and iron level. Monitor these values periodically thereafter.
- Shake oral suspension well before measuring dose.
- Contents of extended-release capsules may be sprinkled over applesauce if patient has difficulty swallowing capsules. Capsules and tablets shouldn't be crushed or chewed, unless labeled as chewable form.
- When giving by nasogastric tube, mix dose with an equal volume of water, normal saline solution, or D_5W. Flush tube with 100 ml of diluent after giving dose.
- Never stop drug suddenly when treating seizures. Notify prescriber immediately if adverse reactions occur.
- Adverse reactions may be minimized by gradually increasing dosage.
- Therapeutic carbamazepine level is 4 to 12 mcg/ml. Monitor level and effects closely. Ask patient when last dose was taken to better evaluate drug level.
- When managing seizures, take appropriate precautions.

!!ALERT Watch for signs of anorexia or subtle appetite changes, which may indicate excessive drug level.
!!ALERT Don't confuse Tegretol with Toradol.
!!ALERT Don't confuse Carbatrol with carvedilol.

Patient teaching

- Instruct patient to take drug with food to minimize GI distress. Tell patient taking suspension form to shake container well before measuring dose.
- Tell patient not to crush or chew extended-release form and not to take broken or chipped tablets.

- Tell patient that Tegretol-XR tablet coating may appear in stool because it isn't absorbed.
- Advise patient to keep tablets in the original container and to keep the container tightly closed and away from moisture. Some formulations may harden when exposed to excessive moisture, so that less is available in the body, decreasing seizure control.
- Inform patient that when drug is used for trigeminal neuralgia, an attempt to decrease dosage or withdraw drug is usually made every 3 months.
- Advise patient to notify prescriber immediately if fever, sore throat, mouth ulcers, or easy bruising or bleeding occurs.
- Tell patient that drug may cause mild to moderate dizziness and drowsiness when first taken. Advise him to avoid hazardous activities until effects disappear, usually within 3 to 4 days.
- Advise patient that periodic eye examinations are recommended.
- Advise woman of risks to fetus if pregnancy occurs while taking carbamazepine.
- Advise woman that breast-feeding isn't recommended during therapy.

carboplatin
Paraplatin, Paraplatin-AQ†

Pregnancy risk category D

Indications & dosages

➲ Advanced ovarian cancer

Adults: 360 mg/m^2 I.V. on day 1 q 4 weeks or 300 mg/m^2 when used with other chemotherapy drugs; doses shouldn't be repeated until platelet count exceeds 100,000/mm^3 and neutrophil count exceeds 2,000/mm^3. Subsequent doses are based on blood counts. Or, refer to package for formula dosing.

If creatinine clearance is 41 to 59 ml/minute, first dose is 250 mg/m^2. If creatinine clearance is 16 to 40 ml/minute, first dose is 200 mg/m^2. Drug isn't recommended for patients with creatinine clearance of 15 ml/minute or less.

Contraindications & cautions

- Contraindicated in patients with severe bone marrow suppression or bleeding or with history of hypersensitivity to cisplatin, platinum-containing compounds, or mannitol.

Adverse reactions

CNS: *asthenia*, dizziness, confusion, ***CVA***, peripheral neuropathy, central neurotoxicity, paresthesia.
CV: ***heart failure***, ***embolism***.
EENT: ototoxicity, visual disturbances.
GI: constipation, diarrhea, *nausea*, *vomiting*, mucositis, change in taste, stomatitis.
Hematologic: **THROMBOCYTOPENIA**, ***leukopenia***, **NEUTROPENIA**, anemia, **BONE MARROW SUPPRESSION**.
Skin: alopecia.
Other: hypersensitivity reactions, *pain*, ***anaphylaxis***.

Interactions

Drug-drug. *Aspirin, NSAIDs:* May increase risk of bleeding. Avoid using together.
Bone marrow suppressants, including radiation therapy: May increase hematologic toxicity. Monitor CBC with differential closely.
Nephrotoxic drugs, especially aminoglycosides and amphotericin B: May enhance nephrotoxicity of carboplatin. Use together cautiously.

Nursing considerations

- Determine electrolyte, creatinine, and BUN levels; CBC; and creatinine clearance before first infusion and before each course of treatment.
- Monitor CBC and platelet count frequently during therapy and, when indicated, until recovery. WBC and platelet count nadirs usually occur by day 21. Levels usually return to baseline by day 28. Dose shouldn't be repeated unless platelet count exceeds 100,000/mm^3.
- Bone marrow suppression may be more severe in patients with creatinine clearance below 60 ml/minute; dosage adjustments are recommended for such patients.

!!ALERT Carefully check ordered dose against laboratory test results. Only one increase in dosage is recommended. Subsequent doses shouldn't exceed 125% of starting dose.

- Therapeutic effects are commonly accompanied by toxicity.

• Carboplatin has less nephrotoxicity and neurotoxicity than cisplatin, but it causes more severe myelosuppression.
• To prevent bleeding, avoid all I.M. injections when platelet count is below 50,000/ mm^3.
• Monitor vital signs during infusion.
• Give antiemetic to reduce nausea and vomiting.
• Anticipate blood transfusions during treatment because of cumulative anemia. Patient may receive injections of RBC colony-stimulating factor to promote cell production.
• Patients older than age 65 are at greater risk for neurotoxicity.
!!ALERT Don't confuse carboplatin with cisplatin.

Patient teaching

• Advise patient of most common adverse reactions: nausea, vomiting, bone marrow suppression, anemia, and reduction in blood platelets.
• Advise patient to watch for signs of infection (fever, sore throat, fatigue) and bleeding (easy bruising, nosebleeds, bleeding gums, tarry stools). Tell patient to take temperature daily.
• Instruct patient to avoid OTC products containing aspirin and NSAIDs.
• Advise women to stop breast-feeding during therapy because of risk of toxicity to infant.
• Because of risk of impotence, sterility, and menstruation cessation, counsel both men and women of childbearing age before starting therapy. Also recommend that women consult prescriber before becoming pregnant.

carisoprodol
Soma, Vanadom

Pregnancy risk category NR

Indications & dosages

➲ **Adjunctive treatment for acute, painful musculoskeletal conditions**
Adults: 350 mg P.O. t.i.d. and h.s.

Contraindications & cautions

• Contraindicated in patients hypersensitive to related compounds (such as meprobamate or tybamate) and in those with intermittent porphyria.
• Use cautiously in patients with impaired hepatic or renal function.
• Safety and efficacy in children younger than age 12 haven't been established.

Adverse reactions

CNS: fever, *drowsiness*, *dizziness*, vertigo, ataxia, tremor, agitation, irritability, headache, depressive reactions, insomnia, syncope.
CV: *orthostatic hypotension*, tachycardia, facial flushing.
GI: nausea, vomiting, epigastric distress.
Hematologic: eosinophilia.
Respiratory: ***asthmatic episodes***, hiccups.
Skin: rash, ***erythema multiforme***, pruritus.
Other: ***angioedema***, ***anaphylaxis***.

Interactions

Drug-drug. *CNS depressants:* May increase CNS depression. Avoid using together.
Drug-lifestyle. *Alcohol use:* May increase CNS depression. Discourage use together.

Nursing considerations

!!ALERT Watch for idiosyncratic reactions after first to fourth doses (weakness, ataxia, visual and speech difficulties, fever, skin eruptions, and mental changes) and for severe reactions, including bronchospasm, hypotension, and anaphylactic shock. After unusual reactions, withhold dose and notify prescriber immediately.
• Record amount of relief to help prescriber determine whether dosage can be reduced.
• Don't stop drug abruptly, which may cause mild withdrawal effects such as insomnia, headache, nausea, or abdominal cramps.
• Drug may be habit forming.

Patient teaching

• Warn patient to avoid activities that require alertness until CNS effects of drug are known. Drowsiness is transient.
• Advise patient to avoid combining drug with alcohol or other CNS depressants.
• Tell patient to ask prescriber before using OTC cold or hay fever remedies.
• Instruct patient to follow prescriber's orders regarding rest and physical therapy.
• Advise patient to avoid sudden changes in posture if dizziness occurs.

• Tell patient to take drug with food or milk if GI upset occurs.

carmustine (BCNU)
BiCNU, Gliadel Wafer

Pregnancy risk category D

Indications & dosages

➲ Brain tumors, Hodgkin's disease, malignant lymphoma, multiple myeloma
Adults: 150 to 200 mg/m² I.V. by slow infusion q 6 weeks; may be divided into daily injections of 75 to 100 mg/m² on two successive days; repeat dose q 6 weeks if platelet count is greater than 100,000/mm³ and WBC count is greater than 4,000/mm³.

Dosage is reduced by 30% when WBC nadir is 2,000 to 2,999/mm³ and platelet nadir is 25,000 to 74,999/mm³. Dosage is reduced by 50% when WBC nadir is less than 2,000/mm³ and platelet nadir is less than 25,000/mm³.

➲ Adjunct to surgery to prolong survival in patients with recurrent glioblastoma multiforme for whom surgical resection is indicated
Adults: 8 wafers placed in the resection cavity if size and shape of cavity allow. If 8 wafers can't be accommodated, use maximum number of wafers allowed. Or, 150 to 200 mg/m² I.V. by slow infusion as single dose, repeated q 6 to 8 weeks.

➲ Cutaneous T-cell lymphoma (mycosis fungoides) ♦
Adults: Apply 0.05% to 0.4% topical solution or ointment once or twice daily. Usual dose is 10 mg daily applied topically for 6 to 8 weeks. If response is inadequate, after a 6-week rest period, apply 20 mg daily topically for 30 days. For persistent papules or small nodules, give intralesionally at a concentration of 0.1% to 0.2%.

➲ Adjunct to surgery and radiation in patients with newly diagnosed high-grade malignant glioma
Adults: 8 wafers placed in the resection cavity if size and shape of cavity allow. If 8 wafers can't be accommodated, use maximum number of wafers allowed.

Contraindications & cautions

• Contraindicated in patients hypersensitive to drug.

Adverse reactions

CNS: ataxia, drowsiness, ***brain edema, seizures***.
EENT: ocular toxicities.
GI: *nausea, vomiting, stomatitis*.
GU: ***nephrotoxicity***, azotemia, ***renal failure***.
Hematologic: ***cumulative bone marrow suppression, leukopenia, thrombocytopenia, acute leukemia or bone marrow dysplasia***, anemia.
Hepatic: ***hepatotoxicity***.
Respiratory: ***pulmonary fibrosis***.
Skin: facial flushing, hyperpigmentation.
Other: *intense pain at infusion site from venous spasm*, ***secondary malignancies***.

Interactions

Drug-drug. *Anticoagulants, aspirin, NSAIDs:* May increase risk of bleeding. Avoid using together.
Cimetidine: May increase carmustine's bone marrow toxicity. Avoid using together.
Digoxin, phenytoin: May decrease levels of these drugs. Monitor patient.
Mitomycin: May increase corneal and conjunctival damage with high doses. Monitor patient.
Myelosuppressives: May increase myelosuppression. Monitor patient.

Nursing considerations

• Pulmonary toxicity appears to be dose-related and may occur 9 days to 15 years after treatment. Obtain pulmonary function tests before and during therapy.
• Bone marrow suppression is delayed with carmustine. Drug shouldn't be given more often than every 6 weeks.
• Give antiemetic before drug, to reduce nausea.
• Avoid contact with skin because carmustine causes a brown stain. If drug contacts skin, wash off thoroughly.
• Perform liver, renal function, and pulmonary function tests periodically.
• Monitor CBC with differential. The absolute neutrophil count may be used to better calculate the patient's immunosuppressive state.
• Monitor uric acid level. To prevent hyperuricemia with resulting uric acid nephropathy, allopurinol may be used with adequate hydration.

- Therapeutic effects are commonly accompanied by toxicity.
- Acute leukemia or bone marrow dysplasia may occur after long-term use.
- To prevent bleeding, avoid all I.M. injections when platelet count is less than 50,000/mm^3.
- Anticipate blood transfusions during treatment because of cumulative anemia. Patient may receive injections of RBC colony-stimulating factor to promote cell production.
- Unopened foil pouches of wafer may be kept at ambient room temperature for a maximum of 6 hours.
- Wafers broken in half may be used; however, discard wafers broken into more than two pieces.

Patient teaching

- Advise patient about common adverse reactions to drug.
- Tell patient to watch for signs and symptoms of infection (fever, sore throat, fatigue) and bleeding (easy bruising, nosebleeds, bleeding gums, tarry stools). Tell him to take temperature daily.
- Instruct patient to avoid OTC products containing aspirin and NSAIDs.
- Advise women to stop breast-feeding during therapy because of possible risk of toxicity to infant.
- Caution woman of childbearing age to avoid becoming pregnant during therapy. Recommend that she consult prescriber before becoming pregnant.

carteolol hydrochloride
Ocupress

Pregnancy risk category C

Indications & dosages

➲ Chronic open-angle glaucoma, intraocular hypertension
Adults: 1 drop into conjunctival sac of affected eye b.i.d.

Contraindications & cautions

- Contraindicated in patients hypersensitive to drug or its components and in those with bronchial asthma, severe COPD, sinus bradycardia, second- or third-degree AV block, overt cardiac failure, or cardiogenic shock.
- Use cautiously in patients hypersensitive to other beta blockers; in those with nonallergic bronchospastic disease, diabetes mellitus, hyperthyroidism, or decreased pulmonary function; and in breast-feeding women.

Adverse reactions

CNS: headache, dizziness, insomnia, asthenia.
CV: ***bradycardia***, hypotension, ***arrhythmias***, palpitations.
EENT: *transient eye irritation, burning, tearing, conjunctival hyperemia, ocular, edema,* blurred and cloudy vision, photophobia, decreased night vision, ptosis, blepharoconjunctivitis, abnormal corneal staining, corneal sensitivity, sinusitis.
GI: taste perversion.
Respiratory: dyspnea.

Interactions

Drug-drug. *Aminophylline, theophylline:* May act antagonistically, reducing the effects of one or both drugs. Elimination of theophylline may also be reduced. Monitor theophylline levels and patient closely.
Catecholamine-depleting drugs such as reserpine, oral beta blockers: May cause additive effects and development of hypotension or bradycardia. Monitor patient closely; monitor vital signs.
Epinephrine: May cause an initial hypertensive episode followed by bradycardia. Stop beta blocker 3 days before anticipated epinephrine use. Monitor patient closely.
Insulin: May mask symptoms of hypoglycemia as a result of beta blockade (such as tachycardia). Use together cautiously in patients with diabetes.
Prazosin: May increase risk of orthostatic hypotension in early phases of use together. Assist patient to stand slowly until effects are known.
Verapamil: May increase effects of both drugs. Monitor cardiac function closely and decrease dosages as necessary.
Drug-lifestyle. *Sun exposure:* May cause photophobia. Advise patient to wear sunglasses.

Nursing considerations

- Monitor vital signs.

!!ALERT Stop drug at first sign of cardiac failure, and notify prescriber.

Patient teaching

- If patient is using more than one topical ophthalmic drug, tell him to apply them at least 10 minutes apart.
- Teach patient how to instill drops. Advise him to wash hands before and after instillation, and warn him not to touch tip of dropper to eye or surrounding tissue.
- Advise patient to apply light finger pressure on lacrimal sac for 1 minute after drug instillation to minimize systemic absorption.
- Tell patient to remove contact lenses before instilling drug.
- Instruct patient to keep bottle tightly closed when not in use and to protect it from light.
- Tell patient that drug is a beta blocker and, although given topically, has the potential to be absorbed systemically.
- Inform patient that adverse reactions from beta blockers can occur with topical administration. Advise him to stop drug and notify prescriber immediately if signs or symptoms of serious adverse reactions or hypersensitivity occur.
- Advise patient to monitor heart rate and blood pressure closely and to report slow heart rate to prescriber.
- Stress importance of compliance with recommended therapy.
- Advise patient to ease sun sensitivity by wearing sunglasses.

carvedilol
Coreg

Pregnancy risk category C

Indications & dosages

➲ Hypertension

Adults: Dosage highly individualized. Initially, 6.25 mg P.O. b.i.d. Measure standing blood pressure 1 hour after first dose. If tolerated, continue dosage for 7 to 14 days. May increase to 12.5 mg P.O. b.i.d. for 7 to 14 days, following same blood pressure monitoring protocol as before. Maximum dose is 25 mg P.O. b.i.d. as tolerated.

➲ Left ventricular dysfunction after MI

Adults: Dosage individualized. Start therapy after patient is hemodynamically stable and fluid retention has been minimized. Initially, 6.25 mg P.O. b.i.d. Increase after 3 to 10 days to 12.5 mg b.i.d., then again to a target dose of 25 mg b.i.d. Or start with 3.25 mg b.i.d., or adjust dosage slower if indicated.

➲ Mild to severe heart failure

Adults: Dosage highly individualized. Initially, 3.125 mg P.O. b.i.d. for 2 weeks; if tolerated, may increase to 6.25 mg P.O. b.i.d. Dosage may be doubled q 2 weeks as tolerated. Maximum dose for patients weighing less than 85 kg (187 lb) is 25 mg P.O. b.i.d.; for those weighing more than 85 kg, dose is 50 mg P.O. b.i.d.

In patient with pulse rate below 55 beats/minute, use reduced dosage.

➲ Angina pectoris♦

Adults: 25 to 50 mg P.O. b.i.d.

➲ Idiopathic cardiomyopathy♦

Adults: 6.25 to 25 mg P.O. b.i.d.

Contraindications & cautions

- Contraindicated in patients hypersensitive to drug and in those with New York Heart Association class IV decompensated cardiac failure requiring I.V. inotropic therapy.
- Contraindicated in those with bronchial asthma or related bronchospastic conditions, second- or third-degree AV block, sick sinus syndrome (unless a permanent pacemaker is in place), cardiogenic shock, severe bradycardia, or symptomatic hepatic impairment.
- Use cautiously in hypertensive patients with left-sided heart failure, perioperative patients who receive anesthetics that depress myocardial function (such as cyclopropane and trichloroethylene), and diabetic patients receiving insulin or oral antidiabetics, and in those subject to spontaneous hypoglycemia.
- Use with caution in patients with thyroid disease (may mask hyperthyroidism; withdrawal may precipitate thyroid storm or exacerbation of hyperthyroidism), pheochromocytoma, Prinzmetal's or variant angina, bronchospastic disease, or peripheral vascular disease (may precipitate or aggravate symptoms of arterial insufficiency).
- Use cautiously in breast-feeding women.
- Safety and efficacy in patients younger than age 18 haven't been established. Don't use drug in these patients.

Adverse reactions

CNS: *asthenia, fatigue,* pain, *dizziness,* headache, malaise, fever, hypesthesia, par-

esthesia, vertigo, somnolence, ***cerebrovascular accident***, depression, insomnia.
CV: *hypotension, postural hypertension,* edema, ***bradycardia***, syncope, angina pectoris, peripheral edema, hypovolemia, fluid overload, ***AV block***, hypertension, palpitations, peripheral vascular disorder, chest pain.
EENT: sinusitis, abnormal vision, blurred vision, pharyngitis, rhinitis.
GI: *diarrhea,* vomiting, nausea, melena, periodontitis, abdominal pain, dyspepsia.
GU: impotence, abnormal renal function, albuminuria, hematuria, UTI.
Hematologic: purpura, anemia, ***thrombocytopenia***.
Metabolic: *hyperglycemia, weight gain,* weight loss, hypercholesterolemia, hyperuricemia, ***hypoglycemia***, hyponatremia, glycosuria, hypervolemia, diabetes mellitus, ***hyperkalemia***, gout, hypertriglyceridemia.
Musculoskeletal: arthralgia, back pain, muscle cramps, hypotonia, arthritis.
Respiratory: bronchitis, *upper respiratory tract infection,* cough, rales, dyspnea, ***lung edema***.
Other: *hypersensitivity reactions,* infection, flulike syndrome, viral infection, injury.

Interactions

Drug-drug. *Amiodarone:* May increase risk of bradycardia, AV block, and myocardial depression. Monitor patient's ECG and vital signs.
Catecholamine-depleting drugs, such as MAO inhibitors, reserpine: May cause bradycardia or severe hypotension. Monitor patient closely.
Cimetidine: May increase bioavailability of carvedilol. Monitor vital signs closely.
Clonidine: May increase blood pressure and heart rate lowering effects. Monitor vital signs closely.
Cyclosporine: May increase cyclosporine level. Monitor cyclosporine level.
Digoxin: May increase digoxin level by about 15% when given together. Monitor digoxin level.
Diltiazem, verapamil: May cause isolated conduction disturbances. Monitor patient's heart rhythm and blood pressure.
Fluoxetine, paroxetine, propafenone, quinidine: May increase level of carvedilol. Monitor patient for hypotension and dizziness.
Insulin, oral antidiabetics: May enhance hypoglycemic properties. Monitor glucose level.
NSAIDs: May decrease antihypertensive effects. Monitor blood pressure.
Rifampin: May reduce carvedilol level by 70%. Monitor vital signs closely.
Drug-herb. *Ma huang:* May decrease antihypertensive effects. Discourage use together.
Drug-food. *Any food:* May delay rate of absorption of carvedilol with no change in bioavailability. Advise patient to take drug with food to minimize orthostatic effects.

Nursing considerations

!!ALERT Patients receiving beta-blocker therapy who have a history of severe anaphylactic reaction to several allergens may be more reactive to repeated challenge (accidental, diagnostic, or therapeutic). They may be unresponsive to dosages of epinephrine typically used to treat allergic reactions.
- Mild hepatocellular injury may occur during therapy. At first sign of hepatic dysfunction, perform tests for hepatic injury or jaundice; if present, stop drug.
- If drug must be stopped, do so gradually over 1 to 2 weeks.
- Monitor patient with heart failure for worsened condition, renal dysfunction, or fluid retention; diuretics may need to be increased.
- Monitor diabetic patient closely; drug may mask signs of hypoglycemia, or hyperglycemia may be worsened.
- Observe patient for dizziness or lightheadedness for 1 hour after giving each new dose.
- Before starting carvedilol, make sure dosages of digoxin, diuretics, and ACE inhibitors are stabilized.
- Monitor elderly patients carefully; drug levels are about 50% higher in elderly patients than in younger patients.

Patient teaching

- Tell patient not to interrupt or stop drug without medical approval.
- Inform patient that improvement of heart failure symptoms might take several weeks of drug therapy.
- Advise patient with heart failure to call prescriber if weight gain or shortness of breath occurs.

- Inform patient that he may experience low blood pressure when standing. If dizziness or fainting (rare) occurs, advise him to sit or lie down and to notify prescriber if symptoms persist.
- Caution patient against performing hazardous tasks during start of therapy.
- Advise diabetic patient to promptly report changes in glucose level.
- Inform patient who wears contact lenses that his eyes may feel dry.

caspofungin acetate
Cancidas

Pregnancy risk category C

Indications & dosages

➲ Invasive aspergillosis in patients who are refractory to or intolerant of other therapies (amphotericin B, lipid formulations of amphotericin B, or itraconazole); candidemia and *Candida*-caused intra-abdominal abscesses, peritonitis, and pleural space infections

Adults: Single 70-mg I.V. loading dose on day 1, followed by 50 mg/day I.V. over about 1 hour. Base treatment duration on severity of patient's underlying disease, recovery from immunosuppression, and clinical response.

➲ Empirical treatment of presumed fungal infections in febrile, neutropenic patients

Adults: Single 70-mg I.V. loading dose on day 1, followed by 50 mg/day I.V. over 1 hour thereafter. Continue empirical therapy until neutropenia resolves. If fungal infection is confirmed, treat for a minimum of 14 days and continue therapy for at least 7 days after neutropenia and symptoms resolve. May increase daily dose to 70 mg if the 50-mg dose is well tolerated but clinical response is suboptimal.

➲ Esophageal candidiasis

Adults: 50 mg I.V. daily over 1 hour.

For patients with Child-Pugh score 7 to 9, after initial 70-mg loading dose (when indicated), give 35 mg/day. Dosage adjustment in patients with Child-Pugh score over 9 is unknown.

Contraindications & cautions

- Contraindicated in patients hypersensitive to drug or its components.
- Safety and efficacy in patients younger than age 18 aren't known.
- It's unknown if drug appears in breast milk. Use cautiously in breast-feeding women.

Adverse reactions

CNS: fever, headache, *paresthesia.*
CV: *tachycardia,* phlebitis, infused vein complications.
GI: nausea, vomiting, diarrhea, abdominal pain, *anorexia.*
GU: proteinuria, hematuria.
Hematologic: eosinophilia, *anemia.*
Metabolic: hypokalemia.
Musculoskeletal: *pain, myalgia.*
Respiratory: *tachypnea.*
Skin: histamine-mediated symptoms including rash, facial swelling, pruritus, sensation of warmth.
Other: *chills, sweating.*

Interactions

Drug-drug. *Cyclosporine:* May increase caspofungin level. Because of increased risk of elevated alanine transaminase level, avoid using together unless benefit outweighs risk.
Inducers of drug clearance or mixed inducer-inhibitors (carbamazepine, dexamethasone, efavirenz, nelfinavir, nevirapine, phenytoin, rifampin): May reduce caspofungin level. May need to adjust dosage.
Tacrolimus: May reduce tacrolimus level. Monitor tacrolimus level; expect to adjust dosage.

Nursing considerations

- Safety information on treatment lasting longer than 2 weeks is limited, but drug continues to be well tolerated with longer courses of therapy.
- Monitor I.V. site carefully for phlebitis.
- Observe patients for histamine-mediated reactions, including rash, facial swelling, pruritus, and a sensation of warmth.

Patient teaching

- Instruct patient to report signs and symptoms of phlebitis.
- Instruct patient to immediately report any signs of a hypersensitivity reaction.

cefaclor

Ceclor, Ceclor CD, Raniclor

Pregnancy risk category B

Indications & dosages

➲ **Respiratory tract infections, UTIs, skin and soft-tissue infections, and otitis media caused by *Haemophilus influenzae, Streptococcus pneumoniae, S. pyogenes, Escherichia coli, Proteus mirabilis, Klebsiella* species, and staphylococci**

Adults: 250 to 500 mg P.O. q 8 hours. For pharyngitis or otitis media, daily dose may be given in two equally divided doses q 12 hours. For extended-release forms in bronchitis, 500 mg P.O. q 12 hours for 7 days; for extended-release forms in pharyngitis or skin and skin-structure infections, 375 mg P.O. q 12 hours for 10 days and 7 to 10 days, respectively.

Children: 20 mg/kg daily P.O. in divided doses q 8 hours. For pharyngitis or otitis media, daily dose may be given in two equally divided doses q 12 hours. In more serious infections, 40 mg/kg daily is recommended, not to exceed 1 g daily.

Contraindications & cautions

- Contraindicated in patients hypersensitive to drug or other cephalosporins.
- Use cautiously in patients hypersensitive to penicillin because of the possibility of cross-sensitivity with other beta-lactam antibiotics.
- Use cautiously in breast-feeding women and in patients with a history of colitis or renal insufficiency.

Adverse reactions

CNS: fever, dizziness, headache, somnolence, malaise.

GI: *nausea*, vomiting, *diarrhea*, anorexia, dyspepsia, abdominal cramps, ***pseudomembranous colitis***, oral candidiasis.

GU: vaginal candidiasis, vaginitis.

Hematologic: ***transient leukopenia***, anemia, eosinophilia, ***thrombocytopenia***, lymphocytosis.

Skin: *maculopapular rash*, dermatitis, pruritus.

Other: hypersensitivity reactions, serum sickness, ***anaphylaxis***.

Interactions

Drug-drug. *Aminoglycosides:* May increase risk of nephrotoxicity. Avoid using together.

Antacids: May decrease absorption of extended-release cefaclor if taken within 1 hour. Separate doses by 1 hour.

Anticoagulants: May increase anticoagulant effects. Monitor PT and INR.

Chloramphenicol: May cause antagonistic effect. Avoid using together.

Probenecid: May inhibit excretion and increase cefaclor level. Monitor patient for increased adverse reactions.

Nursing considerations

- Before administration, ask patient if he is allergic to penicillins or cephalosporins.
- Obtain specimen for culture and sensitivity tests before giving first dose. Therapy may begin while awaiting results.
- If large doses are given, therapy is prolonged, or patient is at high risk, monitor patient for signs and symptoms of superinfection.
- Store reconstituted suspension in refrigerator. Suspension is stable for 14 days if refrigerated. Shake well before use.

!!ALERT Don't confuse drug with other cephalosporins that sound alike.

Patient teaching

- Tell patient to take entire amount of drug exactly as prescribed, even after he feels better.
- Tell patient that drug may be taken with meals. If suspension is used, instruct him to shake container well before measuring dose and to keep the drug refrigerated.
- Advise patient to notify prescriber if rash develops or signs and symptoms of superinfection appear.
- Inform patient not to crush, cut, or chew extended-release tablets.

cefadroxil

Duricef

Pregnancy risk category B

Indications & dosages

➲ **UTIs caused by *Escherichia coli, Proteus mirabilis,* and *Klebsiella* species; skin and soft-tissue infections caused by staphylococci and streptococci; pharyngitis or**

tonsillitis caused by group A beta-hemolytic streptococci
Adults: 1 to 2 g P.O. daily, depending on infection being treated. Usually given once daily or in two divided doses.
Children: 30 mg/kg P.O. daily in two divided doses q 12 hours.

In patients with renal impairment, give first dose of 1 g. Reduce additional doses based on creatinine clearance. If clearance is 25 to 50 ml/minute, give 500 mg P.O. q 12 hours. If clearance is 10 to 25 ml/minute, give 500 mg P.O. q 24 hours; if clearance is less than 10 ml/minute, give 500 mg P.O. q 36 hours.

Contraindications & cautions

- Contraindicated in patients hypersensitive to drug or other cephalosporins.
- Use cautiously in patients with a history of sensitivity to penicillin and in breast-feeding women.
- Use cautiously in patients with impaired renal function; dosage adjustments may be needed.

Adverse reactions

CNS: fever, ***seizures***, dizziness, headache.
GI: ***pseudomembranous colitis***, *nausea*, vomiting, *diarrhea*, glossitis, abdominal cramps, oral candidiasis.
GU: genital pruritus, candidiasis, vaginitis, renal dysfunction.
Hematologic: ***transient neutropenia***, eosinophilia, ***leukopenia***, anemia, ***agranulocytosis***, ***thrombocytopenia***.
Respiratory: dyspnea.
Skin: *maculopapular and erythematous rashes*, urticaria.
Other: hypersensitivity reactions, ***anaphylaxis***, ***angioedema***.

Interactions

Drug-drug. *Aminoglycosides:* May increase risk of nephrotoxicity. Avoid using together.
Probenecid: May inhibit excretion and increase cefadroxil level. Use together cautiously.

Nursing considerations

- Before administration, ask patient if he is allergic to penicillins or cephalosporins.
- Obtain specimen for culture and sensitivity tests before giving first dose. Therapy may begin while awaiting results.
- If creatinine clearance is less than 50 ml/minute, lengthen dosage interval so drug doesn't accumulate. Monitor renal function in patients with renal dysfunction.
- If large doses are given, therapy is prolonged, or patient is high risk, monitor patient for superinfection.

!!ALERT Don't confuse drug with other cephalosporins that sound alike.

Patient teaching

- Instruct patient to take drug with food or milk to lessen GI discomfort.
- Tell patient to take entire amount of drug exactly as prescribed, even after he feels better.
- Advise patient to notify prescriber if rash develops or if signs and symptoms of superinfection appear, such as recurring fever, chills, and malaise.

cefazolin sodium
Ancef

Pregnancy risk category B

Indications & dosages

➲ Perioperative prevention in contaminated surgery
Adults: 1 g I.M. or I.V. 30 to 60 minutes before surgery; then 0.5 to 1 g I.M. or I.V. q 6 to 8 hours for 24 hours. In operations lasting longer than 2 hours, give another 0.5- to 1-g dose I.M. or I.V. intraoperatively. Continue treatment for 3 to 5 days if life-threatening infection is likely.

➲ Infections of respiratory, biliary, and GU tracts; skin, soft-tissue, bone, and joint infections; septicemia; endocarditis caused by *Escherichia coli, Enterobacteriaceae,* gonococci, *Haemophilus influenzae, Klebsiella* species, *Proteus mirabilis, Staphylococcus aureus, Streptococcus pneumoniae,* and group A beta-hemolytic streptococci
Adults: 250 mg to 500 mg I.M. or I.V. q 8 hours for mild infections or 500 mg to 1.5 g I.M. or I.V. q 6 to 8 hours for moderate to severe or life-threatening infections. Maximum 12 g/day in life-threatening situations.
Children older than age 1 month: 25 to 50 mg/kg/day I.M. or I.V. in three or four divided doses. In severe infections, dose may be increased to 100 mg/kg/day.

For patients with creatinine clearance of 35 to 54 ml/minute, give full dose q 8 hours; if clearance is 11 to 34 ml/minute, give 50% usual dose q 12 hours; if clearance is below 10 ml/minute, give 50% of usual dose q 18 to 24 hours.

Contraindications & cautions

- Contraindicated in patients hypersensitive to drug or other cephalosporins.
- Use cautiously in patients hypersensitive to penicillin because of the possibility of cross-sensitivity with other beta-lactam antibiotics.
- Use cautiously in breast-feeding women and in patients with a history of colitis or renal insufficiency.

Adverse reactions

CNS: headache, confusion, ***seizures***.
CV: *phlebitis, thrombophlebitis with I.V. injection.*
GI: ***pseudomembranous colitis***, nausea, anorexia, vomiting, *diarrhea*, glossitis, dyspepsia, abdominal cramps, anal pruritus, oral candidiasis.
GU: genital pruritus, candidiasis, vaginitis.
Hematologic: ***neutropenia***, ***leukopenia***, eosinophilia, ***thrombocytopenia***.
Skin: *maculopapular and erythematous rashes, urticaria, pruritus, pain, induration, sterile abscesses, tissue sloughing at injection site,* ***Stevens-Johnson syndrome***.
Other: hypersensitivity reactions, serum sickness, ***anaphylaxis***, drug fever.

Interactions

Drug-drug. *Aminoglycosides:* May increase risk of nephrotoxicity. Avoid using together.
Anticoagulants: May increase anticoagulant effects. Monitor PT and INR.
Probenecid: May inhibit excretion and increase cefazolin level. Use together cautiously.

Nursing considerations

- Before administration, ask patient if he is allergic to penicillins or cephalosporins.
- Obtain specimen for culture and sensitivity tests before giving first dose. Therapy may begin while awaiting results.
- Expect to adjust dosage and dosing interval if creatinine clearance falls below 55 ml/minute.
- After reconstitution, inject drug I.M. without further dilution. This drug isn't as painful as other cephalosporins. Give injection deep into a large muscle, such as the gluteus maximus or lateral aspect of the thigh.
- If large doses are given, therapy is prolonged, or patient is at high risk, monitor patient for signs and symptoms of superinfection.

!!ALERT Don't confuse drug with other cephalosporins that sound alike.

Patient teaching

- Instruct patient to report adverse reactions promptly.
- Tell patient to report discomfort at I.V. injection site.
- Advise patient to notify prescriber if a rash develops or if signs and symptoms of superinfection appear, such as recurring fever, chills, and malaise.

cefdinir
Omnicef

Pregnancy risk category B

Indications & dosages

➲ Mild to moderate infections caused by susceptible strains of microorganisms in community-acquired pneumonia, acute worsening of chronic bronchitis, acute maxillary sinusitis, acute bacterial otitis media, and uncomplicated skin and skin-structure infections
Adults and children age 12 and older: 300 mg P.O. q 12 hours or 600 mg P.O. q 24 hours for 10 days. Give q 12 hours for pneumonia and skin infections.
Children ages 6 months to 12 years: 7 mg/kg P.O. q 12 hours or 14 mg/kg P.O. q 24 hours, for 10 days, up to maximum dose of 600 mg daily. Give q 12 hours for skin infections.
➲ Pharyngitis, tonsillitis
Adults and children age 12 and older: 300 mg P.O. q 12 hours for 5 to 10 days or 600 mg P.O. q 24 hours for 10 days.
Children ages 6 months to 12 years: 7 mg/kg P.O. q 12 hours for 5 to 10 days; or 14 mg/kg P.O. q 24 hours, for 10 days.

If creatinine clearance is less than 30 ml/minute, reduce dosage to 300 mg P.O. once daily for adults and 7 mg/kg up to 300 mg P.O. once daily for children. In patients receiving long-term hemodialysis, give 300 mg or 7 mg/kg P.O. at end of each dialysis session and then every other day.

Contraindications & cautions

- Contraindicated in patients hypersensitive to drug or other cephalosporins.
- Use cautiously in patients hypersensitive to penicillin because of the possibility of cross-sensitivity with other beta-lactam antibiotics.
- Use cautiously in patients with history of colitis or renal insufficiency.

Adverse reactions

CNS: headache.
GI: abdominal pain, *diarrhea*, nausea, vomiting, ***pseudomembranous colitis***.
GU: vaginal candidiasis; vaginitis; increased urine proteins, WBCs, and RBCs.
Skin: rash, cutaneous candidiasis.
Other: ***hypersensitivity reactions, anaphylaxis***.

Interactions

Drug-drug. *Aminoglycosides:* May increase risk of nephrotoxicity. Avoid using together.
Antacids containing aluminum and magnesium, iron supplements, multivitamins containing iron: May decrease cefdinir rate of absorption and bioavailability. Give such preparations 2 hours before or after cefdinir.
Probenecid: May inhibit renal excretion of cefdinir. Monitor patient for adverse reactions.

Nursing considerations

- Before administration, ask patient if he is allergic to penicillins or cephalosporins.
- Prolonged drug treatment may result in emergence and overgrowth of resistant organisms. Monitor patient for signs and symptoms of superinfection.
- Pseudomembranous colitis has been reported with cefdinir and should be considered in patients with diarrhea after antibiotic therapy and in those with history of colitis.

!!ALERT Don't confuse drug with other cephalosporins that sound alike.

Patient teaching

- Instruct patient to take antacids and iron supplements 2 hours before or after a dose of cefdinir.
- Inform diabetic patient that each teaspoon of suspension contains 2.86 g of sucrose.
- Tell patient that drug may be taken without regard to meals.
- Tell patient to take drug as prescribed, even after he feels better.
- Advise patient to report severe diarrhea or diarrhea accompanied by abdominal pain.
- Tell patient to report adverse reactions or signs and symptoms of superinfection promptly.

cefditoren pivoxil
Spectracef

Pregnancy risk category B

Indications & dosages

➲ Acute bacterial worsening of chronic bronchitis or community-acquired pneumonia caused by *Haemophilus influenzae, H. parainfluenzae, Streptococcus pneumoniae,* or *Moraxella catarrhalis*
Adults and adolescents age 12 and older: 400 mg P.O. b.i.d. with meals for 10 days (chronic bronchitis) or 14 days (community-acquired pneumonia).

➲ Pharyngitis or tonsillitis caused by *Streptococcus pyogenes;* uncomplicated skin and skin-structure infections caused by *S. pyogenes* or *Staphylococcus aureus*
Adults and adolescents age 12 and older: 200 mg P.O. b.i.d. with meals for 10 days.

For patients with creatinine clearance of 30 to 49 ml/minute, don't exceed 200 mg b.i.d. For patients with clearance less than 30 ml/minute, give 200 mg daily.

Contraindications & cautions

- Contraindicated in patients hypersensitive to drug or other cephalosporins.
- Contraindicated in patients with carnitine deficiency or inborn errors of metabolism that may result in clinically significant carnitine deficiency.
- Because cefditoren tablets contain sodium caseinate, a milk protein, don't give drug to patients hypersensitive to milk protein (as distinct from those with lactose intolerance).
- Use cautiously in breast-feeding women because cephalosporins appear in breast milk, and safe use hasn't been established.
- Use cautiously in patients with impaired renal function or penicillin allergy.

Adverse reactions

CNS: headache.
GI: abdominal pain, dyspepsia, *diarrhea*, nausea, vomiting.
GU: vaginal candidiasis, hematuria.
Metabolic: hyperglycemia.

Interactions

Drug-drug. *H_2-receptor antagonists, magnesium, and aluminum antacids:* May decrease cefditoren absorption. Avoid using together.
Probenecid: May increase cefditoren level. Avoid using together.
Drug-food. *Moderate- or high-fat meal:* May increase cefditoren bioavailability. Advise patient to take drug with meals.

Nursing considerations

- Before administration, ask patient if he is allergic to penicillins or cephalosporins.
- Obtain specimen for culture and sensitivity tests before giving first dose. Therapy may begin while awaiting results.
- Give drug with a fatty meal to increase its bioavailability.
- If patient develops diarrhea after receiving cefditoren, keep in mind that this drug may cause pseudomembranous colitis.
- Don't use this drug if patient needs prolonged treatment.
- Monitor patient for overgrowth of resistant organisms.
- Patients with renal or hepatic impairment, in poor nutritional state, receiving a protracted course of antibiotics, or previously stabilized on anticoagulants may be at risk for decreased prothrombin activity. Monitor PT in these patients.

Patient teaching

- Instruct patient to take medication exactly as prescribed.
- Tell patient to take drug with food to increase its absorption.
- Caution patient not to take drug with an H_2-receptor antagonist or an antacid because either may reduce cefditoren absorption.
- Instruct patient not to stop drug before completing treatment and to call prescriber immediately if he experiences any unpleasant adverse reactions.
- Instruct patient to contact prescriber if signs and symptoms of infection don't improve after several days of therapy.
- Inform patient of potential adverse reactions.
- Urge patient not to miss any doses. However, if he does, tell him to take the missed dose as soon as possible unless it's within 4 hours of the next scheduled dose. In that case, tell him to skip the missed dose and go back to the regular dosing schedule. Tell him not to double the dose.

cefepime hydrochloride
Maxipime

Pregnancy risk category B

Indications & dosages

➲ **Mild to moderate UTIs caused by *Escherichia coli, Klebsiella pneumoniae,* or *Proteus mirabilis,* including concurrent bacteremia with these microorganisms**
Adults and children age 12 and older: 0.5 to 1 g I.M. or I.V. infused over 30 minutes q 12 hours for 7 to 10 days. I.M. route used only for *E. coli* infections.
➲ **Severe UTIs, including pyelonephritis, caused by *E. coli* or *K. pneumoniae***
Adults and children age 12 and older: 2 g I.V. infused over 30 minutes q 12 hours for 10 days.
➲ **Moderate to severe pneumonia caused by *Streptococcus pneumoniae, Pseudomonas aeruginosa, K. pneumoniae,* or *Enterobacter* species**
Adults and children age 12 and older: 1 to 2 g I.V. infused over 30 minutes q 12 hours for 10 days.
➲ **Moderate to severe skin infections, uncomplicated skin infections, and skin-structure infections caused by *Streptococcus pyogenes* or methicillin-susceptible strains of *Staphylococcus aureus***
Adults and children age 12 and older: 2 g I.V. infused over 30 minutes q 12 hours for 10 days.
➲ **Complicated intra-abdominal infections caused by *E. coli,* viridans group streptococci, *P. aeruginosa, K. pneumo-***

niae, Enterobacter* species, or *Bacteroides fragilis
Adults: 2 g I.V. infused over 30 minutes q 12 hours for 7 to 10 days. Give with metronidazole.
➲ **Empiric therapy for febrile neutropenia**
Adults: 2 g I.V. q 8 hours for 7 days or until neutropenia resolves.
➲ **Uncomplicated and complicated UTIs (including pyelonephritis), uncomplicated skin and skin-structure infections, pneumonia, empiric therapy for febrile neutropenic children**
Children ages 2 months to 16 years, weighing up to 40 kg (88 lb): 50 mg/kg/dose I.V. infused over 30 minutes q 12 hours, or q 8 hours for febrile neutropenia, for 7 to 10 days. Don't exceed 2 g/dose.

Adjust dosage based on creatinine clearance, as shown in the table. For patients receiving hemodialysis, about 68% of drug is removed after a 3-hour dialysis session. Give a repeat dose, equivalent to the first dose, at the completion of dialysis. For patients receiving continuous ambulatory peritoneal dialysis, give normal dose q 48 hours.

Dosage adjustments for renal impairment

Creatinine clearance (ml/min)	If normal dosage would be			
	500 mg q 12 hr	**1 g q 12 hr**	**2 g q 12 hr**	**2 g q 8 hr**
30–60	500 mg q 24 hr	1 g q 24 hr	2 g q 24 hr	2 g q 12 hr
11–29	500 mg q 24 hr	500 mg q 24 hr	1 g q 24 hr	2 g q 24 hr
< 11	250 mg q 24 hr	250 mg q 24 hr	500 mg q 24 hr	1 g q 24 hr

Contraindications & cautions

- Contraindicated in patients hypersensitive to drug, cephalosporins, beta-lactam antibiotics, or penicillins.
- Use cautiously in patients hypersensitive to penicillin because of possibility of cross-sensitivity with other beta-lactam antibiotics.
- Use cautiously in breast-feeding women and in patients with history of colitis or renal insufficiency.

Adverse reactions

CNS: fever, headache.
CV: phlebitis.
GI: colitis, diarrhea, nausea, vomiting, oral candidiasis.
GU: vaginitis.
Skin: rash, pruritus, urticaria.
Other: pain, inflammation, hypersensitivity reactions, ***anaphylaxis***.

Interactions

Drug-drug. *Aminoglycosides:* May increase risk of nephrotoxicity. Monitor renal function closely.
Potent diuretics: May increase risk of nephrotoxicity. Monitor renal function closely.
Probenecid: May inhibit renal excretion of cefepime. Monitor patient for adverse reactions.

Nursing considerations

- Before administration, ask patient if he is allergic to penicillins or cephalosporins.
- Obtain culture and sensitivity tests before giving first dose. Therapy may begin while awaiting results.
- Adjust dosage in patients with impaired renal function. Serious adverse reactions, including encephalopathy, myoclonus, seizures, and renal failure may occur when dosage isn't adjusted.
- For I.M. administration, reconstitute drug using sterile water for injection, normal saline solution for injection, D_5W injection, 0.5% or 1% lidocaine hydrochloride, or bacteriostatic water for injection with parabens or benzyl alcohol. Follow manufacturer's guidelines for quantity of diluent to use.
- Inspect solution for particulate matter before use. The powder and its solutions tend to darken, depending on storage conditions. Product potency isn't adversely affected when stored as recommended.
- Monitor patient for superinfection. Drug may cause overgrowth of nonsusceptible bacteria or fungi.
- Drug may reduce PT activity. Patients at risk include those with renal or hepatic impairment or poor nutrition and those receiving prolonged cefepime therapy. Monitor PT and INR in these patients, as ordered. Give vitamin K, as indicated.

!!ALERT Don't confuse drug with other cephalosporins that sound alike.

Patient teaching

- Warn patient receiving drug I.M. that pain may occur at injection site.
- Advise patient to notify prescriber if a rash develops or if signs and symptoms of superinfection appear, such as recurring fever, chills, and malaise
- Instruct patient to report adverse reactions promptly.

cefoperazone sodium
Cefobid

Pregnancy risk category B

Indications & dosages

➲ **Serious respiratory tract infections; intra-abdominal, gynecologic, and skin infections; bacteremia; septicemia caused by susceptible microorganisms (*Streptococcus pneumoniae* and *S. pyogenes; Staphylococcus aureus* [penicillinase- and non–penicillinase-producing] and *S. epidermidis;* enterococci; *Escherichia coli; Haemophilus influenzae; Enterobacter, Citrobacter, Klebsiella,* and *Proteus* species; some *Pseudomonas* species, including *P. aeruginosa;* and *Bacteroides fragilis*)**
Adults: Usual dosage is 1 to 2 g q 12 hours I.M. or I.V. In severe infections or in infections caused by less-sensitive organisms, total daily dose or frequency may be increased to 16 g/day.

For patients with hepatic or biliary obstruction, don't exceed total dose of 4 g daily. For patients with hepatic and substantial renal impairment, don't exceed total dose of 2 g daily. Hemodialysis reduces drug's half-life; schedule dose to follow a dialysis session.

Contraindications & cautions

- Contraindicated in patients hypersensitive to drug or other cephalosporins.
- Use cautiously in patients hypersensitive to penicillin because of possibility of cross-sensitivity with other beta-lactam antibiotics.
- Use cautiously in breast-feeding women and in patients with history of colitis or renal insufficiency.
- Give doses of 4 g/day cautiously to patients with hepatic disease or biliary obstruction. Higher dosages require monitoring of drug level.

Adverse reactions

CNS: fever.
CV: *phlebitis, thrombophlebitis.*
GI: ***pseudomembranous colitis***, nausea, vomiting, *diarrhea.*
Hematologic: ***transient neutropenia***, eosinophilia, anemia, hypoprothrombinemia, bleeding.
Skin: *maculopapular and erythematous rashes, urticaria, pain, induration, sterile abscesses, temperature elevation, tissue sloughing at I.M. injection site.*
Other: hypersensitivity reactions, serum sickness, ***anaphylaxis***.

Interactions

Drug-drug. *Aminoglycosides:* May increase risk of nephrotoxicity. Monitor renal function.
Anticoagulants: May increase anticoagulant effects. Monitor PT and INR.
Probenecid: May inhibit excretion and increase cefoperazone level. Use together cautiously.
Drug-lifestyle. *Alcohol use:* May cause a disulfiram-like reaction. Warn patient not to drink alcohol for several days after stopping cefoperazone.

Nursing considerations

- Before administration, ask patient if he is allergic to penicillins or cephalosporins.
- Periodically monitor liver and renal function and compare with baseline.
- Obtain specimen for culture and sensitivity tests before giving first dose. Therapy may begin while awaiting results.
- To prepare drug for I.M. injection using the 1-g vial, dissolve drug with 2 ml of sterile water for injection; then add 0.6 ml of 2% lidocaine hydrochloride for final concentration of 333 mg/ml. Or, dissolve drug with 2.6 ml of sterile water for injection; then add 1 ml of 2% lidocaine hydrochloride for final concentration of 250 mg/ml.
- To prepare drug for I.M. injection using the 2-g vial, dissolve drug with 3.8 ml of sterile water for injection; then add 1.2 ml of 2% lidocaine hydrochloride for final concentration of 333 mg/ml. Or, dissolve drug with 5.4 ml of sterile water for injection; then add

1.8 ml of 2% lidocaine hydrochloride for final concentration of 250 mg/ml.

- For I.M. administration, inject deep into a large muscle, such as the gluteus maximus or the lateral aspect of the thigh.
- If large doses are given, therapy is prolonged, or patient is at high risk, monitor him for signs or symptoms of superinfection.
- Monitor PT and INR regularly. The drug's chemical structure has the methylthiotetrazole side chain that may cause bleeding disorders. Vitamin K promptly reverses bleeding if it occurs.

!!ALERT Don't confuse drug with other cephalosporins that sound alike.

Patient teaching

- Tell patient to report adverse reactions and signs and symptoms of superinfection promptly.
- Instruct patient to report discomfort at I.V. insertion site.

cefotaxime sodium
Claforan

Pregnancy risk category B

Indications & dosages

➲ **Perioperative prevention in contaminated surgery**
Adults: 1 g I.M. or I.V. 30 to 90 minutes before surgery. In patients undergoing bowel surgery, provide preoperative mechanical bowel cleansing and give a nonabsorbable anti-infective drug, such as neomycin. In patients undergoing cesarean delivery, give 1 g I.M. or I.V. as soon as the umbilical cord is clamped; then 1 g I.M. or I.V. 6 and 12 hours later.

➲ **Uncomplicated gonorrhea caused by penicillinase-producing strains or non–penicillinase-producing strains of *Neisseria gonorrhoeae***
Adults and adolescents: 500 mg I.M. as a single dose.

➲ **Rectal gonorrhea**
Men: 1 g I.M. as a single dose.
Women: 500 mg I.M. as a single dose.

➲ **Serious infections of the lower respiratory and urinary tracts, CNS, skin, bone, and joints; gynecologic and intra-abdominal infections; bacteremia; septicemia caused by susceptible microorganisms, such as streptococci (including *Streptococcus pneumoniae* and *S. pyogenes, Staphylococcus aureus* [penicillinase- and non–penicillinase-producing] and *S. epidermidis), Escherichia coli, Klebsiella, Haemophilus influenzae, Serratia marcescens,* and species of *Pseudomonas* (including *P. aeruginosa*), *Enterobacter, Proteus,* and *Peptostreptococcus***
Adults and children weighing 50 kg (110 lb) or more: Usual dose is 1 g I.V. or I.M. q 6 to 8 hours. Up to 12 g daily can be given in life-threatening infections.
Children ages 1 month to 12 years weighing less than 50 kg: 50 to 180 mg/kg/day I.M. or I.V. in four to six divided doses.
Neonates ages 1 to 4 weeks: 50 mg/kg I.V. q 8 hours.
Neonates to age 1 week: 50 mg/kg I.V. q 12 hours.

For patients with creatinine clearance less than 20 ml/minute, give half usual dose at usual interval.

Contraindications & cautions

- Contraindicated in patients hypersensitive to drug or other cephalosporins.
- Use cautiously in patients hypersensitive to penicillin because of possibility of cross-sensitivity with other beta-lactam antibiotics.
- Use cautiously in breast-feeding women and in patients with history of colitis or renal insufficiency.

Adverse reactions

CNS: fever, headache, dizziness.
CV: *phlebitis, thrombophlebitis.*
GI: ***pseudomembranous colitis***, nausea, vomiting, *diarrhea.*
GU: vaginitis, candidiasis, interstitial nephritis.
Hematologic: ***transient neutropenia***, eosinophilia, hemolytic anemia, ***thrombocytopenia, agranulocytosis***.
Skin: *maculopapular and erythematous rashes, urticaria, pain, induration, sterile abscesses, temperature elevation, tissue sloughing at I.M. injection site.*
Other: hypersensitivity reactions, serum sickness, ***anaphylaxis***.

Interactions

Drug-drug. *Aminoglycosides:* May increase risk of nephrotoxicity. Monitor patient's renal function tests.
Probenecid: May inhibit excretion and increase cefotaxime. Use together cautiously.

Nursing considerations

- Before administration, ask patient if he is allergic to penicillins or cephalosporins.
- Obtain specimen for culture and sensitivity tests before giving first dose. Therapy may begin while awaiting results.
- For I.M. administration, inject deep into a large muscle, such as the gluteus maximus or the lateral aspect of the thigh.
- For I.M. doses of 2 g, divide the dose and give at different sites.
- If large doses are given, therapy is prolonged, or patient is at high risk, monitor patient for superinfection.

!!ALERT Don't confuse drug with other cephalosporins that sound alike.

Patient teaching

- Tell patient to report adverse reactions and signs and symptoms of superinfection promptly.
- Instruct patient to report discomfort at I.V. insertion site.

---

cefotetan disodium
Cefotan

Pregnancy risk category B

Indications & dosages

➲ Serious UTIs and lower respiratory tract, gynecologic, skin and skin-structure, intra-abdominal, and bone and joint infections caused by susceptible streptococci, penicillinase- and non-penicillinase-producing *Staphylococcus aureus* and *S. epidermidis, Escherichia coli, Haemophilus influenzae, Neisseria gonorrhoeae,* and species of *Proteus, Klebsiella, Enterobacter,* and *Bacteroides,* including *B. fragilis*
Adults: 1 to 2 g I.V. or I.M. q 12 hours for 5 to 10 days. Up to 6 g daily in life-threatening infections.

➲ Perioperative prevention
Adults: 1 to 2 g I.V. given once 30 to 60 minutes before surgery. In cesarean section, give dose as soon as umbilical cord is clamped.

In patients with creatinine clearance of 10 to 30 ml/minute, give usual dose q 24 hours; if clearance is less than 10 ml/minute, give usual dose q 48 hours. For patients receiving intermittent hemodialysis, give 25% of the usual dose q 24 hours on days between dialysis, and give 50% of the usual dose on days of dialysis.

Contraindications & cautions

- Contraindicated in patients hypersensitive to drug or other cephalosporins.
- Use cautiously in patients hypersensitive to penicillin because of possibility of cross-sensitivity with other beta-lactam antibiotics.
- Use cautiously in breast-feeding women and in patients with history of colitis or renal insufficiency.

Adverse reactions

CNS: fever.
CV: *phlebitis, thrombophlebitis.*
GI: ***pseudomembranous colitis***, nausea, *diarrhea.*
GU: ***nephrotoxicity***.
Hematologic: ***transient neutropenia***, eosinophilia, hemolytic anemia, hypoprothrombinemia, bleeding, thrombocytosis, ***agranulocytosis, thrombocytopenia***.
Skin: *maculopapular and erythematous rashes, urticaria, pain, induration, sterile abscesses, tissue sloughing at injection site.*
Other: hypersensitivity reactions, serum sickness, ***anaphylaxis***.

Interactions

Drug-drug. *Aminoglycosides:* May cause synergistic effect and increased risk of nephrotoxicity. Monitor renal function tests.
Anticoagulants: May increase the risk of bleeding. Monitor PT and INR.
Probenecid: May inhibit excretion and increase cefotetan level. May use together for this effect.
Drug-lifestyle. *Alcohol use:* May cause a disulfiram-like reaction. Strongly discourage use together and for several days after stopping drug.

Nursing considerations

- Before administration, ask patient if he is allergic to penicillins or cephalosporins.
- Obtain specimen for culture and sensitivity tests before giving first dose. Therapy may begin while awaiting results.
- Reconstitute for I.M. injection with sterile water or bacteriostatic water for injection, normal saline solution for injection, or 0.5% or 1% lidocaine hydrochloride. Shake to dissolve and let stand until clear.
- Give I.M. injection deep into the body of a large muscle.
- Reconstituted solution is stable for 24 hours at room temperature or 96 hours refrigerated.
- Patients with renal or hepatic impairment, in poor nutritional state, receiving a protracted course of antibiotics, or previously stabilized on anticoagulants may be at risk for decreased prothrombin activity. Monitor PT in these patients.
- If large doses are given, therapy is prolonged, or patient is at high risk, monitor patient for signs and symptoms of superinfection.

!!ALERT Don't confuse drug with other cephalosporins that sound alike.

Patient teaching

- Tell patient to report adverse reactions and signs and symptoms of superinfection promptly.
- Instruct patient to report discomfort at I.V. site.
- Tell patient to notify prescriber about loose stools or diarrhea.

cefoxitin sodium

Mefoxin

Pregnancy risk category B

Indications & dosages

➲ **Serious infections of the respiratory and GU tracts; skin, soft-tissue, bone, and joint infections; bloodstream and intra-abdominal infections caused by susceptible organisms (such as *Escherichia coli* and other coliform bacteria, penicillinase- and non–penicillinase-producing *Staphylococcus aureus, S. epidermidis,* streptococci, *Klebsiella, Haemophilus influenzae,* and *Bacteroides,* including *B. fragilis*)**

Adults: 1 to 2 g I.V. or I.M. q 6 to 8 hours for uncomplicated infections. Up to 12 g daily in life-threatening infections.

Children older than age 3 months: 80 to 160 mg/kg daily I.V. or I.M., given in four to six equally divided doses. Maximum daily dose is 12 g.

➲ **Uncomplicated gonorrhea**

Adults: 2 g I.M. with 1 g probenecid P.O. as a single dose. Give probenecid within 30 minutes before cefoxitin dose.

➲ **Perioperative prevention**

Adults: 2 g I.M. or I.V. 30 to 60 minutes before surgery; then 2 g I.M. or I.V. q 6 hours for up to 24 hours. For transurethral prostatectomy, give 1 g I.M. or I.V. before surgery; then continue giving 1 g q 8 hours for up to 5 days.

Children age 3 months and older: 30 to 40 mg/kg I.M. or I.V. 30 to 60 minutes before surgery; then 30 to 40 mg/kg q 6 hours for up to 24 hours.

For patients with creatinine clearance of 30 to 50 ml/minute, give 1 to 2 g q 8 to 12 hours; if clearance is 10 to 29 ml/minute, give 1 to 2 g q 12 to 24 hours; if clearance is 5 to 9 ml/minute, give 0.5 to 1 g q 12 to 24 hours; and if clearance is less than 5 ml/minute, give 0.5 to 1 g q 24 to 48 hours. For patients receiving hemodialysis, give a loading dose of 1 to 2 g after each hemodialysis session; then give the maintenance dose based on creatinine level.

Contraindications & cautions

- Contraindicated in patients hypersensitive to drug or other cephalosporins.
- Use cautiously in patients hypersensitive to penicillin because of possibility of cross-sensitivity with other beta-lactam antibiotics.
- Use cautiously in breast-feeding women and in patients with history of colitis or renal insufficiency.

Adverse reactions

CNS: fever.
CV: hypotension, *phlebitis*, *thrombophlebitis*.
GI: ***pseudomembranous colitis***, nausea, vomiting, *diarrhea*.
GU: ***acute renal failure***.

Hematologic: ***transient neutropenia***, eosinophilia, hemolytic anemia, anemia, ***thrombocytopenia***.
Respiratory: dyspnea.
Skin: *maculopapular and erythematous rashes, urticaria*, exfoliative dermatitis, *pain, induration, sterile abscesses, tissue sloughing at injection site.*
Other: hypersensitivity reactions, serum sickness, ***anaphylaxis***.

Interactions

Drug-drug. *Aminoglycosides:* May increase risk of nephrotoxicity. Monitor patient's renal function tests.
Probenecid: May inhibit excretion and increase cefoxitin level. Probenecid may be used for this effect.

Nursing considerations

- Before administration, ask patient if he is allergic to penicillins or cephalosporins.
- Obtain specimen for culture and sensitivity tests before giving first dose. Therapy may begin while awaiting results.

!!ALERT Mefoxin in Galaxy containers is for I.V. use only.

- For I.M. use, reconstitute each 1 g of drug with 2 ml of sterile water for injection or 0.5% or 1% lidocaine hydrochloride (without epinephrine) to minimize pain. Inject deep into a large muscle, such as the gluteus maximus or the lateral aspect of the thigh.
- After reconstitution, drug may be stored for 24 hours at room temperature or 1 week under refrigeration.
- If large doses are given, therapy is prolonged, or patient is at high risk, monitor patient for signs and symptoms of superinfection.

!!ALERT Don't confuse drug with other cephalosporins that sound alike.

Patient teaching

- Tell patient to report adverse reactions and signs and symptoms of superinfection promptly.
- Instruct patient to report discomfort at I.V. site.
- Advise patient to notify prescriber about loose stools or diarrhea.

cefpodoxime proxetil
Vantin

Pregnancy risk category B

Indications & dosages

➲ **Acute, community-acquired pneumonia caused by strains of *Haemophilus influenzae* or *Streptococcus pneumoniae***
Adults and children age 12 and older: 200 mg P.O. q 12 hours for 14 days.

➲ **Acute bacterial worsening of chronic bronchitis caused by *S. pneumoniae* or *H. influenzae* (strains that don't produce beta-lactamase only), or *Moraxella catarrhalis***
Adults and children age 12 and older: 200 mg P.O. q 12 hours for 10 days.

➲ **Uncomplicated gonorrhea in men and women; rectal gonococcal infections in women**
Adults and children age 12 and older: 200 mg P.O. as a single dose. Follow with doxycycline 100 mg P.O. b.i.d. for 7 days.

➲ **Uncomplicated skin and skin-structure infections caused by *Staphylococcus aureus* or *S. pyogenes***
Adults and children age 12 and older: 400 mg P.O. q 12 hours for 7 to 14 days.

➲ **Acute otitis media caused by *S. pneumoniae* (penicillin-susceptible strains only), *S. pyogenes, H. influenzae,* or *M. catarrhalis***
Children age 2 months to 12 years: 5 mg/kg P.O. q 12 hours for 5 days. Don't exceed 200 mg per dose.

➲ **Pharyngitis or tonsillitis caused by *S. pyogenes***
Adults: 100 mg P.O. q 12 hours for 5 to 10 days.
Children ages 2 months to 11 years: 5 mg/kg P.O. q 12 hours for 5 to 10 days. Don't exceed 100 mg per dose.

➲ **Uncomplicated UTIs caused by *Escherichia coli, Klebsiella pneumoniae, Proteus mirabilis,* or *Staphylococcus saprophyticus***
Adults: 100 mg P.O. q 12 hours for 7 days.

➲ **Mild to moderate acute maxillary sinusitis caused by *H. influenzae, S. pneumoniae,* or *M. catarrhalis***
Adults and adolescents age 12 and older: 200 mg P.O. q 12 hours for 10 days.

Children ages 2 months to 11 years: 5 mg/kg P.O. q 12 hours for 10 days; maximum is 200 mg/dose.

For patients with creatinine clearance less than 30 ml/minute, increase dosage interval to q 24 hours. Give to dialysis patients three times weekly after dialysis.

Contraindications & cautions

- Contraindicated in patients hypersensitive to drug or other cephalosporins.
- Use cautiously in patients with a history of penicillin hypersensitivity because of risk of cross-sensitivity.
- Use cautiously in patients receiving nephrotoxic drugs because other cephalosporins have been shown to have nephrotoxic potential.
- Use cautiously in breast-feeding women because drug appears in breast milk.

Adverse reactions

CNS: headache.
GI: *diarrhea*, nausea, vomiting, abdominal pain, ***pseudomembranous colitis***.
GU: vaginal fungal infections.
Skin: rash.
Other: hypersensitivity reactions, ***anaphylaxis***.

Interactions

Drug-drug. *Aminoglycosides:* May increase risk of nephrotoxicity. Monitor renal function tests closely.
Antacids, H_2-receptor antagonists: May decrease absorption of cefpodoxime. Avoid using together.
Probenecid: May decrease excretion of cefpodoxime. Monitor patient for toxicity.
Drug-food. *Any food:* May increase absorption. Give tablets with food to enhance absorption. Oral suspension may be given without regard to food.

Nursing considerations

- Before administration, ask patient if he is allergic to penicillins or cephalosporins.
- Monitor renal function and compare with baseline.
- Obtain specimen for culture and sensitivity tests before giving first dose. Therapy may begin while awaiting results.
- Give drug with food to enhance absorption. Shake suspension well before using.
- Store suspension in the refrigerator (36° to 46° F [2° to 8° C]). Discard unused portion after 14 days.
- Monitor patient for superinfection. Drug may cause overgrowth of nonsusceptible bacteria or fungi.

!!ALERT Don't confuse drug with other cephalosporins that sound alike.

Patient teaching

- Tell patient to take drug as prescribed, even after he feels better.
- Instruct patient to take drug with food. If patient is using suspension, tell him to shake container before measuring dose and to keep container refrigerated.
- Tell patient to call prescriber if rash or signs and symptoms of superinfection occur.
- Instruct patient to notify prescriber about loose stools or diarrhea.

cefprozil
Cefzil

Pregnancy risk category B

Indications & dosages

➲ **Pharyngitis or tonsillitis caused by *Streptococcus pyogenes***
Adults and children age 13 and older: 500 mg P.O. daily for at least 10 days.
➲ **Otitis media caused by *Streptococcus pneumoniae, Haemophilus influenzae,* and *Moraxella catarrhalis***
Infants and children ages 6 months to 12 years: 15 mg/kg P.O. q 12 hours for 10 days.
➲ **Secondary bacterial infections of acute bronchitis and acute bacterial worsening of chronic bronchitis caused by *S. pneumoniae, H. influenzae,* and *M. catarrhalis***
Adults and children age 13 and older: 500 mg P.O. q 12 hours for 10 days.
➲ **Uncomplicated skin and skin-structure infections caused by *Staphylococcus aureus* and *S. pyogenes***
Adults and children age 13 and older: 250 or 500 mg P.O. q 12 hours or 500 mg daily for 10 days.
➲ **Acute sinusitis caused by *S. pneumoniae, H. influenzae* (beta-lactamase– positive and –negative strains), and *M. catar-***

rhalis **(including strains that produce beta-lactamase)**
Adults and children age 13 and older: 250 mg P.O. q 12 hours for 10 days; for moderate to severe infection, 500 mg P.O. q 12 hours for 10 days.
Children ages 6 months to 12 years: 7.5 mg/kg P.O. q 12 hours for 10 days; for moderate to severe infections, 15 mg/kg P.O. q 12 hours for 10 days.

If creatinine clearance is less than 30 ml/minute, give 50% after hemodialysis is completed; drug is removed by hemodialysis.

Contraindications & cautions

- Contraindicated in patients hypersensitive to drug or other cephalosporins.
- Use cautiously in patients hypersensitive to penicillin because of possibility of cross-sensitivity with other beta-lactam antibiotics.
- Use cautiously in breast-feeding women and in patients with history of colitis and renal insufficiency.

Adverse reactions

CNS: dizziness, hyperactivity, headache, nervousness, insomnia, confusion, somnolence.
GI: diarrhea, nausea, vomiting, abdominal pain.
GU: genital pruritus, vaginitis.
Hematologic: eosinophilia.
Skin: rash, urticaria, diaper rash.
Other: superinfection, hypersensitivity reactions, serum sickness, ***anaphylaxis***.

Interactions

Drug-drug. *Aminoglycosides:* May increase risk of nephrotoxicity. Monitor renal function tests closely.
Probenecid: May inhibit excretion and increase cefprozil level. Use together cautiously.

Nursing considerations

- Before administration, ask patient if he is allergic to penicillins or cephalosporins.
- Monitor renal function and liver function test results.
- Obtain specimen for culture and sensitivity tests before giving first dose. Therapy may begin while awaiting results.
- Monitor patient for superinfection. May cause overgrowth of nonsusceptible bacteria or fungi.

!!ALERT Don't confuse drug with other cephalosporins that sound alike.

Patient teaching

- Advise patient to take drug as prescribed, even after he feels better.
- Tell patient to shake suspension well before measuring dose.
- Inform patient or parent that oral suspensions contain the drug in a bubble-gum–flavored form to improve palatability and promote compliance in children. Tell him to refrigerate reconstituted suspension and to discard unused drug after 14 days.
- Instruct patient to notify prescriber if rash or signs and symptoms of superinfection occur.

ceftazidime

Ceptaz, Fortaz, Tazicef, Tazidime

Pregnancy risk category B

Indications & dosages

➲ **Serious UTIs and lower respiratory tract infections; skin, gynecologic, intra-abdominal, and CNS infections; bacteremia; and septicemia caused by susceptible microorganisms, such as streptococci (including *Streptococcus pneumoniae* and *S. pyogenes*), penicillinase- and non-penicillinase-producing *Staphylococcus aureus, Escherichia coli, Klebsiella, Proteus, Enterobacter, Haemophilus influenzae, Pseudomonas,* and some strains of *Bacteroides***
Adults and children age 12 and older: 1 to 2 g I.V. or I.M. q 8 to 12 hours; up to 6 g daily in life-threatening infections.
Children ages 1 month to 11 years: 25 to 50 mg/kg I.V. q 8 hours. Maximum dose is 6 g/day. Use sodium carbonate formulation.
Neonates up to age 4 weeks: 30 mg/kg I.V. q 12 hours. Use sodium carbonate formulation.

➲ **Uncomplicated UTIs**
Adults: 250 mg I.V. or I.M. q 12 hours.

➲ **Complicated UTIs**
Adults and children age 12 and older: 500 mg to 1 g I.V. or I.M. q 8 to 12 hours.

If creatinine clearance is 31 to 50 ml/minute, give 1 g q 12 hours; if clearance is 16 to 30 ml/minute, give 1 g q 24 hours; if clearance is 6 to 15 ml/minute, give 500 mg q 24 hours; if clearance is less than 5 ml/minute, give 500 mg q 48 hours. Ceftazidime is removed by hemodialysis; give a supplemental dose of drug after each dialysis session.

Contraindications & cautions

- Contraindicated in patients hypersensitive to drug or other cephalosporins.
- Use cautiously in patients hypersensitive to penicillin because of possibility of cross-sensitivity with other beta-lactam antibiotics.
- Use cautiously in breast-feeding women and in patients with history of colitis or renal insufficiency.

Adverse reactions

CNS: headache, dizziness, paresthesia, ***seizures***.
CV: *phlebitis, thrombophlebitis.*
GI: ***pseudomembranous colitis***, nausea, vomiting, diarrhea, abdominal cramps.
GU: vaginitis, candidiasis.
Hematologic: eosinophilia, thrombocytosis, ***leukopenia***, hemolytic anemia, ***agranulocytosis***, ***thrombocytopenia***.
Skin: *maculopapular and erythematous rashes, urticaria, pain, induration, sterile abscesses, tissue sloughing at injection site.*
Other: hypersensitivity reactions, serum sickness, ***anaphylaxis***.

Interactions

Drug-drug. *Aminoglycosides:* May cause additive or synergistic effect against some strains of *Pseudomonas aeruginosa* and *Enterobacteriaceae;* may increase risk of nephrotoxicity. Monitor patient for effects and monitor renal function.
Chloramphenicol: May cause antagonistic effect. Avoid using together.

Nursing considerations

- Before administration, ask patient if he is allergic to penicillins or cephalosporins.
- Obtain specimen for culture and sensitivity tests before giving first dose. Therapy may begin while awaiting results.
- For I.M. administration, inject deep into a large muscle, such as the gluteus maximus or the lateral aspect of the thigh.
- If large doses are given, therapy is prolonged, or patient is at high risk, monitor patient for signs and symptoms of superinfection.

!!**ALERT** Commercially available preparations contain either sodium carbonate (Fortaz, Tazicef, Tazidime) or arginine (Ceptaz) to facilitate dissolution of drug. Safety and efficacy of solutions containing arginine in children younger than age 12 haven't been established.

!!**ALERT** Don't confuse drug with other cephalosporins that sound alike.

Patient teaching

- Tell patient to report adverse reactions or signs and symptoms of superinfection promptly.
- Instruct patient to report discomfort at I.V. insertion site.
- Advise patient to notify prescriber about loose stools or diarrhea.

ceftizoxime sodium

Cefizox

Pregnancy risk category B

Indications & dosages

➲ **Serious UTIs, lower respiratory tract infections, gynecologic infections, bacteremia, septicemia, meningitis, intra-abdominal infections, bone and joint infections, and skin infections caused by susceptible microorganisms, such as streptococci (including *Streptococcus pneumoniae* and *S. pyogenes*), *Staphylococcus aureus, S. epidermidis, Escherichia coli, Haemophilus influenzae,* and *Klebsiella, Enterobacter, Proteus, Peptostreptococcus,* and some *Pseudomonas* species**
Adults: Usual dosage is 1 to 2 g I.V. or I.M. q 8 to 12 hours. In life-threatening infections, give up to 2 g q 4 hours.
Children older than age 6 months: 50 mg/kg I.V. q 6 to 8 hours. For serious infections, up to 200 mg/kg/day in divided doses may be used. Don't exceed 12 g/day.
➲ **Uncomplicated gonorrhea**
Adults: 1 g I.M. as a single dose.

If creatinine clearance is 50 to 79 ml/minute, give 500 mg to 1.5 g q 8 hours; if clearance is 5 to 49 ml/minute, give 250 mg to 1 g q 12 hours; if clearance is less than 5 ml/minute or patient undergoes hemodialysis, give 500 mg to 1 g q 48 hours, or 250 to 500 mg q 24 hours.

Contraindications & cautions

- Contraindicated in patients hypersensitive to drug or other cephalosporins.
- Use cautiously in patients hypersensitive to penicillin because of possibility of cross-sensitivity with other beta-lactam antibiotics.
- Use cautiously in breast-feeding women and in patients with history of colitis or renal insufficiency.

Adverse reactions

CNS: fever.
CV: *phlebitis, thrombophlebitis.*
GI: ***pseudomembranous colitis***, nausea, anorexia, vomiting, *diarrhea.*
GU: vaginitis.
Hematologic: ***transient neutropenia***, eosinophilia, hemolytic anemia, ***thrombocytosis***, anemia, ***thrombocytopenia***.
Respiratory: dyspnea.
Skin: *maculopapular and erythematous rashes, urticaria, pain, induration, sterile abscesses, tissue sloughing at injection site.*
Other: hypersensitivity reactions, serum sickness, ***anaphylaxis***.

Interactions

Drug-drug. *Aminoglycosides:* May increase nephrotoxicity. Monitor renal function.
Probenecid: May inhibit excretion and increase ceftizoxime level. Probenecid may be used for this effect.

Nursing considerations

- Before administration, ask patient if he is allergic to penicillins or cephalosporins.
- Obtain specimen for culture and sensitivity tests before giving first dose. Therapy may begin while awaiting results.
- To prepare I.M. injection, mix 1.5 ml of diluent per 500 mg of drug. For I.M. administration, inject deep into a large muscle, such as the gluteus maximus or the lateral aspect of the thigh. Divide larger doses (2 g) and give at two separate sites.
- If large doses are given, therapy is prolonged, or patient is at high risk, monitor patient for signs or symptoms of superinfection.

!! ALERT Don't confuse drug with other cephalosporins that sound alike.

Patient teaching

- Tell patient to report adverse reactions and signs and symptoms of superinfection promptly.
- Instruct patient to report discomfort at I.V. site.
- Tell patient to notify prescriber about loose stools or diarrhea.

ceftriaxone sodium
Rocephin

Pregnancy risk category B

Indications & dosages

➲ Uncomplicated gonococcal vulvovaginitis
Adults: 125 mg I.M. as a single dose, plus azithromycin 1 g P.O. as a single dose or doxycycline 100 mg P.O. b.i.d. for 7 days.

➲ UTIs; lower respiratory tract, gynecologic, bone and joint, intra-abdominal, skin, and skin-structure infections; septicemia
Adults and children older than age 12: 1 to 2 g I.M. or I.V. daily or in equally divided doses q 12 hours. Total daily dose shouldn't exceed 4 g.
Children age 12 and younger: 50 to 75 mg/kg I.M. or I.V., not to exceed 2 g/day, given in divided doses q 12 hours.

➲ Meningitis
Adults and children: Initially, 100 mg/kg I.M. or I.V. Don't exceed 4g; then 100 mg/kg I.M. or I.V., given once daily or in divided doses q 12 hours, not to exceed 4 g, for 7 to 14 days.

➲ Perioperative prevention
Adults: 1 g I.V. as a single dose 30 minutes to 2 hours before surgery.

➲ Acute bacterial otitis media
Children: 50 mg/kg I.M. as a single dose. Don't exceed 1 g.

➲ Neurologic complications, carditis, and arthritis from penicillin G–refractory Lyme disease♦
Adults: 2 g I.V. daily for 14 to 28 days.

Contraindications & cautions

- Contraindicated in patients hypersensitive to drug or other cephalosporins.
- Use cautiously in patients hypersensitive to penicillin because of possibility of cross-sensitivity with other beta-lactam antibiotics.
- Use cautiously in breast-feeding women and in patients with history of colitis and renal insufficiency.

Adverse reactions

CNS: fever, headache, dizziness.
CV: phlebitis.
GI: ***pseudomembranous colitis***, diarrhea.
GU: genital pruritus, candidiasis.
Hematologic: eosinophilia, thrombocytosis, ***leukopenia***.
Skin: pain, induration, tenderness at injection site, *rash*, pruritus.
Other: hypersensitivity reactions, serum sickness, ***anaphylaxis***, chills.

Interactions

Drug-drug. *Aminoglycosides:* May cause synergistic effect against some strains of *P. aeruginosa* and *Enterobacteriaceae* species. Monitor patient.
Probenecid: High doses (1 g or 2 g daily) may enhance hepatic clearance of ceftriaxone and shorten its half-life. Avoid using together.

Nursing considerations

- Before administration, ask patient if he is allergic to penicillins or cephalosporins.
- Obtain specimen for culture and sensitivity tests before giving first dose. Therapy may begin while awaiting results.
- A commercially available I.M. kit containing 1% lidocaine as a diluent is available from the manufacturer.
- For I.M. administration, inject deep into a large muscle, such as the gluteus maximus or the lateral aspect of the thigh.
- If large doses are given, therapy is prolonged, or patient is at high risk, monitor patient for signs and symptoms of superinfection.
- Monitor PT and INR in patients with impaired vitamin K synthesis or low vitamin K stores. Vitamin K therapy may be needed.
- Drug is commonly used in home antibiotic programs for outpatient treatment of serious infections such as osteomyelitis and community-acquired pneumonia.

!!ALERT Don't confuse drug with other cephalosporins that sound alike.

Patient teaching

- Tell patient to report adverse reactions promptly.
- Instruct patient to report discomfort at I.V. insertion site.
- Teach patient and family receiving home care how to prepare and give drug.
- If home care patient is diabetic and is testing his urine for glucose, tell him drug may affect results of cupric sulfate tests; he should use an enzymatic test instead.
- Tell patient to notify prescriber about loose stools or diarrhea.

cefuroxime axetil
Ceftin

cefuroxime sodium
Zinacef

Pregnancy risk category B

Indications & dosages

➲ Pharyngitis, tonsillitis, infections of the urinary and lower respiratory tracts, and skin and skin-structure infections caused by *Streptococcus pneumoniae* and *S. pyogenes, Haemophilus influenzae, Staphylococcus aureus, Escherichia coli, Moraxella catarrhalis* (including beta-lactamase–producing strains), *Neisseria gonorrhoeae*, and *Klebsiella* and *Enterobacter* species
Adults and children age 12 and older: 250 mg cefuroxime axetil P.O. q 12 hours. For severe infections, increase dosage to 500 mg q 12 hours.

➲ Serious lower respiratory tract infections, UTIs, skin and skin-structure infections, bone and joint infections, septicemia, meningitis, and gonorrhea
Adults and children age 12 and older: 750 mg to 1.5 g cefuroxime sodium I.M. or I.V. q 8 hours for 5 to 10 days. For life-threatening infections and infections caused by less susceptible organisms, 1.5 g I.M. or I.V. q 6 hours; for bacterial meningitis, up to 3 g I.V. q 8 hours.

Children and infants older than age 3 months: 50 to 100 mg/kg/day cefuroxime sodium I.M. or I.V. in equally divided doses q 6 to 8 hours. Use higher dosage of 100 mg/kg/day, not to exceed maximum adult dosage, for more severe or serious infections. For bacterial meningitis, 200 to 240 mg/kg cefuroxime sodium I.V. in divided doses q 6 to 8 hours.

➲ **Uncomplicated UTIs**

Adults: 125 to 250 mg P.O. q 12 hours for 7 to 10 days.

➲ **Otitis media**

Children ages 3 months to 12 years: 250 mg P.O. q 12 hours for 10 days for children who can swallow tablets whole. Or, 30 mg/kg/day of oral suspension P.O. in two divided doses for 10 days for children who can't swallow tablets.

➲ **Pharyngitis and tonsillitis**

Children ages 3 months to 12 years: 125 mg P.O. q 12 hours for 10 days, in children who can swallow tablets whole. Or, 20 mg/kg daily of oral suspension in two divided doses for 10 days for children who can't swallow tablets.

➲ **Perioperative prevention**

Adults: 1.5 g I.V. 30 to 60 minutes before surgery; in lengthy operations, 750 mg I.V. or I.M. q 8 hours. For open-heart surgery, 1.5 g I.V. at induction of anesthesia and then q 12 hours for a total dose of 6 g.

➲ **Early Lyme disease (erythema migrans) caused by *Borrelia burgdorferi***

Adults and children age 13 and older: 500 mg P.O. b.i.d. for 20 days.

➲ **Secondary bacterial infection of acute bronchitis**

Adults: 250 to 500 mg tablets P.O. b.i.d. for 5 to 10 days.

➲ **Uncomplicated gonorrhea**

Adults: 1.5 g I.M. with 1 g probenecid P.O. for one dose. Alternatively, 1 g P.O. as a single dose.

➲ **Acute bacterial maxillary sinusitis caused by *Streptococcus pneumoniae* or *Haemophilus influenzae* (only strains that don't produce beta-lactamase)**

Adults and children age 13 and older: 250-mg tablet P.O. b.i.d. for 10 days.

Children ages 3 months to 12 years: 30 mg/kg/day oral suspension P.O. in two divided doses for 10 days.

In patients with creatinine clearance of 10 to 20 ml/minute, give 750 mg I.M. or I.V. q 12 hours; if clearance is less than 10 ml/minute, give 750 mg I.M. or I.V. q 24 hours.

Contraindications & cautions

- Contraindicated in patients hypersensitive to drug or other cephalosporins.
- Use cautiously in patients hypersensitive to penicillin because of possibility of cross-sensitivity with other beta-lactam antibiotics.
- Use cautiously in breast-feeding women and in patients with history of colitis or renal insufficiency.

Adverse reactions

CV: *phlebitis, thrombophlebitis.*

GI: ***pseudomembranous colitis***, nausea, anorexia, vomiting, *diarrhea.*

Hematologic: ***transient neutropenia***, eosinophilia, *hemolytic anemia,* ***thrombocytopenia***.

Skin: *maculopapular and erythematous rashes, urticaria, pain, induration, sterile abscesses, temperature elevation, tissue sloughing at I.M. injection site.*

Other: hypersensitivity reactions, serum sickness, ***anaphylaxis***.

Interactions

Drug-drug. *Aminoglycosides:* May cause synergistic activity against some organisms; may increase nephrotoxicity. Monitor patient's renal function closely.

Loop diuretics: May increase risk of adverse renal reactions. Monitor renal function test results closely.

Probenecid: May inhibit excretion and increase cefuroxime level. Probenecid may be used for this effect.

Drug-food. *Any food:* May increase absorption. Give drug with food.

Nursing considerations

- Before administration, ask patient if he is allergic to penicillins or cephalosporins.
- Obtain specimen for culture and sensitivity tests before giving first dose. Therapy may begin while awaiting results.
- For I.M. administration, inject deep into a large muscle, such as the gluteus maximus or the lateral aspect of the thigh.
- Absorption of cefuroxime axetil is enhanced by food.
- Cefuroxime axetil tablets may be crushed, if absolutely necessary, for patients who

can't swallow tablets. Tablets may be dissolved in small amounts of apple, orange, or grape juice or chocolate milk. However, the drug has a bitter taste that is difficult to mask, even with food.

!!ALERT Cefuroxime axetil film-coated tablet and oral suspension aren't bioequivalent. Don't substitute on a mg/mg basis.

- If large doses are given, therapy is prolonged, or patient is at high risk, monitor patient for signs and symptoms of superinfection.

!!ALERT Don't confuse drug with other cephalosporins that sound alike.

Patient teaching

- Tell patient to take drug as prescribed, even after he feels better.
- Instruct patient to take oral form with food.
- If patient has difficulty swallowing tablets, show him how to dissolve or crush tablets but warn him that the bitter taste is hard to mask, even with food.
- If suspension is being used, tell patient to shake container well before measuring dose.
- Instruct patient to notify prescriber about rash or evidence of superinfection.
- Advise patient receiving drug I.V. to report discomfort at I.V. insertion site.
- Tell patient to notify prescriber about loose stools or diarrhea.

celecoxib
Celebrex

Pregnancy risk category C; D in 3rd trimester

Indications & dosages

➲ Relief from signs and symptoms of osteoarthritis
Adults: 200 mg P.O. daily as a single dose or divided equally b.i.d.

➲ Relief from signs and symptoms of rheumatoid arthritis
Adults: 100 to 200 mg P.O. b.i.d.

➲ Adjunctive treatment for familial adenomatous polyposis to reduce the number of adenomatous colorectal polyps
Adults: 400 mg P.O. b.i.d. with food for up to 6 months.
Elderly: Start at lowest dosage.

➲ Acute pain and primary dysmenorrhea
Adults: 400 mg P.O., initially, followed by an additional 200-mg dose if needed. On subsequent days, 200 mg P.O. b.i.d., p.r.n.
Elderly: Start at lowest dosage.

For patients weighing less than 50 kg (110 lb), start at lowest dosage. For patients with Child-Pugh class II hepatic impairment, start with reduced dosage.

Contraindications & cautions

- Contraindicated in patients hypersensitive to drug, sulfonamides, aspirin, or other NSAIDs.
- Contraindicated in those with severe hepatic impairment.
- Contraindicated in women in the third trimester of pregnancy.
- Use cautiously in patients with history of ulcers or GI bleeding, advanced renal disease, dehydration, anemia, symptomatic liver disease, hypertension, edema, heart failure, or asthma and in poor CYP2C9 metabolizers.
- Use cautiously in elderly or debilitated patients.

Adverse reactions

CNS: dizziness, *headache*, insomnia.
CV: peripheral edema.
EENT: pharyngitis, rhinitis, sinusitis.
GI: abdominal pain, diarrhea, dyspepsia, flatulence, nausea.
Metabolic: hyperchloremia.
Musculoskeletal: back pain.
Respiratory: upper respiratory tract infection.
Skin: rash.
Other: accidental injury.

Interactions

Drug-drug. *ACE inhibitors:* May decrease antihypertensive effects. Monitor patient's blood pressure.
Aluminum- and magnesium-containing antacids: May decrease celecoxib level. Separate doses.
Aspirin: May increase risk of ulcers; low aspirin dosages can be used safely to reduce the risk of CV events. Monitor patient for signs and symptoms of GI bleeding.
Fluconazole: May increase celecoxib level. Reduce dosage of celecoxib to minimal effective dose.

Furosemide, thiazides: May reduce sodium excretion caused by diuretics, leading to sodium retention. Monitor patient for swelling and increased blood pressure.
Lithium: May increase lithium level. Monitor lithium level closely during treatment.
Warfarin: May increase PT and bleeding complications. Monitor PT and INR, and check for signs and symptoms of bleeding.
Drug-herb. *Dong quai, feverfew, garlic, ginger, horse chestnut, red clover:* May increase risk of bleeding. Discourage use together.
White willow: Herb and drug contain similar components. Discourage use together.
Drug-lifestyle. *Long-term alcohol use, smoking:* May cause GI irritation or bleeding. Check for signs and symptoms of bleeding.

Nursing considerations

!!ALERT Patients may be allergic to drug if they are allergic to or have had anaphylactic reactions to sulfonamides, aspirin, or other NSAIDs.

- Patient with history of ulcers or GI bleeding is at higher risk for GI bleeding while taking NSAIDs such as celecoxib. Other risk factors for GI bleeding include treatment with corticosteroids or anticoagulants, longer duration of NSAID treatment, smoking, alcoholism, older age, and poor overall health.
- Although drug may be used with low aspirin dosages, the combination may increase risk of GI bleeding.
- Watch for signs and symptoms of overt and occult bleeding.
- NSAIDs such as celecoxib can cause fluid retention; monitor patient with hypertension, edema, or heart failure.
- Assess patient for CV risk factors before therapy.
- Drug may be hepatotoxic; watch for signs and symptoms of liver toxicity.
- Before starting drug therapy, rehydrate dehydrated patient.
- Drug can be given without regard to meals, but food may decrease GI upset.

!!ALERT Don't confuse Celebrex with Cerebyx or Celexa.

Patient teaching

- Tell patient to report history of allergic reactions to sulfonamides, aspirin, or other NSAIDs before starting therapy.
- Instruct patient to promptly report signs of GI bleeding such as blood in vomit, urine, or stool; or black, tarry stools.
- Advise patient to immediately report rash, unexplained weight gain, or swelling.
- Tell woman to notify prescriber if she becomes pregnant or is planning to become pregnant during drug therapy.
- Instruct patient to take drug with food if stomach upset occurs.
- Teach patient that all NSAIDs, including celecoxib, may harm the liver. Advise patient to stop therapy and notify prescriber immediately if he experiences signs and symptoms of liver toxicity, including nausea, fatigue, lethargy, itching, yellowing of skin or eyes, right upper quadrant tenderness, and flulike syndrome.
- Inform patient that it may take several days before he feels consistent pain relief.
- Advise patient that use of OTC NSAIDs in combination with celecoxib may increase the risk of GI toxicity.

cephalexin hydrochloride
Keftab

cephalexin monohydrate
Apo-Cephalex†, Biocef, Keflex, Novo-Lexin†, Nu-Cephalex†

Pregnancy risk category B

Indications & dosages

➲ **Respiratory tract, GI tract, skin, soft-tissue, bone, and joint infections and otitis media caused by *Escherichia coli* and other coliform bacteria, group A beta-hemolytic streptococci, *Klebsiella* species, *Proteus mirabilis, Streptococcus pneumoniae,* and staphylococci**
Adults: 250 mg to 1 g P.O. q 6 hours or 500 mg q 12 hours. Maximum 4 g daily.
Children: 25 to 50 mg/kg/day P.O. in two to four equally divided doses. In severe infections, dose can be doubled.

For adults with impaired renal function, initial dose is the same. Then, for those with creatinine clearance of 11 to 40 ml/minute, give 500 mg P.O. q 8 to 12 hours; for clearance of 5 to 10 ml/minute, give 250 mg P.O. q 12 hours; and for clearance of less than 5 ml/minute, give 250 mg P.O. q 12 to 24 hours.

Contraindications & cautions

- Contraindicated in patients hypersensitive to cephalosporins.
- Use cautiously in patients hypersensitive to penicillin because of possibility of cross-sensitivity with other beta-lactam antibiotics.
- Use cautiously in breast-feeding women and in patients with history of colitis or renal insufficiency.

Adverse reactions

CNS: dizziness, headache, fatigue, agitation, confusion, hallucinations.
GI: ***pseudomembranous colitis***, *nausea, anorexia*, vomiting, *diarrhea*, gastritis, glossitis, dyspepsia, abdominal pain, anal pruritus, tenesmus, oral candidiasis.
GU: genital pruritus, candidiasis, vaginitis, interstitial nephritis.
Hematologic: ***neutropenia***, eosinophilia, anemia, ***thrombocytopenia***.
Musculoskeletal: arthritis, arthralgia, joint pain.
Skin: *maculopapular and erythematous rashes, urticaria*.
Other: hypersensitivity reactions, serum sickness, ***anaphylaxis***.

Interactions

Drug-drug. *Aminoglycosides:* May increase risk of nephrotoxicity. Avoid using together.
Probenecid: May increase cephalosporin level. Probenecid may be used for this effect.

Nursing considerations

- Ask patient about past reaction to cephalosporin or penicillin therapy before giving first dose.
- Obtain specimen for culture and sensitivity tests before giving first dose. Therapy may begin while awaiting results.
- To prepare oral suspension: Add required amount of water to powder in two portions. Shake well after each addition. After mixing, store in refrigerator. Mixture will remain stable for 14 days. Keep tightly closed and shake well before using.
- If large doses are given or if therapy is prolonged, monitor patient for superinfection, especially if patient is high risk.
- Treat group A beta-hemolytic streptococcal infections for a minimum of 10 days.

!!ALERT Don't confuse drug with other cephalosporins that sound alike.

Patient teaching

- Tell patient to take drug exactly as prescribed, even after he feels better.
- Instruct patient to take drug with food or milk to lessen GI discomfort. If patient is taking suspension form, instruct him to shake container well before measuring dose and to store in refrigerator.
- Tell patient to notify prescriber if rash or signs and symptoms of superinfection develop.

cetirizine hydrochloride
Zyrtec

Pregnancy risk category B

Indications & dosages

➲ Seasonal allergic rhinitis
Adults and children age 6 and older: 5 to 10 mg P.O. once daily.
Children ages 2 to 5: 2.5 mg P.O. once daily. Maximum daily dose is 5 mg.

➲ Perennial allergic rhinitis, chronic urticaria
Adults and children age 6 and older: 5 to 10 mg P.O. once daily.
Children ages 6 months to 5 years: 2.5 mg P.O. once daily; in children ages 1 to 5, increase to maximum of 5 mg daily in two divided doses.

In adults and children age 6 and older receiving hemodialysis, those with hepatic impairment, and those with creatinine clearance less than 31 ml/minute, give 5 mg P.O. daily. Don't use in children younger than age 6 with renal or hepatic impairment.

Contraindications & cautions

- Contraindicated in patients hypersensitive to drug or to hydroxyzine and in breast-feeding women.
- Use cautiously in patients with renal or hepatic impairment.

Adverse reactions

CNS: *somnolence*, fatigue, dizziness, headache.
EENT: pharyngitis.
GI: dry mouth, nausea, vomiting, abdominal distress.

Interactions

Drug-drug. *CNS depressants:* May cause additive effect. Avoid using together.
Theophylline: May decrease cetirizine clearance. Monitor patient closely.
Drug-lifestyle. *Alcohol use:* May cause additive effect. Discourage use together.

Nursing considerations

- Stop drug 4 days before diagnostic skin testing because antihistamines can prevent, reduce, or mask positive skin test response.

!!ALERT Don't confuse Zyrtec with Zyprexa or Zantac.

Patient teaching

- Warn patient not to perform hazardous activities until CNS effects of drug are known. Somnolence is a common adverse reaction.
- Advise patient not to use alcohol or other CNS depressants while taking drug.
- Tell patient that coffee or tea may reduce drowsiness.
- Inform patient that sugarless gum, hard candy, or ice chips may relieve dry mouth.

cetuximab
Erbitux

Pregnancy risk category C

Indications & dosages

➲ **Epidermal growth factor–expressing metastatic colorectal cancer, alone in patients intolerant of irinotecan-based chemotherapy or with irinotecan in patients refractory to irinotecan-based chemotherapy**
Adults: Loading dose, 400 mg/m^2 I.V. over 2 hours (maximum, 5 ml/minute), alone or with irinotecan. Maintenance dosage, 250 mg/m^2 I.V. weekly over 1 hour (maximum, 5 ml/minute). Premedication with an H_1 antagonist (such as 50 mg of diphenhydramine I.V.) is recommended.

If patient develops a grade 1 or 2 infusion reaction, permanently reduce infusion rate by 50%. If patient develops a grade 3 or 4 infusion reaction, stop drug immediately and permanently. If patient develops a severe acneiform rash, follow these guidelines:

- After first occurrence, delay cetuximab infusion 1 to 2 weeks. If patient improves, continue at 250 mg/m^2. If patient doesn't improve, stop drug.
- After second occurrence, delay cetuximab infusion 1 to 2 weeks. If patient improves, reduce dose to 200 mg/m^2. If patient doesn't improve, stop drug.
- After third occurrence, delay cetuximab infusion 1 to 2 weeks. If patient improves, reduce dose to 150 mg/m^2. If patient doesn't improve, stop drug.
- After fourth occurrence, stop drug.

Contraindications & cautions

- Use cautiously in patients hypersensitive to cetuximab, its components, or murine proteins.

Adverse reactions

CNS: *asthenia, depression, fever, headache, insomnia.*
CV: *edema.*
EENT: *conjunctivitis.*
GI: *abdominal pain, anorexia, constipation, diarrhea, dyspepsia, nausea, stomatitis, vomiting.*
GU: ***acute renal failure.***
Hematologic: *anemia,* LEUKOPENIA.
Metabolic: *dehydration, weight loss.*
Musculoskeletal: *back pain.*
Respiratory: *cough, dyspnea,* ***pulmonary embolus.***
Skin: ***acneiform rash,*** *alopecia, maculopapular rash, nail disorder, pruritus.*
Other: *infection,* ***infusion reaction,*** *pain,* ***sepsis.***

Interactions

Drug-lifestyle. *Sun exposure:* May worsen skin reactions. Advise patient to avoid excessive sun exposure.

Nursing considerations

- Premedication with diphenhydramine 50 mg I.V. is recommended.

!!ALERT Severe infusion reactions, including acute airway obstruction, urticaria, and hypotension may occur, usually with the first infusion. If a severe infusion reaction occurs, stop drug immediately and give symptomatic treatment.

- Keep epinephrine, corticosteroids, I.V. antihistamines, bronchodilators, and oxygen available to treat severe infusion reactions.
- Manage mild to moderate infusion reactions by decreasing infusion rate and pre-

medicating with an antihistamine for subsequent infusions.

- Monitor patient for infusion reactions for 1 hour after infusion.
- Assess patient for acute onset or worsening of pulmonary symptoms. If interstitial lung disease is confirmed, stop drug.
- Monitor patient for skin toxicity, which starts most often during first 2 weeks of therapy. Consider treatment with topical and oral antibiotics.
- It's unknown if drug appears in breast milk. Women should stop breast-feeding during therapy and for 60 days after last dose.

Patient teaching

- Tell patient to promptly report adverse reactions.
- Inform patient that skin reactions may occur, typically during the first 2 weeks of treatment.
- Advise patient to avoid prolonged or unprotected sun exposure during treatment.

chlorambucil

Leukeran

Pregnancy risk category D

Indications & dosages

➲ Chronic lymphocytic leukemia; malignant lymphomas, including lymphosarcoma, giant follicular lymphoma, and Hodgkin's disease

Adults: 0.1 to 0.2 mg/kg P.O. daily for 3 to 6 weeks, then adjusted for maintenance (usually 4 to 10 mg daily); or, 3 to 6 mg/m^2 P.O. daily.

Children: 0.1 to 0.2 mg/kg P.O. or 4.5 mg/m^2 P.O. daily for 3 to 6 weeks.

Reduce first dose if given within 4 weeks after a full course of radiation therapy or myelosuppressive drugs, or if pretreatment leukocyte or platelet counts are depressed from bone marrow disease.

➲ Macroglobulinemia♦

Adults: 2 to 10 mg P.O. daily for up to 9 years. Or, 8 mg/m^2 P.O. daily with prednisone for 10 days; repeat q 6 to 8 weeks p.r.n.

➲ Nephrotic syndrome♦

Children: 0.1 to 0.2 mg/kg P.O. daily with prednisone for 8 to 12 weeks.

➲ Intractable idiopathic uveitis, Behçet's syndrome♦

Adults: 6 to 12 mg or 0.1 to 0.2 mg/kg P.O. daily for at least 1 year.

Contraindications & cautions

- Contraindicated in patients with hypersensitivity or resistance to previous therapy. Patients hypersensitive to other alkylating drugs may also be hypersensitive to chlorambucil.
- Use cautiously in patients with history of head trauma or seizures and in patients receiving other drugs that lower the seizure threshold.
- Use cautiously within 4 weeks of a full course of radiation or chemotherapy.

Adverse reactions

CNS: ***seizures***, peripheral neuropathy, tremor, muscle twitching, confusion, agitation, ataxia, flaccid paresis.
GI: *nausea, vomiting*, stomatitis, diarrhea.
GU: *azoospermia, infertility*, sterile cystitis.
Hematologic: ***neutropenia, bone marrow suppression, thrombocytopenia***, anemia, *myelosuppression*.
Hepatic: ***hepatotoxicity***.
Respiratory: interstitial pneumonitis, ***pulmonary fibrosis***.
Skin: rash, ***erythema multiforme***, epidermal necrolysis, ***Stevens-Johnson syndrome***.
Other: drug fever, hypersensitivity reactions, ***secondary malignancies***.

Interactions

Drug-drug. *Anticoagulants, aspirin:* May increase risk of bleeding. Avoid using together.
Myelosuppressives: May increase myelosuppression. Monitor patient.

Nursing considerations

- Monitor CBC with differential.
- Monitor patient for neutropenia, which may not appear until after the third week of treatment. The neutrophil count may continue to decrease for up to 10 days after treatment ends.
- The absolute neutrophil count may be used to better calculate the patient's immunosuppressive state.
- Monitor uric acid level. To prevent hyperuricemia with resulting uric acid nephropathy, allopurinol may be used with adequate hydration.

• If WBC count falls below 2,000/mm^3 or granulocyte count falls below 1,000/mm^3, follow institutional policy for infection control in immunocompromised patients. Patients may receive injections of WBC colony-stimulating factor to increase WBC count recovery. Severe neutropenia is reversible up to cumulative dose of 6.5 mg/kg in a single course.
• Therapeutic effects are frequently accompanied by toxicity.
• To prevent bleeding, avoid all I.M. injections when platelet count is below 50,000/mm^3.
• Anticipate blood transfusions during treatment because of cumulative anemia. Patient may receive injections of RBC colony-stimulating factor to promote RBC production and decrease need for blood transfusions.

Patient teaching

• Advise patient to watch for signs of infection (fever, sore throat, fatigue) and bleeding (easy bruising, nosebleeds, bleeding gums, tarry stools). Tell patient to take temperature daily.
• Instruct patient to avoid OTC products containing aspirin and NSAIDs.
• Advise women to stop breast-feeding during therapy because of risk of toxicity to infant.
• Advise women of childbearing age to avoid becoming pregnant during therapy and to notify prescriber immediately if pregnancy is suspected.

chlordiazepoxide hydrochloride

Apo-Chlordiazepoxide†, Librium, Novo-Poxide†

Pregnancy risk category NR
Controlled substance schedule IV

Indications & dosages

➲ **Mild to moderate anxiety**
Adults: 5 to 10 mg P.O. t.i.d. or q.i.d.
Children older than age 6: 5 mg P.O. b.i.d. to q.i.d. Maximum, 10 mg P.O. b.i.d. or t.i.d.
➲ **Severe anxiety**
Adults: 20 to 25 mg P.O. t.i.d. or q.i.d.
Elderly patients: 5 mg P.O. b.i.d. to q.i.d.
For debilitated patients, 5 mg P.O. b.i.d. to q.i.d.
➲ **Withdrawal symptoms of acute alcoholism**
Adults: 50 to 100 mg P.O., I.M., or I.V. Repeat in 2 to 4 hours, p.r.n. Maximum, 300 mg daily.
➲ **Preoperative apprehension and anxiety**
Adults: 5 to 10 mg P.O. t.i.d. or q.i.d. on day before surgery; or 50 to 100 mg I.M. 1 hour before surgery.

Contraindications & cautions

• Contraindicated in patients hypersensitive to drug and in pregnant women, especially in first trimester.
• Use cautiously in patients with mental depression, porphyria, or hepatic or renal disease.

Adverse reactions

CNS: *drowsiness, lethargy,* ataxia, confusion, extrapyramidal reactions, minor changes in EEG patterns.
CV: edema.
GI: nausea, constipation.
GU: menstrual irregularities.
Hematologic: ***agranulocytosis***.
Hepatic: jaundice.
Skin: *swelling and pain at injection site,* skin eruptions.
Other: altered libido.

Interactions

Drug-drug. *Cimetidine:* May decrease chlordiazepoxide clearance and increases risk of adverse reactions. Monitor patient carefully.
CNS depressants: May increase CNS depression. Use together cautiously.
Digoxin: May increase digoxin level and risk of toxicity. Monitor patient and digoxin level closely.
Disulfiram: May decrease clearance and increase half-life of chlordiazepoxide. Monitor patient for enhanced effects. Consider dosage adjustment.
Fluconazole, itraconazole, ketoconazole, miconazole: May increase and prolong chlordiazepoxide levels, CNS depression, and psychomotor impairment. Avoid using together.
Levodopa: May decrease control of parkinsonian symptoms in patients with Parkinson's disease. Use together cautiously.
Drug-herb. *Kava:* May increase sedation. Discourage use together.

Drug-lifestyle. *Alcohol use:* May cause additive CNS effects. Discourage use together. *Smoking:* May decrease effectiveness of benzodiazepines. Monitor patient closely.

Nursing considerations

!!ALERT Chlordiazepoxide 5-mg and 25-mg unit-dose capsules may look similar in color when viewed through the package. When using unit doses of this or any product, verify contents and read label carefully.
- Long-term effectiveness of drug hasn't been established.
- Injectable form (as hydrochloride) comes in two types of ampules—as diluent and as powdered drug. Read directions carefully.
- Keep powder refrigerated and away from light; mix just before use and discard remainder.
- For I.M. use, add 2 ml of diluent to powder and agitate gently until clear. Use immediately. I.M. form may be absorbed erratically.
- Monitor hepatic, renal, and hematopoietic function periodically in patients receiving repeated or prolonged therapy.

!!ALERT Use of this drug may lead to abuse and addiction. Don't withdraw drug abruptly after long-term administration because withdrawal symptoms may occur.

Patient teaching

- Warn patient to avoid hazardous activities that require alertness and good coordination until effects of drug are known.
- Tell patient to avoid alcohol while taking drug.
- Notify patient that smoking may decrease drug's effectiveness.
- Warn patient not to abruptly stop the drug because withdrawal symptoms may occur.
- Warn woman to avoid use during pregnancy.

chloroquine hydrochloride
Aralen HCl

chloroquine phosphate
Aralen Phosphate

Pregnancy risk category C

Indications & dosages

➲ Acute malarial attacks caused by *Plasmodium vivax, P. malariae, P. ovale,* and susceptible strains of *P. falciparum*
Adults: Initially, 600 mg base P.O.; then 300 mg base at 6, 24, and 48 hours. Or, initially, 160 to 200 mg base I.M., repeated in 6 hours, p.r.n. Switch patient to oral therapy as soon as possible.
Children: Initially, 10 mg/kg base P.O.; then 5 mg/kg base at 6, 24, and 48 hours. Don't exceed adult dose. Or, initially, 5 mg/kg base I.M., repeated in 6 hours, p.r.n. Don't exceed 10 mg/kg base in 24 hours. Switch patient to oral therapy as soon as possible.

➲ To prevent malaria
Adults: 300 mg base P.O. once weekly on the same day each week, for 1 to 2 weeks before entering a malaria-endemic area and continued for 4 weeks after leaving the area. If treatment begins after exposure, give 600 mg base P.O. initially, in two divided doses 6 hours apart, followed by the usual dosing regimen.
Children: 5 mg/kg base P.O. once weekly on the same day each week, for 1 to 2 weeks before entering a malaria-endemic area and continued for 4 weeks after leaving the area. Don't exceed 300 mg. If treatment begins after exposure, give 10 mg/kg base P.O. initially, in two divided doses 6 hours apart, followed by the usual dosing regimen.

➲ Extraintestinal amebiasis
Adults: 600 mg base P.O. once daily for 2 days; then 300 mg base daily for 2 to 3 weeks. Treatment is usually combined with an intestinal amebicide. When oral therapy isn't feasible, give 160 to 200 mg base I.M. daily for 10 to 12 days. Resume oral therapy as soon as possible.
Children: 10 mg/kg base P.O. once daily for 2 to 3 weeks. Maximum dose is 300 mg base daily.

Contraindications & cautions

- Contraindicated in patients hypersensitive to drug and in those with retinal or visual field changes or porphyria.
- Use cautiously in patients with severe GI, neurologic, or blood disorders; hepatic disease or alcoholism; or G6PD deficiency or psoriasis.

Adverse reactions

CNS: mild and transient headache, psychic stimulation, ***seizures***, dizziness, neuropathy.
CV: hypotension, ECG changes.
EENT: blurred vision, difficulty in focusing, reversible corneal changes, typically irreversible, sometimes progressive or delayed retinal changes such as narrowing of arterioles, macular lesions, pallor of optic disk, optic atrophy, patchy retinal pigmentation, typically leading to blindness, ototoxicity, nerve deafness, vertigo, tinnitus.
GI: anorexia, abdominal cramps, diarrhea, nausea, vomiting, stomatitis.
Hematologic: ***agranulocytosis***, ***aplastic anemia***, hemolytic anemia, ***thrombocytopenia***.
Skin: pruritus, lichen planus eruptions, skin and mucosal pigmentary changes, pleomorphic skin eruptions.

Interactions

Drug-drug. *Aluminum salts (kaolin), magnesium:* May decrease GI absorption. Separate dose times.
Cimetidine: May decrease hepatic metabolism of chloroquine. Monitor patient for toxicity.
Drug-lifestyle. *Sun exposure:* May worsen drug-induced dermatoses. Advise patient to avoid excessive sun exposure.

Nursing considerations

!! **ALERT** Drug dosage may be discussed in "mg" or "mg base"; be aware of the difference.
- Ensure that baseline and periodic ophthalmic examinations are performed. Check periodically for ocular muscle weakness after long-term use.
- Help patient obtain audiometric examinations before, during, and after therapy, especially if therapy is long-term.
- Monitor CBC and liver function studies periodically during long-term therapy. If a severe blood disorder not attributable to the disease develops, drug may need to be stopped.

!! **ALERT** Monitor patient for overdose, which can quickly lead to toxic symptoms: headache, drowsiness, visual disturbances, CV collapse, seizures, and then cardiopulmonary arrest. Children are extremely susceptible to toxicity; avoid long-term treatment.

Patient teaching

- Advise patient to take drug immediately before or after a meal on the same day each week, to improve compliance when using drug for prevention.
- Instruct patient to avoid excessive sun exposure to prevent worsening of drug-induced dermatoses.
- Tell patient to report adverse reactions promptly, especially blurred vision, increased sensitivity to light, tinnitus, hearing loss, or muscle weakness.
- Instruct patient to keep drug out of reach of children. Overdose may be fatal.

chlorpheniramine maleate

Aller-Chlor, Allergy, Chlo-Amine, Chlor-Trimeton Allergy 4 hour, Chlor-Trimeton Allergy 8 hour, Chlor-Trimeton Allergy 12 hour, Chlor-Tripolon†

Pregnancy risk category B

Indications & dosages

➲ Rhinitis, allergy symptoms
Adults and children age 12 and older: 4 mg P.O. q 4 to 6 hours, not to exceed 24 mg daily. Or, 8 to 12 mg timed-release P.O. q 8 to 12 hours, not to exceed 24 mg daily.
Children ages 6 to 12: 2 mg P.O. q 4 to 6 hours, not to exceed 12 mg daily. Or, 8 mg timed-release P.O. h.s.
Children ages 2 to 5: 1 mg P.O. q 4 to 6 hours, not to exceed 4 mg daily.
Children younger than age 2: 0.35 mg/kg daily in divided doses q 4 to 6 hours.

Contraindications & cautions

- Contraindicated in patients having acute asthmatic attacks and in those with angle-closure glaucoma, symptomatic prostatic hyperplasia, pyloroduodenal obstruction, or bladder neck obstruction.

• Contraindicated in breast-feeding women and in patients taking MAO inhibitors.
• Use cautiously in elderly patients and in those with increased intraocular pressure, hyperthyroidism, CV or renal disease, hypertension, bronchial asthma, urine retention, prostatic hyperplasia, and stenosing peptic ulcerations.

Adverse reactions

CNS: *stimulation*, sedation, *drowsiness*, excitability in children.
CV: hypotension, palpitations, weak pulse.
GI: epigastric distress, *dry mouth*.
GU: urine retention.
Respiratory: thick bronchial secretions.
Skin: rash, urticaria, pallor.

Interactions

Drug-drug. *CNS depressants:* May increase sedation. Use together cautiously.
MAO inhibitors: May increase anticholinergic effects. Avoid using together.
Drug-lifestyle. *Alcohol use:* May increase CNS depression. Discourage use together.

Nursing considerations

• Stop drug 4 days before diagnostic skin testing because antihistamines can prevent, reduce, or mask positive skin test response.

Patient teaching

• Warn patient to avoid alcohol and hazardous activities that require alertness until CNS effects of drug are known.
• Tell patient that coffee or tea may reduce drowsiness.
• Inform patient that sugarless gum, hard candy, or ice chips may relieve dry mouth.
• Instruct patient to notify prescriber if tolerance develops because a different antihistamine may need to be prescribed.
• Advise patient that extended-release tablets should be swallowed whole and not crushed, chewed, or divided.
• Tell parent that drug (including timed and sustained-release products) shouldn't be used in children younger than age 12 unless directed by prescriber.

chlorpromazine hydrochloride

Chlorpromanyl-20†, Chlorpromanyl-40†, Novo-Chlorpromazin†, Thorazine

Pregnancy risk category C

Indications & dosages

➲ Psychosis, mania
Adults: For hospitalized patients with acute disease, 25 mg I.M.; may give an additional 25 to 50 mg I.M. in 1 hour if needed. Increase over several days to 400 mg q 4 to 6 hours. Switch to oral therapy as soon as possible. Or, 25 mg P.O. t.i.d. initially; then gradually increase to 400 mg daily in divided doses. For outpatients, 30 to 75 mg daily in two to four divided doses. Increase dosage by 20 to 50 mg twice weekly until symptoms are controlled.
Children age 6 months and older: 0.55 mg/kg P.O. q 4 to 6 hours or I.M. q 6 to 8 hours. Or, 1.1 mg/kg P.R. q 6 to 8 hours. Maximum I.M. dose in children younger than age 5 or weighing less than 22.7 kg (50 lb) is 40 mg. Maximum I.M. dose in children ages 5 to 12 or weighing 22.7 to 45.4 kg (50 to 100 lb) is 75 mg.

➲ Nausea and vomiting
Adults: 10 to 25 mg P.O. q 4 to 6 hours, p.r.n. Or, 50 to 100 mg P.R. q 6 to 8 hours, p.r.n. Or, 25 mg I.M. initially. If no hypotension occurs, 25 to 50 mg I.M. q 3 to 4 hours may be given, p.r.n., until vomiting stops.
Children age 6 months and older: 0.55 mg/kg P.O. q 4 to 6 hours or I.M. q 6 to 8 hours. Or, 1.1 mg/kg P.R. q 6 to 8 hours. Maximum I.M. dose in children younger than age 5 or weighing less than 22.7 kg (50 lb) is 40 mg. Maximum I.M. dose in children ages 5 to 12 or weighing 22.7 to 45.4 kg (50 to 100 lb) is 75 mg.

➲ Acute intermittent porphyria, intractable hiccups
Adults: 25 to 50 mg P.O. t.i.d. or q.i.d. If symptoms persist for 2 to 3 days, 25 to 50 mg I.M. For hiccups, if symptoms still persist, 25 to 50 mg diluted in 500 to 1,000 ml of normal saline solution and infused slowly with patient in supine position.

➲ Tetanus
Adults: 25 to 50 mg I.V. or I.M. t.i.d. or q.i.d.

Children age 6 months and older: 0.55 mg/kg I.M. or I.V. q 6 to 8 hours. Maximum parenteral dosage in children weighing less than 22.7 kg (50 lb) is 40 mg daily; for children weighing 22.7 to 45.4 kg (50 to 100 lb), 75 mg, except in severe cases.

➲ **Surgery**

Adults: Preoperatively, 25 to 50 mg P.O. 2 to 3 hours before surgery or 12.5 to 25 mg I.M. 1 to 2 hours before surgery; during surgery, 12.5 mg I.M., repeated in 30 minutes, if needed, or fractional 2-mg doses I.V. at 2-minute intervals to maximum dose of 25 mg; postoperatively, 10 to 25 mg P.O. q 4 to 6 hours or 12.5 to 25 mg I.M., repeated in 1 hour, if needed.

Children age 6 months and older: Preoperatively, 0.55 mg/kg P.O. 2 to 3 hours before surgery or I.M. 1 to 2 hours before surgery. During surgery, 0.275 mg/kg I.M., repeated in 30 minutes if needed, or fractional 1-mg doses I.V. at 2-minute intervals to maximum of 0.275 mg/kg. May repeat fractional I.V. regimen in 30 minutes if needed. Postoperatively, 0.55 mg/kg P.O. or I.M. q 4 to 6 hours (oral dose) or 1 hour (I.M. dose), if needed and if hypotension doesn't occur.

Elderly patients: Lower dosages are sufficient; dosage increments should be more gradual than in adults.

Contraindications & cautions

- Contraindicated in patients hypersensitive to drug; in those with CNS depression, bone marrow suppression, or subcortical damage, and in those in coma.
- Use cautiously in elderly or debilitated patients and in patients with hepatic or renal disease, severe CV disease (may suddenly decrease blood pressure), respiratory disorders, hypocalcemia, glaucoma, or prostatic hyperplasia. Also use cautiously in those exposed to extreme heat or cold (including antipyretic therapy) or organophosphate insecticides.
- Use cautiously in acutely ill or dehydrated children.

Adverse reactions

CNS: *extrapyramidal reactions*, drowsiness, *sedation*, ***seizures***, *tardive dyskinesia*, *pseudoparkinsonism*, dizziness, ***neuroleptic malignant syndrome***.

CV: *orthostatic hypotension*, tachycardia, quinidine-like ECG effects.

EENT: ocular changes, blurred vision, nasal congestion.

GI: *dry mouth, constipation*, nausea.

GU: *urine retention*, menstrual irregularities, inhibited ejaculation, priapism.

Hematologic: ***leukopenia***, ***agranulocytosis***, eosinophilia, hemolytic anemia, ***aplastic anemia***, ***thrombocytopenia***.

Hepatic: jaundice.

Skin: *mild photosensitivity reactions*, allergic reactions, *pain at I.M. injection site*, sterile abscess, skin pigmentation changes.

Other: gynecomastia, lactation, galactorrhea.

Interactions

Drug-drug. *Antacids:* May inhibit absorption of oral phenothiazines. Separate antacid and phenothiazine doses by at least 2 hours.

Anticholinergics such as tricyclic antidepressants, antiparkinsonians: May increase anticholinergic activity, aggravated parkinsonian symptoms. Use together cautiously.

Anticonvulsants: May lower seizure threshold. Monitor patient closely.

Barbiturates, lithium: May decrease phenothiazine effect. Monitor patient.

Centrally acting antihypertensives: May decrease antihypertensive effect. Monitor blood pressure.

CNS depressants: May increase CNS depression. Use together cautiously.

Electroconvulsive therapy, insulin: May cause severe reactions. Monitor patient closely.

Lithium: May increase neurologic effects. Monitor patient closely.

Meperidine: May cause excessive sedation and hypotension. Don't use together.

Propranolol: May increase levels of both propranolol and chlorpromazine. Monitor patient closely.

Warfarin: May decrease effect of oral anticoagulants. Monitor PT and INR.

Drug-herb. *St. John's wort:* May cause photosensitivity reactions. Advise patient to avoid excessive sunlight exposure.

Drug-lifestyle. *Alcohol use:* May increase CNS depression, particularly psychomotor skills. Strongly discourage alcohol use.

Sun exposure: May increase risk of photosensitivity reactions. Advise patient to avoid excessive sunlight exposure.

Nursing considerations

- Obtain baseline blood pressure measurements before starting therapy, and monitor regularly. Watch for orthostatic hypotension, especially with parenteral administration. Monitor blood pressure before and after I.M. administration; keep patient supine for 1 hour afterward and have him get up slowly.
- Wear gloves when preparing solutions and avoid contact with skin and clothing. Oral liquid and parenteral forms can cause contact dermatitis.
- Slight yellowing of injection or concentrate is common and doesn't affect potency. Discard markedly discolored solutions.
- Protect liquid concentrate from light. Dilute with fruit juice, milk, or semisolid food just before administration.
- Give deep I.M. only in upper outer quadrant of buttocks. Consider giving injection by Z-track method. Massage slowly afterward to prevent sterile abscess. Injection stings. Rotate injection sites.
- Monitor patient for tardive dyskinesia, which may occur after prolonged use. It may not appear until months or years later and may disappear spontaneously or persist for life, despite stopping drug.
- After abrupt withdrawal of long-term therapy, gastritis, nausea, vomiting, dizziness, or tremor may occur.

!!ALERT Look for evidence of neuroleptic malignant syndrome (extrapyramidal effects, hyperthermia, autonomic disturbance), which is rare but usually fatal. It may not be related to length of drug use or type of neuroleptic; more than 60% of affected patients are men.

- Withhold dose and notify prescriber if jaundice, symptoms of blood dyscrasia (fever, sore throat, infection, cellulitis, weakness), or persistent extrapyramidal reactions (longer than a few hours) develop, or if such reactions occur in children or pregnant women.
- Don't withdraw drug abruptly unless necessitated by severe adverse reactions.

!!ALERT Don't confuse chlorpromazine with chlorpropamide, a hypoglycemic.

!!ALERT Don't confuse chlorpromazine with clomipramine.

Patient teaching

- Warn patient to avoid activities that require alertness or good coordination until effects of drug are known. Drowsiness and dizziness usually subside after first few weeks.

!!ALERT Advise patient not to crush, chew, or break extended-release capsule form before swallowing.

- Tell patient to avoid alcohol while taking drug.
- Have patient report signs of urine retention or constipation.
- Tell patient to use sunblock and to wear protective clothing to avoid oversensitivity to the sun. Chlorpromazine is more likely to cause sun sensitivity than any other drug in its class.
- Tell patient to relieve dry mouth with sugarless gum or hard candy.
- Advise patient receiving drug by any method other than by mouth to remain lying down for 1 hour afterward and to rise slowly.

chlorpropamide
Apo-Chlorpropamide†, Diabinese

Pregnancy risk category C

Indications & dosages

➲ Adjunct to diet to lower glucose level in patients with type 2 (non–insulin-dependent) diabetes

Adults: Initially, 250 mg P.O. daily with breakfast. Increase first dose after 5 to 7 days because of extended duration of action; then increase q 3 to 5 days by 50 to 125 mg, if needed, to maximum of 750 mg daily. Some patients with mild diabetes respond well to 100 mg daily or less.

Patients older than age 65: Initially, 100 to 125 mg P.O. daily; then increase as with adult dose.

In patients with renal or hepatic impairment, use lower first doses, and increase dosage as tolerated.

➲ To change from insulin to oral therapy

Adults: If insulin dosage is 40 units or less daily, stop insulin and start oral therapy as above. If insulin dosage is more than 40 units daily, start oral therapy as above with insulin reduced by 50%. Further reduce insulin dosage, according to response.

Contraindications & cautions

- Contraindicated in pregnant women, breast-feeding women, patients hypersensitive to drug, and those with type 2 diabetes complicated by ketosis, acidosis, diabetic coma, major surgery, severe infections, or severe trauma.
- Contraindicated for treating type 1 diabetes or diabetes that can be adequately controlled by diet.
- Use cautiously in patients with porphyria or impaired hepatic or renal function, or in debilitated, malnourished, or elderly patients.
- Use cautiously in patients allergic to sulfonamides.

Adverse reactions

CNS: paresthesia, fatigue, dizziness, vertigo, malaise, headache.
CV: ***increased risk of cardiovascular death***.
EENT: tinnitus.
GI: nausea, heartburn, epigastric distress.
GU: tea-colored urine.
Hematologic: ***leukopenia***, ***thrombocytopenia***, ***aplastic anemia***, ***agranulocytosis***, hemolytic anemia.
Hepatic: cholestatic jaundice.
Metabolic: ***prolonged hypoglycemia***, dilutional hyponatremia.
Skin: rash, pruritus, erythema, urticaria.
Other: *disulfiram-like reactions*, hypersensitivity reactions.

Interactions

Drug-drug. *Anabolic steroids, chloramphenicol, clofibrate, guanethidine, MAO inhibitors, salicylates, sulfonamides:* May increase hypoglycemic activity. Monitor glucose level.
Beta blockers: May prolong hypoglycemic effect and mask symptoms of hypoglycemia. Use together cautiously.
Corticosteroids, glucagon, phenytoin, rifampin, thiazide diuretics: May decrease hypoglycemic response. Monitor glucose level.
Oral anticoagulants: May increase hypoglycemic activity or enhance anticoagulant effect. Monitor glucose level, PT, and INR.
Drug-herb. *Bitter melon (karela), burdock, dandelion, eucalyptus, ginkgo biloba, marshmallow:* May increase hypoglycemic effects. Discourage use together.
Drug-lifestyle. *Alcohol use:* May alter glycemic control, most commonly causing hypoglycemia. May also cause a disulfiram-like reaction. Discourage use together.

Nursing considerations

- Elderly patients may be more sensitive to therapeutic and adverse effects.
- Drug may accumulate in patients with renal insufficiency. Watch for and report signs of impending renal insufficiency, such as dysuria, anuria, and hematuria.

!!ALERT Adverse effects of drug, especially hypoglycemia, may be more frequent, prolonged, or severe than with some other sulfonylureas because of drug's long duration of action. If hypoglycemia occurs, monitor patient closely for minimum of 3 to 5 days.

- Patients switching from another oral antidiabetic don't usually need a transition period.
- Patients may need hospitalization during transition from insulin to an oral antidiabetic. Monitor patient's glucose level at least three times daily before meals.

!!ALERT Don't confuse chlorpropamide with chlorpromazine.

Patient teaching

- Instruct patient about nature of disease and importance of following therapeutic regimen, adhering to specific diet, losing weight, getting exercise, following personal hygiene programs, and avoiding infection. Explain how and when to monitor glucose level, and teach recognition of and intervention for both low and high glucose levels.
- Make sure patient understands that therapy relieves symptoms but doesn't cure the disease. He should also understand potential risks and advantages of taking drug and of other treatment methods.
- Advise woman planning pregnancy to consult prescriber before becoming pregnant. Insulin may be needed during pregnancy and breast-feeding.
- Tell patient not to change drug dosage without prescriber's consent and to report abnormal blood or urine glucose test results.
- Teach patient to carry candy or other simple sugars to treat mild low-glucose episodes. Patient experiencing severe episode may need hospital treatment.
- Advise patient not to take other drugs, including OTC drugs, without first checking with prescriber.

!!ALERT Advise patient to avoid alcohol consumption. Signs and symptoms of chlorpropamide-alcohol flush are facial flushing, light-headedness, headache, and occasional breathlessness. Even very small amounts of alcohol can produce this reaction.
- Advise patient to wear or carry medical identification at all times.

!!ALERT Tell patient to report rash, skin eruptions, and other signs and symptoms of hypersensitivity to prescriber immediately.

cholestyramine
LoCHOLEST, LoCHOLEST Light, Prevalite, Questran, Questran Light

Pregnancy risk category C

Indications & dosages
➲ **Primary hyperlipidemia or pruritus caused by partial bile obstruction, adjunct for reduction of increased cholesterol level in patients with primary hypercholesterolemia**

Adults: 4 g once or twice daily. Maintenance dose is 8 to 16 g daily divided into two doses. Maximum daily dose is 24 g.

Contraindications & cautions
- Contraindicated in patients hypersensitive to bile-acid sequestering resins and in those with complete biliary obstruction.
- Use cautiously in patients predisposed to constipation and in those with conditions aggravated by constipation, such as severe, symptomatic coronary artery disease.

Adverse reactions
CNS: *headache*, anxiety, *vertigo*, *dizziness*, insomnia, fatigue, syncope, tinnitus.
GI: *constipation*, *fecal impaction*, hemorrhoids, *abdominal discomfort*, flatulence, *nausea*, vomiting, steatorrhea, GI bleeding, diarrhea, anorexia.
GU: hematuria, dysuria.
Hematologic: anemia, bleeding tendencies, ecchymoses.
Metabolic: hyperchloremic acidosis.
Musculoskeletal: backache, muscle and joint pains, osteoporosis.
Skin: *rash*, irritation of skin, tongue, and perianal area.
Other: *vitamin A, D, E, and K deficiencies from decreased absorption.*

Interactions
Drug-drug. *Acetaminophen, beta blockers, cardiac glycosides, corticosteroids, estrogens, fat-soluble vitamins (A, D, E, and K), iron preparations, niacin, penicillin G, phenobarbital, progestins, tetracycline, thiazide diuretics, thyroid hormones, warfarin and other coumarin derivatives:* May decrease absorption of these drugs. Give other drugs 1 hour before or 4 to 6 hours after cholestyramine.

Nursing considerations
- Monitor cholesterol and triglyceride levels regularly during therapy.
- Monitor levels of cardiac glycosides in patients receiving cardiac glycosides and cholestyramine together. If cholestyramine therapy is stopped, adjust dosage of cardiac glycosides to avoid toxicity.
- Monitor bowel habits. Encourage a diet high in fiber and fluids. If severe constipation develops, decrease dosage, add a stool softener, or stop drug.
- Watch for hyperchloremic acidosis with long-term use or very high doses.
- Long-term use may lead to deficiencies of vitamins A, D, E, and K, and folic acid.

!!ALERT Don't confuse Questran with Quarzan.

Patient teaching
!!ALERT Tell patient never to take drug in its dry form because it may irritate the esophagus or cause severe constipation.
- Tell patient to prepare drug in a large glass containing water, milk, or juice (especially pulpy fruit juice). Powder can be sprinkled on the surface of the preferred beverage; let the mixture stand for a few minutes, and then stir thoroughly. Discourage mixing with carbonated beverages because of excessive foaming. After drinking preparation, patients should swirl a small additional amount of liquid in the same glass and then drink again to make sure they have taken the entire dose.
- Advise patient to take at mealtime, if possible.
- Advise patient to take all other drugs at least 1 hour before or 4 to 6 hours after cholestyramine to avoid blocking their absorption.

• Teach patient about proper dietary management of fats. When appropriate, recommend weight control, exercise, and smoking cessation programs.
• Tell patient that drug may deplete body stores of vitamins A, D, E, and K, and folic acid. Patient should discuss need for supplements with prescriber.

cidofovir
Vistide

Pregnancy risk category C

Indications & dosages

➲ CMV retinitis in patients with AIDS
Adults: Initially, 5 mg/kg I.V. infused over 1 hour once weekly for 2 consecutive weeks; then maintenance dose of 5 mg/kg I.V. infused over 1 hour once q 2 weeks. Give probenecid and prehydration with normal saline solution I.V. concomitantly; may reduce potential for nephrotoxicity.

For patients with creatinine level 0.3 to 0.4 mg/dl above baseline, reduce dosage to 3 mg/kg at same rate and frequency. If creatinine level reaches 0.5 mg/dl or more above baseline, stop drug.

Contraindications & cautions

• Contraindicated in patients hypersensitive to drug or to probenecid or other sulfa-containing drugs.
• Contraindicated in patients receiving drugs with nephrotoxic potential (stop such drugs at least 7 days before starting cidofovir therapy) and in those with creatinine level exceeding 1.5 mg/dl, creatinine clearance of 55 ml/minute or less, or urine protein level of 100 mg/dl or more (equivalent to 2 + proteinuria or more).
• Safety and effectiveness in children haven't been established.
• It's unknown if cidofovir appears in breast milk.
• Use cautiously in patients with renal impairment. Monitor renal function tests and patient's fluid balance.

Adverse reactions

CNS: *asthenia, headache,* amnesia, anxiety, confusion, *fever,* ***seizures***, depression, dizziness, abnormal gait, hallucinations, insomnia, neuropathy, paresthesia, somnolence, malaise.
CV: hypotension, orthostatic hypotension, pallor, syncope, tachycardia, vasodilation.
EENT: amblyopia, conjunctivitis, pharyngitis, eye disorders, *ocular hypotony,* iritis, retinal detachment, uveitis, abnormal vision, rhinitis, sinusitis.
GI: *nausea, vomiting, diarrhea, anorexia, abdominal pain,* dry mouth, colitis, constipation, tongue discoloration, dyspepsia, dysphagia, flatulence, gastritis, melena, oral candidiasis, rectal disorders, stomatitis, aphthous stomatitis, mouth ulcers, taste perversion.
GU: ***nephrotoxicity***, *proteinuria,* glycosuria, hematuria, urinary incontinence, UTI.
Hematologic: ***neutropenia***, *anemia,* ***thrombocytopenia***.
Hepatic: hepatomegaly.
Metabolic: weight loss, fluid imbalance, hyperglycemia, hyperlipemia, hypocalcemia, hypokalemia.
Musculoskeletal: arthralgia, myasthenia, myalgia, pain in back, chest, or neck.
Respiratory: asthma, bronchitis, coughing, *dyspnea,* hiccups, increased sputum, lung disorders, pneumonia.
Skin: *rash, alopecia,* acne, skin discoloration, dry skin, pruritus, sweating, urticaria.
Other: *infections, chills,* allergic reactions, herpes simplex, facial edema, ***sarcoma***, ***sepsis***.

Interactions

Drug-drug. *Nephrotoxic drugs (such as aminoglycosides, amphotericin B, foscarnet, I.V. pentamidine):* May increase nephrotoxicity. Avoid using together.

Nursing considerations

• Don't give as a direct intraocular injection because this may decrease intraocular pressure and impair vision.
• Cidofovir is indicated only for the treatment of CMV retinitis in patients with AIDS. Safety and efficacy of drug haven't been established for treating other CMV infections, congenital or neonatal CMV disease, or CMV disease in patients not infected with HIV.
• Give 1 L normal saline solution I.V. usually over 1- to 2-hour period, immediately before cidofovir infusion.
• Give probenecid with cidofovir.

- Monitor creatinine and urine protein levels and WBC counts with differential before each dose.
- Drug may cause Fanconi syndrome and decreased bicarbonate level with renal tubular damage. Monitor patient closely.
- Drug may cause granulocytopenia.
- Stop zidovudine therapy or reduce dosage by 50% on the days when cidofovir is given; probenecid reduces metabolic clearance of zidovudine.

Patient teaching

- Inform patient that drug doesn't cure CMV retinitis and that regular ophthalmologic follow-up examinations are needed.
- Alert patient taking zidovudine that he'll need to obtain dosage guidelines on days cidofovir is given.
- Tell patient that close monitoring of kidney function will be needed and that abnormalities may require a change in cidofovir therapy.
- Stress importance of completing a full course of probenecid with each cidofovir dose. Tell patient to take probenecid after a meal to decrease nausea.
- Patients with AIDS should use effective contraception, especially during and for 1 month after treatment with cidofovir.
- Advise male patients to practice barrier contraception during and for 3 months after treatment with drug.

cilostazol
Pletal

Pregnancy risk category C

Indications & dosages

➲ To reduce symptoms of intermittent claudication

Adults: 100 mg P.O. b.i.d., at least 30 minutes before or 2 hours after breakfast and dinner.

Decrease dose to 50 mg P.O. b.i.d. when giving with drugs that may interact to cause an increase in cilostazol level.

Contraindications & cautions

- Contraindicated in patients hypersensitive to drug or its components and in those with heart failure of any severity.
- Use cautiously in patients with severe underlying heart disease; also use cautiously with other drugs having antiplatelet activity.

Adverse reactions

CNS: *headache, dizziness,* vertigo.
CV: *palpitations,* tachycardia, peripheral edema.
EENT: *pharyngitis, rhinitis.*
GI: *abnormal stools, diarrhea,* dyspepsia, abdominal pain, flatulence, nausea.
Musculoskeletal: back pain, myalgia.
Respiratory: increased cough.
Other: *infection,* bleeding.

Interactions

Drug-drug. *Diltiazem:* May increase cilostazol level. Reduce cilostazol dosage to 50 mg b.i.d.

Erythromycin, other macrolides: May increase level of cilostazol and its metabolites. Reduce cilostazol dosage to 50 mg b.i.d.

Omeprazole: May increase level of cilostazol metabolite. Reduce cilostazol dosage to 50 mg b.i.d.

Strong inhibitors of CYP3A4 (such as fluconazole, fluoxetine, fluvoxamine, itraconazole, ketoconazole, miconazole, nefazodone, sertraline): May increase level of cilostazol and its metabolites. Reduce cilostazol dosage to 50 mg b.i.d.

Drug-food. *Grapefruit juice:* May increase drug level. Discourage use together.

Drug-lifestyle. *Smoking:* May decrease drug exposure. Discourage smoking.

Nursing considerations

- Give drug at least 30 minutes before or 2 hours after breakfast and dinner.
- Beneficial effects may not be seen for up to 12 weeks after therapy starts.

!!ALERT Cilostazol and similar drugs that inhibit the enzyme phosphodiesterase decrease the likelihood of survival in patients with class III and IV heart failure.

!!ALERT CV risk is unknown in patients who use drug on long-term basis and in those with severe underlying heart disease.

- Dosage can be reduced or stopped without such rebound effects as platelet hyperaggregation.
- Drug may reduce triglyceride levels and increase HDL cholesterol level.

Patient teaching

- Instruct patient to take drug on an empty stomach, at least 30 minutes before or 2 hours after breakfast and dinner.
- Tell patient that beneficial effect of drug on cramping pain isn't likely to be noticed for 2 to 4 weeks and that it may take as long as 12 weeks.
- Advise patient to avoid drinking grapefruit juice during drug therapy.
- Inform patient that CV risk is unknown in patients who use drug on a long-term basis and in those with severe underlying heart disease.
- Tell patient that drug may cause dizziness. Caution patient not to drive or perform other activities that require alertness until response to drug is known.

cimetidine
Tagamet, Tagamet HB ◇

cimetidine hydrochloride
Tagamet

Pregnancy risk category B

Indications & dosages

➲ **To prevent upper GI bleeding in critically ill patients**
Adults: 50 mg/hour by continuous I.V. infusion for up to 7 days; 25 mg/hour to patients with creatinine clearance below 30 ml/minute.

➲ **Short-term treatment of duodenal ulcer; maintenance therapy**
Adults and children age 16 and older: 800 mg P.O. h.s. Or, 400 mg P.O. b.i.d. or 300 mg q.i.d. (with meals and h.s.). Or, 200 mg t.i.d. with a 400-mg h.s. dose. Treatment lasts 4 to 6 weeks unless endoscopy shows healing. For maintenance therapy, 400 mg h.s. For parenteral therapy, 300 mg diluted to 20 ml total volume with normal saline solution or other compatible I.V. solution by I.V. push over at least 5 minutes q 6 to 8 hours; or 300 mg diluted in 50 ml D_5W or other compatible I.V. solution by I.V. infusion over 15 to 20 minutes q 6 to 8 hours; or 300 mg I.M. q 6 to 8 hours (no dilution needed). To increase dosage, give 300-mg doses more frequently to maximum of 2,400 mg daily, p.r.n. Or, 900 mg/day (37.5 mg/hour) I.V. diluted in 100 to 1,000 ml of compatible solution by continuous I.V. infusion.

➲ **Active benign gastric ulceration**
Adults: 800 mg P.O. h.s. or 300 mg P.O. q.i.d. (with meals and h.s.) for up to 8 weeks.

➲ **Pathologic hypersecretory conditions, such as Zollinger-Ellison syndrome, systemic mastocytosis, and multiple endocrine adenomas**
Adults and children age 16 and older: 300 mg P.O. q.i.d. with meals and h.s.; adjusted to patient needs. Maximum oral amount, 2,400 mg daily.

For parenteral therapy, 300 mg diluted to 20 ml with normal saline solution or other compatible I.V. solution by I.V. push over at least 5 minutes q 6 to 8 hours; or 300 mg diluted in 50 ml D_5W or other compatible I.V. solution by I.V. infusion over 15 to 20 minutes q 6 to 8 hours. Increase parenteral dosage by giving 300-mg doses more frequently to maximum of 2,400 mg daily, p.r.n.

➲ **Gastroesophageal reflux disease**
Adults: 800 mg P.O. b.i.d. or 400 mg q.i.d. before meals and h.s. for up to 12 weeks.

In patients with renal impairment, decrease dosage to 300 mg P.O. or I.V. q 12 hours, increasing frequency to q 8 hours with caution. A renally impaired patient who also has liver dysfunction may require even further dose reduction.

➲ **Heartburn**
Adults: 200 mg Tagamet HB P.O. with water as symptoms occur, or as directed, up to b.i.d. Maximum, 400 mg daily. Drug shouldn't be taken daily for longer than 2 weeks.

Contraindications & cautions

- Contraindicated in patients hypersensitive to drug.
- Use cautiously in elderly or debilitated patients because they may be more susceptible to cimetidine-induced confusion.

Adverse reactions

CNS: confusion, dizziness, headache, peripheral neuropathy, somnolence, hallucinations.
GI: mild and transient diarrhea.
GU: impotence.
Musculoskeletal: muscle pain, arthralgia.

Other: mild gynecomastia if used longer than 1 month, hypersensitivity reactions.

Interactions

Drug-drug. *Antacids:* May interfere with cimetidine absorption. Separate doses by at least 1 hour, if possible.
Digoxin, fluconazole, indomethacin, iron salts, ketoconazole, tetracycline: May decrease drug absorption. Separate doses by at least 2 hours.
Fosphenytoin, phenytoin, some benzodiazepines, theophylline, warfarin: May inhibit hepatic microsomal enzyme metabolism of these drugs. Monitor drug level.
I.V. lidocaine: May decrease clearance of lidocaine, increasing the risk of toxicity. Consider using a different H_2 antagonist if possible. Monitor lidocaine level closely.
Metoprolol, propranolol, timolol: May increase the effects of beta-blocker. Consider another H_2 agonist or decrease the dose of beta-blocker.
Procainamide: May increase procainamide level. Avoid this combination if possible. Monitor procainamide level closely and adjust the dose as necessary.
Drug-herb. *Guarana:* May increase caffeine level or prolong caffeine half-life. Monitor patient.
Pennyroyal: May change rate at which toxic metabolites of pennyroyal form. Monitor patient.
Yerba maté: May decrease clearance of yerba maté methylxanthines and cause toxicity. Discourage use together.
Drug-lifestyle. *Alcohol use:* May increase blood alcohol level. Discourage use together.
Smoking: May decrease the ability of cimetidine to inhibit nocturnal gastric secretion. Urge patient to quit smoking.

Nursing considerations

- Assess patient for abdominal pain. Note blood in emesis, stool, or gastric aspirate.
- Identify tablet strength when obtaining a drug history.
- Schedule cimetidine dose at end of hemodialysis treatment because hemodialysis reduces blood levels of cimetidine. Adjust dosage for patients with renal impairment.
- Wait at least 15 minutes after giving Tagamet tablet before drawing sample for Hemoccult or Gastroccult test, and follow test manufacturer's instructions closely.
- I.M. injection may be given undiluted.
- Treatment of gastric ulcer isn't as effective as treatment of duodenal ulcer.
- Overdose of up to 10 g can occur without adverse reactions.

!!**ALERT** Don't confuse cimetidine with simethicone.

Patient teaching

- Remind patient taking cimetidine once daily to take it at bedtime and to take multiple daily doses with meals.
- Instruct patient taking Tagamet HB not to exceed recommended dosage and not to take daily for longer than 14 days.
- Warn patient receiving drug I.M. that injection may be painful.
- Urge patient to avoid cigarette smoking because it may increase gastric acid secretion and worsen disease.
- Advise patient to report abdominal pain and blood in stools or emesis.

cinacalcet hydrochloride
Sensipar

Pregnancy risk category C

Indications & dosages

➲ Secondary hyperparathyroidism in patients with chronic kidney disease undergoing dialysis
Adults: Initially, 30 mg P.O. once daily; adjust no more than q 2 to 4 weeks through sequential doses of 60 mg, 90 mg, 120 mg, and 180 mg P.O. once daily to reach target range of 150 to 300 pg/ml for intact parathyroid hormone (PTH).
➲ Hypercalcemia in patients with parathyroid carcinoma
Adults: Initially, 30 mg P.O. b.i.d.; adjust q 2 to 4 weeks through sequential doses of 30 mg, 60 mg, and 90 mg P.O. b.i.d., and 90 mg P.O. t.i.d. or q.i.d. daily p.r.n. to normalize calcium level.

Contraindications & cautions

- Contraindicated in patients hypersensitive to drug or its components and in patients with calcium level less than 8.4 mg/dl.
- Use cautiously in patients with history of seizures and in those with moderate to severe hepatic impairment.

Adverse reactions

CNS: asthenia, *dizziness.*
CV: chest pain, hypertension.
GI: anorexia, *diarrhea, nausea, vomiting.*
Musculoskeletal: *myalgia.*
Other: access infection.

Interactions

Drug-drug. *Drugs metabolized mainly by CYP2D6 with a narrow therapeutic index (such as flecainide, thioridazine, most tricyclic antidepressants, vinblastine):* May strongly inhibit CYP2D6, causing decreased metabolism and increased levels of these drugs. Adjust dosage of other drugs as needed.
Drugs that strongly inhibit CYP3A4 (such as erythromycin, itraconazole, ketoconazole): May increase cinacalcet level. Use together cautiously, monitoring PTH and calcium level closely and adjusting cinacalcet dosage as needed.

Nursing considerations

!!ALERT Monitor calcium level closely, especially if patient has a history of seizures, because decreased calcium level lowers seizure threshold.
- Patients with moderate to severe hepatic impairment may need dosage adjustment based on PTH and calcium level. Monitor these patients closely.
- Give drug alone or with vitamin D sterols, phosphate binders, or both.
- Measure calcium level within 1 week after starting therapy or adjusting dosage. Once maintenance dose is established, measure calcium level monthly for patients with chronic kidney disease receiving dialysis and every 2 months for those with parathyroid carcinoma.
- Watch carefully for evidence of hypocalcemia: paresthesias, myalgias, cramping, tetany, and seizures.
- If calcium level is 7.5 to 8.4 mg/dl or patient develops symptoms of hypocalcemia, give calcium-containing phosphate binders, vitamin D sterols, or both, to raise calcium level. If calcium level is below 7.5 mg/dl or hypocalcemia symptoms persist and the vitamin D dose can't be increased, withhold cinacalcet until calcium level reaches 8.0 mg/dl, hypocalcemia symptoms resolve, or both. Resume treatment with the next-lowest dose of cinacalcet.
- Measure intact PTH level 1 to 4 weeks after therapy starts or dosage changes. Once the maintenance dose is established, monitor PTH level every 1 to 3 months. Levels in patients with chronic kidney disease receiving dialysis should be 150 to 300 pg/ml.
- Adynamic bone disease may develop if intact PTH levels are suppressed below 100 pg/ml. If this occurs, notify prescriber. The dosage of cinacalcet or vitamin D sterols may need to be reduced or stopped.

!!ALERT Drug isn't approved for patients with chronic kidney disease who aren't receiving dialysis because they have an increased risk of hypocalcemia.

Patient teaching

- Tell patient not to divide tablets but to take them whole, with food or shortly after a meal.
- Advise patient to report to prescriber adverse reactions and signs of hypocalcemia, which include paresthesias, muscle weakness, muscle cramping, and muscle spasm.

ciprofloxacin hydrochloride (ophthalmic)
Ciloxan

Pregnancy risk category C

Indications & dosages

➲ **Corneal ulcers caused by *Pseudomonas aeruginosa, Staphylococcus aureus, Staphylococcus epidermidis, Streptococcus pneumoniae,* and possibly Serratia marcescens and *Streptococcus viridans***
Adults and children older than age 12: 2 drops in affected eye q 15 minutes for first 6 hours; then 2 drops q 30 minutes for remainder of first day. On the second day, 2 drops hourly. On days 3 to 14, 2 drops q 4 hours.
➲ **Bacterial conjunctivitis caused by *Haemophilus influenzae, S. aureus, S. epidermidis,* and possibly *S. pneumoniae***
Adults and children older than age 12: 1 or 2 drops into conjunctival sac of affected eye q 2 hours while awake for first 2 days. Then, 1 or 2 drops q 4 hours while awake for next 5 days.

Contraindications & cautions

- Contraindicated in patients hypersensitive to ciprofloxacin or other fluoroquinolone antibiotics.
- It's unknown if drug appears in breast milk after application to eye; however, ciprofloxacin given systemically has appeared in breast milk. Use cautiously in breastfeeding women.

Adverse reactions

EENT: *local burning or discomfort, white crystalline precipitate in superficial portion of corneal defect in patients with corneal ulcers*, margin crusting, crystals or scales, foreign body sensation, itching, conjunctival hyperemia, allergic reactions.
GI: bad or bitter taste in mouth.

Interactions

None significant.

Nursing considerations

!!ALERT Stop drug at first sign of hypersensitivity, such as rash, and notify prescriber. Serious hypersensitivity reactions, including anaphylaxis, may occur in patients receiving systemic fluoroquinolone therapy.
- A topical overdose may be flushed from eyes with warm tap water.
- If corneal epithelium is still compromised after 14 days of treatment, continue therapy.
- Institute appropriate therapy if superinfection occurs. Prolonged use may result in overgrowth of nonsusceptible organisms, including fungi.

!!ALERT Don't confuse Ciloxan with Cytoxan or cinoxacin.

Patient teaching

- Tell patient to clean eye area of excessive discharge before instilling.
- Teach patient how to instill drops. Advise him to wash hands before and after using solution and not to touch tip of dropper to eye or surrounding tissues.
- Instruct patient to apply light finger pressure on lacrimal sac for 1 minute after drops are instilled.
- Advise patient that drug may cause temporary blurring of vision or stinging after administration. If these symptoms become pronounced or worsen, contact prescriber.
- Tell patient to avoid wearing contacts while treating bacterial conjunctivitis. If approved by prescriber, tell patient to wait at least 15 minutes after instilling drops before inserting contact lenses.
- Tell patient not to share drug, washcloths, or towels with family members and to notify prescriber if anyone develops same signs or symptoms.
- Stress importance of compliance with recommended therapy.

ciprofloxacin (systemic)
Cipro, Cipro I.V., Cipro XR

Pregnancy risk category C

Indications & dosages

➲ **Mild to moderate UTIs caused by *Escherichia coli, Klebsiella pneumoniae, Enterobacter cloacae, Serratia marcescens, Proteus mirabilis, Providencia rettgeri, Morganella morganii, Citrobacter diversus, C. freundii, Pseudomonas aeruginosa, Staphylococcus epidermidis,* and *Enterococcus faecalis***
Adults: 250 mg P.O. or 200 mg I.V. q 12 hours.

➲ **Severe or complicated UTIs; mild to moderate bone and joint infections caused by *E. cloacae, P. aeruginosa,* and *S. marcescens;* mild to moderate respiratory infections caused by *E. coli, K. pneumoniae, E. cloacae, P. mirabilis, P. aeruginosa, Haemophilus influenzae,* and *H. parainfluenzae;* mild to moderate skin and skin-structure infections caused by *E. coli, K. pneumoniae, E. cloacae, P. mirabilis, P. vulgaris, Providencia stuartii, M. morganii, C. freundii, Streptococcus pyogenes, P. aeruginosa, Staphylococcus aureus,* and *S. epidermidis;* infectious diarrhea caused by *E. coli, Campylobacter jejuni, Shigella flexneri,* and *S. sonnei;* typhoid fever**
Adults: 500 mg P.O. or 400 mg I.V. q 12 hours.

➲ **Severe or complicated bone or joint infections, severe respiratory tract infections, severe skin and skin-structure infections**
Adults: 750 mg P.O. q 12 hours or 400 mg I.V. q 8 to 12 hours.

➲ **Chronic bacterial prostatitis caused by *E. coli* or *P. mirabilis***
Adults: 500 mg P.O. q 12 hours or 400 mg I.V. q 12 hours for 28 days.

➲ **Complicated intra-abdominal infections caused by *E. coli, P. aeruginosa, P. mirabilis, K. pneumoniae,* or *Bacteroides fragilis***
Adults: 500 mg P.O. or 400 mg I.V. q 12 hours for 7 to 14 days. Give with metronidazole.

➲ **Acute uncomplicated cystitis**
Adults: 100 mg or 250 mg P.O. q 12 hours for 3 days.

➲ **Uncomplicated UTI**
Adults: 500 mg extended-release tablet P.O. once daily for 3 days.

➲ **Mild to moderate acute sinusitis caused by *H. influenzae, Streptococcus pneumoniae,* or *Moraxella catarrhalis***
Adults: 500 mg P.O. or 400 mg I.V. q 12 hours for 10 days.

➲ **Empirical therapy in febrile neutropenic patients**
Adults: 400 mg I.V. q 8 hours used with piperacillin 50 mg/kg I.V. q 4 hours (not to exceed 24 g/day).

➲ **Inhalation anthrax (postexposure)**
Adults: 400 mg I.V. q 12 hours initially until susceptibility test results are known; then 500 mg P.O. b.i.d.
Children: 10 mg/kg I.V. q 12 hours; then 15 mg/kg P.O. q 12 hours. Don't exceed 800 mg/day I.V. or 1,000 mg/day P.O.
For all patients: Give drug with one or two additional antimicrobials. Switch to oral therapy when appropriate. Treat for 60 days (I.V. and P.O. combined).

➲ **Cutaneous anthrax**♦
Adults: 500 mg P.O. b.i.d. for 60 days.
Children: 10 to 15 mg/kg q 12 hours. Don't exceed 1,000 mg/day. Treat for 60 days.

For patients with a creatinine clearance of 30 to 50 ml/minute, give 250 to 500 mg P.O. q 12 hours or the usual I.V. dose; if clearance is 5 to 29 ml/minute, give 250 to 500 mg P.O. q 18 hours or 200 to 400 mg I.V. q 18 to 24 hours. If patient is receiving hemodialysis, give 250 to 500 mg P.O. q 24 hours after dialysis.

Contraindications & cautions

- Contraindicated in patients sensitive to fluoroquinolones.
- Use cautiously in patients with CNS disorders, such as severe cerebral arteriosclerosis or seizure disorders, and in those at risk for seizures. Drug may cause CNS stimulation.
- Safety in children younger than age 18 hasn't been established; however, drug may be used as recommended by the CDC for inhalational or cutaneous anthrax, as indicated. Drug may cause cartilage erosion.

Adverse reactions

CNS: headache, restlessness, tremor, dizziness, fatigue, drowsiness, insomnia, depression, light-headedness, confusion, hallucinations, ***seizures***, paresthesia.
CV: thrombophlebitis, edema, chest pain.
GI: *nausea, diarrhea,* vomiting, abdominal pain or discomfort, oral candidiasis, ***pseudomembranous colitis***, dyspepsia, flatulence, constipation.
GU: crystalluria, interstitial nephritis.
Hematologic: eosinophilia, ***leukopenia, neutropenia, thrombocytopenia.***
Musculoskeletal: arthralgia, arthropathy, joint or back pain, joint inflammation, joint stiffness, tendon rupture, aching, neck pain.
Skin: *rash,* photosensitivity, ***Stevens-Johnson syndrome, toxic epidermal necrolysis***, exfoliative dermatitis, burning, pruritus, erythema.
Other: hypersensitivity reactions.

Interactions

Drug-drug. *Aluminum hydroxide, calcium carbonate, aluminum-magnesium hydroxide, didanosine (chewable tablets, buffered tablets, or pediatric powder for oral solution), magnesium hydroxide, products containing zinc:* May decrease ciprofloxacin absorption and effects. Give ciprofloxacin 2 hours before or 6 hours after these drugs.
Cyclosporine: May increase risk for cyclosporine toxicity. Monitor cyclosporine serum levels.
Iron salts: May decrease absorption of ciprofloxacin, reducing anti-infective response. Give at least 2 hours apart.
NSAIDs: May increase risk of CNS stimulation. Monitor patient closely.
Probenecid: May elevate level of ciprofloxacin. Monitor patient for toxicity.
Sucralfate: May decrease ciprofloxacin absorption, reducing anti-infective response. If

use together can't be avoided, give at least 6 hours apart.
Theophylline: May increase theophylline level and prolong theophylline half-life. Monitor level of theophylline and watch for adverse effects.
Tizanidine: Increases tizanidine levels, causing low blood pressure, somnolence, dizziness and slowed psychomotor skills. Avoid use together.
Warfarin: May increase anticoagulant effects. Monitor PT and INR closely.
Drug-herb. *Dong quai, St. John's wort:* May cause photosensitivity. Advise patient to avoid excessive sunlight exposure.
Yerba maté: May decrease clearance of yerba maté's methylxanthines and cause toxicity. Discourage use together.
Drug-food. *Caffeine:* May increase effect of caffeine. Monitor patient closely.
Dairy products, other foods: May delay peak drug levels. Advise patient to take drug on an empty stomach.
Orange juice fortified with calcium: May decrease GI absorption of drug, thereby reducing effects. Advise patient to avoid taking drug with calcium-fortified orange juice.
Drug-lifestyle. *Sun exposure:* May cause photosensitivity reactions. Advise patient to avoid excessive sunlight exposure.

Nursing considerations

- Obtain specimen for culture and sensitivity tests before giving first dose. Therapy may begin while awaiting results.
- Be aware of drug interactions. Some require waiting up to 6 hours after ciprofloxacin administration before giving another drug to avoid decreasing drug's effects. Food doesn't affect absorption but may delay peak drug levels.
- Monitor patient's intake and output and observe patient for signs of crystalluria.
- Tendon rupture may occur in patients receiving quinolones. Stop drug if pain or inflammation occurs, or patient ruptures a tendon.
- Long-term therapy may result in overgrowth of organisms resistant to ciprofloxacin.
- Cutaneous anthrax patients with signs of systemic involvement, extensive edema, or lesions on the head or neck need I.V. therapy and a multidrug approach.
- Additional antimicrobials for anthrax multidrug regimens can include rifampin, vancomycin, penicillin, ampicillin, chloramphenicol, imipenem, clindamycin, and clarithromycin.
- Steroids may be used as adjunctive therapy for anthrax patients with severe edema and for meningitis, based on experience with bacterial meningitis from other causes.
- Ciprofloxacin and doxycycline are first-line therapies for anthrax. Amoxicillin 500 mg P.O. t.i.d. for adults and 80 mg/kg daily in divided doses every 8 hours for children is an option for completion of therapy after clinical improvement.
- Follow current CDC recommendations for anthrax.
- Pregnant women and immunocompromised patients should receive the usual doses and regimens for anthrax.

Patient teaching

- Tell patient to take drug as prescribed, even after he feels better.
- Advise patient to drink plenty of fluids to reduce risk of urine crystals.
- Advise patient not to crush, split, or chew the extended-release tablets.
- Warn patient to avoid hazardous tasks that require alertness, such as driving, until effects of drug are known.
- Instruct patient to avoid caffeine while taking drug because of potential for increased caffeine effects.
- Advise patient that hypersensitivity reactions may occur even after first dose. If a rash or other allergic reaction occurs, tell him to stop drug immediately and notify prescriber.
- Tell patient that tendon rupture can occur with drug and to notify prescriber if he experiences pain or inflammation.
- Tell patient to avoid excessive sunlight or artificial ultraviolet light during therapy and to stop drug and call prescriber if phototoxicity occurs.
- Because drug appears in breast milk, advise woman to stop breast-feeding during treatment or to consider treatment with another drug.

cisplatin (CDDP, cisplatinum†)
Platinol AQ

Pregnancy risk category D

Indications & dosages

➲ **Adjunctive therapy in metastatic testicular cancer**
Adults: 20 mg/m^2 I.V. daily for 5 days. Repeat q 3 weeks for three or four cycles.

➲ **Adjunctive therapy in metastatic ovarian cancer**
Adults: 100 mg/m^2 I.V.; repeat q 4 weeks. Or, 50 to 100 mg/m^2 I.V. once q 3 to 4 weeks with cyclophosphamide.

➲ **Advanced bladder cancer**
Adults: 50 to 70 mg/m^2 I.V. q 3 to 4 weeks. Give 50 mg/m^2 q 4 weeks in patients who have received other antineoplastic drugs or radiation therapy.

➲ **Head and neck cancer♦**
Adults: 80 to 120 mg/m^2 I.V. q 3 weeks or 50 mg/m^2 I.V. on days 1 and 8 q 4 weeks. Doses of 50 to 120 mg/m^2 I.V. may be used in combination therapy.

➲ **Cervical cancer**
Adults: 40 to 75 mg/m^2 I.V. weekly or daily as monotherapy, in combination therapy, or with radiation therapy.

➲ **Non–small-cell lung cancer**
Adults: 75 to 100 mg/m^2 I.V. q 3 to 4 weeks in combination therapy.

➲ **Osteogenic sarcoma or neuroblastoma**
Children: 90 mg/m^2 I.V. q 3 weeks, or 30 mg/m^2 I.V. once weekly.

➲ **Recurrent brain tumor**
Children: 60 mg/m^2 I.V. daily for 2 consecutive days q 3 to 4 weeks.

Contraindications & cautions

- Contraindicated in patients hypersensitive to drug or other platinum-containing compounds and in those with severe renal disease, hearing impairment, or myelosuppression.
- Use cautiously in patients previously treated with radiation or cytotoxic drugs and in those with peripheral neuropathies; also use cautiously with other ototoxic and nephrotoxic drugs.

Adverse reactions

CNS: *peripheral neuritis*, ***seizures***.
EENT: *tinnitus, hearing loss, ototoxicity*, vestibular toxicity, optic neuritis, papilledema, cerebral blindness, blurred vision.
GI: loss of taste, *nausea, vomiting*.
GU: PROLONGED RENAL TOXICITY, with repeated courses of therapy.
Hematologic: MYELOSUPPRESSION, ***leukopenia, thrombocytopenia***, anemia.
Metabolic: *hypomagnesemia*, hypokalemia, hypocalcemia, hyponatremia, hypophosphatemia, hyperuricemia.
Other: ***anaphylactoid reaction***.

Interactions

Drug-drug. *Aminoglycosides:* May increase nephrotoxicity. Carefully monitor renal function study results.
Aminoglycosides, bumetanide, ethacrynic acid, furosemide, torsemide: May increase ototoxicity. Avoid using together, if possible.
Aspirin, NSAIDs: May increase risk of bleeding. Avoid using together.
Fosphenytoin, phenytoin: May decrease phenytoin and fosphenytoin levels. Monitor levels.
Myelosuppressives: May increase myelosuppression. Monitor patient.

Nursing considerations

- Monitor CBC, electrolyte levels (especially potassium and magnesium), platelet count, and renal function studies before initial and subsequent doses.
- To detect hearing loss, obtain audiometry tests before initial and subsequent doses.
- Prehydration and mannitol diuresis may significantly reduce renal toxicity and ototoxicity.
- Therapeutic effects are frequently accompanied by toxicity.
- Check current protocol. Some prescribers use I.V. sodium thiosulfate or amifostine to minimize toxicity.
- Patients may experience vomiting 3 to 5 days after treatment, requiring prolonged antiemetic treatment. Some prescribers combine metoclopramide with dexamethasone and antihistamines, or ondansetron or granisetron with dexamethasone to control vomiting. Monitor intake and output. Continue I.V. hydration until patient can tolerate adequate oral intake.
- Renal toxicity is cumulative; don't give next dose until renal function returns to normal.

• Don't repeat dose unless platelet count exceeds 100,000/mm³, WBC count exceeds 4,000/mm³, creatinine level is below 1.5 mg/dl, creatinine clearance is 50 ml/minute or more, and BUN level is below 25 mg/dl.
• To prevent bleeding, avoid all I.M. injections when platelet count is less than 50,000/mm³.
• Anticipate need for blood transfusions during treatment because of cumulative anemia.

!!ALERT Immediately give epinephrine, corticosteroids, or antihistamines for anaphylactoid reactions.
• Safety of drug in children hasn't been established.

!!ALERT Don't confuse cisplatin with carboplatin; they aren't interchangeable.

Patient teaching

• Advise patient to watch for signs and symptoms of infection (fever, sore throat, fatigue) and bleeding (easy bruising, nosebleeds, bleeding gums, tarry stools). Tell patient to take temperature daily.
• Tell patient to immediately report ringing in the ears or numbness in hands or feet.
• Instruct patient to avoid OTC products containing aspirin.
• Advise women to stop breast-feeding during therapy because of risk of toxicity to infant.
• Advise women of childbearing age to consult prescriber before becoming pregnant.

citalopram hydrobromide
Celexa

Pregnancy risk category C

Indications & dosages

➲ Depression
Adults: Initially, 20 mg P.O. once daily, increasing to 40 mg daily after no less than 1 week. Maximum recommended dose is 40 mg daily.
Elderly patients: 20 mg daily P.O. with adjustment to 40 mg daily only for unresponsive patients.

For patients with hepatic impairment, use 20 mg daily P.O. with adjustment to 40 mg daily only for unresponsive patients.

Contraindications & cautions

• Contraindicated in patients hypersensitive to drug or its inactive components, within 14 days of MAO inhibitor therapy, and in patients taking pimozide.
• Use cautiously in patients with history of mania, seizures, suicidal thoughts, or hepatic or renal impairment.
• Use in third trimester of pregnancy may be linked to neonatal complications at birth. Consider the risk versus benefit of treatment during this time.
• Safety and effectiveness of drug haven't been established in children.

Adverse reactions

CNS: tremor, *somnolence*, *insomnia*, anxiety, agitation, dizziness, paresthesia, migraine, impaired concentration, amnesia, depression, apathy, ***suicide attempt***, confusion, fatigue, fever.
CV: tachycardia, orthostatic hypotension, hypotension.
EENT: rhinitis, sinusitis, abnormal accommodation.
GI: *dry mouth*, *nausea*, diarrhea, anorexia, dyspepsia, vomiting, abdominal pain, taste perversion, increased saliva, flatulence, increased appetite.
GU: dysmenorrhea, amenorrhea, ejaculation disorder, impotence, anorgasmia, polyuria.
Metabolic: decreased or increased weight.
Musculoskeletal: arthralgia, myalgia.
Respiratory: upper respiratory tract infection, coughing.
Skin: rash, pruritus, *increased sweating*.
Other: yawning, decreased libido.

Interactions

Drug-drug. *Carbamazepine:* May increase citalopram clearance. Monitor patient for effects.
CNS drugs: May cause additive effects. Use together cautiously.
Drugs that inhibit cytochrome P-450 isoenzymes 3A4 and 2C19: May cause decreased clearance of citalopram. Monitor patient for increased adverse effects.
Imipramine, other tricyclic antidepressants: May increase level of imipramine metabolite desipramine by about 50%. Use together cautiously.

Lithium: May enhance serotonergic effect of citalopram. Use together cautiously, and monitor lithium level.
MAO inhibitors (phenelzine, selegiline, tranylcypromine): May cause serotonin syndrome. Avoid using within 14 days of MAO inhibitor therapy.
Sumatriptan: May cause weakness, hyperreflexia, and incoordination. Monitor patient closely.
Drug-lifestyle. *Alcohol use:* May increase CNS effects. Discourage use together.

Nursing considerations

- Although drug hasn't been shown to impair psychomotor performance, any psychoactive drug has the potential to impair judgment, thinking, or motor skills.
- The possibility of a suicide attempt is inherent in depression and may persist until significant remission occurs. Closely supervise high-risk patients at start of drug therapy. Reduce risk of overdose by limiting amount of drug available per refill.
- At least 14 days should elapse between MAO inhibitor therapy and citalopram therapy.

!!ALERT Don't confuse Celexa with Celebrex or Cerebyx.

Patient teaching

- Tell patient that drug may be taken in the morning or evening without regard to meals. If drowsiness occurs, he should take drug in evening.
- Caution patient against use of MAO inhibitors while taking citalopram.
- Inform patient that, although improvement may take 1 to 4 weeks, he should continue therapy as prescribed.
- Advise patient not to stop medication abruptly.
- Instruct patient to exercise caution when driving or operating hazardous machinery; drug may impair judgment, thinking, and motor skills.
- Advise patient to consult prescriber before taking other prescription or OTC drugs.
- Advise woman of childbearing age to consult prescriber before breast-feeding.
- Warn patient to avoid alcohol during drug therapy.
- Instruct woman of childbearing age to use contraceptives during drug therapy and to notify prescriber immediately if pregnancy is suspected.

clarithromycin
Biaxin, Biaxin XL

Pregnancy risk category C

Indications & dosages

➲ **Pharyngitis or tonsillitis caused by *Streptococcus pyogenes***
Adults: 250 mg P.O. q 12 hours for 10 days.
Children: 15 mg/kg/day P.O. divided q 12 hours for 10 days.

➲ **Acute maxillary sinusitis caused by *S. pneumoniae, Haemophilus influenzae,* or *Moraxella catarrhalis***
Adults: 500 mg P.O. q 12 hours for 14 days or two 500-mg extended-release tablets P.O. daily for 14 days.
Children: 15 mg/kg/day P.O. divided q 12 hours for 10 days.

➲ **Acute worsening of chronic bronchitis caused by *M. catarrhalis, S. pneumoniae;* community-acquired pneumonia caused by *H. influenzae, S. pneumoniae, Mycoplasma pneumoniae,* or *Chlamydia pneumoniae***
Adults: 250 mg P.O. q 12 hours for 7 days (*H. influenzae*) or 7 to 14 days (others).

➲ **Acute worsening of chronic bronchitis caused by *H. influenzae or H. parainfluenzae***
Adults: 500 mg P.O. q 12 hours for 7 days *H. parainfluenzae* or 7 to 14 days *H. influenzae.*

➲ **Acute worsening of chronic bronchitis caused by *M. catarrhalis, S. pneumoniae, H. parainfluenzae,* or *H. influenzae***
Adults: Two 500-mg P.O. extended-release tablets daily for 7 days.

➲ **Mild-to-moderate community-acquired pneumonia, caused by *H. influenzae, H. parainfluenzae, M. catarrhalis, S. pneumoniae, C. pneumoniae,* or *M. pneumoniae***
Adults: Two 500-mg P.O. extended-release tablets daily for 7 days.

➲ **Community-acquired pneumonia from *S. pneumoniae, C. pneumoniae,* and *M. pneumoniae***
Children: 15 mg/kg/day P.O. divided q 12 hours for 10 days.

➲ **Uncomplicated skin and skin-structure infections caused by *Staphylococcus aureus* or *S. pyogenes***
Adults: 250 mg P.O. q 12 hours for 7 to 14 days.
Children: 15 mg/kg/day P.O. divided q 12 hours for 10 days.
➲ **Acute otitis media caused by *H. influenzae, M. catarrhalis,* or *S. pneumoniae***
Children: 15 mg/kg/day P.O. divided q 12 hours for 10 days.
➲ **To prevent and treat disseminated infection caused by *Mycobacterium avium* complex**
Adults: 500 mg P.O. b.i.d.
Children: 7.5 mg/kg P.O. b.i.d., up to 500 mg b.i.d.
➲ ***Helicobacter pylori,* to reduce risk of duodenal ulcer recurrence**
Adults: 500 mg clarithromycin with 30 mg lansoprazole and 1 g amoxicillin, all given q 12 hours for 10 to 14 days. Or, 500 mg clarithromycin with 20 mg omeprazole and 1 g amoxicillin, all given q 12 hours for 10 days. Or, 500 mg clarithromycin b.i.d., 20 mg rabeprazole b.i.d., and 1 g amoxicillin b.i.d., all for 7 days. Or, two-drug regimen with 500 mg clarithromycin q 8 hours and 40 mg omeprazole once daily for 14 days. Continue omeprazole for 14 additional days.

In patients with creatinine clearance less than 30 ml/minute, cut dose in half or double frequency interval.

Contraindications & cautions

- Contraindicated in patients hypersensitive to clarithromycin, erythromycin, or other macrolides and in those receiving pimozide or other drugs that prolong QT interval or cause cardiac arrhythmias.
- Use cautiously in patients with hepatic or renal impairment.

Adverse reactions

CNS: headache.
GI: diarrhea, nausea, taste perversion, abdominal pain or discomfort, ***pseudomembranous colitis***, vomiting (pediatric).
Hematologic: ***leukopenia***, coagulation abnormalities.
Skin: rash (pediatric).

Interactions

Drug-drug. *Alprazolam, midazolam, triazolam:* May decrease clearance of these drugs, causing adverse reactions. Use together cautiously.
Carbamazepine, phenytoin: May inhibit metabolism of these drugs, increasing serum levels and risk of toxicity. Avoid using together.
Cyclosporine: May increase cyclosporine levels. Monitor cyclosporine level.
Digoxin: May increase digoxin level. Monitor patient for digitalis toxicity.
Dihydroergotamine, ergotamine: May cause acute ergot toxicity. Avoid using together.
Fluconazole: May increase clarithromycin level. Monitor patient closely.
HMG-CoA reductase inhibitors: May increase levels of these drugs; may rarely cause rhabdomyolysis. Use together cautiously.
Other drugs that prolong the QTc interval (amiodarone, antipsychotics, disopyramide, fluoroquinolones, procainamide, quinidine, sotalol, tricyclic antidepressants): May have additive effects. Monitor ECG for QTc interval prolongation. Avoid using together if possible.
Pimozide: May cause torsades de pointes. Use together is contraindicated.
Ritonavir: May prolong absorption of clarithromycin.
Sildenafil: May prolong absorption of sildenafil. May need to reduce sildenafil dosage.
Theophylline: May increase theophylline level. Monitor drug level.
Warfarin: May increase PT and INR. Monitor PT and INR carefully.
Zidovudine: May alter zidovudine level. Monitor patient closely.

Nursing considerations

!!ALERT The safety and efficacy of the extended-release formulation haven't been established for treating other infections for which the original formulation has been approved.

- Obtain specimen for culture and sensitivity tests before giving first dose. Therapy may begin pending results.
- Monitor patient for superinfection. Drug may cause overgrowth of nonsusceptible bacteria or fungi.
- Giving clarithromycin with a drug metabolized by CYP3A may increase drug levels

and prolong therapeutic and adverse effects of the drug given concomitantly.

Patient teaching

- Tell patient to take drug as prescribed, even after he feels better.
- Advise patient to report persistent adverse reactions.
- Inform patient that drug may be taken with or without food. Don't refrigerate the suspension form. Discard unused portion after 14 days.

clemastine fumarate

Dayhist-1 ◇, Tavist Allergy ◇

Pregnancy risk category B

Indications & dosages

➲ Rhinitis, allergy symptoms

Adults and children age 12 and older: 1.34 mg P.O. b.i.d.; not to exceed 8.04 mg/day for syrup and 2.68 mg/day for tablets.
Children ages 6 to 11: 0.67 mg syrup P.O. b.i.d.; not to exceed 4.02 mg/day.

➲ Allergic skin manifestation of urticaria and angioedema

Adults and children age 12 and older: 2.68 mg P.O. b.i.d.; not to exceed 8.04 mg daily.
Children ages 6 to 11: 1.34 mg syrup P.O. b.i.d.; not to exceed 4.02 mg/day.

Contraindications & cautions

- Contraindicated in patients hypersensitive to drug or other antihistamines of similar chemical structure, in those taking MAO inhibitors, and in those with acute asthma, angle-closure glaucoma, stenosing peptic ulcer, symptomatic prostatic hyperplasia, bladder neck obstruction, or pyloroduodenal obstruction.
- Contraindicated in neonates, premature infants, and breast-feeding women.
- Use cautiously in elderly patients and in those with increased intraocular pressure, hyperthyroidism, CV disease, hypertension, bronchial asthma, and prostatic hyperplasia.
- Use in children younger than age 12 only as directed by prescriber.

Adverse reactions

CNS: *sedation, drowsiness,* ***seizures****,* nervousness, tremor, confusion, restlessness, vertigo, headache, *sleepiness, dizziness, incoordination,* fatigue.
CV: hypotension, palpitations, tachycardia.
GI: *epigastric distress,* anorexia, diarrhea, nausea, vomiting, constipation, *dry mouth.*
GU: urine retention, urinary frequency.
Hematologic: hemolytic anemia, ***thrombocytopenia***, ***agranulocytosis***.
Respiratory: *thick bronchial secretions.*
Skin: rash, urticaria, photosensitivity, diaphoresis.
Other: ***anaphylactic shock***.

Interactions

Drug-drug. *CNS depressants:* May increase sedation. Use together cautiously.
MAO inhibitors: May increase anticholinergic effects. Avoid using together.
Drug-lifestyle. *Alcohol use:* May increase CNS depression. Discourage use together.
Sun exposure: May cause photosensitivity reactions. Advise patient to avoid extensive sunlight exposure.

Nursing considerations

- Stop drug 4 days before diagnostic skin testing because antihistamines can prevent, reduce, or mask positive skin test result.
- Monitor blood counts during long-term therapy; observe for signs of blood dyscrasias.

Patient teaching

- Warn patient to avoid alcohol and hazardous activities that require alertness until CNS effects of drug are known.
- Tell patient that coffee or tea may reduce drowsiness. Urge caution if palpitations develop.
- Inform patient that sugarless gum, hard candy, or ice chips may relieve dry mouth.
- Warn patient of possible photosensitivity reactions. Advise use of a sunblock.
- Tell patient to notify prescriber if tolerance develops because a different antihistamine may need to be prescribed.

clindamycin hydrochloride
Cleocin HCl

clindamycin palmitate hydrochloride
Cleocin Pediatric, Dalacin C Flavored Granules†

clindamycin phosphate (systemic)
Cleocin Phosphate

Pregnancy risk category B

Indications & dosages

➲ **Infections caused by sensitive staphylococci, streptococci, pneumococci, *Bacteroides, Fusobacterium, Clostridium perfringens* and other sensitive aerobic and anaerobic organisms**
Adults: 150 to 450 mg P.O. q 6 hours; or 300 to 600 mg I.M. or I.V. q 6, 8, or 12 hours.
Children older than age 1 month: 8 to 20 mg/kg P.O. daily, in divided doses q 6 to 8 hours; or 15 to 40 mg/kg I.M. or I.V. daily, in divided doses q 6 or 8 hours.

➲ **Pelvic inflammatory disease**
Adults and adolescents: 900 mg I.V. q 8 hours, with gentamicin. Continue at least 48 hours after symptoms improve; then switch to oral clindamycin 450 mg q.i.d. for total of 10 to 14 days or doxycycline 100 mg P.O. q 12 hours for total of 10 to 14 days.

➲ ***Pneumocystis carinii* pneumonia♦**
Adults: 600 mg I.V. q 6 hours or 900 mg I.V. q 8 hours, with primaquine.

➲ **CNS toxoplasmosis in AIDS patients, as alternative to sulfonamides with pyrimethamine♦**
Adults: 1,200 to 2,400 mg/day in divided doses.

Contraindications & cautions

- Contraindicated in patients hypersensitive to drug or lincomycin.
- Use cautiously in neonates and patients with renal or hepatic disease, asthma, history of GI disease, or significant allergies.

Adverse reactions

CV: thrombophlebitis.
GI: *nausea*, vomiting, abdominal pain, diarrhea, ***pseudomembranous colitis***.
Hematologic: *transient leukopenia*, eosinophilia, ***thrombocytopenia***.
Hepatic: jaundice.
Skin: maculopapular rash, urticaria.
Other: *anaphylaxis*.

Interactions

Drug-drug. *Erythromycin:* May block access of clindamycin to its site of action. Avoid using together.
Kaolin: May decrease absorption of oral clindamycin. Separate dosage times.
Neuromuscular blockers: May increase neuromuscular blockade. Monitor patient closely.
Drug-food. *Diet foods with sodium cyclamate:* May decrease drug level. Discourage use together.

Nursing considerations

- Obtain specimen for culture and sensitivity tests before giving first dose. Therapy may begin pending results.
- For I.M. administration, inject deep into muscle. Rotate sites. Don't exceed 600 mg per injection.
- I.M. injection may raise CK level in response to muscle irritation.
- Don't refrigerate reconstituted oral solution because it will thicken. Drug is stable for 2 weeks at room temperature.
- Monitor renal, hepatic, and hematopoietic functions during prolonged therapy.
- Observe patient for signs and symptoms of superinfection.

!!ALERT Don't give opioid antidiarrheals to treat drug-induced diarrhea; they may prolong and worsen this condition.

- Drug doesn't penetrate blood-brain barrier.

Patient teaching

- Advise patient to take capsule form with a full glass of water to prevent esophageal irritation.
- Warn patient that I.M. injection may be painful.
- Tell patient to report discomfort at I.V. insertion site.
- Instruct patient to notify prescriber of adverse reactions (especially diarrhea). Warn him not to treat such diarrhea himself because clindamycin therapy may cause severe, even life-threatening, colitis.

clindamycin phosphate (topical)

Cleocin, Cleocin T, Clinda-Derm, Clindagel, ClindaMax, Clindesse, Clindets, C/T/S, Evoclin

Pregnancy risk category B

Indications & dosages

➲ **Inflammatory acne vulgaris**

Adults and adolescents: Apply to skin b.i.d., morning and evening or once daily if using Clindagel or Evoclin.

➲ **Bacterial vaginosis**

Adults: 1 applicatorful intravaginally h.s. for 7 days or 1 suppository intravaginally h.s. for 3 days, or one applicatorful of Clindesse intravaginally as a single dose.

Contraindications & cautions

- Contraindicated in patients hypersensitive to drug and in those with history of ulcerative colitis, regional enteritis, or antibiotic-related colitis.

Adverse reactions

CNS: *headache.*
EENT: pharyngitis.
GI: GI upset, diarrhea, bloody diarrhea, abdominal pain, constipation, colitis including pseudomembranous colitis.
GU: *cervicitis, vaginitis,* ***Candida albicans*** *overgrowth, vulvar irritation.*
Skin: *dryness,* rash, *redness,* pruritus, swelling, irritation, contact dermatitis, UTI, vaginal discharge, burning.

Interactions

Drug-drug. *Erythromycin:* May antagonize clindamycin's effect. Separate doses.
Isotretinoin: May cause cumulative dryness, resulting in excessive skin irritation. Use together cautiously.
Neuromuscular blockers: May increase action of neuromuscular blocker. Use together cautiously.
Drug-lifestyle. *Abrasive or medicated soaps or cleansers, acne products, or other preparations containing peeling drugs (benzoyl peroxide, resorcinol, salicylic acid, sulfur, tretinoin), alcohol-containing products (aftershave, cosmetics, perfumed toiletries, shaving creams or lotions), astringent soaps or cosmetics, medicated cosmetics or cover-ups:* May cause cumulative dryness, resulting in excessive skin irritation. Urge caution.

Nursing considerations

- For treating acne, drug may be used with tretinoin or benzoyl peroxide as well as systemic antibiotics.
- Drug can cause excessive dryness.
- Monitor elderly patients for systemic effects.

Patient teaching

- Tell patient to wash area with warm water and soap, rinse, pat dry, and wait 30 minutes after washing or shaving to apply.
- Warn patient to avoid excessive washing of area. Tell patient to cover entire affected area but to avoid contact with eyes, nose, mouth, and other mucous membranes.
- Instruct patient to use other prescribed acne medicines at a different time.
- Tell patient to use only as prescribed.
- Instruct patient to dab, not roll, applicator-tipped bottle. If tip becomes dry, patient should invert bottle and depress tip several times to moisten.
- Warn patient not to smoke while applying topical solution.
- For intravaginal application, make sure patient knows how to use applicators that come with drug.
- Advise patient that the vaginal form contains mineral oil that can weaken latex or rubber products, such as condoms and diaphragms, and that she should use another form of birth control within 5 days of therapy.
- Advise patient to avoid sexual intercourse during intravaginal therapy.
- Instruct patient to notify prescriber immediately if abdominal pain or diarrhea occurs. Inform patient that an antidiarrheal may worsen condition and should only be used as directed by prescriber.
- Tell patient to remove pledgets from foil before use.
- Advise patient to use pledgets only once and then discard. Also, more than 1 pledget may be used per application.
- Advise patient to complete entire course of therapy.

clobetasol propionate
Clobex, Cormax, Dermovate†, Embeline E, Olux, Temovate

Pregnancy risk category C

Indications & dosages

➲ **Inflammation and pruritus from dermatoses responsive to corticosteroids; short-term topical treatment of mild to moderate plaque-type psoriasis of nonscalp regions, excluding the face and intertriginous areas**
Adults: Apply thin layer of Clobex lotion to affected skin areas b.i.d., morning and evening, for maximum of 14 days. For lesions of moderate to severe plaque psoriasis that haven't improved sufficiently, continue treatment for up to 2 more weeks, as long as 10% or less of the body surface area is affected. Total dose shouldn't exceed 50 g (50 ml) of lotion weekly.

➲ **Inflammation and pruritus from dermatoses responsive to corticosteroids; short-term topical treatment of mild to moderate plaque-type psoriasis of nonscalp regions, excluding the face and intertriginous areas**
Adults and children age 12 and older: Apply thin layer to affected skin areas b.i.d., morning and evening, for maximum of 14 days. Total dose shouldn't exceed 50 g of foam, cream, or ointment or 50 ml of lotion or solution weekly.

➲ **Inflammation and pruritus of moderate to severe corticosteroid-responsive dermatoses of the scalp**
Adults: Apply to the affected scalp area b.i.d., morning and evening. Gently massage into affected scalp area until the foam disappears. Repeat until entire affected scalp area is treated. Limit treatment to 14 days, with no more than 50 g of foam weekly.

➲ **Moderate to severe scalp psoriasis**
Adults: Apply Clobex shampoo to affected areas of dry scalp in thin film once daily. Leave in place for 15 minutes before lathering and rinsing. Limit treatment to 4 consecutive weeks.

Contraindications & cautions

- Contraindicated in patients hypersensitive to corticosteroids and in those with primary scalp infections.

Adverse reactions

GU: glycosuria.
Metabolic: hyperglycemia.
Skin: burning, pruritus, irritation, dryness, erythema, folliculitis, perioral dermatitis, allergic contact dermatitis, hypopigmentation, hypertrichosis, acneiform eruptions.
Other: ***hypothalamic-pituitary-adrenal axis suppression***, Cushing's syndrome.

Interactions

None significant.

Nursing considerations

- Gently wash skin before applying. To prevent skin damage, rub medication in gently and completely. When treating hairy sites, part hair and apply directly to lesions.
- Avoid applying near eyes or mucous membranes or in ear canal.

!!ALERT Don't use occlusive dressings or bandages. Don't cover or wrap treated areas unless directed by prescriber.

- If antifungal or antibiotic combined with corticosteroid fails to provide prompt improvement, stop corticosteroid until infection is controlled.
- Stop drug and notify prescriber if skin infection, striae, or atrophy occurs.
- Hypothalamic-pituitary-adrenal axis suppression occurs at doses as low as 2 g daily.

Patient teaching

- Teach patient how to apply drug and to avoid contact with eyes.
- Tell patient to wash hands after application.
- Tell patient to stop drug and report signs of systemic absorption, skin irritation or ulceration, hypersensitivity, or infection.
- Warn patient to use drug for no longer than 14 consecutive days.
- Tell patient using the foam to invert can and dispense a small amount of Olux foam (up to a golf-ball–size dollop) into the cap of the can, onto a saucer or other cool surface, or directly on the lesion, taking care to avoid contact with the eyes. Dispensing directly onto hands isn't recommended because the foam will melt immediately upon contact with warm skin. Tell him to move hair away from affected area of scalp so that foam can be applied to each affected area.
- Tell patient using foam that contents are flammable and under pressure, so he should

avoid smoking during and immediately after application and keep can away from flames. Also tell him not to puncture or incinerate container.

clofarabine
Clolar

Pregnancy risk category D

Indications & dosages

➲ **Relapsed or refractory acute lymphoblastic leukemia (ALL) after at least two previous regimens**
Children ages 1 to 21: 52 mg/m^2 by I.V. infusion over 2 hours daily for 5 consecutive days. Repeat about q 2 to 6 weeks based on recovery or return to baseline of organ function. May also give 100 mg/m^2 hydrocortisone I.V. on days 1 through 3 of cycle to help prevent capillary leak syndrome.

Contraindications & cautions

- No known contraindications.
- Use cautiously in patients with hepatic or renal dysfunction.

Adverse reactions

CNS: *anxiety, depression, dizziness, fatigue, headache, irritability, lethargy, somnolence, tremor.*
CV: *edema, flushing, hypertension, hypotension, left ventricular systolic dysfunction, pericardial effusion, tachycardia.*
EENT: *epistaxis, mucosal inflammation, sore throat.*
GI: *abdominal pain, anorexia, constipation, decreased appetite, decreased weight, diarrhea, gingival bleeding, oral candidiasis, nausea, vomiting.*
GU: *hematuria.*
Hematologic: BONE MARROW SUPPRESSION, FEBRILE NEUTROPENIA, NEUTROPENIA.
Hepatic: *hepatomegaly, jaundice.*
Musculoskeletal: *arthralgia, back pain, limb pain, myalgia.*
Respiratory: *pneumonia, dyspnea, pleural effusion,* RESPIRATORY DISTRESS.
Skin: *contusion, dermatitis, dry skin, erythema, hand-foot syndrome, petechiae, pruritus.*
Other: BACTEREMIA, cellulitis, herpes simplex infection, *injection site pain, pain, pyrexia, rigors,* SEPSIS, ***capillary leak syndrome***, staphylococcal infections, ***systemic inflammatory response syndrome (SIRS)***, transfusion reaction.

Interactions

Drug-drug. *Blood pressure or cardiac drugs:* May increase risk of adverse effects. Monitor patient closely.
Hepatotoxic drugs: May increase the risk of hepatic toxicity. Avoid using together.
Nephrotoxic drugs: May decrease excretion of clofarabine. Avoid using together.

Nursing considerations

- Monitor patient for dehydration. Give I.V. fluids continuously during treatment.
- If you suspect hyperuricemia, give allopurinol.
- Monitor patient's respiratory status and blood pressure closely.
- Assess patient for signs and symptoms of tumor lysis syndrome, cytokine release (tachypnea, tachycardia, hypotension, pulmonary edema) that could develop into SIRS, capillary leak syndrome, and organ dysfunction.
- If patient shows signs and symptoms of SIRS or capillary leak syndrome, stop drug immediately .
- Obtain CBC and platelet count and monitor hepatic and renal function regularly.
- If hypotension develops, stop drug. If hypotension resolves without treatment, restart drug at a lower dose.

Patient teaching

- Tell patient and caregiver that adverse effects are common. Patient will need close monitoring.
- Tell patient and caregiver to immediately report dizziness, light-headedness, fainting, decreased urine output, bruising, flulike symptoms, and infection.
- Urge patient and caregiver to also report yellowing of skin or eyes, darkened urine, and abdominal pain.
- Tell woman of childbearing age not to breast-feed or become pregnant.

clomiphene citrate
Clomid, Milophene, Serophene

Pregnancy risk category X

Indications & dosages
➲ To induce ovulation
Adults: 50 mg P.O. daily for 5 days, starting on day 5 of menstrual cycle (first day of menstrual flow is day 1) if bleeding occurs, or at any time if patient hasn't had recent uterine bleeding. If ovulation doesn't occur, may increase dose to 100 mg P.O. daily for 5 days as soon as 30 days after previous course. Repeat until conception occurs or until three courses of therapy are completed.

Contraindications & cautions
- Contraindicated in pregnant patients and in those with undiagnosed abnormal genital bleeding, ovarian cyst not related to polycystic ovarian syndrome, hepatic disease or dysfunction, uncontrolled thyroid or adrenal dysfunction, or organic intracranial lesion (such as a pituitary tumor).

Adverse reactions
CNS: headache, restlessness, insomnia, dizziness, light-headedness, depression, fatigue.
EENT: blurred vision, diplopia, scotoma, photophobia.
GI: nausea, vomiting, bloating, distention.
GU: urinary frequency and polyuria, abnormal uterine bleeding, *ovarian enlargement,* ovarian cyst that regresses spontaneously when drug is stopped.
Metabolic: weight gain.
Skin: reversible alopecia, urticaria, rash, dermatitis.
Other: *hot flashes, breast discomfort.*

Interactions
None significant.

Nursing considerations
- Monitor patient closely because of potentially serious adverse reactions.
- Long-term cyclic therapy isn't recommended.

!!ALERT Don't confuse clomiphene with clomipramine or clonidine. Don't confuse Serophene with Sarafem.

Patient teaching
- Tell patient about the risk of multiple births, which increases with higher doses.
- Teach patient to take and chart basal body temperature to ascertain if ovulation has occurred.
- Reinforce importance of compliance with medication regimen.
- Reassure patient that ovulation typically occurs after first course of therapy. If pregnancy doesn't occur, therapy may be repeated twice.
- Advise patient to stop drug and contact prescriber immediately if pregnancy is suspected because drug may have teratogenic effect.

!!ALERT Advise patient to stop drug and contact prescriber immediately if abdominal symptoms or pain occur; these symptoms may indicate ovarian enlargement or ovarian cyst. Also tell patient to immediately notify prescriber if signs and symptoms of impending visual toxicity occur, such as blurred vision, double vision, vision defect in one part of the eye (scotoma), or sensitivity to the sun.

- Warn patient to avoid hazardous activities, such as driving or operating machinery, until CNS effects are known. Drug may cause dizziness and visual disturbances.

clomipramine hydrochloride
Anafranil

Pregnancy risk category C

Indications & dosages
➲ Obsessive-compulsive disorder
Adults: Initially, 25 mg P.O. daily with meals, gradually increased to 100 mg daily in divided doses during first 2 weeks. Thereafter, increase to maximum dose of 250 mg daily in divided doses with meals, p.r.n. After adjustment, give total daily dose h.s.
Children and adolescents: Initially, 25 mg P.O. daily with meals, gradually increased over first 2 weeks to daily maximum of 3 mg/kg or 100 mg P.O. in divided doses, whichever is smaller. Maximum daily dose is 3 mg/kg or 200 mg, whichever is smaller; give h.s. after adjustment. Reassess and adjust dosage periodically.

➲ **To manage panic disorder with or without agoraphobia**
Adults: 12.5 to 150 mg P.O. daily (maximum 200 mg).
➲ **Depression, chronic pain♦**
Adults: 100 to 250 mg P.O. daily.
➲ **Cataplexy and related narcolepsy♦**
Adults: 25 to 200 mg P.O. daily.

Contraindications & cautions

- Contraindicated in patients hypersensitive to drug or other tricyclic antidepressants, in those who have taken MAO inhibitors within previous 14 days, and in patients in acute recovery period after MI.
- Use cautiously in patients with history of seizure disorders or with brain damage of varying cause; in patients receiving other seizure threshold-lowering drugs; in patients at risk for suicide; in patients with history of urine retention or angle-closure glaucoma, increased intraocular pressure, CV disease, impaired hepatic or renal function, or hyperthyroidism; in patients with tumors of the adrenal medulla; in patients receiving thyroid drug or electroconvulsive therapy; and in those undergoing elective surgery.

Adverse reactions

CNS: *somnolence, tremor, dizziness, headache, insomnia, nervousness, myoclonus, fatigue,* EEG changes, ***seizures.***
CV: orthostatic hypotension, palpitations, tachycardia.
EENT: *pharyngitis, rhinitis, visual changes.*
GI: *dry mouth, constipation, nausea, dyspepsia, increased appetite,* diarrhea, *anorexia, abdominal pain.*
GU: *urinary hesitancy,* UTI, *dysmenorrhea, ejaculation failure, impotence.*
Hematologic: purpura.
Metabolic: *weight gain.*
Musculoskeletal: *myalgia.*
Skin: *diaphoresis,* rash, pruritus, dry skin.
Other: *altered libido.*

Interactions

Drug-drug. *Barbiturates:* May decrease tricyclic antidepressant level. Watch for decreased antidepressant effect.
Cimetidine, fluoxetine, fluvoxamine, paroxetine, sertraline: May increase tricyclic antidepressant level. Watch for enhanced antidepressant effect.
Clonidine: May cause life-threatening blood pressure elevations. Avoid using together.
CNS depressants: May enhance CNS depression. Avoid using together.
Epinephrine, norepinephrine: May increase hypertensive effect. Use together cautiously.
MAO inhibitors: May cause hyperpyretic crisis, seizures, coma, or death. Avoid using within 14 days of MAO inhibitor therapy.
Drug-herb. *Evening primrose oil:* May cause additive or synergistic effect, resulting in lower seizure threshold and increasing the risk of seizure. Discourage use together.
St. John's wort, SAM-e, yohimbe: May cause serotonin syndrome. Discourage use together.
Drug-lifestyle. *Alcohol use:* May enhance CNS depression. Discourage use together.
Sun exposure: May increase risk of photosensitivity reactions. Advise patient to avoid excessive sunlight exposure.

Nursing considerations

- Monitor mood and watch for suicidal tendencies. Allow patient to have only minimal amount of drug.
- Don't withdraw drug abruptly.
- Because patients using tricyclic antidepressants may suffer hypertensive episodes during surgery, stop drug gradually several days before surgery.
- Relieve dry mouth with sugarless candy or gum. Saliva substitutes may be needed.

!!ALERT Don't confuse clomipramine with chlorpromazine or clomiphene, or Anafranil with enalapril, nafarelin, or alfentanil.

Patient teaching

- Warn patient to avoid hazardous activities requiring alertness and good coordination, especially during adjustment. Daytime sedation and dizziness may occur.
- Tell patient to avoid alcohol during drug therapy.
- Warn patient not to stop drug suddenly.
- Advise patient to use sunblock, wear protective clothing, and avoid prolonged exposure to strong sunlight to prevent oversensitivity to the sun.

clonazepam
Klonopin

Pregnancy risk category D
Controlled substance schedule IV

Indications & dosages

➲ Lennox-Gastaut syndrome, atypical absence seizures, akinetic and myoclonic seizures
Adults: Initially, no more than 1.5 mg P.O. daily in three divided doses. May be increased by 0.5 to 1 mg q 3 days until seizures are controlled. If given in unequal doses, give largest dose h.s. Maximum recommended daily dose is 20 mg.
Children up to age 10 or 30 kg (66 lb): Initially, 0.01 to 0.03 mg/kg P.O. daily (not to exceed 0.05 mg/kg daily) in two or three divided doses. Increase by 0.25 to 0.5 mg q third day to maximum maintenance dose of 0.1 to 0.2 mg/kg daily, p.r.n.
➲ Panic disorder
Adults: Initially, 0.25 mg P.O. b.i.d.; increase to target dose of 1 mg daily after 3 days. Some patients may benefit from dosages up to maximum of 4 mg daily. To achieve 4 mg daily, increase dosage in increments of 0.125 to 0.25 mg b.i.d. q 3 days, as tolerated, until panic disorder is controlled. Taper drug with decrease of 0.125 mg b.i.d. q 3 days until drug is stopped.
➲ Acute manic episodes of bipolar disorder♦
Adults: 0.75 to 16 mg daily P.O.
➲ Adjunct treatment for schizophrenia♦
Adults: 0.5 to 2 mg daily P.O.
➲ Periodic leg movements during sleep♦
Adults: 0.5 to 2 mg P.O. h.s.
➲ Parkinsonian (hypokinetic) dysarthria♦
Adults: 0.25 to 0.5 mg daily P.O.
➲ Multifocal tic disorders♦
Adults: 1.5 to 12 mg daily P.O.
➲ Neuralgias (deafferentation pain syndromes)♦
Adults: 2 to 4 mg daily P.O.

Contraindications & cautions

- Contraindicated in patients hypersensitive to benzodiazepines and in those with significant hepatic disease or acute angle-closure glaucoma.
- Use cautiously in patients with mixed-type seizures because drug may cause generalized tonic-clonic seizures.
- Use cautiously in children and in patients with chronic respiratory disease or open-angle glaucoma.

Adverse reactions

CNS: *drowsiness*, ataxia, behavioral disturbances, slurred speech, tremor, confusion, agitation, depression.
CV: palpitations.
EENT: nystagmus, abnormal eye movements.
GI: sore gums, constipation, gastritis, change in appetite, nausea, vomiting, anorexia, diarrhea.
GU: dysuria, enuresis, nocturia, urine retention.
Hematologic: ***leukopenia***, ***thrombocytopenia***, eosinophilia.
Respiratory: ***respiratory depression***, chest congestion, shortness of breath.
Skin: rash.

Interactions

Drug-drug. *Carbamazepine, phenobarbital, phenytoin:* Lowers clonazepam levels. Monitor patient closely.
CNS depressants: May increase CNS depression. Avoid using together.
Fluconazole, itraconazole, ketoconazole, miconazole: May increase and prolong drug levels, CNS depression, and psychomotor impairment. Avoid using together.
Drug-lifestyle. *Alcohol use:* May cause additive CNS effects. Discourage use together.
Smoking: May increase clearance of clonazepam. Monitor patient for decreased drug effects.

Nursing considerations

- Watch for behavioral disturbances, especially in children.
- Don't stop drug abruptly because this may worsen seizures. Call prescriber at once if adverse reactions develop.
- Assess elderly patient's response closely. Elderly patients are more sensitive to drug's CNS effects.
- Monitor patient for oversedation.
- Monitor CBC and liver function tests.
- Withdrawal symptoms are similar to those of barbiturates.

- To reduce inconvenience of somnolence when drug is used for panic disorder, administration of one dose at bedtime may be desirable.

Patient teaching

- Advise patient to avoid driving and other hazardous activities that require mental alertness until drug's CNS effects are known.
- Instruct parent to monitor child's school performance because drug may interfere with attentiveness.
- Warn patient and parents not to stop drug abruptly because seizures may occur.
- Advise patient that drug isn't for use during pregnancy or breast-feeding.

clonidine
Catapres-TTS

clonidine hydrochloride
Catapres, Duraclon

Pregnancy risk category C

Indications & dosages

➲ **Essential and renal hypertension**
Adults: Initially, 0.1 mg P.O. b.i.d.; then increased by 0.1 to 0.2 mg daily on a weekly basis. Usual range is 0.2 to 0.6 mg daily in divided doses; infrequently, dosages as high as 2.4 mg daily are used.

Or, apply transdermal patch to nonhairy area of intact skin on upper arm or torso once q 7 days, starting with 0.1-mg system and adjusted with another 0.1-mg system or larger system.
Children: 50 to 400 mcg P.O. b.i.d.

➲ **Severe cancer pain that is unresponsive to epidural or spinal opiate analgesia or other more conventional methods of analgesia**
Adults: Initially, 30 mcg/hour by continuous epidural infusion. Experience with rates greater than 40 mcg/hour is limited.
Children: Initially, 0.5 mcg/kg/hour by epidural infusion. Dosage should be cautiously adjusted, based on response.

➲ **Pheochromocytoma diagnosis♦**
Adults: 0.3 mg P.O. for a single dose.

➲ **Migraine prophylaxis♦**
Adults: 0.025 mg P.O. two to four times daily or up to 0.15 mg P.O. daily in divided doses.

➲ **Dysmenorrhea♦**
Adults: 0.025 mg P.O. b.i.d. for 14 days before and during menses.

➲ **Vasomotor symptoms of menopause♦**
Adults: 0.025 to 0.2 mg P.O. b.i.d. or 0.1-mg/24-hour patch applied once q 7 days.

➲ **Opiate dependence♦**
Adults: Initially, 0.005 or 0.006 mg/kg test dose, followed by 0.017 mg/kg P.O. daily in three or four divided doses for 10 days. Or, initially, 0.1 mg P.O. three or four times daily, with dosage adjusted by 0.1 to 0.2 mg daily. Dosage range is 0.3 to 1.2 mg P.O. daily. Stop drug gradually. Follow protocols.

➲ **Alcohol dependence♦**
Adults: 0.5 mg P.O. b.i.d. to t.i.d.

➲ **Smoking cessation♦**
Adults: Initially, 0.1 mg P.O. b.i.d., beginning on or shortly before the day of smoking cessation. Increase dosage q 7 days by 0.1 mg daily, if needed. Or, 0.1-mg/24-hour transdermal patch applied q 7 days. Therapy should begin on or shortly before the day of smoking cessation. Increase dosage by 0.1 mg/24 hour at weekly intervals, if needed.

➲ **Attention deficit hyperactivity disorder♦**
Children: Initially, 0.05 mg P.O. h.s. May increase dosage cautiously over 2 to 4 weeks. Maintenance dosage is 0.05 to 0.4 mg P.O. daily.

Contraindications & cautions

- Contraindicated in patients hypersensitive to drug.
- Transdermal form is contraindicated in patients hypersensitive to any component of the adhesive layer of transdermal system.
- Epidural form is contraindicated in patients receiving anticoagulant therapy, in those with bleeding diathesis, in those with an injection site infection, and in those who are hemodynamically unstable or have severe CV disease.
- Use cautiously in patients with severe coronary insufficiency, recent MI, cerebrovascular disease, chronic renal failure, or impaired liver function.

Adverse reactions

CNS: *drowsiness, dizziness,* fatigue, *sedation, weakness,* malaise, agitation, depression.

CV: orthostatic hypotension, ***bradycardia, severe rebound hypertension.***
GI: *constipation, dry mouth,* nausea, vomiting, anorexia.
GU: urine retention, impotence.
Metabolic: weight gain.
Skin: *pruritus, dermatitis with transdermal patch,* rash.
Other: loss of libido.

Interactions

Drug-drug. *Amitriptyline, amoxapine, clomipramine, desipramine, doxepin, imipramine, nortriptyline, protriptyline, trimipramine:* May cause loss of blood pressure control with life-threatening elevations in blood pressure. Avoid using together.
CNS depressants: May increase CNS depression. Use together cautiously.
Diuretics, other antihypertensives: May increase hypotensive effect. Monitor patient closely.
Levodopa: May reduce effectiveness of levodopa. Monitor patient.
MAO inhibitors, prazosin: May decrease antihypertensive effect. Use together cautiously.
Propranolol, other beta blockers: May cause paradoxical hypertensive response. Monitor patient carefully.
Verapamil: May cause AV block and severe hypotension. Monitor patient.
Drug-herb. *Capsicum:* May reduce antihypertensive effectiveness. Discourage use together.
Ma huang: May decrease antihypertensive effects. Discourage use together.

Nursing considerations

- Drug may be given to lower blood pressure rapidly in some hypertensive emergencies.
- Monitor blood pressure and pulse rate frequently. Dosage is usually adjusted to patient's blood pressure and tolerance.
- Elderly patients may be more sensitive than younger ones to drug's hypotensive effects.
- Observe patient for tolerance to drug's therapeutic effects, which may require increased dosage.
- Noticeable antihypertensive effects of transdermal clonidine may take 2 to 3 days. Oral antihypertensive therapy may have to be continued in the interim.

!!ALERT Remove transdermal patch before defibrillation to prevent arcing.
- When stopping therapy in patients receiving both clonidine and a beta blocker, gradually withdraw the beta blocker first to minimize adverse reactions.
- Don't stop drug before surgery.

!!ALERT Don't confuse clonidine with quinidine or clomiphene; or Catapres with Cetapred or Combipres.
!!ALERT The injection form is for epidural use only.
- The injection form concentrate containing 500 mcg/ml must be diluted before use in normal saline injection to yield 100 mcg/ml.
- When drug is given epidurally, carefully monitor infusion pump and inspect catheter tubing for obstruction or dislodgment.

Patient teaching

- Instruct patient to take drug exactly as prescribed.
- Advise patient that stopping drug abruptly may cause severe rebound high blood pressure. Tell him dosage must be reduced gradually over 2 to 4 days as instructed by prescriber.
- Tell patient to take the last dose immediately before bedtime.
- Reassure patient that the transdermal patch usually remains attached despite showering and other routine daily activities. Instruct him on the use of the adhesive overlay to provide additional skin adherence, if needed. Also tell him to place patch at a different site each week.
- Caution patient that drug may cause drowsiness but that this adverse effect usually diminishes over 4 to 6 weeks.
- Inform patient that dizziness upon standing can be minimized by rising slowly from a sitting or lying position and avoiding sudden position changes.

clopidogrel bisulfate
Plavix

Pregnancy risk category B

Indications & dosages

➲ **To reduce thrombotic events in patients with atherosclerosis documented by**

recent CVA, MI, or peripheral arterial disease
Adults: 75 mg P.O. daily.
➲ **To reduce thrombotic events in patients with acute coronary syndrome (unstable angina and non–Q-wave MI), including those receiving drugs and those having percutaneous coronary intervention (with or without stent) or coronary artery bypass graft (CABG)**
Adults: Initially, a single 300-mg P.O. loading dose; then 75 mg P.O. once daily. Start and continue aspirin (75 to 325 mg once daily) with clopidogrel.

Contraindications & cautions

- Contraindicated in patients hypersensitive to drug or its components and in those with pathologic bleeding (such as peptic ulcer or intracranial hemorrhage).
- Use cautiously in patients at risk for increased bleeding from trauma, surgery, or other pathologic conditions and in those with hepatic impairment.

Adverse reactions

CNS: headache, dizziness, fatigue, depression, pain.
CV: edema, hypertension.
EENT: rhinitis, epistaxis.
GI: ***hemorrhage***, abdominal pain, dyspepsia, gastritis, constipation, diarrhea, ulcers.
GU: UTI.
Hematologic: purpura.
Musculoskeletal: arthralgia.
Respiratory: bronchitis, coughing, dyspnea, upper respiratory tract infection.
Skin: *rash*, pruritus.
Other: flulike syndrome.

Interactions

Drug-drug. *Aspirin, NSAIDs:* May increase risk of GI bleeding. Monitor patient.
Heparin, warfarin: Safety hasn't been established. Use together cautiously.
Drug-herb. *Red clover:* May increase risk of bleeding. Discourage use together.

Nursing considerations

- Platelet aggregation won't return to normal for at least 5 days after drug has been stopped.

!!ALERT Don't confuse Plavix with Paxil.

Patient teaching

- Advise patient it may take longer than usual to stop bleeding. Tell him to refrain from activities in which trauma and bleeding may occur, and encourage him to wear a seatbelt when in a car.
- Instruct patient to notify prescriber if unusual bleeding or bruising occurs.
- Tell patient to inform all health care providers, including dentists, before undergoing procedures or starting new drug therapy, that he is taking drug.
- Inform patient that drug may be taken without regard to meals.

clorazepate dipotassium

Apo-Clorazepate†, Gen-Xene, Novo-Clopate†, Tranxene, Tranxene-SD

Pregnancy risk category D
Controlled substance schedule IV

Indications & dosages

➲ **Acute alcohol withdrawal**
Adults: Day 1, give 30 mg P.O. initially; then 30 to 60 mg P.O. in divided doses. Day 2, give 45 to 90 mg P.O. in divided doses. Day 3, give 22.5 to 45 mg P.O. in divided doses. Day 4, give 15 to 30 mg P.O. in divided doses. Then gradually reduce dosage to 7.5 to 15 mg daily. Maximum dosage is 90 mg daily.
➲ **Anxiety**
Adults: 15 to 60 mg P.O. daily.
Elderly patients: Initially, 7.5 to 15 mg daily in divided doses or as a single dose h.s.

For debilitated patients, initially, 7.5 to 15 mg daily in divided doses or as a single dose h.s.
➲ **Adjunctive treatment for partial seizure disorder**
Adults and children older than age 12: Maximum first dose is 7.5 mg P.O. t.i.d. Dosage increases shouldn't exceed 7.5 mg weekly. Maximum daily dose is 90 mg.
Children ages 9 to 12: Maximum first dose is 7.5 mg P.O. b.i.d. Dosage increases shouldn't exceed 7.5 mg weekly. Maximum daily dose is 60 mg.

Contraindications & cautions

- Contraindicated in patients hypersensitive to drug and in those with acute angle-closure glaucoma.

• Use cautiously in patients with suicidal tendencies, renal or hepatic impairment, pulmonary disease, or history of drug abuse.
• Don't give drug to pregnant women, especially during first trimester.
• Drug isn't recommended for children younger than age 9.

Adverse reactions

CNS: *drowsiness, dizziness,* nervousness, confusion, headache, insomnia, depression, irritability, tremor, minor changes in EEG patterns.
CV: hypotension.
EENT: blurred vision, diplopia.
GI: nausea, vomiting, abdominal discomfort, dry mouth.
GU: urine retention, incontinence.
Skin: rash.

Interactions

Drug-drug. *Cimetidine:* May decrease clorazepate clearance and increase risk of adverse reactions. Monitor patient carefully.
CNS depressants: May increase CNS depression. Use together cautiously.
Digoxin: May increase digoxin level and risk of toxicity. Monitor patient and digoxin level closely.
Levodopa: May decrease effectiveness of levodopa. Monitor patient closely.
Drug-herb. *Kava:* May increase sedation. Discourage use together.
Drug-lifestyle. *Alcohol use:* May cause additive CNS effects. Discourage use together.
Smoking: May decrease benzodiazepine effectiveness. Urge patient to quit smoking, and monitor patient closely.

Nursing considerations

!!ALERT Monitor hepatic, renal, and hematopoietic function periodically in patients receiving repeated or prolonged therapy.
!!ALERT Use of this drug may lead to abuse and addiction. Don't withdraw drug abruptly after prolonged use because withdrawal symptoms may occur.
!!ALERT Don't confuse clorazepate with clofibrate.

Patient teaching

• Warn patient to avoid activities that require alertness and good coordination until effects of drug are known.
!!ALERT Advise patient taking Tranxene-SD to swallow pill whole and not to crush, break, or chew pill before swallowing it.
• Tell patient to avoid alcohol while taking drug.
• Advise patient that smoking may decrease drug's effectiveness.
• Warn patient not to stop drug abruptly because withdrawal symptoms may occur.
• Warn woman of childbearing age to avoid use during pregnancy.
• Inform patient that sugarless chewing gum or hard candy can relieve dry mouth.

clotrimazole

Canesten†, Cruex ◊, Desenex ◊, Gyne-Lotrimin ◊, Lotrimin, Lotrimin AF ◊, Mycelex, Mycelex-7 ◊, Mycelex-G

Pregnancy risk category B; C (for lozenges)

Indications & dosages

➲ **Superficial fungal infections (tinea corporis, tinea cruris, tinea pedis, tinea versicolor, candidiasis)**
Adults and children: Apply thin film and massage into affected and surrounding area, morning and evening, for 2 to 4 weeks. If improvement doesn't occur after 4 weeks, reevaluate patient.
➲ **Vulvovaginal candidiasis**
Adults: One 100-mg vaginal suppository inserted daily h.s. for 7 consecutive days. Or, one 200-mg vaginal suppository h.s. for 3 days. Or, 1 applicatorful of vaginal cream daily h.s. for 7 days.
➲ **Oropharyngeal candidiasis**
Adults and children age 3 and older: Dissolve lozenge in mouth over 15 to 30 minutes five times daily for 14 consecutive days.
➲ **To prevent oropharyngeal candidiasis in patients immunocompromised by chemotherapy, radiotherapy, or corticosteroid therapy in the treatment of leukemia, solid tumors, or renal transplantation**
Adults and children: Dissolve lozenge in mouth over 15 to 30 minutes t.i.d. for duration of chemotherapy or until corticosteroid is reduced to maintenance levels.

Contraindications & cautions

• Contraindicated in patients hypersensitive to drug.

• Contraindicated for ophthalmic use.

Adverse reactions

GI: lower abdominal cramps, nausea and vomiting with lozenges.
GU: *mild vaginal burning or irritation,* urinary frequency.
Skin: blistering, *erythema,* edema, pruritus, burning, stinging, peeling, urticaria, skin fissures, general irritation.

Interactions

None significant.

Nursing considerations

• Clean and dry area before applying drug.
• Watch for and report irritation or sensitivity; stop if irritation occurs, and notify prescriber.
• Improvement usually occurs within 1 week; if no improvement is seen within 4 weeks, review diagnosis.
!!ALERT Don't confuse clotrimazole with co-trimoxazole.

Patient teaching

• Reassure patient that hypopigmentation from tinea versicolor does resolve gradually.
• Warn patient not to use occlusive wrappings or dressings.
• Warn patient to avoid drug contact with eyes.
• Caution patient that frequent or persistent yeast infections may suggest a more serious medical problem.
• Tell patient to refrain from sexual intercourse during intravaginal treatment.
• Warn patient that topical preparation may stain clothing.
• Tell patient that using a sanitary napkin protects clothing when using vaginal preparation.
• Stress need to continue use of vaginal preparations, as prescribed, even if menstruation begins.
• Tell patient with athlete's foot to change shoes and cotton socks daily and to dry between the toes after bathing.
• Tell patient to allow lozenges to dissolve in mouth; for maximum benefit, advise against chewing.
• Stress need to continue treatment for full course and to notify prescriber if no improvement occurs after 4 weeks.

clozapine
Clozaril, Fazaclo

Pregnancy risk category B

Indications & dosages

➲ Schizophrenia in severely ill patients unresponsive to other therapies; to reduce risk of recurrent suicidal behavior in schizophrenia or schizoaffective disorders
Adults: Initially, 12.5 mg P.O. once daily or b.i.d. If using the orally disintegrating tablet, cut in half and discard the unused half. Adjust dose upward by 25 to 50 mg daily (if tolerated) to 300 to 450 mg daily by end of 2 weeks. Individual dosage is based on clinical response, patient tolerance, and adverse reactions. Subsequent dosage shouldn't be increased more than once or twice weekly and shouldn't exceed 50- to 100-mg increments. Many patients respond to dosages of 200 to 600 mg daily, but some may need as much as 900 mg daily. Don't exceed 900 mg daily.

Contraindications & cautions

• Contraindicated in patients with uncontrolled epilepsy, history of clozapine-induced agranulocytosis, WBC count below 3,500/mm^3, severe CNS depression or coma, and myelosuppressive disorders.
• Contraindicated in patients taking other drugs that suppress bone marrow function.
• Use cautiously in patients with prostatic hyperplasia or angle-closure glaucoma because drug has potent anticholinergic effects.

Adverse reactions

CNS: *drowsiness, sedation,* ***seizures,*** *dizziness,* syncope, *vertigo, headache,* tremor, disturbed sleep or nightmares, restlessness, hypokinesia or akinesia, agitation, rigidity, akathisia, confusion, fatigue, insomnia, hyperkinesia, weakness, lethargy, ataxia, slurred speech, depression, myoclonus, anxiety, fever.
CV: *tachycardia,* hypotension, ***cardiomyopathy,*** hypertension, chest pain, ECG changes, orthostatic hypotension, ***myocarditis, pulmonary embolism, cardiac arrest.***
EENT: visual disturbances.

GI: dry mouth, *constipation*, nausea, vomiting, *excessive salivation*, heartburn, diarrhea.
GU: urinary frequency or urgency, urine retention, incontinence, abnormal ejaculation.
Hematologic: ***leukopenia***, ***agranulocytosis***, ***granulocytopenia***, eosinophilia.
Metabolic: weight gain, *hyperglycemia*.
Musculoskeletal: muscle pain or spasm, muscle weakness.
Respiratory: ***respiratory arrest***.
Skin: rash, diaphoresis.

Interactions

Drug-drug. *Anticholinergics:* May potentiate anticholinergic effects of clozapine. Use together cautiously.
Antihypertensives: May potentiate hypotensive effects. Monitor blood pressure.
Benzodiazepines: May increase risk of sedation and CV and respiratory arrest. Use together cautiously.
Bone marrow suppressants: May increase bone marrow toxicity. Avoid using together.
Digoxin, other highly protein-bound drugs, warfarin: May increase levels of these drugs. Monitor patient closely for adverse reactions.
Fluoroquinolones, fluvoxamine, paroxetine, sertraline: May increase clozapine level. Use together cautiously, and monitor patient.
Phenytoin: May decrease clozapine level and cause breakthrough psychosis. Monitor patient for psychosis and adjust clozapine dosage.
Psychoactive drugs: May cause additive effects. Use together cautiously.
Drug-herb. *St. John's wort:* May decrease clozapine level. Discourage use together.
Drug-lifestyle. *Alcohol use:* May increase CNS depression. Discourage use together.
Smoking: May decrease clozapine level. Urge patient to quit smoking. Monitor patient for effectiveness and adjust dosage.

Nursing considerations

!!ALERT Clozapine carries significant risk of agranulocytosis. If possible, give patient at least two trials of standard antipsychotic before starting clozapine. Obtain baseline WBC and differential counts before clozapine therapy. Monitor WBC counts weekly for at least 4 weeks after clozapine therapy ends.

- When giving clozapine, perform WBC counts and blood tests weekly and dispense no more than 1-week supply of drug at a time for first 6 months of therapy. If WBC count stays at 3,000/mm^3 or more and absolute neutrophil count stays at 1,500/mm^3 or more during first 6 months of continuous therapy, frequency of monitoring blood counts may be reduced to every other week.
- If WBC count drops below 3,500/mm^3 after therapy begins or if it drops substantially from baseline, monitor patient closely for signs and symptoms of infection. If WBC count is 3,000 to 3,500/mm^3 and granulocyte count is above 1,500/mm^3, perform WBC and differential count twice weekly. If WBC count drops below 3,000/mm^3 and granulocyte count drops below 1,500/mm^3, interrupt therapy, notify prescriber, and monitor patient for signs and symptoms of infection. Therapy may be restarted cautiously if WBC count returns to above 3,000/mm^3 and granulocyte count returns to above 1,500/mm^3. Continue monitoring WBC and differential counts twice weekly until WBC count exceeds 3,500/mm^3.
- If WBC count drops below 2,000/mm^3 and granulocyte count drops below 1,000/mm^3, patient may need protective isolation. Bone marrow aspiration may be needed to assess bone marrow function. Future clozapine therapy is contraindicated in these patients.

!!ALERT Drug increases the risk of fatal myocarditis especially during, but not limited to, the first month of therapy. In patients in whom myocarditis is suspected (unexplained fatigue, dyspnea, tachypnea, chest pain, tachycardia, fever, palpitations, and other signs or symptoms of heart failure or ECG abnormalities such as ST-T wave abnormalities or arrhythmias), stop clozapine therapy immediately and don't restart.

!!ALERT Drug may cause hyperglycemia. Monitor patients with diabetes regularly. In patients with risk factors for diabetes, obtain fasting blood glucose test results at baseline and periodically.

- Monitor patient for signs and symptoms of cardiomyopathy.
- Seizures may occur, especially in patients receiving high doses.
- Some patients experience transient fever with temperature higher than 100.4° F (38° C), especially in the first 3 weeks of therapy. Monitor these patients closely.

• After abrupt withdrawal of long-term therapy, abrupt recurrence of psychotic symptoms is possible.
• If clozapine therapy must be stopped, withdraw drug gradually over 1 or 2 weeks. If changes in patient's medical condition (including development of leukopenia) require that drug be stopped immediately, monitor patient closely for recurrence of psychotic symptoms.
• If therapy is reinstated in patients withdrawn from drug, follow usual guidelines for dosage increase. Reexposure of patient to drug may increase severity and risk of adverse reactions. If therapy was stopped because WBC counts were below 2,000/mm³ or granulocyte counts were below 1,000/mm³, don't expect drug to be continued.

!!ALERT Don't confuse clozapine with clonidine, clofazimine, or Klonopin.

• Orally disintegrating tablets contain phenylalanine.

Patient teaching

• Tell patient about need for weekly blood tests to check for blood cell deficiency. Advise him to report flulike symptoms, fever, sore throat, lethargy, malaise, or other signs of infection.
• Warn patient to avoid hazardous activities that require alertness and good coordination while taking drug.
• Tell patient to check with prescriber before taking alcohol or nonprescription drugs.
• Advise patient that smoking may decrease drug effectiveness.
• Tell patient to rise slowly to avoid dizziness.
• Tell patient to keep orally disintegrating tablets in the blister package until ready to take it.
• Inform patient that ice chips or sugarless candy or gum may help relieve dry mouth.

codeine phosphate

Paveral†

codeine sulfate

Pregnancy risk category C
Controlled substance schedule II

Indications & dosages

➲ Mild to moderate pain

Adults: 15 to 60 mg P.O. or 15 to 60 mg (phosphate) S.C., I.M., or I.V. q 4 to 6 hours, p.r.n. Maximum daily dose is 360 mg.
Children older than age 1: 0.5 mg/kg P.O., S.C., or I.M. q 4 to 6 hours, p.r.n. Don't give I.V. in children.

➲ Nonproductive cough

Adults: 10 to 20 mg P.O. q 4 to 6 hours. Maximum daily dose is 120 mg.
Children ages 6 to 12: 5 to 10 mg P.O. q 4 to 6 hours. Maximum daily dose is 60 mg.
Children ages 2 to 5: 2.5 to 5 mg P.O. q 4 to 6 hours. Maximum daily dose is 30 mg.

Contraindications & cautions

• Contraindicated in patients hypersensitive to drug.
• I.V. administration contraindicated in children.
• Use cautiously in elderly or debilitated patients and in those with head injury, increased intracranial pressure, increased CSF pressure, hepatic or renal disease, hypothyroidism, Addison's disease, acute alcoholism, seizures, severe CNS depression, bronchial asthma, COPD, respiratory depression, and shock.

Adverse reactions

CNS: *sedation*, *clouded sensorium*, euphoria, dizziness, light-headedness, physical dependence.
CV: hypotension, ***bradycardia***, flushing.
GI: nausea, vomiting, *constipation*, dry mouth, ileus.
GU: urine retention.
Respiratory: ***respiratory depression***.
Skin: pruritus, *diaphoresis*.

Interactions

Drug-drug. *CNS depressants, general anesthetics, hypnotics, MAO inhibitors, other opioid analgesics, sedatives, tranquilizers, tricyclic antidepressants:* May cause additive effects. Use together cautiously; monitor patient response.

Drug-lifestyle. *Alcohol use:* May cause additive effects. Discourage use together.

Nursing considerations

- Reassess patient's level of pain at least 15 and 30 minutes after administration.
- Codeine and aspirin or acetaminophen are commonly prescribed together to provide enhanced pain relief.
- For full analgesic effect, give drug before patient has intense pain.
- Drug is an antitussive and shouldn't be used when cough is a valuable diagnostic sign or is beneficial (as after thoracic surgery).
- Monitor cough type and frequency.
- Monitor respiratory and circulatory status.
- Opiates may cause constipation. Assess bowel function and need for stool softeners or laxatives.
- Codeine may delay gastric emptying, increase biliary tract pressure from contraction of the sphincter of Oddi, and interfere with hepatobiliary imaging studies.

!! ALERT Don't confuse codeine with Cardene, Lodine, or Cordran.

Patient teaching

- Advise patient that GI distress caused by taking drug by mouth can be eased by taking drug with milk or meals.
- Instruct patient to ask for or to take drug before pain is intense.
- Caution ambulatory patient about getting out of bed or walking. Warn outpatient to avoid driving and other hazardous activities that require mental alertness until drug's effects on the CNS are known.
- Advise patient to avoid alcohol during therapy.

colchicine

Pregnancy risk category C; D for I.V.

Indications & dosages

➲ To prevent acute gout attacks

Adults: 0.6 mg P.O. daily. Patients who normally have one attack per year or fewer should receive drug only 3 to 4 days weekly; patients who have more than one attack per year should receive drug daily. In severe cases, 1.2 to 1.8 mg P.O. daily.

➲ To prevent gout attacks in patients undergoing surgery

Adults: 0.6 mg P.O. t.i.d. 3 days before and 3 days after surgery.

➲ Acute gout, acute gouty arthritis

Adults: Initially, 1.2 mg P.O.; then 0.6 mg q 1 hour or 1.2 mg q 2 hours until pain is relieved; nausea, vomiting, or diarrhea ensues; or maximum dose of 8 mg is reached. Wait 3 days before a second oral course to reduce cumulative toxicity. Or, 2 mg I.V.; then 0.5 mg I.V. q 6 hours if needed. (Some prescribers prefer to give a single I.V. injection of 3 mg.) Total I.V. dose over 24 hours (one course of treatment) shouldn't exceed 4 mg. Give no further colchicine (I.V. or P.O.) for at least 7 days.

If creatinine clearance is 10 to 50 ml/minute, reduce dose by 50%. Don't use in patients with creatinine clearance below 10 ml/minute. In patients with hepatic impairment, reduce dose by 50%.

Contraindications & cautions

- Contraindicated in patients hypersensitive to drug and in those with blood dyscrasia, serious CV disease, renal disease, or GI disorders.
- Use cautiously in elderly or debilitated patients and in those with early signs of CV, renal, or GI disease.

Adverse reactions

CNS: peripheral neuritis.
GI: *nausea, vomiting, abdominal pain, diarrhea.*
GU: reversible azoospermia.
Hematologic: ***aplastic anemia, thrombocytopenia, agranulocytosis with long-term use***, nonthrombocytopenic purpura.
Musculoskeletal: myopathy.
Skin: alopecia, urticaria, dermatitis.
Other: severe local irritation if extravasation occurs, hypersensitivity reactions.

Interactions

Drug-drug. *Cyclosporine:* May cause GI, hepatic, renal and neuromuscular toxicity. Use together cautiously.
Vitamin B_{12}: May impair absorption of oral vitamin B_{12}. Avoid using together.

Drug-lifestyle. *Alcohol use:* May impair efficacy of colchicine prophylaxis. Discourage use together.

Nursing considerations

- Obtain baseline laboratory test results, including CBC, before therapy and periodically throughout therapy.

!!ALERT Don't give I.M. or S.C.; severe local irritation occurs.

- As maintenance therapy, give drug with meals to reduce GI effects. Drug may be used with uricosurics.
- Monitor fluid intake and output; keep output at 2 L daily.

!!ALERT After full course of I.V. colchicine (4 mg), don't give colchicine by any route for at least 7 days. Colchicine is a toxic drug, and death has resulted from overdose.

- First sign of acute overdose may be GI symptoms, followed by vascular damage, muscle weakness, and ascending paralysis. Delirium and seizures may occur without patient losing consciousness.
- Stop drug as soon as gout pain is relieved or at first sign of GI symptoms.

Patient teaching

- Teach patient how to take drug, and tell him to drink extra fluids.
- Tell patient to report adverse reactions, especially signs of acute overdose (nausea, vomiting, abdominal pain, diarrhea, unusual bleeding, bruising, tiredness, weakness, numbness, or tingling).
- Advise patient to avoid using alcohol while taking drug.
- Tell patient with gout to limit intake of foods high in purine, such as anchovies, liver, sardines, kidneys, sweetbreads, peas, and lentils.

colesevelam hydrochloride

Welchol

Pregnancy risk category B

Indications & dosages

➲ **Adjunct to diet and exercise, either alone or with an HMG-CoA reductase inhibitor, to reduce elevated LDL cholesterol in patients with primary hypercholesterolemia (Fredrickson type IIa)**

Adults: 3 tablets (1,875 mg) P.O. b.i.d. with meals and liquid, or 6 tablets (3,750 mg) once daily with a meal and liquid. Maximum dosage is 7 tablets (4,375 mg) daily.

Contraindications & cautions

- Contraindicated in patients hypersensitive to drug or any of its components and in patients with bowel obstruction.
- Use cautiously in patients susceptible to vitamin K or fat-soluble vitamin deficiencies and in patients with dysphagia, swallowing disorders, severe GI motility disorders, or major GI tract surgery.
- Use cautiously in patients with triglyceride levels greater than 300 mg/dl.

Adverse reactions

CNS: *headache*, pain, asthenia.
EENT: pharyngitis, rhinitis, sinusitis.
GI: abdominal pain, *constipation*, diarrhea, dyspepsia, *flatulence*, nausea.
Musculoskeletal: myalgia, back pain.
Respiratory: increased cough.
Other: accidental injury, *infection*, flulike syndrome.

Interactions

None reported.

Nursing considerations

- Before starting drug, assess patient for underlying causes of hypercholesterolemia, such as poorly controlled diabetes, hypothyroidism, nephrotic syndrome, dysproteinemias, obstructive liver disease, other drug therapy, and alcoholism.
- Give drug with a meal and a liquid.
- Store tablets at room temperature and protect them from moisture.
- Monitor patient's bowel habits. If severe constipation develops, decrease dosage, add a stool softener, or stop drug.
- Monitor the effects of concurrent drug therapy to identify possible drug interactions.
- Monitor total and LDL cholesterol and triglyceride levels periodically during therapy.
- Use only when clearly needed in breast-feeding patients because it's not known if drug appears in breast milk.

Patient teaching

- Instruct patient to take drug with a meal and a liquid.
- Teach patient to monitor bowel habits. Encourage a diet high in fiber and fluids. Instruct patient to notify prescriber promptly if severe constipation develops.
- Encourage patient to follow prescribed diet, exercise, and monitoring of cholesterol and triglyceride levels.
- Tell patient to notify prescriber if she is pregnant or breast-feeding.

co-trimoxazole (sulfamethoxazole and trimethoprim)

Apo-Sulfatrim†, Apo-Sulfatrim DS†, Bactrim*, Bactrim DS, Bactrim IV, Cotrim, Cotrim D.S, Cotrim Pediatric*, Novo-Trimel†, Novo-Trimel DS†, Nu-Cotrimox†, Roubac†, Septra*, Septra DS, Septra IV, Sulfatrim, Sulfatrim Pediatric

Pregnancy risk category C

Indications & dosages

➲ Shigellosis or UTIs caused by susceptible strains of *Escherichia coli, Proteus* (indole positive or negative), *Klebsiella,* or *Enterobacter* species
Adults: 160 mg trimethoprim/800 mg sulfamethoxazole, 1 double-strength tablet, P.O. q 12 hours for 10 to 14 days in UTIs and for 5 days in shigellosis. If indicated, I.V. infusion is given: 8 to 10 mg/kg/day based on trimethoprim component in two to four divided doses q 6, 8, or 12 hours for 5 days for shigellosis or up to 14 days for severe UTIs. Maximum daily dose is 960 mg trimethoprim (as co-trimoxazole).
Children age 2 months and older: 8 mg/kg/day based on trimethoprim component P.O., in two divided doses q 12 hours for 10 days for UTIs and 5 days for shigellosis. If indicated, I.V. infusion is given: 8 to 10 mg/kg/day based on trimethoprim component, in two to four divided doses q 6, 8, or 12 hours. Don't exceed adult dose.

➲ Otitis media in patients with penicillin allergy or penicillin-resistant infection
Children age 2 months and older: 8 mg/kg/day based on trimethoprim component P.O., in two divided doses q 12 hours for 10 to 14 days.

➲ Chronic bronchitis, upper respiratory tract infections
Adults: 160 mg trimethoprim and 800 mg sulfamethoxazole P.O. q 12 hours for 10 to 14 days.

➲ Traveler's diarrhea
Adults: 160 mg trimethoprim and 800 mg sulfamethoxazole P.O. b.i.d. for 3 to 5 days. Some patients may only need up to 2 days of therapy.

➲ To prevent *Pneumocystis carinii* pneumonia
Adults: 160 mg of trimethoprim and 800 mg sulfamethoxazole P.O. daily; or 80 mg trimethoprim/400 mg sulfamethoxazole P.O. three times weekly.
Children age 2 months and older: 150 mg/m^2 trimethoprim and 750 mg/m^2 sulfamethoxazole P.O. daily in two divided doses on 3 consecutive days each week.

➲ *P. carinii* pneumonia
Adults and children older than age 2 months: 15 to 20 mg/kg/day based on trimethoprim I.V. or P.O. in three or four divided doses for 14 to 21 days.

For patients with creatinine clearance of 15 to 30 ml/minute, reduce daily dose by 50%. Don't give to those with creatinine clearance less than 15 ml/minute.

Contraindications & cautions

- Contraindicated in patients hypersensitive to trimethoprim or sulfonamides.
- Contraindicated in those with creatinine clearance less than 15 ml/minute, porphyria, or megaloblastic anemia from folate deficiency.
- Contraindicated in pregnant women at term, breast-feeding women, and infants younger than age 2 months.
- Use cautiously and in reduced dosages in patients with creatinine clearance of 15 to 30 ml/minute, severe allergy or bronchial asthma, G6PD deficiency, or blood dyscrasia.

Adverse reactions

CNS: headache, depression, aseptic meningitis, tinnitus, apathy, ***seizures***, hallucinations, ataxia, nervousness, fatigue, vertigo, insomnia.
CV: thrombophlebitis.

GI: *nausea, vomiting, diarrhea*, abdominal pain, anorexia, stomatitis, ***pancreatitis, pseudomembranous colitis***.
GU: ***toxic nephrosis with oliguria and anuria***, crystalluria, hematuria, interstitial nephritis.
Hematologic: ***agranulocytosis, aplastic anemia***, megaloblastic anemia, ***thrombocytopenia, leukopenia***, hemolytic anemia.
Hepatic: jaundice, ***hepatic necrosis***.
Musculoskeletal: arthralgia, myalgia, muscle weakness.
Respiratory: pulmonary infiltrates.
Skin: ***erythema multiforme, Stevens-Johnson syndrome***, *generalized skin eruption*, ***toxic epidermal necrolysis***, exfoliative dermatitis, photosensitivity, urticaria, pruritus.
Other: hypersensitivity reactions, serum sickness, drug fever, ***anaphylaxis***.

Interactions

Drug-drug. *Cyclosporine:* May decrease cyclosporine level and increase nephrotoxicity risk. Avoid using together.
Dofetilide: May increase dofetilide level and effects. May increase risk of prolonged QT-interval syndrome and fatal ventricular arrhythmias. Avoid using together.
Hormonal contraceptives: May decrease contraceptive effectiveness and increase risk of breakthrough bleeding. Advise patient to use a nonhormonal contraceptive.
Methotrexate: May increase methotrexate level. Monitor methotrexate level.
Oral anticoagulants: May increase anticoagulant effect. Monitor patient for bleeding; monitor PT and INR.
Oral antidiabetics: May increase hypoglycemic effect. Monitor glucose level.
Phenytoin: May inhibit hepatic metabolism of phenytoin. Monitor phenytoin level.
Drug-herb. *Dong quai, St. John's wort:* May cause photosensitivity reactions. Advise patient to avoid excessive sunlight exposure.
Drug-lifestyle. *Sun exposure:* May cause photosensitivity reactions. Advise patient to avoid excessive sunlight exposure.

Nursing considerations

- Before giving drug, ask patient if he is allergic to sulfa drugs.
- Obtain specimen for culture and sensitivity tests before first dose. Therapy may begin while awaiting results.

!!ALERT Double-check dosage, which may be written as trimethoprim component.
!!ALERT "DS" product means "double strength."

- Never give drug I.M.
- Monitor renal and liver function test results.
- Promptly report rash, sore throat, fever, cough, mouth sores, or iris lesions—early signs and symptoms of erythema multiforme, which may progress to Stevens-Johnson syndrome, which is sometimes fatal. These symptoms may also represent early signs of blood dyscrasias.
- Watch for signs and symptoms of superinfection, such as fever, chills, and increased pulse.

!!ALERT Adverse reactions, especially hypersensitivity reactions, rash, and fever, occur much more frequently in patients with AIDS.

Patient teaching

- Tell patient to take drug as prescribed, even if he feels better.
- Encourage patient to drink plenty of fluids.
- Tell patient to report adverse reactions promptly.
- Instruct patient receiving drug I.V. to report discomfort at I.V. insertion site.
- Advise patient to avoid prolonged sun exposure, wear protective clothing, and use sunscreen.
- Instruct patient to take oral form with 8 ounces (240 ml) of water on an empty stomach.

cyclobenzaprine hydrochloride
Flexeril

Pregnancy risk category B

Indications & dosages

➲ Adjunct to rest and physical therapy to relieve muscle spasm from acute, painful musculoskeletal conditions
Adults: 5 mg P.O. t.i.d. Based on response, dose may be increased to 10 mg t.i.d. Don't exceed 60 mg/day. Use for longer than 2 or 3 weeks isn't recommended.

In elderly patients and in those with mild hepatic impairment, start with 5 mg and adjust slowly upward. Drug isn't recommended in patients with moderate to severe hepatic impairment.

Contraindications & cautions

- Contraindicated in patients hypersensitive to drug; in those with hyperthyroidism, heart block, arrhythmias, conduction disturbances, or heart failure; in those who have received MAO inhibitors within 14 days; and in and those in the acute recovery phase of an MI.
- Use cautiously in elderly or debilitated patients and in those with a history of urine retention, acute angle-closure glaucoma, or increased intraocular pressure.
- Safety and efficacy in children younger than age 15 haven't been established.

Adverse reactions

CNS: *drowsiness*, headache, insomnia, fatigue, asthenia, nervousness, confusion, paresthesia, *dizziness*, depression, ***seizures***, dysarthria, ataxia, syncope.
CV: tachycardia, ***arrhythmias***, palpitations, hypotension, vasodilation.
EENT: visual disturbances, blurred vision.
GI: dyspepsia, abnormal taste, constipation, *dry mouth*, nausea.
GU: urine retention, urinary frequency.
Skin: rash, urticaria, pruritus.

Interactions

Drug-drug. *Anticholinergics:* May have additive anticholinergic effects. Avoid using together.
CNS depressants: May increase CNS depression. Avoid using together.
MAO inhibitors: May cause hyperpyretic crisis, seizures, and death when MAO inhibitors are used with tricyclic antidepressants; may also occur with cyclobenzaprine. Avoid using within 2 weeks of MAO inhibitor therapy.
Drug-lifestyle. *Alcohol use:* May increase CNS depression. Discourage use together.

Nursing considerations

- Cyclobenzaprine may cause toxic reactions similar to those of tricyclic antidepressants. Observe same precautions as when giving tricyclic antidepressants.
- Monitor patient for nausea, headache, and malaise, which may occur if drug is stopped abruptly after long-term use.

!!**ALERT** Notify prescriber immediately of signs and symptoms of overdose, including cardiac toxicity.
!!**ALERT** Don't confuse Flexeril with Floxinl.

Patient teaching

- Advise patient to report urinary hesitancy or urine retention. If constipation is a problem, suggest that patient increase fluid intake and use a stool softener.
- Warn patient to avoid activities that require alertness until CNS effects of drug are known.
- Warn patient not to combine with alcohol or other CNS depressants, including OTC cold or allergy remedies.
- Instruct patient not to attempt splitting the generic 10-mg tablets because of a high potential for inconsistent doses.

cyclophosphamide

Cytoxan, Cytoxan Lyophilized, Neosar, Procytox†

Pregnancy risk category D

Indications & dosages

➲ Breast and ovarian cancers, Hodgkin's disease, chronic lymphocytic leukemia, chronic myelocytic leukemia, acute lymphoblastic leukemia, acute myelocytic and monocytic leukemia, neuroblastoma, retinoblastoma, malignant lymphoma, multiple myeloma, mycosis fungoides, sarcoma
Adults: Initially for induction, 40 to 50 mg/kg I.V. in divided doses over 2 to 5 days. Or, 10 to 15 mg/kg I.V. q 7 to 10 days, 3 to 5 mg/kg I.V. twice weekly, or 1 to 5 mg/kg P.O. daily, based on patient tolerance.
Children: Initially for induction, 2 to 8 mg/kg or 60 to 250 mg/m^2 P.O. or I.V. daily. Maintenance dose is 2 to 5 mg/kg P.O. or 50 to 150 mg/m^2 P.O. twice weekly.

Adjust subsequent doses according to evidence of antitumor activity or leukopenia.

➲ Minimal-change nephrotic syndrome in children
Children: 2 to 3 mg/kg P.O. daily for 60 to 90 days.

Contraindications & cautions

- Contraindicated in patients hypersensitive to drug and in those with severe bone marrow suppression.
- Use cautiously in patients with leukopenia, thrombocytopenia, malignant cell infiltration of bone marrow, or hepatic or renal disease and in those who have recently undergone radiation therapy or chemotherapy.

Adverse reactions

CV: ***cardiotoxicity with very high doses and with doxorubicin***, flushing.
GI: anorexia, *nausea and vomiting*, abdominal pain, stomatitis, mucositis.
GU: HEMORRHAGIC CYSTITIS, impaired fertility.
Hematologic: ***leukopenia, thrombocytopenia***, anemia.
Hepatic: ***hepatotoxicity***.
Metabolic: hyperuricemia, SIADH.
Respiratory: ***pulmonary fibrosis with high doses***.
Skin: *reversible alopecia*, rash, pigmentation, nail changes, itching.
Other: ***secondary malignant disease, anaphylaxis***, hypersensitivity reactions.

Interactions

Drug-drug. *Allopurinol, myelosuppressives:* May increase myelosuppression. Monitor patient for toxicity.
Anticoagulants: May increase anticoagulant effect. Monitor patient for bleeding.
Aspirin, NSAIDs: May increase risk of bleeding. Avoid using together.
Barbiturates: May enhance cyclophosphamide toxicity. Monitor patient closely.
Cardiotoxic drugs: May increase adverse cardiac effects. Monitor patient for toxicity.
Chloramphenicol, corticosteroids: May reduce activity of cyclophosphamide. Use together cautiously.
Ciprofloxacin: May decrease antimicrobial effect. Monitor patient for effect.
Digoxin: May decrease digoxin level. Monitor level closely.
Succinylcholine: May prolong neuromuscular blockade. Avoid using together.

Nursing considerations

- Don't give drug at bedtime; infrequent urination during the night may increase possibility of cystitis. If cystitis occurs, stop drug and notify prescriber. Cystitis can occur months after therapy ends. Mesna may be given to reduce frequency and severity of bladder toxicity. Test urine for blood.
- Adequately hydrate patients before and after dose to decrease risk of cystitis.
- Use caution to ensure correct dose to decrease risk of cardiac toxicity.
- Monitor CBC and renal and liver function test results.
- Monitor patient closely for leukopenia (nadir between days 8 and 15, recovery in 17 to 28 days).
- Monitor uric acid level. To prevent hyperuricemia with resulting uric acid nephropathy, allopurinol may be used with adequate hydration.

!!ALERT Monitor patient for cyclophosphamide toxicity (leukopenia, thrombocytopenia, cardiotoxicity) if patient's corticosteroid therapy is stopped.

- To prevent bleeding, avoid all I.M. injections when platelet count is less than $50,000/mm^3$.
- Anticipate blood transfusions because of cumulative anemia. Patients may receive injections of RBC colony–stimulating factor to promote RBC production and decrease need for blood transfusions.
- Therapeutic effects are often accompanied by toxicity.
- Use of drug to treat nephrotic syndrome in boys for more than 60 days increases the incidence of oligospermia and azoospermia. Use for more than 90 days increases the risk of sterility.
- Drug may be used to treat non-oncologic disorders such as lupus, nephritis, and rheumatoid arthritis.

Patient teaching

- Warn patient that hair loss is likely to occur but is reversible.
- Advise patient to watch for signs and symptoms of infection (fever, sore throat, fatigue) and bleeding (easy bruising, nosebleeds, bleeding gums, tarry stools). Tell patient to take temperature daily.
- Instruct patient to avoid OTC products that contain aspirin.
- To minimize risk of hemorrhagic cystitis, encourage patient to urinate every 1 to 2 hours while awake and to drink at least 3 L of fluid daily. If patient is taking oral form of drug, tell him not to take it at bedtime

because infrequent urination increases risk of cystitis.

- Advise both men and women to practice contraception during therapy and for 4 months afterward; drug may cause birth defects.
- Advise women to stop breast-feeding during therapy because of risk of toxicity to infant.
- Drug can cause irreversible sterility in both men and women. Counsel patients of childbearing potential before starting therapy. Also recommend that women consult prescriber before becoming pregnant.

cycloserine

Seromycin

Pregnancy risk category C

Indications & dosages

➲ **Adjunctive treatment for pulmonary or extrapulmonary tuberculosis (TB)**

Adults: Initially, 250 mg P.O. q 12 hours for 2 weeks; then, if blood levels are below 25 to 30 mcg/ml and no toxicity has developed, increase dosage to 250 mg q 8 hours for 2 weeks. If optimum blood levels still aren't achieved and no toxicity has developed, then increase dosage to 250 mg q 6 hours. Maximum dosage is 1 g daily. If CNS toxicity occurs, stop drug for 1 week, then resume at 250 mg daily for 2 weeks. If no serious toxic effects occur, increase dosage by 250-mg increments q 10 days until blood level of 25 to 30 mcg/ml is obtained.

Children♦*:* 10 to 20 mg/kg/day P.O. in two divided doses. Maximum dosage is 1 g daily.

➲ **Acute UTIs**

Adults: 250 mg P.O. q 12 hours for 2 weeks.

Contraindications & cautions

- Contraindicated in patients hypersensitive to drug, in those who use alcohol excessively, and in those with seizure disorders, depression, severe anxiety, psychosis, or severe renal insufficiency.
- Use cautiously in patients with impaired renal function; reduce dosage in these patients.

Adverse reactions

CNS: ***seizures***, drowsiness, somnolence, headache, tremor, dysarthria, vertigo, confusion, loss of memory, ***possible suicidal tendencies***, psychosis, hyperirritability, paresthesia, paresis, hyperreflexia, ***coma***.

CV: ***sudden heart failure***.

Other: ***hypersensitivity reactions***.

Interactions

Drug-drug. *Ethionamide:* May potentiate neurotoxic adverse reactions. Monitor patient closely.

Isoniazid: May increase risk of CNS toxicity, including dizziness or drowsiness. Monitor patient closely.

Drug-lifestyle. *Alcohol use:* May increase risk of CNS toxicity, including seizures. Discourage use together.

Nursing considerations

- Obtain specimen for culture and sensitivity tests before therapy begins and then periodically to detect possible resistance.
- Cycloserine is considered a second-line drug in TB treatment and should always be given with other antituberculotics to prevent the development of resistant organisms.
- Use cycloserine to treat UTIs only when better alternatives are contraindicated and susceptibility to cycloserine is confirmed.
- Monitor cycloserine level periodically, especially in patients receiving high dosages (more than 500 mg daily), because toxic reactions may occur with blood levels above 30 mcg/ml.
- Observe patient receiving dosages of more than 500 mg daily for signs and symptoms of CNS toxicity, such as seizures, anxiety, and tremor.
- Monitor results of hematologic tests and renal and liver function tests.
- Observe patient for psychotic symptoms, hallucinations, and possible suicidal tendencies.
- Monitor patient for hypersensitivity reactions, such as allergic dermatitis.
- Give anticonvulsant, tranquilizer, or sedative to relieve adverse reactions.

Patient teaching

- Warn patient to avoid alcohol, which may cause serious neurologic reactions.
- Advise patient not to perform hazardous activities if drowsiness occurs.
- Tell patient to report adverse reactions promptly; dosage may need to be adjusted

or other drugs prescribed to relieve adverse reactions.

cyclosporine
Neoral, Sandimmune

cyclosporine, modified
Gengraf

Pregnancy risk category C

Indications & dosages

➲ To prevent organ rejection in renal, hepatic, or cardiac transplantation

Adults and children: 15 mg/kg P.O. 4 to 12 hours before transplantation and continue daily for 1 to 2 weeks postoperatively. Then reduce dosage by 5% each week to maintenance level of 5 to 10 mg/kg daily. Or, 5 to 6 mg/kg I.V. concentrate 4 to 12 hours before transplantation as a continuous infusion. Postoperatively, repeat dose daily until patient can tolerate P.O. forms.

For conversion from Sandimmune to Gengraf or Neoral, use same daily dose as previously used for Sandimmune. Monitor blood levels q 4 to 7 days after conversion, and monitor blood pressure and creatinine level q 2 weeks during the first 2 months.

➲ Severe, active rheumatoid arthritis (RA) that hasn't adequately responded to methotrexate

Adults: 2.5 mg/kg Gengraf and Neoral daily P.O., taken b.i.d. as divided dose. Dosage may be increased by 0.5 to 0.75 mg/kg daily after 8 weeks and again after 12 weeks to a maximum of 4 mg/kg daily. If no response is seen after 16 weeks, stop therapy.

➲ Psoriasis

Adults: 1.25 mg/kg Gengraf and Neoral daily P.O. b.i.d. for at least 4 weeks. Dosage may be increased by 0.5 mg/kg daily once q 2 weeks p.r.n. to a maximum of 4 mg/kg daily.

For patients with adverse effects such as hypertension, creatinine level 30% above pretreatment level, abnormal CBC count, or liver function test results, decrease dosage by 25% to 50%.

Contraindications & cautions

- Contraindicated in patients hypersensitive to drug or polyoxyethylated castor oil (found in injectable form).
- Contraindicated in patients with RA or psoriasis with abnormal renal function, uncontrolled hypertension, or malignancies (Neoral or Gengraf).
- Psoriasis patients shouldn't receive psoralen plus ultraviolet A (PUVA) or ultraviolet B (UVB) therapy, methotrexate, other immunosuppressants, coal tar, or radiation (Neoral or Gengraf).

Adverse reactions

CNS: *tremor*, *headache*, confusion, paresthesia.
CV: *hypertension*, flushing.
EENT: *gum hyperplasia*, sinusitis.
GI: *nausea*, *vomiting*, diarrhea, oral thrush, abdominal discomfort.
GU: NEPHROTOXICITY.
Hematologic: anemia, ***leukopenia***, ***thrombocytopenia***.
Hepatic: ***hepatotoxicity***.
Metabolic: hyperglycemia.
Skin: *hirsutism*, acne.
Other: ***infections***, ***anaphylaxis***, gynecomastia.

Interactions

Drug-drug. *Acyclovir, aminoglycosides, amphotericin B, cimetidine, co-trimoxazole, diclofenac, gentamicin, ketoconazole, melphalan, NSAIDs, ranitidine, sulfamethoxazole/trimethoprim, tacrolimus, tobramycin, vancomycin:* May increase risk of nephrotoxicity. Avoid using together.

Allopurinol, bromocriptine, cimetidine, clarithromycin, danazol, diltiazem, erythromycin, fluconazole, imipenem-cilastatin, itraconazole, ketoconazole, methylprednisolone, metoclopramide, nicardipine, prednisolone, verapamil: May increase cyclosporine level. Monitor patient for increased toxicity.

Azathioprine, corticosteroids, cyclophosphamide, verapamil: May increase immunosuppression. Monitor patient closely.

Carbamazepine, isoniazid, nafcillin, octreotide, phenobarbital, phenytoin, rifabutin, rifampin, ticlopidine: May decrease immunosuppressant effect from low cyclosporine level. Cyclosporine dosage may need to be increased.

Digoxin, lovastatin, prednisolone: May decrease clearance of these drugs. Use together cautiously.

Mycophenolate mofetil: May decrease mycophenolate level. Monitor patient closely when cyclosporine is either added or deleted from therapy.
Potassium-sparing diuretics: May induce hyperkalemia. Monitor patient closely.
Sirolimus: May increase sirolimus level. Take sirolimus at least 4 hours after cyclosporine dose. If separating doses isn't possible, monitor patient for increased adverse effects.
Vaccines: May decrease immune response. Delay routine immunization.
Drug-herb. *Alfalfa sprouts, astragalus, echinacea, licorice:* May interfere with immunosuppressive effect. Discourage use together.
St. John's wort: May reduce cyclosporine level, resulting in transplant failure. Discourage use together.
Drug-food. *Grapefruit and grapefruit juices:* May increase drug level and cause toxicity. Advise patient to avoid grapefruit or grapefruit juice.
High-fat meals: May decrease Neoral absorption. Urge patient to be consistent in how he takes cyclosporine in relation to meals.
Drug-lifestyle. *Sunlight:* May increase risk of sensitivity to sunlight. Advise patient to avoid excessive sunlight exposure.

Nursing considerations

- Cyclosporine can cause nephrotoxicity and hepatotoxicity.
- Measure oral solution doses carefully in an oral syringe. To improve the taste of conventional oral solution, mix it with milk, chocolate milk, or orange juice. Oral solution for emulsion may be mixed with orange or apple juice (avoid grapefruit juice). Emulsion solution is less palatable when mixed with milk. Use a glass container to mix, and have patient drink at once. Don't rinse dosing syringe with water. If syringe is cleaned, it must be completely dry before reuse.
- Monitor elderly patient for renal impairment and hypertension.
- Monitor cyclosporine blood levels at regular intervals. Absorption of cyclosporine oral solution can be erratic.

!!ALERT Don't confuse cyclosporine with cyclophosphamide or cycloserine.

!!ALERT Don't confuse Sandimmune with Sandoglobulin or Sandostatin.

- Neoral has greater bioavailability than Sandimmune. A lower dose of Neoral may be needed to provide blood level similar to that achieved with Sandimmune. Monitor blood level when switching patients between these two brands.
- Gengraf and Sandimmune aren't bioequivalent and can't be interchanged without prescriber supervision. Convert Gengraf to Sandimmune only with increased monitoring to prevent underdosing.
- Gengraf is bioequivalent to and interchangeable with Neoral capsules.
- Always give cyclosporine with corticosteroids.
- Use Neoral or Gengraf to treat RA or psoriasis.

RA patients

- Before starting treatment, measure blood pressure at least twice and obtain two creatinine levels to estimate baseline.
- Evaluate blood pressure and creatinine level every 2 weeks during first 3 months and then monthly if patient is stable.
- Monitor blood pressure and creatinine level after an increase in NSAID dosage or introduction of a new NSAID. Monitor CBC and liver function tests monthly if patient also receives methotrexate.
- If hypertension occurs, decrease dosage of Gengraf or Neoral by 25% to 50%. If hypertension persists, decrease dosage further or control blood pressure with antihypertensives.

Psoriasis patients

- First measure blood pressure at least twice to achieve a baseline.
- Evaluate patient for occult infection and tumors initially and throughout treatment.
- Obtain baseline creatinine level (on two occasions), CBC, and BUN, magnesium, uric acid, potassium, and lipid levels.
- Evaluate creatinine and BUN levels every 2 weeks during first 3 months and then monthly thereafter if patient is stable.
- If creatinine level is 25% above pretreatment levels, repeat creatinine level measurement within 2 weeks. If creatinine level stays 25% to 50% above baseline, reduce dosage by 25% to 50%. If creatinine level is ever 50% above baseline, reduce dosage by 25% to 50%. Stop therapy if creatinine

level isn't reversed after two dosage modifications.

- Monitor creatinine level after increasing NSAID dose or starting a new NSAID.
- Evaluate blood pressure, CBC, and uric acid, potassium, lipid, and magnesium levels every 2 weeks for the first 3 months and then monthly if patient is stable, or more frequently if a dosage is adjusted.
- Reduce dosage by 25% to 50% for an abnormality of clinical concern.
- Improvement in psoriasis takes 12 to 16 weeks of therapy.

Patient teaching

- Encourage patient to take drug at same time each day, and teach him how to measure dosage and mask taste of oral solution, if prescribed. Tell him not to take cyclosporine with grapefruit juice.
- Instruct patient to fill glass with water after dose and drink it to make sure he consumes all of drug.
- Advise patient to take drug with meals if nausea occurs.
- Advise patient to take Neoral or Gengraf on an empty stomach.
- Tell patient being treated for psoriasis that improvement may not occur until after 12 to 16 weeks of therapy.
- Stress that drug shouldn't be stopped without prescriber's approval.
- Explain to patient the importance of frequent laboratory monitoring while receiving therapy.
- Tell patient to avoid people with infections because drug lowers resistance to infection.
- Advise patient to perform careful oral care and to see a dentist regularly because drug can cause gum disease.
- Advise woman to use barrier contraception during therapy, not hormonal contraceptives. Advise her of the potential risk during pregnancy and the increased risk of tumors, high blood pressure, and renal problems.
- Warn patient to wear protection in the sun and to avoid excessive sun exposure.

cytarabine (ara-C, cytosine arabinoside)

Cytosar†, Cytosar-U, Tarabine PFS

Pregnancy risk category D

Indications & dosages

➲ Acute nonlymphocytic leukemia, acute lymphocytic leukemia

Adults and children: For single-agent therapy, 200 mg/m^2 daily by continuous I.V. infusion for 5 days at 2-week intervals. For combination therapy, 100 to 200 mg/m^2 I.V. daily by continuous I.V. infusion or in two or three divided doses by rapid I.V. injection or I.V. infusion for 5 to 10 days in a course of therapy or daily until remission is attained. For maintenance, 1 to 1.5 mg/kg I.M. or S.C. q 1 to 4 weeks.

➲ Refractory acute leukemia; refractory non-Hodgkin's lymphoma♦

Adults: 3 g/m^2 I.V. over 1 to 3 hours q 12 hours for 4 to 12 doses. Repeat at 2- to 3-week intervals or after patient recovers from toxicity.

➲ Meningeal leukemia

Adults and children: Highly variable from 5 to 75 mg/m^2 intrathecally. Frequency varies from once daily for 4 days to once q 2 to 7 days. The most frequently used dose is 30 mg/m^2 q 4 days until CSF fluid is normal; then one additional dose.

Contraindications & cautions

- Contraindicated in patients hypersensitive to drug.
- Use cautiously in patients with hepatic or renal compromise, gout, or myelosuppression.

Adverse reactions

CNS: neurotoxicity, malaise, dizziness, headache, cerebellar syndrome, *fever*.
CV: *thrombophlebitis*, edema.
EENT: conjunctivitis.
GI: *nausea, vomiting, diarrhea, anorexia, anal ulceration*, abdominal pain, oral ulcers in 5 to 10 days, projectile vomiting, bowel necrosis with high doses given rapid I.V.
GU: urine retention, renal dysfunction.
Hematologic: ***leukopenia***, anemia, reticulocytopenia, ***thrombocytopenia***, *megaloblastosis*.
Hepatic: ***hepatotoxicity***, jaundice.

Metabolic: hyperuricemia.
Musculoskeletal: myalgia, bone pain.
Respiratory: pulmonary edema, shortness of breath, pulmonary hypersensitivity.
Skin: *rash*, pruritus, alopecia, freckling.
Other: flulike syndrome, infection, ***anaphylaxis***.

Interactions

Drug-drug. *Digoxin, except oral liquid and liquid-filled capsules:* May decrease oral digoxin absorption. Monitor digoxin level closely.
Flucytosine: May decrease flucytosine activity. Avoid using together.
Gentamicin: May decrease activity against *Klebsiella pneumoniae*. Avoid using together.

Nursing considerations

- For intrathecal administration, use preservative-free normal saline solution. Add 5 ml to 100-mg vial or 10 ml to 500-mg vial. Use immediately after reconstitution. Discard unused drug.
- Monitor fluid intake and output carefully. Maintain high fluid intake and give allopurinol to avoid urate nephropathy in leukemia-induction therapy. Monitor uric acid level.
- Monitor hepatic and renal function studies and CBC.
- Therapy may be modified or stopped if granulocyte count is below 1,000/mm^3 or platelet count is below 50,000/mm^3.
- Corticosteroid eyedrops are prescribed to prevent drug-induced conjunctivitis.
- Provide diligent mouth care to help prevent stomatitis.

!! ALERT Assess patient receiving high doses for neurotoxicity, which may first appear as nystagmus but can progress to ataxia and cerebellar dysfunction.

- To prevent bleeding, avoid all I.M. injections when platelet count is below 50,000/mm^3.
- Anticipate blood transfusions because of cumulative anemia. Patient may receive RBC colony–stimulating factors to promote RBC production and decrease need for blood transfusions.
- Therapeutic effects are frequently accompanied by toxicity.
- In leukopenia, initial WBC count nadir occurs 7 to 9 days after drug is stopped. A second, more severe nadir occurs 15 to 24 days after drug is stopped. In thrombocytopenia, platelet count nadir occurs on days 12 to 15.

Patient teaching

- Instruct patient to watch for signs and symptoms of infection (fever, sore throat, fatigue) and bleeding (easy bruising, nosebleeds, bleeding gums, tarry stools). Tell patient to take temperature daily.
- Advise patient to report visual changes, blurred vision, or eye pain to prescriber.
- Advise breast-feeding woman to stop breast-feeding during therapy because of risk of toxicity to infant.
- Caution woman of childbearing age to consult prescriber before becoming pregnant because drug may harm fetus.

cytomegalovirus immune globulin (human), intravenous (CMV-IGIV)

CytoGam

Pregnancy risk category C

Indications & dosages

➲ To attenuate primary cytomegalovirus (CMV) disease in seronegative kidney transplant recipients who receive a kidney from a CMV-seropositive donor
Adults: Give an initial dose of 150 mg/kg I.V. within 72 hours after transplant. Then give 100 mg/kg once every 2 weeks at 2, 4, 6, and 8 weeks after transplant, followed by 50 mg/kg given at 12 and 16 weeks after transplant. Maximum dose per infusion is 150 mg/kg.

Give first dose at 15 mg/kg/hour. Increase infusion rate to 30 mg/kg/hour after 30 minutes if no adverse reactions occur, and then to 60 mg/kg/hour after another 30 minutes if no reactions occur. Don't exceed volume of 75 ml/hour. Subsequent doses may be given at 15 mg/kg/hour for 15 minutes, increasing q 15 minutes in a stepwise fashion to 60 mg/kg/hour.

➲ To prevent CMV disease caused by lung, liver, pancreas, and heart transplantations
Adults: Give an initial dose of 150 mg/kg I.V. within 72 hours after transplant. Additional doses of 150 mg/kg should be given every 2 weeks at 2, 4, 6, and 8 weeks after trans-

plant, followed by 100 mg/kg given at 12 and 16 weeks after transplant.

Give first dose at 15 mg/kg/hour. If no adverse reactions occur after 30 minutes, increase infusion rate to 30 mg/kg/hour. If no adverse reactions occur after another 30 minutes, increase rate to 60 mg/kg/hour (don't exceed 75 ml/hour). Subsequent doses may be given at 15 mg/kg/hour for 15 minutes, increasing q 15 minutes in a stepwise fashion to maximum rate of 60 mg/kg/hour (don't exceed 75 ml/hour). Monitor patient closely during and after each rate change.

Contraindications & cautions

- Contraindicated in patients sensitive to other human immunoglobulin preparations or with selective immunoglobulin A deficiency.

Adverse reactions

CNS: fever, aseptic meningitis syndrome.
CV: hypotension, *flushing*.
GI: *nausea, vomiting*.
Musculoskeletal: muscle cramps, *back pain*.
Respiratory: *wheezing*.
Other: ***anaphylaxis***, *chills*.

Interactions

Drug-drug. *Live-virus vaccines:* May interfere with immune response to live-virus vaccines. Postpone vaccination for at least 3 months.

Nursing considerations

- Monitor patient's vital signs closely before, during, and after infusion and before and after infusion rate increases.

!!ALERT If anaphylaxis occurs or blood pressure drops, stop infusion, notify prescriber, and be prepared to give cardiopulmonary resuscitation and such drugs as diphenhydramine and epinephrine.

- Refrigerate drug at 36° to 46° F (2° to 8° C).

Patient teaching

- Review drug therapy regimen with patient, and stress importance of compliance in follow-up visits.
- Instruct patient to report adverse reactions promptly.

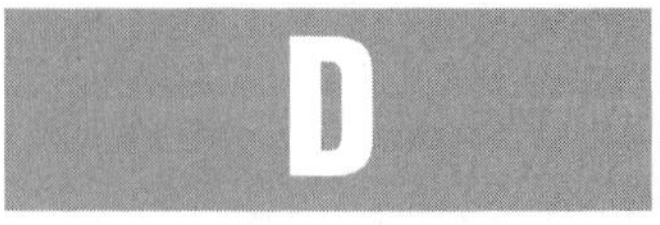

dacarbazine (DTIC)

DTIC†, DTIC-Dome

Pregnancy risk category C

Indications & dosages

➲ Metastatic malignant melanoma
Adults: 2 to 4.5 mg/kg I.V. daily for 10 days; repeat q 4 weeks, as tolerated. Or, 250 mg/m² I.V. daily for 5 days; repeat q 3 weeks.

➲ Hodgkin's disease
Adults: 150 mg/m² I.V. daily (with other drugs) for 5 days; repeat q 4 weeks. Or, 375 mg/m² on first day of combination regimen; repeat q 15 days.

Contraindications & cautions

- Contraindicated in patients hypersensitive to drug.
- Use cautiously in patients with impaired bone marrow function and those with severe renal or hepatic dysfunction.

Adverse reactions

CNS: facial paresthesia.
GI: *severe nausea and vomiting, anorexia*, stomatitis.
Hematologic: ***leukopenia, thrombocytopenia***.
Skin: phototoxicity, alopecia, rash, facial flushing.
Other: tissue damage, *flulike syndrome*, ***anaphylaxis***, severe pain with infiltration or a too-concentrated solution.

Interactions

Drug-lifestyle. *Sun exposure:* May cause photosensitivity reaction, especially during first 2 days of therapy. Advise patient to avoid excessive sunlight exposure.

Nursing considerations

- Give antiemetics before giving dacarbazine. Nausea and vomiting may subside after several doses.
- To prevent bleeding, avoid all I.M. injections when platelet count is below 50,000/mm³.

• Anticipate need for blood transfusions to combat anemia. Patient may receive injections of RBC colony-stimulating factors to promote RBC production and decrease need for blood transfusions.
• Therapeutic effects are commonly accompanied by toxicity. Monitor CBC and platelet count.
• For Hodgkin's disease, drug is usually given with bleomycin, vinblastine, and doxorubicin.
!!ALERT Don't confuse dacarbazine with Dicarbosil or procarbazine.

Patient teaching

• Tell patient to watch for evidence of infection (fever, sore throat, fatigue) and bleeding (easy bruising, nosebleeds, bleeding gums, tarry stools). Tell him to take temperature daily.
• Tell patient to avoid people with upper respiratory tract infections.
• Instruct patient to avoid OTC products that contain aspirin or NSAIDs.
• Advise patient to avoid sunlight and sunlamps for first 2 days after treatment.
• Reassure patient that fever, malaise, and muscle pain, beginning 7 days after treatment ends and possibly lasting 7 to 21 days, may be treated with mild fever reducers such as acetaminophen.
• Advise woman to avoid pregnancy and breast-feeding during therapy.

daclizumab
Zenapax

Pregnancy risk category C

Indications & dosages

➲ To prevent acute organ rejection in patients receiving renal transplants with an immunosuppressive regimen that includes cyclosporine and corticosteroids
Adults: 1 mg/kg I.V. Standard course of therapy is five doses. Give first dose no more than 24 hours before transplantation; remaining four doses are given at 14-day intervals.

Contraindications & cautions

• Contraindicated in patients hypersensitive to drug or its components.
• Use cautiously and only under supervision of prescriber experienced in immunosuppressive therapy and management of organ transplantation.

Adverse reactions

CNS: tremor, headache, fever, dizziness, insomnia, generalized weakness, prickly sensation, fatigue, depression, anxiety.
CV: tachycardia, hypertension, hypotension, aggravated hypertension, edema, chest pain.
EENT: blurred vision, pharyngitis, rhinitis.
GI: constipation, nausea, diarrhea, vomiting, abdominal pain, dyspepsia, pyrosis, abdominal distention, epigastric pain, flatulence, gastritis, hemorrhoids.
GU: ***oliguria***, dysuria, ***renal tubular necrosis***, renal damage, urine retention, hydronephrosis, urinary tract bleeding, urinary tract disorder, renal insufficiency.
Hematologic: lymphocele, platelet, bleeding, and clotting disorders.
Metabolic: diabetes mellitus, dehydration, fluid overload.
Musculoskeletal: musculoskeletal or back pain, arthralgia, myalgia, leg cramps.
Respiratory: dyspnea, coughing, atelectasis, congestion, ***hypoxia***, crackles, abnormal breath sounds, pleural effusion, ***pulmonary edema***.
Skin: acne, impaired wound healing without infection, pruritus, hirsutism, rash, night sweats, increased sweating.
Other: shivering, limb edema, pain.

Interactions

Drug-drug. *Corticosteroids, cyclosporine, mycophenolate mofetil:* May increase mortality, especially in patients taking antilymphocyte antibody therapy, and in those in whom severe infections develop. Monitor patient closely.

Nursing considerations

• Protect undiluted solution from direct light.
!!ALERT Concomitant cyclosporine, mycophenolate mofetil, and corticosteroids may be associated with an increase in mortality. Monitor patients for increased risk of lymphoproliferative disorders and opportunistic infections.
!!ALERT Monitor patient for severe, acute hypersensitivity reactions when giving each dose. Reactions may include anaphylaxis,

hypotension, bronchospasm, loss of consciousness, injection site reactions, edema, and arrhythmias. Stop if severe reaction occurs. Keep immediately available drugs used to treat anaphylactic reactions

Patient teaching

- Tell patient to consult prescriber before taking other drugs during therapy.
- Advise patient to practice infection prevention precautions.
- Inform patient that neither he nor any household member should receive vaccinations unless medically approved.
- Urge patient to immediately report wounds that fail to heal, unusual bruising or bleeding, or fever.
- Advise patient to drink plenty of fluids during drug therapy and to report painful urination, bloody urine, or decreased urine volume.
- Instruct woman of childbearing age to use effective contraception before therapy starts and to continue for 4 months after therapy stops.

dalteparin sodium
Fragmin

Pregnancy risk category B

Indications & dosages

➲ **To prevent deep vein thrombosis (DVT) in patients undergoing abdominal surgery who are at risk for thromboembolic complications**
Adults: 2,500 IU S.C. daily, starting 1 to 2 hours before surgery and repeated once daily for 5 to 10 days postoperatively.

➲ **To prevent DVT in patients undergoing hip replacement surgery**
Adults: 2,500 IU S.C. within 2 hours before surgery and second dose 2,500 IU S.C. in the evening after surgery (at least 6 hours after first dose). If surgery is performed in the evening, omit second dose on day of surgery. Starting on first postoperative day, give 5,000 IU S.C. once daily for 5 to 10 days. Or, give 5,000 IU S.C. on the evening before surgery; then 5,000 IU S.C. once daily starting in the evening of surgery for 5 to 10 days postoperatively.

➲ **Unstable angina non–Q-wave MI**
Adults: 120 IU/kg S.C. every 12 hours with aspirin P.O., unless contraindicated. Maximum dose, 10,000 IU. Treatment usually lasts 5 to 8 days.

➲ **To prevent DVT in patients at risk for thromboembolic complications because of severely restricted mobility during acute illness**
Adults: 5,000 IU S.C. once daily for 12 to 14 days.

Contraindications & cautions

- Contraindicated in patients hypersensitive to drug, heparin, or pork products; in those with active major bleeding; and in those with thrombocytopenia and antiplatelet antibodies in presence of drug.
- Use with caution in patients with history of heparin-induced thrombocytopenia and in patients at increased risk for hemorrhage, such as those with severe uncontrolled hypertension, bacterial endocarditis, congenital or acquired bleeding disorders, active ulceration, angiodysplastic GI disease, or hemorrhagic CVA; also use with caution shortly after brain, spinal, or ophthalmic surgery. Monitor vital signs.
- Use with caution in patients with bleeding diathesis, thrombocytopenia, platelet defects, severe hepatic or renal insufficiency, hypertensive or diabetic retinopathy, or recent GI bleeding.

Adverse reactions

CNS: fever.
Hematologic: ***thrombocytopenia***, ***hemorrhage***, ecchymoses, bleeding complications.
Skin: pruritus, rash, *hematoma at injection site*, injection site pain.
Other: ***anaphylaxis***.

Interactions

Drug-drug. *Antiplatelet drugs, oral anticoagulants, thrombolytics:* May increase risk of bleeding. Use together cautiously.

Nursing considerations

!!ALERT Patients receiving low-molecular-weight heparins or heparinoids who have epidural or spinal anesthesia or spinal puncture are at risk for developing epidural or spinal hematoma that can result in long-term paralysis. Risk increases with use of epidural catheters, drugs affecting hemostasis, or traumatic or repeated epidural or spinal punctures. Monitor these patients frequently for signs of neurologic impairment. Urgent treatment is needed.

- DVT is a risk factor in patients who are candidates for therapy, including those older than age 40, those who are obese, those undergoing surgery under general anesthesia lasting longer than 30 minutes, and those who have additional risk factors (such as malignancy or history of DVT or pulmonary embolism).
- Have patient sit or lie supine when giving drug. Give S.C. injection deeply. Injection sites include a U-shaped area around the navel, upper outer side of thigh, and upper outer quadrangle of buttock. Rotate sites daily. When area around the navel or thigh is used, use thumb and forefinger to lift up a fold of skin while giving injection. Insert the entire length of needle at a 45- to 90-degree angle.
- Never give drug I.M.
- Don't mix with other injections or infusions unless specific compatibility data support such mixing.
- Multidose vial shouldn't be used in pregnant women.

!!ALERT Drug isn't interchangeable (unit for unit) with unfractionated heparin or other low-molecular-weight heparin.

- Periodic, routine CBC and fecal occult blood tests are recommended during therapy. Patients don't need regular monitoring of PT or activated PTT.
- Monitor patient closely for thrombocytopenia.
- Stop drug if a thromboembolic event occurs despite dalteparin prophylaxis. May use alternative therapy, or may have been inadequate dose.

Patient teaching

- Instruct patient and family to watch for and report signs of bleeding (bruising and blood in stools).
- Tell patient to avoid OTC drugs containing aspirin or other salicylates unless ordered by prescriber.

dantrolene sodium

Dantrium, Dantrium Intravenous

Pregnancy risk category C

Indications & dosages

➲ Spasticity and sequelae from severe chronic disorders, such as multiple sclerosis, cerebral palsy, spinal cord injury, CVA

Adults: 25 mg P.O. daily. Increase by 25-mg increments, up to 100 mg b.i.d. to q.i.d. Maintain each dosage level for 4 to 7 days to determine response. Maximum, 400 mg daily.

Children: Initially, 0.5 mg/kg P.O. q.d. for 7 days; then 0.5 mg/kg t.i.d. for 7 days, 1 mg/kg t.i.d. for 7 days, and finally, 2 mg/kg, t.i.d. for 7 days. May increase up to 3 mg/kg b.i.d. to q.i.d. if necessary. Maximum, 100 mg q.i.d.

➲ To manage malignant hyperthermic crisis

Adults and children: Initially, 1 mg/kg I.V. push. Repeat, p.r.n., up to cumulative dose of 10 mg/kg.

➲ To prevent or attenuate malignant hyperthermic crisis in susceptible patients who need surgery

Adults and children: 4 to 8 mg/kg P.O. daily in three or four divided doses for 1 or 2 days before procedure. Give final dose 3 or 4 hours before procedure. Or, 2.5 mg/kg I.V. about 1 hour before anesthesia; infuse over 1 hour.

➲ To prevent recurrence of malignant hyperthermic crisis

Adults: 4 to 8 mg/kg P.O. daily in four divided doses for up to 3 days after hyperthermic crisis.

Contraindications & cautions

- Contraindicated for spasms in rheumatic disorders and when spasticity is used to maintain motor function.
- Contraindicated in breast-feeding patients and patients with upper motor neuron disorders or active hepatic disease.
- Use cautiously in women, patients older than age 35, and patients with hepatic disease or severely impaired cardiac or pulmonary function.

Adverse reactions

CNS: *drowsiness, dizziness,* headache, lightheadedness, *malaise, fatigue,* confusion, nervousness, insomnia, *seizures,* fever, depression.
CV: tachycardia, blood pressure changes, phlebitis, thrombophlebitis.
EENT: excessive lacrimation, speech disturbance, diplopia, visual disturbances.
GI: anorexia, constipation, cramping, dysphagia, metallic taste, severe diarrhea, GI bleeding, vomiting.
GU: urinary frequency, hematuria, incontinence, nocturia, dysuria, crystalluria, difficult erection, urine retention.
Hepatic: ***hepatitis.***
Musculoskeletal: myalgia, back pain, *muscle weakness.*
Respiratory: pleural effusion with pericarditis, pulmonary edema.
Skin: eczematous eruption, pruritus, urticaria, abnormal hair growth, diaphoresis.
Other: chills.

Interactions

Drug-drug. *Clofibrate, warfarin:* May decrease plasma protein binding of dantrolene. Use together cautiously.
CNS depressants: May increase CNS depression. Avoid using together.
Estrogens: May increase risk of hepatotoxicity. Use together cautiously.
I.V. verapamil and other calcium channel blockers: May result in CV collapse. Stop verapamil before giving I.V. dantrolene.
Vecuronium: May increase neuromuscular blockade effect. Use together cautiously.
Drug-lifestyle. *Alcohol use:* May increase CNS depression. Discourage use together.
Sun exposure: May cause photosensitivity reactions. Advise patient to avoid excessive sunlight exposure.

Nursing considerations

- Because of risk of liver damage with long-term use, stop therapy within 45 days if benefits don't occur.
- Obtain liver function test results at start of therapy.
- Prepare oral suspension for single dose by dissolving capsule contents in juice or other liquid. For multiple doses, use acid vehicle, and refrigerate. Use within several days.

!!ALERT Watch for hepatitis (fever and jaundice), severe diarrhea, severe weakness, and sensitivity reactions (fever or skin eruptions). Withhold dose and notify prescriber.

- The amount of relief obtained determines whether dosage (and drowsiness) can be reduced.

!!ALERT Don't confuse Dantrium with Daraprim.

Patient teaching

- Instruct patient to take drug with meals or milk in four divided doses.
- Tell patient to eat cautiously to avoid choking. Some patients may have trouble swallowing during therapy.
- Warn patient to avoid driving and other hazardous activities until CNS effects of drug are known.
- Advise patient to avoid combining drug with alcohol or other CNS depressants.
- Advise patient to notify prescriber if skin or eyes turn yellow, skin itches, or fever develops.
- Tell patient to avoid photosensitivity reactions by using sunblock and wearing protective clothing, to report abdominal discomfort or GI problems immediately, and to follow prescriber's orders regarding rest and physical therapy.

daptomycin
Cubicin

Pregnancy risk category B

Indications & dosages

➲ **Complicated skin and skin-structure infections caused by susceptible strains of *Staphylococcus aureus* (including methicillin-resistant strains), *Streptococcus pyogenes, Streptococcus agalactiae, Streptococcus dysgalactiae,* and *Enterococcus faecalis* (vancomycin-susceptible strains only)**
Adults: 4 mg/kg I.V. over 30 minutes q 24 hours for 7 to 14 days.

In patients with creatinine clearance less than 30 ml/minute, including those receiving hemodialysis or continuous ambulatory peritoneal dialysis, give 4 mg/kg I.V. q 48 hours. When possible, give drug after hemodialysis.

Contraindications & cautions

- Contraindicated in patients hypersensitive to drug.
- Use cautiously in those with renal insufficiency and those who are older than age 65, pregnant, or breast-feeding.
- Safety and efficacy haven't been established in patients younger than age 18.

Adverse reactions

CNS: anxiety, confusion, dizziness, fever, headache, insomnia.
CV: ***cardiac failure***, chest pain, edema, hypertension, hypotension.
EENT: sore throat.
GI: abdominal pain, constipation, decreased appetite, diarrhea, nausea, ***pseudomembranous colitis***, vomiting.
GU: ***renal failure***, urinary tract infection.
Hematologic: anemia.
Metabolic: hyperglycemia, ***hypoglycemia***, hypokalemia.
Musculoskeletal: limb and back pain, myopathy.
Respiratory: cough, dyspnea.
Skin: cellulitis, injection site reactions, pruritus, rash.
Other: fungal infections.

Interactions

Drug-drug. *HMG-CoA reductase inhibitors:* May increase risk of myopathy. Consider stopping these drugs while giving daptomycin.
Tobramycin: May affect levels of both drugs. Use together cautiously.
Warfarin: May alter anticoagulant activity. Monitor PT and INR for the first several days of daptomycin therapy.

Nursing considerations

- Obtain specimen for culture and sensitivity tests before giving first dose.
- Monitor CBC and renal and liver function tests periodically.

!! ALERT Because drug may increase the risk of myopathy, monitor CK level weekly. If CK level rises, monitor it more often. Stop drug in patients with myopathy and CK level over 1,000 units/L or more than 10 times the upper limit of normal. Consider stopping all other drugs linked with myopathy (such as HMG-CoA reductase inhibitors) while giving daptomycin.

- Monitor patient for superinfection because drug may cause overgrowth of nonsusceptible organisms.
- Watch for evidence of pseudomembranous colitis and treat accordingly.

Patient teaching

- Advise patient to immediately report muscle weakness and infusion site irritation.
- Tell patient to report severe diarrhea, rash, and infection.
- Inform patient about possible adverse reactions.

darbepoetin alfa
Aranesp

Pregnancy risk category C

Indications & dosages

➲ Anemia from chronic renal failure
Adults: 0.45 mcg/kg I.V. or S.C. once weekly. Adjust doses so that hemoglobin level doesn't exceed 12 g/dl. Don't increase dose more often than once a month. In patients converting from epoetin alfa, base starting dose on the previous epoetin alfa dose (see table).

Previous epoetin alfa dose (units/wk)	Darbepoetin alfa dose (mcg/wk)
< 2,500	6.25
2,500–4,999	12.5
5,000–10,999	25
11,000–17,999	40
18,000–33,999	60
34,000–89,999	100
≥ 90,000	200

Give darbepoetin alfa less often than epoetin alfa. If patient was receiving epoetin alfa two to three times weekly, give darbepoetin alfa once weekly. If patient was receiving epoetin alfa once weekly, give darbepoetin alfa once q 2 weeks.

If increasing hemoglobin level approaches 12 g/dl, reduce dose by 25%. If hemoglobin level continues to increase, withhold dose until hemoglobin level begins to decrease; then restart therapy at a dose 25% below the previous dose. If hemoglobin level increases more than 1 g/dl over 2 weeks, decrease dose by 25%. If hemoglobin level increases less than 1 g/dl over 4 weeks and iron stores are adequate, increase dose by 25% of previous dose. Make further increases at 4-week intervals until target hemoglobin level is reached. Patients who don't need dialysis may need lower maintenance doses.

➲ **Anemia from chemotherapy in patients with nonmyeloid malignancies**

Adults: 2.25 mcg/kg S.C. weekly.

If hemoglobin level increases less than 1 g/dl after 6 weeks of therapy, increase dose up to 4.5 mcg/kg. If hemoglobin level increases by more than 1 g/dl in a 2-week period or if hemoglobin level exceeds 12 g/dl, reduce dose by about 25%. If hemoglobin level exceeds 13 g/dl, withhold drug until hemoglobin level drops to 12 g/dl. Therapy can then be restarted at a dose about 25% below the previous dose.

Contraindications & cautions

- Contraindicated in patients hypersensitive to the drug or its components and in those with uncontrolled hypertension.
- Safety and effectiveness haven't been established in patients with underlying hematologic disease, such as hemolytic anemia, sickle cell anemia, thalassemia, or porphyria. Use with caution.

Adverse reactions

CNS: *headache, fever, dizziness, fatigue,* asthenia, ***seizures***.

CV: *hypertension, hypotension,* CARDIAC ARRHYTHMIA, CARDIAC ARREST, angina, ***heart failure, thrombosis****, edema,* chest pain, ***acute MI***.

GI: *diarrhea, vomiting, nausea, abdominal pain, constipation,* ***GI hemorrhage***.

Metabolic: dehydration.

Musculoskeletal: *myalgia, arthralgia, limb pain,* back pain.

Respiratory: *upper respiratory tract infection, dyspnea, cough,* bronchitis, pneumonia, ***pulmonary embolism***.

Skin: pruritus, rash.

Other: *infection,* fluid overload, flulike symptoms, ***hemorrhage at access site***.

Interactions

None reported.

Nursing considerations

- Some patients are treated successfully with a S.C. dose given once every 2 weeks.
- Hemoglobin level may not increase until 2 to 6 weeks after starting therapy.
- Darbepoetin alfa may increase the risk of CV events. Control blood pressure and monitor carefully.

!!ALERT Monitor hemoglobin level weekly until stabilized. Don't exceed the target of 12 g/dl.

- Monitor renal function and electrolytes in predialysis patients.
- Monitor iron status before and during treatment. Give iron supplements to patients whose ferritin level is less than 100 mcg/L and transferrin saturation is less than 20%.
- Patients who are marginally dialyzed may need adjustments in dialysis prescriptions.
- Serious allergic reactions, including skin rash and urticaria, may occur. If an anaphylactic reaction occurs, stop the drug and give appropriate therapy.
- Store drug in the refrigerator; don't freeze. Protect drug from light.

!!ALERT Decrease dosage if hemoglobin level increases 1 g/dl in 2 weeks.

Patient teaching

- Instruct patients on proper administration and use and disposal of needles.
- Advise patient of possible side effects and allergic reactions.
- Inform patient of the need for frequent monitoring of blood pressure and hemoglobin level; stress compliance with his treatment for high blood pressure.
- Instruct patient how to take drug correctly at home, including how to dispose of supplies properly.

darifenacin hydrobromide

Enablex

Pregnancy risk category C

Indications & dosages

➲ **Urge incontinence, urgency, and frequency from an overactive bladder**

Adults: Initially, 7.5 mg P.O. once daily.After 2 weeks,may increase to 15 mg P.O. once daily if needed.

If patient has a Child-Pugh score of B or takes a potent CYP3A4 inhibitor, such as clarithromycin, itraconazole, ketoconazole, nefazodone, nelfinavir, ritonavir, don't exceed 7.5 mg P.O. once daily.

Contraindications & cautions

- Contraindicated in patients hypersensitive to drug or its ingredients.
- Contraindicated in patients who have or who are at risk for urine retention, gastric retention, or uncontrolled narrow-angle glaucoma.
- Avoid use in patients with a Child-Pugh score of C.
- Use cautiously in patients with bladder outflow or GI obstruction, ulcerative colitis, myasthenia gravis, severe constipation, controlled narrow-angle glaucoma, decreased GI motility, or a Child-Pugh score of B.

Adverse reactions

CNS: asthenia, dizziness.
CV: hypertension.
EENT: abnormal vision, dry eyes, pharyngitis, rhinitis, sinusitis.
GI: abdominal pain, diarrhea, *dry mouth, constipation*, dyspepsia, nausea, vomiting.
GU: urinary tract disorder, UTI, vaginitis.
Metabolic: weight gain.
Musculoskeletal: arthralgia, back pain.
Respiratory: bronchitis.
Skin: dry skin, pruritus, rash.
Other: accidental injury, flulike syndrome, pain, peripheral edema.

Interactions

Drug-drug. *Anticholinergics:* May increase anticholinergic effects, such as dry mouth, blurred vision, and constipation. Monitor patient closely.
Digoxin: May increase digoxin level. Monitor digoxin level.
Drugs metabolized by CYP2D6 (such as flecainide, thioridazine, tricyclic antidepressants): May increase levels of these drugs. Use together cautiously.
Midazolam: May increase midazolam level. Monitor patient carefully.
Potent CYP3A4 inhibitors (such as clarithromycin, itraconazole, ketoconazole, nefazodone, nelfinavir, ritonavir): May increase darifenacin level. Maintain dosage no higher than 7.5 mg P.O. daily.
Drug-lifestyle. *Hot weather:* May cause heat prostration from decreased sweating. Urge caution.

Nursing considerations

- Assess bladder function, and monitor drug effects.
- If patient has bladder outlet obstruction, watch for urine retention.
- Assess patient for decreased gastric motility and constipation.
- Use during pregnancy only if maternal benefit outweighs fetal risk.
- It's unknown if drug appears in breast milk.

Patient teaching

- Tell patient to swallow tablet whole with plenty of liquid; caution against crushing or chewing tablet.
- Inform patient that drug may be taken with or without food.
- Explain that drug may cause blurred vision. Tell patient to use caution, especially when performing hazardous tasks, until drug effects are known.
- Tell patient to report blurred vision, constipation, and urine retention.
- Discourage use of other drugs that may cause dry mouth, constipation, urine retention, or blurred vision.
- Tell patient that drug decreases sweating, and advise cautious use in hot environments and during strenuous activity.

daunorubicin citrate liposomal
DaunoXome

Pregnancy risk category D

Indications & dosages

➲ **First-line cytotoxic therapy for advanced HIV-related Kaposi's sarcoma**
Adults: 40 mg/m^2 I.V. over 60 minutes once q 2 weeks. Continue treatment until progressive disease becomes evident or until other complications of HIV infection preclude continuation of therapy.

For patients with impaired hepatic and renal function, if bilirubin level is 1.2 to 3 mg/dl, give three-fourths normal dose; if bilirubin or creatinine level exceeds 3 mg/dl, give one-half normal dose.

Contraindications & cautions

- Contraindicated in patients who have experienced severe hypersensitivity reaction to drug or its components.
- Use cautiously in patients with myelosuppression, cardiac disease, previous radiotherapy encompassing the heart, previous anthracycline use (doxorubicin cumulative dose is 300 mg/m^2 or above), or hepatic or renal dysfunction.

Adverse reactions

CNS: *headache, neuropathy,* depression, dizziness, syncope, insomnia, amnesia, anxiety, ataxia, confusion, ***seizures,*** hallucination, tremor, hypertonia, ***meningitis,*** *fatigue,* malaise, emotional lability, abnormal gait, hyperkinesia, somnolence, abnormal thinking, *fever.*
CV: ***dose-related cardiomyopathy,*** chest pain, hypertension, palpitations, ***arrhythmias, pericardial effusion, pericardial tamponade, cardiac arrest,*** angina pectoris, ***pulmonary hypertension,*** flushing, edema, tachycardia, ***MI.***
EENT: *rhinitis,* stomatitis, sinusitis, abnormal vision, conjunctivitis, tinnitus, eye pain, deafness, earache.
GI: taste disturbances, dry mouth, gingival bleeding, *nausea, diarrhea, abdominal pain, vomiting, anorexia,* constipation, thirst, ***GI hemorrhage,*** gastritis, dysphagia, stomatitis, increased appetite, melena, hemorrhoids, tenesmus.
GU: dysuria, nocturia, polyuria.
Hematologic: NEUTROPENIA, THROMBOCYTOPENIA.
Hepatic: hepatomegaly.
Metabolic: dehydration.
Musculoskeletal: *rigors, back pain,* arthralgia, myalgia.
Respiratory: *cough, dyspnea,* hemoptysis, hiccups, pulmonary infiltration, increased sputum.
Skin: alopecia, pruritus, *increased sweating,* dry skin, seborrhea, folliculitis, injection site inflammation.
Other: splenomegaly, lymphadenopathy, tooth caries, *opportunistic infections,* allergic reactions, flulike symptoms.

Interactions

None significant.

Nursing considerations

- Liposomal daunorubicin causes less nausea, vomiting, alopecia, neutropenia, thrombocytopenia, and potentially less cardiotoxicity than conventional daunorubicin.
- Give only under supervision of prescriber specializing in chemotherapy.
- Monitor cardiac function regularly. Assess patient before giving each dose because of risk of cardiac toxicity and heart failure. Determine left ventricular ejection fraction at total cumulative doses of 320 mg/m^2 and every 160 mg/m^2 thereafter. Total cumulative doses generally shouldn't exceed 550 mg/m^2.
- Provide careful hematologic monitoring because severe myelosuppression may occur. Repeat blood counts and evaluate before giving each dose. Withhold treatment if absolute granulocyte count is below 750 cells/mm^3.
- Monitor patient closely for signs and symptoms of opportunistic infection, especially because patients with HIV infection are immunocompromised.

!!ALERT Don't confuse daunorubicin citrate liposomal with daunorubicin hydrochloride.

Patient teaching

- Inform patient that hair loss may occur, but that it's usually reversible.
- Instruct patient to call prescriber if sore throat, fever, or other signs or symptoms of infection occur. Tell patient to avoid exposure to people with infections.
- Advise woman to report suspected or confirmed pregnancy during therapy.
- Tell patient to report back pain, flushing, or chest tightness during infusion.

daunorubicin hydrochloride
Cerubidine

Pregnancy risk category D

Indications & dosages

Dosages vary. Check treatment protocol with prescriber.

➲ **To induce remission in acute nonlymphocytic (myelogenous, monocytic, erythroid) leukemia**

Adults age 60 and older: In combination, 30 mg/m^2 per day I.V. on days 1, 2, and 3

of first course and on days 1 and 2 of subsequent courses with cytarabine infusions.
Adults younger than age 60: In combination, 45 mg/m^2 per day I.V. on days 1, 2, and 3 of first course and on days 1 and 2 of subsequent courses with cytarabine infusions.

➲ **To induce remission in acute lymphocytic leukemia (with combination therapy)**

Adults: 45 mg/m^2 per day I.V. on days 1, 2, and 3 of first course.
Children age 2 and older: 25 mg/m^2 I.V. on day 1 q week for up to 6 weeks, if needed.
Children younger than age 2 or with body surface area less than 0.5 m^2: Dose based on body weight, not surface area.

For patients with impaired hepatic and renal function, reduce dosage as follows: If bilirubin level is 1.2 to 3 mg/dl, give three-fourths normal dose; if bilirubin or creatinine level exceeds 3 mg/dl, give one-half normal dose.

Contraindications & cautions

- Contraindicated in patients hypersensitive to the drug.
- Use cautiously in patients with myelosuppression or impaired cardiac, renal, or hepatic function.

Adverse reactions

CNS: fever.
CV: IRREVERSIBLE CARDIOMYOPATHY, ECG changes.
GI: *nausea, vomiting,* diarrhea, stomatitis.
GU: red urine.
Hematologic: ***bone marrow suppression.***
Hepatic: ***hepatotoxicity.***
Metabolic: hyperuricemia.
Skin: rash, *reversible alopecia,* darkening or redness of previously irradiated areas, *severe cellulitis and tissue sloughing with drug extravasation.*
Other: ***anaphylactoid reaction,*** chills.

Interactions

Drug-drug. *Doxorubicin:* May cause additive cardiotoxicity. Monitor patient for toxicity.
Hepatotoxic drugs: May increase risk of additive hepatotoxicity. Monitor hepatic function closely.
Myelosuppressive drugs: May increase risk of myelosuppression. Monitor patient closely.

Nursing considerations

- Take preventive measures (including adequate hydration) before starting treatment. Hyperuricemia may result from rapid lysis of leukemic cells. Allopurinol may be ordered.
- Perform cardiac function studies, including ECG and ejection fraction, before treatment and then periodically throughout therapy.
- Never give drug I.M. or S.C.

!! ALERT Cumulative adult dosage is limited to 400 to 550 mg/m^2 (450 mg/m^2 when patient is also receiving or has received cyclophosphamide or radiation therapy to cardiac area).

- Therapeutic effects are commonly accompanied by toxicity.
- Monitor CBC and hepatic function tests; monitor ECG every month during therapy.
- Monitor pulse rate closely. Notify prescriber if light resting pulse rate (a sign of cardiac adverse reactions) occurs.

!! ALERT Stop drug immediately and notify prescriber if signs of heart failure, cardiomyopathy, or arrhythmia develop.

- Watch for nausea and vomiting, which may last 24 to 48 hours.
- Anticipate need for blood transfusions to combat anemia. Patient may receive injected RBC colony–stimulating factor to promote RBC production and decrease need for blood transfusions.

!! ALERT Reddish color of drug is similar to that of doxorubicin; don't confuse the two.

- Lowest blood counts occur 10 to 14 days after administration.

!! ALERT Don't confuse daunorubicin hydrochloride with daunorubicin citrate liposomal.

Patient teaching

- Advise patient to report any pain or burning at site of injection during or after administration.
- Advise patient to watch for signs and symptoms of infection (fever, sore throat, fatigue) and bleeding (easy bruising, nosebleeds, bleeding gums, tarry stools) and to take temperature daily.
- Inform patient that red urine for 1 to 2 days is normal and doesn't indicate the presence of blood in urine.
- Advise patient that hair loss may occur, but that it's usually reversible.

• Caution woman of childbearing age to avoid becoming pregnant during therapy. Recommend that she consult prescriber before becoming pregnant.

delavirdine mesylate
Rescriptor

Pregnancy risk category C

Indications & dosages
➲ HIV-1 infection when therapy is warranted
Adults: 400 mg P.O. t.i.d. with other appropriate antiretrovirals.

Contraindications & cautions
• Contraindicated in patients hypersensitive to drug or its components.
• Use cautiously in patients with impaired hepatic function.

Adverse reactions
CNS: pain, fever, depression, *fatigue, headache,* insomnia, *asthenia.*
EENT: pharyngitis, sinusitis.
GI: diarrhea, *nausea,* vomiting, abdominal cramps, distention, or pain.
GU: epididymitis, hematuria, hemospermia, impotence, renal calculi, renal pain, metrorrhagia, nocturia, polyuria, proteinuria, vaginal candidiasis.
Respiratory: bronchitis, cough, upper respiratory tract infection.
Skin: *rash.*
Other: flulike syndrome.

Interactions
Drug-drug. *Amphetamines, nonsedating antihistamines, benzodiazepines, calcium channel blockers, clarithromycin, dapsone, ergot alkaloid preparations, indinavir, quinidine, rifabutin, sedative-hypnotics, warfarin:* May increase or prolong therapeutic and adverse effects of these drugs. Avoid using together, or, if use together is unavoidable, reduce doses of indinavir and clarithromycin.
Antacids: May reduce absorption of delavirdine. Separate doses by at least 1 hour.
Carbamazepine, phenobarbital, phenytoin: May decrease delavirdine level. Use together cautiously.
Clarithromycin, fluoxetine, ketoconazole: May cause a 50% increase in delavirdine bioavailability. Monitor patient and reduce dose of clarithromycin.
Didanosine: May decrease absorption of both drugs by 20%. Separate doses by at least 1 hour.
H_2-receptor antagonists: May increase gastric pH and reduce absorption of delavirdine. Long-term use together isn't recommended.
HMG-CoA reductase inhibitors, such as atorvastatin, lovastatin, simvastatin: May increase levels of these drugs, which increases risk of myopathy, including rhabdomyolysis. Avoid using together.
Rifabutin, rifampin: May decrease delavirdine level. May increase rifabutin level by 100%. Avoid using together.
Saquinavir: May increase bioavailability of saquinavir fivefold. Monitor AST and ALT levels frequently when used together.
Sildenafil: May increase sildenafil level and may increase sildenafil adverse events, including hypotension, visual changes, and priapism. Tell patient not to exceed 25 mg of sildenafil in 48 hours.
Drug-herb. *St. John's wort:* May decrease delavirdine level. Discourage use together.

Nursing considerations
• Because drug's effects in patients with hepatic or renal impairment haven't been studied, monitor renal and liver function test results carefully.
• Drug-induced diffuse, maculopapular, erythematous, pruritic rash occurs most commonly on upper body and arms of patients with lower CD4 cell counts, usually within first 3 weeks of treatment. Dosage adjustment doesn't seem to affect rash. Treat symptoms with diphenhydramine, hydroxyzine, or topical corticosteroids.
• Drug doesn't reduce risk of transmission of HIV-1.
• Because resistance develops rapidly when used as monotherapy, always use drug with appropriate antiretrovirals.
• Monitor patient's fluid balance and weight.

Patient teaching
• Tell patient to stop drug and call prescriber if severe rash or such symptoms as fever, fa-

tigue, headache, nausea, abdominal pain, or cough occur.

- Inform patient that drug doesn't cure HIV-1 infection and that he may continue to acquire illnesses related to HIV-1 infection, including opportunistic infections. Therapy hasn't been shown to reduce the risk or frequency of such illnesses. Drug hasn't been shown to reduce transmission of HIV.
- Advise patient to remain under medical supervision when taking drug because the long-term effects aren't known.
- Tell patient to take drug as prescribed and not to alter doses without prescriber's approval. If a dose is missed, tell patient to take the next dose as soon as possible; he shouldn't double the next dose.
- Inform patient that drug may be dispersed in water before ingestion. Add tablets to at least 5 ounces (148 ml) of water, allow to stand for a few minutes, and stir until a uniform dispersion occurs. Tell patient to drink dispersion promptly, rinse glass, and swallow the rinse to ensure that entire dose is consumed.
- Tell patient that drug may be taken without regard to food.
- Instruct patient with absence of hydrochloric acid in the stomach to take drug with an acidic beverage, such as orange or cranberry juice.
- Instruct patient to take drug and antacids at least 1 hour apart.
- Advise patient to report use of other prescription or nonprescription drugs, including herbal remedies.
- Advise patient taking sildenafil about an increased risk of sildenafil-related adverse events, including low blood pressure, visual changes, and painful penile erection. Tell him to promptly report any symptoms to his prescriber. Tell patient not to exceed 25 mg of sildenafil in a 48-hour period.

desipramine hydrochloride

Apo-Desipramine†, Norpramin, Novo-Desipramine†

Pregnancy risk category NR

Indications & dosages

➲ Depression

Adults: 100 to 200 mg P.O. daily in divided doses; increase to maximum of 300 mg daily. Or, give entire dose h.s.

Adolescents and elderly patients: 25 to 100 mg P.O. daily in divided doses; increase gradually to maximum of 150 mg daily, if needed.

Contraindications & cautions

- Contraindicated in patients hypersensitive to drug, in those who have taken MAO inhibitors within previous 14 days.
- Contraindicated during acute recovery phase after MI.
- Use with extreme caution in patients with CV disease; in those with history of urine retention, glaucoma, seizure disorders, or thyroid disease; and in those taking thyroid drug.
- Avoid use in children.

Adverse reactions

CNS: *drowsiness, dizziness*, excitation, tremor, weakness, confusion, anxiety, restlessness, agitation, headache, nervousness, EEG changes, ***seizures***, extrapyramidal reactions.

CV: orthostatic hypotension, *tachycardia*, ECG changes, hypertension.

EENT: *blurred vision*, tinnitus, mydriasis.

GI: *dry mouth*, constipation, nausea, vomiting, anorexia, paralytic ileus.

GU: urine retention.

Metabolic: ***hypoglycemia***, hyperglycemia.

Skin: rash, urticaria, photosensitivity reactions, diaphoresis.

Other: hypersensitivity reactions, ***sudden death in children***.

Interactions

Drug-drug. *Barbiturates, CNS depressants:* May enhance CNS depression. Avoid using together.

Cimetidine, fluvoxamine, fluoxetine, paroxetine, sertraline: May increase desipramine level. Monitor patient for adverse reactions.

Clonidine: May cause life-threatening blood pressure elevations. Avoid using together.
Epinephrine, norepinephrine: May increase hypertensive effect. Use together cautiously.
MAO inhibitors: May cause severe excitation, hyperpyrexia, or seizures, usually with high doses. Avoid using within 14 days of MAO inhibitor therapy.
Drug-herb. *Evening primrose oil:* May cause additive or synergistic effect, resulting in lower seizure threshold and increasing the risk of seizure. Discourage use together.
St. John's wort, SAM-e, yohimbe: May cause serotonin syndrome. Discourage use together.
Drug-lifestyle. *Alcohol use:* May enhance CNS depression. Discourage use together.
Smoking: May lower desipramine level. Monitor patient for lack of effect.
Sun exposure: May increase risk of photosensitivity reactions. Advise patient to avoid excessive sunlight exposure.

Nursing considerations

- Monitor patient for nausea, headache, and malaise after abrupt withdrawal of long-term therapy; these symptoms don't indicate addiction.
- Don't withdraw drug abruptly.
- Because patients using tricyclic antidepressants may suffer hypertensive episodes during surgery, stop drug gradually several days before surgery.
- If signs or symptoms of psychosis occur or increase, expect prescriber to reduce dosage. Record mood changes. Monitor patient for suicidal tendencies, and allow only a minimum supply of drug.
- Because desipramine produces fewer anticholinergic effects than other tricyclic antidepressants, it's often prescribed for cardiac patients.
- Recommend sugarless hard candy or gum to relieve dry mouth. Saliva substitutes may be needed.

!!ALERT Norpramin may contain tartrazine.
!!ALERT Don't confuse desipramine with disopyramide or imipramine.

Patient teaching

- Advise patient to take full dose at bedtime, whenever possible.
- Warn patient to avoid hazardous activities that require alertness and good coordination until effects of drug are known. Drowsiness and dizziness usually subside after a few weeks.
- Advise patient to call prescriber if fever and sore throat occur. Blood counts may need to be obtained.
- Tell patient to avoid alcohol during drug therapy because it may antagonize effects of desipramine.
- Tell patient to consult prescriber before taking other prescription or OTC drugs.
- Warn patient not to stop drug suddenly.
- To prevent sensitivity to the sun, advise patient to use sunblock, wear protective clothing, and avoid prolonged exposure to strong sunlight.

desirudin
Iprivask

Pregnancy risk category C

Indications & dosages

➲ To prevent deep vein thrombosis in patients undergoing hip replacement surgery
Adults: 15 mg S.C. every 12 hours for 9 to 12 days. Give first injection 5 to 15 minutes before surgery, after induction of regional block anesthesia, if used.

If creatinine clearance is 31 to 60 ml/minute, give 5 mg S.C. q 12 hours. If creatinine clearance is less than 31 ml/minute, give 1.7 mg S.C. q 12 hours. Check activated PTT and creatinine daily. If activated PTT exceeds two times control, stop therapy until it's within two times control; then resume at a reduced dose.

Contraindications & cautions

- Contraindicated in patients hypersensitive to natural or recombinant hirudins and in patients with active bleeding or irreversible coagulation disorders.
- Use cautiously in patients with a creatinine clearance less than 60 ml/minute; patients undergoing spinal or epidural anesthesia; patients with hepatic insufficiency or injury; patients with GI or pulmonary bleeding within 3 months; patients with severe uncontrolled hypertension, bacterial endocarditis, or a hemostatic disorder; and patients with an increased risk of bleeding, such as those with recent major surgery, organ biopsy, puncture of a noncompressible

vessel (within 1 month), intracranial or intraocular bleeding, or hemorrhagic or ischemic CVA.

Adverse reactions

CNS: cerebrovascular disorder, dizziness, fever.
CV: deep thrombophlebitis, hypotension, ***thrombosis***.
EENT: epistaxis.
GI: ***hematemesis***, nausea, vomiting.
GU: hematuria.
Hematologic: anemia, ***hemorrhage***.
Other: ***anaphylaxis***, impaired healing, injection site mass, leg edema, leg pain, wound seeping.

Interactions

Drug-drug. *Abciximab, acetylsalicylic acid, clopidogrel, dipyridamole, glycoprotein IIb/IIIa antagonists, ketorolac, salicylates, sulfinpyrazone, ticlopidine:* May increase the risk of bleeding. Use together cautiously.
Anticoagulants, dextran 40, glucocorticoids, thrombolytics: May increase the risk of bleeding. Avoid using together.
Epidural or spinal anesthesia: May increase risk of neuraxial hematoma and paralysis. Catheter may be placed before desirudin is started and removed when anticoagulant effect is low.
Drug-herb. *Alfalfa, anise:* May increase the risk of bleeding because of coumarin constituents. Discourage use together.
Black currant, cat's claw, evening primrose oil: May inhibit platelet function and prolong bleeding time. Discourage use together.

Nursing considerations

- Reconstitute each 15-mg vial with 0.5 ml of provided diluent (mannitol 3%).
- Shake vial gently until powder is dissolved. Once reconstituted, each 0.5 ml contains 15.75 mg of desirudin.
- Inspect vial. If solution contains visible particles, don't use it.
- Use reconstituted solutions immediately or store them at room temperature for up to 24 hours protected from light.
- Use a syringe with a ½ -inch 26G or 27G needle to withdraw all of the reconstituted solution.
- With the patient lying down, inject entire contents of syringe by deep S.C. injection. Insert entire length of needle into a skinfold held between thumb and forefinger.
- Rotate sites between the right and left thigh or right and left anterolateral and posterolateral abdominal walls.
- Don't give this drug I.M.
- Don't mix other drugs with desirudin before or during administration.

!!ALERT If the patient has an unexplained decline in hematocrit or blood pressure or has other unexplained symptoms, consider the possibility of hemorrhage.

- Monitor coagulation tests, hemoglobin level, hematocrit, and renal function throughout therapy.
- Watch venipuncture sites for bleeding, hematoma, or inflammation.
- If drug is given with epidural or spinal anesthesia, consider the risk of epidural or spinal hematoma, which may cause long-term or permanent paralysis. Watch for evidence of neurologic impairment, such as back pain, numbness or weakness in lower limbs, and bowel or bladder dysfunction.

Patient teaching

- Advise patient that this drug can cause bleeding. Stress the need to report unusual bruising or bleeding (nosebleeds, blood in urine, tarry stools) immediately.
- Caution patient not to take any other drugs that increase the risk of bleeding, such as aspirin or NSAIDs, while receiving desirudin.
- Advise against activities risk injury.
- Tell patient to use a soft toothbrush and electric razor while receiving desirudin.

---

desloratadine

Clarinex, Clarinex Reditabs

Pregnancy risk category C

Indications & dosages

➲ Seasonal allergic rhinitis (patients age 2 and older); perennial allergic rhinitis; chronic idiopathic urticaria
Adults and children age 12 and older: 5 mg P.O. tablets or syrup once daily.
Children ages 6 to 11: 5 ml syrup (2.5 mg) P.O. once daily.
Children ages 12 months to 5 years: 2.5 ml syrup (1.25 mg) P.O. once daily.

Infants ages 6 to 11 months: 2 ml syrup (1 mg) P.O. once daily.

In patients with hepatic or renal impairment, start dosage at 5 mg P.O. every other day.

Contraindications & cautions

- Contraindicated in breast-feeding women and in patients hypersensitive to drug, to any of its components, or to loratadine.
- Use cautiously in elderly patients because of the greater likelihood of decreased hepatic, renal, or cardiac function, and concomitant disease or other drug therapy.
- Safety and effectiveness haven't been established in children younger than age 12.

Adverse reactions

CNS: *headache*, somnolence, fatigue, dizziness.
EENT: pharyngitis, dry throat.
GI: nausea, dry mouth.
Musculoskeletal: myalgia.
Other: flulike symptoms.

Interactions

None reported.

Nursing considerations

- Stop drug 4 days before diagnostic skin testing because antihistamines can prevent, reduce, or mask positive skin test response.
- Store tablets at 36° to 86° F (2° to 30° C); store orally disintegrating tablets at 59° to 86° F (15° to 30° C).

Patient teaching

- Advise patient not to exceed recommended dosage. Higher doses don't increase effectiveness and may cause somnolence.
- Tell patient that drug can be taken without regard to meals.
- Instruct patient to remove orally disintegrating tablets from blister pack and place on tongue immediately to dissolve.
- Orally disintegrating tablets may be taken with or without water.
- Tell patient to report adverse effects.

desmopressin acetate
DDAVP, Stimate

Pregnancy risk category B

Indications & dosages

➲ **Nonnephrogenic diabetes insipidus, temporary polyuria, and polydipsia related to pituitary trauma**
Adults and children older than age 12: 0.1 to 0.4 ml intranasally daily in one to three doses. Most adults need 0.2 ml daily in two divided doses. Or, give 0.5 to 1 ml I.V. or S.C. daily, usually in two divided doses. Or, give 0.05 mg P.O. b.i.d.; adjust dosage to patient response. If patient previously received the drug intranasally, begin oral therapy 12 hours after last intranasal dose.
Children ages 3 months to 12 years: 0.05 to 0.3 ml intranasally daily in one or two doses.

➲ **Hemophilia A and von Willebrand's disease**
Adults and children: 0.3 mcg/kg diluted in normal saline solution and infused I.V. over 15 to 30 minutes. Repeat dose, if needed, as indicated by laboratory response and patient's condition. Or, 300 mcg (one spray in each nostril) of solution containing 1.5 mcg/ml. Dose of 150 mcg (one spray of solution containing 1.5 mg/ml into a single nostril) may be adequate for patients weighing less than 50 kg (110 lb). Give drug 2 hours before surgery.

➲ **Primary nocturnal enuresis**
Children age 6 and older: Initially, 20 mcg (0.2 ml) intranasally h.s. (10 mcg in each nostril). Adjust dosage based on response; maximum recommended dosage is 40 mcg daily. Or, initially 0.2 mg P.O. h.s., and adjust dose up to 0.6 mg to achieve desired response. For patients previously on intranasal DDAVP therapy, start tablet 24 hours after last intranasal dose in the nighttime.

Contraindications & cautions

- Contraindicated in patients hypersensitive to drug and in those with type IIB von Willebrand's disease.
- Use cautiously in patients with coronary artery insufficiency, hypertensive CV disease, and conditions linked to fluid and electrolyte imbalances, such as cystic fibrosis, because these patients are susceptible to hyponatremia.

• Use cautiously in breast-feeding women; it's unknown if drug appears in breast milk.

Adverse reactions

CNS: headache.
CV: flushing, slight rise in blood pressure.
EENT: rhinitis, epistaxis, sore throat.
GI: nausea, abdominal cramps.
GU: vulvar pain.
Respiratory: cough.
Skin: local erythema, swelling, or burning after injection.

Interactions

Drug-drug. *Carbamazepine, chlorpropamide:* May increase ADH; may increase desmopressin effect. Avoid using together.
Clofibrate: May enhance and prolong effects of desmopressin. Monitor patient closely.
Demeclocycline, epinephrine, heparin, lithium: May increase risk of adverse effects. Monitor patient closely.
Pressor agents: May enhance pressor effects with large doses of desmopressin. Monitor patient closely.
Drug-lifestyle. *Alcohol use:* May increase risk of adverse effects. Discourage use together.

Nursing considerations

• Morning and evening doses are adjusted separately for adequate diurnal rhythm of water turnover.
• Don't use desmopressin injection in patients with hemophilia A with factor VIII of up to 5% or severe von Willebrand's disease.
• Ensure nasal passages are intact, clean, and free of obstruction before giving intranasally.
• Intranasal use can cause changes in the nasal mucosa, resulting in erratic, unreliable absorption. Report worsening condition to prescriber, who may recommend injectable DDAVP.
• Adjust fluid intake to reduce risk of water intoxication and sodium depletion, especially in children or elderly patients.
!!ALERT Overdose may cause oxytocic or vasopressor activity. Withhold drug and notify prescriber. Use furosemide if fluid retention is excessive.
!!ALERT Don't confuse desmopressin with vasopressin.
• Nasal spray pump only delivers doses of 10 mcg DDAVP or 150 mcg Stimate. If doses other than those are required, use the nasal tube delivery system or injection.

Patient teaching

• Some patients may have trouble measuring and inhaling drug into nostrils. Teach patient and caregivers correct administration method.
• Instruct patient to clear nasal passages before giving drug.
• Instruct patient to press down four times to prime pump. Tell him to discard the bottle after 25 (150 mcg/spray) or 50 doses (10 mcg/spray), depending on the strength, because the amount left may be less than desired dose.
• Advise patient to report nasal congestion, allergic rhinitis, or upper respiratory tract infection to prescriber; dosage adjustment may be needed.
• Teach patient using S.C. desmopressin to rotate injection sites to prevent tissue damage.
• Warn patient to drink only enough water to satisfy thirst.
• Inform patient with hemophilia A or von Willebrand's disease that taking desmopressin may prevent hazards of using blood products.
• Advise patient to carry or wear medical identification indicating use of drug.

dexamethasone (ophthalmic)
Maxidex

dexamethasone sodium phosphate
AK-Dex, Decadron

Pregnancy risk category C

Indications & dosages

➲ **Uveitis; iridocyclitis; inflammatory conditions of eyelids, conjunctiva, cornea, anterior segment of globe; corneal injury from chemical or thermal burns, or penetration of foreign bodies; allergic conjunctivitis; suppression of graft rejection after keratoplasty**
Adults and children: 1 or 2 drops of suspension or solution or 1.25 to 2.5 cm of ointment into conjunctival sac. In severe dis-

ease, give drops q 1 to 2 hours, tapering to end as condition improves. In mild conditions, give drops up to four to six times daily or apply ointment t.i.d. or q.i.d. As condition improves, taper dosage to b.i.d.; then once daily. Treatment may extend from a few days to several weeks.

Contraindications & cautions

- Contraindicated in patients hypersensitive to any component of drug.
- Contraindicated in those with ocular tuberculosis or acute superficial herpes simplex (dendritic keratitis), vaccinia, varicella, or other fungal or viral diseases of cornea and conjunctiva; in patients with acute, purulent, untreated infections of eye; and in those who have had uncomplicated removal of superficial corneal foreign body.
- Use cautiously in patients with corneal abrasions that may be infected (especially with herpes).
- Use cautiously in patients with glaucoma (any form) because intraocular pressure may increase. Dosage of glaucoma drugs may need to be increased to compensate.
- Safe use in pregnant and breast-feeding women hasn't been established.

Adverse reactions

EENT: increased intraocular pressure, thinning of cornea, interference with corneal wound healing, increased susceptibility to viral or fungal corneal infection, corneal ulceration, glaucoma worsening, cataracts, defects in visual acuity and visual field, optic nerve damage with excessive or long-term use, mild blurred vision, burning, stinging, or redness of eyes, dry eyes, discharge, discomfort, ocular pain, foreign body sensation, photophobia.
Other: systemic effects, adrenal suppression with excessive or long-term use.

Interactions

None significant.

Nursing considerations

- Drug isn't for long-term use.
- Watch for corneal ulceration; which may require stopping drug.
- Corneal viral and fungal infections may be worsened by corticosteroid application.

!!ALERT Don't confuse dexamethasone with desoximetasone.

!!ALERT Don't confuse Maxidex with Maxzide.

Patient teaching

- Tell patient to shake suspension well before use.
- Teach patient how to instill drops or apply ointment. Advise him to wash hands before and after applying ointment or solution, and warn him not to touch tip of dropper to eye or surrounding tissue.
- Tell patient to apply light finger pressure on lacrimal sac for 1 minute after instillation.
- Advise patient that he may use eye pad with ointment.
- Warn patient not to use leftover drug for new eye inflammation; doing so may cause serious problems.

!!ALERT Warn patient to call prescriber immediately and to stop drug if visual acuity changes or visual field diminishes.

- Tell patient not to share drug, washcloths, or towels with family members and to notify prescriber if anyone develops same signs or symptoms.
- Stress importance of compliance with recommended therapy.
- Tell patient who wears contact lenses to check with prescriber before using lenses again.

dexamethasone (systemic)

Decadron*, Dexameth, Dexone, Hexadrol

dexamethasone acetate

Cortastat LA, Dalalone D.P., Decaject LA, Dexasone LA, Dexone LA, Solurex LA

dexamethasone sodium phosphate

Cortastat, Dalalone, Decadron Phosphate, Decaject, Dexasone, Hexadrol Phosphate, Solurex

Pregnancy risk category C

Indications & dosages

➲ **Cerebral edema**

Adults: Initially, 10 mg phosphate I.V.; then 4 to 6 mg I.M. q 6 hours until symptoms subside (usually 2 to 4 days); then tapered over 5 to 7 days.

➲ **Inflammatory conditions, allergic reactions, neoplasias**

Adults: 0.75 to 9 mg/day P.O. or 0.5 to 9 mg/day phosphate I.M. Or, 8 to 16 mg acetate I.M. into joint or soft tissue q 1 to 3 weeks. Or, 0.8 to 1.6 mg acetate into lesions q 1 to 3 weeks.

➲ **Shock**

Adults: 20 mg phosphate as single first dose; then 3 mg/kg/24 hours via continuous I.V. infusion. Or, 1 to 6 mg/kg phosphate I.V. as single dose. Or, 40 mg phosphate I.V. q 2 to 6 hours, p.r.n., continued only until patient is stabilized (usually not longer than 48 to 72 hours).

➲ **Dexamethasone suppression test for Cushing's syndrome**

Adults: Determine baseline 24-hour urine levels of 17-hydroxycorticosteroids; then, give 0.5 mg P.O. q 6 hours for 48 hours. Repeat 24-hour urine collection to determine 17-hydroxycorticosteroid excretion during second 24 hours of dexamethasone administration. Or, 1 mg P.O. as single dose at 11:00 p.m. with determination of plasma cortisol at 8 a.m. the next morning.

➲ **Adrenocortical insufficiency**

Children: 0.024 to 0.34 mg/kg or 0.66 to 10 mg/m P.O. daily, in four divided doses.

Contraindications & cautions

- Contraindicated in patients hypersensitive to drug or its ingredients, in those with systemic fungal infections, and in those receiving immunosuppressive doses together with live virus vaccines.
- Use with caution in patient with recent MI.
- Use cautiously in patients with GI ulcer, renal disease, hypertension, osteoporosis, diabetes mellitus, hypothyroidism, cirrhosis, diverticulitis, nonspecific ulcerative colitis, recent intestinal anastomoses, thromboembolic disorders, seizures, myasthenia gravis, heart failure, tuberculosis, active hepatitis, lactation, ocular herpes simplex, emotional instability, or psychotic tendencies.
- Because some formulations contain sulfite preservatives, also use cautiously in patients sensitive to sulfites.

Adverse reactions

CNS: *euphoria, insomnia*, psychotic behavior, ***pseudotumor cerebri***, vertigo, headache, paresthesia, ***seizures***.

CV: ***heart failure***, hypertension, edema, ***arrhythmias***, thrombophlebitis, ***thromboembolism***.

EENT: cataracts, glaucoma.

GI: *peptic ulceration*, GI irritation, increased appetite, ***pancreatitis***, nausea, vomiting.

GU: menstrual irregularities, increased urine glucose and calcium levels.

Metabolic: hypokalemia, hyperglycemia, carbohydrate intolerance, hypercholesterolemia, hypocalcemia.

Musculoskeletal: growth suppression in children, muscle weakness, osteoporosis.

Skin: hirsutism, delayed wound healing, acne, various skin eruptions, atrophy at I.M. injection site.

Other: cushingoid state, susceptibility to infections, acute adrenal insufficiency after increased stress or abrupt withdrawal after long-term therapy.

After abrupt withdrawal: rebound inflammation; fatigue; weakness; arthralgia; fever; dizziness; lethargy; depression; fainting; orthostatic hypotension; dyspnea; anorexia; ***hypoglycemia. After prolonged use, sudden withdrawal may be fatal.***

Interactions

Drug-drug. *Aminoglutethimide:* May cause loss of dexamethasone-induced adrenal suppression. Use together cautiously.

Antidiabetics, including insulin: May decrease response. May need dosage adjustment.

Aspirin, indomethacin, other NSAIDs: May increase risk of GI distress and bleeding. Use together cautiously.

Barbiturates, carbamazepine, phenytoin, rifampin: May decrease corticosteroid effect. Increase corticosteroid dosage.

Cardiac glycosides: May increase risk of arrhythmia resulting from hypokalemia. May need dosage adjustment.

Cyclosporine: May increase toxicity. Monitor patient closely.

Ephedrine: May cause decreased half-life and increased clearance of dexamethasone. Monitor patient.

Oral anticoagulants: May alter dosage requirements. Monitor PT and INR closely.

Potassium-depleting drugs such as thiazide diuretics: May enhance potassium-wasting effects of dexamethasone. Monitor potassium level.
Salicylates: May decrease salicylate level. Monitor patient for lack of salicylate effectiveness.
Skin-test antigens: May decrease response. Postpone skin testing until therapy is completed.
Toxoids, vaccines: May decrease antibody response and may increase risk of neurologic complications. Avoid using together.
Drug-herb. *Echinacea:* May increase herb's action. Discourage use together.
Ginseng: May increase immunomodulating response. Discourage use together.
Drug-lifestyle. *Alcohol use:* May increase risk of gastric irritation and GI ulceration. Discourage use together.

Nursing considerations

- Determine whether patient is sensitive to other corticosteroids.
- Most adverse reactions to corticosteroids are dose- or duration-dependent.
- For better results and less toxicity, give once-daily dose in morning.
- Give oral dose with food when possible. Patient may need medication to prevent GI irritation.
- Give I.M. injection deeply into gluteal muscle. Rotate injection sites to prevent muscle atrophy. Avoid S.C. injection because atrophy and sterile abscesses may occur.
- Always adjust to lowest effective dose.
- Monitor patient's weight, blood pressure, and electrolyte levels.
- Monitor patient for cushingoid effects, including moon face, buffalo hump, central obesity, thinning hair, hypertension, and increased susceptibility to infection.
- Watch for depression or psychotic episodes, especially in high-dose therapy.
- Diabetic patient may need increased insulin; monitor glucose levels.
- Drug may mask or worsen infections, including latent amebiasis.
- Elderly patients may be more susceptible to osteoporosis with long-term use.
- Inspect patient's skin for petechiae.
- Gradually reduce dosage after long-term therapy.

!!ALERT Don't confuse dexamethasone with desoximetasone.

Patient teaching

- Tell patient not to stop drug abruptly or without prescriber's consent.
- Instruct patient to take drug with food or milk.
- Teach patient signs and symptoms of early adrenal insufficiency: fatigue, muscle weakness, joint pain, fever, anorexia, nausea, shortness of breath, dizziness, and fainting.
- Instruct patient to carry or wear medical identification indicating his need for supplemental systemic glucocorticoids during stress, especially when dosage is decreased. This card should contain prescriber's name and name and dosage of drug.
- Warn patient on long-term therapy about cushingoid effects (moon face, buffalo hump) and the need to notify prescriber about sudden weight gain or swelling.
- Warn patient about easy bruising.
- Advise patient receiving long-term therapy to consider exercise or physical therapy. Tell him to ask prescriber about vitamin D or calcium supplement.
- Instruct patient receiving long-term therapy to have periodic eye examinations.
- Advise patient to avoid exposure to infections (such as measles and chickenpox) and to notify prescriber if such exposure occurs.

dexamethasone (topical)

Aeroseb-Dex, Decaspray

dexamethasone sodium phosphate

Decadron Phosphate

Pregnancy risk category C

Indications & dosages

➲ Inflammation from dermatoses responsive to corticosteroids
Adults and children: Clean area; apply cream or aerosol sparingly t.i.d. or q.i.d. For aerosol use on scalp, shake can well but gently, and apply to dry scalp after sham-

pooing. Hold can upright or inverted and 6 inches (15 cm) away from area. Spray while moving container to all affected areas, which should take about 2 seconds. Don't massage drug into scalp or spray forehead or near eyes. When result is obtained, reduce dose gradually, then stop use.

Contraindications & cautions

- Contraindicated in patients hypersensitive to drug or its components.

Adverse reactions

GU: glycosuria.
Metabolic: hyperglycemia.
Skin: burning, pruritus, irritation, dryness, erythema, folliculitis, hypertrichosis, acneiform eruptions, perioral dermatitis, hypopigmentation, allergic contact dermatitis, *maceration, secondary infection, atrophy, striae, miliaria with occlusive dressings.*
Other: ***hypothalamic-pituitary-adrenal axis suppression***, Cushing's syndrome, altered growth and development in children.

Interactions

None significant.

Nursing considerations

- Gently wash skin before applying. To prevent skin damage, rub cream in gently, leaving a thin coat. When treating hairy sites, part hair and apply directly to lesions.
- Avoid applying near eyes or mucous membranes or in ear canal, groin, or axillae.
- For patients with eczematous dermatitis whose skin may be irritated by adhesive material, hold dressing in place with gauze, stockings, or stockinette.
- Change dressing as prescribed. Stop drug and tell prescriber if skin infection, striae, or atrophy occurs.
- If an occlusive dressing has been applied and a fever develops, notify prescriber and remove dressing.
- When using aerosol around face, cover patient's eyes and warn against inhalation of spray. Aerosol preparation contains alcohol and may cause irritation or burning when used on open lesions. To avoid freezing tissues, don't spray longer than 1 to 2 seconds or from less than 6 inches (15 cm) away.
- If antifungal or antibiotic combined with corticosteroid fails to provide prompt improvement, stop corticosteroid until infection is controlled.
- Systemic absorption is likely with use of occlusive dressings, prolonged treatment, or extensive body surface treatment. Watch for symptoms.
- Avoid using plastic pants or tight-fitting diapers on treated areas in young children. Children may absorb larger amounts of drug and be more susceptible to systemic toxicity.
- Continue treatment for a few days after lesions clear.

!! ALERT Don't confuse dexamethasone with desoximetasone.

Patient teaching

- Teach patient and family how to apply drug.
- If an occlusive dressing is used, advise patient to leave it in place for no longer than 12 hours each day and not to use dressing on infected or weeping lesions.
- Tell patient to stop drug and report signs of systemic absorption, skin irritation or ulceration, hypersensitivity, or infection.
- Tell patient to avoid scratching.

dexmedetomidine hydrochloride
Precedex

Pregnancy risk category C

Indications & dosages

➲ To sedate initially intubated and mechanically ventilated patients in intensive care unit (ICU)
Adults: Loading infusion of 1 mcg/kg I.V. over 10 minutes; then maintenance infusion of 0.2 to 0.7 mcg/kg/hour for up to 24 hours, titrated to achieve desired level of sedation.

Contraindications & cautions

- Contraindicated in patients hypersensitive to dexmedetomidine hydrochloride.
- Use cautiously in patients with advanced heart block or renal or hepatic impairment and in elderly patients.

Adverse reactions

CNS: pain.
CV: *hypotension*, ***bradycardia***, ***arrhythmias***, *hypertension*, atrial fibrillation.
GI: *nausea*, vomiting, thirst.
GU: oliguria.
Hematologic: anemia, leukocytosis.
Respiratory: ***hypoxia***, pleural effusion, ***pulmonary edema***.
Other: infection, rigors.

Interactions

Drug-drug. *Anesthetics, hypnotics, opioids, sedatives:* May enhance effects of dexmedetomidine. May need to reduce dexmedetomidine dose.

Nursing considerations

- Only health care professionals skilled in managing patients in the intensive care unit, where cardiac status can be continuously monitored, should give drug.

!!ALERT Give using controlled infusion device at rate calculated for body weight.

- Determine renal and hepatic function before administration, and consider dosage adjustments in patients with renal or hepatic impairment and in elderly patients.
- Some patients receiving drug can awaken when stimulated. This alone shouldn't be considered evidence of lack of efficacy in absence of other signs and symptoms.
- Drug may be continuously infused in mechanically ventilated patients before, during, and after extubation. It isn't necessary to stop drug before extubation.

Patient teaching

- Tell patient he will be sedated while drug is being given but that he may awaken when stimulated.
- Reassure patient that he will be closely monitored and attended while sedated.

dexmethylphenidate hydrochloride

Focalin, Focalin XR

Pregnancy risk category C
Controlled substance schedule II

Indications & dosages

➲ **Attention deficit hyperactivity disorder (ADHD)**
immediate-release tablets
Adults and children ages 6 and older: For patients who aren't now taking methylphenidate, initially, 2.5 mg immediate-release tablets P.O. b.i.d., given at least 4 hours apart. Increase weekly by 2.5 to 5 mg daily, up to a maximum of 20 mg daily in divided doses.

For patients who are now taking methylphenidate, initially give half the current methylphenidate dosage, up to a maximum of 20 mg P.O. daily in divided doses.
extended-release capsules
Adults: For patients who aren't now taking dexmethylphenidate or methylphenidate, or who are on stimulants other than methylphenidate, give 10 mg P.O. extended-release capsules once daily in the morning. May adjust in weekly increments of 10 mg to a maximum dose of 20 mg daily.

For patients who are now taking methylphenidate, initially give half the total daily dose of methylphenidate. Patients who are now taking the immediate-release form of dexmethylphenidate may be switched to the same daily dose of extended-release form. Maximum daily dose is 20 mg.
Children ages 6 and older: For patients who aren't now taking dexmethylphenidate or methylphenidate, or who are on stimulants other than methylphenidate, give 5 mg P.O. extended-release capsules once daily in the morning. May adjust in weekly increments of 5 mg to a maximum daily dose of 20 mg.

For patients who are now taking methylphenidate, initially give half the total daily dose of methylphenidate. Patients who are now taking the immediate-release form of dexmethylphenidate may be switched to the same daily dose of extended-release form. Maximum daily dose is 20 mg.

Contraindications & cautions

- Contraindicated in patients hypersensitive to methylphenidate or other components.

- Contraindicated in patients with severe anxiety, tension, or agitation; glaucoma; or motor tics or a family history or diagnosis of Tourette syndrome.
- Contraindicated within 14 days of MAO inhibitor therapy.
- Use cautiously in patients with a history of drug abuse or alcoholism.
- Use cautiously in patients with psychosis, seizures, hypertension, hyperthyroidism, heart failure, or recent MI.
- Use in pregnant women only if the benefits outweigh the risks; drug may delay skeletal ossification, suppress weight gain, and impair organ development in the fetus.
- Use cautiously in breast-feeding women. It's unknown if drug appears in breast milk.

Adverse reactions

CNS: fever, insomnia, nervousness, *headache, anxiety, feeling jittery,* dizziness.
CV: tachycardia.
EENT: throat pain.
GI: *anorexia, abdominal pain,* nausea, dyspepsia, dry mouth.
Musculoskeletal: twitching (motor or vocal tics).
Other: hypersensitivity reactions.

Interactions

Drug-drug. *Antacids, acid suppressants:* May alter the release of extended-release formulation. Avoid using together.
Anticoagulants, phenobarbital, phenytoin, primidone, tricyclic antidepressants: May inhibit metabolism of these drugs. May need to decrease dosage of these drugs; monitor drug levels.
Antihypertensives: May decrease effectiveness of these drugs. Use together cautiously; monitor blood pressure.
Clonidine, other centrally acting alpha agonists: May cause serious adverse effects. Use together cautiously.
MAO inhibitors: May increase risk of hypertensive crisis. Using together within 14 days of MAO inhibitor therapy is contraindicated.

Nursing considerations

- Diagnosis of ADHD must be based on complete history and evaluation of the patient by psychological and educational experts.
- Refer patient for psychological, educational, and social support.
- Periodically reevaluate the long-term usefulness of the drug.
- Monitor CBC and differential and platelet counts during prolonged therapy.
- Don't use for severe depression or normal fatigue states.
- Stop treatment or reduce dosage if symptoms worsen or adverse reactions occur.
- Long-term stimulant use may temporarily suppress growth. Monitor children for growth and weight gain. If growth slows or weight gain is lower than expected, stop drug.
- Routinely monitor blood pressure and pulse.
- Monitor patient for signs of drug dependence or abuse.
- If seizures occur, stop drug.

Patient teaching

- Stress the importance of taking the correct dose of drug at the same time every day. Report accidental overdose immediately.
- Advise patients unable to swallow capsules to empty the contents of the capsule onto a spoonful of applesauce and eat immediately.

!!ALERT Tell patient not to cut, crush, or chew the contents of the extended-release beaded capsule.

- Advise parents to monitor child for medication abuse or sharing.
- Advise parents to monitor child's height and weight and to tell the prescriber if they suspect growth is slowing.
- Advise patient to report blurred vision to the prescriber.

dextroamphetamine sulfate

Dexedrine*, Dexedrine Spansule, DextroStat

Pregnancy risk category C
Controlled substance schedule II

Indications & dosages

➲ Narcolepsy
Adults: 5 to 60 mg P.O. daily in divided doses.
Children ages 6 to 12: 5 mg P.O. daily. Increase by 5 mg at weekly intervals p.r.n.
Children age 12 and older: 10 mg P.O. daily. Increase by 10 mg at weekly intervals, p.r.n. Give first dose on awakening; additional

doses (one or two) given at intervals of 4 to 6 hours.

➲ **Attention deficit hyperactivity disorder (ADHD)**

Children age 6 and older: 5 mg P.O. once daily or b.i.d. Increase by 5 mg at weekly intervals, p.r.n. It's rarely necessary to exceed 40 mg/day.

Children ages 3 to 5: 2.5 mg P.O. daily. Increase by 2.5 mg at weekly intervals, p.r.n.

➲ **Short-term adjunct in exogenous obesity♦**

Adults and children age 12 and older: 5 to 30 mg P.O. daily 30 to 60 minutes before meals in divided doses of 5 to 10 mg. Or, 10- or 15-mg extended-release capsule daily in the morning.

Contraindications & cautions

- Contraindicated in patients hypersensitive to or with idiosyncratic reactions to sympathomimetic amines, and in those with hyperthyroidism, moderate to severe hypertension, symptomatic CV disease, glaucoma, advanced arteriosclerosis, or history of drug abuse.
- Contraindicated within 14 days of MAO inhibitor therapy.
- Contraindicated as first-line treatment for obesity. Use as an anorexigenic is prohibited in some states.
- Use cautiously in agitated patients and patients with motor tics, phonic tics, or Tourette syndrome.

Adverse reactions

CNS: *restlessness*, tremor, *insomnia*, dizziness, headache, chills, overstimulation, dysphoria, euphoria, *nervousness*.

CV: *tachycardia*, *palpitations*, hypertension, ***arrhythmias***.

GI: dry mouth, taste perversion, diarrhea, constipation, anorexia, other GI disturbances.

GU: impotence.

Metabolic: weight loss.

Skin: urticaria.

Other: increased libido.

Interactions

Drug-drug. *Acetazolamide, alkalizing drugs, antacids, sodium bicarbonate:* May increase renal reabsorption. Monitor patient for enhanced amphetamine effects.

Acidifying drugs, ammonium chloride, ascorbic acid: May decrease level and increase renal clearance of dextroamphetamine. Monitor patient for decreased amphetamine effects.

Adrenergic blockers: May inhibit adrenergic blocking effects. Avoid using together.

Chlorpromazine: May inhibit central stimulant effects of amphetamines. May use to treat amphetamine poisoning.

Insulin, oral antidiabetics: May decrease antidiabetic requirements. Monitor glucose level.

MAO inhibitors: May cause severe hypertension or hypertensive crisis. Avoid using within 14 days of MAO inhibitor therapy.

Meperidine: May potentiate analgesic effect. Use together cautiously.

Methenamine: May increase urinary excretion of amphetamines and reduce efficacy. Monitor drug effects.

Norepinephrine: May enhance adrenergic effect of norepinephrine. Monitor patient.

Phenobarbital, phenytoin: May delay absorption of these drugs. Monitor patient closely.

Drug-food. *Caffeine:* May increase amphetamine and related amine effects. Urge caution.

Nursing considerations

- Drug shouldn't be used to prevent fatigue.
- Obese patients should follow a weight-reduction program.
- Drug has a high abuse potential and may cause dependence.
- Certain formulations may contain tartrazine.

!!ALERT Overdose may cause seizures.

- If tolerance to anorexigenic effect develops, stop drug and notify prescriber.

!!ALERT Don't confuse Dexedrine with dextran or Excedrin.

Patient teaching

- Tell patient to take drug 30 to 60 minutes before meals if used for weight reduction and at least 6 hours before bedtime to avoid sleep interference.
- Warn patient to avoid activities that require alertness or good coordination until CNS effects of drug are known.
- Tell patient he may get tired as drug effects wear off.

• Ask patient to report signs and symptoms of excessive stimulation.
• Advise patient to consume caffeine-containing products cautiously.
• Warn patient with a seizure disorder that drug may decrease seizure threshold. Instruct him to notify prescriber if seizures occur.

dextromethorphan hydrobromide

Balminil DM ◊, Benylin DM ◊, Broncho-Grippol-DM†, Buckley's DM, Children's Hold ◊, Delsym, Hold ◊, Koffex DM†, Pertussin CS ◊, Pertussin ES ◊, Robitussin Pediatric ◊, St. Joseph Cough Suppressant for Children ◊, Trocal ◊, Vicks Formula 44e Pediatric ◊

Commonly available in combination products, such as
Anti-Tuss DM Expectorant ◊, Benylin Expectorant ◊, Cheracol D Cough ◊, DexAlone ◊, Glycotuss-dM, Guiamid D.M. Liquid ◊, Guiatuss-DM ◊, Halotussin-DM ◊, Kolephrin GG/DM ◊, Mytussin DM ◊, Naldecon Senior DX ◊, Pertussin CS ◊, Rhinosyn-DMX Expectorant ◊, Robitussin-DM ◊, Scot-Tussin DM Cough Chasers ◊, Tolu-Sed DM ◊, Tuss-DM ◊, Unproco ◊, Vicks Pediatric 44E ◊

Pregnancy risk category C

Indications & dosages

➲ Nonproductive cough
Adults and children age 12 and older: 10 to 20 mg P.O. q 4 hours, or 30 mg q 6 to 8 hours. Or, 60 mg extended-release liquid b.i.d. Maximum, 120 mg daily.
Children ages 6 to 11: 5 to 10 mg P.O. q 4 hours, or 15 mg q 6 to 8 hours. Or, 30 mg extended-release liquid b.i.d. Maximum, 60 mg daily.
Children ages 2 to 5: 2.5 to 5 mg P.O. q 4 hours, or 7.5 mg q 6 to 8 hours. Or, 15 mg extended-release liquid b.i.d. Maximum, 30 mg daily.
Children younger than age 2: Individualize dosages.

Contraindications & cautions

• Contraindicated in patients currently taking MAO inhibitors or within 2 weeks of stopping MAO inhibitors.
• Use cautiously in atopic children, sedated or debilitated patients, and patients confined to the supine position.
• Use cautiously in patients sensitive to aspirin or tartrazine dyes.

Adverse reactions

CNS: drowsiness, dizziness.
GI: nausea, vomiting, stomach pain.

Interactions

Drug-drug. *MAO inhibitors:* May cause risk of hypotension, coma, hyperpyrexia, and death. Avoid using together.
Quinidine: May increase the risk of dextromethorphan adverse effects. Consider decreasing dextromethorphan dose if needed.
Selegiline: May cause risk of confusion, coma, hyperpyrexia. Avoid using together.
Drug-herb. *Parsley:* May promote or produce serotonin syndrome. Discourage use together.

Nursing considerations

• Don't use dextromethorphan when cough is a valuable diagnostic sign or is beneficial (as after thoracic surgery).
• Dextromethorphan 15 to 30 mg is equivalent to 8 to 15 mg codeine as an antitussive.
• Drug produces no analgesia or addiction and little or no CNS depression.
• Use drug with chest percussion and vibration.
• Monitor cough type and frequency.

Patient teaching

• Instruct patient to take drug exactly as prescribed.
• Tell patient to report adverse reactions.
!!ALERT Make sure patient understands that persistent cough may indicate a serious condition and that he should contact his prescriber if cough lasts longer than 1 week, recurs frequently, or is accompanied by high fever, rash, or severe headache.

diazepam

Apo-Diazepam†, Diastat, Diazepam Intensol, Novo-Dipam†, PMS-Diazepam†, Valium, Vivol†

Pregnancy risk category D
Controlled substance schedule IV

Indications & dosages

➲ **Anxiety**
Adults: Depending on severity, 2 to 10 mg P.O. b.i.d. to q.i.d. or 15 to 30 mg extended-release capsules P.O. once daily. Or, 2 to 10 mg I.M. or I.V. q 3 to 4 hours, p.r.n.
Children age 6 months and older: 1 to 2.5 mg P.O. t.i.d. or q.i.d., increase gradually, as needed and tolerated.
Elderly patients: Initially, 2 to 2.5 mg once daily or b.i.d.; increase gradually.

➲ **Acute alcohol withdrawal**
Adults: 10 mg P.O. t.i.d. or q.i.d. first 24 hours; reduce to 5 mg P.O. t.i.d. or q.i.d., p.r.n. Or, initially, 10 mg I.M. or I.V. Then, 5 to 10 mg I.M. or I.V. q 3 to 4 hours, p.r.n.

➲ **Before endoscopic procedures**
Adults: Adjust I.V. dose to desired sedative response (up to 20 mg). Or, 5 to 10 mg I.M. 30 minutes before procedure.

➲ **Muscle spasm**
Adults: 2 to 10 mg P.O. b.i.d. to q.i.d. Or, 15 to 30 mg extended-release capsules once daily. Or, 5 to 10 mg I.M. or I.V. initially; then 5 to 10 mg I.M. or I.V. q 3 to 4 hours, p.r.n. For tetanus, larger doses up to 20 mg q 2 to 8 hours may be needed.
Children age 5 and older: 5 to 10 mg I.M. or I.V. q 3 to 4 hours, p.r.n.
Children ages 1 month to 5 years: 1 to 2 mg I.M. or I.V. slowly, repeat q 3 to 4 hours, p.r.n.

➲ **Preoperative sedation**
Adults: 10 mg I.M. (preferred) or I.V. before surgery.

➲ **Cardioversion**
Adults: 5 to 15 mg I.V. within 5 to 10 minutes before procedure.

➲ **Adjunct treatment for seizure disorders**
Adults: 2 to 10 mg P.O. b.i.d. to q.i.d.
Children age 6 months and older: 1 to 2.5 mg P.O. t.i.d. or q.i.d. initially; increase as needed and as tolerated.

➲ **Status epilepticus, severe recurrent seizures**
Adults: 5 to 10 mg I.V. or I.M. initially. Use I.M. route only if I.V. access is unavailable. Repeat q 10 to 15 minutes, p.r.n., up to maximum dose of 30 mg. Repeat q 2 to 4 hours, if needed.
Children age 5 and older: 1 mg I.V. q 2 to 5 minutes up to maximum of 10 mg. Repeat q 2 to 4 hours, if needed.
Children ages 1 month to 5 years: 0.2 to 0.5 mg I.V. slowly q 2 to 5 minutes up to maximum of 5 mg. Repeat q 2 to 4 hours, if needed.

➲ **Patients on stable regimens of antiepileptic drugs who need diazepam intermittently to control bouts of increased seizure activity**
Adults and children age 12 and older: 0.2 mg/kg P.R., rounding up to the nearest available dose form. A second dose may be given 4 to 12 hours later.
Children ages 6 to 11: 0.3 mg/kg P.R., rounding up to the nearest available dose form. A second dose may be given 4 to 12 hours later.
Children ages 2 to 5: 0.5 mg/kg P.R., rounding up to the nearest available dose form. A second dose may be given 4 to 12 hours later.

For elderly and debilitated patients, reduce dosage to decrease the likelihood of ataxia and oversedation.

Contraindications & cautions

- Contraindicated in patients hypersensitive to drug or soy protein; in patients experiencing shock, coma, or acute alcohol intoxication (parenteral form); in pregnant women, especially in first trimester; and in children younger than age 6 months (oral form).
- Diastat rectal gel is contraindicated in patients with acute angle-closure glaucoma.
- Use cautiously in patients with liver or renal impairment, depression, or chronic open-angle glaucoma. Use cautiously in elderly and debilitated patients.

Adverse reactions

CNS: *drowsiness*, dysarthria, slurred speech, tremor, transient amnesia, fatigue, ataxia, headache, insomnia, paradoxical anxiety, hallucinations, minor changes in EEG patterns.

CV: hypotension, ***CV collapse, bradycardia***.
EENT: diplopia, blurred vision, nystagmus.
GI: nausea, constipation, diarrhea with rectal form.
GU: incontinence, urine retention.
Hematologic: ***neutropenia***.
Hepatic: jaundice.
Respiratory: ***respiratory depression, apnea***.
Skin: rash.
Other: altered libido, physical or psychological dependence, *pain, phlebitis at injection site.*

Interactions

Drug-drug. *Cimetidine, disulfiram, fluoxetine, fluvoxamine, hormonal contraceptives, isoniazid, metoprolol, propoxyphene, propranolol, valproic acid:* May decrease clearance of diazepam and increase risk of adverse effects. Monitor patient for excessive sedation and impaired psychomotor function.
CNS depressants: May increase CNS depression. Use together cautiously.
Digoxin: May increase digoxin level and risk of toxicity. Monitor patient and digoxin level closely.
Diltiazem: May increase CNS depression and prolong effects of diazepam. Reduce dose of diazepam.
Fluconazole, itraconazole, ketoconazole, miconazole: May increase and prolong diazepam level, CNS depression, and psychomotor impairment. Avoid using together.
Levodopa: May decrease levodopa effectiveness. Monitor patient.
Phenobarbital: May increase effects of both drugs. Use together cautiously.
Drug-herb. *Kava:* May increase sedation. Discourage use together.
Drug-lifestyle. *Alcohol use:* May cause additive CNS effects. Discourage use together.
Smoking: May decrease effectiveness of benzodiazepines. Monitor patient closely.

Nursing considerations

- Use Diastat rectal gel to treat no more than five episodes per month and no more than one episode every 5 days because tolerance may develop.
- When using oral concentrate solution, dilute dose just before giving.

!!ALERT Only caregivers who can distinguish the distinct cluster of seizures or events from the patient's ordinary seizure activity, who have been instructed and can give the treatment competently, who understand which seizures may or may not be treated with Diastat, and who can monitor the clinical response and recognize when immediate professional medical evaluation is needed should give Diastat rectal gel.

- Monitor periodic hepatic, renal, and hematopoietic function studies in patients receiving repeated or prolonged therapy.

!!ALERT Use of this drug may lead to abuse and addiction. Don't withdraw drug abruptly after long-term use; withdrawal symptoms may occur.

!!ALERT Don't confuse diazepam with diazoxide.

Patient teaching

- Warn patient to avoid activities that require alertness and good coordination until effects of drug are known.
- Tell patient to avoid alcohol while taking drug.
- Notify patient that smoking may decrease drug's effectiveness.
- Warn patient not to abruptly stop drug because withdrawal symptoms may occur.
- Warn woman to avoid use during pregnancy.
- Instruct patient's caregiver on the proper administration of Diastat rectal gel.

---

diclofenac potassium
Cataflam

diclofenac sodium (systemic)
Voltaren, Voltaren-XR, Voltaren Rapide†, Voltaren SR†

Pregnancy risk category B; D in 3rd trimester

Indications & dosages

➲ **Ankylosing spondylitis**
Adults: 25 mg delayed-release diclofenac sodium P.O. q.i.d.; may add another 25-mg dose h.s.

➲ **Osteoarthritis**
Adults: 50 mg P.O. b.i.d. or t.i.d., or 75 mg P.O. b.i.d. diclofenac potassium or delayed-release diclofenac sodium only. Or, 100 mg P.O. daily or b.i.d. extended-release diclofenac sodium only.

➲ Rheumatoid arthritis
Adults: 50 mg P.O. t.i.d. or q.i.d., or 75 mg P.O. b.i.d. diclofenac potassium or delayed-release diclofenac sodium only. Or, 100 mg P.O. daily or b.i.d. extended-release diclofenac sodium only, or 50 to 100 mg diclofenac sodium P.R. h.s. as substitute for last P.O. dose of the day. Don't exceed 150 mg daily.
➲ Analgesia, primary dysmenorrhea
Adults: 50 mg diclofenac potassium P.O. t.i.d. For some patients, the first dose on the first day may be 100 mg, followed by 50 mg for the second and third doses; maximum dose for first day is 200 mg. Don't exceed 150 mg daily after the first day.

Contraindications & cautions

- Contraindicated in patients hypersensitive to drug and in those with hepatic porphyria or history of asthma, urticaria, or other allergic reactions after taking aspirin or other NSAIDs.
- Drug isn't recommended for use during late pregnancy or breast-feeding.
- Use cautiously in patients with history of peptic ulcer disease, hepatic dysfunction, cardiac disease, hypertension, fluid retention, or impaired renal function.

Adverse reactions

CNS: anxiety, depression, dizziness, drowsiness, insomnia, irritability, headache, ***aseptic meningitis***.
CV: ***heart failure***, hypertension, edema, fluid retention.
EENT: tinnitus, ***laryngeal edema***, swelling of the lips and tongue, blurred vision, eye pain, night blindness, epistaxis, reversible hearing loss.
GI: abdominal pain or cramps, constipation, diarrhea, indigestion, nausea, abdominal distention, flatulence, taste disorder, peptic ulceration, bleeding, melena, bloody diarrhea, appetite change, colitis.
GU: proteinuria, ***acute renal failure***, oliguria, interstitial nephritis, papillary necrosis, *nephrotic syndrome*, fluid retention.
Hepatic: jaundice, ***hepatitis***, ***hepatotoxicity***.
Metabolic: ***hypoglycemia***, hyperglycemia.
Musculoskeletal: back, leg, or joint pain.
Respiratory: asthma.
Skin: rash, pruritus, urticaria, eczema, dermatitis, alopecia, photosensitivity reactions, bullous eruption, ***Stevens-Johnson syndrome***, allergic purpura.
Other: ***anaphylaxis***, ***anaphylactoid reactions***, ***angioedema***.

Interactions

Drug-drug. *Anticoagulants, including warfarin:* May cause bleeding. Monitor patient closely.
Aspirin: May decrease effectiveness of diclofenac and increase GI toxicity. Avoid using together.
Beta blockers: May decrease antihypertensive effects. Monitor patient closely.
Cyclosporine, digoxin, lithium, methotrexate: May reduce renal clearance of these drugs and increase risk of toxicity. Monitor patient closely.
Diuretics: May decrease effectiveness of diuretics. Avoid using together.
Insulin, oral antidiabetics: May alter requirements for antidiabetics. Monitor patient closely.
Potassium-sparing diuretics: May enhance retention and increase level of potassium. Monitor potassium level.
Drug-herb. *Dong quai, feverfew, garlic, ginger, horse chestnut, red clover:* May cause bleeding based on the known effects or components. Discourage use together.
White willow: Herb contains components similar to those of aspirin. Discourage use together.
Drug-lifestyle. *Sun exposure:* May cause photosensitivity reactions. Advise patient to avoid excessive sunlight exposure.

Nursing considerations

- Because NSAIDs impair the synthesis of renal prostaglandins, they can decrease renal blood flow and lead to reversible renal impairment, especially in patients with renal or heart failure or liver dysfunction, in elderly patients, and in those taking diuretics. Monitor these patients closely.
- Liver function test values may increase during therapy. Monitor transaminase, especially ALT levels, periodically in patients undergoing long-term therapy. Make first transaminase measurement no later than 8 weeks after therapy begins.
- Because of their antipyretic and anti-inflammatory actions, NSAIDs may mask the signs and symptoms of infection.

- Serious GI toxicity, including peptic ulcers and bleeding, can occur in patient taking NSAIDs, despite lack of symptoms.

!!ALERT Don't confuse diclofenac with Diflucan or Duphalac.

Patient teaching

- Tell patient to take drug with milk, meals, or antacids to minimize GI distress.
- Instruct patient not to crush, break, or chew enteric-coated tablets.
- Advise patient not to take this drug with any other diclofenac-containing products (such as Arthrotec).
- Teach patient signs and symptoms of GI bleeding, including blood in vomit, urine, or stool; coffee-ground vomit; and black, tarry stool. Tell him to notify prescriber immediately if any of these occurs.
- Teach patient the signs and symptoms of damage to the liver, including nausea, fatigue, lethargy, itching, yellowed skin or eyes, right upper quadrant tenderness, and flulike symptoms. Tell patient to contact prescriber immediately if these symptoms occur.
- Advise patient to avoid consuming alcohol or aspirin during drug therapy.
- Tell patient to wear sunscreen or protective clothing because drug may cause sensitivity to sunlight.
- Warn patient to avoid hazardous activities that require alertness until it is known whether the drug causes CNS symptoms.
- Tell pregnant woman to avoid use of drug during last trimester.
- Advise patient that use of OTC NSAIDs and diclofenac may increase the risk of GI toxicity.

diclofenac sodium (ophthalmic)

Voltaren Ophthalmic

Pregnancy risk category B

Indications & dosages

➲ Postoperative inflammation after removal of cataract

Adults: 1 drop in conjunctival sac q.i.d., beginning 24 hours after surgery and continuing throughout first 2 weeks of postoperative period.

➲ Corneal refractive surgery

Adults: 1 or 2 drops to operative eye 1 hour before surgery. Within 15 minutes after surgery, instill 1 or 2 drops into operative eye. Then 1 drop q.i.d. beginning 4 to 6 hours after surgery up to 3 days.

Contraindications & cautions

- Contraindicated in patients hypersensitive to any component of drug and in those wearing soft contact lenses. Because of known effects of prostaglandin-inhibiting drugs on fetal CV system (closure of ductus arteriosus), avoid use of drug during late pregnancy.
- Use cautiously in patients hypersensitive to acetylsalicylic acid, phenylacetic acid derivatives, and other NSAIDs; potential for cross-sensitivity exists.
- Use cautiously in surgical patients with known bleeding tendencies and in those receiving drugs that may prolong bleeding time.

Adverse reactions

EENT: *transient stinging and burning, increased intraocular pressure, keratitis,* anterior chamber reaction, ocular allergy, increased bleeding of ocular tissue, including hyphemas with ocular surgery.

GI: nausea, vomiting.

Other: viral infection.

Interactions

None significant.

Nursing considerations

- Drug may slow or delay healing.
- Most cases of increased intraocular pressure have occurred postoperatively and before drug administration.

!!ALERT Don't confuse diclofenac with Diflucan or Duphalac.

!!ALERT Don't confuse Voltaren with Verelan.

Patient teaching

- Teach patient how to instill drops. Advise him to wash hands before and after instilling solution and not to touch tip of dropper to eye or surrounding tissue.
- Advise patient to apply light finger pressure on lacrimal sac for 1 minute after instilling drops.

• Stress importance of compliance with recommended therapy.
• Warn patient not to use leftover drug for new eye inflammation.
• Remind patient to discard drug when no longer needed.

diclofenac sodium (topical)
Solaraze

Pregnancy risk category B

Indications & dosages

➲ Actinic keratosis
Adults: Apply gently to lesion b.i.d. for 60 to 90 days. Use enough gel to cover the lesion; for example, use 0.5 g of gel on a 5-cm × 5-cm lesion.

Contraindications & cautions

• Contraindicated in patients hypersensitive to diclofenac, benzyl alcohol, polyethylene glycol monomethyl ether 350, or hyaluronic acid.
• Use cautiously in patients with the aspirin triad; these patients are usually asthmatics who develop rhinitis, with or without nasal polyps, after taking aspirin or other NSAIDs.
• Use cautiously in patients with active GI bleeding or ulceration and in those with severe renal or hepatic impairment.
• Use cautiously in breast-feeding women; it's unknown if drug appears in breast milk. Patient should either stop breast-feeding or stop treatment, taking into account importance of drug to mother.

Adverse reactions

CNS: headache, pain, asthenia, migraine, hypokinesia, *paresthesia.*
CV: chest pain, hypertension.
EENT: sinusitis, pharyngitis, rhinitis, conjunctivitis, eye pain.
GI: diarrhea, dyspepsia, abdominal pain.
GU: hematuria, renal impairment.
Hepatic: liver impairment.
Metabolic: hypercholesterolemia, hyperglycemia.
Musculoskeletal: arthralgia, arthrosis, back pain, myalgia, neck pain.
Respiratory: asthma, dyspnea, pneumonia.
Skin: *reaction at application site, contact dermatitis, dry skin, pruritus, rash,* localized edema, *exfoliation,* acne, alopecia, *localized pain,* photosensitivity, skin carcinoma, skin ulcer.
Other: ***anaphylaxis,*** *flulike syndrome,* infection, allergic reaction.

Interactions

Drug-drug. *Oral NSAIDs:* May increase drug effects. Minimize use together.
Drug-lifestyle. *Sun exposure:* May increase risk of photosensitivity reactions. Advise patient to avoid excessive sun exposure.

Nursing considerations

• Don't apply to open wounds or broken skin.
• Avoid contact with eyes.
• Safety and effectiveness of sunscreens, cosmetics, or other topical medications used with drug are unknown.
• Complete healing or optimal therapeutic effect may not be seen until 30 days after therapy is complete.
• Reevaluate lesions that don't respond to therapy.
• Because of the risk of premature closure of the ductus arteriosus, avoid diclofenac in late pregnancy.

Patient teaching

• Inform patient about risk of skin reactions (rash, itchiness, pain, irritation) at the application site. Urge patient to seek medical attention if adverse reactions persist or worsen.
• Encourage patient to minimize sun exposure during therapy. Explain that sunscreen may be helpful but that the safety of using sunscreen with diclofenac is unknown.
• Caution patient not to apply gel to open wounds or broken skin.
• Instruct patient to avoid contact with eyes.
• Instruct patient not to apply other topical drugs or cosmetics to affected area while using drug, unless directed.
• Tell patient to notify prescriber if she's pregnant or breast-feeding.

dicyclomine hydrochloride

Antispas, Bentyl, Bentylol†, Byclomine, Dibent, Di-Spaz, Formulex†, Lomine†, Or-Tyl, Spasmoban†

Pregnancy risk category NR

Indications & dosages

➲ Irritable bowel syndrome, other functional GI disorders
Adults: Initially, 20 mg P.O. q.i.d., increased to 40 mg q.i.d. Or, 20 mg I.M. q.i.d.

Contraindications & cautions

- Contraindicated in patients hypersensitive to anticholinergics and in those with obstructive uropathy, obstructive disease of the GI tract, reflux esophagitis, severe ulcerative colitis, toxic megacolon, myasthenia gravis, unstable CV status in acute hemorrhage, tachycardia secondary to cardiac insufficiency or thyrotoxicosis, or glaucoma.
- Contraindicated in breast-feeding patients and in children younger than age 6 months.
- Use cautiously in patients with autonomic neuropathy, hyperthyroidism, coronary artery disease, arrhythmias, heart failure, hypertension, hiatal hernia, hepatic or renal disease, prostatic hyperplasia, known or suspected GI infection, and ulcerative colitis.
- Use cautiously in patients in hot or humid environments; drug can cause heatstroke.

Adverse reactions

CNS: *headache, dizziness,* fever, insomnia, light-headedness, drowsiness, nervousness, confusion, and excitement in elderly patients.
CV: *palpitations,* tachycardia.
EENT: blurred vision, increased intraocular pressure, mydriasis, photophobia.
GI: nausea, vomiting, *constipation, dry mouth, thirst,* abdominal distention, heartburn, paralytic ileus.
GU: *urinary hesitancy, urine retention,* impotence.
Skin: urticaria, decreased sweating or inability to sweat, local irritation.
Other: allergic reactions.

Interactions

Drug-drug. *Amantadine, antihistamines, antiparkinsonians, disopyramide, glutethimide, meperidine, phenothiazines, procainamide, quinidine, tricyclic antidepressants:* May have additive adverse effects. Avoid using together.

Nursing considerations

- Give drug 30 to 60 minutes before meals and at bedtime. Bedtime dose can be larger; give at least 2 hours after last meal of day.

!!ALERT Don't give S.C. or I.V.

- Adjust dosage based on patient's needs and response. Dosages up to 40 mg P.O. q.i.d. have been used in adults, but safety and efficacy for longer than 2 weeks haven't been established.
- Dicyclomine is a synthetic tertiary derivative that may have atropine-like adverse reactions.

!!ALERT Overdose may cause curarelike effects such as respiratory paralysis. Keep emergency equipment available.

- Monitor patient's vital signs and urine output carefully.

!!ALERT The dicyclomine labeling may be misleading. The ampule label reads 10 mg/ml but doesn't indicate that the ampule contains 2 ml of solution (20 mg of drug).

!!ALERT Don't confuse dicyclomine with dyclonine or doxycycline; don't confuse Bentyl with Aventyl or Benadryl.

Patient teaching

- Tell patient when to take drug, and stress importance of doing so on time and at evenly spaced intervals.
- Advise patient to avoid driving and other hazardous activities if drowsiness, dizziness, or blurred vision occurs; to drink plenty of fluids to help prevent constipation; and to report rash or other skin eruption.

didanosine (ddI)
Videx, Videx EC

Pregnancy risk category B

Indications & dosages

➲ HIV infection when antiretroviral therapy is warranted

Adults weighing 60 kg (132 lb) or more: 200 mg tablets P.O. q 12 hours or 400 mg P.O. once daily; or 250 mg buffered powder P.O. q 12 hours; or 400 mg capsule P.O. daily.

Adults weighing less than 60 kg: 125 mg tablets P.O. q 12 hours or 250 mg P.O. once daily; or 167 mg buffered powder P.O. q 12 hours; or 250 mg capsule P.O. daily.

Children: 120 mg/m^2 P.O. q 12 hours; Videx EC hasn't been studied in children.

Dialysis patients should receive 25% of usual Videx dose once daily. If patient weighs 60 kg or more, give 125 mg of Videx EC once daily. Don't use in patients who weigh less than 60 kg. If creatinine clearance is less than 10 ml/minute, don't give a supplemental dose after hemodialysis for either drug.

In adults who weigh 60 kg or more with creatinine clearance of 30 to 59 ml/minute, give 100-mg tablet b.i.d., 200-mg tablet or 200-mg capsule once daily, or 100-mg buffered powder b.i.d. If clearance is 10 to 29 ml/minute, give 150-mg tablet, 125-mg capsule, or 167-mg buffered powder once daily. If clearance is less than 10 ml/minute, give 100-mg tablet, 125-mg capsule, or 100-mg buffered powder once daily.

In adults who weigh less than 60 kg and have a clearance of 30 to 59 ml/minute, give 75-mg tablet b.i.d., 150-mg tablet or 125-mg capsule once daily, or 100-mg buffered powder b.i.d. If clearance is 10 to 29 ml/minute, give 100-mg tablet, 125-mg capsule, or 100-mg buffered powder once daily. For clearance less than 10 ml/minute, give 75-mg tablet or 100-mg buffered powder once daily; capsule not indicated for these patients.

Contraindications & cautions

- Contraindicated in patients hypersensitive to drug or its components.
- Use cautiously in patients with history of pancreatitis; deaths have occurred. Also use cautiously in patients with peripheral neuropathy, renal or hepatic impairment, or hyperuricemia. Monitor liver and renal function tests.

Adverse reactions

CNS: *headache*, ***seizures***, confusion, anxiety, pain, *fever*, nervousness, abnormal thinking, twitching, depression, *peripheral neuropathy, dizziness*, asthenia, insomnia.
CV: hypertension, edema, ***heart failure***.
EENT: retinal changes, optic neuritis.
GI: *diarrhea, nausea, vomiting, abdominal pain*, ***pancreatitis***, anorexia, dry mouth.
Hematologic: ***leukopenia***, granulocytosis, ***thrombocytopenia***, anemia.
Hepatic: ***hepatic failure***.
Metabolic: hyperuricemia.
Musculoskeletal: myopathy.
Respiratory: dyspnea, pneumonia.
Skin: rash, pruritus, alopecia.
Other: infection, ***sarcoma***, allergic reactions, *chills*.

Interactions

Drug-drug. *Amprenavir, delavirdine, indinavir, nelfinavir, ritonavir, saquinavir:* May alter pharmacokinetics of didanosine or these drugs. Separate dosage times.

Antacids containing magnesium or aluminum hydroxides: May enhance adverse effects of the antacid component (including diarrhea or constipation) when given with didanosine tablets or pediatric suspension. Avoid using together.

Co-trimoxazole, pentamidine, other drugs linked to pancreatitis: May increase risk of pancreatic toxicity. Use together cautiously; consider temporarily stopping didanosine during administration of these drugs.

Dapsone, drugs that require gastric acid for adequate absorption, ketoconazole: May decrease absorption from buffering action. Give these drugs 2 hours before didanosine.

Fluoroquinolones, tetracyclines: May decrease absorption from buffering products in didanosine tablets or antacids in pediatric suspension. Separate dosage times by at least 2 hours.

Itraconazole: May decrease itraconazole level. Avoid using together.

Drug-herb. *St. John's wort:* May decrease drug level, decreasing therapeutic effects. Discourage use together.

Drug-food. *Any food:* May decrease rate of absorption. Advise patient to take drug on an empty stomach at least 30 minutes before a meal.

Nursing considerations

- Give didanosine on an empty stomach, at least 30 minutes before or 2 hours after eating, regardless of dosage form used; giving drug with meals can decrease absorption by 50%.
- To give single-dose packets containing buffered powder for oral solution, pour contents into 4 ounces (120 ml) of water. Don't use fruit juice or other beverages that may be acidic. Stir for 2 or 3 minutes until the powder dissolves completely. Give immediately.
- The powder for oral solution may cause diarrhea. The manufacturer suggests switching to the tablet formulation if diarrhea is a problem.

!!ALERT The pediatric powder for oral solution must be prepared by a pharmacist before dispensing. It must be constituted with purified USP water and then diluted with an antacid (Mylanta Double Strength Liquid, Extra Strength Maalox Plus Suspension, or Maalox TC Suspension) to a final concentration of 10 mg/ml. The admixture is stable for 30 days at 36° to 46° F (2° to 8° C). Shake the solution well before measuring dose.

- Because of a high rate of early virologic failure and emergence of resistance, therapy with tenofovir in combination with didanosine and lamivudine isn't recommended as a new treatment regimen for therapy-naïve or experienced patients with HIV infection. Patients on this regimen should be considered for treatment modification.

!!ALERT Don't confuse drug with other antivirals that use abbreviations for identification.

Patient teaching

- Instruct patient to take drug on an empty stomach, 30 minutes before or 2 hours after eating.
- Because the tablets contain buffers that raise stomach pH to levels that prevent degradation of the active drug, instruct patient to chew tablets thoroughly before swallowing and to drink at least 1 ounce (30 ml) of water with each dose. Teach patient how to prepare crushed tablets or buffered powder form for ingestion, if appropriate.
- Inform patient that drug doesn't cure HIV infection, that opportunistic infections and other complications of HIV infection may continue to occur, and that transmission of HIV to others through sexual contact or blood contamination is still possible.
- To reduce the risk of GI adverse effects from excess antacid, advise patient to take no more than 4 didanosine buffered tablets at each dose.
- Inform patient on a sodium-restricted diet that each 2-tablet dose of didanosine contains 529 mg of sodium; each single packet of buffered powder for oral solution contains 1.38 g of sodium.
- Tell patient to report symptoms of inflammation of the pancreas, such as abdominal pain, nausea, vomiting, diarrhea, or symptoms of peripheral neuropathy.

diflunisal

Dolobid

Pregnancy risk category C

Indications & dosages

➲ Osteoarthritis, rheumatoid arthritis

Adults: 500 to 1,000 mg P.O. daily in two divided doses, usually q 12 hours. Maximum, 1,500 mg daily.

Elderly patients: In patients older than age 65, one-half usual adult dosage.

➲ Mild to moderate pain

Adults: 1 g P.O., then 500 mg q 8 to 12 hours. A lower dosage of 500 mg P.O., then 250 mg q 8 to 12 hours may be appropriate.

Contraindications & cautions

- Contraindicated in patients hypersensitive to drug and in those for whom acute asthmatic attacks, urticaria, or rhinitis are precipitated by aspirin or other NSAIDs.
- Use cautiously in patients with GI bleeding, history of peptic ulcer disease, renal impairment, compromised cardiac function, hypertension, or other conditions predisposing patient to fluid retention.

Adverse reactions

CNS: dizziness, somnolence, insomnia, headache, fatigue.
EENT: tinnitus.
GI: nausea, dyspepsia, GI pain, diarrhea, vomiting, constipation, flatulence, stomatitis.
GU: renal impairment, hematuria, ***interstitial nephritis***.
Skin: rash, pruritus, sweating, ***erythema multiforme, Stevens-Johnson syndrome***.

Interactions

Drug-drug. *Acetaminophen, hydrochlorothiazide, indomethacin:* May substantially increase levels of these drugs, increasing risk of toxicity. Avoid using together.
Antacids, aspirin: May decrease diflunisal level. Monitor patient for reduced therapeutic effect.
Anticoagulants, thrombolytics: May enhance effects of these drugs. Use together cautiously.
Cyclosporine: May enhance the nephrotoxicity of cyclosporine. Avoid using together.
Methotrexate: May enhance the toxicity of methotrexate. Avoid using together.
Sulindac: May decrease level of sulindac's metabolite. Monitor patient for reduced effect.

Nursing considerations

!!ALERT Because of the epidemiologic link to Reye's syndrome, the Centers for Disease Control and Prevention recommend not giving salicylates to children and teenagers with chickenpox or flulike illness.

Patient teaching

- Advise patient to take with water, milk, or meals.
- Tell patient that tablets must be swallowed whole.
- Instruct patient to avoid aspirin or acetaminophen while using diflunisal, unless prescribed.
- Inform breast-feeding woman that drug appears in breast milk and that she should stop either breast-feeding or taking drug.

digoxin

Digitek, Digoxin, Lanoxicaps, Lanoxin*

Pregnancy risk category C

Indications & dosages

➲ Heart failure, paroxysmal supraventricular tachycardia, atrial fibrillation and flutter

Capsules

Adults: For rapid digitalization, give 0.4 to 0.6 mg P.O. initially, followed by 0.1 to 0.3 mg q 6 to 8 hours, as needed and tolerated, for 24 hours. For slow digitalization, give 0.05 to 0.35 mg daily in two divided doses for 7 to 22 days, p.r.n., until therapeutic levels are reached. Maintenance dose is 0.05 to 0.35 mg daily in one or two divided doses.
Children: Digitalizing dose is based on child's age and is given in three or more divided doses over the first 24 hours. First dose is 50% of the total dose; subsequent doses are given q 4 to 8 hours as needed and tolerated.
Children age 10 and older: For rapid digitalization, give 8 to 12 mcg/kg P.O. over 24 hours, divided as above. Maintenance dose is 25% to 35% of total digitalizing dose, given daily as a single dose.
Children ages 5 to 10: For rapid digitalization, give 15 to 30 mcg/kg P.O. over 24 hours, divided as above. Maintenance dose is 25% to 35% of total digitalizing dose, divided and given in two or three equal portions daily.
Children ages 2 to 5: For rapid digitalization, give 25 to 35 mcg/kg P.O. over 24 hours, divided as above. Maintenance dose is 25% to 35% of total digitalizing dose, divided and given in two or three equal portions daily.

Elixir, tablets

Adults: For rapid digitalization, give 0.75 to 1.25 mg P.O. over 24 hours in two or more divided doses q 6 to 8 hours. For slow digitalization, give 0.125 to 0.5 mg daily for 5 to 7 days. Maintenance dose is 0.125 to 0.5 mg daily.
Children age 10 and older: 10 to 15 mcg/kg P.O. over 24 hours in two or more divided doses q 6 to 8 hours. Maintenance dose is 25% to 35% of total digitalizing dose.

Children ages 5 to 10: 20 to 35 mcg/kg P.O. over 24 hours in two or more divided doses q 6 to 8 hours. Maintenance dose is 25% to 35% of total digitalizing dose.
Children ages 2 to 5: 30 to 40 mcg/kg P.O. over 24 hours in two or more divided doses q 6 to 8 hours. Maintenance dose is 25% to 35% of total digitalizing dose.
Infants ages 1 month to 2 years: 35 to 60 mcg/kg P.O. over 24 hours in two or more divided doses q 6 to 8 hours. Maintenance dose is 25% to 35% of total digitalizing dose.
Neonates: 25 to 35 mcg/kg P.O. over 24 hours in two or more divided doses q 6 to 8 hours. Maintenance dose is 25% to 35% of total digitalizing dose.
Premature infants: 20 to 30 mcg/kg P.O. over 24 hours in two or more divided doses q 6 to 8 hours. Maintenance dose is 20% to 30% of total digitalizing dose.
Injection
Adults: For rapid digitalization, give 0.4 to 0.6 mg I.V. initially, followed by 0.1 to 0.3 mg I.V. q 4 to 8 hours, as needed and tolerated, for 24 hours. For slow digitalization, give appropriate daily maintenance dose for 7 to 22 days p.r.n. until therapeutic levels are reached. Maintenance dose is 0.125 to 0.5 mg I.V. daily in one or two divided doses.
Children: Digitalizing dose is based on child's age; give in three or more divided doses over the first 24 hours. First dose is 50% of total dose; subsequent doses are given q 4 to 8 hours as needed and tolerated.
Children age 10 and older: For rapid digitalization, give 8 to 12 mcg/kg I.V. over 24 hours, divided as above. Maintenance dose is 25% to 35% of total digitalizing dose, given daily as a single dose.
Children ages 5 to 10: For rapid digitalization, give 15 to 30 mcg/kg I.V. over 24 hours, divided as above. Maintenance dose is 25% to 35% of total digitalizing dose, divided and given in two or three equal portions daily.
Children ages 2 to 5: For rapid digitalization, give 25 to 35 mcg/kg I.V. over 24 hours, divided as above. Maintenance dose is 25% to 35% of total digitalizing dose, divided and given in two or three equal portions daily.
Infants ages 1 month to 2 years: For rapid digitalization, give 30 to 50 mcg/kg I.V. over 24 hours, divided as above. Maintenance dose is 25% to 35% of total digitalizing dose, divided and given in two or three equal portions daily.
Neonates: For rapid digitalization, give 20 to 30 mcg/kg I.V. over 24 hours, divided as above. Maintenance dose is 25% to 35% of the total digitalizing dose, divided and given in two or three equal portions daily.
Premature infants: For rapid digitalization, give 15 to 25 mcg/kg I.V. over 24 hours, divided as above. Maintenance dose is 20% to 30% of the total digitalizing dose, divided and given in two or three equal portions daily.

Give smaller loading and maintenance doses to patients with impaired renal function.

Contraindications & cautions

- Contraindicated in patients hypersensitive to drug and in those with digitalis-induced toxicity, ventricular fibrillation, or ventricular tachycardia unless caused by heart failure.
- Use with extreme caution in elderly patients and in those with acute MI, incomplete AV block, sinus bradycardia, PVCs, chronic constrictive pericarditis, hypertrophic cardiomyopathy, renal insufficiency, severe pulmonary disease, or hypothyroidism.

Adverse reactions

CNS: *fatigue, generalized muscle weakness, agitation, hallucinations*, headache, malaise, dizziness, vertigo, stupor, paresthesia.
CV: ***arrhythmias***.
EENT: yellow-green halos around visual images, blurred vision, light flashes, photophobia, diplopia.
GI: *anorexia, nausea*, vomiting, diarrhea.

Interactions

Drug-drug. *Amiloride:* May decrease digoxin effect and increase digoxin excretion. Monitor patient for altered digoxin effect.
Amiodarone, diltiazem, indomethacin, nifedipine, quinidine, verapamil: May increase digoxin level. Monitor patient for toxicity.
Amphotericin B, carbenicillin, corticosteroids, diuretics (such as chlorthalidone, loop diuretics, metolazone, thiazides), ticarcillin:

May cause hypokalemia, predisposing patient to digitalis toxicity. Monitor potassium level.
Antacids, kaolin-pectin: May decrease absorption of oral digoxin. Separate doses as much as possible.
Antibiotics: May increase risk of toxicity because of altered intestinal flora. Monitor patient for toxicity.
Anticholinergics: May increase digoxin absorption of oral digoxin tablets. Monitor drug level and observe for toxicity.
Cholestyramine, colestipol, metoclopramide: May decrease absorption of oral digoxin. Monitor patient for decreased digoxin level and effect. Give digoxin 1½ hours before or 2 hours after other drugs.
Parenteral calcium, thiazides: May cause hypercalcemia and hypomagnesemia, predisposing patient to digitalis toxicity. Monitor calcium and magnesium levels.
Drug-herb. *Betel palm, fumitory, goldenseal, hawthorn, lily of the valley, motherwort, rue, shepherd's purse:* May increase cardiac effects. Discourage use together.
Gossypol, horsetail, licorice, oleander, Siberian ginseng, squill: May increase toxicity. Monitor patient closely.
Plantain, St. John's wort: May decrease effectiveness of digoxin. Discourage use together.

Nursing considerations

- Drug-induced arrhythmias may increase the severity of heart failure and hypotension.
- In children, cardiac arrhythmias, including sinus bradycardia, are usually early signs of toxicity.
- Patients with hypothyroidism are extremely sensitive to cardiac glycosides and may need lower doses.
- Before giving loading dose, obtain baseline data (heart rate and rhythm, blood pressure, and electrolytes) and ask patient about use of cardiac glycosides within the previous 2 to 3 weeks.
- Loading dose is usually divided over the first 24 hours with approximately half the loading dose given in the first dose.
- Before giving drug, take apical-radial pulse for 1 minute. Record and notify prescriber of significant changes (sudden increase or decrease in pulse rate, pulse deficit, irregular beats and, particularly, regularization of a previously irregular rhythm). If these occur, check blood pressure and obtain a 12-lead ECG.
- Toxic effects on the heart may be life-threatening and require immediate attention.
- Absorption of digoxin from liquid-filled capsules is superior to absorption from tablets or elixir. Expect dosage reduction of 20% to 25% when changing from tablets or elixir to liquid-filled capsules or parenteral therapy.
- Monitor digoxin level. Therapeutic level ranges from 0.8 to 2 ng/ml. Obtain blood for digoxin level at least 6 to 8 hours after last oral dose, preferably just before next scheduled dose.

!!ALERT Excessive slowing of the pulse rate (60 beats/minute or less) may be a sign of digitalis toxicity. Withhold drug and notify prescriber.
- Monitor potassium level carefully. Take corrective action before hypokalemia occurs.
- Reduce drug dose for 1 to 2 days before elective cardioversion. Adjust dosage after cardioversion.

!!ALERT Don't confuse digoxin with doxepin.

Patient teaching

- Teach patient and a responsible family member about drug action, dosage regimen, how to take pulse, reportable signs, and follow-up care.
- Tell patient to report pulse less than 60 beats/minute or more than 110 beats/minute, or skipped beats or other rhythm changes.
- Instruct patient to report adverse reactions promptly. Nausea, vomiting, diarrhea, appetite loss, and visual disturbances may be early indicators of toxicity.
- Encourage patient to eat potassium-rich foods.
- Tell patient not to substitute one brand of digoxin for another.
- Advise patient to avoid the use of herbal drugs or to consult his prescriber before taking one.

digoxin immune Fab (ovine)
Digibind, DigiFab

Pregnancy risk category C

Indications & dosages

➲ Potentially life-threatening digitalis toxicity

Adults and children: Base dosage on ingested amount or level of digoxin. When calculating amount of antidote, round up to the nearest whole number.

For digoxin tablets, calculate number of antidote vials as follows: multiply ingested amount by 0.8; then divide answer by 0.5. For example, if patient takes 25 tablets of 0.25 mg digoxin, the ingested amount is 6.25 mg. Multiply 6.25 mg by 0.8 and divide answer by 0.5 to obtain 10 vials of antidote.

For digoxin capsules, divide the ingested dose in mg by 0.5. For example, if patient takes 50 capsules of 0.2 mg, the ingested amount is 10 mg. Divide 10 mg by 0.5 to obtain 20 vials of antidote.

If digoxin level is known, determine the number of antidote vials as follows: multiply the digoxin level in nanograms per milliliter by patient's weight in kg; then divide by 100. For example, if digoxin level is 4 nanograms/ml, and patient weighs 60 kg, multiply together to obtain 240. Divide answer by 100 to obtain 2.4 vials; then round up to 3 vials.

➲ Acute toxicity, or if estimated ingested amount or digoxin level is unknown

Adults and children: Consider giving 10 vials of digoxin immune Fab and observing patient's response. Follow with another 10 vials if indicated. Dosage should be effective in most life-threatening cases in adults and children but may cause volume overload in young children.

Contraindications & cautions

- Use cautiously in patients allergic to sheep proteins and in those who have previously received antibodies.

Adverse reactions

CV: ***heart failure***, rapid ventricular rate, worsening low cardiac output.
Metabolic: hypokalemia.
Other: hypersensitivity reactions, ***anaphylaxis***.

Interactions

None significant.

Nursing considerations

- In patients allergic to sheep proteins and in those who have previously received antibodies, skin testing is recommended because drug is derived from digoxin-specific antibody fragments obtained from immunized sheep.
- Drug is used for life-threatening overdose in patients with anaphylaxis, severe hypotension, or cardiac arrest and in those with ventricular arrhythmias (such as ventricular tachycardia or fibrillation), progressive bradycardia (such as severe sinus bradycardia), or second- or third-degree AV block not responsive to atropine.
- Heart failure and rapid ventricular rate may result by reversal of cardiac glycoside's therapeutic effects.
- Monitor potassium level closely.
- In most patients, signs of digitalis toxicity disappear within a few hours.

Patient teaching

- Explain use and administration of drug to patient and family.
- Instruct patient to report adverse reactions promptly.

diltiazem hydrochloride
Apo-Diltiaz†, Cardizem, Cardizem CD, Cardizem LA, Cardizem SR, Cartia XT, Dilacor XR, Diltia XT, Tiazac

Pregnancy risk category C

Indications & dosages

➲ To manage Prinzmetal's or variant angina or chronic stable angina pectoris

Adults: 30 mg P.O. q.i.d. before meals and h.s. Increase dose gradually to maximum of 360 mg/day divided into three to four doses, as indicated. Or, give 120 or 180 mg (extended-release) P.O. once daily. Adjust over a 7- to 14-day period as needed and tolerated up to a maximum dose of 360 mg/day (Cardizem LA), 480 mg/day (Cardizem CD, Cartia XT, Dilacor XR, Dilacor XT), or 540 mg/day (Tiazac).

➲ **Hypertension**
Adults: 60 to 120 mg P.O. b.i.d. (sustained-release). Adjust up to maximum recommended dose of 360 mg/day, p.r.n. Or, give 180 to 240 mg (extended-release) P.O. once daily. Adjust dosage based on patient response to a maximum dose of 480 mg/day. Or 120 to 240 mg P.O. (Cardizem LA) once daily. Dosage can be adjusted about every 2 weeks to a maximum of 540 mg daily.
➲ **Atrial fibrillation or flutter; paroxysmal supraventricular tachycardia**
Adults: 0.25 mg/kg I.V. as a bolus injection over 2 minutes. Repeat after 15 minutes if response isn't adequate with a dose of 0.35 mg/kg I.V. over 2 minutes. Follow bolus with continuous I.V. infusion at 5 to 15 mg/hour (for up to 24 hours).

Contraindications & cautions

- Contraindicated in patients hypersensitive to drug and in those with sick sinus syndrome or second- or third-degree AV block in the absence of an artificial pacemaker, ventricular tachycardia, systolic blood pressure below 90 mm Hg, acute MI, or pulmonary congestion (documented by X-ray).
- I.V. preparations are contraindicated in patients who have atrial fibrillation or flutter with an accessory bypass tract, as in Wolff-Parkinson-White syndrome or short PR interval syndrome.
- Use cautiously in elderly patients and in those with heart failure or impaired hepatic or renal function.

Adverse reactions

CNS: *headache*, dizziness, asthenia, somnolence.
CV: *edema*, ***arrhythmias***, flushing, ***bradycardia***, hypotension, conduction abnormalities, ***heart failure***, ***AV block***, abnormal ECG.
GI: nausea, constipation, abdominal discomfort.
Hepatic: ***acute hepatic injury***.
Skin: rash.

Interactions

Drug-drug. *Anesthetics:* May increase effects of anesthetics. Monitor patient.
Carbamazepine: May increase level of carbamazepine. Monitor carbamazepine level, and watch for signs and symptoms of toxicity.
Cimetidine: May inhibit diltiazem metabolism, increasing additive AV node conduction slowing. Monitor patient for toxicity.
Cyclosporine: May increase cyclosporine level, possibly by decreasing its metabolism, leading to increased risk of cyclosporine toxicity. Monitor cyclosporine level with each dosage change.
Diazepam, midazolam, triazolam: May increase CNS depression and prolonged effects of these drugs. Use lower dose of these benzodiazepines.
Digoxin: May increase digoxin level. Monitor patient for digoxin toxicity.
Furosemide: May form a precipitate when mixed with diltiazem injection. Give through separate I.V. lines.
Propranolol, other beta blockers: May precipitate heart failure or prolong conduction time. Use together cautiously.
Sirolimus, tacrolimus: May increase level of these drugs. Monitor drug level and patient for toxicity.

Nursing considerations

- Patients controlled on diltiazem alone or in combination with other medications may be switched to Cardizem LA tablets once a day at the nearest equivalent total daily dose.
- Monitor blood pressure and heart rate when starting therapy and during dosage adjustments.
- Maximum antihypertensive effect may not be seen for 14 days.
- If systolic blood pressure is below 90 mm Hg or heart rate is below 60 beats/minute, withhold dose and notify prescriber.

!! **ALERT** Don't confuse Cardizem SR with Cardene SR.

Patient teaching

- Instruct patient to take medication as prescribed, even when feeling better.
- Advise patient to avoid hazardous activities during start of therapy.
- Stress patient compliance if nitrate therapy is prescribed during adjustment of diltiazem dosage. Tell patient that S.L. nitroglycerin may be taken with drug, as needed, when angina symptoms are acute.

!! **ALERT** Tell patient to swallow extended-release capsules whole, and not to open, crush, or chew them.

dimenhydrinate

Apo-Dimenhydrinate†, Calm-X ◇, Children's Dramamine ◇ *, Dramamine ◇ *, Dramamine Liquid ◇ *, Dramanate, Dymenate, Gravol†, Gravol L/A†, Hydrate, PMS-Dimenhydrinate†, Triptone Caplets ◇

Pregnancy risk category B

Indications & dosages

➲ To prevent and treat motion sickness
Adults and children age 12 and older: 50 to 100 mg P.O. q 4 to 6 hours; 50 mg I.M., p.r.n.; or 50 mg I.V. diluted in 10 ml normal saline solution for injection, injected over 2 minutes. Maximum, 400 mg daily. For prevention, use drug 30 minutes before motion exposure.
Children ages 6 to 11: 25 to 50 mg P.O. q 6 to 8 hours, not to exceed 150 mg in 24 hours. Or, 1.25 mg/kg or 37.5 mg/m^2 I.M. or P.O. q.i.d. Maximum, 300 mg daily.
Children ages 2 to 5: 12.5 to 25 mg P.O. q 6 to 8 hours, not to exceed 75 mg in 24 hours. Or, 1.25 mg/kg or 37.5 mg/m^2 I.M. or P.O. q.i.d. Maximum, 300 mg daily.

Contraindications & cautions

- Contraindicated in patients hypersensitive to drug or its components.
- Use cautiously in elderly patients, patients receiving ototoxic drugs, and patients with seizures, acute angle-closure glaucoma, or enlarged prostate gland.

Adverse reactions

CNS: *drowsiness*, headache, dizziness, confusion, nervousness, vertigo, tingling and weakness of hands, lassitude, excitation, insomnia.
CV: palpitations, hypotension, tachycardia.
EENT: blurred vision, dry respiratory passages, diplopia, nasal congestion.
GI: dry mouth, nausea, vomiting, diarrhea, epigastric distress, constipation, anorexia.
GU: urine retention.
Respiratory: wheezing, thickened bronchial secretions.
Skin: photosensitivity, urticaria, rash.
Other: ***anaphylaxis***, tightness of chest.

Interactions

Drug-drug. *CNS depressants:* May cause additive CNS depression. Avoid using together.
Ototoxic drugs: Dimenhydrinate may mask symptoms of ototoxicity. Use together cautiously.
Tricyclic antidepressants, other anticholinergics: May increase anticholinergic activity. Monitor patient.
Drug-lifestyle. *Alcohol use:* May cause additive CNS depression. Discourage use together.

Nursing considerations

- Elderly patients may be more susceptible to adverse CNS effects.
- Undiluted solution irritates veins and may cause sclerosis.
- Drug may alter or confuse test results for xanthines (caffeine, aminophylline) because of its 8-chlorotheophylline content.
- Stop drug 4 days before diagnostic skin tests to prevent falsifying test response.
- Dramamine may contain tartrazine.

!!ALERT Drug may mask symptoms of ototoxicity, brain tumor, or intestinal obstruction.

!!ALERT Don't confuse dimenhydrinate with diphenhydramine.

Patient teaching

- Advise patient to avoid activities that require alertness until CNS effects of drug are known.
- Instruct patient to report adverse reactions promptly.

dimercaprol

BAL in Oil

Pregnancy risk category C

Indications & dosages

➲ Severe arsenic or gold poisoning
Adults and children: 3 mg/kg deep I.M. q 4 hours for 2 days; then q.i.d. on third day; then b.i.d. for 10 days.

➲ Mild arsenic or gold poisoning
Adults and children: 2.5 mg/kg deep I.M. q.i.d. for 2 days; then b.i.d. on third day; then once daily for 10 days.

➲ Mercury poisoning
Adults and children: Initially, 5 mg/kg deep I.M.; then 2.5 mg/kg daily or b.i.d. for 10 days.
➲ Acute lead encephalopathy or lead level greater than 100 mcg/ml
Adults and children: 4 mg/kg deep I.M.; then q 4 hours with edetate calcium disodium for 2 to 7 days. Use separate sites. For less severe poisoning, reduce dose to 3 mg/kg after first dose.

Contraindications & cautions

- Contraindicated in patients with hepatic dysfunction (except postarsenical jaundice) or iron, cadmium, or selenium poisoning; also contraindicated in those allergic to peanuts.
- Don't use in pregnant patient except to treat life-threatening acute poisoning.
- Use cautiously in patients with hypertension, G6PD deficiency, or oliguria.

Adverse reactions

CNS: headache, *fever*, paresthesia, anxiety.
CV: *transient increase in blood pressure, tachycardia.*
EENT: blepharospasm, conjunctivitis, lacrimation, rhinorrhea.
GI: *nausea, vomiting*, excessive salivation, *abdominal pain, burning sensation in lips, mouth, and throat.*
Musculoskeletal: muscle pain or weakness.
Other: pain or tightness in throat, chest, or hands.

Interactions

Drug-drug. *Iron:* May cause toxic metal complex. Take iron 24 hours after last dimercaprol dose.

Nursing considerations

!!ALERT Don't give drug I.V.; give by deep I.M. route only.
- Don't let drug contact skin because it may cause a skin reaction.
- Drug has an unpleasant, garlicky odor.
- Solution with slight sediment is usable.
- Use antihistamine to prevent or relieve mild adverse reactions.
- Keep urine alkaline to prevent renal damage.

Patient teaching

- Explain use and administration of drug to patient and family.
- Instruct patient to report adverse reactions promptly.

diphenhydramine hydrochloride

Allerdryl † ◇, AllerMax Allergy and Cough Formula, AllerMax Caplets ◇, Aller-med ◇, Banophen ◇, Banophen Caplets ◇, Benadryl ◇, Benadryl Allergy, Benylin Cough ◇, Bydramine Cough ◇, Compoz ◇, Diphen Cough ◇, Diphenadryl ◇, Diphenhist ◇, Diphenhist Captabs ◇, Dormarex 2 ◇, Genahist ◇, Hydramine ◇, Hydramine Cough ◇, Nervine Nighttime Sleep-Aid ◇, Nordryl Cough ◇, Sleep-eze 3 ◇, Sominex ◇, Tusstat ◇, Twilite Caplets ◇, Uni-Bent Cough ◇

Pregnancy risk category B

Indications & dosages

➲ Rhinitis, allergy symptoms, motion sickness, Parkinson's disease
Adults and children age 12 and older: 25 to 50 mg P.O. t.i.d. or q.i.d. Maximum, 300 mg P.O. daily. Or, 10 to 50 mg deep I.M. or I.V. Maximum by I.M. or I.V. route, 400 mg daily.
Children younger than age 12: 5 mg/kg/day P.O., deep I.M., or I.V., in divided doses q.i.d. Maximum, 300 mg daily.
➲ Sedation
Adults: 25 to 50 mg P.O. or deep I.M., p.r.n.
➲ Nighttime sleep aid
Adults: 25 to 50 mg P.O. h.s.
➲ Nonproductive cough (syrup only)
Adults and children age 12 and older: 25 mg P.O. q 4 to 6 hours. Don't exceed 150 mg daily.
Children ages 6 to 11: 12.5 mg P.O. q 4 to 6 hours. Don't exceed 75 mg daily.
Children ages 2 to 5: 6.25 mg P.O. q 4 to 6 hours. Don't exceed 25 mg daily.

Contraindications & cautions

- Contraindicated in patients hypersensitive to drug; newborns; premature neonates; breast-feeding women; patients with angle-closure glaucoma, stenosing peptic ulcer, symptomatic prostatic hyperplasia, bladder neck obstruction, or pyloroduodenal ob-

struction; and those having an acute asthmatic attack.
- Avoid use in patients taking MAO inhibitors.
- Use with caution in patients with prostatic hyperplasia, asthma, COPD, increased intraocular pressure, hyperthyroidism, CV disease, and hypertension.
- Children younger than age 12 should use drug only as directed by prescriber.

Adverse reactions

CNS: *drowsiness*, confusion, insomnia, headache, vertigo, *sedation*, *sleepiness*, *dizziness*, *incoordination*, fatigue, restlessness, tremor, nervousness, ***seizures***.
CV: palpitations, hypotension, tachycardia.
EENT: diplopia, blurred vision, nasal congestion, tinnitus.
GI: *nausea*, vomiting, diarrhea, *dry mouth*, constipation, *epigastric distress*, anorexia.
GU: dysuria, urine retention, urinary frequency.
Hematologic: hemolytic anemia, ***thrombocytopenia***, ***agranulocytosis***.
Respiratory: *thickening of bronchial secretions.*
Skin: urticaria, photosensitivity, rash.
Other: ***anaphylactic shock***.

Interactions

Drug-drug. *CNS depressants:* May increase sedation. Use together cautiously.
MAO inhibitors: May increase anticholinergic effects. Avoid using together.
Other products that contain diphenhydramine (including topical therapy): May increase risk of adverse reactions. Avoid using together.
Drug-lifestyle. *Alcohol use:* May increase CNS depression. Discourage use together.
Sun exposure: May cause photosensitivity reactions. Advise patient to avoid extensive sunlight exposure.

Nursing considerations

- Stop drug 4 days before diagnostic skin testing because antihistamines can prevent, reduce, or mask positive skin test response.
- Alternate injection sites to prevent irritation. Give I.M. injection deep into large muscle.

!!ALERT Don't confuse diphenhydramine with dimenhydrinate; don't confuse Benadryl with Bentyl, or benazepril.

Patient teaching

- Warn patient not to take this drug with any other products that contain diphenhydramine (including topical therapy) because of increased adverse reactions.
- Instruct patient to take drug 30 minutes before travel to prevent motion sickness.
- Tell patient to take diphenhydramine with food or milk to reduce GI distress.
- Warn patient to avoid alcohol and hazardous activities that require alertness until CNS effects of drug are known.
- Tell patient that coffee or tea may reduce drowsiness. Urge caution if palpitations develop.
- Inform patient that sugarless gum, hard candy, or ice chips may relieve dry mouth.
- Tell patient to notify prescriber if tolerance develops because a different antihistamine may need to be prescribed.
- Diphenhydramine is in many OTC sleep and cold products. Advise patient to consult prescriber before using these products.
- Warn patient of possible photosensitivity reactions. Advise use of a sunblock.

diphenoxylate hydrochloride and atropine sulfate

Logen, Lomanate, Lomotil*, Lonox

Pregnancy risk category C
Controlled substance schedule V

Indications & dosages

➲ Acute, nonspecific diarrhea
Adults and children older than age 12: Initially, 5 mg P.O. q.i.d.; then adjusted, p.r.n. Maximum dosage 20 mg/day.
Children ages 2 to 12: 0.3 to 0.4 mg/kg liquid form P.O. daily in four divided doses. For maintenance, reduce first dose p.r.n., up to 75%. Maximum dosage 20 mg/day.

Contraindications & cautions

- Contraindicated in patients hypersensitive to diphenoxylate or atropine, in those with obstructive jaundice, and in children younger than age 2.
- Contraindicated in those with acute diarrhea resulting from poison (until toxic material is eliminated from GI tract), from organisms that penetrate intestinal mucosa, or from antibiotic-induced pseudomembranous enterocolitis.

- Use cautiously in children age 2 and older; in patients with hepatic disease, opioid dependence, or acute ulcerative colitis; and in pregnant patients.

Adverse reactions

CNS: *sedation, dizziness,* headache, drowsiness, lethargy, restlessness, depression, euphoria, malaise, confusion, numbness in limbs.
CV: tachycardia.
EENT: blurred vision.
GI: *dry mouth,* nausea, vomiting, abdominal discomfort or distention, ***paralytic ileus***, anorexia, fluid retention in bowel or megacolon, ***pancreatitis***, swollen gums.
GU: urine retention.
Respiratory: ***respiratory depression***.
Skin: pruritus, rash, dry skin.
Other: ***angioedema***, ***anaphylaxis***, possible physical dependence with long-term use.

Interactions

Drug-drug. *Barbiturates, CNS depressants, opioids, tranquilizers:* May enhance CNS depression. Monitor patient closely.
MAO inhibitors: May cause hypertensive crisis. Avoid using together.
Drug-lifestyle. *Alcohol use:* May enhance CNS depression. Discourage use together.

Nursing considerations

!!ALERT Monitor fluid and electrolyte balance. Correct fluid and electrolyte disturbances before starting drug. Dehydration, especially in young children, may increase risk of delayed toxicity. Fluid retention in bowel or megacolon may occur with drug use and may mask depletion of extracellular fluid and electrolytes, especially in young children treated for acute gastroenteritis.
- Stop therapy immediately and notify prescriber if abdominal distention or other signs or symptoms of toxic megacolon develop.
- Don't use to treat antibiotic-induced diarrhea.
- Drug is unlikely to be effective if no response occurs within 48 hours.
- Risk of physical dependence increases with high dosage and long-term use. Atropine sulfate helps discourage abuse.
- Monitor for signs of overdose, which may include restlessness, flushing, hyperthermia, and tachycardia, initially, followed by lethargy, coma, pinpoint pupils, hypotonicity, and respiratory depression.

!!ALERT Don't confuse Lomotil with Lamictal.

Patient teaching

- Tell patient not to exceed recommended dosage.
- Warn patient not to use drug to treat acute diarrhea for longer than 2 days and to seek medical attention if diarrhea continues.
- Advise patient to avoid hazardous activities, such as driving, until CNS effects of drug are known.

diphtheria and tetanus toxoids and acellular pertussis vaccine adsorbed (DTaP)

Certiva, Daptacel, Infanrix, Tripedia

Pregnancy risk category C

Indications & dosages

➲ Primary immunization
Children ages 6 weeks to 7 years: Give 0.5 ml I.M. 4 to 8 weeks apart for three doses (6 to 8 weeks for Daptacel) and a fourth dose at least 6 months after the third dose.

➲ Booster immunization
Children ages 6 weeks to 7 years: If Tripedia was used for the first four doses, a fifth dose is recommended at age 4 to 6 before entering school. If the fourth dose was given after age 4, a fifth dose isn't needed.

Certiva is recommended as a fourth dose at ages 15 to 20 months in children who received their first three doses as whole-cell diphtheria, tetanus, and pertussis (DTP) vaccine. A fifth dose is recommended at age 4 to 6 in children who received four doses of whole-cell DTP vaccine or three doses of whole-cell vaccine followed by one dose of DTaP, unless the fourth dose was given after the fourth birthday.

Infanrix is indicated as a fifth dose in children ages 4 to 6 before entering school in those who received at least one dose of whole-cell DTP vaccine, unless the fourth dose was given after the fourth birthday.

Daptacel may be given to complete the immunization series in children who have received at least one dose of whole-cell DTP vaccine.

Contraindications & cautions

- Contraindicated in adults or children older than age 7, immunosuppressed patients, those on corticosteroid therapy, and those with history of seizures.
- Pertussis component of vaccine is contraindicated in children who have neurologic disorders or who exhibited neurologic signs after previous injection. Give these children diphtheria and tetanus toxoids (DT) vaccine instead. Postpone vaccination in patients with acute febrile illness.

!!ALERT Give vaccine to patients age 7 and older only in special circumstances, never routinely.

Adverse reactions

CNS: ***seizures***, *fever, drowsiness.*
GI: *anorexia*, vomiting.
Skin: *tenderness, redness, and swelling at injection site.*
Other: *hypersensitivity reactions, fretfulness,* irritability, crying longer than 1 hour.

Interactions

Drug-drug. *Immunosuppressants:* May reduce response to DTP vaccine. Avoid using together.

Nursing considerations

- Children whose seizures are well controlled or who had an explainable single-episode seizure may receive the acellular vaccine.
- Obtain history of allergies and reaction to immunization, especially to pertussis vaccine.
- Keep epinephrine 1:1,000 available to treat anaphylaxis.
- If an immediate allergic reaction occurs after giving the vaccine, withhold subsequent vaccination and refer patient to an allergist for evaluation. Documentation of a specific allergy may warrant desensitization to tetanus toxoid.
- Give only by deep I.M. injection, preferably in thigh or deltoid muscle. Don't give S.C.
- In infants, give I.M. injection in the anterolateral thigh.
- Vaccine may be given at same time as polio vaccine and, if indicated, when the patient receives vaccines against *Haemophilus influenzae* type b, measles, mumps, and rubella.
- Acellular vaccine may be linked to a lower risk of local pain and fever.

!!ALERT DTP preparations usually aren't interchangeable. It's recommended to use the vaccine from the same manufacturer, if possible, for at least the first three doses.

Patient teaching

- Explain risks and benefits of vaccine to parents before it's given.
- Tell parents to report systemic reactions promptly; remind them that local reactions are common. Acetaminophen in age-appropriate doses will decrease occurrence of postvaccination fever in children susceptible to febrile seizure activity.
- Stress importance of keeping scheduled appointments for subsequent doses. Full immunization requires a series of injections.

diphtheria and tetanus toxoids, acellular pertussis adsorbed, hepatitis B (recombinant), and inactivated poliovirus vaccine combined

Pediarix

Pregnancy risk category C

Indications & dosages

➲ Active immunization
Children ages 6 weeks to 7 years: Primary series is three 0.5-ml doses I.M. at 6- to 8-week intervals (preferably 8), usually starting at age 2 months; may start at age 6 weeks.

Contraindications & cautions

- Contraindicated in patients hypersensitive to any component of vaccine, including yeast, neomycin, and polymyxin B.
- Contraindicated if a previous dose of vaccine or its components caused a serious allergic reaction.
- Contraindicated in patient with progressive neurologic disorder, including infantile spasms, uncontrolled epilepsy, progressive encephalopathy, or encephalopathy within 7 days of a previous dose of pertussis-containing vaccine that can't be attributed to another cause.

• Use cautiously in children with bleeding disorders, such as hemophilia or thrombocytopenia, and take steps to reduce the risk of hematoma after injection.
• Avoid giving drug to an infant younger than 6 weeks, to a child age 7 or older, or to a child receiving anticoagulant therapy, unless the potential benefit outweighs the risk.
• Drug isn't indicated for adults.

Adverse reactions

CNS: *fever, fussiness, increased sleeping, restlessness, unusual cry.*
GI: *anorexia.*
Skin: *injection site reactions,* (pain, *redness, swelling).*

Interactions

Drug-drug. *Immunosuppressive therapies, such as alkylating agents, antimetabolites, corticosteroids, cytotoxic drugs, radiation:* May reduce immune response to the vaccine. If immunosuppressive therapy will end soon, postpone immunization until 3 months after immunosuppressive therapy; otherwise, vaccinate patient during immunosuppressive therapy, but expect inadequate response.

Nursing considerations

• Inject vaccine into the anterolateral aspect of the thigh or the deltoid muscle of the upper arm. Don't inject in the gluteal area or any area that may contain a major nerve trunk.
!!ALERT The tip cap and plunger of the needleless prefilled syringe contain latex and may cause allergic reactions in sensitive persons.
• Combined vaccine is more likely to cause fever than vaccines given separately.
• For children at high risk of seizures, give an antipyretic with vaccination and for 24 hours afterward to reduce risk of fever.
• Postpone vaccination if patient has a moderate or severe illness with or without fever.
• If patient has seizures within 3 days after being vaccinated, a temperature higher than 105° F (40.50° C), collapse or shocklike state, or persistent, inconsolable crying lasting 3 hours or more within 48 hours of the vaccine, postpone future doses of this drug or any vaccine containing pertussis until potential benefits and possible risks are reviewed.
• Interrupting the recommended schedule doesn't alter final immunity. The series need not be started over, regardless of the time elapsed between doses.
• Don't give drug as a booster dose after the main three-dose series. Instead, give a DTaP vaccine at age 15 to 18 months (Infanrix, because its pertussis antigen components match those in Pediarix) and IPV at age 4 to 6.

Patient teaching

• Tell parent to expect some redness, soreness, swelling, and hardness at the injection site.
• Tell parent that a nodule may form at the injection site and may persist for several weeks.
• Recommend acetaminophen to relieve discomfort.
• Stress the importance of keeping scheduled appointments for subsequent doses.

diphtheria antitoxin, equine

Pregnancy risk category C

Indications & dosages

➲ Diphtheria prevention
Adults and children: 5,000 to 10,000 units I.M.
➲ Pharyngeal or laryngeal diphtheria lasting 48 hours
Adults and children: 20,000 to 40,000 units I.M. or slow I.V. infusion.
➲ Nasopharyngeal lesions
Adults and children: 40,000 to 60,000 units I.M. or slow I.V. infusion.
➲ Extensive disease lasting 3 or more days or disease with neck swelling
Adults and children: 80,000 to 120,000 units by slow I.V. infusion.

Contraindications & cautions

• Contraindicated in patients hypersensitive to drug or its components.
• Use antitoxin with extreme caution in patients with history of allergic disorders.

Adverse reactions

Skin: erythema, urticaria.
Other: pain, hypersensitivity reactions, ***anaphylaxis***, serum sickness.

Interactions

None significant.

Nursing considerations

- Obtain history of allergies, especially to horses, and reactions to immunizations. Have epinephrine 1:1,000 available in case of anaphylaxis.
- Test for sensitivity before giving drug.

!! ALERT If patient has signs or symptoms of diphtheria (sore throat, fever, tonsillar membrane), start therapy immediately, without waiting for culture reports.

- For storage, refrigerate antitoxin at 36° to 50° F (2° to 10° C). Before giving, warm to 90° to 95° F (32° to 35° C), never higher.
- Begin appropriate antimicrobial therapy.
- Monitor patient for serum sickness (urticaria, pruritus, fever, malaise, arthralgia), which may occur in 7 to 12 days.

Patient teaching

- Explain to patient and family that test dose will be given first to check for sensitivity to drug.
- Tell patient to report adverse reactions promptly.

dipyridamole

Apo-Dipyridamole FC†, Novo-Dipiradol†, Persantine

Pregnancy risk category B

Indications & dosages

➲ To inhibit platelet adhesion in prosthetic heart valves (given together with warfarin)
Adults: 75 to 100 mg P.O. q.i.d.
➲ Alternative to exercise in evaluation of coronary artery disease during thallium myocardial perfusion scintigraphy
Adults: 0.57 mg/kg as an I.V. infusion at a constant rate over 4 minutes (0.142 mg/kg/minute).

Contraindications & cautions

- Contraindicated in patients hypersensitive to drug.
- Use cautiously in patients with hypotension.

Adverse reactions

CNS: *headache, dizziness*, syncope.
CV: flushing, hypotension, *angina pectoris, chest pain*, ***ECG abnormalities***, blood pressure lability, hypertension.
GI: *nausea*, vomiting, diarrhea, abdominal distress.

Interactions

Drug-drug. *Heparin:* May increase risk of bleeding. Monitor patient closely.
Theophylline: May prevent coronary vasodilation by I.V. dipyridamole, causing a false-negative thallium-imaging result. Avoid using together.

Nursing considerations

- If GI distress develops, give drug 1 hour before meals or with meals.
- Observe for adverse reactions, especially with large doses. Monitor blood pressure.
- Observe for signs and symptoms of bleeding; note prolonged bleeding time (especially with large doses or long-term therapy).
- The value of dipyridamole as part of an antithrombotic regimen is controversial; its use may not provide significantly better results than aspirin alone.

!! ALERT Don't confuse dipyridamole with disopyramide.

!! ALERT Don't confuse Persantine with Periactin.

- Persantine may contain tartrazine.

Patient teaching

- Instruct patient to take drug exactly as prescribed.
- Tell patient to report adverse reactions promptly.
- Tell patient receiving drug I.V. to report discomfort at insertion site.

disopyramide

disopyramide phosphate

Norpace, Norpace CR, Rythmodan-LA†

Pregnancy risk category C

Indications & dosages

➲ **Ventricular tachycardia; life-threatening ventricular arrhythmias**

Adults weighing more than 50 kg (110 lb): 150 mg P.O. q 6 hours with regular-release formulation or 300 mg q 12 hours with extended-release preparations.

Adults weighing 50 kg or less: 100 mg P.O. q 6 hour with regular-release formulation or 200 mg P.O. q 12 hours with extended-release preparations.

Children ages 12 to 18: 6 to 15 mg/kg P.O. daily, divided into four doses (q 6 hours).

Children ages 4 to 12: 10 to 15 mg/kg P.O. daily, divided into four doses (q 6 hours).

Children ages 1 to 4: 10 to 20 mg/kg P.O. daily, divided into four doses (q 6 hours).

Children younger than age 1: 10 to 30 mg/kg P.O. daily, divided into four doses (q 6 hours).

If creatinine clearance is 30 to 40 ml/minute, give 100 mg q 8 hours; if clearance is 15 to 30 ml/minute, give 100 mg q 12 hours; if clearance is less than 15 ml/minute, give 100 mg q 24 hours.

Contraindications & cautions

- Contraindicated in patients hypersensitive to drug.
- Contraindicated in those with sick sinus syndrome, cardiogenic shock, congenital QT interval prolongation, or second- or third-degree heart block in the absence of an artificial pacemaker.
- Use cautioously or avoid, if possible, in patients with heart failure.
- Use cautiously in patients with underlying conduction abnormalities, urinary tract diseases (especially prostatic hyperplasia), hepatic or renal impairment, myasthenia gravis, or acute angle-closure glaucoma.

Adverse reactions

CNS: dizziness, ***agitation***, depression, fatigue, headache, nervousness, acute psychosis, syncope.

CV: ***hypotension***, ***heart failure***, ***heart block***, edema, ***arrhythmias***, shortness of breath, chest pain.

EENT: blurred vision, dry eyes or nose.

GI: *dry mouth*, nausea, vomiting, anorexia, bloating, gas, weight gain, abdominal pain, *constipation*, diarrhea.

GU: *urinary hesitancy*, urine retention, urinary frequency, urinary urgency, impotence.

Hepatic: cholestatic jaundice.

Musculoskeletal: muscle weakness, aches, pain.

Skin: rash, pruritus, dermatosis.

Interactions

Drug-drug. *Antiarrhythmics:* May increase QRS complex or QT interval, which may lead to other arrhythmias. Monitor ECG closely.

Clarithromycin, erythromycin: May increase disopyramide level, resulting in arrhythmias. Monitor ECG closely.

Phenytoin: May increase metabolism of disopyramide. Watch for decreased antiarrhythmic effect.

Rifampin: May decrease disopyramide level. Monitor patient for lack of effect.

Thioridazine: May cause life-threatening arrhythmias including torsades de pointes. Avoid using together.

Verapamil: May cause additive effects and impairment of left ventricular function. Don't give disopyramide 48 hours before starting verapamil therapy or 24 hours after verapamil is stopped.

Drug-herb. *Jimsonweed:* May adversely affect CV function. Discourage use together.

Nursing considerations

- Correct electrolyte abnormalities before starting therapy.
- Digitalize patients with atrial fibrillation or flutter before starting disopyramide because of the risk of enhancing AV conduction.
- Check apical pulse before giving drug. Notify prescriber if pulse rate is slower than 60 beats/minute or faster than 120 beats/minute.
- Don't use sustained- or controlled-release preparations to control ventricular arrhythmias when therapeutic drug level must be rapidly attained, in patients with cardiomyopathy or possible cardiac decompensation, or in those with severe renal impairment.

!!ALERT Don't open the extended-release capsules.
- For use in young children, pharmacist may prepare disopyramide suspension using 100-mg capsules and cherry syrup. Pharmacist should dispense suspension in amber glass bottles. Protect suspension from light.
- Watch for recurrence of arrhythmias and check for adverse reactions; notify prescriber if any occur.
- Stop drug if heart block develops, if QRS complex widens by more than 25%, or if QT interval lengthens by more than 25% above baseline.

!!ALERT Don't confuse disopyramide with desipramine or dipyridamole.

Patient teaching
- Teach patient importance of taking drug on time and exactly as prescribed.
- If transferring patient from immediate-release to sustained-release capsules, advise him to take the first sustained-release capsule 6 hours after taking the last immediate-release capsule.
- Tell patient not to crush or chew sustained-release capsules or tablets.
- If not contraindicated, advise patient to chew gum or hard candy to relieve dry mouth and to increase fiber and fluid intake to relieve constipation.

dobutamine hydrochloride
Dobutrex

Pregnancy risk category B

Indications & dosages
➲ Increased cardiac output in short-term treatment of cardiac decompensation caused by depressed contractility, such as during refractory heart failure; adjunctive therapy in cardiac surgery
Adults: 0.5 to 1 mcg/kg/minute I.V. infusion, titrating to optimal dosage of 2 to 20 mcg/kg/minute. Usual effective range to increase cardiac output is 2 to 10 mcg/kg/minute. Rarely, rates up to 40 mcg/kg/minute may be needed.

Contraindications & cautions
- Contraindicated in patients hypersensitive to drug or its components and in those with idiopathic hypertrophic subaortic stenosis.
- Use cautiously in patients with history of hypertension because drug may increase pressor response.
- Use cautiously in patients with history of sulfite sensitivity.

Adverse reactions
CNS: headache.
CV: angina, *hypertension, increased heart rate,* PVCs, phlebitis, nonspecific chest pain, palpitations, hypotension.
GI: nausea, vomiting.
Respiratory: shortness of breath, ***asthma attacks***.
Other: hypersensitivity reactions, ***anaphylaxis***.

Interactions
Drug-drug. *Beta blockers:* May antagonize dobutamine effects. Avoid using together.
General anesthetics: May have greater risk of ventricular arrhythmias. Monitor ECG closely.
Guanethidine, oxytocic drugs: May increase pressor response, causing severe hypertension. Monitor blood pressure closely.
Tricyclic antidepressants: May potentiate pressor response and cause arrhythmias. Use together cautiously.
Drug-herb. *Rue:* May increase inotropic potential. Discourage use together.

Nursing considerations
- Before starting dobutamine therapy, give a plasma volume expander to correct hypovolemia.
- Before starting dobutamine therapy, give a cardiac glycoside. Because drug increases AV node conduction, patients with atrial fibrillation may develop a rapid ventricular rate.
- Continuously monitor ECG, blood pressure, pulmonary artery wedge pressure, cardiac output, and urine output.
- Monitor electrolyte levels. Drug may lower potassium level.

!!ALERT Don't confuse dobutamine with dopamine.

Patient teaching
- Tell patient to report adverse reactions promptly, especially labored breathing and drug-induced headache.
- Instruct patient to report discomfort at I.V. insertion site.

docetaxel
Taxotere

Pregnancy risk category D

Indications & dosages

➲ **Locally advanced or metastatic breast cancer after failure of previous chemotherapy**

Adults: 60 to 100 mg/m^2 I.V. over 1 hour q 3 weeks.

In patients receiving 100 mg/m^2 who experience febrile neutropenia, neutrophil count of less than 500/mm^3 for longer than 1 week, severe or cumulative cutaneous reactions, or severe peripheral neuropathy, reduce subsequent dose by 25%, to 75 mg/m^2. In patients who continue to experience reactions with decreased dose, either decrease it further to 55 mg/m^2 or stop drug.

➲ **Locally advanced or metastatic non–small-cell lung cancer after failure of previous cisplatin-based chemotherapy**

Adults: 75 mg/m^2 I.V. over 1 hour q 3 weeks.

In patients who experience febrile neutropenia, neutrophil count of less than 500/mm^3 for longer than 1 week, severe or cumulative cutaneous reactions, or severe peripheral neuropathy, withhold drug until toxicity resolves; then restart at 55 mg/m^2. In patients who develop grade 3 peripheral neuropathy or above, stop drug.

➲ **Unresectable, locally advanced, or metastatic non–small-cell lung cancer not previously treated with chemotherapy**

Adults: 75 mg/m^2 docetaxel I.V. over 1 hour, immediately followed by cisplatin 75 mg/m^2 I.V. over 30 to 60 minutes every 3 weeks.

In patients whose nadir platelet count during the previous course of therapy is less than 25,000 cells/mm^3, those with febrile neutropenia, and those with serious nonhematologic toxicities, decrease docetaxel dosage to 65 mg/m^2. For patients who require a further dose reduction, a dose of 50 mg/m^2 is recommended. For cisplatin dosage adjustments, see manufacturers' prescribing information.

➲ **Androgen-independent metastatic prostate cancer, with prednisone**

Adults: 75 mg/m^2 I.V., as a 1-hour infusion q 3 weeks, given with 5 mg prednisone P.O. b.i.d. continuously. Premedicate with dexamethasone 8 mg P.O. at 12 hours, 3 hours, and 1 hour before docetaxel infusion.

In patients who experience febrile neutropenia, neutrophil count less than 500 cells/mm^3 for more than 1 week, severe or cumulative cutaneous reactions or moderate neurosensory sign or symptoms, reduce subsequent dose to 60 mg/m^2. In patients who continue to experience reactions with the decreased dose, stop treatment.

➲ **Adjuvant postsurgery treatment of operable, node-positive breast cancer**

Adults: 75 mg/m^2 I.V. as a 1-hour infusion given 1 hour after doxorubicin 50 mg/m^2 and cyclophosphamide 500 mg/m^2 q 3 weeks for six cycles. Patient's neutrophil count should be 1,500 cells/mm^3 or higher.

Patients who experience febrile neutropenia should receive granulocyte colony–stimulating factor (G-CSF) in all subsequent cycles. If febrile neutropenia doesn't resolve, continue G-CSF and reduce docetaxel dose to 60 mg/m^2. For patients who experience severe or cumulative cutaneous reactions or moderate neurosensory signs and symptoms, reduce dose to 60 mg/m^2. If these reactions persist at the reduced dosage, stop treatment.

Contraindications & cautions

- Contraindicated in patients severely hypersensitive to drug or to other formulations containing polysorbate 80 and in those with neutrophil counts below 1,500 cells/mm^3.
- Patients with severe hepatic impairment shouldn't receive this drug. Don't give drug to patients with bilirubin levels exceeding upper limit of normal (ULN) or those with ALT or AST levels above 1½ times ULN and alkaline phosphatase levels over 2½ times ULN or with baseline neutrophil count less than 1,500/mm^3.
- Safety and effectiveness in children haven't been established.

Adverse reactions

CNS: *asthenia*, paresthesia, peripheral neuropathy.

CV: *fluid retention, peripheral edema*, hypotension, flushing, chest tightness.

GI: *stomatitis, nausea, vomiting, diarrhea*.

Hematologic: *anemia*, NEUTROPENIA, FEBRILE NEUTROPENIA, MYELOSUPPRESSION, LEUKOPENIA, THROMBOCYTOPENIA.

Hepatic: ***hepatotoxicity***.

Musculoskeletal: *myalgia*, arthralgia, back pain.
Respiratory: dyspnea, ***pulmonary edema***.
Skin: *alopecia*, skin eruptions, desquamation, nail pigmentation alterations, nail pain, rash, reaction at injection site.
Other: hypersensitivity reactions, *infection*, drug fever, chills, ***death***.

Interactions

Drug-drug. *Compounds that induce, inhibit, or are metabolized by CYP3A4, such as cyclosporine, erythromycin, ketoconazole, troleandomycin:* May modify metabolism of docetaxel. Use together cautiously.

Nursing considerations

- Give oral corticosteroid such as dexamethasone 16 mg P.O. (8 mg b.i.d.) daily for 3 days, starting 1 day before docetaxel administration, to reduce risk or severity of fluid retention and hypersensitivity reactions.
- Bone marrow toxicity is the most frequent and dose-limiting toxicity. Frequent blood count monitoring is needed during therapy.
- Monitor patient closely for hypersensitivity reactions, especially during first and second infusions.
- Contact between undiluted docetaxel concentrate and polyvinyl chloride equipment or devices isn't recommended.
- Fluid retention is dose-related and may be severe. Monitor patient closely.

!!ALERT Don't confuse Taxotere with Taxol.

Patient teaching

- Caution woman of childbearing age to avoid pregnancy or breast-feeding during therapy.
- Advise patient to report any pain or burning at site of injection during or after administration.
- Warn patient that hair loss occurs in almost 80% of patients but is reversible when treatment stops.
- Tell patient to promptly report sore throat, fever, or unusual bruising or bleeding, as well as signs and symptoms of fluid retention, such as swelling or shortness of breath.

docusate calcium (dioctyl calcium sulfosuccinate)

DC Softgels ◇, DC Softgels, Surfak ◇

docusate sodium (dioctyl sodium sulfosuccinate)

Colace ◇, Diocto ◇, Dioeze ◇, D.O.S ◇, D-S-S ◇, Duosol ◇, Ex-Lax Stool Softener Caplets, Modane Soft ◇, Phillips' Liqui-Gels, Regulax SS ◇, Regulex† ◇

Pregnancy risk category C

Indications & dosages

➲ Stool softener
Adults and children older than age 12: 50 to 500 mg docusate calcium or sodium P.O. daily until bowel movements are normal. Or, give enema. Dilute 1:24 with sterile water before use, and give 100 to 150 ml retention enema, 300 to 500 ml evacuation enema, or 0.5 to 1.5 L flushing enema P.R.
Children ages 7 to 12: 40 to 120 mg docusate sodium P.O. daily.
Children ages 3 to 6: 20 to 60 mg docusate sodium P.O. daily.
Children younger than age 3: 10 to 40 mg docusate sodium P.O. daily.

Higher dosage is used for initial therapy. Adjust dosage to individual response.

Contraindications & cautions

- Contraindicated in patients hypersensitive to drug and in those with intestinal obstruction or signs and symptoms of appendicitis, fecal impaction, or acute surgical abdomen, such as undiagnosed abdominal pain or vomiting.

Adverse reactions

GI: bitter taste, mild abdominal cramping, diarrhea.
Other: laxative dependence with long-term or excessive use.

Interactions

Drug-drug. *Mineral oil:* May increase mineral oil absorption and cause toxicity and lipid pneumonia. Separate doses.

Nursing considerations

- Drug isn't used to treat existing constipation but prevents constipation from developing.
- Before giving drug, determine whether patient has adequate fluid intake, exercise, and diet.
- Give liquid (not syrups) in milk, fruit juice, or infant formula to mask bitter taste.
- Drug is laxative of choice for patients who shouldn't strain during defecation, including patients recovering from MI or rectal surgery, those with rectal or anal disease that makes passage of firm stools difficult, and those with postpartum constipation.
- Store drug at 59° to 86° F (15° to 30° C), and protect liquid from light.

Patient teaching

- Teach patient about dietary sources of bulk, including bran and other cereals, fresh fruit, and vegetables.
- Instruct patient to use drug only occasionally and not for longer than 1 week without prescriber's knowledge.
- Tell patient to stop drug and notify prescriber if severe cramping occurs.
- Notify patient that it may take from 1 to 3 days to soften stools.

dofetilide
Tikosyn

Pregnancy risk category C

Indications & dosages

➲ To maintain normal sinus rhythm in patients with symptomatic atrial fibrillation or atrial flutter lasting longer than 1 week who have been converted to normal sinus rhythm; to convert atrial fibrillation and atrial flutter to normal sinus rhythm

Adults: Individualized dosage based on creatinine clearance and baseline QTc interval (or QT interval if heart rate is below 60 beats/minute), determined before first dose; usually 500 mcg P.O. b.i.d. for patients with creatinine clearance greater than 60 ml/minute.

If creatinine clearance is 40 to 60 ml/minute, starting dose is 250 mcg P.O. b.i.d.; if clearance is 20 to 39 ml/minute, starting dose is 125 mcg P.O. b.i.d. Don't use drug at all if clearance is less than 20 ml/minute.

Determine QTc interval 2 to 3 hours after first dose. If QTc interval has increased by more than 15% above baseline or if it's more than 500 msec (550 msec in patients with ventricular conduction abnormalities), adjust dosage as follows: If starting dose based on creatinine clearance was 500 mcg P.O. b.i.d., give 250 mcg P.O. b.i.d. If starting dose based on clearance was 250 mcg b.i.d., give 125 mcg b.i.d. If starting dose based on clearance was 125 mcg b.i.d., give 125 mcg once a day.

Determine QTc interval 2 to 3 hours after each subsequent dose while patient is in hospital. If at any time after second dose the QTc interval exceeds 500 msec (550 msec in patients with ventricular conduction abnormalities), stop drug.

Contraindications & cautions

- Contraindicated in patients hypersensitive to drug, in those with congenital or acquired long QT interval syndromes or with baseline QTc interval greater than 440 msec (500 msec in patients with ventricular conduction abnormalities), and in those with creatinine clearance less than 20 ml/minute.
- Contraindicated for use with verapamil and with cation transport system inhibitors (cimetidine, ketoconazole, megestrol, prochlorperazine, trimethoprim with or without sulfamethoxazole).
- Use cautiously in patients with severe hepatic impairment.

Adverse reactions

CNS: *headache*, dizziness, insomnia, anxiety, migraine, cerebral ischemia, ***CVA***, asthenia, paresthesia, syncope.
CV: ***ventricular fibrillation***, ***ventricular tachycardia***, ***torsades de pointes***, ***AV block***, bundle-branch block, ***heart block***, *chest pain*, angina, atrial fibrillation, hypertension, palpitations, ***bradycardia***, edema, ***cardiac arrest***, ***MI***.
GI: nausea, diarrhea, abdominal pain.
GU: UTI.
Hepatic: liver damage.
Musculoskeletal: back pain, arthralgia, facial paralysis.
Respiratory: respiratory tract infection, dyspnea, increased cough.
Skin: rash, sweating.

Other: flu syndrome, ***angioedema***, peripheral edema.

Interactions

Drug-drug. *Antiarrhythmics (classes I and III):* May increase dofetilide level. Withhold other antiarrhythmics for at least three plasma half-lives before giving dofetilide.
Drugs secreted by renal tubular cationic transport (amiloride, metformin, triamterene): May increase dofetilide level. Use together cautiously; monitor patient for adverse effects.
Drugs that prolong QT interval: May increase risk of QT interval prolongation. Avoid using together.
Inhibitors of CYP3A4 (amiodarone, azole antifungals, cannabinoids, diltiazem, macrolides, nefazodone, norfloxacin, protease inhibitors, quinine, SSRIs, zafirlukast): May decrease metabolism and increase dofetilide level. Use together cautiously.
Inhibitors of renal cationic secretion (cimetidine, ketoconazole, megestrol, prochlorperazine, trimethoprim with or without sulfamethoxazole), verapamil: May increase dofetilide level. Use together is contraindicated.
Potassium-depleting diuretics: May increase risk of hypokalemia or hypomagnesemia. Monitor potassium and magnesium levels.
Drug-food. *Grapefruit juice:* May decrease hepatic metabolism and increase drug level. Discourage use together.

Nursing considerations

- Provide continuous ECG monitoring for at least 3 days.
- Don't discharge patient within 12 hours of conversion to normal sinus rhythm.
- Monitor patient for prolonged diarrhea, sweating, and vomiting. Report these signs to prescriber because electrolyte imbalance may increase potential for arrhythmia development.
- Monitor renal function and QTc interval every 3 months.
- Use of potassium-depleting diuretics may cause hypokalemia and hypomagnesemia, increasing the risk of torsades de pointes. Give dofetilide after potassium level reaches and stays in normal range.
- If patient doesn't convert to normal sinus rhythm within 24 hours of starting dofetilide, consider electrical conversion.
- Before starting dofetilide, stop previous antiarrhythmics while carefully monitoring patient for a minimum of three plasma half-lives. Don't give drug after amiodarone therapy until amiodarone level falls below 0.3 mcg/ml or until amiodarone has been stopped for at least 3 months.
- If dofetilide must be stopped to allow dosing with interacting drugs, allow at least 2 days before starting other drug therapy.

Patient teaching

- Tell patient to report any change in OTC or prescription drug use, or supplement or herb use.
- Inform patient that drug can be taken without regard to meals or antacid administration.
- Tell patient to immediately report excessive or prolonged diarrhea, sweating, vomiting, or loss of appetite or thirst.
- Advise patient not to take drug with grapefruit juice.
- Advise patient to use antacids, such as Zantac 75 mg, Pepcid, Prilosec, Axid, or Prevacid instead of Tagamet HB if needed for ulcers or heartburn.
- Instruct patient to tell prescriber if she becomes pregnant.
- Advise patient not to breast-feed while taking dofetilide because drug appears in breast milk.
- If a dose is missed, tell patient not to double a dose but to skip that dose and take the next regularly scheduled dose.

dolasetron mesylate

Anzemet

Pregnancy risk category B

Indications & dosages

➲ To prevent nausea and vomiting from cancer chemotherapy
Adults: 100 mg P.O. given as a single dose 1 hour before chemotherapy. Or, 1.8 mg/kg or a fixed dose of 100 mg as a single I.V. dose given 30 minutes before chemotherapy.
Children ages 2 to 16: 1.8 mg/kg P.O. given 1 hour before chemotherapy. Or, 1.8 mg/kg as a single I.V. dose given 30 minutes before chemotherapy. Injectable formulation

can be mixed with apple juice and given P.O. Maximum dose is 100 mg.

➲ To prevent postoperative nausea and vomiting

Adults: 100 mg P.O. within 2 hours before surgery. Or, 12.5 mg as a single I.V. dose about 15 minutes before cessation of anesthesia or as soon as nausea or vomiting presents.

Children ages 2 to 16: 1.2 mg/kg P.O. given within 2 hours before surgery, to maximum of 100 mg. Or, 0.35 mg/kg, up to 12.5 mg given as a single I.V. dose about 15 minutes before cessation of anesthesia or as soon as nausea or vomiting presents. Injectable formulation can be mixed with apple juice and given P.O.

➲ Postoperative nausea and vomiting

Adults: 12.5 mg as a single I.V. dose as soon as nausea or vomiting occurs.

Children ages 2 to 16: 0.35 mg/kg, to maximum dosage of 12.5 mg, given as a single I.V. dose as soon as nausea or vomiting occurs.

Contraindications & cautions

- Contraindicated in patients hypersensitive to drug.

!!ALERT Give with caution in patients who have or may develop prolonged cardiac conduction intervals, such as those with electrolyte abnormalities, history of arrhythmia, and cumulative high-dose anthracycline therapy.

- Drug isn't recommended for use in children younger than age 2. Use cautiously in breast-feeding women.

Adverse reactions

CNS: fever, *headache*, dizziness, drowsiness, fatigue.
CV: ***arrhythmias***, ECG changes, edema, hypotension, hypertension, tachycardia.
GI: *diarrhea*, dyspepsia, abdominal pain, constipation, anorexia.
GU: polyuria, hematuria, urine retention.
Skin: pruritus, rash.
Other: chills, pain at injection site.

Interactions

Drug-drug. *Drugs that prolong ECG intervals, such as antiarrhythmics:* May increase risk of arrhythmia. Monitor patient closely.
Drugs that inhibit CYP enzymes, such as cimetidine: May increase level of hydrodolasetron, an active metabolite of dolasetron. Monitor patient for adverse effects.
Drugs that induce CYP enzymes, such as rifampin: May decrease level of hydrodolasetron, an active metabolite of dolasetron. Monitor patient for decreased efficacy of antiemetic.

Nursing considerations

- Injection for oral use is stable in apple or apple-grape juice for 2 hours at room temperature.

!!ALERT Don't confuse Anzemet with Aldomet or Avandamet.

Patient teaching

- Tell patient about possible adverse effects.
- Instruct patient not to mix injection in juice for oral use until just before dosing.
- Tell patient to report nausea or vomiting.

donepezil hydrochloride
Aricept

Pregnancy risk category C

Indications & dosages

➲ Mild to moderate Alzheimer's dementia

Adults: Initially, 5 mg P.O. daily h.s. After 4 to 6 weeks, increase to 10 mg daily.

Contraindications & cautions

- Contraindicated in patients hypersensitive to drug or piperidine derivatives and in breast-feeding patients.
- Use cautiously in pregnant patients and in those who take NSAIDs or have CV disease, asthma, obstructive pulmonary disease, urinary outflow impairment, or history of ulcer disease.

Adverse reactions

CNS: *headache*, *insomnia*, dizziness, fatigue, depression, abnormal dreams, somnolence, ***seizures***, tremor, irritability, paresthesia, aggression, vertigo, ataxia, restlessness, abnormal crying, nervousness, aphasia, syncope, pain.
CV: chest pain, hypertension, vasodilation, atrial fibrillation, hot flashes, hypotension.
EENT: cataract, blurred vision, eye irritation, sore throat.

GI: *nausea, diarrhea,* vomiting, anorexia, fecal incontinence, GI bleeding, bloating, epigastric pain.
GU: urinary frequency.
Metabolic: weight loss, dehydration.
Musculoskeletal: muscle cramps, arthritis, bone fracture.
Respiratory: dyspnea, bronchitis.
Skin: pruritus, urticaria, diaphoresis, ecchymoses.
Other: toothache, influenza, increased libido.

Interactions

Drug-drug. *Anticholinergics:* May decrease donepezil effects. Avoid using together.
Anticholinesterases, cholinomimetics: May cause synergistic effect. Monitor patient closely.
Bethanechol, succinylcholine: May have additive effects. Monitor patient closely.
Carbamazepine, dexamethasone, phenobarbital, phenytoin, rifampin: May increase rate of donepezil elimination. Monitor patient.

Nursing considerations

- Monitor patient for evidence of active or occult GI bleeding.

!!ALERT Don't confuse Aricept with Ascriptin.

Patient teaching

- Stress that drug doesn't alter underlying degenerative disease but can temporarily stabilize or relieve symptoms. Effectiveness depends on taking drug at regular intervals.
- Tell caregiver to give drug just before patient's bedtime.
- Advise patient and caregiver to report immediately significant adverse effects or changes in overall health status and to inform health care team that patient is taking drug before he receives anesthesia.
- Tell patient to avoid OTC cold or sleep remedies because of risk of increased anticholinergic effects.

dopamine hydrochloride

Intropin, Revimine†

Pregnancy risk category C

Indications & dosages

➲ **To treat shock and correct hemodynamic imbalances, to improve perfusion to vital organs, to increase cardiac output, to correct hypotension**
Adults: Initially, 1 to 5 mcg/kg/minute by I.V. infusion. Titrate dosage to desired hemodynamic or renal response. Infusion may be increased by 1 to 4 mcg/kg/minute at 10- to 30-minute intervals.

Contraindications & cautions

- Contraindicated in patients with uncorrected tachyarrhythmias, pheochromocytoma, or ventricular fibrillation.
- Use cautiously in patients with occlusive vascular disease, cold injuries, diabetic endarteritis, and arterial embolism; in pregnant patients; in those with a history of sulfite sensitivity; and in those taking MAO inhibitors.

Adverse reactions

CNS: headache.
CV: ectopic beats, tachycardia, angina, palpitations, *hypotension.*
GI: nausea, vomiting.
Metabolic: azotemia, hyperglycemia.
Respiratory: dyspnea, ***asthmatic episodes.***
Skin: necrosis and tissue sloughing with extravasation, piloerection.
Other: ***anaphylactic reactions.***

Interactions

Drug-drug. *Alpha blockers, beta blockers:* May antagonize dopamine effects. Monitor patient closely.
Ergot alkaloids: May cause extremely high blood pressure. Avoid using together.
Inhaled anesthetics: May increase risk of arrhythmias or hypertension. Monitor patient closely.
MAO inhibitors (phenelzine, tranylcypromine): May cause severe headache, hypertension, fever and hypertensive crisis. Avoid using together.
Oxytocics: May cause severe, persistent hypertension. Use together cautiously.

Phenytoin: May cause seizures, severe hypotension, and bradycardia. Monitor patient carefully.
Tricyclic antidepressants: May decrease pressor response. Monitor patient closely.

Nursing considerations

- Drug isn't a substitute for blood or fluid volume deficit. If deficit exists, replace fluid before giving vasopressors.
- During infusion, frequently monitor ECG, blood pressure, cardiac output, central venous pressure, pulmonary artery wedge pressure, pulse rate, urine output, and color and temperature of limbs.
- If diastolic pressure rises disproportionately (a significant decrease in pulse pressure) in a patient receiving dopamine, decrease infusion rate, and watch carefully for further evidence of predominant vasoconstrictor activity, unless such an effect is desired.
- Observe patient closely for adverse reactions; dosage may need to be adjusted or drug stopped.
- Check urine output often. If urine flow decreases without hypotension, notify prescriber because dosage may need to be reduced.

!!ALERT After drug is stopped, watch closely for sudden drop in blood pressure. Taper dosage slowly to evaluate stability of blood pressure.

- Acidosis decreases effectiveness of dopamine.

!!ALERT Don't confuse dopamine with dobutamine.

Patient teaching

- Tell patient to report adverse reactions promptly.
- Instruct patient to report discomfort at I.V. insertion site.

dornase alfa
Pulmozyme

Pregnancy risk category B

Indications & dosages

➲ To improve pulmonary function and decrease the frequency of moderate to severe respiratory tract infections in patients with cystic fibrosis
Adults and children age 5 and older: 1 ampule or 2.5 mg inhaled once daily. Treatment usually takes 10 to 15 minutes. Use drug only with an approved nebulizer.

Contraindications & cautions

- Contraindicated in patients hypersensitive to drug or to products derived from Chinese hamster ovary cells.
- Safety and efficacy haven't been established for use longer than 12 months, for children younger than age 5, and for children with forced vital capacity below 40% of normal value.

Adverse reactions

CV: *chest pain.*
EENT: *pharyngitis, voice alteration,* laryngitis, conjunctivitis.
Skin: *rash,* urticaria.

Interactions

None significant.

Nursing considerations

- Drug is used with other standard therapies for cystic fibrosis.
- Patients older than age 21 and those with a forced vital capacity over 85% may benefit from twice-daily use.

!!ALERT Give only with the Hudson T Updraft II disposable jet nebulizer, the Marquest Acorn II disposable jet nebulizer along with Pulmo-Aide compressor, or the LC Jet+ reusable nebulizer or the Pari Baby along with the Pari Proneb compressor, or the Durable sidestream with either the Mobilairé or Porta Neb compressors.

- Discard cloudy or discolored solution.
- Don't mix with other drugs in the nebulizer. Mixing could lead to a physical or chemical reaction that may inactivate dornase alfa.
- Refrigerate drug in its protective foil pouch to protect it from strong light.
- Once opened, the entire ampule must be used or discarded.

Patient teaching

- Teach patient how to use drug at home.
- Remind patient to breathe only through his mouth when using the nebulizer. If this is difficult, suggest that he use a nose clip.

• Tell patient that if he begins coughing during treatment, he should turn off nebulizer without spilling drug. To resume, he should turn on nebulizer and continue breathing through the mouthpiece until the nebulizer cup is empty or mist is no longer produced.

dorzolamide hydrochloride
Trusopt

Pregnancy risk category C

Indications & dosages

➲ Increased intraocular pressure (IOP) in patients with ocular hypertension or open-angle glaucoma
Adults and children: 1 drop into conjunctival sac of affected eye t.i.d.

Contraindications & cautions

• Contraindicated in patients hypersensitive to drug or its components.
• Use cautiously in patients with hepatic or renal impairment.

Adverse reactions

CNS: headache, asthenia, fatigue.
EENT: *ocular burning, stinging, and discomfort, superficial punctate keratitis, ocular allergic reaction, blurred vision, lacrimation, dryness, photophobia,* iridocyclitis.
GI: nausea, *bitter taste.*
GU: urolithiasis.
Skin: rash.

Interactions

Drug-drug. *Oral carbonic anhydrase inhibitors:* May cause additive effects. Avoid using together.

Nursing considerations

• If more than one topical ophthalmic drug is used, give drugs at least 10 minutes apart.

Patient teaching

• Teach patient how to instill drops. Advise him to wash hands before and after instillation, and warn him not to touch tip of dropper to eye or surrounding tissue.
• Tell patient that drug is a sulfonamide and, although it's given topically, it can be absorbed systemically. Advise patient to apply light finger pressure on lacrimal sac for 1 minute after drug instillation to minimize systemic absorption.
• Tell patient to stop drug and notify prescriber immediately if signs or symptoms of serious adverse reactions or hypersensitivity occur, including eye inflammation and eyelid reactions.
• Tell patient not to wear soft contact lenses during therapy.
• Stress importance of compliance with recommended therapy.

doxapram hydrochloride
Dopram

Pregnancy risk category B

Indications & dosages

➲ Postanesthesia respiratory stimulation
Adults: 0.5 to 1 mg/kg as a single I.V. injection (not to exceed 1.5 mg/kg) or as multiple injections q 5 minutes, total not to exceed 2 mg/kg. Or, 250 mg in 250 ml of normal saline solution or D_5W infused at initial rate of 5 mg/minute I.V. until satisfactory response is achieved. Maintain at 1 to 3 mg/minute. Don't exceed total dose for infusion of 4 mg/kg.
➲ Drug-induced CNS depression
Adults: For injection, priming dose of 2 mg/kg I.V., repeated in 5 minutes and again q 1 to 2 hours until patient awakens (and if relapse occurs). Maximum daily dose is 3 g.

For infusion, priming dose of 2 mg/kg I.V., repeated in 5 minutes and again in 1 to 2 hours, if needed. If response occurs, give I.V. infusion (1 mg/ml) at 1 to 3 mg/minute until patient awakens. Don't infuse for longer than 2 hours or give more than 3 g/day. May resume I.V. infusion after rest period of 30 minutes to 2 hours, if needed.
➲ Chronic pulmonary disease related to acute hypercapnia
Adults: 1 to 2 mg/minute by I.V. infusion using 2 mg/ml solution. Maximum, 3 mg/minute for up to 2 hours.

Contraindications & cautions

• Contraindicated in patients with seizure disorders; head injury; CV disorders; frank, uncompensated heart failure; severe hypertension; CVA; respiratory failure or incompetence secondary to neuromuscular disor-

ders, muscle paresis, flail chest, obstructed airway, pulmonary embolism, pneumothorax, restrictive respiratory disease, acute bronchial asthma, or extreme dyspnea; or hypoxia unrelated to hypercapnia.
- Use cautiously in patients with bronchial asthma, severe tachycardia or arrhythmias, cerebral edema, increased intracranial pressure, hyperthyroidism, pheochromocytoma, or metabolic disorders.

Adverse reactions

CNS: ***seizures***, *headache, dizziness*, apprehension, disorientation, hyperactivity, bilateral Babinski's signs, paresthesia.
CV: *chest pain and tightness, variations in heart rate, hypertension,* ***arrhythmias***, T-wave depression on ECG, flushing.
EENT: sneezing, ***laryngospasm***.
GI: nausea, vomiting, diarrhea.
GU: urine retention, bladder stimulation with incontinence, albuminuria.
Musculoskeletal: muscle spasms.
Respiratory: cough, ***bronchospasm***, dyspnea, rebound hypoventilation, hiccups.
Skin: pruritus, diaphoresis.

Interactions

Drug-drug. *General anesthetics:* May cause self-limiting arrhythmias. Avoid using doxapram within 10 minutes of an anesthetic that sensitizes the myocardium to catecholamines.
MAO inhibitors, sympathomimetics: May potentiate adverse CV effects. Use together cautiously.

Nursing considerations

- Drug is used only in surgical or emergency department situations.
- Separate end of anesthetic treatment and start of doxapram by at least 10 minutes.

!!ALERT Establish an adequate airway before giving drug. Prevent patient from aspirating vomitus by placing him on his side.
- Monitor blood pressure, heart rate, deep tendon reflexes, and arterial blood gases before giving drug and every 30 minutes afterward.
- Monitor patient for evidence of overdose, such as hypertension, tachycardia, arrhythmias, skeletal muscle hyperactivity, and dyspnea. Hold drug and notify prescriber if patient needs mechanical ventilation or shows signs of increased arterial carbon dioxide or oxygen tension.

!!ALERT Don't confuse doxapram with doxorubicin, doxepin, doxacurium, or doxazosin.

Patient teaching

- Inform family and patient about need for drug.
- Answer patient's questions and address his concerns.

doxazosin mesylate
Cardura

Pregnancy risk category C

Indications & dosages

Essential hypertension
Adults: Initially, 1 mg P.O. daily; determine effect on standing and supine blood pressure at 2 to 6 hours and 24 hours after dose. May increase at 2-week intervals to 2 mg and, thereafter, 4 mg and 8 mg once daily, p.r.n. Maximum daily dose is 16 mg, but doses over 4 mg daily increase the risk of adverse reactions.
BPH
Adults: Initially, 1 mg P.O. once daily in the morning or evening; may increase at 1- or 2-week intervals to 2 mg and, thereafter, 4 mg and 8 mg once daily, p.r.n.

Contraindications & cautions

- Contraindicated in patients hypersensitive to drug and quinazoline derivatives (including prazosin and terazosin).
- Use cautiously in patients with impaired hepatic function.

Adverse reactions

CNS: *dizziness*, vertigo, somnolence, drowsiness, *asthenia, headache*, pain.
CV: *orthostatic hypotension*, hypotension, edema, palpitations, ***arrhythmias***, tachycardia.
EENT: rhinitis, pharyngitis, abnormal vision.
GI: nausea, vomiting, diarrhea, constipation.
Hematologic: ***leukopenia, neutropenia***.
Musculoskeletal: arthralgia, myalgia.
Respiratory: dyspnea.
Skin: rash, pruritus.

Interactions

Drug-drug. *Midodrine:* May decrease the effectiveness of midodrine. Monitor patient for therapeutic effect.
Drug-herb. *Butcher's broom:* May decrease effect of doxazosin. Discourage use together. *Ma huang:* May decrease antihypertensive effects. Discourage use together.

Nursing considerations

- Monitor blood pressure closely.
- If syncope occurs, place patient in a recumbent position and treat supportively. A transient hypotensive response isn't considered a contraindication to continued therapy.

!!ALERT Don't confuse doxazosin with doxapram, doxorubicin, or doxepin.
!!ALERT Don't confuse Cardura with Coumadin, K-Dur, Cardene, or Cordarone.

Patient teaching

- Instruct patient to take drug exactly as prescribed.

!!ALERT Advise patient that he is susceptible to a first-dose effect (marked low blood pressure on standing up with dizziness or fainting) similar to that produced by other alpha blockers. This is most common after first dose but also can occur during dosage adjustment or interruption of therapy.
- Warn patient that dizziness or fainting may occur during therapy. Advise him to avoid driving and other hazardous activities until drug's effects on the CNS are known.

doxepin hydrochloride
Novo-Doxepin†, Sinequan, Triadapin†

Pregnancy risk category C

Indications & dosages

➲ Depression
Adults: Initially, 75 mg P.O. daily. Usual dosage range is 75 to 150 mg daily to maximum of 300 mg daily in divided doses. Or, entire maintenance dose may be given once daily with maximum dose of 150 mg.

Contraindications & cautions

- Contraindicated in patients hypersensitive to drug and in those with glaucoma or tendency toward urine retention; also contraindicated in those who have received an MAO inhibitor within past 14 days and during acute recovery phase of an MI.

Adverse reactions

CNS: *drowsiness, dizziness,* confusion, numbness, hallucinations, paresthesia, ataxia, weakness, headache, ***seizures***, extrapyramidal reactions.
CV: *orthostatic hypotension, tachycardia,* ECG changes.
EENT: *blurred vision,* tinnitus.
GI: *dry mouth, constipation,* nausea, vomiting, anorexia.
GU: urine retention.
Metabolic: ***hypoglycemia***, hyperglycemia.
Skin: rash, urticaria, photosensitivity reactions, *diaphoresis.*
Other: hypersensitivity reactions.

Interactions

Drug-drug. *Barbiturates, CNS depressants:* May enhance CNS depression. Avoid using together.
Cimetidine, fluoxetine, fluvoxamine, paroxetine, sertraline: May increase doxepin level. Watch for increased adverse reactions.
Clonidine: May cause life-threatening blood pressure elevations. Avoid using together.
Epinephrine, norepinephrine: May increase hypertensive effect. Use together cautiously.
MAO inhibitors: May cause severe excitation, hyperpyrexia, or seizures, usually with high dosage. Avoid using within 14 days of MAO inhibitor therapy.
Drug-herb. *Evening primrose oil:* May cause additive or synergistic effect, resulting in lower seizure threshold and increasing the risk of seizure. Discourage use together.
St. John's wort, SAM-e, yohimbe: May cause serotonin syndrome. Discourage use together.
Drug-lifestyle. *Alcohol use:* May enhance CNS depression. Discourage use together.
Sun exposure: May increase risk of photosensitivity reactions. Advise patient to avoid excessive sunlight exposure.

Nursing considerations

- Don't withdraw drug abruptly.
- Monitor patient for nausea, headache, and malaise after abrupt withdrawal of long-term therapy; these symptoms don't indicate addiction.

!!ALERT Because hypertensive episodes may occur during surgery in patients receiving tricyclic antidepressants, stop drug gradually several days before surgery.
- If signs or symptoms of psychosis occur or increase, expect prescriber to reduce dosage. Record mood changes. Monitor patient for suicidal tendencies and allow only a minimum supply of drug.
- Doxepin has strong anticholinergic effects and is one of the most sedating tricyclic antidepressants. Adverse anticholinergic effects can occur rapidly.
- Recommend use of sugarless hard candy or gum to relieve dry mouth.

!!ALERT Don't confuse doxepin with doxazosin, digoxin, doxapram, or Doxidan; don't confuse Sinequan with saquinavir.

Patient teaching
- Tell patient to dilute oral concentrate with 4 ounces (120 ml) of water, milk, or juice (orange, grapefruit, tomato, prune, or pineapple, but not grape); preparation shouldn't be mixed with carbonated beverages.
- Tell patient to take full dose at bedtime whenever he can, but warn him of possible morning dizziness on standing up quickly.
- Advise patient to consult prescriber before taking other prescription or OTC drugs.
- Warn patient to avoid hazardous activities that require alertness and good psychomotor coordination until effects of drug are known. Drowsiness and dizziness usually subside after a few weeks.
- Tell patient to avoid alcohol during drug therapy.
- Tell patient that maximum antidepressant effect may not be evident for 2 to 3 weeks.
- Warn patient not to stop drug suddenly.
- To prevent sensitivity to the sun, advise patient to use sunblock, wear protective clothing, and avoid prolonged exposure to strong sunlight.

doxorubicin hydrochloride
Adriamycin PFS, Adriamycin RDF, Rubex

Pregnancy risk category D

Indications & dosages
➲ **Bladder, breast, lung, ovarian, stomach, and thyroid cancers; non-Hodgkin's disease; Hodgkin's disease; acute lymphoblastic and myeloblastic leukemia; Wilms' tumor; neuroblastoma; lymphoma; sarcoma**

Adults: 60 to 75 mg/m² I.V. as single dose q 3 weeks; or 30 mg/m² I.V. in single daily dose, days 1 to 3 of 4-week cycle.

Or, 20 mg/m² I.V. once weekly. Maximum cumulative dose is 550 mg/m².

Elderly patients: May need reduced dosages.

Reduce dosage for patients with myelosuppression or impaired cardiac or liver function. Be prepared to decrease dosage if bilirubin level rises: Give 50% of dose when bilirubin level is 1.2 to 3 mg/100 ml; 25% when it's 3.1 to 5 mg/100 ml.

Contraindications & cautions
- Contraindicated in patients with a history of sensitivity reactions to doxorubicin or its components.
- Contraindicated in patients with marked myelosuppression induced by previous treatment with other antitumor drugs or radiotherapy and in those who have received a lifetime cumulative dose of 550 mg/m² of doxorubicin or daunorubicin.

Adverse reactions
CV: cardiac depression, ***arrhythmias, acute left ventricular failure, irreversible cardiomyopathy***.
EENT: conjunctivitis.
GI: *nausea, vomiting*, diarrhea, *stomatitis*, esophagitis, anorexia.
GU: transient red urine.
Hematologic: ***leukopenia, thrombocytopenia***, **MYELOSUPPRESSION**.
Metabolic: hyperuricemia.
Skin: *severe cellulitis and tissue sloughing with drug extravasation*, urticaria, facial flushing, *complete alopecia within 3 to 4 weeks*, hyperpigmentation of nail beds and dermal creases, radiation recall effect.
Other: chills, ***anaphylaxis***.

Interactions
Drug-drug. *Aminophylline, cephalothin, dexamethasone, fluorouracil, heparin, hydrocortisone:* May form a precipitate. Don't mix together.
Calcium channel blockers: May increase cardiotoxic effects. Monitor patient's ECG closely.

Cyclosporine: May increase doxorubicin concentration. Monitor patient for toxicity.
Digoxin: May decrease digoxin level. Monitor digoxin level closely.
Fosphenytoin, phenytoin: May decrease level of phenytoin or fosphenytoin. Monitor drug level.
Paclitaxel: May decrease doxorubicin clearance. Monitor patient for toxicity.
Phenobarbital: May increase doxorubicin clearance. Monitor patient closely.
Streptozocin: May increase and prolong doxorubicin level. Dosage may have to be adjusted.

Nursing considerations

- Perform cardiac function studies, including ECG and ejection fraction, before treatment and then periodically throughout therapy. Dexrazoxane may be given within 30 minutes of doxorubicin if the accumulated dose of doxorubicin has reached 300 mg/m^2.
- Take preventive measures, including adequate hydration of the patient, before starting treatment. Rapid lysis of leukemic cells may cause hyperuricemia. Allopurinol may be ordered.
- Premedicate with antiemetic to reduce nausea.
- If skin or mucosal contact occurs, immediately wash with soap and water.
- Never give drug I.M. or S.C.
- Dosage modification may be needed in patients with myelosuppression or impaired cardiac or hepatic function and in elderly patients.
- Monitor CBC with differential and hepatic function tests; monitor ECG monthly during therapy. If WBC count falls below 2,000/mm^3 or granulocyte count falls below 1,000/mm^3, follow institutional policy for infection control in immunocompromised patients.
- Monitor ECG for changes such as sinus tachycardia, T-wave flattening, ST-segment depression, and voltage reduction.
- Leukopenia may occur during days 10 to 15, with recovery by day 21.
- Be prepared to stop drug or slow rate of infusion, and notify prescriber if tachycardia develops.

!!ALERT If signs of heart failure develop, stop drug and notify prescriber. Heart failure can often be prevented by limiting cumulative dose to 550 mg/m^2 (400 mg/m^2 when patient is also receiving or has received cyclophosphamide or radiation therapy to cardiac area).

- Reddish color of drug is similar to that of daunorubicin; don't confuse the two drugs.
- Esophagitis is common in patients who also have received radiation therapy.

!!ALERT If patient has previously received radiation therapy, he is susceptible to radiation recall effect.

!!ALERT Don't confuse doxorubicin with doxorubicin liposomal.

Patient teaching

- Advise patient to report any pain or burning at site of injection during or after administration.
- Advise patient to watch for signs and symptoms of infection (fever, sore throat, fatigue) and bleeding (easy bruising, nosebleeds, bleeding gums, tarry stools) and to take temperature daily.
- Advise patient that orange to red urine for 1 to 2 days is normal and doesn't indicate presence of blood.
- Inform patient that hair loss may occur, but it's usually reversible. Hair may regrow 2 to 5 months after drug is stopped.

doxorubicin hydrochloride liposomal

Doxil

Pregnancy risk category D

Indications & dosages

➲ Metastatic ovarian carcinoma refractory to both paclitaxel- and platinum-based chemotherapy regimens

Women: 50 mg/m^2 I.V. initially at 1 mg/minute once q 4 weeks for minimum of four courses. Continue as long as condition doesn't progress, patient shows no evidence of cardiotoxicity, and patient continues to tolerate treatment. If no infusion-related adverse reactions develop, increase infusion rate to complete administration over 1 hour.

➲ AIDS-related Kaposi's sarcoma refractory to previous combination chemotherapy and in patients intolerant of such therapy

Adults: 20 mg/m^2 I.V. over 30 minutes once q 3 weeks. Continue as long as patient responds satisfactorily and tolerates treatment.

For patients with impaired hepatic function, reduce dosage as follows: If bilirubin level is 1.2 to 3 mg/dl, give one-half normal dose; if bilirubin level is more than 3 mg/dl, give one-fourth normal dose. Consult package insert for dose modifications for stomatitis, myelosuppression, and hand-foot syndrome.

Contraindications & cautions

- Contraindicated in patients hypersensitive to conventional formulation of doxorubicin hydrochloride or any component in the liposomal formulation.
- Contraindicated in patients with marked myelosuppression and those who have received a lifetime cumulative dose of 550 mg/m^2 (400 mg/m^2 in patients who have received radiotherapy to the mediastinal area or therapy with other cardiotoxic drugs such as cyclophosphamide).
- Use cautiously in patients who have received other anthracyclines.

Adverse reactions

CNS: *asthenia*, paresthesia, headache, somnolence, dizziness, depression, insomnia, anxiety, malaise, emotional lability, fatigue, fever.
CV: chest pain, hypotension, tachycardia, peripheral edema, ***cardiomyopathy***, ***heart failure***, ***arrhythmias***, pericardial effusion.
EENT: pharyngitis, rhinitis, conjunctivitis, retinitis, optic neuritis.
GI: *nausea*, *vomiting*, *constipation*, *anorexia*, *diarrhea*, abdominal pain, dyspepsia, oral candidiasis, enlarged abdomen, esophagitis, dysphagia, *stomatitis*, taste perversion, glossitis.
GU: albuminuria.
Hematologic: LEUKOPENIA, NEUTROPENIA, THROMBOCYTOPENIA, *anemia*.
Hepatic: hyperbilirubinemia.
Metabolic: dehydration, weight loss, hypocalcemia, hyperglycemia.
Musculoskeletal: myalgia, back pain.
Respiratory: dyspnea, increased cough, pneumonia.
Skin: *rash*, *alopecia*, dry skin, pruritus, skin discoloration, skin disorder, exfoliative dermatitis, sweating, *palmar-plantar erythrodysesthesia*.
Other: allergic reaction, chills, *herpes zoster*, infection, infusion-related reactions.

Interactions

None reported. However, drug may interact with drugs that interact with conventional form of doxorubicin hydrochloride.

Nursing considerations

- Consider previous or current therapy with related compounds such as daunorubicin when calculating total dose of drug to be given. Heart failure and cardiomyopathy may occur after stopping therapy.
- Give drug to patient with history of CV disease only when benefit outweighs risk to patient.
- Don't give I.M. or S.C.

!!ALERT Monitor patient for signs and symptoms of palmar-plantar erythrodysesthesia, hematologic toxicity, or stomatitis. These adverse reactions may be managed with dosage delays and adjustments.

- Evaluate patient's hepatic function before therapy, and adjust dosage accordingly.
- Drug exhibits pharmacokinetic properties different from those of conventional doxorubicin hydrochloride and shouldn't be substituted on a milligram-per-milligram basis.
- Drug may potentiate toxicity of other antineoplastic therapies.
- Closely monitor cardiac function by endomyocardial biopsy, echocardiography, or gated radionuclide scans. If results indicate possible cardiac injury, the benefit of continued therapy must be weighed against the risk of myocardial injury.
- Monitor CBC, including platelets, before each dose and frequently throughout therapy. Leukopenia is usually transient. Persistent severe myelosuppression may result in superinfection or hemorrhage. Patient may need G-CSF (or GM-CSF) to support blood counts.

Patient teaching

- Tell patient to notify prescriber if he experiences signs and symptoms of hand-foot syndrome (such as tingling or burning, redness, flaking, bothersome swelling, small blisters, or small sores on palms of hands or soles of feet).
- Advise patient to report signs and symptoms of mouth inflammation (such as painful redness, swelling, or sores in mouth).
- Warn patient to avoid exposure to people with infections. Tell patient to report temperature of 100.5° F (38° C) or higher.

• Tell patient to report nausea, vomiting, tiredness, weakness, rash, or mild hair loss.
• Advise woman of childbearing age to avoid pregnancy during therapy.

doxycycline calcium
Vibramycin

doxycycline hyclate
Apo-Doxy†, Doryx, Doxy 100, Doxy 200, Doxycin†, Doxytec†, Novo-Doxylin†, Nu-Doxycycline†, Periostat, Vibramycin, Vibra-Tabs

doxycycline hydrochloride‡

doxycycline monohydrate
Adoxa, Monodox, Vibramycin

Pregnancy risk category D

Indications & dosages

➲ **Infections caused by susceptible gram-positive and gram-negative organisms (including *Haemophilus ducreyi, Yersinia pestis,* and *Campylobacter fetus*), *Rickettsiae* species, *Mycoplasma pneumoniae, Chlamydia trachomatis*), and *Borrelia burgdorferi* (Lyme disease); psittacosis; granuloma inguinale**
Adults and children older than age 8, weighing at least 45 kg (99 lb): 100 mg P.O. q 12 hours on first day; then 100 mg P.O. daily as a single dose or divided b.i.d. Or, 200 mg I.V. on first day in one or two infusions; then 100 to 200 mg I.V. daily. Daily doses of 200 mg I.V. can be given as a single dose or divided into two infusions.
Children older than age 8, weighing less than 45 kg: 4.4 mg/kg P.O. or I.V. daily, in divided doses q 12 hours on first day; then 2.2 to 4.4 mg/kg daily in one or two divided doses.

Give I.V. infusion slowly (minimum 1 hour). Infusion must be completed within 12 hours (within 6 hours in lactated Ringer's solution or dextrose 5% in lactated Ringer's solution).

➲ **Gonorrhea in patients allergic to penicillin**
Adults: 100 mg P.O. b.i.d. for 7 days. Use for 10 days for epididymitis.

➲ **Syphilis in patients allergic to penicillin (except Adoxa, Doryx, Monodox)**
Adults: 100 mg P.O. b.i.d. for 14 days (early). If more than 1 year duration, 100 mg P.O. daily for 4 weeks.

➲ **Primary or secondary syphilis in patients allergic to penicillin (Adoxa, Doryx, Monodox only)**
Adults: 300 mg P.O. daily in divided doses for at least 10 days.

➲ **Uncomplicated urethral, endocervical, or rectal infections caused by *C. trachomatis* or *Ureaplasma urealyticum***
Adults: 100 mg P.O. b.i.d. for at least 7 days. In those with epididymitis, treat for 10 days.

➲ **To prevent malaria**
Adults: 100 mg P.O. daily beginning 1 to 2 days before travel to endemic area and continued for 4 weeks after travel.
Children older than age 8: 2 mg/kg P.O. once daily beginning 1 to 2 days before travel to endemic area and continued for 4 weeks after travel. Don't exceed daily dose of 100 mg.

➲ **Pelvic inflammatory disease**
Adults: 100 mg I.V. q 12 hours with cefoxitin or cefotetan and continued for at least 2 days after symptomatic improvement; then 100 mg P.O. q 12 hours for a total course of 14 days.

➲ **Adjunct to other antibiotics for inhalation, GI, and oropharyngeal anthrax**
Adults: 100 mg q 12 hours I.V. initially until susceptibility test results are known. Switch to 100 mg P.O. b.i.d. when appropriate. Treat for 60 days total.
Children older than age 8, weighing more than 45 kg (99 lb): 100 mg q 12 hours I.V.; then switch to 100 mg P.O. b.i.d. when appropriate. Treat for 60 days total.
Children older than age 8, weighing 45 kg or less: 2.2 mg/kg q 12 hours I.V.; then switch to 2.2 mg/kg P.O. b.i.d. when appropriate. Treat for 60 days total.
Children age 8 and younger: 2.2 mg/kg q 12 hours I.V.; then switch to 2.2 mg/kg P.O. b.i.d. when appropriate. Treat for 60 days total.

➲ **Cutaneous anthrax**
Adults: 100 mg P.O. q 12 hours for 60 days.
Children older than age 8, weighing more than 45 kg (99 lb): 100 mg P.O. q 12 hours for 60 days.
Children older than age 8, weighing 45 kg or less: 2.2 mg/kg q 12 hours P.O. for 60 days.

Children age 8 and younger: 2.2 mg/kg P.O. q 12 hours for 60 days.

➲ **Adjunct to scaling and root planing to improve attachment and reduce pocket depth in patients with adult periodontitis**
Adults: 20 mg P.O. Periostat b.i.d., more than 1 hour before or 2 hours after the morning and evening meals and after scaling and root planing. Effective for 9 months.

➲ **Adjunctive treatment for severe acne**
Adults: 200 mg Adoxa P.O. on the first day of treatment (100 mg given q 12 hours or 50 mg q 6 hours), followed by a maintenance dose of 100 mg/day in single or divided doses.

➲ **To prevent traveler's diarrhea caused by *Escherichia coli*♦**
Adults: 100 mg P.O. daily.

Contraindications & cautions

- Contraindicated in patients hypersensitive to drug or other tetracyclines.
- Use cautiously in patients with impaired renal or hepatic function. Use of these drugs during last half of pregnancy and in children younger than age 8 may cause permanent discoloration of teeth, enamel defects, and bone growth retardation in children.

Adverse reactions

CNS: ***intracranial hypertension***.
CV: pericarditis, thrombophlebitis.
GI: anorexia, glossitis, dysphagia, *epigastric distress, nausea,* vomiting, *diarrhea,* oral candidiasis, enterocolitis, anogenital inflammation.
Hematologic: ***neutropenia***, eosinophilia, ***thrombocytopenia***, hemolytic anemia.
Musculoskeletal: bone growth retardation in children younger than age 8.
Skin: *maculopapular and erythematous rashes, photosensitivity, increased pigmentation, urticaria.*
Other: hypersensitivity reactions, ***anaphylaxis***, superinfection, permanent discoloration of teeth, enamel defects.

Interactions

Drug-drug. *Antacids (including sodium bicarbonate) and laxatives containing aluminum, magnesium, or calcium, antidiarrheals:* May decrease antibiotic absorption. Give antibiotic 1 hour before or 2 hours after any of these drugs.
Carbamazepine, phenobarbital, rifamycins: May decrease antibiotic effect. Avoid using together.
Ferrous sulfate and other iron products, zinc: May decrease antibiotic absorption. Give drug 2 hours before or 3 hours after iron administration.
Hormonal contraceptives: May decrease contraceptive effectiveness and increase risk of breakthrough bleeding. Advise use of a nonhormonal contraceptive.
Methoxyflurane: May cause nephrotoxicity with tetracyclines. Avoid using together.
Oral anticoagulants: May increase anticoagulant effect. Monitor PT and INR, and adjust dosage.
Penicillins: May interfere with bactericidal action of penicillins. Avoid using together.
Drug-lifestyle. *Alcohol use:* May decrease antibiotic effect. Discourage use together.
Sun exposure: May cause photosensitivity reactions. Advise patient to avoid excessive sunlight exposure.

Nursing considerations

- Obtain specimen for culture and sensitivity tests before giving first dose. Therapy may begin while awaiting test results.

!!ALERT Check expiration date. Outdated or deteriorated tetracyclines have been linked to reversible nephrotoxicity (Fanconi's syndrome).

- Give drug with milk or food if adverse GI reactions occur.
- If large doses are given, therapy is prolonged, or patient is at high risk, monitor patient for signs and symptoms of superinfection.
- Cutaneous anthrax with signs of systemic involvement, extensive edema, or lesions on the head or neck requires I.V. therapy and a multidrug approach.
- Additional antimicrobials for anthrax multidrug regimens may include rifampin, vancomycin, penicillin, ampicillin, chloramphenicol, imipenem, clindamycin, and clarithromycin.
- Steroids may be considered as adjunctive therapy for anthrax patients with severe edema and for meningitis, based on experience with bacterial meningitis of other etiologies.
- If meningitis is suspected, doxycycline would be less optimal because of poor CNS penetration.

• Ciprofloxacin or doxycycline is the first-line therapy for anthrax. Amoxicillin 500 mg P.O. t.i.d. for adults and 80 mg/kg/day in divided doses every 8 hours for children is an option for completion of therapy after clinical improvement.
• Give pregnant women and immunocompromised patients the usual dosage schedule used for anthrax. In pregnant women, adverse effects on developing teeth and bones are dose-limited; therefore, doxycycline might be used for a short time (7 to 14 days) before 6 months of gestation.
• Check patient's tongue for signs of fungal infection. Stress good oral hygiene.
• Photosensitivity reactions may occur within a few minutes to several hours after exposure. Photosensitivity lasts after therapy ends.
!!ALERT Don't confuse doxycycline, doxylamine, and dicyclomine.

Patient teaching

• Tell patient to take entire amount of drug exactly as prescribed, even after he feels better.
• Instruct patient to report adverse reactions promptly. If drug is being given I.V., tell him to report discomfort at I.V site.
• Advise patient to take oral form of drug with food or milk if stomach upset occurs.
• Advise patient to increase fluid intake and not to take oral tablets or capsules within 1 hour of bedtime because of possible esophageal irritation or ulceration.
• Advise parent giving drug to a child that tablets may be crushed and mixed with low-fat milk, chocolate milk, chocolate pudding, or apple juice mixed equally with sugar. Tell parent to store mixtures in refrigerator (except apple juice mixture, which can be stored at room temperature) and to discard after 24 hours.
• Warn patient to avoid direct sunlight and ultraviolet light, wear protective clothing, and use sunscreen.
• Tell patient to report signs and symptoms of superinfection to prescriber.

dronabinol (delta-9-tetrahydrocannabinol)
Marinol

Pregnancy risk category C
Controlled substance schedule III

Indications & dosages

➲ Nausea and vomiting from cancer chemotherapy
Adults: 5 mg/m^2 P.O. 1 to 3 hours before chemotherapy session. Then same dose q 2 to 4 hours after chemotherapy, for total of four to six doses daily. If needed, increase dosage in 2.5-mg/m^2 increments to maximum of 15 mg/m^2 per dose.
➲ Anorexia and weight loss in patients with AIDS
Adults: 2.5 mg P.O. b.i.d. before lunch and dinner. If patient can't tolerate it, decrease to 2.5 mg P.O. given as a single dose daily in evening or h.s. May gradually increase to maximum of 20 mg daily given in divided doses.

Contraindications & cautions

• Contraindicated in patients hypersensitive to sesame oil or cannabinoids.
• Use cautiously in elderly, pregnant, or breast-feeding patients and in those with heart disease, psychiatric illness, or history of drug abuse.

Adverse reactions

CNS: *dizziness, drowsiness, euphoria, ataxia*, depersonalization, hallucinations, somnolence, headache, muddled thinking, asthenia, amnesia, confusion, *paranoia*.
CV: tachycardia, orthostatic hypotension, palpitations, vasodilation.
EENT: visual disturbances.
GI: *dry mouth, nausea, vomiting, abdominal pain*, diarrhea.

Interactions

Drug-drug. *CNS depressants, psychomimetic substances, sedatives:* May cause additive CNS depression. Avoid using together.
Drug-lifestyle. *Alcohol use:* May cause additive CNS depression. Discourage use together.

Nursing considerations

- Expect drug to be prescribed only for patients who haven't responded satisfactorily to other antiemetics.

!!ALERT Dronabinol is the principal active substance in *Cannabis sativa* (marijuana), which can produce both physiological and psychological dependence and has a high risk of abuse.

- CNS effects are intensified at higher dosages.
- Drug effects may persist for days after treatment ends.

!!ALERT Don't confuse dronabinol with droperidol.

Patient teaching

- Tell patient that drug may induce unusual changes in mood or other adverse behavioral effects.
- Advise patient against performing activities that require alertness until CNS effects of drug are known.
- Warn caregivers to supervise patient during and immediately after treatment.
- Advise patient to take drug 1 to 3 hours before chemotherapy use.

droperidol
Inapsine

Pregnancy risk category C

Indications & dosages

➲ To prevent nausea and vomiting from surgical or diagnostic procedures

Adults and children older than age 12: Maximum first dose, 2.5 mg I.M. or slow I.V. Give additional 1.25 mg cautiously, if needed. Give additional doses only if benefit outweighs risk.

Children ages 2 to 12: Maximum first dose, 0.1 mg/kg, considering patient's age and other factors. Give additional doses cautiously and only if benefit outweighs risk.

In elderly or debilitated patients and those who have received other CNS depressant drugs, give reduced dosage.

Contraindications & cautions

- Contraindicated in patients hypersensitive to drug.
- Contraindicated in patients with prolonged QT interval, including patients with congenital long QT-interval syndrome.
- Use cautiously in those at risk for prolonged QT-interval syndrome (those with heart failure, bradycardia, cardiac hypertrophy, hypokalemia, or hypomagnesemia and those taking drugs that prolong QT interval or worsen hypokalemia or hypomagnesemia).
- Use cautiously in patients with hepatic or renal dysfunction and in breast-feeding patients.
- Use with caution in patients with suspected or diagnosed pheochromocytoma because severe hypertension and tachycardia can occur.

Adverse reactions

CNS: *drowsiness*, restlessness, hyperactivity, anxiety, extrapyramidal symptoms, dizziness, hallucinations, dysphoria, ***neuroleptic malignant syndrome***.

CV: hypotension, tachycardia.

Respiratory: ***laryngospasm***, ***bronchospasm***.

Other: chills, shivering.

Interactions

Drug-drug. *CNS depressants:* May cause additive CNS effects. Adjust dosage, as needed.

Cyclobenzaprines: May have additive effects on prolonging QT interval. Monitor patient closely.

Fentanyl citrate: May cause hypertension and respiratory depression. Use together cautiously.

Nursing considerations

- When used for induction of general anesthesia, give drug with an analgesic.
- If used in procedures such as bronchoscopy, appropriate topical anesthesia is still needed.

!!ALERT Keep fluids and other measures to manage hypotension readily available.

- Monitor patient for signs and symptoms of neuroleptic malignant syndrome (fever, altered consciousness, extrapyramidal symptoms, tachycardia).

!!ALERT Don't confuse droperidol with dronabinol.

Patient teaching

- Warn patient to rise slowly to minimize dizziness.

• Advise patient to avoid alcohol for 24 hours after receiving droperidol.

drospirenone and ethinyl estradiol
Yasmin

Pregnancy risk category X

Indications & dosages

➲ Contraception

Women: 1 yellow tablet P.O. daily for 21 days beginning on day 1 of menstrual cycle or the first Sunday after the onset of menstruation. Then take 1 white inert tablet P.O. daily on days 22 through 28. Begin the next and all subsequent 28-day regimens on the same day of the week that the first regimen began, following the same schedule. Restart taking yellow tablets on the next day after taking the last white tablet.

Contraindications & cautions

• Contraindicated in women with hepatic dysfunction, tumor, or disease; renal or adrenal insufficiency; thrombophlebitis, thromboembolic disorders, or history of deep vein thrombosis or thromboembolic disorders; cerebrovascular or coronary artery disease; known or suspected breast cancer, endometrial cancer, or other estrogen-dependent neoplasia; abnormal genital bleeding; or cholestatic jaundice of pregnancy or jaundice with other contraceptive pill use.

• Contraindicated in women who are or may be pregnant and in women older than age 35 who smoke 15 or more cigarettes daily.

• Use cautiously in patients with risk factors for CV disease, such as hypertension, hyperlipidemias, obesity, and diabetes.

• Use cautiously in patients with conditions aggravated by fluid retention.

Adverse reactions

CNS: asthenia, ***cerebral hemorrhage***, ***cerebral thrombosis***, depression, dizziness, emotional lability, headache, migraine, nervousness.

CV: ***arterial thromboembolism***, hypertension, ***mesenteric thrombosis***, ***MI***, thrombophlebitis.

EENT: cataracts, steepening of corneal curvature, intolerance to contact lenses, pharyngitis, retinal thrombosis, sinusitis.

GI: abdominal pain, abdominal cramping, bloating, changes in appetite, colitis, diarrhea, gastroenteritis, nausea, vomiting, gallbladder disease.

GU: amenorrhea, breakthrough bleeding, change in cervical erosion and secretion, change in menstrual flow, cystitis, cystitis-like syndrome, dysmenorrhea, ***hemolytic-uremic syndrome***, impaired renal function, leukorrhea, menstrual disorder, premenstrual syndrome, spotting, temporary infertility after discontinuing treatment, UTI, vaginal candidiasis, vaginitis.

Hepatic: ***Budd-Chiari syndrome***, cholestatic jaundice, ***hepatic adenomas***, benign liver tumors.

Metabolic: reduced tolerance to carbohydrates, porphyria, weight change.

Musculoskeletal: back pain.

Respiratory: bronchitis, ***pulmonary embolism***, upper respiratory tract infection.

Skin: acne, ***erythema multiforme***, erythema nodosum, hemorrhagic eruption, hirsutism, loss of scalp hair, melasma, pruritus, rash.

Other: changes in libido.

Interactions

Drug-drug. *ACE inhibitors, aldosterone antagonists, angiotensin II receptor antagonists, NSAIDs, potassium-sparing diuretics:* May increase risk of hyperkalemia. Monitor potassium level.

Acetaminophen: May increase level of contraceptive and decrease effectiveness of acetaminophen. Monitor patient for adverse effects. Adjust acetaminophen dose p.r.n.

Ampicillin, griseofulvin, tetracycline: May decrease contraceptive effect. Encourage use of additional method of birth control while taking the antibiotic.

Ascorbic acid, atorvastatin: May increase level of contraceptive. Monitor patient for adverse effects.

Carbamazepine, phenobarbital, phenytoin: May increase metabolism of ethinyl estradiol and decrease contraceptive effectiveness. Encourage use of alternative method of birth control.

Clofibrate, morphine, salicylic acid, temazepam: May decrease levels and increase

clearance of these drugs. Monitor patient for effectiveness.
Cyclosporine, prednisolone, theophylline: May increase levels of these drugs. Monitor patient for adverse effects and toxicity.
Phenylbutazone, rifampin: May decrease contraceptive effectiveness and increase menstrual irregularities. Advise patient to use alternative method of birth control.
Drug-herb. *St. John's wort:* May decrease contraceptive effectiveness and increase breakthrough bleeding. Discourage use together, or advise use of additional method of birth control.
Drug-lifestyle. *Smoking:* May increase risk of CV adverse effects. Advise patient to avoid smoking.

Nursing considerations

- The use of contraceptives causes increased risk of MI, thromboembolism, stroke, hepatic neoplasia, gallbladder disease, and hypertension. Risk increases in patients with hypertension, diabetes, hyperlipidemia, and obesity.
- Smoking increases the risk of serious CV adverse effects. The risk increases with age (especially age older than 35 years) and in patients who smoke 15 or more cigarettes daily.
- The relationship between the use of hormonal contraceptives and breast and cervical cancers is unclear. Encourage women to schedule a complete gynecologic examination at least yearly and to perform breast self-examinations monthly.
- In patients scheduled to have elective surgery that may increase the risk of thromboembolism, stop contraceptive use from at least 4 weeks before until 2 weeks after surgery. Also stop use during and after prolonged immobilization.
- Because of increased risk of thromboembolism in the postpartum period, don't start contraceptive earlier than 4 to 6 weeks after delivery.
- Stop use and evaluate patient if loss of vision, proptosis, diplopia, papilledema, or retinal vascular lesions occur. Recommend that contact lens wearers be evaluated by an ophthalmologist if visual changes or lens intolerance occurs.
- If patient misses two consecutive periods, she should obtain a negative pregnancy test result before continuing use of contraceptive.
- Immediately stop use if pregnancy is confirmed.
- Closely monitor patient with diabetes. Glucose intolerance may occur.
- Closely monitor patient with hypertension or a history of depression. Stop drug if these events occur.
- In patient taking medications that may increase potassium, check potassium level during the first treatment cycle.
- Stop drug and evaluate patient if persistent, severe headaches occur or if migraines occur or are worsened.
- Evaluate patient for malignancy or pregnancy if she experiences breakthrough bleeding or spotting.
- Closely monitor patient with hyperlipidemias.
- Stop use if jaundice occurs.

Patient teaching

- Advise patient to use additional method of birth control during the first 7 days of the first cycle of hormonal contraceptive.
- Inform patient that pills don't protect against sexually transmitted diseases, such as HIV.
- Advise patient of the dangers of smoking while taking hormonal contraceptives. Suggest smokers choose a different form of birth control.
- Tell patient to schedule gynecologic examinations yearly and perform breast self-examination monthly.
- Inform patient that spotting, light bleeding, or stomach upset may occur during the first 1 to 3 packs of pills. Tell her to continue taking the pills and to notify her health care provider if these symptoms persist.
- Tell patient to take the pill at the same time each day.
- Tell patient to immediately report sharp chest pain; coughing of blood or sudden shortness of breath; calf pain; crushing chest pain or chest heaviness; sudden severe headache or vomiting, dizziness or fainting, visual or speech disturbances, weakness or numbness in an arm or leg; vision loss; breast lumps; severe stomach pain or tenderness; difficulty sleeping, lack of energy, fatigue, or change in mood; jaundice with fever, fatigue, loss of appetite, dark urine, or light-colored bowel movements.

• Tell patient to notify health care provider if she wears contact lenses and notices a change in vision or has trouble wearing the lenses.
• Tell patient that the risk of pregnancy increases with each active yellow tablet she forgets to take. Inform patient what to do if she misses pills.
• Tell patient to use an additional method of birth control and to notify health care provider if she isn't sure what to do about missed pills.
• Small amounts of hormonal contraceptives appear in breast milk. Yellow skin and eyes (jaundice) and breast enlargement may occur in breast-feeding infants.

drotrecogin alfa (activated)

Xigris

Pregnancy risk category C

Indications & dosages

➲ To reduce the risk of death in patients with severe sepsis from acute organ dysfunction

Adults: 24 mcg/kg/hour I.V. infusion for a total of 96 hours.

Contraindications & cautions

• Contraindicated in patients hypersensitive to drug or any of its components, those with active internal bleeding, and those who have had hemorrhagic CVA in the past 3 months or intracranial or intraspinal surgery in the past 2 months.
• Contraindicated in patients with severe head trauma, trauma with increased risk of life-threatening bleeding, an epidural catheter, intracranial neoplasm or mass lesion, or cerebral herniation.

!!ALERT Use only after assessing the risk versus benefit in patients with single organ dysfunction and recent surgery because these patients may not be at a high risk of death.

• Use cautiously in patients taking other drugs that affect hemostasis such as heparin (at least 15 units/kg/hour) and in those with a platelet count less than 30,000 × 10^6/L (even if the platelet count is increased after transfusions) or an INR greater than 3.
• Use cautiously in patients who have had GI bleeding in the past 6 weeks; thrombolytic therapy in the past 3 days; oral anticoagulants, glycoprotein IIb/IIIa inhibitors, or aspirin (more than 650 mg/day) or other platelet inhibitors in the past week; ischemic CVA in the past 3 months; or intracranial arteriovenous malformation or aneurysm, bleeding diathesis, chronic severe hepatic disease, or any condition in which bleeding poses a significant hazard or would be difficult to manage because of its location.

Adverse reactions

Hematologic: *hemorrhage*.

Interactions

Drug-drug. *Drugs that affect hemostasis:* May increase risk of bleeding. Use together cautiously.

Nursing considerations

• Use aseptic technique during preparation.
• If the infusion is interrupted, restart at the 24-mcg/kg/hour infusion rate.
• Monitor patient closely for bleeding. Notify prescriber if bleeding occurs.
• Stop drug 2 hours before an invasive surgical procedure. After hemostasis has been achieved, drug may be restarted 12 hours after major invasive procedure or immediately after uncomplicated less invasive procedure.
• Because drug has minimal effect on the PT, this value can be used to monitor the patient's coagulopathy status.

Patient teaching

• Inform patient of the potential adverse reactions.
• Instruct patient to promptly report signs of bleeding.
• Advise patient that bleeding may occur for up to 28 days after treatment.

duloxetine hydrochloride

Cymbalta

Pregnancy risk category C

Indications & dosages

➲ Major depressive disorder

Adults: Initially, 20 mg P.O. b.i.d.; then, 60 mg P.O. once daily or divided in two equal doses. Maximum, 60 mg daily.

➲ Neuropathic pain related to diabetic peripheral neuropathy
Adults: 60 mg P.O. once daily.

In patients with impaired renal function, reduce starting dose and increase gradually.

Contraindications & cautions

- Contraindicated in patients hypersensitive to drug or its ingredients, patients taking MAO inhibitors, patients with uncontrolled angle-closure glaucoma, and patients with a creatinine clearance less than 30 ml/ minute. Drug isn't recommended for patients with hepatic dysfunction or end-stage renal disease.
- Use cautiously in patients with a history of mania or seizures, patients who drink substantial amounts of alcohol, patients with hypertension, patients with controlled angle-closure glaucoma, and patients with conditions that slow gastric emptying.

Adverse reactions

CNS: anxiety, asthenia, *dizziness*, *fatigue*, fever, *headache*, hypoesthesia, initial insomnia, *insomnia*, irritability, lethargy, nervousness, nightmares, restlessness, sleep disorder, *somnolence*, ***suicidal thoughts***, tremor.
CV: hot flushes, hypertension, increased heart rate.
EENT: blurred vision, nasopharyngitis, pharyngolaryngeal pain.
GI: *constipation*, *diarrhea*, *dry mouth*, dyspepsia, gastritis, *nausea*, vomiting.
GU: abnormal orgasm, abnormally increased frequency of urinating, delayed or dysfunctional ejaculation, dysuria, erectile dysfunction, urinary hesitation.
Metabolic: *decreased appetite*, ***hypoglycemia***, increased appetite, weight gain or loss.
Musculoskeletal: muscle cramps, myalgia.
Respiratory: cough.
Skin: increased sweating, night sweats, pruritus, rash.
Other: decreased libido, rigors.

Interactions

Drug-drug. *Antiarrhythmics of type 1C (flecainide, propafenone), phenothiazines (except thioridazine):* May increase levels of these drugs. Use together cautiously.
CNS drugs: May increase adverse effects. Use together cautiously.
CYP1A2 inhibitors (cimetidine, fluvoxamine, certain quinolones): May increase duloxetine level. Avoid using together.
CYP2D6 inhibitors (fluoxetine, paroxetine, quinidine): May increase duloxetine level. Use together cautiously.
Drugs that reduce gastric acidity: May cause premature breakdown of duloxetine's protective coating and early release of the drug. Monitor patient for effects.
MAO inhibitors: May cause hyperthermia, rigidity, myoclonus, autonomic instability, rapid fluctuations of vital signs, agitation, delirium, and coma. Avoid use within 2 weeks after MAO inhibitor therapy; wait at least 5 days after stopping duloxetine before starting MAO inhibitor.
Thioridazine: May prolong the QT interval and increase risk of serious ventricular arrhythmias and sudden death. Avoid using together.
Tricyclic antidepressants (amitriptyline, nortriptyline, imipramine): May increase levels of these drugs. Reduce tricyclic antidepressant dose, and monitor drug levels closely.
Drug-lifestyle. *Alcohol use:* May increase risk of liver damage. Discourage use together.

Nursing considerations

- Monitor patient for worsening of depression or suicidal behavior, especially when therapy starts or dosage changes.
- Treatment of overdose is symptomatic. Don't induce emesis; gastric lavage or activated charcoal may be performed soon after ingestion or if patient is still symptomatic. Because drug undergoes extensive distribution, forced diuresis, dialysis, hemoperfusion, and exchange transfusion aren't useful. Contact a poison control center for information.
- If taken with tricyclic antidepressants, duloxetine metabolism will be prolonged, and patient will need extended monitoring.
- Periodically reassess patient to determine the need for continued therapy.
- Decrease duloxetine dosage gradually, and watch for symptoms that may arise when drug is stopped, such as dizziness, nausea, headache, paresthesia, vomiting, irritability, and nightmares.
- If intolerable symptoms arise when decreasing or stopping drug, restart at previ-

ous dose and decrease even more gradually.
- Monitor blood pressure periodically during treatment.
- Use during the third trimester of pregnancy may cause neonatal complications including respiratory distress, cyanosis, apnea, seizures, vomiting, hypoglycemia, and hyperreflexia, which may require prolonged hospitalization, respiratory support, and tube feeding. Consider potential benefit of drug to the mother versus risks to the fetus.
- Older patients may be more sensitive to drug effects than younger adults.

Patient teaching

!!ALERT Warn families or caregivers to report signs of worsening depression (such as agitation, irritability, insomnia, hostility, impulsivity) and signs of suicidal behavior to prescriber immediately.
- Tell patient to consult his prescriber or pharmacist if he plans to take other prescription or OTC drugs or an herbal or other dietary supplement.
- Instruct patient to swallow capsules whole and not to chew, crush, or open them because they have an enteric coating.
- Urge patient to avoid activities that are hazardous or require mental alertness until he knows how the drug affects him.
- Warn against drinking amounts of alcohol while taking duloxetine.
- If patient takes duloxetine for depression, explain that it may take 1 to 4 weeks to notice an effect.

dutasteride
Avodart

Pregnancy risk category X

Indications & dosages

To improve the symptoms of BPH, reduce the risk of acute urine retention, and reduce the need for BPH-related surgery
Adults: 0.5 mg P.O. once daily.

Contraindications & cautions

- Contraindicated in women and children and in patients hypersensitive to dutasteride or its ingredients or to other 5-alpha-reductase inhibitors.
- Use cautiously in patients with hepatic disease and in those taking long-term potent cytochrome P-450 inhibitors.

Adverse reactions

GU: impotence, decreased libido, ejaculation disorder.
Other: gynecomastia.

Interactions

Drug-drug. *Cytochrome P-450 inhibitors (such as cimetidine, ciprofloxacin, diltiazem, ketoconazole, ritonavir, verapamil):* May increase dutasteride level. Use together cautiously.

Nursing considerations

- Because dutasteride may be absorbed through the skin, women who are or may become pregnant shouldn't handle the drug.
- If contact is made with leaking capsules, wash the contact area immediately with soap and water.
- Carefully monitor patients with a large residual urine volume or severely diminished urine flow, or both, for obstructive uropathy.
- Patients should wait at least 6 months after their last dose before donating blood.
- Establish a new baseline PSA level in men treated for 3 to 6 months and use it to assess potentially cancer-related changes in PSA level.
- To interpret PSA values in men treated for 6 months or more, double the PSA value for comparison with normal values in untreated men.

Patient teaching

- Tell patient to swallow the capsule whole.
- Inform patient that ejaculate volume may decrease but that sexual function should remain normal.
- Teach women who are pregnant or may become pregnant not to handle drug. A male fetus exposed to dutasteride by the mother's swallowing or absorbing the drug through her skin may be born with abnormal sex organs.

!!ALERT Tell patient not to donate blood for at least 6 months after final dose.
- Tell patient he'll need periodic blood tests to monitor therapeutic effects.

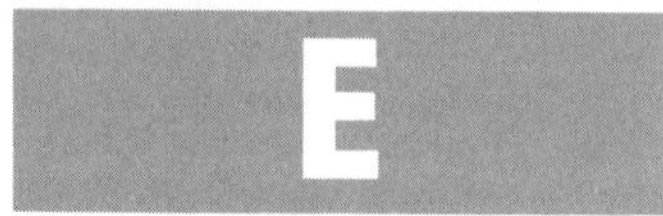

econazole nitrate

Ecostatin†, Spectazole

Pregnancy risk category C

Indications & dosages

➲ **Tinea corporis, tinea cruris, tinea pedis, tinea versicolor**

Adults and children: Rub into affected areas daily for at least 2 weeks.

➲ **Cutaneous candidiasis**

Adults and children: Rub into affected areas b.i.d.

Contraindications & cautions

- Contraindicated in patients hypersensitive to drug or its components.

Adverse reactions

Skin: burning, pruritus, stinging, erythema.

Interactions

Drug-drug. *Corticosteroids:* May inhibit antifungal activity against certain organisms. Monitor patient for clinical effect.

Nursing considerations

- Clean and dry affected area before applying.
- Don't use occlusive dressings.

Patient teaching

- Tell patient to use drug for entire treatment period, even if signs and symptoms improve. Instruct him to notify prescriber if no improvement occurs after 2 weeks in fungal infection on hairless skin (tinea corporis), jock itch, or fungal skin infection (tinea versicolor), or after 4 weeks for athlete's foot.
- Reassure patient that lack of pigmentation from tinea versicolor resolves gradually.
- Tell patient to stop drug and notify prescriber if condition persists or worsens or if irritation occurs.
- Warn patient that drug may stain clothing.
- Tell patient with athlete's foot to change shoes and cotton socks daily and to dry between toes after bathing.
- Tell patient to keep drug out of eyes.

edetate calcium disodium

Calcium Disodium Versenate, Calcium EDTA

Pregnancy risk category B

Indications & dosages

➲ **Acute lead encephalopathy or lead levels greater than 70 mcg/dl**

Adults and children: 1 to 1.5 g/m^2 I.V. or I.M. daily in divided doses at 8- to 12-hour intervals for 5 days, usually with dimercaprol. A second course may be given after at least a 2-day drug-free interval.

➲ **Lead poisoning without encephalopathy or asymptomatic with lead levels less than 70 mcg/dl**

Children: 1 g/m^2 I.V. or I.M. daily in divided doses for 5 days.

Contraindications & cautions

- Contraindicated in patients with anuria, hepatitis, or acute renal disease.
- Use with caution in patients with mild renal disease. Expect dosages to be reduced.

Adverse reactions

CNS: fever, tremors, headache, paresthesia, malaise, fatigue.
CV: hypotension, rhythm irregularities.
EENT: histamine-like reactions (including, sneezing, congestion, and lacrimation).
GI: cheilosis, nausea, vomiting, anorexia, excessive thirst.
GU: proteinuria, hematuria, ***nephrotoxicity with renal tubular necrosis leading to fatal nephrosis***.
Hematologic: ***transient bone marrow suppression***, anemia.
Metabolic: zinc deficiency, hypercalcemia.
Musculoskeletal: myalgia, arthralgia.
Skin: rash.
Other: pain at I.M. injection site, chills.

Interactions

Drug-drug. *Insulin:* May interfere with action of insulin by binding with zinc. Adjust insulin dosage as directed.

Nursing considerations

- Add procaine hydrochloride to I.M. solution to minimize pain. Watch for local reactions.

!!ALERT Because rapid I.V. use may increase intracranial pressure, I.M. route may be preferred for treating lead encephalopathy.

- Although I.M. route may be preferred for children and patients with lead encephalopathy, most experts recommend I.V. infusion whenever possible.
- Monitor fluid intake and output, urinalysis, BUN level, and ECG daily.
- To avoid toxicity, use with dimercaprol; don't mix in same syringe.

!!ALERT Don't confuse edetate calcium disodium with edetate disodium.

Patient teaching

- Explain use and administration of drug to patient and family.
- Tell patients with lead encephalopathy to avoid excess fluids.

edetate disodium

Disodium EDTA, Endrate

Pregnancy risk category C

Indications & dosages

➲ Hypercalcemic crisis

Adults: 50 mg/kg/day by slow I.V. infusion over at least 3 hours. Maximum dose is 3 g/day.

Children♦: 40 mg/kg/day by slow I.V. infusion over at least 3 hours. Maximum dose is 70 mg/kg/day. Alternatively, a dose of 1.5 g/m^2 may be used as a single dose.

Contraindications & cautions

- Contraindicated in patients hypersensitive to drug and in those with anuria, known or suspected hypocalcemia, significant renal disease, active or healed tubercular lesions, or history of seizures or intracranial lesions.
- Use cautiously in patients with limited cardiac reserve, heart failure, or hypokalemia.

Adverse reactions

CNS: circumoral paresthesia, numbness, headache.
CV: hypotension, thrombophlebitis.
EENT: erythema.
GI: nausea, vomiting, diarrhea.
GU: ***nephrotoxicity with urinary urgency***, nocturia, dysuria, polyuria, proteinuria, renal insufficiency, ***renal failure, tubular necrosis***.
Metabolic: severe hypocalcemia.
Skin: exfoliative dermatitis.
Other: pain at infusion site.

Interactions

None significant.

Nursing considerations

- Keep I.V. calcium available to treat hypocalcemia.
- Keep patients in bed for 15 minutes after infusion to avoid effects of orthostatic hypotension. Monitor blood pressure closely.
- Monitor ECG and renal function tests frequently.
- Obtain calcium level after each dose.
- Don't use to treat lead toxicity; use edetate calcium disodium instead.

!!ALERT Don't confuse edetate disodium with edetate calcium disodium.

Patient teaching

- Explain use and administration of drug to patient and family.
- Instruct patient to report adverse reactions promptly.

efalizumab

Raptiva

Pregnancy risk category C

Indications & dosages

➲ Chronic moderate to severe plaque psoriasis when systemic therapy or phototherapy is appropriate

Adults: A single dose of 0.7 mg/kg S.C. followed by weekly doses of 1 mg/kg S.C., beginning 1 week after first dose. Maximum single dose, 200 mg.

Contraindications & cautions

- Contraindicated in patients hypersensitive to efalizumab or its components and in patients with significant infection.
- Use cautiously in patients with chronic infection or history of recurrent infection.
- Use cautiously in patients with history of or high risk for malignancy.

• It isn't known whether efalizumab appears in breast milk. Breast-feeding patients should consider stopping breast-feeding during therapy.

Adverse reactions

CNS: ***CVA***, fever, *headache, pain.*
GI: *nausea.*
Musculoskeletal: back pain, myalgia.
Skin: acne.
Other: *chills*, flulike syndrome, ***hypersensitivity reaction***, *infection.*

Interactions

Drug-drug. *Other immunosuppressants:* May increase risk of infection and malignancy. Avoid using together.
Vaccines: May decrease or negate immune response to vaccine. Avoid using together.

Nursing considerations

• Reconstitute the drug immediately before use.
• To reconstitute, inject 1.3 ml of sterile water for injection into the vial. Swirl gently to dissolve the powder, which takes less than 5 minutes. Don't shake the vial.
• Don't use any other diluent besides sterile water, and use a vial only once.
• The reconstituted solution should be colorless to pale yellow and free of particulates. Don't use the solution if it contains particulates or is discolored.
• If not used immediately, the reconstituted solution may be stored at room temperature for up to 8 hours. Keep efalizumab powder refrigerated, and protect vials from light.
• Rotate injection sites.
• Don't add other drugs to reconstituted solution.
• Notify prescriber if patient develops a severe infection or malignancy is suspected.
• Watch for evidence of thrombocytopenia. Check patient's platelet count monthly during initial treatment and then every 3 months.
• Monitor patient for worsening of psoriasis during or after therapy.

Patient teaching

• Tell patient to take the drug exactly as prescribed.
• Explain that platelet counts will be monitored during therapy.
• Urge patient to immediately report evidence of severe thrombocytopenia, such as bleeding gums, bruising, or petechiae.
• Tell patient to report weight changes because dose may need to be changed.
• Advise patient to report any infection or worsening psoriasis.
• Advise patient to hold off receiving vaccines during therapy because the immune response may be inadequate.
• Caution patient to immediately report pregnancy or suspected pregnancy.

efavirenz

Sustiva

Pregnancy risk category D

Indications & dosages

➲ **HIV-1 infection, with a protease inhibitor or nucleoside analogue reverse transcriptase inhibitors**
Adults and children age 3 and older, weighing 40 kg (88 lb) or more: 600 mg (three 200-mg capsules or one 600-mg tablet) P.O. once daily on an empty stomach, preferably h.s.
Children age 3 and older, weighing 33 to less than 40 kg (72 to under 88 lb): 400 mg P.O. once daily on an empty stomach, preferably h.s.
Children age 3 and older, weighing 25 to less than 33 kg (55 to under 72 lb): 350 mg P.O. once daily on an empty stomach, preferably h.s.
Children age 3 and older, weighing 20 to less than 25 kg (44 to under 55 lb): 300 mg P.O. once daily on an empty stomach, preferably h.s.
Children age 3 and older, weighing 15 to less than 20 kg (33 to under 44 lb): 250 mg P.O. once daily on an empty stomach, preferably h.s.
Children age 3 and older, weighing 10 to less than 15 kg (22 to under 33 lb): 200 mg P.O. once daily on an empty stomach, preferably h.s.

Contraindications & cautions

• Contraindicated in patients hypersensitive to drug or its components.
• Use cautiously in patients with hepatic impairment and in those receiving hepatotoxic drugs. Monitor liver function test results in

patients with history of hepatitis B or C and in those taking ritonavir.

Adverse reactions

CNS: abnormal dreams or thinking, agitation, amnesia, confusion, depersonalization, depression, *dizziness*, euphoria, fever, fatigue, hallucinations, headache, hypoesthesia, impaired concentration, insomnia, somnolence, nervousness.
GI: abdominal pain, anorexia, *diarrhea*, dyspepsia, flatulence, *nausea*, vomiting.
GU: hematuria, renal calculi.
Skin: increased sweating, ***erythema multiforme, Stevens-Johnson syndrome, toxic epidermal necrolysis***, *rash*, pruritus.

Interactions

Drug-drug. *Amprenavir, clarithromycin, indinavir, lopinavir:* May decrease levels of these drugs. Consider alternative therapy or dosage adjustment.
Drugs that induce the cytochrome P-450 enzyme system (such as phenobarbital, rifampin): May increase clearance of efavirenz, resulting in lower drug level. Avoid using together.
Ergot derivatives, midazolam, triazolam: May inhibit metabolism of these drugs and cause serious or life-threatening adverse events (such as arrhythmias, prolonged sedation, or respiratory depression). Avoid using together.
Estrogens, ritonavir: May increase drug levels. Monitor patient.
Hormonal contraceptives: May increase ethinyl estradiol level; no data on progesterone component. Advise use of a reliable method of barrier contraception in addition to use of hormonal contraceptives.
Psychoactive drugs: May cause additive CNS effects. Avoid using together.
Rifabutin: May decrease rifabutin level. Increase rifabutin dosage to 450 to 600 mg once daily or 600 mg two to three times a week.
Ritonavir: May increase levels of both drugs. Monitor patient and liver function closely.
Saquinavir: May decrease saquinavir level and efavirenz exposure to the body. Don't use with saquinavir as sole protease inhibitor.
Voriconazole: Efavirenz significantly decreases voriconazole levels while efavirenz levels significantly increase. Avoid using together.
Warfarin: May increase or decrease level and effects of warfarin. Monitor INR.
Drug-herb. *St. John's wort:* May decrease efavirenz level. Discourage use together.
Drug-food. *High-fat meals:* May increase absorption of drug. Instruct patient to maintain a proper low-fat diet.
Drug-lifestyle. *Alcohol use:* May enhance CNS effects. Discourage use together.

Nursing considerations

- Monitor cholesterol level.

!!ALERT Drug shouldn't be used as monotherapy or added on as a single drug to a regimen failing because of viral resistance.

- Using drug with ritonavir may increase liver enzyme levels and adverse effects (such as dizziness, nausea, paresthesia).
- Give drug at bedtime to decrease CNS adverse effects.
- Pregnancy must be ruled out before starting therapy in women of childbearing age.
- Children may be more prone to adverse reactions, especially diarrhea, nausea, vomiting, and rash.

Patient teaching

- Instruct patient to take drug with water, preferably at bedtime and on an empty stomach.
- Inform patient about need for scheduled blood tests to monitor liver function and cholesterol level.
- Tell patient to use a barrier contraceptive with a hormonal contraceptive and to notify prescriber immediately if pregnancy is suspected; drug is a known risk to the fetus.
- Inform patient that drug doesn't cure HIV infection, that opportunistic infections and other complications of HIV infection may continue to occur, and that transmission of HIV to others through sexual contact or blood contamination is still possible.
- Instruct patient to take drug at the same time daily and always with other antiretrovirals.
- Tell patient to take drug exactly as prescribed and not to stop it without medical approval. Also instruct patient to report adverse reactions.
- Inform patient that rash is the most common adverse effect. Tell patient to report

rash immediately because it may be serious (in rare cases).
- Advise patient to report use of other drugs.
- Advise patient that dizziness, difficulty sleeping or concentrating, drowsiness, or unusual dreams may occur during the first few days of therapy. Reassure him that these symptoms typically resolve after 2 to 4 weeks and may be less problematic if drug is taken at bedtime.
- Tell patient to avoid alcohol, driving, or operating machinery until the drug's effects are known.

eletriptan hydrobromide
Relpax

Pregnancy risk category C

Indications & dosages

➲ Acute migraine with or without aura
Adults: 20 to 40 mg P.O. at first migraine symptom. If headache recurs, dose may be repeated at least 2 hours later to a maximum of 80 mg daily.

Contraindications & cautions

- Contraindicated in patients hypersensitive to drug or its components and in those with severe hepatic impairment; ischemic heart disease, such as angina pectoris, a history of MI, or silent ischemia; coronary artery vasospasm, including Prinzmetal's variant angina; and other significant CV conditions.
- Contraindicated in patients with cerebrovascular syndromes, such as CVA or transient ischemic attack; peripheral vascular disease, including ischemic bowel disease; uncontrolled hypertension; or hemiplegic or basilar migraine.
- Contraindicated within 24 hours of another 5-HT_1 agonist, drugs containing ergotamine, or ergot-type drug.
- Contraindicated in patients with risk factors for coronary artery disease (CAD) such as hypertension, hypercholesterolemia, smoking, obesity, diabetes, strong family history of CAD, postmenopausal women, or men older than age 40, unless patient is free from cardiac disease. Monitor patient closely after first dose.

Adverse reactions

CNS: *asthenia*, dizziness, headache, hypertonia, hypesthesia, pain, paresthesia, somnolence, vertigo.
CV: chest tightness, pain, and pressure, flushing, palpitations.
EENT: pharyngitis.
GI: abdominal pain, discomfort, or cramps, dry mouth, dyspepsia, dysphagia, nausea.
Musculoskeletal: back pain.
Skin: increased sweating.
Other: chills.

Interactions

Drug-drug. *CYP3A4 inhibitors (such as clarithromycin, itraconazole, ketoconazole, nefazodone, nelfinavir, ritonavir, troleandomycin):* May decrease eletriptan metabolism. Avoid use within 72 hours of these drugs.
Ergotamine-containing or ergot-type drugs (such as dihydroergotamine or methysergide), other 5-HT_1 agonists: May prolong vasospastic reactions. Avoid use within 24 hours of these drugs.
SSRIs: May increase the risk of serotonin syndrome (weakness, hyperreflexia, and incoordination). If used together, observe patient closely.

Nursing considerations

- Drug isn't intended for migraine prevention.
- Safety of treating more than three migraine headaches in 30 days hasn't been established
- Use drug only when patient has a clear diagnosis of migraine. If the first use produces no response, reconsider the migraine diagnosis.

!!ALERT Serious cardiac events including acute MI, arrhythmias, and death occur rarely within a few hours after use of 5-HT_1 agonists.

- Ophthalmologic effects may occur with long-term use.
- Older patients may develop higher blood pressure than younger patients after taking drug.

Patient teaching

- Instruct patient to take dose at the first sign of a migraine headache. If the headache comes back after the first dose, he may take a second dose after 2 hours. Caution

patient not to take more than 80 mg in 24 hours.
- Warn patient to avoid driving and operating machinery if he feels dizzy or fatigued after taking the drug.
- Tell patient to immediately report pain, tightness, heaviness, or pressure in the chest, throat, neck, or jaw.

emtricitabine
Emtriva

Pregnancy risk category B

Indications & dosages
➲ **HIV-1 infection, with other antiretrovirals**
Adults: 200 mg P.O. once daily.

In patients with creatinine clearance of 30 to 49 ml/minute, give 200 mg P.O. q 48 hours; if clearance is 15 to 29 ml/minute, give 200 mg P.O. q 72 hours; if clearance is less than 15 ml/minute or patient is receiving dialysis, give 200 mg P.O. q 96 hours. If dose is due on dialysis day, give after dialysis session ends.

Contraindications & cautions
- Contraindicated in patients hypersensitive to drug or its ingredients.
- Don't use drug for treating chronic hepatitis B virus (HBV); safety and efficacy haven't been established in patients infected with both HBV and HIV.
- Use cautiously in elderly patients because of the increased likelihood of concurrent disease or drug therapy, and decreased hepatic, renal, or cardiac function.
- Use cautiously in patients with impaired renal function.

Adverse reactions
CNS: *abnormal dreams, asthenia,* depressive disorders, *dizziness, headache, insomnia,* neuritis, paresthesia, peripheral neuropathy.
EENT: *rhinitis.*
GI: *abdominal pain, diarrhea,* dyspepsia, *nausea,* vomiting.
Hepatic: ***hepatotoxicity.***
Musculoskeletal: arthralgia, myalgia.
Respiratory: *increased cough.*
Skin: *allergic skin reaction, discoloration, maculopapular rash, pruritus, urticarial and purpuric lesions, vesiculobullous rash.*

Interactions
None reported.

Nursing considerations
- Test all patients for HBV before starting drug.
- Hepatitis B may worsen after emtricitabine therapy stops. Patients with both HIV and HBV need close clinical and laboratory follow-up for several months or longer after stopping drug.
- Like other antiretrovirals, emtricitabine may cause changes or increases in body fat, including central obesity, buffalo hump, peripheral wasting, facial wasting, breast enlargement, and a cushingoid appearance.

!!ALERT Notify prescriber immediately if lactic acidosis or pronounced hepatotoxicity occurs.
- Use drug only if clearly needed in pregnant women.

Patient teaching
- Remind patient that anti-HIV medicine must be taken for life.
- Inform patient that drug doesn't cure HIV infection, that opportunistic infections and other complications of HIV infection may continue to occur, and that transmission of HIV to others through sexual contact or blood contamination is still possible.
- Explain possible adverse reactions, including lactic acidosis, hepatotoxicity, and changes or increases in body fat.
- Tell patient to notify prescriber immediately if she is or could be pregnant.
- Inform patient the drug may be taken with or without food.

enalaprilat

enalapril maleate
Vasotec

Pregnancy risk category C; D in 2nd and 3rd trimesters

Indications & dosages

➲ Hypertension

Adults: In patients not taking diuretics, initially, 5 mg P.O. once daily; then adjusted based on response. Usual dosage range is 10 to 40 mg daily as a single dose or two divided doses. Or, 1.25 mg I.V. infusion over 5 minutes q 6 hours.

If patient is taking diuretics or creatinine clearance is 30 ml/minute or less, initially, 2.5 mg P.O. once daily. Or, 0.625 mg I.V. over 5 minutes, and repeat in 1 hour, if needed; then 1.25 mg I.V. q 6 hours.

➲ To convert from I.V. therapy to oral therapy

Adults: Initially, 2.5 mg P.O. once daily; if patient was receiving 0.625 mg I.V. q 6 hours, then 2.5 mg P.O. once daily. Adjust dosage based on response.

➲ To convert from oral therapy to I.V. therapy

Adults: 1.25 mg I.V. over 5 minutes q 6 hours. Higher dosages aren't more effective.

If creatinine level is more than 1.6 mg/dl or sodium level below 130 mEq/L, initially, 2.5 mg P.O. daily and adjust slowly.

➲ To manage symptomatic heart failure

Adults: Initially, 2.5 mg P.O. daily or b.i.d., increased gradually over several weeks. Maintenance is 5 to 20 mg daily in two divided doses. Maximum daily dose is 40 mg in two divided doses.

➲ Asymptomatic left ventricular dysfunction

Adults: Initially, 2.5 mg P.O. b.i.d. Increase as tolerated to target daily dose of 20 mg P.O. in divided doses.

Contraindications & cautions

- Contraindicated in patients hypersensitive to drug and in those with a history of angioedema related to previous treatment with an ACE inhibitor.
- Use cautiously in renally impaired patients or those with aortic stenosis or hypertrophic cardiomyopathy.

Adverse reactions

CNS: headache, dizziness, fatigue, vertigo, *asthenia*, syncope.
CV: hypotension, chest pain, angina pectoris.
GI: diarrhea, nausea, abdominal pain, vomiting.
GU: decreased renal function (in patients with bilateral renal artery stenosis or heart failure).
Hematologic: bone marrow depression.
Respiratory: dyspnea; *dry, persistent, tickling, nonproductive cough.*
Skin: rash.
Other: ***angioedema***.

Interactions

Drug-drug. *Azathioprine:* May increase risk of anemia or leukopenia. Monitor hematologic studies if used together.
Diuretics: May excessively reduce blood pressure. Use together cautiously.
Insulin, oral antidiabetics: May cause hypoglycemia, especially at start of enalapril therapy. Monitor patient closely.
Lithium: May cause lithium toxicity. Monitor lithium level.
NSAIDs: May reduce antihypertensive effect. Monitor blood pressure.
Potassium-sparing diuretics, potassium supplements: May cause hyperkalemia. Avoid using together unless hypokalemia is confirmed.
Drug-herb. *Capsaicin:* May cause cough. Discourage use together.
Ma huang: May decrease antihypertensive effects. Discourage use together.
Drug-food. *Salt substitutes containing potassium:* May cause hyperkalemia. Monitor patient closely.

Nursing considerations

- Closely monitor blood pressure response to drug.

!!ALERT Similar packaging and labeling of enalaprilat injection and pancuronium, a paralyzing drug, could result in a fatal medication error. Check all labeling carefully.

- Monitor CBC with differential counts before and during therapy.
- Diabetic patients, those with impaired renal function or heart failure, and those receiving drugs that can increase potassium level may develop hyperkalemia. Monitor potassium intake and potassium level.

!!ALERT Don't confuse enalapril with Anafranil or Eldepryl.

Patient teaching

- Instruct patient to report breathing difficulty or swelling of face, eyes, lips, or tongue. Swelling of the face and throat (including swelling of the larynx) may occur, especially after first dose.
- Advise patient to report signs of infection, such as fever and sore throat.
- Inform patient that light-headedness can occur, especially during first few days of therapy. Tell him to rise slowly to minimize this effect and to notify prescriber if symptoms develop. If he faints, he should stop taking drug and call prescriber immediately.
- Tell patient to use caution in hot weather and during exercise. Inadequate fluid intake, vomiting, diarrhea, and excessive perspiration can lead to light-headedness and fainting.
- Advise patient to avoid salt substitutes; these products may contain potassium, which can cause high potassium levels in patients taking this drug.
- Tell woman of childbearing age to notify prescriber if pregnancy occurs. Drug will need to be stopped.

enfuvirtide
Fuzeon

Pregnancy risk category B

Indications & dosages

➲ To help control HIV-1 infection, with other antiretrovirals, in patients who have continued HIV-1 replication despite antiretroviral therapy
Adults: 90 mg/1 ml S.C. b.i.d., injected into the upper arm, anterior thigh, or abdomen.
Children ages 6 to 16: 2 mg/kg S.C. b.i.d.; maximum 90 mg per dose.

Contraindications & cautions

- Contraindicated in patients hypersensitive to drug and in those not infected with HIV.
- Use in pregnant patients only if clearly needed. Pregnant patients can be registered in the Antiretroviral Pregnancy Registry by phoning 1-800-258-4263.
- Safety and efficacy haven't been established in patients younger than age 6.

Adverse reactions

CNS: anxiety, asthenia, depression, *fatigue, insomnia,* peripheral neuropathy.
EENT: conjunctivitis, sinusitis, taste disturbance.
GI: abdominal pain, constipation, *diarrhea, nausea,* ***pancreatitis***.
Metabolic: anorexia, weight decrease.
Musculoskeletal: myalgia.
Respiratory: ***bacterial pneumonia***, cough.
Skin: *injection site reactions*, pruritus, skin papilloma.
Other: herpes simplex, influenza, influenza-like illness, lymphadenopathy.

Interactions

None reported.

Nursing considerations

!!ALERT Drug is available only through a progressive distribution program. Information may be obtained by calling 866-694-6670.

- For S.C. administration, reconstitute vial with 1.1 ml sterile water for injection. Tap vial for 10 seconds and then gently roll to prevent foaming. Let drug stand for up to 45 minutes to ensure reconstitution. Or, gently roll vial between hands until product is completely dissolved. Then draw up correct dose and inject drug.
- If you won't be using drug immediately after reconstitution, refrigerate in original vial and use within 24 hours. Don't inject drug until it's at room temperature.
- Store unreconstituted vials at room temperature.
- Vial is for single use; discard unused portion.
- Rotate injection sites. Don't inject into the same site for two consecutive doses, and don't inject into moles, scar tissue, bruises, or the navel.
- Injection site reactions (pain, discomfort, induration, erythema, pruritus, nodules, cysts, ecchymosis) are common and may require analgesics or rest.

!!ALERT Monitor patient closely for evidence of bacterial pneumonia. Patients at high risk include those with a low initial CD4 count or high initial viral load, those who use I.V. drugs or smoke, and those with history of lung disease.

- Hypersensitivity may occur with the first dose or later doses. If symptoms occur, stop drug.

Patient teaching

- Teach patient how to prepare and give drug and how to safely dispose of used needles and syringes.
- Tell patient to rotate injection sites and to watch for cellulitis or local infection.
- Urge patient to immediately report evidence of pneumonia, such as cough with fever, rapid breathing, or shortness of breath.
- Tell patient to stop taking drug and seek medical attention if evidence of hypersensitivity develops, such as rash, fever, nausea, vomiting, chills, rigors, and hypotension.
- Teach patient that drug doesn't cure HIV infection and that it must be taken with other antiretroviral drugs.
- Tell patient to inform prescriber if she's pregnant, plans to become pregnant, or is breast-feeding while taking this drug. Because HIV could be transmitted to the infant, HIV-infected mothers shouldn't breast-feed.
- Tell patient that drug may impair the ability to drive or operate machinery.

enoxaparin sodium
Lovenox

Pregnancy risk category B

Indications & dosages

➲ To prevent pulmonary embolism and deep vein thrombosis (DVT) after hip or knee replacement surgery
Adults: 30 mg S.C. every 12 hours for 7 to 10 days. Give initial dose between 12 and 24 hours postoperatively, as long as hemostasis has been established. Continue treatment during postoperative period until risk of DVT has diminished. Hip replacement patients may receive 40 mg S.C. given 12 hours preoperatively. After initial phase of therapy, hip replacement patients should continue with 40 mg S.C. daily for 3 weeks.

➲ To prevent pulmonary embolism and DVT after abdominal surgery
Adults: 40 mg S.C. daily with initial dose 2 hours before surgery. Give subsequent dose, as long as hemostasis has been established, 24 hours after initial preoperative dose and continue once daily for 7 to 10 days. Continue treatment during postoperative period until risk of DVT has diminished.

➲ To prevent pulmonary embolism and DVT in patients with acute illness who are at increased risk because of decreased mobility
Adults: 40 mg once daily S.C. for 6 to 11 days. Treatment for up to 14 days has been well tolerated.

In patients with creatinine clearance less than 30 ml/minute receiving drug as prophylaxis after abdominal surgery or hip or knee replacement surgery, and in medical patients for prophylaxis during acute illness, give 30 mg S.C. once daily.

➲ To prevent ischemic complications of unstable angina and non–Q-wave MI with oral aspirin therapy
Adults: 1 mg/kg S.C. every 12 hours until clinical stabilization (minimum 2 days) with aspirin 100 to 325 mg P.O. once daily.

➲ Inpatient treatment of acute DVT with and without pulmonary embolism when given with warfarin sodium
Adults: 1 mg/kg S.C. q 12 hours; or, 1.5 mg/kg S.C. once daily (at same time daily) for 5 to 7 days until therapeutic oral anticoagulant effect (INR 2 to 3) is achieved. Warfarin sodium therapy is usually started within 72 hours of enoxaparin injection.

➲ Outpatient treatment of acute DVT without pulmonary embolism when given with warfarin sodium
Adults: 1 mg/kg S.C. q 12 hours for 5 to 7 days until therapeutic oral anticoagulant effect (INR 2 to 3) is achieved. Warfarin sodium therapy is usually started within 72 hours of enoxaparin injection.

In patients with creatinine clearance less than 30 ml/minute receiving drug for acute DVT or prophylaxis of ischemic complications of unstable angina and non–Q-wave MI, give 1 mg/kg S.C. once daily.

Contraindications & cautions

- Contraindicated in patients hypersensitive to drug, heparin, or pork products; in those with active major bleeding; and in those with thrombocytopenia and antiplatelet antibodies in presence of drug.
- Use cautiously in patients with history of heparin-induced thrombocytopenia, aneurysms, cerebrovascular hemorrhage, spinal or epidural punctures (as with anesthesia), uncontrolled hypertension, or threatened abortion.

• Use cautiously in elderly patients and in those with conditions that place them at increased risk for hemorrhage, such as bacterial endocarditis, congenital or acquired bleeding disorders, ulcer disease, angiodysplastic GI disease, hemorrhagic CVA, or recent spinal, eye, or brain surgery.
• Use cautiously in patients with regional or lumbar block anesthesia, blood dyscrasias, recent childbirth, pericarditis or pericardial effusion, renal insufficiency, or severe CNS trauma.

Adverse reactions

CNS: fever, pain.
CV: edema, peripheral edema.
GI: nausea.
Hematologic: hypochromic anemia, ***thrombocytopenia***, ***hemorrhage***, ecchymoses, bleeding complications.
Skin: irritation, pain, hematoma, and erythema at injection site, *rash*, *urticaria*.
Other: ***angioedema***, ***anaphylaxis***.

Interactions

Drug-drug. *Anticoagulants, antiplatelet drugs, NSAIDs:* May increase risk of bleeding. Use together cautiously. Monitor PT and INR.

Nursing considerations

• The vascular access sheath for instrumentation should remain in place for 6 to 8 hours after a dose; give next dose no sooner than 6 to 8 hours after sheath removal. Monitor vital signs.
• Drug isn't recommended for thromboprophylaxis in patients with prosthetic heart valves because they may be at higher risk for thromboembolism.
• Monitor closely pregnant women receiving drug. Warn pregnant women and women of childbearing age about the potential hazard to the fetus and the mother if drug is given during pregnancy.
• Women who received enoxaparin during pregnancy may give birth to infants with congenital anomalies, such as cerebral and limb anomalies, hypospadias, peripheral vascular malformation, fibrotic dysplasia, and cardiac defect.
!!ALERT Patients receiving low-molecular-weight heparins or heparinoids who have epidural or spinal anesthesia or spinal puncture are at risk for developing epidural or spinal hematoma that can result in long-term paralysis. Risk increases with use of epidural catheters, drugs affecting hemostasis, or traumatic or repeated epidural or spinal punctures. Monitor these patients frequently for signs of neurologic impairment. Urgent treatment is needed.
• Draw blood to establish baseline coagulation parameters before therapy.
• Never give drug I.M.
!!ALERT Don't try to expel the air bubble from the 30- or 40-mg prefilled syringes. This may lead to loss of drug and an incorrect dose.
• With patient lying down, give by deep S.C. injection, alternating doses between left and right anterolateral and posterolateral abdominal walls.
• Don't massage after S.C. injection. Watch for signs of bleeding at site. Rotate sites and keep record.
• Avoid excessive I.M. injections of other drugs to prevent or minimize hematomas. If possible, don't give I.M. injections at all.
• Monitor platelet counts regularly. Patients with normal coagulation won't need close monitoring of PT or PTT.
• Regularly inspect patient for bleeding gums, bruises on arms or legs, petechiae, nosebleeds, melena, tarry stools, hematuria, hematemesis.
• To treat severe overdose, give protamine sulfate (a heparin antagonist) by slow I.V. infusion at concentration of 1% to equal dose of drug injected.
!!ALERT Enoxaparin isn't interchangeable with heparin or other low-molecular-weight heparins.

Patient teaching

• Instruct patient and family to watch for signs of bleeding or abnormal bruising and to notify prescriber immediately if any occur.
• Tell patient to avoid OTC drugs containing aspirin or other salicylates unless ordered by prescriber.

entacapone
Comtan

Pregnancy risk category C

Indications & dosages

➲ **Adjunct to levodopa and carbidopa for treatment of idiopathic Parkinson's disease in patients with signs and symptoms of end-of-dose wearing off**

Adults: 200 mg P.O. with each dose of levodopa and carbidopa, up to eight times daily. Maximum, 1,600 mg daily. May need to reduce daily levodopa dose or extend the interval between doses to optimize patient's response.

Contraindications & cautions

- Contraindicated in patients hypersensitive to drug.
- Use cautiously in patients with hepatic impairment, biliary obstruction, or orthostatic hypotension.

Adverse reactions

CNS: *dyskinesia, hyperkinesia,* hypokinesia, dizziness, anxiety, somnolence, agitation, fatigue, asthenia, hallucinations.
GI: *nausea, diarrhea,* abdominal pain, constipation, vomiting, dry mouth, dyspepsia, flatulence, gastritis, taste perversion.
GU: *urine discoloration.*
Hematologic: purpura.
Musculoskeletal: back pain.
Respiratory: dyspnea.
Skin: sweating.
Other: bacterial infection.

Interactions

Drug-drug. *Ampicillin, chloramphenicol, cholestyramine, erythromycin, probenecid:* May block biliary excretion, resulting in higher levels of entacapone. Use together cautiously.
CNS depressants: May cause additive effect. Use together cautiously.
Drugs metabolized by COMT (dobutamine, dopamine, epinephrine, isoetharine, isoproterenol, norepinephrine): May cause higher levels of these drugs, resulting in increased heart rate, changes in blood pressure, or arrhythmias. Use together cautiously.
Nonselective MAO inhibitors (such as phenelzine, tranylcypromine): May inhibit normal catecholamine metabolism. Avoid using together.
Drug-lifestyle. *Alcohol use:* May cause additive CNS effects. Discourage use together.

Nursing considerations

- Use drug only with levodopa and carbidopa; no antiparkinsonian effects occur when drug is given as monotherapy.
- Levodopa and carbidopa dosage requirements are usually lower when drug is given with entacapone; lower levodopa and carbidopa dose or increase dosing interval to avoid adverse effects.
- Drug may cause or worsen dyskinesia, even if levodopa dose is lowered.
- Hallucinations may occur or worsen during therapy with this drug.
- Monitor blood pressure closely, and watch for orthostatic hypotension.
- Diarrhea most often begins within 4 to 12 weeks of starting therapy but may begin as early as 1 week or as late as many months after starting treatment.
- Drug may discolor urine.
- Rarely, rhabdomyolysis has occurred with drug use.
- Rapid withdrawal or abrupt reduction in dose could lead to signs and symptoms of Parkinson's disease; it may also lead to hyperpyrexia and confusion, a group of symptoms resembling neuroleptic malignant syndrome. Stop drug gradually, and monitor patient closely. Adjust other dopaminergic treatments, as needed.
- Drug can be given with immediate or sustained-release levodopa and carbidopa and can be taken with or without food.

Patient teaching

- Instruct patient not to crush or break tablet and to take it at same time as levodopa and carbidopa.
- Warn patient to avoid hazardous activities until CNS effects of drug are known.
- Advise patient to avoid alcohol during treatment.
- Instruct patient to use caution when standing after a prolonged period of sitting or lying down because dizziness may occur. This effect is more common during initial therapy.
- Warn patient that hallucinations, increased difficulty with voluntary movements, nausea, and diarrhea could occur.

• Inform patient that drug may turn urine brownish orange.
• Advise patient to notify prescriber about planned, suspected, or known pregnancy, and to notify prescriber if she's breast-feeding.

entecavir
Baraclude

Pregnancy risk category C

Indications & dosages

➲ **Chronic hepatitis B virus (HBV) infection in patients with active viral replication and either persistently increased aminotransferase levels or histologically active disease**

Adults and adolescents age 16 and older who have had no previous nucleoside treatment: 0.5 mg P.O. once daily at least 2 hours before or after a meal.

If creatinine clearance is 30 to 49 ml/minute, give 0.25 mg P.O. once daily. If clearance is 10 to 30 ml/minute, give 0.15 mg P.O. once daily. If clearance is less than 10 ml/minute or patient is undergoing hemodialysis or continuous ambulatory peritoneal analysis, give 0.05 mg P.O. once daily.

Adults and adolescents age 16 and older who have a history of viremia and are taking lamivudine or have resistance mutations: 1 mg P.O. once daily at least 2 hours before or after a meal.

If creatinine clearance is 30 to 49 ml/minute, give 0.5 mg P.O. once daily. If clearance is 10 to 30 ml/minute, give 0.3 mg P.O. once daily. If clearance is less than 10 ml/minute or patient is undergoing hemodialysis or continuous ambulatory peritoneal dialysis, give 0.1 mg P.O. once daily.

Contraindications & cautions

• Contraindicated in patients hypersensitive to drug or its components.
• Use cautiously in patients with renal impairment and in patients who have had a liver transplant.

Adverse reactions

CNS: dizziness, fatigue, headache.
GI: diarrhea, dyspepsia, nausea.
GU: hematuria, glycosuria.

Interactions

Drug-drug. *Cyclosporine, tacrolimus:* May further decrease renal function. Monitor renal function carefully.
Drugs that reduce renal function or compete for active tubular secretion: May increase level of either drug. Monitor renal function, and watch for adverse effects.
Drug-food. *All foods:* Delays absorption and decreases drug level. Give drug on an empty stomach, at least 2 hours before or after a meal.

Nursing considerations

!!ALERT Drug may cause life-threatening lactic acidosis and severe hepatomegaly with steatosis.
!!ALERT HBV infection may worsen severely after therapy stops.
• Monitor hepatic function for several months in patients who stop therapy. If appropriate, start therapy for HBV infection.
• Use cautiously in pregnant women only if maternal benefit outweighs fetal risk. To monitor fetal outcome data,, call the pregnancy registry at 1-800-258-4263.
• It's unknown if drug appears in breast milk. Avoid use in breast-feeding women.
• In elderly patients, adjust dosage for age-related decrease in renal function.

Patient teaching

• Tell patient that drug should be taken on an empty stomach at least 2 hours before or after a meal.
• Caution against mixing or diluting oral solution with any other substance. Teach proper use of dosing spoon.
• Tell patient to report to prescriber any new adverse effects from this drug and any new drugs he's taking.
• Explain that drug doesn't reduce the risk of HBV transmission to others.
• Teach patient the signs and symptoms of lactic acidosis, such as muscle pain, weakness, dyspnea, GI distress, cold hands and feet, dizziness, or fast or irregular heartbeat.
• Teach patient the signs and symptoms of hepatotoxicity, such as jaundice, dark urine, light-colored stool, loss of appetite, nausea, and lower stomach pain.
• Warn patient not to stop drug abruptly.

ephedrine sulfate

Pretz-D ◇

Pregnancy risk category C

Indications & dosages

➲ Hypotension

Adults: 25 mg one to four times daily P.O. Or, 25 to 50 mg I.M. or S.C. Or, 10 to 25 mg I.V., p.r.n., to maximum of 150 mg/24 hours.

Children: 3 mg/kg or 25 to 100 mg/m^2 S.C. or I.V. daily, in four to six divided doses.

➲ Bronchodilation, nasal decongestion

Adults and children older than age 12: 12.5 to 50 mg P.O. q 3 to 4 hours, p.r.n., not to exceed 150 mg in 24 hours. As a nasal decongestant, 2 to 3 sprays in each nostril q 4 hours.

Children age 2 to 12: 2 to 3 mg/kg or 100 mg/m^2 P.O. daily in four to six divided doses. Or, for children ages 6 to 12, 6.25 to 12.5 mg P.O. q 4 hours, not to exceed 75 mg in 24 hours. As a nasal decongestant, 1 to 2 sprays in each nostril q 4 hours.

Contraindications & cautions

- Contraindicated in patients hypersensitive to ephedrine and other sympathomimetics and in those with porphyria, severe coronary artery disease, arrhythmias, angle-closure glaucoma, psychoneurosis, angina pectoris, substantial organic heart disease, or CV disease.
- Contraindicated in those receiving MAO inhibitors or general anesthesia with cyclopropane or halothane.
- Use with caution in elderly patients and in those with hypertension, hyperthyroidism, nervous or excitable states, diabetes, or prostatic hyperplasia.

Adverse reactions

CNS: *insomnia, nervousness,* dizziness, headache, muscle weakness, euphoria, confusion, delirium, tremor, ***cerebral hemorrhage***.

CV: *palpitations,* tachycardia, hypertension, precordial pain, ***arrhythmias***.

EENT: dry nose and throat.

GI: nausea, vomiting, anorexia.

GU: urine retention, painful urination from visceral sphincter spasm.

Skin: diaphoresis.

Interactions

Drug-drug. *Acetazolamide:* May increase ephedrine level. Monitor patient for toxicity.

Alpha blockers: May reduce vasopressor response. Monitor patient closely.

Antihypertensives: May decrease effects. Monitor blood pressure.

Beta blockers: May block the effects of ephedrine. Monitor patient closely.

Cardiac glycosides, general anesthetics (halogenated hydrocarbons): May increase risk of ventricular arrhythmias. Monitor ECG closely.

Guanethidine: May decrease pressor effects of ephedrine. Monitor patient closely.

MAO inhibitors (phenelzine, tranylcypromine): May cause severe headache, hypertension, fever, and hypertensive crisis. Avoid using together.

Methyldopa, reserpine: May inhibit ephedrine effects. Use together cautiously.

Oxytocics: May cause severe hypertension. Avoid using together.

Tricyclic antidepressants: May decrease pressor response. Monitor patient closely.

Nursing considerations

!!ALERT Hypoxia, hypercapnia, and acidosis must be identified and corrected before or during ephedrine therapy because they may reduce effectiveness or increase adverse reactions.

- Drug isn't a substitute for blood or fluid volume replenishment. Volume deficit must be corrected before giving vasopressors.
- To prevent insomnia, avoid giving drug within 2 hours of bedtime.
- Effectiveness decreases after 2 to 3 weeks as tolerance develops. Prescriber may increase dosage. Drug isn't addictive.
- Use ephedrine in children younger than age 12 only under direction of prescriber.
- Rebound congestion and tachyphylaxis may occur with topical decongestant formulations.

!!ALERT Don't confuse ephedrine with epinephrine.

Patient teaching

- Tell patient taking oral form of drug at home to take last dose of day at least 2 hours before bedtime.

- Warn patient not to take OTC drugs or herbs that contain ephedrine without consulting prescriber.

epinastine hydrochloride
Elestat

Pregnancy risk category C

Indications & dosages

➲ To prevent itching from allergic conjunctivitis

Adults and children age 3 and older: Instill 1 drop into each eye b.i.d. Continue treatment as long as allergen is present, even if symptoms resolve.

Contraindications & cautions

- Contraindicated in patients hypersensitive to drug or its components.
- Contraindicated for irritation related to contact lenses.
- Use cautiously in pregnant or breast-feeding women.
- Safety and effectiveness haven't been established in children younger than age 3.

Adverse reactions

CNS: headache.
EENT: burning eyes, hyperemia, increased lymph nodes near eyes, *cold symptoms*, pharyngitis, pruritus, rhinitis, sinusitis.
Respiratory: increased cough, *upper respiratory tract infection.*

Interactions

None reported.

Nursing considerations

- Drug is for ophthalmic use only. Don't inject or give orally.
- Monitor patient for signs and symptoms of infection.
- Soft contact lenses may absorb the preservative benzalkonium.

Patient teaching

- Teach patient proper instillation technique. Instruct him not to touch any surface, eyelid, or surrounding areas with tip of dropper.
- Caution patient not to use drops to treat contact lens–related eye irritation and not to wear contact lenses if eyes are red.
- Warn patient that soft contact lenses may absorb the preservative benzalkonium.
- Advise patient to report adverse reactions to drug.
- Tell patient to keep bottle tightly closed when not in use.
- Instruct patient who wears soft contact lenses and whose eyes aren't red to wait at least 10 minutes after instilling drug before inserting contact lenses.

epinephrine (adrenaline)
Bronkaid Mistometer†, Primatene Mist ◇

epinephrine bitartrate
AsthmaHaler Mist ◇, Primatene Mist*

epinephrine hydrochloride (systemic)
Adrenalin Chloride, AsthmaNefrin ◇, EpiPen, EpiPen Jr, MicroNefrin ◇, Nephron ◇, Sus-Phrine, Vaponefrin

Pregnancy risk category C

Indications & dosages

➲ Bronchospasm, hypersensitivity reactions, anaphylaxis

Adults: 0.1 to 0.5 ml of 1:1,000 solution S.C. or I.M. Repeat q 10 to 15 minutes, p.r.n. Or, 0.1 to 0.25 ml of 1:1,000 solution I.V. slowly over 5 to 10 minutes (1 to 2.5 ml of a commercially available 1:10,000 injection or of a 1:10,000 dilution prepared by diluting 1 ml of a commercially available 1:1,000 injection with 10 ml of water for injection or normal saline solution for injection). May repeat q 5 to 15 minutes, p.r.n., or follow with a continuous I.V. infusion, starting at 1 mcg/minute and increasing to 4 mcg/minute, p.r.n.

Children: 0.01 ml/kg (10 mcg) of 1:1,000 solution S.C.; repeat q 20 minutes to 4 hours, p.r.n. Maximum single dose shouldn't exceed 0.5 mg. Or, 0.004 to 0.005 ml/kg of 1:200 Sus-Phrine S.C.; repeat q 8 to 12 hours, p.r.n. Maximum single dose shouldn't exceed 0.75 mg.

➲ Hemostasis

Adults: 1:50,000 to 1:1,000, sprayed or applied topically.

➲ Acute asthma attacks
Adults and children age 4 and older: 1 inhalation, repeated once if needed after at least 1 minute; don't give subsequent doses for at least 3 hours. Or, 1 to 3 deep inhalations using a hand-bulb nebulizer containing 1% (1:100) solution of epinephrine or 2.25% solution of racepinephrine, repeated q 3 hours, p.r.n.

➲ To prolong local anesthetic effect
Adults and children: With local anesthetics, may be used in concentrations of 1:500,000 to 1:50,000; most commonly, 1:200,000.

➲ To restore cardiac rhythm in cardiac arrest
Adults: 0.5 to 1 mg I.V., repeated q 3 to 5 minutes, if needed. Higher-dose epinephrine may be used if 1-mg doses fail: 3- to 5-mg (about 0.1 mg/kg) doses of epinephrine, repeated q 3 to 5 minutes.
Children: 0.01 mg/kg (0.1 ml/kg of 1:10,000 injection) I.V. First endotracheal dose is 0.1 mg/kg (0.1 ml/kg of a 1:1,000 injection) diluted in 1 to 2 ml of half-normal or normal saline solution. Give subsequent I.V. or intratracheal doses from 0.1 to 0.2 mg/kg (0.1 to 0.2 ml/kg of a 1:1,000 injection), repeated q 3 to 5 minutes, if needed.

Contraindications & cautions

- Contraindicated in patients with angle-closure glaucoma, shock (other than anaphylactic shock), organic brain damage, cardiac dilation, arrhythmias, coronary insufficiency, or cerebral arteriosclerosis.
- Contraindicated in patients receiving general anesthesia with halogenated hydrocarbons or cyclopropane and in patients in labor (may delay second stage).
- Commercial products containing sulfites contraindicated in patients with sulfite allergies, except when epinephrine is being used to treat serious allergic reactions or other emergency situations.
- Contraindicated for use in fingers, toes, ears, nose, or genitalia when used with local anesthetic.
- Use cautiously in patients with long-standing bronchial asthma or emphysema who have developed degenerative heart disease.
- Use cautiously in elderly patients and in those with hyperthyroidism, CV disease, hypertension, psychoneurosis, and diabetes.

Adverse reactions

CNS: *nervousness, tremor*, vertigo, pain, *headache*, disorientation, agitation, *drowsiness*, fear, dizziness, weakness, ***cerebral hemorrhage, CVA***.
CV: *palpitations*, widened pulse pressure, hypertension, tachycardia, ***ventricular fibrillation, shock***, anginal pain, altered ECG (including a decreased T-wave amplitude).
GI: *nausea, vomiting.*
Respiratory: dyspnea.
Skin: urticaria, hemorrhage at injection site, pallor.
Other: tissue necrosis.

Interactions

Drug-drug. *Alpha blockers:* May cause hypotension from unopposed beta-adrenergic effects. Avoid using together.
Antihistamines, thyroid hormones: When given with sympathomimetics, may cause severe adverse cardiac effects. Avoid using together.
Cardiac glycosides, general anesthetics (halogenated hydrocarbons): May increase risk of ventricular arrhythmias. Monitor ECG closely.
Carteolol, nadolol, penbutolol, pindolol, propranolol, timolol: May cause hypertension followed by bradycardia. Stop beta blocker 3 days before starting epinephrine.
Doxapram, mazindol, methylphenidate: May enhance CNS stimulation or pressor effects. Monitor patient closely.
Ergot alkaloids: May decrease vasoconstrictor activity. Monitor patient closely.
Guanadrel, guanethidine: May enhance pressor effects of epinephrine. Monitor patient closely.
Levodopa: May enhance risk of arrhythmias. Monitor ECG closely.
MAO inhibitors: May increase risk of hypertensive crisis. Monitor blood pressure closely.
Tricyclic antidepressants: May potentiate the pressor response and cause arrhythmias. Use together cautiously.

Nursing considerations

- Drug increases rigidity and tremor in patients with Parkinson's disease.
- Epinephrine therapy interferes with tests for urinary catecholamines.
- One mg equals 1 ml of 1:1,000 solution or 10 ml of 1:10,000 solution.

- Epinephrine is drug of choice in emergency treatment of acute anaphylactic reactions.
- Discard epinephrine solution after 24 hours, or if it's discolored or contains precipitate. Keep solution in light-resistant container, and don't remove before use.

!!ALERT Avoid I.M. use of parenteral suspension into buttocks. Gas gangrene may occur because epinephrine reduces oxygen tension of the tissues, encouraging growth of contaminating organisms.

- Massage site after I.M. injection to counteract possible vasoconstriction. Repeated local injection can cause necrosis caused by vasoconstriction at injection site.
- Observe patient closely for adverse reactions. Notify prescriber if adverse reactions develop; dosage adjustment or drug discontinuation may be necessary.
- If blood pressure increases sharply, rapid-acting vasodilators such as nitrates or alpha blockers can be given to counteract the marked pressor effect of large doses of epinephrine.
- Epinephrine is rapidly destroyed by oxidizing products, such as iodine, chromates, nitrites, oxygen, and salts of easily reducible metals (such as iron).

!!ALERT Don't confuse epinephrine with ephedrine or norepinephrine.

- When treating patient with reactions caused by other drugs given I.M. or S.C., inject epinephrine into the site where the other drug was given to minimize further absorption.

Patient teaching

- Teach patient to perform oral inhalation correctly. Give the following instructions for using a metered-dose inhaler (MDI):
  - Shake canister.
  - Clear nasal passages and throat.
  - Breathe out, expelling as much air from lungs as possible.
  - Place mouthpiece well into mouth, and inhale deeply as you release dose from inhaler. Or, hold inhaler about 1 inch (two fingerwidths) from open mouth, and inhale while releasing dose.
  - Hold breath for several seconds, remove mouthpiece, and exhale slowly.
- If more than one inhalation is prescribed, advise patient to wait at least 2 minutes before repeating procedure.
- Tell patient that use of a spacer device may improve drug delivery to lungs.
- If patient is also using a corticosteroid inhaler, instruct him to use the bronchodilator first and then to wait about 5 minutes before using the corticosteroid. This lets the bronchodilator open the air passages for maximum effectiveness.
- Instruct patient to remove canister and wash inhaler with warm, soapy water at least once weekly.
- If patient has acute hypersensitivity reactions (such as to bee stings), you may need to teach him to self-inject epinephrine.

epinephrine hydrochloride (nasal)

Adrenalin Chloride

Pregnancy risk category C

Indications & dosages

➲ Nasal congestion, local superficial nasal bleeding

Adults and children age 6 and older: Instill 1 or 2 drops of solution into each nostril.

Contraindications & cautions

- Contraindicated in patients hypersensitive to drug.
- Use cautiously in patients with hyperthyroidism, coronary artery disease, hypertension, or diabetes mellitus.

Adverse reactions

CNS: nervousness, excitation.
CV: *tachycardia.*
EENT: rebound nasal congestion, slight stinging on application.

Interactions

None significant.

Nursing considerations

- Monitor heart rate.

!!ALERT Don't confuse epinephrine with ephedrine.

Patient teaching

- Teach patient how to instill nose drops.
- Caution patient not to share product to prevent spread of infection.
- Tell patient not to exceed recommended dosage and to use only when needed.

epinephrine hydrochloride (ophthalmic)
Epifrin, Glaucon

epinephryl borate
Epinal

Pregnancy risk category C

Indications & dosages
➲ Open-angle glaucoma
Adults: 1 or 2 drops of 1% or 2% solution once daily or b.i.d. Adjust dosage based on tonometric readings.

Contraindications & cautions
- Contraindicated in patients hypersensitive to drug or sulfites and in those with hypertensive CV disease or coronary artery disease.
- Contraindicated in patients with aphakia, those with angle-closure glaucoma, and those with glaucoma of unknown cause.
- Use cautiously in elderly patients and in those with diabetes mellitus, hypertension, Parkinson's disease, hyperthyroidism, cardiac disease, cerebral arteriosclerosis, or bronchial asthma.

Adverse reactions
CNS: browache, headache, light-headedness.
CV: palpitations, tachycardia, ***arrhythmias***, hypertension.
EENT: corneal or conjunctival pigmentation, corneal edema with long-term use, follicular hypertrophy, chemosis, conjunctivitis, iritis, hyperemic conjunctiva, eye stinging, burning, tearing on instillation, eye pain, allergic lid reaction, ocular irritation.
Skin: maculopapular rash.

Interactions
Drug-drug. *Antihistamines (dexchlorpheniramine, diphenhydramine), tricyclic antidepressants:* May increase cardiac effects of epinephrine. Monitor patient closely.
Beta blockers, osmotic drugs, systemic carbonic anhydrase inhibitors, topical miotics: May cause additive lowering of intraocular pressure. Use together cautiously.
Cardiac glycosides: May increase risk of arrhythmias. Monitor patient closely.
Cyclopropane, halogenated hydrocarbons: May cause arrhythmias, tachycardia. Use together cautiously, if at all.
Local or systemic sympathomimetics: May have additive toxic effects. Avoid using together.
MAO inhibitors: May exaggerate adrenergic effects. Adjust dosage of epinephrine carefully.

Nursing considerations
- Drug can be injected into anterior chamber to produce rapid mydriasis during cataract removal or can be used to control local bleeding during surgery.

!!ALERT The hydrochloride and borate formulations aren't interchangeable.
- Monitor blood pressure and other vital signs.

!!ALERT Don't confuse epinephrine with ephedrine, or Glaucon with glucagon.

Patient teaching
- Teach patient how to instill drug. Advise him to wash hands before and after instillation and to apply light finger pressure on lacrimal sac for 1 minute after drops are instilled. Warn him not to touch tip of dropper to eye or surrounding tissue.
- Urge patient to immediately report any decrease in visual acuity.
- Advise patient not to use drug while wearing soft contact lenses because lenses may discolor.
- Tell patient not to use darkened solution.

epirubicin hydrochloride
Ellence

Pregnancy risk category D

Indications & dosages
➲ Adjuvant therapy in patients with evidence of axillary node tumor involvement after resection of primary breast cancer
Adults: 100 to 120 mg/m^2 I.V. infusion over 3 to 5 minutes through a free-flowing I.V. solution on day 1 of each cycle, or divided equally in two doses on days 1 and 8 of each cycle; cycle repeated q 3 to 4 weeks for six cycles; used with regimens containing cyclophosphamide and fluorouracil.

Dosage modification after first cycle is based on toxicity. For patients with platelet count nadir below 50,000/mm^3, absolute neutrophil count (ANC) below 250/mm^3, neutropenic fever, or grade 3 or 4 nonhematologic toxicity, reduce day 1 dose in subsequent cycles to 75% of day 1 dose given in current cycle. Delay day 1 therapy in subsequent cycles until platelet count is at least 100,000/mm^3, ANC is at least 1,500/mm^3, and nonhematologic toxicities recover to grade 1.

For patients receiving divided doses (days 1 and 8), day 8 dose should be 75% of day 1 dose if platelet count is 75,000 to 100,000/mm^3 and ANC is 1,000 to 1,499/mm^3. If day 8 platelet count is below 75,000/mm^3, ANC is below 1,000/mm^3, or grade 3 or 4 nonhematologic toxicity has occurred, omit day 8 dose.

For patients with bone marrow dysfunction (heavily pretreated patients, patients with bone marrow depression, or those with neoplastic bone marrow infiltration), start at lower doses of 75 to 90 mg/m^2. For patients with hepatic dysfunction, if bilirubin is 1.2 to 3 mg/dl or AST is two to four times upper limit of normal, give one-half recommended starting dose. If bilirubin level is above 3 mg/dl or AST is more than four times upper limit of normal, give one-fourth recommended starting dose. For patients with severe renal dysfunction (creatinine level over 5 mg/dl), consider lower doses.

Contraindications & cautions

- Contraindicated in patients hypersensitive to drug, other anthracyclines, or anthracenediones, and in patients with baseline neutrophil counts below 1,500 cells/mm^3, severe myocardial insufficiency, recent MI, serious arrhythmias, or severe hepatic dysfunction.
- Contraindicated in patients who have had previous treatment with anthracyclines to total cumulative doses.
- Use cautiously in patients with active or dormant cardiac disease, previous or current radiotherapy to mediastinal and pericardial areas, or previous therapy with other anthracyclines or anthracenediones.
- Use cautiously in patients receiving other cardiotoxic drugs.

Adverse reactions

CNS: *lethargy*, fever.
CV: ***cardiomyopathy, heart failure***, hot flashes.
EENT: *conjunctivitis, keratitis.*
GI: *nausea, vomiting, diarrhea*, anorexia, *mucositis.*
GU: *amenorrhea*, red urine.
Hematologic: LEUKOPENIA, NEUTROPENIA, *febrile neutropenia, anemia*, THROMBOCYTOPENIA.
Skin: *alopecia*, rash, itch, skin changes, local toxicity.
Other: *infection.*

Interactions

Drug-drug. *Calcium channel blockers, other cardioactive compounds:* May increase risk of heart failure. Monitor cardiac function closely.
Cimetidine: May increase epirubicin level by 50%. Avoid using together.
Cytotoxic drugs: May cause additive toxicities (especially hematologic and GI). Monitor patient closely.

Nursing considerations

- Give drug under supervision of prescriber experienced in cancer chemotherapy. Don't handle drug if you are pregnant.
- Give patients receiving 120 mg/m^2 of epirubicin prophylactic antibiotic therapy with co-trimoxazole or a fluoroquinolone.
- Consider giving antiemetic before epirubicin to reduce nausea and vomiting.
- Before therapy starts, obtain total bilirubin, AST, and creatinine levels; CBC including ANC; and left ventricular ejection fraction (LVEF).
- Monitor LVEF regularly during therapy. Stop drug at first sign of impaired cardiac function. Early signs of cardiac toxicity include sinus tachycardia, ECG abnormalities, tachyarrhythmias, bradycardia, AV block, and bundle-branch block.
- Delayed cardiac toxicity may occur 2 to 3 months after treatment ends; indications include reduced LVEF and signs and symptoms of heart failure (tachycardia, dyspnea, pulmonary edema, dependent edema, hepatomegaly, ascites, pleural effusion, and gallop rhythm). Delayed cardiac toxicity depends on cumulative dose of epirubicin. Don't exceed cumulative dose of 900 mg/m^2.

• Obtain total and differential WBC, CBC, platelet counts, and liver function tests before and during each cycle of therapy.
• WBC nadir is usually reached 10 to 14 days after drug administration, and returns to normal by day 21.
• Monitor uric acid, potassium, calcium phosphate, and creatinine levels immediately after initial chemotherapy administration in patients susceptible to tumor lysis syndrome. Hydration, urine alkalinization, and prophylaxis with allopurinol may prevent hyperuricemia and minimize potential complications of tumor lysis syndrome.
• Epirubicin may enhance the effects of radiation therapy or cause an inflammatory cell reaction at irradiation site. Monitor patient closely.

Patient teaching

• Advise patient to report any pain or burning at site of injection during or after administration.
• Advise patient to report nausea, vomiting, mouth inflammation, dehydration, fever, evidence of infection, or symptoms of heart failure (rapid heartbeat, labored breathing, swelling).
• Tell patient that urine will be reddish-pink for 1 to 2 days after treatment.
• Inform patient of risk of heart damage and treatment-related leukemia with use of drug.
• Advise men to use effective contraception during treatment.
• Advise women that irreversible cessation of menstruation or premature menopause may occur.
• Tell patient that hair usually regrows within 2 to 3 months after therapy stops.

eplerenone
Inspra

Pregnancy risk category B

Indications & dosages

➲ Hypertension
Adults: 50 mg P.O. once daily. If response is inadequate after 4 weeks, increase dosage to 50 mg P.O. b.i.d. Maximum daily dose 100 mg.

In patients taking weak CYP3A4 inhibitors (erythromycin, fluconazole, saquinavir, verapamil), reduce eplerenone starting dose to 25 mg P.O. once daily.

➲ Heart failure after an MI
Adults: Initially, 25 mg P.O. once daily. Increase within 4 weeks, as tolerated and according to potassium level, to 50 mg P.O. once daily.

If potassium level is less than 5 mEq/L, increase dosage from 25 mg every other day to 25 mg daily; or increase dosage from 25 mg daily to 50 mg daily. If potassium level is 5 to 5.4 mEq/L, don't adjust dosage. If potassium level is 5.5 to 5.9 mEq/L, decrease dosage from 50 mg daily to 25 mg daily; or decrease dosage from 25 mg daily to 25 mg every other day; or if dosage was 25 mg every other day, withhold drug. If potassium level is greater than 6 mEq/L, withhold drug. May restart drug at 25 mg every other day when potassium level is less than 5.5 mEq/L. In patients taking weak CYP3A4 inhibitors (erythromycin, fluconazole, saquinavir, verapamil), reduce eplerenone starting dose to 25 mg P.O. once daily.

Contraindications & cautions

• When used for hypertension, contraindicated in patients with type 2 diabetes with microalbuminuria, creatinine level greater than 2 mg/dl in men or greater than 1.8 mg/dl in women, or creatinine clearance less than 50 ml/minute and in patients taking potassium supplements or potassium-sparing diuretics (amiloride, spironolactone, or triamterene).
• Contraindicated in patients with potassium level greater than 5.5 mEq/ml or creatinine clearance 30 ml/minute or less, and in patients taking strong CYP3A4 inhibitors, such as ketoconazole, clarithromycin, ritonavir, nefazodone, or itraconazole.
• Use cautiously in patient with mild to moderate hepatic impairment.
• Use in pregnant woman only if the potential benefits justify the potential risk to the fetus. Use cautiously in breast-feeding women; it's unknown if drug appears in breast milk.

Adverse reactions

CNS: dizziness, fatigue.
GI: diarrhea, abdominal pain.
GU: albuminuria, abnormal vaginal bleeding.
Metabolic: ***hyperkalemia***.

Respiratory: cough.
Other: flulike symptoms, gynecomastia.

Interactions

Drug-drug. *ACE inhibitors, angiotensin II receptor antagonists:* May increase risk of hyperkalemia. Use together cautiously.
Lithium: May increase risk of lithium toxicity. Monitor lithium level.
NSAIDs: May reduce the antihypertensive effect and cause severe hyperkalemia in patients with impaired renal function. Monitor blood pressure and potassium level.
Potassium supplements, potassium-sparing diuretics (amiloride, spironolactone, triamterene): May increase risk of hyperkalemia and sometimes-fatal arrhythmias. Avoid using together.
Strong CYP3A4 inhibitors (itraconazole, ketoconazole): May increase eplerenone level. Avoid using together.
Weak CYP3A4 inhibitors (erythromycin, fluconazole, saquinavir, verapamil): May increase eplerenone level. Reduce eplerenone starting dose to 25 mg P.O. once daily.
Drug-herb. *St. John's wort:* May decrease eplerenone level over time. Discourage use together.

Nursing considerations

- Drug may be used alone or with other antihypertensives.
- Full therapeutic effect of the drug occurs in 4 weeks.
- In patients with heart failure, measure potassium level at baseline, within the first week, at 1 month after starting therapy, and periodically thereafter.
- Monitor patient for signs and symptoms of hyperkalemia.

Patient teaching

- Inform patient that drug may be taken with or without food.
- Advise patient to avoid potassium supplements and salt substitutes during treatment.
- Tell patient to report adverse reactions.

epoetin alfa (erythropoietin)

Epogen, Procrit

Pregnancy risk category C

Indications & dosages

➲ Anemia from reduced production of endogenous erythropoietin caused by end-stage renal disease
Adults: Dosage is individualized. Starting dose is 50 to 100 units/kg I.V. three times weekly. Nondialysis patients with chronic renal failure or patients receiving continuous peritoneal dialysis may receive drug by S.C. injection or I.V. Maintenance dosage is highly individualized.

Reduce dosage when target hematocrit is reached or if hematocrit rises more than 4 points in 2 weeks. Increase dosage if hematocrit doesn't increase by 5 to 6 points after 8 weeks of therapy.

➲ Adjunctive treatment of HIV-infected patients with anemia from zidovudine therapy
Adults: 100 units/kg I.V. or S.C. three times weekly for 8 weeks or until target hemoglobin level is reached. If response isn't satisfactory after 8 weeks, increase dosage by 50 to 100 units/kg I.V. or S.C. three times weekly. After 4 to 8 weeks, further increase dosage in increments of 50 to 100 units/kg three times weekly, up to maximum of 300 units/kg I.V. or S.C. three times weekly.

➲ Anemia from cancer chemotherapy
Adults: 150 units/kg S.C. three times weekly for 8 weeks or until target hemoglobin level is reached. If response isn't satisfactory after 8 weeks, increase dosage up to 300 units/kg S.C. three times weekly.

If hematocrit exceeds 40%, withhold drug until hematocrit falls to 36%.

➲ Reduce need for allogenic blood transfusion in anemic patients scheduled to have elective, noncardiac, nonvascular surgery
Adults: 300 units/kg daily S.C. daily for 10 days before surgery, on day of surgery, and for 4 days after surgery. Or, 600 units/kg S.C. in once-weekly doses (21, 14, and 7 days before surgery), plus one-fourth dose on day of surgery.

➲ Anemia in pediatric patients with chronic renal failure who are having dialysis

Infants and children ages 1 month to 16 years: 50 units/kg I.V. or S.C. three times weekly. Maintenance dosage is highly individualized to keep hematocrit within target range.

Reduce dosage when target hematocrit is reached or if hematocrit increases more than 4 points in 2 weeks. Increase dosage if hematocrit doesn't increase by 5 to 6 points after 8 weeks of therapy and is below target range.

Contraindications & cautions

- Contraindicated in patients hypersensitive to products derived from mammal cells or albumin (human) and in those with uncontrolled hypertension.
- Use cautiously in breast-feeding women.

Adverse reactions

CNS: *headache*, ***seizures***, *paresthesia*, *fatigue*, dizziness, *asthenia*.
CV: *hypertension*, *edema*, increased clotting of arteriovenous grafts.
GI: *nausea*, *vomiting*, *diarrhea*.
Metabolic: hyperuricemia, ***hyperkalemia***, hyperphosphatemia.
Musculoskeletal: *arthralgia*.
Respiratory: *cough*, *shortness of breath*.
Skin: *rash*, *injection site reactions*, urticaria.
Other: *pyrexia*.

Interactions

None significant.

Nursing considerations

- Monitor blood pressure before therapy. Up to 80% of patients with chronic renal failure have hypertension. Blood pressure may increase, especially when hematocrit is increasing in the early part of therapy.
- If hematocrit is increasing and approaching 36%, reduce dosage to maintain target hematocrit range. If hematocrit remains unchanged after reducing dosage, withhold dose temporarily until hematocrit decreases.
- When used in HIV-infected patients, be prepared to individualize dosage based on response. Dosage recommendations are for patients with endogenous erythropoietin levels of 500 units/L or less and cumulative zidovudine doses of 4.2 g/week or less.
- Patient treated with epoetin alfa may need additional heparin to prevent clotting during dialysis treatments.
- Monitor blood count; increasing hematocrit may cause excessive clotting.
- Institute diet restrictions or drug therapy to control blood pressure. Reduce dosage in patients who exhibit rapid increase in hematocrit (more than 4 points in a 2-week period), to prevent hypertension.
- Patient's response to epoetin alfa depends on amount of endogenous erythropoietin in the plasma. Patients with levels of 500 units/L or more usually have transfusion-dependent anemia and probably won't respond to drug. Those with levels below 500 units/L usually respond well.
- Patient should receive adequate iron supplementation beginning no later than when epoetin alfa treatment starts and continuing throughout therapy. Patient also may need vitamin B_{12} and folic acid.

!! ALERT Don't confuse Epogen with Neupogen.

Patient teaching

- Inform patient that pain or discomfort in limbs (long bones) and pelvis, and coldness and sweating aren't uncommon after injection (usually occurring within 2 hours). Symptoms may last for 12 hours and then disappear.
- Advise patient that blood specimens will be drawn weekly for blood counts and that dosage adjustments may be made based on results.
- Advise patient to avoid driving or operating heavy machinery at start of therapy. There may be a relationship between excessively rapid hematocrit rise and seizures.
- Tell patient to monitor blood pressure at home and to adhere to dietary restrictions.
- Instruct patient to check that syringes used to give drug are in tenths-of-milliliter increments.

eprosartan mesylate
Teveten

Pregnancy risk category C; D in 2nd and 3rd trimesters

Indications & dosages

➲ **Hypertension (alone or with other antihypertensives)**
Adults: Initially, 600 mg P.O. daily. Dosage ranges from 400 to 800 mg daily, given as single daily dose or two divided doses.

Contraindications & cautions

- Contraindicated in patients hypersensitive to eprosartan or its components.
- Use cautiously in patients with renal artery stenosis; in patients with an activated renin-angiotensin system, such as volume- or salt-depleted patients; and in patients whose renal function may depend on the renin-angiotensin-aldosterone system, such as those with severe heart failure.
- Safety and effectiveness in children haven't been established.

Adverse reactions

CNS: depression, fatigue, headache, dizziness.
CV: chest pain, dependent edema.
EENT: pharyngitis, rhinitis, sinusitis.
GI: abdominal pain, dyspepsia, diarrhea.
GU: UTI.
Hematologic: ***neutropenia***.
Musculoskeletal: arthralgia, myalgia.
Respiratory: cough, upper respiratory tract infection, bronchitis.
Other: injury, viral infection.

Interactions

Drug-drug. *NSAIDs:* May decrease antihypertensive effects. Monitor blood pressure.
Drug-herb. *Ma huang:* May decrease antihypertensive effects. Discourage use together.

Nursing considerations

- Correct hypovolemia and hyponatremia before starting therapy to reduce risk of symptomatic hypotension.
- Monitor blood pressure closely for 2 hours at start of treatment. If hypotension occurs, place patient in a supine position and, if needed, give an I.V. infusion of normal saline solution.
- A transient episode of hypotension isn't a contraindication to continued treatment. Drug may be restarted once patient's blood pressure has stabilized.
- Drug may be used alone or with other antihypertensives, such as diuretics and calcium channel blockers. Maximal blood pressure response may take 2 or 3 weeks.
- Monitor patient for facial or lip swelling because angioedema has occurred with other angiotensin II antagonists.
- Closely observe infants exposed to eprosartan in utero for hypotension, oliguria, and hyperkalemia.

Patient teaching

- Advise woman of childbearing age to use a reliable form of contraception and to notify her prescriber immediately if pregnancy is suspected. Treatment may need to be stopped under medical supervision.
- Advise patient to report facial or lip swelling and signs and symptoms of infection, such as fever and sore throat.
- Tell patient to notify prescriber before taking OTC medication to treat a dry cough.
- Inform patient that drug may be taken without regard to meals.
- Advise breast-feeding woman to either stop therapy or stop breast-feeding because of potential for adverse reactions in infant.
- Tell patient to store drug at 68°to 77° F (20° to 25°C).

eptifibatide
Integrilin

Pregnancy risk category B

Indications & dosages

➲ **Acute coronary syndrome (unstable angina or non–Q-wave MI) in patients receiving drug therapy and in those having percutaneous coronary intervention (PCI)**
Adults: 180 mcg/kg I.V. bolus as soon as possible after diagnosis, followed by a continuous I.V. infusion at a rate of 2 mcg/kg/minute until hospital discharge or initiation of coronary artery bypass graft (CABG) surgery, for up to 72 hours. If patient is having PCI, continue infusion until hospital discharge or for 18 to 24 hours after the pro-

cedure, whichever comes first, for up to 96 hours. Patients weighing more than 121 kg (266 lb) should receive a bolus not to exceed 22.6 mg, followed by a maximum infusion rate of 15 mg/hour.

If creatinine clearance is less than 50 ml/minute or creatinine level is greater than 2 mg/dl, give 180 mcg/kg I.V. bolus as soon as possible after diagnosis, followed by a continuous I.V. infusion at a rate of 1 mcg/kg/minute. Patients with this creatinine clearance who weigh more than 121 kg should receive a bolus not to exceed 22.6 mg, followed by a maximum infusion rate of 7.5 mg/hour.

➲ **Patients having PCI**

Adults: 180 mcg/kg I.V. bolus given just before the procedure, immediately followed by an infusion of 2 mcg/kg/minute and a second I.V. bolus of 180 mcg/kg given 10 minutes after the first bolus. Continue infusion until hospital discharge or for 18 to 24 hours, whichever comes first; the minimum duration of infusion is 12 hours. Patients weighing more than 121 kg should receive a bolus not to exceed 22.6 mg, followed by a maximum infusion rate of 15 mg/hour.

If creatinine clearance is less than 50 ml/minute or creatinine level is greater than 2 mg/dl, give 180 mcg/kg I.V. bolus just before the procedure, immediately followed by a continuous I.V. infusion at 1 mcg/kg/minute and a second bolus of 180 mcg/kg given 10 minutes after the first bolus. Patients with this creatinine clearance who weigh more than 121 kg should receive a bolus not to exceed 22.6 mg, followed by a maximum infusion rate of 7.5 mg/hour.

Contraindications & cautions

- Contraindicated in patients hypersensitive to drug or its ingredients and in those with history of bleeding diathesis or evidence of active abnormal bleeding within previous 30 days; severe hypertension (systolic blood pressure higher than 200 mm Hg or diastolic blood pressure higher than 110 mm Hg) not adequately controlled with antihypertensives; major surgery within previous 6 weeks; history of CVA within 30 days or history of hemorrhagic CVA; current or planned use of another parenteral GP IIb/IIIa inhibitor; or platelet count less than 100,000/mm^3.
- Contraindicated in patients with creatinine level 4 mg/dl or higher and in patients dependent on renal dialysis.
- Use cautiously in patients at increased risk for bleeding, in those with platelet count less than 150,000/mm^3, in those with hemorrhagic retinopathy, and in those weighing more than 143 kg (315 lb).

Adverse reactions

CV: hypotension.
GU: hematuria.
Hematologic: *bleeding*, ***thrombocytopenia***.
Other: bleeding at femoral artery access site.

Interactions

Drug-drug. *Clopidogrel, dipyridamole, NSAIDs, oral anticoagulants (warfarin), thrombolytics, ticlopidine:* May increase risk of bleeding. Monitor patient closely.
Other inhibitors of platelet receptor IIb/IIIa: May cause serious bleeding. Avoid using together.

Nursing considerations

- Drug is intended for use with heparin and aspirin.
- Stop eptifibatide and heparin and achieve sheath hemostasis by standard compressive techniques at least 4 hours before hospital discharge.
- Remove sheath during eptifibatide infusion only after heparin has been stopped and its effects largely reversed.
- If patient is to undergo CABG surgery, stop infusion before surgery.
- Minimize use of arterial and venous punctures, I.M. injections, urinary catheters, and nasotracheal and nasogastric tubes.
- When obtaining I.V. access, avoid use of noncompressible sites (such as subclavian or jugular veins).
- Monitor patient for bleeding.

!!ALERT If patient's platelet count is less than 100,000/mm^3, stop eptifibatide and heparin.

- Perform baseline laboratory tests before start of drug therapy; also determine hemoglobin, hematocrit, PT, INR, APTT, platelet count, and creatinine level.

Patient teaching

- Explain that drug is a blood thinner used to prevent chest pain and heart attack.

• Explain that benefits of drug far outweigh risk of serious bleeding.
• Tell patient to report to prescriber chest discomfort or other adverse effects immediately.

erlotinib
Tarceva

Pregnancy risk category D

Indications & dosages

➲ Locally advanced or metastatic non-small-cell lung cancer after failure of at least one chemotherapy regimen.
Adults: 150 mg P.O. once daily taken at least 1 hour before or 2 hours after meals. Continue until disease progresses or intolerable toxicity occurs.

In patients with severe skin reactions or severe diarrhea refractory to loperamide, reduce dose in 50-mg decrements or stop therapy.

Contraindications & cautions

• None reported
• Use cautiously in patients with pulmonary disease or liver impairment. Also use cautiously in patients who have received or are receiving chemotherapy because it may worsen adverse pulmonary effects.

Adverse reactions

CNS: *fatigue.*
EENT: *conjunctivitis, keratoconjuctivitis sicca.*
GI: *abdominal pain, anorexia, diarrhea, nausea, stomatitis, vomiting.*
Respiratory: *cough, dyspnea,* ***pulmonary toxicity.***
Skin: *dry skin, pruritus, rash.*
Other: *infection.*

Interactions

Drug-drug. *Anticoagulants, such as warfarin:* May increase risk of bleeding. Monitor PT and INR.
Atazanavir, clarithromycin, indinavir, itraconazole, ketoconazole, nefazodone, nelfinavir, ritonavir, saquinavir, telithromycin, troleandomycin, voriconazole: May decrease erlotinib metabolism. Use together cautiously, and consider reducing erlotinib dosage.
Carbamazepine, phenobarbital, phenytoin, rifampicin, rifabutin: May increase erlotinib metabolism. Erlotinib dosage may need to be increased.
Drug-herb. *St. John's wort:* May increase erlotinib metabolism. Drug dosage may need to be increased. Discourage use together.

Nursing considerations

• Monitor liver function tests periodically during therapy. Notify prescriber if values change dramatically. Dose may need to be reduced or drug stopped.
!!ALERT Rarely, serious interstitial lung disease may occur. If patient develops dyspnea, cough, and fever, notify prescriber. Therapy may need to be interrupted. Stop drug if interstitial lung disease has developed.
• Monitor patient for severe diarrhea, and give loperamide if needed.
• Women of childbearing potential should use contraception while taking this drug and for 2 weeks afterward.
• If patient becomes pregnant during therapy, drug may harm fetus and increase risk of miscarriage.
• Women shouldn't breast-feed while taking this drug.

Patient teaching

!!ALERT Tell patient to immediately report new or worsened cough, shortness of breath, eye irritation, or severe or persistent diarrhea, nausea, anorexia, or vomiting.
• Instruct patient to take drug 1 hour before or 2 hours after food.
• Advise women of childbearing potential to use contraception while taking this drug and for 2 weeks afterward.
• Explain the likelihood of serious interactions with other drugs and herbal supplements and the need to tell prescriber about any change in drugs and supplements taken.

ertapenem sodium
Invanz

Pregnancy risk category B

Indications & dosages

➲ **Complicated intra-abdominal infections caused by *Escherichia coli, Clostridium clostridiiforme, Eubacterium lentum, Peptostreptococcus* species, *Bacteroides fragilis, B. distasonis, B. ovatus, B. thetaiotaomicron,* or *B. uniformis***
Adults and children age 13 and older: 1 g I.V. or I.M. once daily for 5 to 14 days.
Infants and children age 3 months to 13 years: 15 mg/kg I.V. or I.M. q 12 hours for 5 to 14 days. Don't exceed 1 g daily.

➲ **Complicated skin and skin-structure infections caused by *Staphylococcus aureus* (methicillin-susceptible strains), *Streptococcus pyogenes, E. coli,* or *Peptostreptococcus* species**
Adults and children age 13 and older: 1 g I.V. or I.M. once daily for 7 to 14 days.
Infants and children age 3 months to 13 years: 15 mg/kg I.V. or I.M. q 12 hours for 7 to 14 days. Don't exceed 1 g daily.

➲ **Community-acquired pneumonia from *S. pneumoniae* (penicillin-susceptible strains), *Haemophilus influenzae* (beta-lactamase–negative strains), or *Moraxella catarrhalis;* complicated UTIs, including pyelonephritis, caused by *E. coli* or *Klebsiella pneumoniae***
Adults and children age 13 and older: 1 g I.V. or I.M. once daily for 10 to 14 days. If patient improves after at least 3 days of treatment, use appropriate oral therapy to complete the full course of therapy.
Infants and children age 3 months to 13 years: 15 mg/kg I.V. or I.M. q 12 hours for 10 to 14 days. Don't exceed 1 g daily. If patient improves after at least 3 days of treatment, use appropriate oral therapy to complete the full course of therapy.

➲ **Acute pelvic infections including postpartum endomyometritis, septic abortion, and postsurgical gynecologic infections caused by *S. agalactiae, E. coli, B. fragilis, Porphyromonas asaccharolyticus, Peptostreptococcus* species, or *Prevotella bivia***
Adults and children age 13 and older: 1 g I.V. or I.M. once daily for 3 to 10 days.
Infants and children age 3 months to 13 years: 15 mg/kg I.V. or I.M. q 12 hours for 3 to 10 days. Don't exceed 1 g daily.

In adult patients with creatinine clearance of 30 ml/minute or less, give 500 mg/day. In hemodialysis patients receiving daily 500-mg dose less than 6 hours before hemodialysis, give supplementary 150-mg dose afterward. In hemodialysis patients receiving dose 6 hours or more before hemodialysis, no supplementary dose is needed.

Contraindications & cautions

- Contraindicated in patients hypersensitive to any component of the drug or to other drugs in the same class and in patients who have had anaphylactic reactions to beta-lactams. I.M. use is contraindicated in patients hypersensitive to local anesthetics of the amide type (because of the diluent lidocaine hydrochloride).
- Use cautiously in patients with CNS disorders, compromised renal function, or both, as seizures may occur in these patients.

Adverse reactions

CNS: fever, asthenia, fatigue, anxiety, altered mental status, dizziness, headache, insomnia.
CV: edema, swelling, chest pain, hypertension, hypotension, tachycardia, infused vein complication, phlebitis, thrombophlebitis.
EENT: pharyngitis.
GI: abdominal pain, acid regurgitation, oral candidiasis, constipation, *diarrhea*, dyspepsia, nausea, vomiting.
GU: vaginitis, renal dysfunction.
Hematologic: coagulation abnormalities, eosinophilia, anemia, ***neutropenia, leukopenia, thrombocytopenia***, thrombocytosis.
Hepatic: jaundice.
Metabolic: hyperglycemia, ***hyperkalemia***.
Musculoskeletal: leg pain.
Respiratory: cough, dyspnea, rales, rhonchi, respiratory distress.
Skin: erythema, pruritus, rash, extravasation, infusion site pain and redness.
Other: hypersensitivity reactions.

Interactions

Drug-drug. *Probenecid:* May reduce renal clearance and may increase half-life. Don't give together with probenecid to extend half-life.

Nursing considerations

- Check for previous penicillin, cephalosporin, or other beta-lactam hypersensitivity before giving first dose.
- Check for hypersensitivity to local anesthetics of the amide type if giving dose I.M.
- Obtain specimens for culture and sensitivity testing before giving first dose. Therapy may start pending results.
- To give I.M., reconstitute 1-g vial with 3.2 ml of 1% lidocaine hydrochloride injection (without epinephrine). Shake vial thoroughly to form solution. Immediately withdraw the contents of the vial and give by deep I.M. injection into a large muscle, such as the gluteal muscles or lateral part of the thigh. Use the reconstituted I.M. solution within 1 hour after preparation. Don't give reconstituted solution I.V.
- Don't store lyophilized powder above 77° F (25° C). The reconstituted solution, immediately diluted in normal saline, may be stored at room temperature (25° C) and used within 6 hours or refrigerated for 24 hours at 41° F (5° C) and used within 4 hours after removal from refrigeration. Don't freeze solutions of ertapenem.
- If diarrhea persists during therapy, notify prescriber and collect stool specimen for culture to rule out pseudomembranous colitis.
- Vomiting occurs more frequently in children than adults. Monitor children closely for signs and symptoms of dehydration and electrolyte imbalance.
- If allergic reaction occurs, stop drug immediately.
- Anaphylactic reactions require immediate emergency treatment with epinephrine, oxygen, I.V. steroids, and airway management.
- Anticonvulsants may continue in patients with seizure disorders. If focal tremors, myoclonus, or seizures occur, notify prescriber. The dosage of ertapenem may need to be decreased or stopped.
- Monitor renal, hepatic, and hematopoietic function during prolonged therapy.
- Methicillin-resistant staphylococci and *Enterococcus* species are resistant to ertapenem.

!!ALERT Don't confuse Invanz (ertapenem) with Avinza (morphine sulfate)

Patient teaching

- Inform patient of potential adverse reactions.
- Tell patient to alert nurse if discomfort occurs at injection site.

erythromycin (ophthalmic)

Ilotycin

Pregnancy risk category B

Indications & dosages

➲ Acute and chronic conjunctivitis, other eye infections

Adults and children: Apply a ribbon of ointment about 1 cm long directly to infected eye up to six times daily, depending on severity of infection.

➲ Chlamydial ophthalmic infections (trachoma)

Adults and children: Apply small amount to each eye b.i.d. for 2 months or b.i.d. on first 5 days of each month for 6 months.

➲ To prevent ophthalmia neonatorum caused by *Neisseria gonorrhoeae* or *Chlamydia trachomatis*

Neonates: Apply a ribbon of ointment about 1 cm long in lower conjunctival sac of each eye shortly after birth.

Contraindications & cautions

- Contraindicated in patients hypersensitive to drug.
- Use cautiously in breast-feeding women.

Adverse reactions

EENT: slowed corneal wound healing, blurred vision, itching and burning eyes.
Skin: urticaria, dermatitis.
Other: overgrowth of nonsusceptible organisms with long-term use.

Interactions

None significant.

Nursing considerations

- To prevent ophthalmia neonatorum, apply ointment no later than 1 hour after birth. Drug is used in neonates born either vaginally or by cesarean section. Gently massage eyelids for 1 minute to spread ointment.
- Use drug only when sensitivity studies show it's effective against infecting orga-

nisms; don't use in infections of unknown cause.
• Store drug at room temperature in tightly closed, light-resistant container.

Patient teaching

• Tell patient to clean eye area of excessive discharge before application.
• Teach patient how to apply drug. Advise him to wash hands before and after applying ointment, and warn him not to touch tip of applicator to eye or surrounding tissue.
• Tell patient that vision may be blurred for a few minutes after applying ointment.
• Advise patient to watch for and report signs and symptoms of sensitivity (itching lids, redness, swelling, or constant burning).
• Tell patient not to share drug, washcloths, or towels with family members and to notify prescriber if anyone develops same signs or symptoms.
• Stress importance of compliance with recommended therapy.

erythromycin (topical)

Akne-mycin, A/T/S, Del-Mycin, Emgel, Erycette, EryDerm, Erygel, Erymax, EryPads, Ery-Sol†, ETS†, Sans-Acne†, Staticin, T-Stat†

Pregnancy risk category C; B (for EryDerm, Erygel)

Indications & dosages

➲ Inflammatory acne vulgaris
Adults and children: Apply to affected areas b.i.d., morning and evening.

Contraindications & cautions

• Contraindicated in patients hypersensitive to drug or its components.

Adverse reactions

Skin: sensitivity reactions, erythema, *burning, dryness, pruritus*, irritation, peeling, oily skin.

Interactions

Drug-drug. *Clindamycin:* May antagonize clindamycin's effect. Avoid using together. *Isotretinoin:* May cause cumulative dryness, resulting in excessive skin irritation. Use together cautiously.

Drug-lifestyle. *Abrasive or medicated soaps or cleansers, acne products, or other preparations containing peeling drugs (benzoyl peroxide, resorcinol, salicylic acid, sulfur, tretinoin), alcohol-containing products (aftershave, cosmetics, perfumed toiletries, shaving creams or lotions), astringent soaps or cosmetics, medicated cosmetics or coverups:* May cause cumulative dryness, resulting in excessive skin irritation. Urge caution.

Nursing considerations

• Wash, rinse, and dry affected areas before application.
• Prolonged use may be needed when treating acne vulgaris, which may result in overgrowth of nonsusceptible organisms.

Patient teaching

• Advise patient to wash, rinse, and dry face thoroughly before each use.
• Advise patient to avoid use near eyes, nose, mouth, or other mucous membranes.
• Tell patient to wash hands after each application.
• Tell patient to stop using drug and notify prescriber if no improvement occurs or if condition worsens in 3 to 12 weeks.
• Advise patient not to share towels or washcloths.
• Instruct patient to use each pledget once, then discard.
• Caution patient to keep drug away from heat and open flame.

erythromycin base

Apo-Erythro Base†, E-Base, E-Mycin, Erybid†, Eryc, Ery-Tab, Erythromycin Base Filmtab, Erythromycin Delayed-Release, PCE Dispertab

erythromycin estolate

Ilosone, Ilosone Pulvules

erythromycin ethylsuccinate

Apo-Erythro-ES†, E.E.S, EES Granules, EryPed, EryPed 200, EryPed 400

erythromycin lactobionate

Erythrocin

erythromycin stearate
Apo-Erythro-S†, Erythrocin Stearate

Pregnancy risk category B

Indications & dosages

➲ **Acute pelvic inflammatory disease caused by *Neisseria gonorrhoeae***
Adults: 500 mg I.V. lactobionate q 6 hours for 3 days; then 250 mg base or stearate or 400 mg ethylsuccinate P.O. q 6 hours for 7 days.

➲ **Intestinal amebiasis caused by *Entamoeba histolytica***
Adults: 250 mg P.O. q.i.d. or 333 mg P.O. q 8 hours, or 500 mg delayed-release tablets P.O. q 12 hours for 10 to 14 days.
Children: 30 to 50 mg/kg P.O. daily, in divided doses, for 10 to 14 days.

➲ **Erythrasma**
Adults: 250 mg P.O. t.i.d. for 21 days.

➲ **To prevent rheumatic fever**
Adults: 250 mg base, estolate, or stearate P.O. b.i.d; or, 400 mg ethylsuccinate P.O. b.i.d.

➲ **Mild to moderately severe respiratory tract, skin, and soft-tissue infections from sensitive group A beta-hemolytic streptococci, *Streptococcus pneumoniae, Mycoplasma pneumoniae, Corynebacterium diphtheriae,* or *Bordetella pertussis***
Adults: 250 to 500 mg base, estolate, or stearate P.O. q 6 hours; or 400 to 800 mg ethylsuccinate P.O. q 6 hours; or 15 to 20 mg/kg I.V. daily, as continuous infusion or in divided doses q 6 hours for 10 days (3 weeks for *Mycoplasma* species infection).
Children: 30 to 50 mg/kg oral erythromycin salts P.O. daily, in divided doses q 6 hours; or 15 to 20 mg/kg I.V. daily, in divided doses q 4 to 6 hours for 10 days (3 weeks for *Mycoplasma* species infection).

➲ ***Listeria monocytogenes* infection**
Adults: 250 mg P.O. q 6 hours or 500 mg P.O. q 12 hours.

➲ **Nongonococcal urethritis caused by *Ureaplasma urealyticum***
Adults: 500 mg P.O. q 6 hours for at least 7 days or 250 mg P.O. q.i.d. for 14 days if patient can't tolerate higher doses.

➲ **Syphilis in patients allergic to penicillin**
Adults: 500 mg P.O. q.i.d. for 2 weeks.

➲ **Legionnaires' disease**
Adults: 1 to 4 g P.O. daily in divided doses for 10 to 14 days alone or with rifampin. I.V. route may be used initially in severe cases.

➲ **Uncomplicated urethral, endocervical, or rectal infections caused by *Chlamydia trachomatis,* when tetracyclines are contraindicated**
Adults: 500 mg base P.O. q.i.d. for at least 7 days, or 666 mg P.O. q 8 hours for at least 7 days, or 250 mg P.O. q.i.d. for 14 days if patient can't tolerate higher doses.

➲ **Urogenital *C. trachomatis* infections during pregnancy**
Adults: 500 mg base, estolate, or stearate P.O. q.i.d. for at least 7 days or 250 mg base, estolate, or stearate or 400 mg ethylsuccinate P.O. q.i.d. for at least 14 days.

➲ **Conjunctivitis caused by *C. trachomatis* in neonates**
Neonates: 50 mg/kg base, estolate, or stearate P.O. daily in four divided doses for 14 days.

➲ **Pneumonia in infants caused by *C. trachomatis***
Infants: 50 mg/kg/day base, estolate, or stearate P.O. in four divided doses for 21 days, or 15 to 20 mg/kg/day lactobionate I.V. as a continuous infusion or in four divided doses.

➲ **Chancroid caused by *Haemophilus ducreyi*♦**
Adults: 500 mg base P.O. q.i.d. for 7 days.

➲ **Diarrhea caused by *Campylobacter jejuni* enteritis or enterocolitis**
Adults: 500 mg base P.O. q.i.d. for 7 days.

Contraindications & cautions

- Contraindicated in pregnant patients and those hypersensitive to drug or other macrolides.
- Erythromycin estolate is contraindicated in patients with hepatic disease.
- Use erythromycin salts cautiously in patients with impaired hepatic function. Monitor liver function test results.
- Erythromycin estolate isn't recommended during pregnancy because of the potential adverse effects on the mother and fetus.
- Drug appears in breast milk. Use cautiously in breast-feeding women.
- Don't use drug to treat neurosyphilis.

Adverse reactions

CNS: fever.

CV: ***ventricular arrhythmias***, *vein irritation or thrombophlebitis after I.V. injection.*
EENT: hearing loss (with high I.V. doses).
GI: *abdominal pain and cramping, nausea, vomiting, diarrhea.*
Hepatic: cholestatic jaundice (with erythromycin estolate).
Skin: urticaria, rash, eczema.
Other: overgrowth of nonsusceptible bacteria or fungi, ***anaphylaxis***.

Interactions

Drug-drug. *Carbamazepine:* May inhibit metabolism of carbamazepine, increasing blood level and risk of toxicity. Avoid using together.
Clindamycin, lincomycin: May be antagonistic. Avoid using together.
Cyclosporine: May increase cyclosporine level. Monitor drug level.
Digoxin: May increase digoxin level. Monitor patient for digoxin toxicity.
Disopyramide: May increase disopyramide level, which may cause arrhythmias and prolonged QT intervals. Monitor ECG.
Midazolam, triazolam: May increase effects of these drugs. Monitor patient closely.
Oral anticoagulants: May increase anticoagulant effect. Monitor PT and INR closely.
Other drugs that prolong the QTc interval (amiodarone, antipsychotics, fluoroquinolones, procainamide, quinidine, sotalol, tricyclic antidepressants): May have additive effects. Monitor ECG for QTc interval prolongation. Avoid using together, if possible.
Strong CYP3A inhibitors (such as diltiazem, verapamil, troleandomycin): May increase the risk of sudden death from cardiac causes. Don't use together.
Theophylline: May decrease erythromycin level and increase theophylline toxicity. Use together cautiously.
Drug-herb. *Pill-bearing spurge:* May inhibit CYP3A enzymes, affecting drug metabolism. Urge caution.

Nursing considerations

- Obtain urine specimen for culture and sensitivity tests before giving first dose. Therapy may begin pending results.
- When giving suspension, note the concentration.
- Monitor patient for superinfection. Drug may cause overgrowth of nonsusceptible bacteria or fungi.
- Monitor hepatic function. Erythromycin estolate may cause serious hepatotoxicity in adults (reversible cholestatic jaundice). Other erythromycin salts cause less serious hepatotoxicity.
- Ototoxicity may occur, especially in patients with renal or hepatic insufficiency and in those receiving high doses of drug.
- Coated tablets or encapsulated pellets cause less GI upset, so they may be better tolerated by patients who can't tolerate erythromycin.

Patient teaching

- Tell patient to take drug as prescribed, even after he feels better.
- Instruct patient to take oral form of drug with full glass of water 1 hour before or 2 hours after meals for best absorption.
- Drug may be taken with food if GI upset occurs. Tell patient not to take drug with fruit juice or to swallow whole chewable erythromycin tablets.
- Instruct patient to report adverse reactions, especially nausea, abdominal pain, vomiting, and fever.

escitalopram oxalate
Lexapro

Pregnancy risk category C

Indications & dosages

➲ Treatment and maintenance therapy for patients with major depressive disorder
Adults: Initially, 10 mg P.O. once daily, increasing to 20 mg if necessary after at least 1 week.

For elderly patients and those with hepatic impairment, 10 mg P.O. daily, initially and as maintenance dosages.

Contraindications & cautions

- Contraindicated in patients taking MAO inhibitors or within 14 days of MAO inhibitor therapy and in those hypersensitive to escitalopram, citalopram, or any of its inactive ingredients.
- Use cautiously in patients with a history of mania, seizure disorders, suicidal thoughts, or renal or hepatic impairment.

- Use cautiously in patients with diseases that produce altered metabolism or hemodynamic responses.
- Use with caution in elderly patients because they may have greater sensitivity to drug.
- Use in third trimester of pregnancy may be associated with neonatal complications at birth. Consider the risk versus benefit of treatment during this time.
- Drug appears in breast milk. Patient should either stop breast-feeding or stop taking drug.

Adverse reactions

CNS: fever, insomnia, dizziness, somnolence, paresthesia, light-headedness, migraine, tremor, vertigo, abnormal dreams, irritability, impaired concentration, fatigue, lethargy, ***suicidal behavior***.
CV: palpitations, hypertension, flushing, chest pain.
EENT: rhinitis, sinusitis, blurred vision, tinnitus, earache.
GI: *nausea*, diarrhea, constipation, indigestion, abdominal pain, vomiting, increased or decreased appetite, dry mouth, flatulence, heartburn, cramps, gastroesophageal reflux.
GU: ejaculation disorder, impotence, anorgasmia, menstrual cramps, UTI, urinary frequency.
Metabolic: weight gain or loss.
Musculoskeletal: arthralgia, myalgia, muscle cramps, pain in arms or legs.
Respiratory: bronchitis, cough.
Skin: rash, increased sweating.
Other: decreased libido, yawning, flulike symptoms.

Interactions

Drug-drug. *Carbamazepine:* May increase escitalopram clearance. Monitor patient for expected antidepressant effect and adjust dose as needed.
Cimetidine: May increase escitalopram level. Monitor patient for increased adverse reactions to escitalopram.
Citalopram: May cause additive effects. Avoid using together.
CNS drugs: May cause additive effects. Use together cautiously.
Desipramine, other drugs metabolized by CYP2D6: May increase levels of these drugs. Use together cautiously.
Lithium: May enhance serotonergic effect of escitalopram. Use together cautiously, and monitor lithium level.
MAO inhibitors: May cause serious, sometimes fatal, serotonin syndrome. Avoid using within 14 days of MAO inhibitor therapy.
Sumatriptan: May increase serotonergic effects, leading to weakness, enhanced reflex response, and incoordination. Use together cautiously.
Drug-lifestyle. *Alcohol use:* May increase CNS effects. Discourage use together.

Nursing considerations

- Closely monitor patients at high risk of suicide.
- Evaluate patient for history of drug abuse and observe for signs of misuse or abuse.
- Periodically reassess patient to determine need for maintenance treatment and appropriate dosing.

Patient teaching

- Inform patient that symptoms should improve gradually over several weeks, rather than immediately.
- Tell patient that although improvement may occur within 1 to 4 weeks, he should continue drug should as prescribed.
- Tell patient to use caution while driving or operating hazardous machinery because of drug's potential to impair judgment, thinking, or motor skills.
- Advise patient to consult health care provider before taking other prescription or OTC drugs.
- Tell patient that drug may be taken in the morning or evening without regard to meals.
- Encourage patient to avoid alcohol while taking drug.
- Tell patient to notify health care provider if she's pregnant or breast-feeding.

esmolol hydrochloride
Brevibloc

Pregnancy risk category C

Indications & dosages

➲ **Supraventricular tachycardia; postoperative tachycardia or hypertension; noncompensatory sinus tachycardias**

Adults: 500 mcg/kg/minute as loading dose by I.V. infusion over 1 minute; then 4-minute maintenance infusion of 50 mcg/kg/minute. If adequate response doesn't occur within 5 minutes, repeat loading dose and follow with maintenance infusion of 100 mcg/kg/minute for 4 minutes. Repeat loading dose and increase maintenance infusion by increments of 50 mcg/kg/minute. Maximum maintenance infusion for tachycardia is 200 mcg/kg/minute.

➲ **Intraoperative tachycardia or hypertension**

Adults: For intraoperative treatment of tachycardia or hypertension, 80 mg (about 1 mg/kg) I.V. bolus over 30 seconds; then 150 mcg/kg/minute I.V. infusion, if needed. Titrate infusion rate, p.r.n., to maximum of 300 mcg/kg/minute.

Contraindications & cautions

- Contraindicated in patients with sinus bradycardia, second- or third-degree heart block, cardiogenic shock, or overt heart failure.
- Use cautiously if patient has renal impairment, diabetes, or bronchospasm.

Adverse reactions

CNS: anxiety, depression, dizziness, somnolence, headache, agitation, fatigue, confusion.
CV: HYPOTENSION, peripheral ischemia.
GI: nausea, vomiting.
Skin: inflammation or induration at infusion site.

Interactions

Drug-drug. *Digoxin:* May increase digoxin level by 10% to 20%. Monitor digoxin level.
Morphine: May increase esmolol level. Adjust esmolol dosage carefully.
Prazosin: May increase risk of orthostatic hypotension. Help patient to stand slowly until effects are known.
Reserpine, other catecholamine-depleting drugs: May increase bradycardia and hypotension. Adjust esmolol dosage carefully.
Succinylcholine: May prolong neuromuscular blockade. Monitor patient closely.
Verapamil: May increase the effects of both drugs. Monitor cardiac function closely and decrease dosages as necessary.

Nursing considerations

- Dosage for postoperative treatment of tachycardia and hypertension is same as for supraventricular tachycardia.

!!ALERT Monitor ECG and blood pressure continuously during infusion. Up to 50% of all patients treated with esmolol develop hypotension. Diaphoresis and dizziness may accompany hypotension. Monitor patient closely, especially if he had low blood pressure before treatment.

- Hypotension can usually be reversed within 30 minutes by decreasing the dose or, if needed, by stopping the infusion. Notify prescriber if this becomes necessary.
- If a local reaction develops at the infusion site, change to another site. Avoid using butterfly needles.
- Esmolol should be used for no longer than 48 hours. Watch infusion site carefully for signs of extravasation; if they occur, stop infusion immediately and call prescriber.
- When patient's heart rate becomes stable, esmolol will be replaced by alternative (longer-acting) antiarrhythmics, such as propranolol, digoxin, or verapamil. A half-hour after the first dose of the alternative drug is given, reduce infusion rate by 50%. Monitor patient response and, if heart rate is controlled for 1 hour after administration of the second dose of the alternative drug, stop esmolol infusion.

Patient teaching

- Instruct patient to report adverse reactions promptly.
- Tell patient to report discomfort at I.V. site.

esomeprazole magnesium
Nexium

esomeprazole sodium
Nexium I.V.

Pregnancy risk category B

Indications & dosages

➲ **Gastroesophageal reflux disease (GERD), healing erosive esophagitis**
Adults: 20 or 40 mg P.O. daily for 4 to 8 weeks. Maintenance dose for healing erosive esophagitis is 20 mg P.O. for no longer than 6 months.

➲ **Symptomatic GERD**
Adults: 20 mg P.O. daily for 4 weeks. If symptoms are unresolved, may continue treatment for 4 more weeks.

➲ **Short-term therapy (up to 10 days) of GERD in patients with a history of erosive esophagitis who are unable to take drug orally.**
Adult: Reconstitute 20 or 40 mg with 5 ml of D_5W, normal saline solution, or lactated Ringer's injection and give by I.V. bolus over 3 minutes. Or, further dilute to a total volume of 50 ml and give I.V. over 10 to 30 minutes. Switch patient to oral therapy as soon as he can tolerate it.

➲ **To reduce the risk of gastric ulcers in patients receiving continuous NSAID therapy**
Adults: 20 or 40 mg P.O. once daily for up to 6 months.

➲ ***Helicobacter pylori* eradication**
Adults: 40 mg esomeprazole magnesium P.O. daily, 1,000 mg amoxicillin P.O. b.i.d., and 500 mg clarithromycin P.O. b.i.d., given together for 10 days to reduce duodenal ulcer recurrence.

For patient with severe hepatic failure, maximum daily dose is 20 mg.

Contraindications & cautions

- Contraindicated in patients hypersensitive to drug or components of esomeprazole or omeprazole.
- Use cautiously in patients with hepatic insufficiency and in pregnant or breast-feeding women.
- Patients receiving continuous NSAID therapy who are at increased risk for gastric ulcers include those age 60 and older or those with a history of gastric ulcers.

Adverse reactions

CNS: headache.
GI: dry mouth, diarrhea, abdominal pain, nausea, flatulence, vomiting, constipation.

Interactions

Drug-drug. *Amoxicillin, clarithromycin:* May increase levels of esomeprazole. Monitor patient for toxicity.
Diazepam: May decrease clearance of diazepam. Monitor patient for diazepam toxicity.
Drugs metabolized by CYP2C19: May alter clearance of esomeprazole, especially in elderly patients or patients with hepatic insufficiency. Monitor patient for toxicity.
Warfarin: May prolong PT and INR causing abnormal bleeding. Monitor the patient and his PT and INR.
Drug-food. *Any food:* May reduce drug level. Advise patient to take drug 1 hour before food.

Nursing considerations

- Give drug at least 1 hour before meals. If patient has difficulty swallowing the capsule, contents of the capsule can be emptied and mixed with 1 tablespoon of applesauce and swallowed (without chewing the enteric-coated pellets).
- Antacids can be used while taking drug, unless otherwise directed by prescriber.
- Monitor patient for rash or signs and symptoms of hypersensitivity. Monitor GI symptoms for improvement or worsening. Monitor liver function tests, especially in patients with preexisting hepatic disease.
- Long-term therapy with omeprazole, a drug similar to esomeprazole, may cause atrophic gastritis.
- It's unknown if drug appears in breast milk. Because omeprazole does appear in breast milk, use esomeprazole cautiously in breast-feeding women.

Patient teaching

- Instruct patient to take drug exactly as prescribed.
- Tell patient to take drug at least 1 hour before a meal.

- Advise patient that antacids can be used while taking drug unless otherwise directed by prescriber.
- Warn patient not to chew or crush drug pellets because this makes the drug ineffective.
- If patient has difficulty swallowing capsule, tell him to mix contents of capsule with 1 tablespoon of soft applesauce and swallow immediately.
- Advise patient to store capsules at room temperature in a tight container.
- Tell patient to inform prescriber of worsening signs and symptoms or pain.
- Instruct patient to alert prescriber if rash or other signs and symptoms of allergy occur.

estazolam
ProSom

Pregnancy risk category X
Controlled substance schedule IV

Indications & dosages

➲ Insomnia

Adults: 1 mg P.O. h.s. Some patients may need 2 mg.
Elderly patients: 1 mg P.O. h.s. Use higher doses with extreme care. Frail, elderly, or debilitated patients may take 0.5 mg, but this low dose may be only marginally effective.

Contraindications & cautions

- Contraindicated in pregnant patients and in those hypersensitive to drug.
- Use cautiously in patients with depression, suicidal tendencies, or hepatic, renal, or pulmonary disease.

Adverse reactions

CNS: fatigue, dizziness, daytime drowsiness, *somnolence, asthenia*, hypokinesia, abnormal thinking.
GI: dyspepsia, abdominal pain.
Musculoskeletal: back pain, stiffness.
Respiratory: cold symptoms, pharyngitis.

Interactions

Drug-drug. *Cimetidine, disulfiram, hormonal contraceptives, isoniazid:* May impair metabolism and clearance of benzodiazepines and prolong their half-life. Watch for increased CNS depression.
CNS depressants, including antihistamines, opioid analgesics, other benzodiazepines: May increase CNS depression. Avoid using together.
Digoxin: May increase digoxin level, resulting in toxicity. Monitor patient closely.
Fluconazole, itraconazole, ketoconazole, miconazole: May increase drug level, CNS depression, and psychomotor impairment. Avoid using together.
Phenytoin: May increase phenytoin level, resulting in toxicity. Monitor patient closely.
Rifampin: May increase metabolism and clearance and decrease drug half-life of estazolam. Watch for decreased effectiveness.
Theophylline: May have antagonistic effect. Watch for decreased effectiveness of estazolam.
Drug-herb. *Calendula, hops, kava, lemon balm, passion flower, skullcap, valerian:* May enhance sedative effect of drug. Discourage use together.
Drug-lifestyle. *Alcohol use:* May cause additive CNS effects. Discourage use together.
Smoking: May increase metabolism and clearance. Advise patient to watch for signs of decreased effectiveness.

Nursing considerations

- Check liver and renal function and CBC before and periodically during long-term therapy.
- Take precautions to prevent depressed, suicidal, or drug-dependent patients or those with history of drug abuse from hoarding drug.
- Patients who receive prolonged treatment with benzodiazepines may experience withdrawal symptoms if drug is suddenly stopped (possibly after 6 weeks of continuous therapy).

!! ALERT Don't confuse ProSom with Proscar, Prozac, or Psorcon E.

Patient teaching

- Advise patient to notify prescriber about planned, suspected, or known pregnancy during therapy.
- Tell patient not to increase dosage but to inform prescriber if he thinks that drug is no longer effective.

• Caution patient to avoid performing activities that require mental alertness or physical coordination.
• Warn patient that drinking alcohol while taking drug or within 24 hours after taking drug can increase depressant effects.
• Warn patient not to abruptly stop use after taking drug for 1 month or longer.
• Tell breast-feeding patient to avoid using drug.

esterified estrogens

Estratab, Menest, Neo-Estrone†

Pregnancy risk category X

Indications & dosages

➲ Inoperable prostate cancer
Men: 1.25 to 2.5 mg P.O. t.i.d.

➲ Breast cancer
Men and postmenopausal women: 10 mg P.O. t.i.d. for 3 or more months.

➲ Female hypogonadism
Women: 2.5 to 7.5 mg daily in divided doses in cycles of 20 days on, 10 days off.

➲ Castration, primary ovarian failure
Women: 1.25 mg daily in cycles of 3 weeks on, 1 week off. Adjust for symptoms. Can be given continuously.

➲ Vasomotor menopausal symptoms
Women: 1.25 mg P.O. daily in cycles of 3 weeks on, 1 week off. Dosage may be increased to 2.5 to 3.75 mg P.O. daily if needed.

➲ Atrophic vaginitis, atrophic urethritis
Women: 0.3 to 1.25 mg or more P.O. daily in cycles of 3 weeks on, 1 week off.

Contraindications & cautions

• Contraindicated in pregnant patients, in patients hypersensitive to drug, and in patients with breast cancer (except metastatic disease), estrogen-dependent neoplasia, active thrombophlebitis, thromboembolic disorders, undiagnosed abnormal genital bleeding, or history of thromboembolic disease.
• Use cautiously in patients with history of hypertension, mental depression, cardiac or renal dysfunction, liver impairment, bone disease, migraine, seizures, or diabetes.

Adverse reactions

CNS: headache, dizziness, chorea, depression, ***CVA***, ***seizures***.
CV: thrombophlebitis, ***thromboembolism***, hypertension, *edema*, ***pulmonary embolism***, ***MI***.
EENT: worsening myopia or astigmatism, intolerance of contact lenses.
GI: *nausea*, vomiting, abdominal cramps, bloating, anorexia, increased appetite, ***pancreatitis***, increased risk of gallbladder disease.
GU: breakthrough bleeding, altered menstrual flow, dysmenorrhea, amenorrhea, ***increased risk of endometrial cancer***, cervical erosion, altered cervical secretions, enlargement of uterine fibromas, vaginal candidiasis, testicular atrophy, impotence.
Hepatic: cholestatic jaundice, ***hepatic adenoma***.
Metabolic: hypercalcemia, weight changes.
Skin: melasma, rash, hirsutism or hair loss, erythema nodosum, dermatitis.
Other: *breast tenderness, enlargement, or secretion, gynecomastia,* ***increased risk of breast cancer***.

Interactions

Drug-drug. *Carbamazepine, fosphenytoin, phenobarbital, phenytoin, rifampin:* May decrease effectiveness of estrogen therapy. Monitor patient closely.
Corticosteroids: May enhance effects. Monitor patient closely.
Cyclosporine: May increase risk of toxicity. Use together with caution, and monitor cyclosporine level frequently.
Dantrolene, hepatotoxic drugs: May increase risk of hepatotoxicity. Monitor liver function closely.
Oral anticoagulants: May decrease anticoagulant effects. Dosage adjustments may be needed. Monitor PT and INR.
Tamoxifen: May interfere with tamoxifen effectiveness. Avoid using together.
Drug-herb. *Black cohosh:* May increase adverse effects of estrogens. Discourage use together.
Saw palmetto: May have antiestrogenic effects. Discourage use together.
St. John's wort: May decrease effects of estrogens. Discourage use together.
Drug-food. *Caffeine:* May increase caffeine level. Urge caution.
Drug-lifestyle. *Smoking:* May increase risk of CV effects. If smoking continues, may need alternative form of therapy.

Nursing considerations

- When used for vasomotor symptoms in menstruating women, cyclic administration is started on day 5 of bleeding.
- Make sure patient has thorough physical examination before starting estrogen therapy. Patients receiving long-term therapy should have annual examinations. Periodically monitor body weight, blood pressure, lipid levels, and hepatic function.
- Notify pathologist about patient's estrogen therapy when sending specimens to laboratory for evaluation.
- Because of risk of thromboembolism, stop therapy at least 1 month before procedures that cause prolonged immobilization or increased risk of thromboembolism, such as knee or hip surgery.
- Glucose tolerance may be impaired. Monitor glucose level closely in patients with diabetes.

!! ALERT Don't confuse Estratab with Estratest.

Patient teaching

- Tell patient to read package insert describing estrogen's adverse effects; also, give patient verbal explanation.
- Emphasize importance of regular physical examinations. Postmenopausal women who use estrogen replacement for longer than 5 years to treat menopausal symptoms may be at increased risk for endometrial cancer. This risk is reduced by using cyclic rather than continuous therapy and the lowest possible estrogen dosage. Adding progestins to the regimen decreases risk of endometrial hyperplasia; but it's unknown whether progestins affect risk of endometrial cancer.

!! ALERT Warn patient to immediately report abdominal pain; pain, numbness, or stiffness in legs or buttocks; pressure or pain in chest or shortness of breath; severe headaches; visual disturbances such as blind spots, flashing lights, or blurriness; vaginal bleeding or discharge; breast lumps; swelling of hands or feet; yellow skin or sclera; dark urine; or light-colored stools.

- Tell diabetic patient to report elevated glucose level so that antidiabetic dosage can be adjusted.
- Explain to patient receiving cyclic therapy for postmenopausal symptoms that she may experience withdrawal bleeding during week off drug. Tell her to report unusual vaginal bleeding.
- Teach woman to perform routine breast self-examination.
- Advise woman of childbearing age to consult prescriber before taking drug and to advise prescriber immediately if she becomes pregnant.
- Teach patient methods to decrease risk of blood clots.
- Encourage patient to stop smoking or reduce number of cigarettes smoked because of the risk of CV complications.

estradiol and norethindrone acetate transdermal system

CombiPatch

Pregnancy risk category X

Indications & dosages

➲ Moderate to severe vasomotor symptoms from menopause; vulvar and vaginal atrophy; hypoestrogenemia from hypogonadism, castration, or primary ovarian failure in women with intact uterus

Continuous combined regimen

Women: Wear 9-cm^2 patch continuously on lower abdomen. Replace system twice weekly during 28-day cycle. May increase to 16-cm^2 patch.

Continuous sequential regimen

Women: For use in sequential regimen with an estradiol transdermal system (such as Alora, Esclim, Estraderm, Vivelle), wear 0.05-mg estradiol transdermal patch for first 14 days of 28-day cycle; replace system twice weekly. Wear 9-cm^2 patch system on lower abdomen for rest of 28-day cycle. May increase to 16-cm^2 patch, p.r.n.

Contraindications & cautions

- Contraindicated in women hypersensitive to estrogen, progestin, or any component of the patch; in pregnant patients; and in patients with known or suspected breast cancer, known or suspected estrogen-dependent neoplasia, undiagnosed abnormal genital bleeding, active thrombophlebitis, thromboembolic disorders, or CVA.
- Use cautiously in breast-feeding women and in patients with impaired liver func-

tion, asthma, epilepsy, migraine, or cardiac or renal dysfunction.

Adverse reactions

CNS: *asthenia*, ***increased risk of CVA***, depression, insomnia, nervousness, dizziness, *headache*.
CV: ***thromboembolism***, thrombophlebitis, hypertension, *edema*, **pulmonary embolism**, ***MI***.
EENT: pharyngitis, *rhinitis, sinusitis*.
GI: *abdominal pain, diarrhea*, dyspepsia, flatulence, *nausea*, constipation.
GU: *dysmenorrhea, leukorrhea, menstrual disorder*, suspicious Papanicolaou smears, *vaginitis*, menorrhagia, vaginal hemorrhage.
Musculoskeletal: arthralgia, *back pain*.
Respiratory: *respiratory disorder*, bronchitis.
Skin: application site reactions, acne.
Other: *accidental injury, flulike syndrome, pain, breast pain*, tooth disorder, peripheral edema, breast enlargement, infection.

Interactions

Drug-drug. *Carbamazepine, fosphenytoin, phenobarbital, phenytoin, rifampin:* May decrease estrogen therapy effectiveness. Monitor patient closely.
Corticosteroids: May enhance effects of corticosteroids. Monitor patient closely.
Cyclosporine: May increase risk of toxicity. Use together with caution; monitor cyclosporine level frequently.
Dantrolene, hepatotoxic drugs: May increase risk of hepatotoxicity. Monitor liver function closely.
Oral anticoagulants: May decrease effect of anticoagulant. May need to adjust dose. Monitor PT and INR.
Tamoxifen: May interfere with tamoxifen effectiveness. Avoid using together.
Drug-herb. *Black cohosh:* May increase adverse effects of estrogens. Discourage use together.
Saw palmetto: May cause antiestrogenic effects. Discourage use together.
St. John's wort: May decrease effects of estrogens. Discourage use together.
Drug-food. *Caffeine:* May increase caffeine level. Advise patient to avoid caffeine.
Grapefruit juice: May elevate estrogen level. Advise patient to take with liquid other than grapefruit juice.
Drug-lifestyle. *Smoking:* May increase risk of adverse CV effects. If smoking continues, may need alternative therapy.

Nursing considerations

- Women not receiving continuous estrogen or combined estrogen and progestin therapy may start therapy at any time.
- Women receiving continuous hormone replacement therapy should complete the current cycle before starting therapy. Women commonly have withdrawal bleeding at completion of cycle; first day of withdrawal bleeding is appropriate time to start therapy.
- Store norethindrone patches in refrigerator before dispensing. Patient may then store patches at room temperature for up to 3 months.
- Reevaluate therapy at 3- to 6-month intervals.
- A combined estrogen and progestin regimen is indicated for a woman with an intact uterus. Progestins taken with estrogen significantly reduce, but don't eliminate, risk of endometrial cancer linked to use of estrogen alone.
- Blood pressure increases have been linked to estrogen use. Monitor patient's blood pressure regularly.
- Treatment of postmenopausal symptoms usually starts during menopausal stage when vasomotor symptoms occur.
- Apply patch system to a smooth (fold-free), clean, dry, nonirritated area of skin on lower abdomen, avoiding the waistline. Rotate application sites, with an interval of at least 1 week between applications to same site.
- Don't apply patch on or near breasts.
- Avoid applying to areas that may get prolonged sun exposure.
- Reapply patch, if needed, to another area of lower abdomen. If patch fails to adhere, replace with a new one.
- Monitor glucose level closely in patients with diabetes.

!!ALERT Don't interchange CombiPatch with other estrogen patches. Verify therapy before application.

Patient teaching

- Teach patient how to apply patch properly. She should wear only one patch at any

time during therapy. Tell her to apply patch immediately after opening protective cover.
- Tell patient an oil-based cream or lotion may help remove adhesive from the skin once patch has been removed and the area allowed to dry for 15 minutes.
- Advise patient not to use patch if she's pregnant or plans to become pregnant.
- Urge woman of childbearing age to consult prescriber before applying patch and to advise prescriber immediately if she becomes pregnant.
- Instruct patient that the continuous combined regimen may lead to irregular bleeding, particularly in the first 6 months, but that it usually decreases with time, and often stops completely.
- Tell patient that, for the continuous sequential regimen, monthly withdrawal bleeding is common.
- Advise patient to alert prescriber and remove patch at first sign of clotting disorders (thrombophlebitis, cerebrovascular disorders, and pulmonary embolism).
- Instruct patient to stop using patch and call prescriber about any loss of vision, sudden onset of protrusion of the eyeball (proptosis), double vision, or migraine.
- Encourage patient to stop or reduce smoking because of the risk of CV complications.
- Advise patient not to store patches where extreme temperatures can occur.

estradiol (oestradiol)

Alora, Climara, Esclim, Estrace, Estrace Vaginal Cream, Estraderm, Estring Vaginal Ring, FemPatch, Femring, Gynodiol, Menostar, Vivelle, Vivelle-Dot

estradiol cypionate

depGynogen, Depo-Estradiol Cypionate, Depogen

estradiol hemihydrate

Estrasorb, Vagifem

estradiol valerate (oestradiol valerate)

Delestrogen, Estra-L 40, Gynogen L.A, Valergen

Pregnancy risk category X

Indications & dosages

➲ Vasomotor menopausal symptoms, female hypogonadism, female castration, primary ovarian failure

Women: 0.5 to 2 mg P.O. estradiol daily in cycles of 21 days on and 7 days off or cycles of 5 days on and 2 days off. Or, for vasomotor symptoms, 1 to 5 mg cypionate I.M. once q 3 to 4 weeks; for female hypogonadism, 1.5 to 2 mg cypionate I.M. once q month.

Transdermal patch

Women: Esclim 0.025 mg/24 hours, Estraderm 0.05 mg/24 hours, Vivelle 0.0375 mg/24 hours, Vivelle 0.05 mg/24 hours twice weekly, Climara 0.05 mg/24 hours, or FemPatch 0.025 mg/24 hours once weekly. Apply to clean, dry area of the trunk. Adjust dose if necessary after the first 2 or 3 weeks of therapy; then q 3 to 6 months, p.r.n. Rotate application sites weekly, with an interval of at least 1 week between particular sites used. Adjust dosage, p.r.n.

➲ Postmenopausal urogenital symptoms

Women: One ring inserted into the upper third of the vagina. Ring is kept in place for 3 months.

➲ Atrophic vaginitis, kraurosis vulvae

Women: 0.05 mg/24 hours Estraderm applied twice weekly in a cyclic regimen. Or, 0.05 mg/24 hours Climara applied weekly in a cyclic regimen. Or, 2 to 4 g intravaginal applications of cream daily for 1 to 2 weeks. When vaginal mucosa is restored, maintenance dose is 1 g one to three times weekly in a cyclic regimen. If using Vagifem for atrophic vaginitis, give 1 tablet vaginally once daily for 2 weeks. Maintenance dose is 1 tablet inserted vaginally twice weekly. Or, 10 to 20 mg valerate I.M. q 4 weeks, p.r.n. Or, 1 to 5 mg estradiol cypionate I.M. once q 3 to 4 weeks.

➲ Palliative treatment of advanced, inoperable breast cancer

Men and postmenopausal women: 10 mg P.O. estradiol t.i.d. for 3 months.

➲ **Palliative treatment of advanced, inoperable prostate cancer**
Men: 30 mg valerate I.M. q 1 to 2 weeks, or 1 to 2 mg P.O. estradiol t.i.d.
➲ **To prevent postmenopausal osteoporosis**
Women: Place a 6.5-cm^2 (0.025 mg/24 hours) Climara patch once weekly on clean, dry skin of lower abdomen or upper quadrant of buttock. Or, place a 3.25 cm^2 (0.014 mg/24 hours) Menostar patch once weekly to clean, dry area of the lower abdomen. For each system, press firmly in place for about 10 seconds; ensure complete contact, especially around edges. Or, 0.025-mg/24 hours Vivelle, Vivelle-Dot, or Alora system applied to a clean, dry area of the trunk twice weekly.
➲ **Moderate to severe vasomotor symptoms from menopause**
Women: Apply contents of two 1.74-g foil pouches (total 3.48 g) of Estrasorb daily. Open each pouch individually and use contents of one pouch for each leg. Rub emulsion into thigh and calf for 3 minutes until thoroughly absorbed; rub excess emulsion remaining on hands onto the buttocks. Allow areas to dry before covering with clothing. Wash hands with soap and water to remove excess drug.

Contraindications & cautions

- Contraindicated in pregnant patients and patients with thrombophlebitis or thromboembolic disorders, estrogen-dependent neoplasia, breast or reproductive organ cancer (except for palliative treatment), undiagnosed abnormal genital bleeding, or history of thrombophlebitis or thromboembolic disorders linked to previous estrogen use (except for palliative treatment of breast and prostate cancer).
- Contraindicated in patients with liver dysfunction or disease.
- Use cautiously in patients with cerebrovascular or coronary artery disease, asthma, bone disease, migraine, seizures, or cardiac or renal dysfunction.
- Use cautiously in women who have a strong family history (grandmother, mother, sister) of breast cancer, breast nodules, fibrocystic breasts, or abnormal mammogram findings.

!!ALERT Postmenopausal women age 50 to 79 years old who are taking estrogen and progestin have an increased risk of MI, CVA, invasive breast cancer, PE, and DVT. Postmenopausal women age 65 or older also have an increased risk of dementia.

Adverse reactions

CNS: ***increased risk of CVA***, *headache*, dizziness, chorea, depression, ***seizures***, insomnia (Vagifem).
CV: thrombophlebitis, ***thromboembolism***, hypertension, *edema*, ***pulmonary embolism, MI***.
EENT: worsening myopia or astigmatism, intolerance of contact lenses, sinusitis (Vagifem).
GI: *nausea*, vomiting, abdominal cramps, bloating, increased appetite, ***pancreatitis***, anorexia, gallbladder disease, dyspepsia (Vagifem).
GU: breakthrough bleeding, altered menstrual flow, dysmenorrhea, amenorrhea, ***increased risk of endometrial cancer***, cervical erosion, altered cervical secretions, enlargement of uterine fibromas, vaginal candidiasis in women, testicular atrophy, impotence in men, genital pruritus, hematuria, vaginal discomfort, vaginitis (Vagifem).
Hepatic: cholestatic jaundice, ***hepatic adenoma***.
Metabolic: weight changes.
Respiratory: *upper respiratory tract infection*, allergy, bronchitis (Vagifem).
Skin: melasma, urticaria, erythema nodosum, dermatitis, hair loss.
Other: *gynecomastia*, ***increased risk of breast cancer***, hot flashes, pain (Vagifem), *breast tenderness, enlargement, or secretion*.

Interactions

Drug-drug. *Carbamazepine, fosphenytoin, phenobarbital, phenytoin, rifampin:* May decrease effectiveness of estrogen therapy. Monitor patient closely.
Corticosteroids: May enhance effects of corticosteroids. Monitor patient closely.
Cyclosporine: May increase risk of toxicity. Use together with caution and monitor cyclosporine level frequently.
Dantrolene, other hepatotoxic drugs: May increase risk of hepatotoxicity. Monitor liver function closely.
Oral anticoagulants: May decrease anticoagulant effect. Dosage adjustments may be needed. Monitor PT and INR.

Tamoxifen: May interfere with tamoxifen effectiveness. Avoid using together.
Drug-herb. *Black cohosh:* May increase estrogen adverse effects. Discourage use together.
Saw palmetto: May have antiestrogenic effects. Discourage use together.
St. John's wort: May decrease effects of estrogens. Discourage use together.
Drug-food. *Caffeine:* May increase caffeine level. Advise patient to avoid or minimize use of caffeine.
Grapefruit juice: May elevate estrogen level. Tell patient to take drug with liquid other than grapefruit juice.
Drug-lifestyle. *Smoking:* May increase risk of adverse CV effects. If smoking continues, may need alternative therapy.
Sunscreen use: May increase absorption of estradiol topical emulsion (Estrasorb). Separate application times.

Nursing considerations

- Ensure that patient has physical examination before starting therapy. Patients receiving long-term therapy should have yearly examinations. Monitor lipid levels, blood pressure, body weight, and hepatic function.
- Ask patient about allergies, especially to foods and plants. Estradiol is available as an aqueous solution or as a solution in peanut oil; estradiol cypionate, as a solution in cottonseed oil; estradiol valerate, as a solution in castor oil or sesame oil.
- To give I.M. injection, make sure drug is well dispersed by rolling vial between palms. Inject deep into large muscle. Rotate injection sites to prevent muscle atrophy. Never give drug I.V.
- Apply transdermal patch to clean, dry, hairless, intact skin on abdomen or buttock. Don't apply it to breasts, waistline, or other areas where clothing can loosen patch. When applying, ensure thorough contact between patch and skin, especially around edges, and hold in place for about 10 seconds. Apply patch immediately after opening and removing protective cover. Rotate application sites.
- In women also taking oral estrogen, treatment with the Estraderm transdermal patch can begin 1 week after withdrawal of oral therapy, or sooner if menopausal symptoms appear before the end of the week.
- Transdermal systems may be used continually rather than cyclically. Other alternative regimens are 1 to 5 mg (cypionate) I.M. q 3 to 4 weeks and 10 to 20 mg (valerate) I.M. q 4 weeks, p.r.n.
- Instruct patients using Vagifem who have severely atrophic vaginal mucosa to be careful when inserting the applicator. After gynecologic surgery, tell patient to use any vaginal applicator cautiously and only if clearly indicated.
- The prescriber should assess the patient's need to continue Vagifem therapy. Make attempts to stop or taper at 3- to 6-month intervals.
- Because of risk of thromboembolism, stop therapy at least 1 month before high-risk procedures or those that cause prolonged immobilization, such as knee or hip surgery.
- Glucose tolerance may be impaired. Monitor glucose level closely in patients with diabetes.
- Notify pathologist about estrogen therapy when sending specimens to laboratory for evaluation.
- Estrace may contain tartrazine.

Patient teaching

- Tell patient to read package insert describing estrogen's adverse effects and give verbal explanation.
- Emphasize importance of regular physical examinations. Postmenopausal women who use estrogen replacement for longer than 5 years may be at increased risk for endometrial cancer. Risk is reduced by using cyclic rather than continuous therapy and the lowest possible dosages of estrogen. Adding progestins to the regimen decreases risk of endometrial hyperplasia; however, it isn't known whether progestins affect risk of endometrial cancer. No increased risk of breast cancer has been reported.
- Teach patient how to use cream. Patient should wash vaginal area with soap and water before applying and insert cream high into the vagina (about two-thirds the length of the applicator). Patient should take drug at bedtime, or lie flat for 30 minutes after instillation to minimize drug loss.
- Tell patient using Estrasorb emulsion not to apply it with sunscreen.

• Tell patient to use transdermal system correctly, to rotate sites, to avoid breasts and waistline, and to reapply patch if it falls off.
• Tell patient to insert Vagifem by the applicator as far into vagina as it can comfortably go, without using force.
!! ALERT Warn patient to immediately report abdominal pain, pressure or pain in chest, shortness of breath, severe headaches, visual disturbances, vaginal bleeding or discharge, breast lumps, swelling of hands or feet, yellow skin or sclera, dark urine, light-colored stools, and pain, numbness, or stiffness in legs or buttocks.
• Explain to patient receiving cyclic therapy for postmenopausal symptoms that withdrawal bleeding may occur during week off drug. Tell her to report unusual vaginal bleeding.
• Tell diabetic patient to report elevated glucose level so that antidiabetic dosage can be adjusted.
• Teach woman how to perform routine breast self-examination.
• Teach patient methods to decrease risk of blood clots.
• Advise woman not to become pregnant during estrogen therapy.
• Advise woman of childbearing age to consult prescriber before taking drug and to advise prescriber immediately if she becomes pregnant.
• Encourage patient to stop or reduce smoking because of the risk of CV complications.

estrogens, conjugated (estrogenic substances, conjugated; oestrogens, conjugated)

C.E.S†, Cenestin, Premarin, Premarin Intravenous

Pregnancy risk category X

Indications & dosages

➲ Abnormal uterine bleeding (hormonal imbalance)
Adults: 25 mg I.V. or I.M. Repeat dose in 6 to 12 hours, if necessary.
➲ Vulvar or vaginal atrophy
Adults: 0.5 to 2 g cream intravaginally once daily in cycles of 3 weeks on, 1 week off.
➲ Castration and primary ovarian failure
Adults: Initially, 1.25 mg Premarin P.O. daily in cycles of 3 weeks on, 1 week off. Adjust dose p.r.n.
➲ Female hypogonadism
Adults: 0.3 to 0.625 mg Premarin P.O. daily, given cyclically 3 weeks on, 1 week off.
➲ Moderate to severe vasomotor symptoms with or without moderate to severe symptoms of vulvar and vaginal atrophy associated with menopause
Adults: Initially, 0.3 mg Premarin P.O. daily, or cyclically 25 days on, 5 days off. Adjust dosage based on patient response.
➲ Moderate to severe vasomotor symptoms from menopause
Adults: 0.45 mg Cenestin P.O. daily. Adjust dose based on patient response.
➲ Moderate to severe symptoms of vulvar and vaginal atrophy from menopause
Adults: 0.3 mg Cenestin P.O. daily.
➲ To prevent osteoporosis
Adults: 0.3 mg Premarin P.O. daily, or cyclically, 25 days on, 5 days off. Adjust dose based on response of bone mineral density testing.
➲ Palliative treatment of inoperable prostatic cancer
Adults: 1.25 to 2.5 mg Premarin P.O. t.i.d.
➲ Palliative treatment of breast cancer
Adults: 10 mg Premarin P.O. t.i.d. for at least 3 months.

Contraindications & cautions

• Contraindicated in pregnant patients and in patients with thrombophlebitis, thromboembolic disorders, estrogen-dependent neoplasia, breast or reproductive cancer (except for palliative treatment), or undiagnosed abnormal genital bleeding.
• Use cautiously in patients with cerebrovascular or coronary artery disease, asthma, bone disease, migraine, seizures, or cardiac, hepatic, or renal dysfunction.
• Use cautiously in women who have a strong family history (mother, grandmother, sister) of breast or genital tract cancer, breast nodules, fibrocystic breasts, or abnormal mammogram findings.

Adverse reactions

CNS: headache, dizziness, chorea, depression, ***increased risk of CVA, seizures.***

CV: flushing with rapid I.V. administration, thrombophlebitis, ***thromboembolism***, hypertension, *edema*, ***pulmonary embolism***, ***MI***.
EENT: worsening myopia or astigmatism, intolerance of contact lenses.
GI: *nausea*, vomiting, abdominal cramps, bloating, anorexia, increased appetite, ***pancreatitis***, gallbladder disease.
GU: breakthrough bleeding, altered menstrual flow, dysmenorrhea, amenorrhea, ***increased risk of endometrial cancer***, cervical erosion, altered cervical secretions, enlargement of uterine fibromas, vaginal candidiasis, testicular atrophy, impotence.
Hepatic: cholestatic jaundice, ***hepatic adenoma***.
Metabolic: weight changes.
Skin: melasma, urticaria, hirsutism or hair loss, erythema nodosum, dermatitis.
Other: *breast tenderness, enlargement, or secretion, gynecomastia*, **INCREASED RISK OF BREAST CANCER**.

Interactions

Drug-drug. *Carbamazepine, fosphenytoin, phenobarbital, phenytoin, rifampin:* May decrease effectiveness of estrogen therapy. Monitor patient closely.
Corticosteroids: May enhance corticosteroid effects. Monitor patient closely.
Cyclosporine: May increase risk of toxicity. Use together with caution, and monitor cyclosporine level frequently.
Dantrolene, other hepatotoxic drugs: May increase risk of hepatotoxicity. Monitor liver function closely.
Oral anticoagulants: May decrease anticoagulant effects. May need to adjust dosage. Monitor PT and INR.
Tamoxifen: May interfere with tamoxifen effectiveness. Avoid using together.
Drug-herb. *Black cohosh:* May increase adverse effects of estrogens. Discourage use together.
Red clover: May interfere with hormonal therapies. Discourage use together.
Saw palmetto: May have antiestrogenic effects. Discourage use together.
St. John's wort: May decrease effects of estrogens. Discourage use together.
Drug-food. *Caffeine:* May increase caffeine level. Advise caution.
Drug-lifestyle. *Smoking:* May increase risk of adverse CV effects. If smoking continues, may need alternative therapy.

Nursing considerations

- Make sure patient has thorough physical examination before starting estrogen therapy. Patients receiving long-term therapy should have annual examinations. Periodically monitor lipid levels, blood pressure, body weight, and hepatic function.
- Rapid treatment of dysfunctional uterine bleeding or reduction of surgical bleeding usually requires delivery by I.V. or I.M. route.

!!ALERT Estrogens and progestins shouldn't be used to prevent CV disease. The Women's Health Initiative (WHI) study reported increased risks of MI, stroke, invasive breast cancer, pulmonary emboli, and deep vein thrombosis in postmenopausal women during 5 years of combination therapy. Because of these risks, estrogens and progestins should be prescribed at the lowest effective doses and for the shortest duration consistent with treatment goals and risks for the individual woman.

!!ALERT Postmenopausal women who use estrogen replacement for longer than 5 years to treat menopausal symptoms may be at increased risk for endometrial cancer. This risk is reduced by using cyclic rather than continuous therapy and lowest possible estrogen dosage. Adding progestins to the regimen decreases risk of endometrial hyperplasia; but it's unknown whether progestins affect risk of endometrial cancer.

- When giving by I.M. injection, inject deep into large muscle. Rotate injection sites to prevent muscle atrophy.
- When used solely for the treatment of vulvar and vaginal atrophy, topical products should be considered.
- Notify pathologist about estrogen therapy when sending specimens to laboratory for evaluation.
- Because of thromboembolism risk, stop therapy at least 1 month before procedures that prolong immobilization or raise the risk of thromboembolism, such as knee or hip surgery.
- Glucose tolerance may be impaired. Monitor glucose level closely in patients with diabetes.

!!**ALERT** Don't confuse Premarin with Primaxin.

Patient teaching

- Tell patient to read package insert describing estrogen's adverse effects and explain effects verbally.
- Emphasize importance of regular physical examinations.
- Teach patient how to use vaginal cream. Patient should wash the vaginal area with soap and water before applying and insert cream high into the vagina (about two thirds the length of the applicator). Tell her to use drug at bedtime or to lie flat for 30 minutes after instillation to minimize drug loss.
- Explain to patient that cyclic therapy for postmenopausal symptoms may cause withdrawal bleeding during week off drug. Tell her to report unusual vaginal bleeding.

!!**ALERT** Warn patient to immediately report abdominal pain; pain, numbness, or stiffness in legs or buttocks; pressure or pain in chest; shortness of breath; severe headaches; visual disturbances, such as blind spots, flashing lights, or blurriness; vaginal bleeding or discharge; breast lumps; swelling of hands or feet; yellow skin or sclera; dark urine; and light-colored stools.

- Tell diabetic patient to report elevated glucose level so that antidiabetic dosage can be adjusted.
- Teach woman how to perform routine breast self-examination.
- Advise patient not to become pregnant during estrogen therapy.
- Advise woman of childbearing age to consult prescriber before taking drug and to advise prescriber immediately if she becomes pregnant.
- Encourage patient to stop smoking or reduce number of cigarettes smoked because of the risk of CV complications.

estropipate (piperazine estrone sulfate)

Ogen, Ortho-Est

Pregnancy risk category X

Indications & dosages

➲ Vulvar and vaginal atrophy

Women: 0.75 to 6 mg P.O. daily, 3 weeks on and 1 week off; or 2 to 4 g vaginal cream daily. Drug usually given on a cyclic, short-term basis but can be given continuously.

➲ Primary ovarian failure, female castration, female hypogonadism

Women: 1.5 to 9 mg P.O. daily for first 3 weeks; then a rest period of 8 to 10 days. If bleeding doesn't occur by end of rest period, cycle is repeated. Can be given continuously.

➲ Vasomotor menopausal symptoms

Women: 0.75 to 6 mg P.O. daily in cyclic method, 3 weeks on and 1 week off. Can be given continuously.

➲ To prevent osteoporosis

Women: 0.75 mg P.O. daily for 25 days of a 31-day cycle.

Contraindications & cautions

- Contraindicated in pregnant patients and those with active thrombophlebitis, thromboembolic disorders, estrogen-dependent neoplasia, undiagnosed genital bleeding, and breast, reproductive organ, or genital cancer.
- Use cautiously in patients with cerebrovascular or coronary artery disease, asthma, mental depression, bone disease, migraine, seizures, or cardiac, hepatic, or renal dysfunction.
- Use cautiously in women who have a family history (mother, grandmother, sister) of breast or genital tract cancer, breast nodules, fibrocystic breasts, or abnormal mammogram findings.

Adverse reactions

CNS: depression, headache, dizziness, migraine, ***seizures, increased risk of CVA.***

CV: *edema,* thrombophlebitis, ***increased risk of pulmonary embolism and MI, thromboembolism.***

GI: nausea, vomiting, gallbladder disease, abdominal cramps, bloating.

GU: increased size of uterine fibromas, ***increased risk of endometrial cancer***, vaginal candidiasis, cystitis-like syndrome, dysmenorrhea, amenorrhea, breakthrough bleeding, condition resembling premenstrual syndrome.
Hepatic: cholestatic jaundice, ***hepatic adenoma***.
Metabolic: weight changes.
Skin: hemorrhagic eruption, erythema nodosum, ***erythema multiforme***, hirsutism or hair loss, melasma.
Other: breast engorgement or enlargement, ***possible increased risk of breast cancer***.

Interactions

Drug-drug. *Carbamazepine, fosphenytoin, phenobarbital, phenytoin, rifampin:* May decrease estrogen effect. Monitor patient closely.
Corticosteroids: May enhance corticosteroid effect. Monitor patient closely.
Cyclosporine: May increase risk of toxicity. Use together with caution; frequently monitor cyclosporine level.
Dantrolene, other hepatotoxic drugs: May increase risk of hepatotoxicity. Monitor liver function closely.
Oral anticoagulants: May decrease anticoagulant effect. Dosage adjustments may be needed. Monitor PT and INR.
Tamoxifen: May interfere with tamoxifen effect. Avoid using together.
Drug-herb. *Black cohosh:* May increase adverse effects of estrogen. Discourage use together.
Red clover: May interfere with hormonal therapies. Discourage use together.
Saw palmetto: May have antiestrogenic effect. Discourage use together.
St. John's wort: May decrease estrogen effect. Discourage use together.
Drug-food. *Caffeine:* May increase caffeine level. Advise caution.
Drug-lifestyle. *Smoking:* May increase risk of adverse CV effects. If smoking continues, may need alternative therapy.

Nursing considerations

• Make sure patient has thorough physical examination before starting estrogen therapy. Patients receiving long-term therapy should have examinations yearly. Periodically monitor lipid levels, blood pressure, body weight, and hepatic function.

!! ALERT Estrogens and progestins shouldn't be used to prevent CV disease. The Women's Health Initiative (WHI) study reported increased risks of MI, CVA, invasive breast cancer, pulmonary emboli, and deep vein thrombosis in postmenopausal women during 5 years of combination therapy. Because of these risks, estrogens and progestins should be prescribed at the lowest effective doses and for the shortest duration consistent with treatment goals and risks for the individual woman.

• When used to treat hypogonadism, duration of therapy needed to produce withdrawal bleeding depends on patient's endometrial response to drug. If satisfactory withdrawal bleeding doesn't occur, an oral progestin is added to the regimen. Explain to patient that, despite return of withdrawal bleeding, pregnancy can't occur because she doesn't ovulate.

• Estropipate–estrone equivalents are:
0.75 mg estropipate = 0.625 mg estrone 1.5 mg estropipate = 1.25 mg estrone 3 mg estropipate = 2.5 mg estrone 6 mg estropipate = 5 mg estrone.

• May give with meals to minimize GI upset.

• Because of risk of thromboembolism, stop therapy at least 1 month before procedures that prolong immobilization or raise the risk of thromboembolism, such as knee or hip surgery.

• Glucose tolerance may be impaired. Monitor glucose level closely in patients with diabetes.

Patient teaching

• Tell patient to read package insert describing estrogen's adverse effects; also explain effects verbally.

• Teach patient how to use vaginal cream. Patient should wash the vaginal area with soap and water and then insert vaginal cream high into the vagina (about two-thirds the length of the applicator). Tell her to use drug at bedtime or to lie flat for 30 minutes after application to minimize drug loss.

• Tell diabetic patient to report elevated glucose level to prescriber.

• Stress importance of regular physical examinations. Postmenopausal women who use estrogen replacement for longer than 5 years may have increased risk of endometrial cancer. Using cyclic therapy and lowest possible estrogen dosage reduces risk. Adding progestins to regimen decreases risk of endometrial hyperplasia; however, it isn't known whether progestins affect risk of endometrial cancer.

!!ALERT Warn patient to immediately report abdominal pain; pain, stiffness, or numbness in legs or buttocks; pressure or pain in chest; shortness of breath; severe headaches; visual disturbances, such as blind spots or flashing lights; vaginal bleeding or discharge; breast lumps; swelling of hands or feet; yellow skin or sclera; dark urine; and light-colored stools.

- Teach woman how to perform routine breast self-examination.
- Advise patient not to become pregnant while on estrogen therapy.
- Encourage patient to stop or reduce smoking because of the risk of CV complications.
- Advise woman of childbearing age to consult prescriber before taking drug and to tell prescriber immediately if she becomes pregnant.

eszopiclone
Lunesta

Pregnancy risk category C
Controlled substance schedule IV

Indications & dosages

Insomnia

Adults: 2 mg P.O. immediately before bed. Increase to 3 mg if needed.
Elderly patients having trouble falling asleep: 1 mg P.O. immediately before bed. Increase to 2 mg if needed.
Elderly patients having trouble staying asleep: 2 mg P.O. immediately before bed.

In patients with severe hepatic impairment, start with 1 mg P.O. In patients who also take a potent CYP3A4 inhibitor, start with 1 mg and increase to 2 mg if needed.

Contraindications & cautions

- There are no known contraindications.
- Use cautiously in patients with diseases or conditions that could affect metabolism or hemodynamic responses. Also use cautiously in patients with compromised respiratory function, severe hepatic impairment, or signs and symptoms of depression.

Adverse reactions

CNS: abnormal dreams, anxiety, confusion, decreased libido, depression, dizziness, hallucinations, *headache*, nervousness, pain, *somnolence*, neuralgia.
EENT: *unpleasant taste.*
GI: diarrhea, dry mouth, dyspepsia, nausea, vomiting.
GU: UTI.
Respiratory: *respiratory infection.*
Skin: pruritus, rash.
Other: accidental injury, viral infection.

Interactions

Drug-drug. *CNS depressants:* May have additive CNS effects. Adjust dosage of either drug as needed.
CYP3A4 inhibitors (clarithromycin, itraconazole, ketoconazole, nefazodone, nelfinavir, ritonavir, troleandomycin): May decrease eszopiclone elimination, increasing the risk of toxicity. Use together cautiously.
Olanzapine: May impair cognitive function or memory. Use together cautiously.
Rifampicin: May decrease eszopiclone activity. Don't use together.
Drug-food. *High-fat meals:* May decrease drug absorption and effects. Discourage high-fat meals with or just before taking drug.
Drug-lifestyle. *Alcohol use:* May decrease psychomotor ability. Discourage use together.

Nursing considerations

- Evaluate patient for physical and psychiatric disorders before treatment.
- Use the lowest effective dose.

!!ALERT Give drug immediately before patient goes to bed or after patient has gone to bed and has trouble falling asleep.

- Use only for short periods (for example, 7 to 10 days). If patient still has trouble sleeping, check for other psychological disorders.
- Monitor patient for changes in behavior, including those that suggest depression or suicidal thinking.

Patient teaching

- Urge patient to take drug immediately before going to bed because drug may cause dizziness or light-headedness.
- Caution patient not to take drug unless he can get a full night's sleep.

- Advise patient to avoid taking drug after a high-fat meal.
- Tell patient to avoid activities that require mental alertness until the drug's effects are known.
- Advise patient to avoid alcohol while taking drug.
- Urge patient to immediately report changes in behavior and thinking.
- Warn patient not to stop drug abruptly or change dose without consulting the prescriber.
- Inform patient that tolerance or dependence may develop if drug is taken for a prolonged period.

etanercept
Enbrel

Pregnancy risk category B

Indications & dosages

➲ **To reduce signs and symptoms of moderately to severely active polyarticular-course juvenile rheumatoid arthritis (RA) in patients whose response to one or more disease-modifying antirheumatic drugs has been inadequate**

Children ages 4 to 17: 0.8 mg/kg S.C. weekly (maximum 50 mg/week). For pediatric patients weighing 63 kg (138 lb) or more, give weekly dose using the prefilled syringe. For pediatric patients weighing 31 to 62 kg (68 to 136 lb), give total weekly dose as two S.C. injections, either on the same day or 3 or 4 days apart using the multi-use vial. For pediatric patients weighing less than 31 kg (68 lb), give weekly dose as single S.C. injection using the correct volume from the multi-use vial. Glucocorticoids, NSAIDs, or analgesics may be continued during treatment. Use with methotrexate hasn't been studied in pediatric patients.

➲ **RA, psoriatic arthritis, ankylosing spondylitis**

Adults: 50 mg S.C. once weekly using the 50 mg/ml single-use prefilled syringe. Methotrexate, glucocorticoids, salicylates, NSAIDs, or analgesics may be continued during treatment.

➲ **Chronic moderate to severe plaque psoriasis in patients who are candidates for systemic therapy or phototherapy**

Adults: 50 mg S.C. twice weekly, 3 to 4 days apart for 3 months. Then, reduce dose to 50 mg S.C. once weekly. Give dose using 50 mg/ml single-use prefilled syringes.

Contraindications & cautions

- Contraindicated in patients hypersensitive to drug or its components, in those with sepsis, and in those receiving a live vaccine.
- Drug isn't indicated for use in children younger than age 4.
- Use cautiously in patients with underlying diseases that predispose them to infection, such as diabetes, heart failure, or history of active or chronic infections.
- Use cautiously in RA patients with preexisting or recent onset of demyelinating disorders, including multiple sclerosis, myelitis, and optic neuritis.

Adverse reactions

CNS: asthenia, *headache*, dizziness.
EENT: *rhinitis*, pharyngitis, sinusitis.
GI: abdominal pain, dyspepsia.
Respiratory: *upper respiratory tract infections*, cough, respiratory disorder.
Skin: *injection site reaction*, rash.
Other: *infections*, malignancies.

Interactions

Drug-drug. *Vaccines:* May affect normal immune response. Postpone live-virus vaccine until therapy stops.

Nursing considerations

- Methotrexate, glucocorticoids, salicylates, NSAIDs, or analgesics may be continued during treatment in adults.

!!ALERT Anti-TNF therapies, including etanercept, may affect defenses against infection. Notify prescriber and stop therapy if serious infection occurs.

!!ALERT Don't give live vaccines during therapy.

- If possible, bring patients with juvenile RA up-to-date with all immunizations before starting treatment.

!!ALERT Give a 50-mg dose as one S.C. injection using a 50-mg/ml single-use prefilled syringe or as two 25-mg S.C injections using multiple-use vial. Give the two 25-mg injections on the same day or 3 to 4 days apart.

- Store prefilled syringe at 36° to 46° F (2° to 8° C), but let it reach room temperature (15 to 30 minutes) before use. Don't remove the needle shield while syringe is being allowed to reach room temperature.
- Reconstitute multiple-use vial aseptically with 1 ml of supplied sterile bacteriostatic water for injection (0.9% benzyl alcohol). Use a 25G needle rather than the supplied vial adapter if the vial will be used for multiple doses. Don't filter reconstituted solution when preparing or giving drug. Inject diluent slowly into vial.
- Minimize foaming by gently swirling during dissolution rather than shaking. Dissolution takes less than 10 minutes.
- Visually check solution for particulates and discoloration before use. Don't use solution if it's discolored or cloudy, or if it contains particulate matter.
- Don't add other drugs or diluents to reconstituted solution.
- Reconstituted solution prepared with sterile bacteriostatic water for injection (0.9% benzyl alcohol) using a 25G needle may be refrigerated in vial for up to 14 days at 36° to 46° F (2° to 8° C).
- Make injection sites at least 1 inch apart; never use areas where skin is tender, bruised, red, or hard. Recommended sites include the thigh, abdomen, and upper arm. Rotate sites regularly.
- Needle cover of diluent syringe and prefilled syringe contains dry natural rubber (latex) and shouldn't be handled by persons sensitive to latex.

Patient teaching

- If patient will be giving drug, advise him about mixing and injection techniques, including rotation of injection sites.
- Instruct patient to use puncture-resistant container for disposal of needles and syringes.
- Tell patient that injection site reactions generally occur within first month of therapy and decrease thereafter.
- Inform patient of importance of avoiding live vaccine administration during therapy.
- Stress importance of alerting other health care providers of etanercept use.
- Instruct patient to promptly report signs and symptoms of infection to prescriber.
- Advise breast-feeding woman to stop breast-feeding during therapy.

ethambutol hydrochloride

Etibit†, Myambutol

Pregnancy risk category B

Indications & dosages

➲ Adjunctive treatment for pulmonary tuberculosis

Adults and children older than age 13: In patients who haven't received previous antitubercular therapy, 15 mg/kg P.O. daily as a single dose, combined with other antituberculotics. For retreatment, 25 mg/kg P.O. daily as a single dose for 60 days (or until bacteriologic smears and cultures become negative) with at least one other antituberculotic; then decreased to 15 mg/kg/day as a single dose.

Contraindications & cautions

- Contraindicated in children younger than age 13, patients hypersensitive to drug, and patients with optic neuritis.
- Use cautiously in patients with impaired renal function, cataracts, recurrent eye inflammation, gout, or diabetic retinopathy.

Adverse reactions

CNS: headache, dizziness, fever, mental confusion, hallucinations, malaise, peripheral neuritis.
EENT: optic neuritis.
GI: anorexia, nausea, vomiting, abdominal pain, GI upset.
Hematologic: ***thrombocytopenia***.
Metabolic: hyperuricemia.
Musculoskeletal: joint pain.
Respiratory: bloody sputum.
Skin: dermatitis, pruritus, ***toxic epidermal necrolysis***.
Other: ***anaphylactoid reactions***, precipitation of acute gout.

Interactions

Drug-drug. *Aluminum salts:* May delay and reduce absorption of ethambutol. Separate doses by several hours.

Nursing considerations

- Perform visual acuity and color discrimination tests before and during therapy.

- Ensure that any changes in vision don't result from an underlying condition.
- Obtain AST and ALT levels before therapy, and monitor these levels every 3 to 4 weeks.
- Anticipate dosage reduction in patients with impaired renal function.
- Always give ethambutol with other antituberculotics to prevent development of resistant organisms.
- Monitor uric acid level; observe patient for signs and symptoms of gout.

Patient teaching

- Reassure patient that visual disturbances usually disappear several weeks to months after drug is stopped. Inflammation of the optic nerve is related to dosage and duration of treatment.
- Inform patient that drug is given with other antituberculotics.
- Stress importance of compliance with drug therapy.
- Advise patient to report adverse reactions to prescriber.

ethinyl estradiol and desogestrel

monophasic
Apri, Desogen, Ortho-Cept

biphasic
Kariva, Mircette

triphasic
Cyclessa, Velivet

ethinyl estradiol and ethynodiol diacetate

monophasic
Demulen 1/35, Demulen 1/50, Zovia 1/35E, Zovia 1/50E

ethinyl estradiol and levonorgestrel

monophasic
Alesse-21, Alesse-28, Aviane, Lessina, Levlen, Levlite, Levora-21, Levora-28, Nordette-21, Nordette-28, Portia-21, Portia-28, Seasonale

biphasic
Preven Emergency Contraceptive Kit

triphasic
Enpresse, Tri-Levlen, Triphasil, Trivora-28

ethinyl estradiol and norethindrone

monophasic
Brevicon, Genora 0.5/35, Genora 1/35, Junel 21-1/20, Junel 21-1.5/30, ModiCon, N.E.E. 1/35, Necon 1/35-21, Necon 1/35-28, Necon 0.5/35-21, Necon 0.5/35-28, Nelova 0.5/35E, Nelova 1/35E, Norethin 1/35E, Norinyl 1 + 35, Ortho-Novum 1/35, Ovcon-35, Ovcon-50

biphasic
Necon 10/11-21, Necon 10/11-28, Ortho-Novum 10/11

triphasic
Necon 7/7/7, Nortel 7/7/7, Ortho-Novum 7/7/7, Tri-Norinyl

ethinyl estradiol and norethindrone acetate

monophasic
Junel 21-1/20, Junel 21-1.5/30, Loestrin 1/20, Loestrin 1.5/30

triphasic
Estrostep 21

ethinyl estradiol and norgestimate

monophasic
MonoNessa, Ortho-Cyclen, Sprintec

triphasic
Ortho Tri-Cyclen, Ortho Tri-Cyclen Lo, Tri-Sprintec

ethinyl estradiol and norgestrel

monophasic
Cryselle, Lo/Ovral, Lo-Ogestrel, Ogestrel, Ovral

ethinyl estradiol, norethindrone acetate, and ferrous fumarate

monophasic
Loestrin Fe 1/20, Loestrin Fe 1.5/30, Microgesin Fe 1/20, Microgesin Fe 1.5/30

triphasic
Estrostep Fe

mestranol and norethindrone

monophasic
Genora 1/50, Necon 1/50-21, Necon 1/50-28, Nelova 1/50M, Norethin 1/50M, Norinyl 1+50, Ortho-Novum 1/50

Pregnancy risk category X

Indications & dosages

➲ Contraception

Monophasic hormonal contraceptives

Women: 1 tablet P.O. daily beginning on the first day of menstrual cycle or the first Sunday after menstrual cycle begins. With 20- and 21-tablet package, new cycle begins 7 days after last tablet taken. With 28-tablet package, dosage is 1 tablet daily without interruption; extra tablets taken on days 22 to 28 are placebos or contain iron. Or, for Seasonale, 1 pink tablet P.O. daily beginning on the first Sunday after menstrual cycle begins, for 84 consecutive days, followed by 7 days of white (inert) tablets.

Biphasic hormonal contraceptives

Women: 1 color tablet P.O. daily for 10 days; then next color tablet for 11 days. With 21-tablet packages, new cycle begins 7 days after last tablet taken. With 28-tablet packages, dosage is 1 tablet daily without interruption.

Triphasic hormonal contraceptives

Women: 1 tablet P.O. daily in the sequence specified by the brand. With 21-tablet packages, new dosing cycle begins 7 days after last tablet taken. With 28-tablet packages, dosage is 1 tablet daily without interruption.

➲ To prevent pregnancy after unprotected intercourse

Women: For Preven Emergency Contraceptive Kit, 2 tablets P.O. within 72 hours of unprotected intercourse; take second dose 12 hours after the first dose.

➲ Moderate acne vulgaris in women age 15 and older who have no known contraindications to hormonal contraceptive therapy, who want oral contraception for at least 6 months, who have reached menarche, and who are unresponsive to topical antiacne drugs

Women age 15 and older: 1 tablet Estrostep or Ortho Tri-Cyclen P.O. daily (21 tablets contain active ingredients and 7 are inert).

Contraindications & cautions

- Contraindicated in patients with thromboembolic disorders, cerebrovascular or coronary artery disease, diplopia or ocular lesions arising from ophthalmic vascular disease, classic migraine, MI, known or suspected breast cancer, known or suspected estrogen-dependent neoplasia, benign or malignant liver tumors, active liver disease or history of cholestatic jaundice with pregnancy or previous use of hormonal contraceptives, and undiagnosed abnormal vaginal bleeding.
- Contraindicated in women who are or may be pregnant and in breast-feeding women.
- Use cautiously in patients with hyperlipidemia, hypertension, migraines, seizure disorders, asthma, or cardiac, renal, or hepatic insufficiency.

Adverse reactions

CNS: *headache, dizziness*, depression, lethargy, migraine, ***CVA***.
CV: ***thromboembolism***, hypertension, edema, ***pulmonary embolism***.
EENT: worsening myopia or astigmatism, intolerance of contact lenses, exophthalmos, diplopia.
GI: *nausea*, vomiting, abdominal cramps, bloating, anorexia, changes in appetite, gallbladder disease, ***pancreatitis***.
GU: *breakthrough bleeding, spotting*, granulomatous colitis, dysmenorrhea, amenorrhea, cervical erosion or abnormal secretions, enlargement of uterine fibromas, vaginal candidiasis.
Hepatic: cholestatic jaundice, ***liver tumors***.
Metabolic: weight gain.
Skin: rash, acne, ***erythema multiforme***.
Other: breast tenderness, enlargement, or secretion.

Interactions

Drug-drug. *Beta blockers:* May increase beta-blocker level. Dosage adjustment may be necessary.
Carbamazepine, fosphenytoin, phenobarbital, phenytoin, rifampin: May decrease estrogen effect. Use together cautiously.
Corticosteroids: May enhance corticosteroid effect. Monitor patient closely.
Griseofulvin, penicillins, sulfonamides, tetracyclines: May decrease hormonal contraceptive effect. Avoid using together, if possible.
Insulin, sulfonylureas: Glucose intolerance may decrease antidiabetic effects. Monitor these effects.
Oral anticoagulants: May decrease anticoagulant effect. Dosage adjustments may be needed. Monitor PT and INR.
Tamoxifen: May inhibit tamoxifen effect. Avoid using together.
Drug-herb. *Black cohosh:* May increase adverse effects of estrogen. Discourage use together.
Red clover: May interfere with hormonal therapy. Discourage use together.
Saw palmetto: May have antiestrogenic effect. Discourage use together.
St. John's wort: May decrease hormonal contraceptive effect because of increased hepatic metabolism. Discourage use together, or advise patient to use an additional method of contraception.
Drug-food. *Caffeine:* May increase caffeine level. Urge caution.
Grapefruit juice: May increase estrogen level. Advise patient to take with liquid other than grapefruit juice.
Drug-lifestyle. *Smoking:* May increase risk of adverse CV effects. If smoking continues, may need alternative therapy.

Nursing considerations

- Use estrogen-containing hormonal contraceptives with caution in patients who smoke.
- Triphasic hormonal contraceptives may cause fewer adverse reactions, such as breakthrough bleeding and spotting.
- The Centers for Disease Control and Prevention reports that use of hormonal contraceptives may decrease risk of ovarian and endometrial cancers and doesn't seem to increase risk of breast cancer. However, the FDA reports that hormonal contraceptives may be linked to an increase in cervical cancer.
- Monitor lipid levels, blood pressure, body weight, and hepatic function.

!!ALERT Many hormonal contraceptives share similar names. Make sure to check the hormone strength for verification.

- Estrogens and progestins may alter glucose tolerance, thus changing dosage requirements for antidiabetics. Monitor glucose level.
- Stop hormonal contraceptives for a few weeks before adrenal function tests.
- Stop hormonal contraceptive and notify prescriber if patient develops granulomatous colitis.
- Stop drug at least 1 week before surgery to decrease risk of thromboembolism. Tell patient to use an alternative method of birth control.

Patient teaching

- Tell patient to take tablets at same time each day; nighttime doses may reduce nausea and headaches.
- Advise patient to use an additional method of birth control, such as condoms or a diaphragm with spermicide, for the first week of the first cycle.
- Tell patient that missing doses in midcycle greatly increases likelihood of pregnancy.
- Tell patient that missing a dose may cause spotting or light bleeding.
- Tell patient that hormonal contraceptives don't protect against HIV or other sexually transmitted diseases.
- Tell patient using Seasonale that there will be four planned menses per year, but spotting or bleeding between menses may occur.
- If 1 pill is missed, tell patient to take it as soon as possible (2 pills if remembered on the next day), and then to continue regular schedule. Advise an additional method of contraception for remainder of cycle. If 2 consecutive pills are missed, tell patient to take 2 pills a day for next 2 days and then resume regular schedule. Advise an additional method of contraception for the next 7 days or preferably for the remainder of cycle. If 2 consecutive pills are missed in the 3rd week or if patient misses 3 consecutive pills, tell patient to contact prescriber for instructions.

- Warn patient of common adverse effects, such as headache, nausea, dizziness, breast tenderness, spotting, and breakthrough bleeding, which usually diminish after 3 to 6 months.
- Instruct patient to weigh herself at least twice a week and to report any sudden weight gain or swelling to prescriber.
- Warn patient to avoid exposure to ultraviolet light or prolonged exposure to sunlight.

!!ALERT Warn patient to immediately report abdominal pain; numbness, stiffness, or pain in legs or buttocks; pressure or pain in chest; shortness of breath; severe headache; visual disturbances such as blind spots, blurriness, or flashing lights; undiagnosed vaginal bleeding or discharge; two consecutive missed menstrual periods; lumps in the breast; swelling of hands or feet; or severe pain in the abdomen (tumor rupture in liver).

- Advise patient of increased risks created by simultaneous use of cigarettes and hormonal contraceptives.
- If one menstrual period is missed and tablets have been taken on schedule, tell patient to continue taking them. If two consecutive menstrual periods are missed, tell patient to stop drug and have pregnancy test. Progestins may cause birth defects if taken early in pregnancy.
- Advise patient not to take same drug for longer than 12 months without consulting prescriber. Stress importance of Pap tests and annual gynecologic examinations.
- Advise patient to check with prescriber about how soon pregnancy may be attempted after hormonal therapy is stopped. Many prescribers recommend that women not become pregnant within 2 months after stopping drug.
- Warn patient of possible delay in achieving pregnancy when drug is stopped.
- Teach woman how to perform routine breast self-examination.
- Teach patient methods to decrease risk of thromboembolism.
- Advise patient taking hormonal contraceptives to use additional form of birth control during concurrent treatment with certain antibiotics.
- Advise patient that hormonal contraceptives may change the fit of contact lenses.

etodolac

Lodine, Lodine XL

Pregnancy risk category C; D in 3rd trimester

Indications & dosages

➲ Acute pain

Adults: 200 to 400 mg P.O. q 6 to 8 hours, p.r.n., not to exceed 1,200 mg daily. In patients weighing 60 kg (132 lb) or less, don't exceed total daily dose of 20 mg/kg.

➲ Short- and long-term management of osteoarthritis and rheumatoid arthritis

Adults: 600 to 1,000 mg P.O. daily, divided into two or three doses. Maximum daily dose is 1,200 mg. For extended-release tablets, 400 to 1,000 mg P.O. daily. Maximum daily dose is 1,200 mg.

Contraindications & cautions

- Contraindicated in patients hypersensitive to drug and in those with history of aspirin- or NSAID-induced asthma, rhinitis, urticaria, or other allergic reactions.
- Use cautiously in patients with history of renal or hepatic impairment, preexisting asthma, or GI bleeding, ulceration, and perforation.

Adverse reactions

CNS: asthenia, malaise, dizziness, depression, drowsiness, nervousness, insomnia, syncope, fever.
CV: hypertension, ***heart failure***, flushing, palpitations, edema, fluid retention.
EENT: blurred vision, tinnitus, photophobia.
GI: *dyspepsia*, flatulence, abdominal pain, diarrhea, nausea, constipation, gastritis, melena, vomiting, anorexia, ***peptic ulceration with or without GI bleeding or perforation***, ulcerative stomatitis, thirst, dry mouth.
GU: dysuria, urinary frequency, ***renal failure***.
Hematologic: anemia, ***leukopenia***, hemolytic anemia.
Hepatic: ***hepatitis***.
Metabolic: weight gain.
Respiratory: asthma.
Skin: pruritus, rash, cutaneous vasculitis, ***Stevens-Johnson syndrome***.
Other: chills.

Interactions

Drug-drug. *Antacids:* May decrease etodolac's peak level. Watch for decreased effect of etodolac.
Aspirin: May decrease protein-binding of etodolac without altering its clearance. May increase GI toxicity. Avoid using together.
Beta blockers, diuretics: May blunt effects of these drugs. Monitor patient closely.
Cyclosporine: May increase risk of nephrotoxicity. Avoid using together.
Digoxin, lithium, methotrexate: May impair elimination of these drugs, increasing risk of toxicity. Monitor drug levels.
Phenylbutazone: May increase etodolac level. Avoid using together.
Phenytoin: May increase phenytoin level. Monitor patient for toxicity.
Warfarin: May decrease the protein binding of warfarin but doesn't change its clearance. Although no dosage adjustment is needed, monitor INR closely and watch for bleeding.
Drug-herb. *Dong quai, feverfew, garlic, ginger, horse chestnut, red clover:* May increase risk of bleeding. Discourage use together.
White willow: Herb and drug contain similar components. Discourage use together.
Drug-lifestyle. *Alcohol use:* May increase risk of adverse effects. Discourage use together.
Sun exposure: May cause photosensitivity reactions. Advise patient to avoid excessive sunlight exposure.

Nursing considerations

- Because NSAIDs impair the synthesis of renal prostaglandins, they can decrease renal blood flow and lead to reversible renal impairment, especially in patients with renal or heart failure or liver dysfunction, in elderly patients, and in those taking diuretics. Monitor these patients closely.
- Serious GI toxicity, including peptic ulcers and bleeding, can occur in patient taking NSAIDs, despite lack of symptoms.

!!ALERT Don't confuse Lodine with codeine, iodine, or Iopidine.

Patient teaching

- Tell patient to take drug with milk or meals to minimize GI discomfort.
- Teach patient signs and symptoms of GI bleeding, including blood in vomit, urine, or stool; coffee-ground vomit; and black, tarry stool. Tell him to notify prescriber immediately if any of these occurs.
- Advise patient to avoid consuming alcohol or aspirin while taking drug.
- Warn patient to avoid hazardous activities that require alertness until harmful CNS effects of drug are known.
- Teach patient signs and symptoms of liver damage, including nausea, fatigue, lethargy, itching, yellowed skin or eyes, right upper quadrant tenderness, and flulike symptoms. Tell him to contact prescriber immediately if any of these symptoms occur.
- Advise patient to use a sunblock, wear protective clothing, and avoid prolonged exposure to sunlight because of possible sensitivity to sunlight.
- Tell pregnant woman to avoid use of drug during last trimester.
- Advise patient that use of OTC NSAIDs and etodolac may increase the risk of GI toxicity.

etonogestrel and ethinyl estradiol vaginal ring

NuvaRing

Pregnancy risk category X

Indications & dosages

➲ Contraception
Women: Insert one ring into the vagina and leave in place for 3 weeks. Insert new ring 1 week after the previous ring is removed.

Contraindications & cautions

- Contraindicated in patients hypersensitive to any component of drug, patients who are or may be pregnant, patients older than age 35 who smoke 15 or more cigarettes daily, and patients with thrombophlebitis, thromboembolic disorder, history of deep vein thrombophlebitis, cerebral vascular or coronary artery disease (current or previous), valvular heart disease with complications, severe hypertension, diabetes with vascular complications, headache with focal neurologic symptoms, major surgery with prolonged immobilization, known or suspected cancer of the endometrium or breast, estrogen-dependent neoplasia, abnormal undiagnosed genital bleeding, jaundice related to pregnancy or previous use of hor-

monal contraceptive, active liver disease, or benign or malignant hepatic tumors.
• Use cautiously in patients with hypertension, hyperlipidemias, obesity, or diabetes.
• Use cautiously in patients with conditions that could be aggravated by fluid retention, and in patients with a history of depression.

Adverse reactions

CNS: *headache*, emotional lability, ***cerebral thrombosis***.
CV: hypertension, ***thromboembolic events***, coagulation abnormalities.
EENT: *sinusitis*.
GI: *nausea*.
GU: *vaginitis, leukorrhea*, device-related events (for example, foreign body sensation, coital difficulties, device expulsion), vaginal discomfort.
Hepatic: ***hepatic adenomas***, benign liver tumors.
Metabolic: weight gain.
Respiratory: *upper respiratory tract infection*.

Interactions

Drug-drug. *Acetaminophen:* May decrease acetaminophen level and increase ethinyl estradiol level. Monitor patient for effects.
Ampicillin, barbiturates, carbamazepine, felbamate, griseofulvin, oxcarbazepine, phenylbutazone, phenytoin, rifampin, tetracyclines, topiramate: May decrease contraceptive effect and increase risk of pregnancy, breakthrough bleeding, or both. Tell patient to use an additional form of contraception while taking these drugs.
Ascorbic acid, atorvastatin, itraconazole: May increase ethinyl estradiol level. Monitor patient for adverse effects.
Clofibric acid, morphine, salicylic acid, temazepam: May increase clearance of these drugs. Monitor patient for effectiveness.
Cyclosporine, prednisolone, theophylline: May increase levels of these drugs. Monitor levels if appropriate and adjust dosage.
HIV protease inhibitors: May affect contraceptive effect. Refer to the specific protease inhibitor drug literature. May need to use a backup method of contraception.
Drug-herb. *St. John's wort:* May reduce contraceptive effectiveness and increase the risk of breakthrough bleeding and pregnancy. Discourage use together.
Drug-lifestyle. *Smoking:* May increase risk of serious CV adverse effects, especially in those older than age 35 who smoke 15 or more cigarettes daily. Urge patient to avoid smoking.

Nursing considerations

!!ALERT Drug may increase the risk of MI, thromboembolism, CVA, hepatic neoplasia, and gallbladder disease.
• Cigarette smoking increases the risk of serious adverse cardiac effects. The risk increases with age and in patients who smoke 15 or more cigarettes daily.
• Stop drug at least 4 weeks before and for 2 weeks after procedures that may increase the risk of thromboembolism, and during and after prolonged immobilization.
• Stop drug and notify prescriber if patient develops unexplained partial or complete loss of vision, proptosis, diplopia, papilledema, retinal vascular lesions, migraines, depression, or jaundice.
• Monitor blood pressure closely if patient has hypertension or renal disease.
• Ring should remain in place continuously for a full 3 weeks to maintain efficacy. It is then removed for 1 week. During this time, withdrawal bleeding occurs (usually starting 2 or 3 days after removal). A new ring should be inserted 1 week after removal of the previous one, regardless of whether the patient is still menstruating.
• Rule out pregnancy if patient hasn't adhered to the prescribed regimen and a period is missed, if prescribed regimen is adhered to and two periods are missed, or if the patient has retained the ring for longer than 4 weeks.

Patient teaching

• Stress importance of having regular annual physical examinations to check for adverse effects or developing contraindications.
• Tell patient that drug doesn't protect against HIV and other sexually transmitted diseases.
• Advise patient not to smoke while using contraceptive.
• Tell patient not to use a diaphragm if a back-up method of birth control is needed.
• Tell patient who wears contact lenses to contact an ophthalmologist if vision or lens tolerance changes.

- Advise patient to follow the manufacturer's instructions for use if switching from a different form of hormonal contraceptive.
- Tell patient to insert ring into the vagina (using fingers) and keep it in place continuously for 3 weeks to maintain efficacy, saving the foil package for later disposal. Explain that it is then removed for 1 full week and that, during this time, withdrawal bleeding occurs (usually starting 2 or 3 days after removal). Tell patient to insert a new ring 1 week after removing the previous one, regardless of menstrual bleeding. Tell patient to reseal the ring in the package after removing it from the vagina.
- Advise patient that, if the ring is removed or expelled (such as while removing a tampon, straining, or moving bowels), it should be washed with cool to lukewarm (not hot) water and reinserted immediately. Stress that contraceptive efficacy may be compromised if the ring stays out for longer than 3 hours and that she should use a backup method of contraception until the newly reinserted ring is used continuously for 7 days.

etoposide (VP-16, VP-16-213)

Toposar, VePesid

etoposide phosphate

Etopophos

Pregnancy risk category D

Indications & dosages

Testicular cancer

Adults: 50 to 100 mg/m^2 daily I.V. on five consecutive days q 3 to 4 weeks. Or, 100 mg/m^2 daily I.V. on days 1, 3, and 5 q 3 to 4 weeks for three or four courses of therapy.

Small-cell carcinoma of the lung

Adults: 35 mg/m^2 daily I.V. for 4 days. Or, 50 mg/m^2 daily I.V. for 5 days. P.O. dose is two times I.V. dose, rounded to nearest 50 mg.

For patients with creatinine clearance of 15 to 50 ml/minute, reduce dose by 25%.

Kaposi's sarcoma♦

Adults: 150 mg/m^2 I.V. daily for 3 days q 4 weeks. Repeat p.r.n., based on response.

Contraindications & cautions

- Contraindicated in patients hypersensitive to drug.
- Use cautiously in patients who have had cytotoxic or radiation therapy and in those with hepatic impairment.

Adverse reactions

CNS: peripheral neuropathy.
CV: hypotension.
GI: *nausea, vomiting, anorexia, diarrhea,* abdominal pain, stomatitis.
Hematologic: *anemia,* ***myelosuppression,*** LEUKOPENIA, THROMBOCYTOPENIA, NEUTROPENIA.
Hepatic: ***hepatotoxicity.***
Skin: *reversible alopecia,* rash.
Other: hypersensitivity reactions, ***anaphylaxis.***

Interactions

Drug-drug. *Phosphatase inhibitors, such as levamisole hydrochloride:* May decrease etoposide effectiveness. Monitor drug effects. *Warfarin:* May further prolong PT. Monitor PT and INR closely.

Nursing considerations

- Obtain baseline blood pressure before starting therapy.
- Anticipate need for antiemetics.
- Have diphenhydramine, hydrocortisone, epinephrine, and emergency equipment available to establish an airway in case anaphylaxis occurs.
- Store capsules in refrigerator.
- Monitor CBC. Watch for evidence of bone marrow suppression.
- Observe patient's mouth for signs of ulceration.
- To prevent bleeding, avoid all I.M. injections when platelet count is below 50,000/mm^3.
- Anticipate need for blood transfusions to combat anemia. Patient may receive injections of RBC colony–stimulating factors to promote RBC production and decrease need for blood transfusions.
- Etoposide phosphate dose is expressed as etoposide equivalents; 119.3 mg of etoposide phosphate is equivalent to 100 mg of etoposide.

Patient teaching

- Tell patient to watch for signs and symptoms of infection (fever, sore throat, fatigue) and bleeding (easy bruising, nosebleeds, bleeding gums, tarry stools). Tell patient to take temperature daily.
- Inform patient of need for frequent blood pressure readings during I.V. administration.
- Caution woman of childbearing age to avoid pregnancy and breast-feeding during therapy.

exemestane
Aromasin

Pregnancy risk category D

Indications & dosages

➲ **Advanced breast cancer in postmenopausal women whose disease has progressed after treatment with tamoxifen**
Adults: 25 mg P.O. once daily after food.

Contraindications & cautions

- Contraindicated in patients hypersensitive to drug or its components.

Adverse reactions

CNS: *depression, insomnia, anxiety, fatigue, pain,* dizziness, headache, paresthesia, generalized weakness, asthenia, confusion, hypoesthesia, fever.
CV: hypertension, edema, chest pain, *hot flashes.*
EENT: sinusitis, rhinitis, pharyngitis.
GI: *nausea,* vomiting, abdominal pain, anorexia, constipation, diarrhea, increased appetite, dyspepsia.
GU: UTI.
Hematologic: *lymphopenia.*
Musculoskeletal: pathologic fractures, arthritis, back pain, skeletal pain.
Respiratory: *dyspnea,* bronchitis, cough, upper respiratory tract infection.
Skin: rash, increased sweating, alopecia, itching.
Other: infection, flulike syndrome, lymphedema.

Interactions

Drug-drug. *Drugs that induce CYP3A4, estrogenics:* May decrease exemestane level. Monitor patient closely.

Nursing considerations

- Use drug only in postmenopausal women. Pregnancy must be ruled out before starting drug therapy.
- Continue treatment until tumor progression is apparent.

Patient teaching

- Direct patient to take drug after a meal.
- Tell patient that she may need to take drug for a long time.
- Advise patient to report adverse effects, especially fever or swelling of arms or legs.

ezetimibe
Zetia

Pregnancy risk category C

Indications & dosages

➲ **Adjunct to diet and exercise to reduce total cholesterol, LDL cholesterol, and apolipoprotein B levels in patients with primary hypercholesterolemia, alone or combined with HMG-CoA reductase inhibitors (statins) or bile acid sequestrants; adjunct to other lipid-lowering drugs (combined with atorvastatin or simvastatin) in patients with homozygous familial hypercholesterolemia; adjunct to diet in patients with homozygous sitosterolemia to reduce sitosterol and campesterol levels**
Adults and children age 10 and older: 10 mg P.O. daily.

Contraindications & cautions

- Contraindicated in patients allergic to any component of the drug.
- Contraindicated with HMG-CoA reductase inhibitor in pregnant or breast-feeding patients and in patients with active hepatic disease or unexplained increased transaminase level.
- Use cautiously in elderly patients.

Adverse reactions

CNS: dizziness, headache, fatigue.
CV: chest pain.
EENT: pharyngitis, sinusitis.
GI: abdominal pain, diarrhea.
Musculoskeletal: back pain, arthralgia, myalgia.
Respiratory: cough, *upper respiratory tract infection.*

Other: viral infection.

Interactions

Drug-drug. *Bile acid sequestrant (cholestyramine):* May decrease ezetimibe level. Give ezetimibe at least 2 hours before or 4 hours after cholestyramine.
Cyclosporine, fenofibrate, gemfibrozil: May increase ezetimibe level. Monitor patient closely for adverse reactions.
Fibrates: May increase excretion of cholesterol into the gallbladder bile. Avoid using together.

Nursing considerations

- Before starting treatment, assess patient for underlying causes of dyslipidemia.
- Obtain baseline triglyceride and total, LDL, and HDL cholesterol levels.
- When ezetimibe is used with an HMG-CoA reductase inhibitor, check liver function test values at start of therapy and thereafter according to the HMG-CoA reductase inhibitor manufacturer's recommendations.
- Use of ezetimibe with an HMG-CoA reductase inhibitor significantly reduces total and LDL cholesterol, apolipoprotein B, and triglyceride levels and (except with pravastatin) increases HDL cholesterol level more than use of an HMG-CoA reductase inhibitor alone.
- Patient should maintain a cholesterol-lowering diet during treatment.

Patient teaching

- Emphasize importance of following a cholesterol-lowering diet during drug therapy.
- Tell patient he may take drug without regard to meals.
- Advise patient to notify prescriber of unexplained muscle pain, weakness, or tenderness.
- Urge patient to tell his prescriber about any herbal or dietary supplements he's taking.
- Advise patient to visit his prescriber for routine follow-up and blood tests.
- Tell patient to notify prescriber if she becomes pregnant.

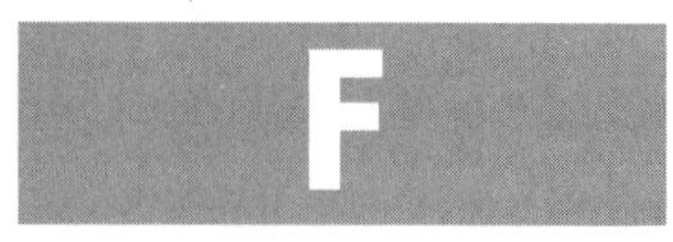

famciclovir
Famvir

Pregnancy risk category B

Indications & dosages

➲ **Acute herpes zoster infection (shingles)**
Adults: 500 mg P.O. q 8 hours for 7 days.
For patients with creatinine clearance of 40 to 59 ml/minute, give 500 mg P.O. q 12 hours; if clearance is 20 to 39 ml/minute, give 500 mg P.O. q 24 hours; and if it's less than 20 ml/minute, give 250 mg P.O. q 24 hours. For hemodialysis patients, give 250 mg P.O. after each hemodialysis session.

➲ **Recurrent genital herpes**
Adults: 125 mg P.O. b.i.d. for 5 days. Begin therapy as soon as symptoms occur.
For patients with creatinine clearance of 39 ml/minute or less, give 125 mg P.O. q 24 hours. For hemodialysis patients, give 125 mg P.O. after each hemodialysis session.

➲ **Suppression of recurrent genital herpes**
Adults: 250 mg P.O. b.i.d. for up to 1 year.
For patients with creatinine clearance of 20 to 39 ml/minute, give 125 mg P.O. q 12 hours; if clearance is less than 20 ml/minute, give 125 mg P.O. q 24 hours. For hemodialysis patients, give 125 mg P.O. after each hemodialysis session.

➲ **Recurrent mucocutaneous herpes simplex infections in HIV-infected patients**
Adults: 500 mg P.O. b.i.d. for 7 days.
For patients with creatinine clearance of 20 to 39 ml/minute, give 500 mg P.O. q 24 hours; if clearance is less than 20 ml/minute, give 250 mg P.O. q 24 hours. For hemodialysis patients, give 250 mg P.O. after each hemodialysis session.

Contraindications & cautions

- Contraindicated in patients hypersensitive to drug.
- Use cautiously in patients with renal or hepatic impairment.

Adverse reactions
CNS: *headache*, fatigue, fever, dizziness, paresthesia, somnolence.
EENT: pharyngitis, sinusitis.
GI: diarrhea, *nausea*, vomiting, constipation, anorexia, abdominal pain.
Musculoskeletal: back pain, arthralgia.
Skin: pruritus.
Other: zoster-related signs, symptoms, and complications.

Interactions
Drug-drug. *Probenecid:* May increase level of penciclovir, the active metabolite of famciclovir. Monitor patient for increased adverse reactions.

Nursing considerations
- Drug may be taken without regard to meals.
- Dosage adjustment may be needed in patients with renal or hepatic impairment.
- Monitor renal and liver function tests in these patients.

Patient teaching
- Inform patient that drug doesn't cure genital herpes but can decrease the length and severity of symptoms.
- Teach patient how to avoid spreading infection to others.
- Urge patient to recognize the early signs and symptoms of herpes infection, such as tingling, itching, and pain, and to report them. Treatment is more effective if therapy is started within 48 hours of rash onset.

famotidine
Mylanta-AR ◇, Pepcid, Pepcid AC ◇, Pepcid RPD

Pregnancy risk category B

Indications & dosages
➲ Short-term treatment for duodenal ulcer
Adults: For acute therapy, 40 mg P.O. once daily h.s. or 20 mg P.O. b.i.d. Healing usually occurs within 4 weeks. For maintenance therapy, 20 mg P.O. once daily h.s.
➲ Short-term treatment for benign gastric ulcer
Adults: 40 mg P.O. daily h.s. for 8 weeks.
Children ages 1 to 16: 0.5 mg/kg/day P.O. at h.s. or divided b.i.d., up to 40 mg daily.
➲ Pathologic hypersecretory conditions (such as Zollinger-Ellison syndrome)
Adults: 20 mg P.O. q 6 hours, up to 160 mg q 6 hours.
➲ Hospitalized patients who can't take oral drug or who have intractable ulcers or hypersecretory conditions
Adults: 20 mg I.V. q 12 hours.
➲ Gastroesophageal reflux disease (GERD)
Adults: 20 mg P.O. b.i.d. for up to 6 weeks. For esophagitis caused by GERD, 20 to 40 mg b.i.d. for up to 12 weeks.
Children ages 1 to 16: 1 mg/kg/day P.O. divided twice daily up to 40 mg b.i.d.
➲ To prevent or treat heartburn
Adults: 10 mg Pepcid AC P.O. 1 hour before meals to prevent symptoms, or 10 mg Pepcid AC P.O. with water when symptoms occur. Maximum daily dose is 20 mg. Drug shouldn't be taken daily for longer than 2 weeks.

For patients with creatinine clearance below 50 ml/minute, give half the dose, or increase dosing interval to q 36 to 48 hours.

Contraindications & cautions
- Contraindicated in patients hypersensitive to drug.

Adverse reactions
CNS: *headache*, fever, dizziness, vertigo, malaise, paresthesia.
CV: palpitations, flushing.
EENT: tinnitus, orbital edema.
GI: diarrhea, constipation, anorexia, taste perversion, dry mouth.
Musculoskeletal: bone and muscle pain.
Skin: acne, dry skin.
Other: transient irritation at I.V. site.

Interactions
None significant.

Nursing considerations
- Assess patient for abdominal pain. Note blood in emesis, stool, or gastric aspirate.
- Oral suspension must be reconstituted and shaken before use.
- Store reconstituted oral suspension below 86° F (30° C). Discard after 30 days.

Patient teaching

- Instruct patient in proper use of OTC product, if appropriate.
- Tell patient to take prescription drug with a snack, if desired.
- Remind patient that prescription drug is most effective if taken at bedtime. Tell patient taking 20 mg twice daily to take one dose at bedtime.
- Advise patient to limit use of prescription drug to no longer than 8 weeks, unless ordered by prescriber, and OTC drug to no longer than 2 weeks.
- With prescriber's knowledge, let patient take antacids together, especially at beginning of therapy when pain is severe.
- Urge patient to avoid cigarette smoking because it may increase gastric acid secretion and worsen disease.
- Advise patient to report abdominal pain or blood in stools or vomit.

felodipine

Plendil, Renedil†

Pregnancy risk category C

Indications & dosages

➲ Hypertension

Adults: Initially, 5 mg P.O. daily. Adjust dosage based on patient response, usually at intervals not less than 2 weeks. Usual dose is 2.5 to 10 mg daily; maximum dosage is 10 mg daily.

Elderly patients: 2.5 mg P.O. daily; adjust dosage as for adults. Maximum dosage is 10 mg daily.

For patients with impaired hepatic function, 2.5 mg P.O. daily; adjust dosage as for adults. Maximum daily dose is 10 mg.

Contraindications & cautions

- Contraindicated in patients hypersensitive to drug.
- Use cautiously in patients with heart failure, particularly those receiving beta blockers, and in patients with impaired hepatic function.

Adverse reactions

CNS: *headache*, dizziness, paresthesia, asthenia.

CV: *peripheral edema*, chest pain, palpitations, flushing.

EENT: rhinorrhea, pharyngitis.

GI: abdominal pain, nausea, constipation, diarrhea.

Musculoskeletal: muscle cramps, back pain.

Respiratory: upper respiratory tract infection, cough.

Skin: rash.

Interactions

Drug-drug. *Anticonvulsants:* May decrease felodipine level. Avoid using together.

CYP3A4 inhibitors such as azole antifungals, cimetidine, erythromycin: May decrease clearance of felodipine. Reduce doses of felodipine; monitor patient for toxicity.

Metoprolol: May alter pharmacokinetics of metoprolol. Monitor patient for adverse reactions.

NSAIDs: May decrease antihypertensive effects. Monitor blood pressure.

Theophylline: May slightly decrease theophylline level. Monitor patient response closely.

Drug-herb. *Ma huang:* May decrease antihypertensive effects. Discourage use together.

Drug-food. *Grapefruit, lime:* May increase drug's level and adverse effects. Discourage use together.

Nursing considerations

- Monitor blood pressure for response.
- Monitor patient for peripheral edema, which appears to be both dose- and age-related. It's more common in patients taking higher doses, especially those older than age 60.

!! ALERT Don't confuse Plendil with pindolol.

Patient teaching

- Tell patient to swallow tablets whole and not to crush or chew them.
- Tell patient to take drug without food or with a light meal.
- Advise patient not to take drug with grapefruit juice.
- Advise patient to continue taking drug even when he feels better, to watch his diet, and to check with prescriber or pharmacist before taking other drugs, including OTC drugs, nutritional supplements, or herbal remedies.

• Advise patient to observe good oral hygiene and to see a dentist regularly; use of drug may cause mild gum problems.

fenofibrate (micronized)
Lofibra, Tricor

Pregnancy risk category C

Indications & dosages

➲ Adjunct to diet to reduce very high triglyceride levels (type IV and V hyperlipidemia) in patients at high risk for pancreatitis who don't respond adequately to diet alone

Adults: 67- to 200-mg capsule or 54- to 160-mg tablet P.O. daily. Based on response, increase dose if necessary after repeating triglyceride level check at 4- to 8-week intervals to maximum dose of 200-mg capsule or 160-mg tablet daily.

If creatinine clearance is less than 50 ml/minute or patient is elderly, initially, 67-mg capsule or 54-mg tablet daily; increase only after evaluating effects on renal function and triglyceride levels at this dose.

➲ Adjunct to diet to reduce LDL, total cholesterol, triglyceride, and apolipoprotein B levels and to increase HDL cholesterol levels in patients with primary hypercholesterolemia or mixed dyslipidemia (Fredrickson types IIa and IIb)

Adults: 200-mg capsule or 160-mg tablet P.O. daily.

If creatinine clearance is less than 50 ml/minute or patient is elderly, initially, 67-mg capsule or 54-mg tablet daily; increase only after evaluating effects on renal function and triglyceride levels at this dose.

Contraindications & cautions

• Contraindicated in patients hypersensitive to drug and in those with gallbladder disease, hepatic dysfunction, primary biliary cirrhosis, severe renal dysfunction, or unexplained persistent liver function abnormalities.

• Use cautiously in patients with a history of pancreatitis.

Adverse reactions

CNS: *dizziness*, localized pain, asthenia, fatigue, paresthesia, insomnia, *headache*.
CV: ***arrhythmias***.
EENT: eye discomfort, eye floaters, earache, conjunctivitis, blurred vision, rhinitis, sinusitis.
GI: dyspepsia, eructation, flatulence, nausea, vomiting, abdominal pain, constipation, diarrhea, increased appetite.
GU: polyuria, vaginitis.
Musculoskeletal: arthralgia.
Respiratory: cough.
Skin: pruritus, rash.
Other: decreased libido, hypersensitivity reactions, *infection*, flulike syndrome.

Interactions

Drug-drug. *Bile-acid sequestrants:* May bind and inhibit absorption of fenofibrate. Give drug 1 hour before or 4 to 6 hours after bile-acid sequestrants.

Coumarin-type anticoagulants: May potentiate anticoagulant effect, prolonging PT and INR. Monitor PT and INR closely. May need to reduce anticoagulant dosage.

Cyclosporine, immunosuppressants, nephrotoxic drugs: May induce renal dysfunction that may affect fenofibrate elimination. Use together cautiously.

HMG-CoA reductase inhibitors: May increase risk of adverse musculoskeletal effects. Avoid using together, unless potential benefit outweighs risk.

Drug-food. *Any food:* May increase fenofibrate absorption. Advise patient to take drug with meals.

Drug-lifestyle. *Alcohol use:* May increase triglyceride levels. Discourage use together.

Nursing considerations

• Obtain baseline lipid levels and liver function test results before starting therapy. Monitor liver function periodically during drug therapy. Stop drug if enzyme levels persist above three times normal limit.

• Watch for signs and symptoms of pancreatitis, myositis, rhabdomyolysis, cholelithiasis, and renal failure. Monitor patient for muscle pain, tenderness, or weakness, especially with malaise or fever.

• If an adequate response hasn't been obtained after 2 months of treatment with maximum daily dose, therapy must be stopped.

• Drug lowers uric acid level by increasing uric acid excretion in patients with or without hyperuricemia.

- Beta blockers, estrogens, and thiazide diuretics may increase triglyceride levels; evaluate need for continued use of these drugs.
- Hemoglobin level, hematocrit, and WBC count may decrease when therapy starts but stabilize with long-term administration.

Patient teaching

- Inform patient that drug therapy doesn't reduce need for following a triglyceride-lowering diet.
- Advise patient to promptly report unexplained muscle weakness, pain, or tenderness, especially if accompanied by malaise or fever.
- Inform patient to take drug with meals for best drug absorption.
- Advise patient to continue weight control measures, including diet and exercise, and to drink less alcohol before starting drug therapy.
- Instruct patient who is also taking a bile-acid resin to take fenofibrate 1 hour before or 4 to 6 hours after taking resin.
- Advise patient about potential for tumor growth.
- Tell breast-feeding woman to either stop breast-feeding or stop taking drug.

fentanyl citrate
Sublimaze

fentanyl transdermal system
Duragesic-12, Duragesic-25, Duragesic-50, Duragesic-75, Duragesic-100

fentanyl transmucosal
Actiq

Pregnancy risk category C
Controlled substance schedule II

Indications & dosages

➲ Adjunct to general anesthetic
Adults: For low-dose therapy, 2 mcg/kg I.V. For moderate-dose therapy, 2 to 20 mcg/kg I.V.; then 25 to 100 mcg I.V., p.r.n. For high-dose therapy, 20 to 50 mcg/kg I.V.; then 25 mcg to one-half initial loading dose I.V., p.r.n.

➲ Adjunct to regional anesthesia
Adults: 50 to 100 mcg I.M. or slowly I.V. over 1 to 2 minutes, p.r.n.

➲ Induce and maintain anesthesia
Children ages 2 to 12: 2 to 3 mcg/kg I.V.

➲ Postoperative pain, restlessness, tachypnea, and emergence delirium
Adults: 50 to 100 mcg I.M. q 1 to 2 hours, p.r.n.

➲ Preoperative medication
Adults: 50 to 100 mcg I.M. 30 to 60 minutes before surgery.

➲ To manage chronic pain
Adults: Apply 1 transdermal system to a portion of the upper torso on an area of skin that isn't irritated and hasn't been irradiated. Start therapy with the 25-mcg/hour system; adjust dosage as needed and tolerated. Each system may be worn for 72 hours, although some patients may need systems to be applied q 48 hours. May increase dose q 3 days after first dose; thereafter, don't increase more often than q 6 days.

➲ To manage breakthrough cancer pain in patients already receiving and tolerating an opioid
Adults: 200 mcg Actiq initially; may give second dose 15 minutes after completion of the first (30 minutes after first lozenge placed in mouth). Maximum dose is 2 lozenges per breakthrough episode. If several episodes of breakthrough pain requiring 2 lozenges occur, dose may be increased to the next available strength. Once a successful dosage has been reached, patient should limit use to no more than 4 lozenges daily.

Contraindications & cautions

- Contraindicated in patients intolerant to drug.
- Fentanyl patch is contraindicated in patients hypersensitive to adhesives, for pain management after surgery, mild or intermittent pain that can be managed with nonopioid drugs, and in initial doses over 25 mcg/hour.
- Actiq is contraindicated in children and in management of acute or postoperative pain.
- Don't give transdermal fentanyl to patients younger than age 12 or those younger than age 18 who weigh less than 110 lb (50 kg) or for postoperative pain.
- Use with caution in patients with head injury, increased CSF pressure, COPD, de-

creased respiratory reserve, potentially compromised respirations, hepatic or renal disease, or cardiac bradyarrhythmias.
- Use with caution in elderly or debilitated patients.

Adverse reactions

CNS: *sedation, somnolence, clouded sensorium, euphoria,* dizziness, headache, *confusion, asthenia,* nervousness, hallucinations, anxiety, depression, ***seizures***.
CV: hypotension, hypertension, ***arrhythmias***, chest pain.
GI: nausea, vomiting, constipation, ileus, abdominal pain, dry mouth, anorexia, diarrhea, dyspepsia.
GU: urine retention.
Musculoskeletal: skeletal muscle rigidity (dose-related).
Respiratory: ***respiratory depression***, hypoventilation, dyspnea, ***apnea***.
Skin: erythema at application site (transdermal), *pruritus, diaphoresis.*
Other: physical dependence.

Interactions

Drug-drug. *CNS depressants, general anesthetics, hypnotics, MAO inhibitors, other opioid analgesics, sedatives, tricyclic antidepressants:* May cause additive effects. Use together cautiously. Reduce dosages of these drugs and reduce fentanyl dose by one-fourth to one-third.
CYP3A4 inhibitors (erythromycin, ketoconazole, protease inhibitors such as ritonavir): May cause increased analgesia, CNS depression, and hypotensive effects. Monitor patient's respiratory status and vital signs.
CYP3A4 inducers (carbamazepine, phenytoin, rifampin): May decrease analgesic effects. Monitor patient for adequate pain relief.
Diazepam: May cause CV depression when given with high doses of fentanyl. Monitor patient closely.
Droperidol: May cause hypotension and decreases pulmonary arterial pressure. Use together cautiously.
Drug-lifestyle. *Alcohol use:* May cause additive effects. Discourage use together.

Nursing considerations

- For better analgesic effect, give drug before patient has intense pain.

!!ALERT High doses can produce muscle rigidity, which can be reversed with neuromuscular blockers; however, patient must be artificially ventilated.
- Monitor circulatory and respiratory status and urinary function carefully. Drug may cause respiratory depression, hypotension, urine retention, nausea, vomiting, ileus, or altered level of consciousness no matter how it is given.
- Periodically monitor postoperative vital signs and bladder function. Because drug decreases both rate and depth of respirations, monitoring of arterial oxygen saturation (SaO_2) may help assess respiratory depression. Immediately report respiratory rate below 12 breaths/minute, decreased respiratory volume, or decreased SaO_2.

Transdermal form
- Dosage equivalent charts are available to calculate the fentanyl transdermal dose based on the daily morphine intake; for example, for every 90 mg of oral morphine or 15 mg of I.M. morphine per 24 hours, 25 mcg/hour of transdermal fentanyl is needed.
- Make dosage adjustments gradually in patient using the transdermal system. Reaching steady-state level of a new dosage may take up to 6 days; delay dosage adjustment until after at least two applications.
- Monitor patient who develops adverse reactions to the transdermal system for at least 12 hours after removal. Fentanyl level drops gradually and may take as long as 17 hours to decline by 50%.
- Most patients experience good control of pain for 3 days while wearing the transdermal system, but a few may need a new application after 48 hours.
- Because the fentanyl level rises for the first 24 hours after application, analgesic effect can't be evaluated on the first day. Make sure patient has adequate supplemental analgesic to prevent breakthrough pain.
- When reducing opiate therapy or switching to a different analgesic, withdraw the transdermal system gradually. Because the fentanyl level drops gradually after removal, give half of the equianalgesic dose of the new analgesic 12 to 18 hours after removal.

Transmucosal form

!!ALERT Actiq is used only to manage breakthrough cancer pain in patients who are al-

ready receiving and tolerating an opioid for their persistent cancer pain.
- Remove foil overwrap of Actiq just before giving.
- The lozenge is placed between the cheek and gum and may occasionally be moved from side to side using the stick. The Actiq lozenge shouldn't be chewed and should be consumed over about 15 minutes. Discard the stick in the trash after use or, if any drug matrix remains on the stick, place under hot running tap water until dissolved or place in child-resistant container provided, and dispose as appropriate for schedule II drugs.

!!ALERT Don't confuse fentanyl with alfentanil.

Patient teaching

- When drug is used for pain control, instruct patient to request drug before pain becomes intense.
- When drug is used after surgery, encourage patient to turn, cough, and breathe deeply to prevent lung problems.
- Instruct patient to avoid hazardous activities until CNS effects subside.
- Tell home care patient to avoid drinking alcohol or taking other CNS-type drugs while receiving fentanyl because additive effects can occur.
- Advise patient not to stop drug abruptly.
- Teach patient about proper application of prescribed transdermal patch. Tell patient to clip hair at application site, but not to use a razor, which may irritate skin. Wash area with clear water, if needed, but not with soaps, oils, lotions, alcohol, or other substances that may irritate skin or prevent adhesion. Dry area completely before application.
- Tell patient to remove transdermal system from package just before applying, hold in place for 30 seconds, and be sure the edges of patch stick to skin.
- Teach patient not to alter the transdermal system (such as by cutting) in any way before application.
- Teach patient to dispose of the transdermal patch by folding it so the adhesive side adheres to itself and then flushing it down the toilet.
- Tell patient that, if another patch is needed after 48 to 72 hours, he should apply it to a different skin site.
- Inform patient that heat from fever or environment, such as from heating pads, electric blankets, heat lamps, hot tubs, or water beds, may increase transdermal delivery and cause toxicity requiring dosage adjustment. Instruct patient to notify prescriber if fever occurs or if he'll be spending time in a hot climate.

!!ALERT Warn patient and patient's family that the amount of fentanyl in one Actiq lozenge can be fatal to a child. Keep well secured and out of children's reach.

ferrous fumarate

Femiron ◇, Feostat ◇, Hemocyte ◇, Ircon ◇, Nephro-Fer ◇, Novofumar†, Palafer†, Palafer Pediatric Drops†, Vitron-C

Pregnancy risk category A

Indications & dosages

➲ Iron deficiency

Adults: 100 to 200 mg (2 to 3 mg/kg) P.O. elemental iron daily in three divided doses.
Children ages 2 to 12: 50 to 100 mg (1 to 1.5 mg/kg) P.O. elemental iron daily in three or four divided doses.
Children ages 6 months to 2 years: 3 to 6 mg/kg P.O. elemental iron daily in three divided doses.
Infants younger than age 6 months: 10 to 25 mg P.O. elemental iron daily in three or four divided doses.

➲ As a supplement during pregnancy

Women: 15 to 30 mg elemental iron P.O. daily during last two trimesters.

Contraindications & cautions

- Contraindicated in patients with primary hemochromatosis or hemosiderosis, hemolytic anemia (unless patient also has iron-deficiency anemia), peptic ulcer disease, regional enteritis, or ulcerative colitis.
- Contraindicated in those receiving repeated blood transfusions.
- Use cautiously on long-term basis.

Adverse reactions

GI: *nausea*, epigastric pain, vomiting, *constipation*, diarrhea, *black stools*, anorexia.
Other: temporarily stained teeth from suspension and drops.

Interactions

Drug-drug. *Antacids, cholestyramine resin, cimetidine:* May decrease iron absorption. Separate doses by at least 2 hours.
Chloramphenicol: May delay response to iron therapy. Monitor patient.
Fluoroquinolones, penicillamine, tetracyclines: May decrease GI absorption of these drugs, possibly causing decreased levels or effect. Separate doses by 2 to 4 hours.
Levodopa, methyldopa: May decrease absorption and efficacy of levodopa and methyldopa. Watch for decreased effect of these drugs.
L-Thyroxine: May decrease L-thyroxine absorption. Separate doses by at least 2 hours. Monitor thyroid function.
Vitamin C: May increase iron absorption. Use together for therapeutic effect.
Drug-herb. *Black cohosh, chamomile, feverfew, gossypol, hawthorn, nettle, plantain, St. John's wort:* May decrease iron absorption. Discourage use together.
Oregano: May decrease iron absorption. Tell patient to separate ingestion of oregano from ingestion of food containing iron or iron supplement by at least 2 hours.
Drug-food. *Cereals, cheese, coffee, eggs, milk, tea, whole-grain breads, yogurt:* May decrease iron absorption. Discourage use together.

Nursing considerations

- GI upset may be related to dose.
- Between-meal doses are preferable, but drug can be given with some foods, although absorption may be decreased.
- Enteric-coated products reduce GI upset but also reduce amount of iron absorbed.
- Check for constipation; record color and amount of stools.

!!ALERT Oral iron may turn stools black. Although this unabsorbed iron is harmless, it could mask presence of melena.

- Monitor hemoglobin level, hematocrit, and reticulocyte count during therapy.
- Combination products such as Ferro-Sequels contain stool softeners, which help prevent constipation, a common adverse reaction.

Patient teaching

- Tell patient to take tablets with juice (preferably orange juice) or water but not with milk or antacids.
- Tell patient to take suspension with straw and place drops at back of throat to avoid staining teeth.
- Caution patient not to crush tablets or chew extended-release forms.
- Advise patient not to substitute one iron salt for another; the amount of elemental iron may vary.

!!ALERT Inform parents that as few as 3 or 4 tablets can cause serious poisoning in children.

- Advise patient to report constipation and change in stool color or consistency.

ferrous gluconate

Fergon ◇, Fertinic†, Novoferrogluc†

Pregnancy risk category A

Indications & dosages

➲ Iron deficiency
Adults: 100 to 200 mg (2 to 3 mg/kg) P.O. elemental iron daily in three divided doses.
Children ages 2 to 12: 50 to 100 mg (1 to 1.5 mg/kg) P.O. elemental iron daily in three or four divided doses.
Children ages 6 months to 2 years: 3 to 6 mg/kg P.O. elemental iron daily in three divided doses.
Infants younger than age 6 months: 10 to 25 mg P.O. elemental iron daily in three or four divided doses.
➲ As a supplement during pregnancy
Adults: 15 to 30 mg elemental iron P.O. daily during last two trimesters.

Contraindications & cautions

- Contraindicated in patients with peptic ulceration, regional enteritis, ulcerative colitis, hemosiderosis, primary hemochromatosis, or hemolytic anemia (unless patient also has iron-deficiency anemia) and in those receiving repeated blood transfusions.
- Use cautiously on long-term basis.

Adverse reactions

GI: *nausea*, epigastric pain, vomiting, *constipation*, diarrhea, *black stools*, anorexia.

Interactions

Drug-drug. *Antacids, cholestyramine resin, cimetidine:* May decrease iron absorption. Separate doses by at least 2 hours.

Chloramphenicol: Delays response to iron therapy. Monitor patient.
Fluoroquinolones, penicillamine, tetracyclines: May decrease GI absorption of these drugs, possibly causing decreased level or effect. Separate doses by 2 to 4 hours.
Levodopa, methyldopa: May decrease levodopa and methyldopa absorption and effect. Watch for decreased effect of these drugs.
L-Thyroxine: May decrease L-thyroxine absorption. Separate doses by at least 2 hours. Monitor thyroid function.
Vitamin C: May increase iron absorption. Use together for therapeutic effect.
Drug-herb. *Black cohosh, chamomile, feverfew, gossypol, hawthorn, nettle, plantain, St. John's wort:* May decrease iron absorption. Discourage use together.
Oregano: May decrease iron absorption. Tell patient to separate ingestion of oregano from ingestion of food containing iron or iron supplement by at least 2 hours.
Drug-food. *Cereals, cheese, coffee, eggs, milk, tea, whole-grain breads, yogurt:* May decrease iron absorption. Discourage use together.

Nursing considerations

- GI upset may be related to dose.
- Between-meal doses are preferable, but drug can be given with some foods, although absorption may be decreased.
- Enteric-coated products reduce GI upset but also reduce amount of iron absorbed.
- Check for constipation; record color and amount of stools.

!!ALERT Oral iron may turn stools black. Although this unabsorbed iron is harmless, it could mask melena.

- Monitor hemoglobin level, hematocrit, and reticulocyte count during therapy.

Patient teaching

- Tell patient to take tablets with juice (preferably orange juice) or water, but not with milk or antacids.

!!ALERT Inform parents that as few as 3 or 4 tablets can cause serious iron poisoning in children.

- Caution patient not to substitute one iron salt for another because the amounts of elemental iron vary.
- Advise patient to report constipation and change in stool color or consistency.

ferrous sulfate

Apo-Ferrous Sulfate†, ED-IN-SOL, Feosol ◇ *, Fer-Gen-Sol ◇ *, Fer-In-Sol ◇ *, Fer-Iron ◇ *

ferrous sulfate, dried

Fe50 ◇, Feosol ◇, Feratab ◇, Novoferrosulfate†, PMS-Ferrous Sulfate†, Slow FE ◇

Pregnancy risk category A

Indications & dosages

➲ Iron deficiency
Adults: 100 to 200 mg (2 to 3 mg/kg) P.O. elemental iron daily in three divided doses.
Children ages 2 to 12: 50 to 100 mg (1 to 1.5 mg/kg) P.O. elemental iron daily in three or four divided doses.
Children ages 6 months to 2 years: 3 to 6 mg/kg P.O. elemental iron daily in three divided doses.
Infants younger than age 6 months: 10 to 25 mg P.O. elemental iron daily in three or four divided doses.
➲ As a supplement during pregnancy
Adults: 15 to 30 mg elemental iron P.O. daily during last two trimesters.

Contraindications & cautions

- Contraindicated in patients with hemosiderosis, primary hemochromatosis, hemolytic anemia (unless patient also has iron-deficiency anemia), peptic ulceration, ulcerative colitis, or regional enteritis and in those receiving repeated blood transfusions.
- Use cautiously on long-term basis.

Adverse reactions

GI: *nausea,* epigastric pain, vomiting, *constipation, black stools,* diarrhea, anorexia.
Other: temporarily stained teeth from liquid forms.

Interactions

Drug-drug. *Antacids, cholestyramine resin, cimetidine:* May decrease iron absorption. Separate doses if possible.
Chloramphenicol: May delay response to iron therapy. Monitor patient.
Fluoroquinolones, penicillamine, tetracyclines: May decrease GI absorption of these drugs, possibly resulting in decreased lev-

els or efficacy. Separate doses by 2 to 4 hours.
Levodopa, methyldopa: May decrease absorption and efficacy of levodopa and methyldopa. Watch for decreased effect of these drugs.
L-Thyroxine: May decrease L-thyroxine absorption. Separate doses by at least 2 hours. Monitor thyroid function.
Vitamin C: May increase iron absorption. Use together for therapeutic effect.
Drug-herb. *Black cohosh, chamomile, feverfew, gossypol, hawthorn, nettle, plantain, St. John's wort:* May decrease iron absorption. Discourage use together.
Oregano: May decrease iron absorption. Tell patient to separate ingestion of oregano from ingestion of food containing iron or iron supplement by at least 2 hours.
Drug-food. *Cereals, cheese, coffee, eggs, milk, tea, whole-grain breads, yogurt:* May decrease iron absorption. Discourage use together.

Nursing considerations

- GI upset may be related to dose.
- Between-meal doses are preferable. Drug can be given with some foods, although absorption may be decreased.
- Enteric-coated products reduce GI upset but also reduce amount of iron absorbed.

!!ALERT Oral iron may turn stools black. Although this unabsorbed iron is harmless, it could mask melena.

- Monitor hemoglobin level, hematocrit, and reticulocyte count during therapy.

!!ALERT Don't confuse different iron salts; elemental content may vary.

Patient teaching

- Tell patient to take tablets with juice (preferably orange juice) or water, but not with milk or antacids.
- Instruct patient not to crush or chew extended-release forms.

!!ALERT Inform parents that as few as 3 to 4 tablets can cause serious iron poisoning in children.

- Caution patient not to substitute one iron salt for another because amounts of elemental iron vary.
- Advise patient to report constipation and change in stool color or consistency.

fexofenadine hydrochloride
Allegra

Pregnancy risk category C

Indications & dosages

➲ **Seasonal allergic rhinitis**
Adults and children age 12 and older: 60 mg P.O. b.i.d. or 180 mg P.O. once daily.
Children ages 6 to 11: 30 mg P.O. b.i.d.

➲ **Chronic idiopathic urticaria**
Adults and children age 12 and older: 60 mg P.O. b.i.d.
Children ages 6 to 11: 30 mg P.O. b.i.d.

For patients with impaired renal function or a need for dialysis, give adults 60 mg daily and children 30 mg daily.

Contraindications & cautions

- Contraindicated in patients hypersensitive to drug or its components.
- Use cautiously in patients with impaired renal function.

Adverse reactions

CNS: fatigue, drowsiness, headache.
GI: nausea, dyspepsia.
GU: dysmenorrhea.
Other: viral infection.

Interactions

Drug-drug. *Aluminum or magnesium antacids:* May decrease fexofenadine level. Separate dosage times.
Erythromycin, ketoconazole: May increase fexofenadine level. Monitor patient for side effects.
Drug-food. *Apple juice, grapefruit juice, orange juice:* May decrease fexofenadine effects. Patients should take drug with liquid other than these juices.
Drug-lifestyle. *Alcohol use:* May increase CNS depression. Discourage use together.

Nursing considerations

- Stop drug 4 days before patient undergoes diagnostic skin tests because drug can prevent, reduce, or mask positive skin test response.
- No data exist to demonstrate whether drug appears in breast milk; use caution when giving drug to breast-feeding woman. Advise woman taking drug to avoid breast-feeding.

Patient teaching

- Instruct patient not to exceed prescribed dosage and to take drug only when needed.
- Warn patient to avoid alcohol and hazardous activities that require alertness until CNS effects of drug are known. Explain that drug may cause drowsiness.
- Tell patient to avoid taking antacids within 2 hours of fexofenadine.
- Inform patient that sugarless gum, hard candy, or ice chips may relieve dry mouth.

filgrastim (G-CSF; granulocyte-colony stimulating factor)

Neupogen

Pregnancy risk category C

Indications & dosages

➲ To decrease risk of infection in patients with nonmyeloid malignant disease receiving myelosuppressive antineoplastics
Adults and children: 5 mcg/kg daily I.V. or S.C. as single dose given no sooner than 24 hours after cytotoxic chemotherapy. Doses may be increased in increments of 5 mcg/kg for each chemotherapy cycle depending on duration and severity of the nadir of absolute neutrophil count (ANC).

➲ To decrease risk of infection in patients with nonmyeloid malignant disease receiving myelosuppressive antineoplastics followed by bone marrow transplantation
Adults and children: 10 mcg/kg daily I.V. infusion of 4 or 24 hours or as continuous 24-hour S.C. infusion at least 24 hours after cytotoxic chemotherapy and bone marrow infusion. Adjust subsequent dosages based on neutrophil response.

For patients with ANC over 1,000/mm^3 for 3 consecutive days, reduce dosage to 5 mcg/kg daily; if ANC remains over 1,000/mm^3 for 3 more consecutive days, stop drug. If ANC decreases to below 1,000/mm^3, resume therapy at 5 mcg/kg daily.

➲ Congenital neutropenia
Adults: 6 mcg/kg S.C. b.i.d. Adjust dosage based on patient response.

For patients with an ANC persistently above 10,000/mm^3, reduce dosage, as directed.

➲ Idiopathic or cyclic neutropenia
Adults: 5 mcg/kg S.C. daily. Adjust dosage based on patient response.

➲ Peripheral blood progenitor cell collection and therapy in cancer patients
Adults: 10 mcg/kg S.C. daily. Give 4 days before leukapheresis and continue until last leukapheresis.

Patients with WBC count over 100,000/mm^3 may need dosage adjustment.

➲ To reduce the risk of bacterial infection in patients with HIV♦
Adults and adolescents: 5 to 10 mcg/kg S.C. once daily for 2 to 4 weeks.

Contraindications & cautions

- Contraindicated in patients hypersensitive to drug or its components or to proteins derived from ***Escherichia coli***.
- Use cautiously in breast-feeding women.

Adverse reactions

CNS: *fever*, headache, weakness, *fatigue*.
CV: ***MI, arrhythmias***, chest pain, hypotension.
GI: *nausea, vomiting, diarrhea, mucositis*, stomatitis, constipation.
Hematologic: ***thrombocytopenia***, leukocytosis.
Metabolic: hyperuricemia.
Musculoskeletal: *bone pain*.
Respiratory: dyspnea, cough.
Skin: *alopecia*, rash, cutaneous vasculitis.
Other: hypersensitivity reactions.

Interactions

Drug-drug. *Chemotherapeutic drugs:* Rapidly dividing myeloid cells may be sensitive to cytotoxic drugs. Don't use within 24 hours before or after a dose of one of these drugs.

Nursing considerations

- Obtain baseline CBC and platelet count before therapy.
- Once a dose is withdrawn, don't reuse vial. Discard unused portion. Vials are for single-dose use and contain no preservatives.
- Obtain CBC and platelet count two to three times weekly during therapy. Patients who receive drug also may receive high doses of chemotherapy, which may increase risk of toxicities.
- A transiently increased neutrophil count is common 1 or 2 days after therapy starts. Give daily for up to 2 weeks or until ANC has returned to 10,000/mm^3 after the ex-

pected chemotherapy-induced neutrophil nadir.

!!ALERT Don't confuse Neupogen with Epogen or Neumega.

Patient teaching

- If patient will give drug, teach him how to do so and how to dispose of used needles, syringes, drug containers, and unused medicine.

!!ALERT Rarely, splenic rupture may occur. Advise patient to immediately report upper left abdominal or shoulder tip pain.

- Instruct patient to report persistent or serious adverse reactions promptly.

finasteride
Propecia, Proscar

Pregnancy risk category X

Indications & dosages

➲ Male pattern hair loss (androgenetic alopecia) in men only
Adults: 1 mg P.O. Propecia daily.

➲ To improve symptoms of BPH and reduce risk of acute urine retention and need for surgery, including transurethral resection of prostate and prostatectomy
Adults: 5 mg P.O. Proscar daily.

➲ With doxazosin, to reduce the risk of BPH symptom progression (Proscar)
Adults: 5 mg P.O. daily.

Contraindications & cautions

- Contraindicated in patients hypersensitive to drug or to other 5-alpha-reductase inhibitors, such as dutasteride. Although drug isn't used in women or children, manufacturer indicates pregnancy as a contraindication.
- Use cautiously in patients with liver dysfunction.

Adverse reactions

GU: impotence, decreased volume of ejaculate, decreased libido.

Interactions

None significant.

Nursing considerations

- Before therapy, evaluate patient for conditions that mimic BPH, including hypotonic bladder, prostate cancer, infection, or stricture.
- Carefully monitor patients who have a large residual urine volume or severely diminished urine flow.
- Sustained increase in PSA level could indicate noncompliance with therapy.
- A minimum of 6 months of therapy may be needed for treatment of BPH.

Patient teaching

- Tell patient that drug may be taken without regard to meals.
- Warn woman who is or may become pregnant not to handle crushed tablets because of risk of adverse effects on male fetus.
- Inform patient that signs of improvement may require at least 3 months of daily use when drug is used to treat hair loss or at least 6 months when taken for BPH.
- Reassure patient that drug may decrease volume of ejaculate without impairing normal sexual function.

flecainide acetate
Tambocor

Pregnancy risk category C

Indications & dosages

➲ Paroxysmal supraventricular tachycardia, including AV nodal re-entrant tachycardia and AV re-entrant tachycardia or paroxysmal atrial fibrillation or flutter in patients without structural heart disease; life-threatening ventricular arrhythmias such as sustained ventricular tachycardia
Adults: For paroxysmal supraventricular tachycardia, 50 mg P.O. q 12 hours. Increase in increments of 50 mg b.i.d. q 4 days. Maximum dose is 300 mg/day. For life-threatening ventricular arrhythmias, 100 mg P.O. q 12 hours. Increase in increments of 50 mg b.i.d. q 4 days until desired effect occurs. Maximum dose for most patients is 400 mg/day. Or, where available for emergency treatment,‡ 2 mg/kg I.V. push over not less than 10 minutes to maximum dose of 150 mg; or dilute dose and give as an infusion over 10 to 30 minutes.

If creatinine clearance is 35 ml/minute or less, first dose is 100 mg P.O. once daily or 50 mg P.O. b.i.d.

Contraindications & cautions

- Contraindicated in patients hypersensitive to drug and in those with second- or third-degree AV block or right bundle-branch block with a left hemiblock (in the absence of an artificial pacemaker), recent MI, or cardiogenic shock.
- Use cautiously in patients with heart failure, cardiomyopathy, severe renal or hepatic disease, prolonged QT interval, sick sinus syndrome, or blood dyscrasia.

Adverse reactions

CNS: *dizziness, headache,* fatigue, fever, tremor, anxiety, insomnia, depression, malaise, paresthesia, ataxia, vertigo, *lightheadedness, syncope,* asthenia.
CV: ***new or worsened arrhythmias,*** chest pain, ***heart failure, cardiac arrest,*** palpitations, edema, flushing.
EENT: eye pain, eye irritation, *blurred vision and other visual disturbances.*
GI: nausea, constipation, abdominal pain, dyspepsia, vomiting, diarrhea, anorexia.
Respiratory: *dyspnea.*
Skin: rash.

Interactions

Drug-drug. *Amiodarone, cimetidine:* May increase level of flecainide. Watch for toxicity.
Digoxin: May increase digoxin level by 15% to 25%. Monitor digoxin level.
Disopyramide, verapamil: May increase negative inotropic properties. Avoid using together.
Propranolol, other beta blockers: May increase flecainide and propranolol levels by 20% to 30%. Watch for propranolol and flecainide toxicity.
Urine-acidifying and urine-alkalinizing drugs: May cause extremes of urine pH, which may alter flecainide excretion. Monitor patient for flecainide toxicity or decreased effectiveness.
Drug-lifestyle. *Smoking:* May decrease flecainide level. Monitor patient closely.

Nursing considerations

- When used to prevent ventricular arrhythmias, reserve drug for patients with documented life-threatening arrhythmias.
- Check that pacing threshold was determined 1 week before and after starting therapy in a patient with a pacemaker; flecainide can alter endocardial pacing thresholds.
- Correct hypokalemia or hyperkalemia before giving flecainide because these electrolyte disturbances may alter drug's effect.
- Monitor ECG rhythm for proarrhythmic effects.
- Most patients can be adequately maintained on an every-12-hour dosing schedule, but some need to receive flecainide every 8 hours.
- Adjust dosage only once every 3 to 4 days.
- Monitor flecainide level, especially if patient has renal or heart failure. Therapeutic flecainide levels range from 0.2 to 1 mcg/ml. Risk of adverse effects increases when trough blood level exceeds 1 mcg/ml.

Patient teaching

- Stress importance of taking drug exactly as prescribed.
- Instruct patient to report adverse reactions promptly and to limit fluid and sodium intake to minimize fluid retention.
- Tell patient receiving drug I.V. to report discomfort at insertion site.

fluconazole

Diflucan

Pregnancy risk category C

Indications & dosages

➲ **Oropharyngeal candidiasis**
Adults: 200 mg P.O. or I.V. on first day, then 100 mg once daily for at least 2 weeks.
Children: 6 mg/kg P.O. or I.V. on first day, then 3 mg/kg daily for 2 weeks.
➲ **Esophageal candidiasis**
Adults: 200 mg P.O. or I.V. on first day, then 100 mg once daily. Up to 400 mg daily has been used, depending on patient's condition and tolerance of treatment. Patients should receive drug for at least 3 weeks and for 2 weeks after symptoms resolve.
Children: 6 mg/kg P.O. or I.V. on first day, then 3 mg/kg daily for at least 3 weeks and for at least 2 weeks after symptoms resolve. Maximum daily dose 12 mg/kg.
➲ **Vulvovaginal candidiasis**
Adults: 150 mg P.O. for one dose only.
➲ **Systemic candidiasis**
Adults: 400 mg P.O. or I.V. on first day, then 200 mg once daily for at least 4 weeks and

for 2 weeks after symptoms resolve. Doses up to 400 mg/day may be used.
Children: 6 to 12 mg/kg/day P.O. or I.V.

➲ Cryptococcal meningitis
Adults: 400 mg P.O. or I.V. on first day, then 200 mg once daily for 10 to 12 weeks after CSF culture result is negative. Doses up to 400 mg/day may be used.
Children: 12 mg/kg/day P.O. or I.V. on first day, then 6 mg/kg/day for 10 to 12 weeks after CSF culture result is negative.

➲ To prevent candidiasis in bone marrow transplant
Adults: 400 mg P.O. or I.V. once daily. Start treatment several days before anticipated agranulocytosis, and continue for 7 days after neutrophil count exceeds 1,000 cells/mm^3.

➲ To suppress relapse of cryptococcal meningitis in patients with AIDS
Adults: 200 mg P.O. or I.V. daily.
Children: 3 to 6 mg/kg/day P.O. or I.V.

If creatinine clearance is 11 to 50 ml/minute, reduce dosage by 50%. Patients receiving regular hemodialysis treatment should receive usual dose after each dialysis session.

Contraindications & cautions

- Contraindicated in patients hypersensitive to drug and breast-feeding patients.
- Use cautiously in patients hypersensitive to other antifungal azole compounds.

Adverse reactions

CNS: *headache*, dizziness.
GI: nausea, vomiting, abdominal pain, diarrhea, dyspepsia, taste perversion.
Hematologic: ***leukopenia, thrombocytopenia***.
Skin: rash.
Other: ***anaphylaxis***.

Interactions

Drug-drug. *Alprazolam, chlordiazepoxide, clonazepam, clorazepate, diazepam, estazolam, flurazepam, midazolam, quazepam, triazolam:* May increase and prolong levels of these drugs, CNS depression, and psychomotor impairment. Avoid using together.
Cimetidine: May decrease fluconazole level. Monitor patient response to fluconazole.
Cyclosporine, phenytoin, theophylline: May increase levels of these drugs. Monitor cyclosporine, theophylline, and phenytoin levels.
HMG-CoA reductase inhibitors (atorvastatin, fluvastatin, lovastatin, pravastatin, simvastatin): May increase levels and adverse effects of these drugs. Avoid using together, or reduce dosage of HMG-CoA reductase inhibitor.
Isoniazid, oral sulfonylureas, phenytoin, rifampin, valproic acid: May increase hepatic transaminase level. Monitor liver function test results closely.
Oral sulfonylureas (such as glipizide, glyburide, tolbutamide): May increase levels of these drugs. Monitor patient for enhanced hypoglycemic effect.
Rifampin: May enhance fluconazole metabolism. Monitor patient for lack of response to fluconazole.
Tacrolimus: May cause increased tacrolimus level and nephrotoxicity. Monitor patient carefully.
Warfarin: May increase risk of bleeding. Monitor PT and INR.
Zidovudine: May increase zidovudine activity. Monitor patient closely.

Nursing considerations

- Serious hepatotoxicity has occurred in patients with underlying medical conditions.
- If patient develops mild rash, monitor him closely. Stop drug if lesions progress.
- Risk of adverse reactions appears to be greater in HIV-infected patients.

Patient teaching

- Tell patient to take drug as directed, even after he feels better.
- Instruct patient to report adverse reactions promptly.

flucytosine (5-FC, 5-fluorocytosine)

Ancobon

Pregnancy risk category C

Indications & dosages

➲ Severe fungal infections from susceptible strains of *Candida* (including septicemia, endocarditis, and urinary tract or pulmonary infection), and of *Cryptococ-*

cus **(including meningitis and urinary tract or pulmonary infection)**
Adults: 50 to 150 mg/kg daily P.O. in four equally divided doses q 6 hours.

Contraindications & cautions

- Contraindicated in patients hypersensitive to drug.
- Use with extreme caution in patients with impaired hepatic or renal function or bone marrow suppression.

Adverse reactions

CNS: headache, vertigo, sedation, fatigue, weakness, confusion, hallucinations, psychosis, ataxia, hearing loss, paresthesia, parkinsonism, peripheral neuropathy.
CV: ***cardiac arrest***, chest pain.
GI: nausea, vomiting, diarrhea, ***hemorrhage***, abdominal pain, dry mouth, duodenal ulcer, ulcerative colitis, anorexia.
GU: azotemia, crystalluria, ***renal failure***.
Hematologic: anemia, ***leukopenia***, ***bone marrow suppression***, ***thrombocytopenia***, eosinophilia, ***agranulocytosis***, ***aplastic anemia***.
Hepatic: jaundice.
Metabolic: ***hypoglycemia***, hypokalemia.
Respiratory: ***respiratory arrest***, dyspnea.
Skin: occasional rash, pruritus, urticaria, photosensitivity.

Interactions

Drug-drug. *Amphotericin B:* May cause synergistic effects and may increase risk of toxicity. Monitor patient for increased adverse reactions and toxicity.

Nursing considerations

- Patient should take capsules over 15 minutes to reduce adverse GI reactions.
- Monitor blood, liver, and renal function studies frequently during therapy; obtain susceptibility tests weekly to monitor drug resistance.
- If possible, regularly perform blood level assays of drug to maintain therapeutic flucytosine level of 40 to 60 mcg/ml. Blood levels of drug above 100 mcg/ml may be toxic.
- Monitor fluid intake and output; report marked changes.

Patient teaching

- Tell patient that therapeutic response may take weeks or months.
- Advise patient to report adverse reactions promptly.
- Instruct patient to take capsules over 15 minutes to reduce adverse GI reactions.

fludarabine phosphate

Fludara

Pregnancy risk category D

Indications & dosages

➲ **B-cell chronic lymphocytic leukemia in patients with no or inadequate response to at least one standard alkylating drug regimen**
Adults: 25 mg/m^2 I.V. daily over 30 minutes for 5 consecutive days. Repeat cycle q 28 days.

In patients with creatinine clearance of 30 to 70 ml/minute, decrease dose by 20%. Don't use drug in patients with clearance less than 30 ml/minute.

Contraindications & cautions

- Contraindicated in patients hypersensitive to drug or its components and in those with creatinine clearance less than 30 ml/minute.
- Use cautiously in patients with renal insufficiency.

Adverse reactions

CNS: *fatigue*, *malaise*, *weakness*, *paresthesia*, peripheral neuropathy, ***CVA***, headache, sleep disorder, depression, cerebellar syndrome, ***transient ischemic attack***, agitation, *confusion*, *fever*, ***coma***.
CV: *edema*, angina, phlebitis, ***arrhythmias***, ***heart failure***, ***MI***, supraventricular tachycardia, ***deep vein thrombosis***, ***aneurysm***, ***hemorrhage***.
EENT: *visual disturbances*, hearing loss, delayed blindness, sinusitis, pharyngitis, epistaxis.
GI: *nausea*, *vomiting*, *diarrhea*, constipation, *anorexia*, stomatitis, ***GI bleeding***, esophagitis, mucositis.
GU: dysuria, *UTI*, urinary hesitancy, proteinuria, hematuria, ***renal failure***.
Hematologic: ***hemolytic anemia***, **MYELOSUPPRESSION**.
Hepatic: ***liver failure***, cholelithiasis.
Metabolic: hypocalcemia, hyperkalemia, hyperglycemia, dehydration, hyperuricemia, hyperphosphatemia.

Musculoskeletal: *myalgia.*
Respiratory: *cough, pneumonia, dyspnea, upper respiratory tract infection,* allergic pneumonitis, hemoptysis, hypoxia, bronchitis.
Skin: *rash,* pruritus, alopecia, seborrhea, diaphoresis.
Other: *chills, pain,* tumor lysis syndrome, INFECTION, ***anaphylaxis.***

Interactions

Drug-drug. *Cytarabine:* May decrease metabolism of subsequently given fludarabine and inhibition of fludarabine activity. Monitor patient closely.
Myelosuppressives: May increase toxicity. Avoid using together, if possible.
Pentostatin: May increase risk of pulmonary toxicity, which can be fatal. Avoid using together.

Nursing considerations

!!ALERT Monitor patient closely and expect modified dosage based on toxicity. Most toxic effects are dose-dependent. Advanced age, renal insufficiency, and bone marrow impairment may predispose patients to increased or excessive toxicity.
!!ALERT Careful hematologic monitoring is needed, especially of neutrophil and platelet counts. Bone marrow suppression can be severe.
- To prevent bleeding, avoid all I.M. injections when platelet count is below 50,000/mm^3.
- Anticipate blood transfusions because of cumulative anemia. Patients may receive RBC colony–stimulating factors to promote RBC production and decrease need for blood transfusions.
- Take preventive measures before starting drug treatment. Hyperuricemia, hypocalcemia, hyperkalemia, and renal failure may result from rapid lysis of tumor cells.

!!ALERT Don't confuse fludarabine with floxuridine, fluorouracil, or flucytosine.

Patient teaching

- Instruct patient to watch for signs and symptoms of infection (fever, sore throat, fatigue) and bleeding (easy bruising, nosebleeds, bleeding gums, tarry stools). Tell patient to take temperature daily.
- Advise woman of childbearing age to consult prescriber before becoming pregnant.
- Caution woman to stop breast-feeding during therapy because of risk of toxicity to infant.

fludrocortisone acetate
Florinef Acetate

Pregnancy risk category C

Indications & dosages

➲ Salt-losing adrenogenital syndrome
Adults: 0.1 to 0.2 mg P.O. daily.
➲ Addison's disease (adrenocortical insufficiency)
Adults: 0.1 mg P.O. daily. Usual dosage range is 0.1 mg three times weekly to 0.2 mg daily. Decrease dosage to 0.05 mg daily if transient hypertension develops as a result of drug therapy.

Contraindications & cautions

- Contraindicated in patients hypersensitive to drug and in those with systemic fungal infections.
- Use cautiously in patients with hypothyroidism, recent MI, cirrhosis, ocular herpes simplex, emotional instability, psychotic tendencies, diverticulitis, fresh intestinal anastomoses, active or latent peptic ulcer, renal insufficiency, hypertension, osteoporosis, myasthenia gravis, active hepatitis, lactation, or nonspecific ulcerative colitis.

Adverse reactions

CV: hypertension, cardiac hypertrophy, edema, ***heart failure.***
Hematologic: bruising.
Metabolic: *sodium and water retention,* hypokalemia.
Skin: diaphoresis, urticaria, allergic rash.

Interactions

Drug-drug. *Barbiturates, carbamazepine, fosphenytoin, phenytoin, rifampin:* May increase clearance of fludrocortisone acetate. Monitor patient for possible diminished effect of corticosteroid. Corticosteroid dosage may need to be increased.
Potassium-depleting drugs such as amphotericin B, thiazide diuretics: May enhance potassium-wasting effects of fludrocortisone. Monitor potassium level.

Drug-food. *Sodium-containing drugs or foods:* May increase blood pressure. Sodium intake may need adjustment.

Nursing considerations

- Drug is used with cortisone or hydrocortisone in adrenal insufficiency.
- Perform glucose tolerance tests only if needed because addisonian patients tend to develop severe hypoglycemia within 3 hours of the test.

!!ALERT Monitor patient's blood pressure and electrolyte levels. If hypertension occurs, notify prescriber and expect dosage to be decreased by 50%.

- Weigh patient daily; notify prescriber about sudden weight gain.
- Unless contraindicated, give low-sodium diet that is high in potassium and protein. Potassium supplements may be needed.
- Drug may cause adverse effects similar to those of glucocorticoids.

Patient teaching

- Tell patient to notify prescriber if low blood pressure, weakness, cramping, or palpitations worsen, or if changes in mental status occur.
- Warn patient that mild swelling is common.

flumazenil
Romazicon

Pregnancy risk category C

Indications & dosages

➲ Complete or partial reversal of sedative effects of benzodiazepines after anesthesia or conscious sedation
Adults: Initially, 0.2 mg I.V. over 15 seconds. If patient doesn't reach desired level of consciousness after 45 seconds, repeat dose. Repeat at 1-minute intervals, if needed, until cumulative dose of 1 mg has been given (first dose plus four more doses). Most patients respond after 0.6 to 1 mg of drug. In case of resedation, dosage may be repeated after 20 minutes, but never give more than 1 mg at any one time or exceed 3 mg/hour.
Children age 1 year and older: 0.01 mg/kg I.V. over 15 seconds. If patient doesn't reach desired level of consciousness after 45 seconds, repeat dose. Repeat at 1-minute intervals, if needed, until cumulative dose of 0.05 mg/kg or 1 mg, whichever is lower, has been given (first dose plus four more doses).

➲ Suspected benzodiazepine overdose
Adults: Initially, 0.2 mg I.V. over 30 seconds. If patient doesn't reach desired level of consciousness after 30 seconds, give 0.3 mg over 30 seconds. If patient still doesn't respond adequately, give 0.5 mg over 30 seconds. Repeat 0.5-mg doses, p.r.n., at 1-minute intervals until cumulative dose of 3 mg has been given. Most patients with benzodiazepine overdose respond to cumulative doses between 1 and 3 mg; rarely, patients who respond partially after 3 mg may need additional doses, up to 5 mg total. If patient doesn't respond in 5 minutes after receiving 5 mg, sedation is unlikely to be caused by benzodiazepines. In case of resedation, dosage may be repeated after 20 minutes, but never give more than 1 mg at any one time or exceed 3 mg/hour.

Contraindications & cautions

- Contraindicated in patients hypersensitive to flumazenil or benzodiazepines, in those with evidence of serious tricyclic antidepressant overdose, and in those who have received benzodiazepines to treat a potentially life-threatening condition, such as status epilepticus.
- Use cautiously in patients with head injury, psychiatric disorders, or alcohol dependence.
- Use cautiously in patients at high risk for developing seizures and in those who have recently received multiple doses of a parenteral benzodiazepine, who display signs of seizure activity, or who may be at risk for benzodiazepine dependence, such as intensive care unit patients.

Adverse reactions

CNS: *dizziness, abnormal or blurred vision, headache,* ***seizures***, agitation, emotional lability, tremor, insomnia.
CV: ***arrhythmias***, cutaneous vasodilation, palpitations.
GI: *nausea, vomiting.*
Respiratory: dyspnea, hyperventilation.
Skin: *diaphoresis.*
Other: *pain at injection site.*

Interactions

Drug-drug. *Antidepressants, drugs that may cause seizures or arrhythmias:* May increase risk of seizures or arrhythmias. Don't use flumazenil when overdose involves more than one drug, especially when seizures (from any cause) are likely to occur.

Nursing considerations

- Monitor patient closely for resedation that may occur after reversal of benzodiazepine effects because flumazenil's duration of action is shorter than that of all benzodiazepines. Duration of monitoring period depends on specific drug being reversed. Monitor patient closely after doses of long-acting benzodiazepines, such as diazepam, or after high doses of short-acting benzodiazepines, such as 10 mg of midazolam. In most cases, severe resedation is unlikely in patients who fail to show signs of resedation 2 hours after a 1-mg dose of flumazenil.

Patient teaching

- Warn patient not to perform hazardous activities within 24 hours of procedure because of resedation risk.
- Tell patient to avoid alcohol, CNS depressants, and OTC drugs for 24 hours.
- Give family necessary instructions or provide patient with written instructions. Patient won't recall information given after the procedure; drug doesn't reverse amnesic effects of benzodiazepines.

---

flunisolide

AeroBid, AeroBid-M, Bronalide†, Nasalide, Nasarel

Pregnancy risk category C

Indications & dosages

➲ Chronic asthma

Adults and adolescents older than age 15: 2 inhalations (500 mcg) b.i.d. Maximum, 8 inhalations (2,000 mcg) daily.
Children ages 6 to 15: 2 inhalations (500 mcg) b.i.d. Maximum, 1,000 mcg daily.

➲ Seasonal or perennial rhinitis

Adults and adolescents older than age 14: 2 sprays (50 mcg) in each nostril b.i.d. May be increased to t.i.d. if necessary. Maximum dose is 8 sprays in each nostril daily (400 mcg).
Children ages 6 to 14: 1 spray (25 mcg) in each nostril t.i.d. or 2 sprays (50 mcg) in each nostril b.i.d. Maximum dose is 4 sprays in each nostril daily (200 mcg).

Contraindications & cautions

- Contraindicated in patients hypersensitive to drug and in those with status asthmaticus or respiratory tract infections.
- Drug isn't recommended in patients with nonasthmatic bronchial diseases or with asthma controlled by bronchodilator or other noncorticosteroid alone.

Adverse reactions

CNS: fever, dizziness, irritability, nervousness, *headache.*
CV: palpitations, chest pain, edema.
EENT: throat irritation, hoarseness, nasopharyngeal fungal infections, *sore throat, nasal congestion*, nasal irritation, nasal burning or stinging.
GI: *nausea, vomiting*, dry mouth, *unpleasant taste, diarrhea, upset stomach*, abdominal pain, decreased appetite.
Respiratory: *upper respiratory tract infection, cold symptoms.*
Skin: rash, pruritus.
Other: *influenza.*

Interactions

None significant.

Nursing considerations

- A spacer device may help to ensure proper administration and decrease oral adverse effects.
- Store drug between 59° and 86° F (15° and 30° C).
- Stop nasal spray after 3 weeks if symptoms don't improve.

!!ALERT Withdraw drug slowly in patients who have received long-term oral corticosteroid therapy.

- After withdrawing systemic corticosteroids, patient may need supplemental systemic corticosteroids if stress (trauma, surgery, or infection) causes adrenal insufficiency.

!!ALERT Don't confuse flunisolide with fluocinonide.

Patient teaching

Oral inhalant

- Warn patient that flunisolide doesn't relieve acute asthma attacks.
- Advise patient to ensure delivery of proper dose by gently warming the canister to room temperature before using. Some patients carry the canister in a pocket to keep it warm.
- Tell patient who also is using a bronchodilator to use it several minutes before beginning flunisolide treatment.
- Instruct patient to allow 1 minute to elapse before repeating inhalations and to hold his breath for a few seconds to enhance drug action.
- Teach patient to keep inhaler clean and unobstructed. He should wash it with warm water and dry it thoroughly after use.
- Teach patient to check mucous membranes frequently for signs and symptoms of fungal infection.
- Advise patient to prevent oral fungal infections by gargling or rinsing mouth with water after each inhaler use. Caution him not to swallow the water.
- Warn patient to avoid exposure to chickenpox or measles. If exposed, contact prescriber immediately.
- Advise parents of a child receiving long-term therapy that the child should have periodic growth measurements and be checked for evidence of hypothalamic-pituitary-adrenal axis suppression.

Nasal spray

- Tell patient to prime the nasal inhaler (5 to 6 sprays) before first use and after long periods of no use.
- Advise patient to clear nasal passageways before use.
- Patient should follow manufacturer's instructions for use and cleaning. Discard open containers after 3 months.
- Advise patient that therapeutic results may take several weeks.

fluorometholone

Flarex, Fluor-Op, FML, FML Forte, FML S.O.P.

Pregnancy risk category C

Indications & dosages

➲ **Inflammatory and allergic conditions of cornea, conjunctiva, sclera, anterior uvea**

Adults and children: 1 or 2 drops in conjunctival sac b.i.d. to q.i.d. May be given q 2 hours during first 1 to 2 days, if needed. Or, apply 1.25-cm ribbon of ointment to conjunctival sac q 4 hours, decreased to once daily to t.i.d. as inflammation subsides.

Contraindications & cautions

- Contraindicated in patients with vaccinia, varicella, acute superficial herpes simplex (dendritic keratitis), other fungal or viral eye diseases, ocular tuberculosis, or acute, purulent, untreated eye infections.
- Use cautiously in patients with corneal abrasions that may be contaminated (especially with herpes).
- Safety and efficacy of drug in children younger than age 2 haven't been established.

Adverse reactions

EENT: increased intraocular pressure, thinning of cornea, interference with corneal wound healing, corneal ulceration, increased susceptibility to viral or fungal corneal infections, glaucoma worsening, discharge, discomfort, ocular pain, foreign body sensation, cataracts, decreased visual acuity, diminished visual field, optic nerve damage with excessive or long-term use.
Other: systemic effects, adrenal suppression with excessive or long-term use.

Interactions

None significant.

Nursing considerations

- Treatment may last from a few days to several weeks, but avoid long-term use. Monitor intraocular pressure.
- Drug is less likely to cause increased intraocular pressure with extended use than

other ophthalmic anti-inflammatories (except medrysone).

- In chronic conditions, withdraw treatment by gradually decreasing frequency of applications.

Patient teaching

- Tell patient to shake container well before use.
- Teach patient how to instill drops or apply ointment. Advise him to wash hands before and after using either form, and warn him not to touch tip of dropper to eye or surrounding tissue.
- Advise patient to apply light finger pressure on lacrimal sac for 1 minute after instillation.
- Urge patient to call prescriber immediately and to stop drug if visual acuity decreases or visual field diminishes.
- Tell patient not to share drug, washcloths, or towels with family members and to notify prescriber if anyone develops same signs or symptoms.
- Warn patient not to use leftover drug for new eye inflammation; it may cause serious problems.
- Advise patient to consult prescriber if condition doesn't improve after 2 days. Don't stop treatment prematurely.
- Tell patient to store drug in tightly covered, light-resistant container.

fluorouracil (5-fluorouracil, 5-FU)
Adrucil, Carac, Efudex, Fluoroplex

Pregnancy risk category D (injection); X (topical form)

Indications & dosages

➲ **Colon, rectal, breast, stomach, and pancreatic cancers**

Adults: Initially, 12 mg/kg I.V. daily for 4 days; if no toxicity, give 6 mg/kg on days 6, 8, 10, and 12; then give a single weekly maintenance dose of 10 to 15 mg/kg I.V. begun after toxicity (if any) from first course has subsided. (Recommended dosages are based on actual body weight unless patient is obese or retaining fluid.) Maximum single recommended dose is 800 mg daily.

➲ **Palliative treatment of advanced colorectal cancer**

Adults: 425 mg/m^2 I.V. daily for 5 consecutive days. Give with 20 mg/m^2 of leucovorin I.V. Repeat at 4-week intervals for two additional courses; then repeat at 4- to 5-week intervals if tolerated.

➲ **Early breast cancer**

Adults: 600 mg/m^2 I.V. on days 1 and 8 of each cycle, combined with cyclophosphamide 100 mg/m^2 on days 1 through 14 of each cycle and methotrexate 40 mg/m^2 on days 1 and 8 of each cycle. Repeat monthly for 6 to 12 months, allowing for a 2-week rest period between cycles. In adults older than age 60, first fluorouracil dose is 400 mg/m^2 and methotrexate dose is 30 mg/m^2.

➲ **Multiple actinic (solar) keratoses**

Adults: Apply Carac cream once daily for up to 4 weeks. Or, apply Efudex or Fluoroplex cream or topical solution b.i.d. for 2 to 6 weeks.

➲ **Superficial basal cell carcinoma**

Adults: Apply 5% Efudex cream or topical solution b.i.d. usually for 3 to 6 weeks, maximum, 12 weeks.

Contraindications & cautions

- Contraindicated in patients hypersensitive to drug and in those with bone marrow suppression (WBC counts of 5,000/mm^3 or less or platelet counts of 100,000/mm^3 or less) or potentially serious infections.
- Contraindicated in patients in a poor nutritional state and those who have had major surgery within previous month.
- Topical formulations contraindicated in pregnant women.
- Use cautiously in patients who have received high-dose pelvic radiation or alkylating drugs and in those with impaired hepatic or renal function or widespread neoplastic infiltration of bone marrow.

Adverse reactions

CNS: acute cerebellar syndrome, confusion, disorientation, euphoria, ataxia, headache, *weakness, malaise.*

CV: ***myocardial ischemia***, angina, thrombophlebitis.

EENT: epistaxis, photophobia, lacrimation, lacrimal duct stenosis, nystagmus, visual changes, eye irritation.

GI: *stomatitis, GI ulcer, nausea, vomiting, diarrhea, anorexia,* ***GI bleeding***.
Hematologic: ***leukopenia, thrombocytopenia, agranulocytosis***, *anemia*.
Skin: *dermatitis, erythema, scaling, pruritus,* nail changes, pigmented palmar creases, erythematous contact dermatitis, desquamative rash of hands and feet, hand-and-foot syndrome with long-term use, photosensitivity, *reversible alopecia, pain, burning,* soreness, suppuration, *swelling, dryness, erosion with topical use.*
Other: ***anaphylaxis***.

Interactions

Drug-drug. *Leucovorin calcium:* May increase cytotoxicity and toxicity of fluorouracil. Monitor patient closely.
Drug-lifestyle. *Sun exposure:* May cause photosensitivity reactions. Advise patient to avoid excessive sunlight exposure.

Nursing considerations

- Apply topical form cautiously near patient's eyes, nose, and mouth.
- Avoid occlusive dressings with topical form because they increase risk of inflammatory reactions in adjacent normal skin.
- Apply topical form with a nonmetal applicator or suitable gloves. Wash hands immediately after handling topical form.
- The 1% topical strength is used on patient's face. Higher strengths, such as 5%, are used for thicker-skinned areas or resistant lesions, such as superficial basal cell carcinoma.
- Ingestion and systemic absorption of topical form may cause leukopenia, thrombocytopenia, stomatitis, diarrhea, or GI ulceration, bleeding, and hemorrhage. Application to large ulcerated areas may cause systemic toxicity.
- Watch for stomatitis or diarrhea (signs of toxicity). Consider using topical oral anesthetic to soothe lesions. Stop drug and notify prescriber if diarrhea occurs.
- Encourage diligent oral hygiene to prevent superinfection of denuded mucosa.
- Monitor WBC and platelet counts daily. Watch for ecchymoses, petechiae, easy bruising, and anemia.
- Monitor fluid intake and output, CBC, and renal and hepatic function tests.
- Long-term use may cause erythematous, desquamative rash of the hands and feet, which may be treated with pyridoxine 50 to 150 mg P.O. daily for 5 to 7 days.
- Dermatologic adverse effects are reversible when drug is stopped.
- To prevent bleeding, avoid I.M. injections when platelet count is below 50,000/mm^3.
- Anticipate blood transfusions because of cumulative anemia. Patient may receive injections of RBC colony–stimulating factors to promote RBC production and decrease need for blood transfusions.

!! ALERT Fluorouracil toxicity may be delayed for 1 to 3 weeks.

- The WBC count nadir occurs 9 to 14 days after first dose; the platelet count nadir occurs in 7 to 14 days.

!! ALERT Drug may be ordered as "5-fluorouracil" or "5-FU." The numeral 5 is part of drug name and shouldn't be confused with dosage units.

!! ALERT Don't confuse fluorouracil with floxuridine, fludarabine, or flucytosine.

Patient teaching

- Warn patient that hair loss may occur but is reversible.
- Caution patient to avoid prolonged exposure to sunlight or ultraviolet light when topical form is used.
- Tell patient to use highly protective sunblock to avoid inflammatory skin irritation.
- Warn patient that topically treated area may be unsightly during therapy and for several weeks afterward. Complete healing may take 1 or 2 months.
- Caution woman of childbearing age to consult prescriber before becoming pregnant.
- Advise woman to stop breast-feeding during therapy because of risk of toxicity to infant.

fluoxetine hydrochloride

Prozac, Prozac Weekly, Sarafem

Pregnancy risk category C

Indications & dosages

➲ **Depression, obsessive-compulsive disorder (OCD)**
Adults: Initially, 20 mg P.O. in the morning; increase dosage based on patient response. Maximum daily dose is 80 mg.

Children ages 7 to 17 (OCD): 10 mg P.O. daily. After 2 weeks, increase to 20 mg daily. Dosage is 20 to 60 mg daily.
Children ages 8 to 18 (depression): 10 mg P.O. once daily for 1 week; then increase to 20 mg daily.

➲ **Depression in elderly patients**
Adults age 65 and older: Initially, 20 mg P.O. daily in the morning. Increase dose based on response. Doses may be given b.i.d., morning and noon. Maximum daily dose is 80 mg. Consider using a lower dosage or less-frequent dosing in these patients, especially those with systemic illness and those who are receiving drugs for other illnesses.

➲ **Maintenance therapy for depression in stabilized patients (not for newly diagnosed depression)**
Adults: 90 mg Prozac Weekly P.O. once weekly. Start once-weekly dosing 7 days after the last daily dose of Prozac 20 mg.

➲ **Short-term and long-term treatment of bulimia nervosa**
Adults: 60 mg P.O. daily in the morning.

➲ **Short-term treatment of panic disorder with or without agoraphobia**
Adults: 10 mg P.O. once daily for 1 week, then increase dose as needed to 20 mg daily. Maximum daily dose is 60 mg.

For patients with renal or hepatic impairment, reduce dose or increase dosing interval.

➲ **Anorexia nervosa in weight-restored patients♦**
Adults: 40 mg P.O. daily.

➲ **Depression caused by bipolar disorder♦**
Adults: 20 to 60 mg P.O. daily.

➲ **Cataplexy♦**
Adults: 20 mg P.O. once or twice daily with CNS stimulant therapy.

➲ **Alcohol dependence♦**
Adults: 60 mg P.O. daily.

➲ **Premenstrual dysphoric disorder**
Sarafem
Adults: 20 mg P.O. daily continuously (every day of the menstrual cycle) or intermittently (daily dose starting 14 days before the anticipated onset of menstruation through the first full day of menses and repeating with each new cycle). Maximum daily dose is 80 mg P.O.

For patients with renal or hepatic impairment and those taking several drugs at the same time, reduce dose or increase dosing interval.

Contraindications & cautions

- Contraindicated in patients hypersensitive to drug and in those taking MAO inhibitors within 14 days of starting therapy. MAO inhibitors shouldn't be started within 5 weeks of stopping fluoxetine therapy. Avoid using thioridazine with fluoxetine or within a minimum of 5 weeks after stopping fluoxetine.
- Use cautiously in patients at high risk for suicide and in those with history of diabetes mellitus; seizures; mania; or hepatic, renal, or CV disease.
- Use in third trimester of pregnancy may be associated with neonatal complications at birth. Consider the risk versus benefit of treatment during this time.

Adverse reactions

CNS: *nervousness, somnolence, anxiety, insomnia, headache, drowsiness,* fatigue, *tremor, dizziness, asthenia,* fever, ***suicidal behavior.***
CV: palpitations, hot flashes.
EENT: nasal congestion, pharyngitis, sinusitis.
GI: *nausea, diarrhea, dry mouth, anorexia,* dyspepsia, constipation, abdominal pain, vomiting, flatulence, increased appetite.
GU: sexual dysfunction.
Metabolic: weight loss.
Musculoskeletal: muscle pain.
Respiratory: upper respiratory tract infection, cough, respiratory distress.
Skin: rash, pruritus, diaphoresis.
Other: flulike syndrome.

Interactions

Drug-drug. *Benzodiazepines, lithium, tricyclic antidepressants:* May increase CNS effects. Monitor patient closely.
Beta blockers, carbamazepine, flecainide, vinblastine: May increase levels of these drugs. Monitor drug levels and monitor patient for adverse reactions.
Cyproheptadine: May reverse or decrease fluoxetine effect. Monitor patient closely.
Dextromethorphan: May cause unusual side effects, such as visual hallucinations. Advise use of cough suppressant that doesn't contain dextromethorphan while taking fluoxetine.

Insulin, oral antidiabetics: May alter glucose level and antidiabetic requirements. Adjust dosage.
Lithium, tricyclic antidepressants: May increase adverse CNS effects. Monitor patient closely.
MAO inhibitors (phenelzine, selegiline, tranylcypromine): May cause serotonin syndrome. Avoid using with fluoxetine or within a minimum of 5 weeks after stopping fluoxetine.
Phenytoin: May increase phenytoin level and risk of toxicity. Monitor phenytoin level and adjust dosage.
Sumatriptan: May cause weakness, hyperreflexia, and incoordination. Monitor patient closely.
Thioridazine: May increase thioridazine level, increasing risk of serious ventricular arrhythmias and sudden death. Avoid using with fluoxetine or within a minimum of 5 weeks after stopping fluoxetine.
Tramadol: May cause serotonin syndrome. Avoid using together.
Tryptophan: May increase agitation, restlessness, and GI adverse effects. Use together cautiously.
Warfarin, other highly protein-bound drugs: May increase level of fluoxetine or other highly protein-bound drugs. Monitor patient closely.
Drug-herb. *St. John's wort:* May increase sedative and hypnotic effects; may cause serotonin syndrome. Discourage use together.
Drug-lifestyle. *Alcohol use:* May increase CNS depression. Discourage use together.

Nursing considerations

- Use antihistamines or topical corticosteroids to treat rashes or pruritus.
- Watch for weight change during therapy, particularly in underweight or bulimic patients.
- Record mood changes. Watch for suicidal tendencies.

!!ALERT Don't confuse fluoxetine with fluvoxamine or fluvastatin
!!ALERT Don't confuse Prozac with Proscar, Prilosec, or ProSom.

Patient teaching

- Tell patient to avoid taking drug in the afternoon whenever possible because fluoxetine commonly causes nervousness and insomnia.
- Drug may cause dizziness or drowsiness. Warn patient to avoid driving and other hazardous activities that require alertness and good psychomotor coordination until effects of drug are known.
- Tell patient to consult prescriber before taking other prescription or OTC drugs.
- Advise patient that full therapeutic effect may not be seen for 4 weeks or longer.

fluphenazine decanoate
Modecate Concentrate†, Prolixin Decanoate

fluphenazine hydrochloride
Apo-Fluphenazine†, Moditen HCl†, Permitil†*, Permitil Concentrate, Prolixin†*, Prolixin Concentrate

Pregnancy risk category C

Indications & dosages

➲ Psychotic disorders
Adults: Initially, 0.5 to 10 mg fluphenazine hydrochloride P.O. daily in divided doses q 6 to 8 hours; may increase cautiously to 20 mg. Maintenance dose is 1 to 5 mg P.O. daily. I.M. doses are one-third to one-half of P.O. doses. Usual I.M. dose is 1.25 mg. Give more than 10 mg daily with caution.

Or, 12.5 to 25 mg of fluphenazine decanoate I.M. or S.C. q 1 to 6 weeks; maintenance dose is 25 to 100 mg, p.r.n.
Elderly patients: 1 to 2.5 mg fluphenazine hydrochloride P.O daily.

Contraindications & cautions

- Contraindicated in patients hypersensitive to drug and in those with coma, CNS depression, bone marrow suppression or other blood dyscrasia, subcortical damage, or liver damage.
- Use cautiously in elderly or debilitated patients and in those with pheochromocytoma, severe CV disease (may cause sudden drop in blood pressure), peptic ulcer, respiratory disorder, hypocalcemia, seizure disorder (may lower seizure threshold), severe reactions to insulin or electroconvulsive therapy, mitral insufficiency, glaucoma, or prostatic hyperplasia.
- Use cautiously in those exposed to extreme heat or cold (including antipyretic therapy) or phosphorus insecticides.

• Use parenteral form cautiously in patients who have asthma or are allergic to sulfites.

Adverse reactions

CNS: *extrapyramidal reactions, tardive dyskinesia,* sedation, *pseudoparkinsonism,* EEG changes, drowsiness, ***seizures,*** dizziness, ***neuroleptic malignant syndrome.***
CV: orthostatic hypotension, tachycardia, ECG changes.
EENT: ocular changes, *blurred vision,* nasal congestion.
GI: *dry mouth, constipation,* increased appetite.
GU: *urine retention,* dark urine, menstrual irregularities, inhibited ejaculation.
Hematologic: ***leukopenia, agranulocytosis,*** eosinophilia, hemolytic anemia, ***aplastic anemia, thrombocytopenia.***
Hepatic: cholestatic jaundice.
Metabolic: weight gain.
Skin: *mild photosensitivity reactions,* allergic reactions.
Other: gynecomastia, galactorrhea.

Interactions

Drug-drug. *Antacids:* May inhibit absorption of oral phenothiazines. Separate antacid and phenothiazine doses by at least 2 hours.
Anticholinergics: May increase anticholinergic effects. Use together cautiously.
Barbiturates, lithium: May decrease phenothiazine effect and increase neurologic adverse effects. Monitor patient.
Centrally acting antihypertensives: May decrease antihypertensive effect. Monitor blood pressure.
CNS depressants: May increase CNS depression. Use together cautiously.
Drug-herb. *St. John's wort:* May increase risk of photosensitivity reactions. Advise patient to avoid excessive sunlight exposure.
Drug-lifestyle. *Alcohol use:* May increase CNS depression, especially that involving psychomotor skills. Strongly discourage alcohol use.
Sun exposure: May increase risk of photosensitivity reactions. Advise patient to avoid excessive sunlight exposure.

Nursing considerations

• Prolixin Concentrate and Permitil Concentrate are 10 times more concentrated than Prolixin elixir (5 mg/ml versus 0.5 mg/ml). Check dosage order carefully.
• Oral liquid and parenteral forms can cause contact dermatitis. Wear gloves when preparing solutions, and avoid contact with skin and clothing.
• Protect drug from light. Slight yellowing of injection or concentrate is common and doesn't affect potency. Discard markedly discolored solutions.
• Dilute liquid concentrate with water, fruit juice, milk, or semisolid food just before administration.
• For long-acting form (decanoate), which is an oil preparation, use a dry needle of at least 21G. Allow 24 to 96 hours for onset of action. Note and report to prescriber adverse reactions in patients taking this drug form.
• Monitor patient for tardive dyskinesia, which may occur after prolonged use. It may not appear until months or years later and may disappear spontaneously or persist for life, despite ending drug.
!!ALERT Watch for signs and symptoms of neuroleptic malignant syndrome (extrapyramidal effects, hyperthermia, autonomic disturbance), which is rare but commonly fatal. It may not be related to length of drug use or type of neuroleptic; more than 60% of affected patients are men.
• Withhold dose and notify prescriber if patient—especially child or pregnant woman—develops signs or symptoms of blood dyscrasia (fever, sore throat, infection, cellulitis, weakness) or extrapyramidal reactions persisting longer than a few hours.
• Don't withdraw drug abruptly unless serious adverse reactions occur.
• Abrupt withdrawal of long-term therapy may cause gastritis, nausea, vomiting, dizziness, tremor, feeling of warmth or cold, diaphoresis, tachycardia, headache, or insomnia.
!!ALERT Permitil and Prolixin may contain tartrazine.

Patient teaching

• Warn patient to avoid activities that require alertness and good coordination until effects of drug are known. Drowsiness and dizziness usually subside after first few weeks.
• Warn patient to avoid alcohol while taking drug.

- Tell patient to relieve dry mouth with sugarless gum or hard candy.
- Have patient report signs of urine retention or constipation.
- Advise patient to use sunblock and wear protective clothing to avoid sensitivity to the sun.
- Tell patient that drug may discolor urine.

flurazepam hydrochloride
Apo-Flurazepam†, Dalmane, Novo-Flupam†

Pregnancy risk category X
Controlled substance schedule IV

Indications & dosages
➲ Insomnia
Adults: 15 to 30 mg P.O. h.s. May repeat dose once, p.r.n.
Elderly patients: 15 mg P.O. h.s. initially, until response is determined.

Contraindications & cautions
- Contraindicated in patients hypersensitive to drug and during pregnancy.
- Use cautiously in patients with impaired hepatic or renal function, chronic pulmonary insufficiency, mental depression, suicidal tendencies, or history of drug abuse.

Adverse reactions
CNS: *daytime sedation, dizziness, drowsiness, disturbed coordination*, lethargy, confusion, physical or psychological dependence, *headache*, light-headedness, nervousness, hallucinations, staggering, ataxia, disorientation, ***coma***.
GI: nausea, vomiting, heartburn, diarrhea, abdominal pain.

Interactions
Drug-drug. *Cimetidine:* May increase sedation. Monitor patient carefully.
CNS depressants, including opioid analgesics: May cause excessive CNS depression. Use together cautiously.
Digoxin: May increase digoxin level, resulting in toxicity. Monitor patient closely.
Disulfiram, hormonal contraceptives, isoniazid: May decrease metabolism of benzodiazepines, leading to toxicity. Monitor patient closely.
Fluconazole, itraconazole, ketoconazole, miconazole: May increase and prolong drug level, CNS depression, and psychomotor impairment. Avoid using together.
Phenytoin: May increase phenytoin level. Watch for toxicity.
Rifampin: May enhance metabolism of benzodiazepines. Watch for decreased effectiveness of benzodiazepine.
Theophylline: May act as antagonist with flurazepam. Watch for decreased effectiveness of flurazepam.
Drug-herb. *Calendula, hops, kava, lemon balm, passion flower, skullcap, valerian:* May enhance sedative effect of drug. Discourage use together.
Drug-lifestyle. *Alcohol use:* May cause additive CNS effects. Discourage use together.
Smoking: May increase metabolism and clearance and decrease drug half-life. Advise patient to watch for signs of decreased effectiveness.

Nursing considerations
- Check hepatic and renal function and CBC before and periodically during long-term therapy.
- Minor changes in EEG patterns (usually low-voltage, fast activity) may occur during and after flurazepam therapy.
- Assess mental status before starting therapy. Elderly patients are more sensitive to drug's adverse CNS reactions.
- Take precautions to prevent hoarding or self-overdosing by depressed, suicidal, or drug-dependent patients and those with history of drug abuse.
- Patient may become physically and psychologically dependent with long-term use.

!!ALERT Don't confuse Dalmane with Dialume or Demulen.

Patient teaching
- Inform patient that drug is more effective on second, third, and fourth nights of treatment because drug builds up in the body.
- Warn patient not to abruptly stop drug after taking it for 1 month or longer.
- Tell patient to avoid alcohol use while taking drug.
- Caution patient to avoid performing activities that require mental alertness or physical coordination.

• Warn patient that prolonged use of this drug may produce psychological and physical dependence.
• Advise patient to warn prescriber about planned, suspected, or known pregnancy.

flutamide
Euflex†, Eulexin

Pregnancy risk category D

Indications & dosages
➲ **Metastatic locally confined prostate cancer (stages B_2, C, D_2), combined with luteinizing hormone–releasing hormone analogues such as leuprolide acetate or goserelin**
Adults: 250 mg P.O. q 8 hours.

Contraindications & cautions
• Contraindicated in patients hypersensitive to drug and in those with severe liver dysfunction.

Adverse reactions
CNS: drowsiness, ***encephalopathy***, confusion, depression, anxiety, nervousness, paresthesia.
CV: peripheral edema, hypertension, *hot flashes.*
GI: *diarrhea, nausea, vomiting,* anorexia.
GU: *impotence.*
Hematologic: anemia, ***leukopenia, thrombocytopenia***, hemolytic anemia.
Hepatic: ***hepatitis***.
Skin: rash, photosensitivity reactions.
Other: *loss of libido,* gynecomastia.

Interactions
Drug-drug. *Warfarin:* May increase PT. Monitor PT and INR.
Drug-lifestyle. *Sun exposure:* May cause photosensitivity reactions. Advise patient to avoid excessive sunlight exposure.

Nursing considerations
• Monitor liver function tests and CBC periodically.
• Flutamide must be taken continuously with drug used for medical castration (such as leuprolide) to allow full therapeutic benefit. Leuprolide suppresses testosterone production, whereas flutamide inhibits testosterone action at cellular level; together, they can impair growth of androgen-responsive tumors.

Patient teaching
• Advise patient not to stop drug without consulting prescriber.
• Instruct patient to report adverse reactions promptly, especially dark yellow or brown urine, vomiting, or yellowing of the eyes or skin.

fluticasone propionate
Flonase, Flovent Diskus†, Flovent HFA

Pregnancy risk category C

Indications & dosages
➲ **As preventative in maintenance of chronic asthma in patients requiring oral corticosteroid**
Flovent Diskus
Adults and children ages 12 and older: In patients previously taking bronchodilators alone, initially, inhaled dose of 100 mcg b.i.d. to maximum of 500 mcg b.i.d.
Adults and children age 12 and older previously taking inhaled corticosteroids: Initially, inhaled dose of 100 to 250 mcg b.i.d. to maximum of 500 mcg b.i.d.
Adults and children ages 12 and older previously taking oral corticosteroids: Inhaled dose of 500 to 1,000 mcg b.i.d. Maximum dose, 1,000 mcg b.i.d.
Children ages 4 to 11: For patients previously on bronchodilators alone or on inhaled corticosteroids, initially, inhaled dose of 50 mcg b.i.d. to maximum of 100 mcg b.i.d.
Flovent HFA
Adults and children age 12 and older: In those previously taking bronchodilators alone, initially, inhaled dose of 88 mcg b.i.d. to maximum of 440 mcg b.i.d.
Adults and children age 12 and older previously taking inhaled corticosteroids: Initially, inhaled dose of 88 to 220 mcg b.i.d. to maximum of 440 mcg b.i.d.
Adults and children age 12 and older previously taking oral corticosteroids: Initially, inhaled dose of 440 mcg b.i.d. to maximum of 880 mcg b.i.d.

➲ Nasal symptoms of seasonal and perennial allergic and nonallergic rhinitis
Flonase
Adults: Initially, 2 sprays (100 mcg) in each nostril daily or 1 spray b.i.d. Once symptoms are controlled, decrease to 1 spray in each nostril daily. Or, for seasonal allergic rhinitis, 2 sprays in each nostril once daily, as needed, for symptom control.
Adolescents and children age 4 and older: Initially, 1 spray (50 mcg) in each nostril daily. If not responding, increase to 2 sprays in each nostril daily. Once symptoms are controlled, decrease to 1 spray in each nostril daily. Maximum dose is 2 sprays in each nostril daily.

Contraindications & cautions

- Contraindicated in patients hypersensitive to ingredients in these preparations.
- Contraindicated as primary treatment of patients with status asthmaticus or other acute episodes of asthma requiring more intensive measures.
- Use cautiously in breast-feeding patients.

Adverse reactions

CNS: fever, *headache*, dizziness, migraine, nervousness.
EENT: *pharyngitis*, blood in nasal mucous, sinusitis, dysphonia, rhinitis, nasal discharge, laryngitis, epistaxis, hoarseness, conjunctivitis, eye irritation, nasal burning or irritation, dry eye, cataracts.
GI: mouth irritation, *oral candidiasis*, diarrhea, abdominal pain, viral gastroenteritis, abdominal discomfort, nausea, vomiting.
GU: UTI.
Metabolic: hyperglycemia, cushingoid features, growth retardation in children, weight gain.
Musculoskeletal: osteoporosis, joint pain, aches and pains, disorder or symptoms of neck sprain or strain, muscular soreness.
Respiratory: *upper respiratory tract infection*, bronchitis, chest congestion, dyspnea, ***bronchospasm***, asthma symptoms, cough.
Skin: dermatitis, urticaria.
Other: influenza, ***eosinophilic conditions***, viral infections, ***angioedema***.

Interactions

Drug-drug. *Ketoconazole and other cytochrome P-450 3A4 inhibitors:* May increase mean fluticasone level. Use together cautiously.
Ritonavir: May cause systemic corticosteroid effects such as Cushing syndrome and adrenal suppression. Avoid use together.

Nursing considerations

- Because of risk of systemic absorption of inhaled corticosteroids, observe patient carefully for evidence of systemic corticosteroid effects.
- Monitor patient, especially postoperatively or during periods of stress, for evidence of inadequate adrenal response.
- During withdrawal from oral corticosteroids, some patients may experience signs and symptoms of systemically active corticosteroid withdrawal, such as joint or muscle pain, lassitude, and depression, despite maintenance or even improvement of respiratory function.
- For patients starting therapy who are currently receiving oral corticosteroid therapy, reduce dose of prednisone to no more than 2.5 mg/day on a weekly basis, beginning after at least 1 week of therapy with fluticasone.

!!ALERT As with other inhaled asthma drugs, bronchospasm may occur with an immediate increase in wheezing after a dose. If bronchospasm occurs after a dose of fluticasone inhalation aerosol, treat immediately with a fast-acting inhaled bronchodilator.

Patient teaching

- Tell patient that drug isn't indicated for the relief of acute bronchospasm.
- For proper use of drug and to attain maximum improvement, tell patient to carefully follow the accompanying patient instructions.
- Advise patient to use drug at regular intervals, as directed.
- Instruct patient to contact prescriber if nasal spray doesn't improve condition after 4 days of treatment.
- Instruct patient to immediately contact prescriber if asthma episodes unresponsive to bronchodilators occur during treatment with fluticasone. During such episodes, patient may need therapy with oral corticosteroids.
- Warn patient to avoid exposure to chickenpox or measles and, if exposed, to consult prescriber immediately.

- Tell patient to carry or wear medical identification indicating that he may need supplementary corticosteroids during stress or a severe asthma attack.
- During periods of stress or a severe asthma attack, instruct patient who has been withdrawn from systemic corticosteroids to resume oral corticosteroids (in prescribed doses) immediately and to contact prescriber for further instruction. Instruct him to rinse his mouth and spit water out after inhalation.
- Tell patient to prime inhaler with 4 test sprays (away from his face) before first use, shaking well before each spray. Also, prime with 1 spray if inhaler has been dropped or not used for 1 week or longer.
- Advise patient to avoid spraying inhalation aerosol into eyes.
- Instruct patient to shake canister well before using inhalation aerosol.
- Advise patient to store fluticasone powder in a dry place.

Flonase nasal spray

- Tell patient to prime the nasal inhaler before first use or after 1 week or longer of nonuse.
- Have patient clear nasal passages before use.
- Advise patient to follow manufacturer's recommendations for use and cleaning.
- Advise patient to use at regular intervals for full benefit.
- Tell patient to contact provider if signs or symptoms don't improve within 4 days or if signs or symptoms worsen.
- Tell patient that the correct amount of spray can't be guaranteed after 120 sprays even though the bottle may not be completely empty.

fluticasone propionate
Cutivate

Pregnancy risk category C

Indications & dosages

➲ **Inflammation and pruritus from dermatoses responsive to corticosteroids**

Adults: Apply sparingly to affected area b.i.d.; rub in gently and completely.

Children age 3 months and older: Apply a thin film (0.05%) to affected areas b.i.d. Rub in gently. Don't use for longer than 4 weeks.

➲ **Inflammation and pruritus from atopic dermatitis**

Children age 3 months and older: Apply thin film (0.05%) to affected areas once daily or b.i.d. Rub in gently. Don't use for longer than 4 weeks.

Contraindications & cautions

- Contraindicated in patients hypersensitive to drug or its components and in those with viral, fungal, herpetic, or tubercular skin lesions.

Adverse reactions

CNS: light-headedness.
GU: glycosuria.
Metabolic: hyperglycemia.
Skin: urticaria, burning, hypertrichosis, pruritus, irritation, erythema.
Other: ***hypothalamic-pituitary-adrenal axis suppression***, Cushing's syndrome.

Interactions

None significant.

Nursing considerations

- Don't mix drug with other bases or vehicles because doing so may affect potency.
- If adverse reactions occur, prescriber may order less potent drug.
- Stop drug if local irritation or systemic infection, absorption, or hypersensitivity occurs.
- Absorption of corticosteroid is increased when drug is applied to inflamed or damaged skin, eyelids, or scrotal area; it's lowest when applied to intact normal skin, palms of hands, or soles of feet.
- Don't use drug with an occlusive dressing or in diaper area.

!!ALERT Don't confuse fluticasone with fluconazole.

Patient teaching

- Teach patient or family member how to apply drug using gloves, sterile applicator, or after careful hand washing.
- Tell patient to wash hands after application.
- Tell patient to avoid prolonged use and contact with eyes. Warn him not to apply to face, in skin creases, or around eyes, genitals, underarms, or rectum.

• Instruct patient to notify prescriber if condition persists or worsens or if burning or irritation develops.

fluticasone propionate and salmeterol inhalation powder

Advair Diskus 100/50, Advair Diskus 250/50, Advair Diskus 500/50

Pregnancy risk category C

Indications & dosages

➲ Long-term maintenance of asthma

Adults and children age 12 and older: 1 inhalation b.i.d., at least 12 hours apart.

Adults and children age 12 and older not currently taking an inhaled corticosteroid: 1 inhalation of Advair Diskus 100/50 b.i.d.

Adults and children age 12 and older currently taking beclomethasone dipropionate: If beclomethasone dipropionate daily dose is 420 mcg or less, start with 1 inhalation of Advair Diskus 100/50 b.i.d. If beclomethasone dipropionate daily dose is 462 to 840 mcg, start with 1 inhalation of Advair Diskus 250/50 b.i.d.

Adults and children age 12 and older currently taking budesonide: If budesonide daily dose is 400 mcg or less, start with 1 inhalation of Advair Diskus 100/50 b.i.d. If budesonide daily dose is 800 to 1,200 mcg, start with 1 inhalation of Advair Diskus 250/50 b.i.d. If budesonide daily dose is 1,600 mcg, start with 1 inhalation of Advair Diskus 500/50 b.i.d.

Adults and children age 12 and older currently taking flunisolide: If flunisolide daily dose is 1,000 mcg or less, start with 1 inhalation of Advair Diskus 100/50 b.i.d. If flunisolide daily dose is 1,250 to 2,000 mcg, start with 1 inhalation of Advair Diskus 250/50 b.i.d.

Adults and children age 12 and older currently taking fluticasone propionate inhalation aerosol: If fluticasone propionate inhalation aerosol daily dose is 176 mcg or less, start with 1 inhalation of Advair Diskus 100/50 b.i.d. If fluticasone propionate inhalation aerosol daily dose is 440 mcg, start with 1 inhalation of Advair Diskus 250/50 b.i.d. If fluticasone propionate inhalation aerosol daily dose is 660 to 880 mcg, start with 1 inhalation of Advair Diskus 500/50 b.i.d.

Adults and children age 12 and older currently taking fluticasone propionate inhalation powder: If fluticasone propionate inhalation powder daily dose is 200 mcg or less, start with 1 inhalation of Advair Diskus 100/50 b.i.d. If fluticasone propionate inhalation powder daily dose is 500 mcg, start with 1 inhalation of Advair Diskus 250/50 b.i.d. If fluticasone propionate inhalation powder daily dose is 1,000 mcg, start with 1 inhalation of Advair Diskus 500/50 b.i.d.

Adults and children age 12 and older currently taking triamcinolone acetonide: If triamcinolone acetonide dose is 1,000 mcg daily or less, start with 1 inhalation of Advair Diskus 100/50 b.i.d. If triamcinolone acetonide daily dose is 1,100 to 1,600 mcg, start with 1 inhalation of Advair Diskus 250/50 b.i.d.

For patients already using an inhaled corticosteroid: Maximum inhalation of Advair Diskus is 500/50 b.i.d.

➲ Asthma in children who remain symptomatic while taking an inhaled corticosteroid

Children ages 4 to 11: 1 inhalation (100 mg fluticasone and 50 mg salmeterol) b.i.d., morning and evening, about 12 hours apart.

➲ Maintenance therapy for airflow obstruction in patients with COPD from chronic bronchitis

Adults: 1 inhalation of Advair Diskus 250/50 only, b.i.d., about 12 hours apart.

Contraindications & cautions

• Contraindicated in patients hypersensitive to drug or its components.

• Contraindicated as primary treatment of status asthmaticus or other acute asthmatic episodes.

• Use cautiously, if at all, in patients with active or quiescent respiratory tuberculosis infection; untreated systemic fungal, bacterial, viral, or parasitic infection; or ocular herpes simplex.

• Use cautiously in patients with CV disorders, seizure disorders or thyrotoxicosis; in patients unusually responsive to sympathomimetic amines; and in patients with hepatic impairment.

Adverse reactions

CNS: sleep disorders, tremors, hypnagogic effects, compressed nerve syndromes, *headache.*

CV: palpitations, pain.
EENT: *pharyngitis*, sinusitis, hoarseness or dysphonia, oral candidiasis, dental discomfort and pain, rhinorrhea, rhinitis, sneezing, nasal irritation, blood in nasal mucosa, keratitis, conjunctivitis, eye redness, viral eye infections, congestion.
GI: nausea, vomiting, abdominal pain and discomfort, diarrhea, gastroenteritis, oral discomfort and pain, constipation, oral ulcerations, oral erythema and rashes, appendicitis, unusual taste.
Musculoskeletal: muscle pain, arthralgia, articular rheumatism, muscle stiffness, tightness, rigidity, bone and cartilage disorders.
Respiratory: *upper respiratory tract infection*, lower respiratory tract infections, bronchitis, cough, pneumonia.
Skin: infection, urticaria, skin flakiness, disorders of sweat and sebum, sweating.
Other: viral or bacterial infections, chest symptoms, fluid retention, allergic reactions.

Interactions

Drug-drug. *Beta blockers:* Blocked pulmonary effect of salmeterol may produce severe bronchospasm in patients with asthma. Avoid using together. If necessary, use a cardioselective beta blocker cautiously.
Ketoconazole, other inhibitors of cytochrome P-450: May increase fluticasone level and adverse effects. Use together cautiously.
Loop diuretics, thiazide diuretics: Potassium-wasting diuretics may cause or worsen ECG changes or hypokalemia. Use together cautiously.
MAO inhibitors, tricyclic antidepressants: May potentiate the action of salmeterol on the vascular system. Separate doses by 2 weeks.

Nursing considerations

!!ALERT Patient shouldn't be switched from systemic corticosteroids to Advair Diskus because of hypothalamic-pituitary-adrenal axis suppression. Death from adrenal insufficiency can occur. Several months are required for recovery of hypothalamic-pituitary-adrenal function after withdrawal of systemic corticosteroids.
- Don't start therapy during rapidly deteriorating or potentially life-threatening episodes of asthma. Serious acute respiratory events, including fatality, can occur.
- The benefit of Advair 250/50 in treating patients with COPD for more than 6 months is unknown. If drug is used for longer than 6 months, periodically reevaluate patient to assess for benefits or risks of therapy.
- Monitor patient for urticaria, angioedema, rash, bronchospasm, or other signs of hypersensitivity.
- Don't use Advair Diskus to stop an asthma attack. Patients using Advair Diskus should carry an inhaled, short-acting beta$_2$ agonist (such as albuterol) for acute symptoms.
- If Advair Diskus causes paradoxical bronchospasm, treat immediately with a short-acting inhaled bronchodilator (such as albuterol), and notify prescriber.

!!ALERT Rare, serious asthma episodes or asthma-related deaths have occurred in patients taking salmeterol; black patients may be at a greater risk.
- Monitor patient for increased use of inhaled short-acting beta$_2$-agonist. The dose of Advair Diskus may need to be increased.
- Closely monitor children for growth suppression.

Patient teaching

- Instruct patient on proper use of the dry-powder multidose inhaler to provide effective treatment.
- Tell patient to avoid exhaling into the dry-powder multidose inhaler; to activate and use the dry-powder multidose inhaler in a level, horizontal position; and not to use Advair Diskus with a spacer device.
- Instruct patient to keep the dry-powder multidose inhaler in a dry place, away from direct heat or sunlight, to avoid washing the mouthpiece or other parts of the device. Patient should discard device 1 month after removal from the moisture-protective overwrap pouch or after every blister has been used, whichever comes first. He shouldn't attempt to take device apart.
- Instruct patient to rinse mouth after inhalation to prevent oral candidiasis.
- Inform patient that improvement may occur within 30 minutes after an Advair dose, but the full benefit may not occur for 1 week or more.
- Advise patient not to exceed recommended prescribing dose.
- Instruct patient not to relieve acute symptoms with Advair Diskus. Treat acute symp-

toms with an inhaled short-acting $beta_2$ agonist.

- Instruct patient to report decreasing effects or use of increasing doses of their short-acting inhaled $beta_2$ agonist.
- Tell patient to report palpitations, chest pain, rapid heart rate, tremor, or nervousness.
- Instruct patient to call immediately if exposed to chickenpox or measles.

fluvastatin sodium
Lescol, Lescol XL

Pregnancy risk category X

Indications & dosages

➲ To reduce LDL and total cholesterol levels in patients with primary hypercholesterolemia (types IIa and IIb); to slow progression of coronary atherosclerosis in patients with coronary artery disease; elevated triglyceride and apolipoprotein B levels in patients with primary hypercholesterolemia and mixed dyslipidemia whose response to dietary restriction and other nonpharmacologic measures has been inadequate

Adults: Initially, 20 to 40 mg P.O. h.s., increasing p.r.n. to maximum of 80 mg daily in divided doses or 80 mg Lescol XL P.O. h.s.

➲ To reduce the risk of undergoing coronary revascularization procedures

Adults: In patients who must reduce LDL cholesterol level by at least 25%, initially, 40 mg P.O. once daily or b.i.d.; or one 80-mg extended-release tablet as a single dose in the evening. In patients who must reduce LDL cholesterol level by less than 25%, initially, 20 mg P.O. daily. Dosages range from 20 to 80 mg daily.

Contraindications & cautions

- Contraindicated in patients hypersensitive to drug and in those with active liver disease or unexplained persistent elevations of transaminase levels; also contraindicated in pregnant and breast-feeding women and in women of childbearing age.
- Use cautiously in patients with severe renal impairment and history of liver disease or heavy alcohol use.

Adverse reactions

CNS: headache, fatigue, dizziness, insomnia.
EENT: sinusitis, rhinitis, pharyngitis.
GI: dyspepsia, diarrhea, nausea, vomiting, abdominal pain, constipation, flatulence.
Hematologic: ***thrombocytopenia***, hemolytic anemia, ***leukopenia***.
Musculoskeletal: arthralgia, back pain, myalgia.
Respiratory: *upper respiratory tract infection*, cough, bronchitis.
Other: hypersensitivity reactions.

Interactions

Drug-drug. *Cholestyramine, colestipol:* May bind with fluvastatin in the GI tract and decrease absorption. Separate doses by at least 4 hours.
Cimetidine, omeprazole, ranitidine: May decrease fluvastatin metabolism. Monitor patient for enhanced effects.
Cyclosporine and other immunosuppressants, erythromycin, gemfibrozil, niacin: May increase risk of polymyositis and rhabdomyolysis. Avoid using together.
Digoxin: May alter digoxin pharmacokinetics. Monitor digoxin level carefully.
Fluconazole, itraconazole, ketoconazole: May increase fluvastatin level and adverse effects. Avoid using together, or, if they must be given together, reduce dose of fluvastatin.
Phenytoin: May increase phenytoin levels. Monitor phenytoin levels.
Rifampin: May enhance fluvastatin metabolism and decrease levels. Monitor patient for lack of effect.
Warfarin: May increase anticoagulant effect with bleeding. Monitor patient.
Drug-herb. *Eucalyptus, jin bu huan, kava:* May increase risk of hepatotoxicity. Discourage use together.
Red yeast rice: May increase risk of adverse reactions because herb contains compounds similar to those of statin drugs. Discourage use together.
Drug-lifestyle. *Alcohol use:* May increase risk of hepatotoxicity. Discourage use together.

Nursing considerations

- Use only after diet and other nondrug therapies prove ineffective. Patient should

follow a standard low-cholesterol diet during therapy.
• Test liver function at start of therapy, at 12 weeks after start of therapy, 12 weeks after an increase in dose, and then periodically. Stop drug if there is a persistent increase in ALT or AST levels of at least three times the upper limit of normal.
• Watch for signs of myositis.
!!ALERT Don't confuse fluvastatin with fluoxetine.

Patient teaching
• Tell patient that drug may be taken without regard to meals, but it will work better if it's taken in the evening.
• Advise the patient who is also taking a bile-acid resin such as cholestyramine to take fluvastatin at bedtime, at least 4 hours after taking the resin.
• Teach patient about proper dietary management, weight control, and exercise. Explain their importance in controlling elevated cholesterol and triglyceride levels.
• Warn patient to avoid alcohol.
• Tell patient to notify prescriber of adverse reactions, particularly muscle aches and pains.
• Advise patient that it may take up to 4 weeks for the drug to be completely effective.
!!ALERT Tell woman of childbearing age to stop drug and notify prescriber immediately if she is or may be pregnant or if she's breast-feeding.

fluvoxamine maleate
Luvox

Pregnancy risk category C

Indications & dosages
➲ Obsessive-compulsive disorder (OCD)
Adults: Initially, 50 mg P.O. daily h.s.; increase by 50 mg q 4 to 7 days. Maximum, 300 mg daily. Give total daily amounts above 100 mg in two divided doses.
Children ages 8 to 17: Initially, 25 mg P.O. daily h.s.; increase by 25 mg q 4 to 7 days. Maximum, 200 mg daily for children ages 8 to 11 and 300 mg daily for children ages 11 to 17. Give total daily amounts over 50 mg in two divided doses.

In elderly patients and those with hepatic impairment, give lower first dose and adjust dose more slowly.

Contraindications & cautions
• Contraindicated in patients hypersensitive to drug or to other phenyl piperazine antidepressants, in those receiving pimozide or thioridazine therapy, and within 2 weeks of MAO inhibitor.
• Use cautiously in patients with hepatic dysfunction, other conditions that may affect hemodynamic responses or metabolism, or history of mania or seizures.

Adverse reactions
CNS: *headache, asthenia, somnolence, insomnia, nervousness, dizziness,* tremor, anxiety, hypertonia, *agitation,* depression, CNS stimulation.
CV: palpitations, vasodilation.
EENT: amblyopia.
GI: *nausea, diarrhea, constipation, dyspepsia,* anorexia, *vomiting,* flatulence, dysphagia, *dry mouth,* taste perversion.
GU: abnormal ejaculation, urinary frequency, impotence, anorgasmia, urine retention.
Respiratory: upper respiratory tract infection, dyspnea, yawning.
Skin: sweating.
Other: tooth disorder, flulike syndrome, chills, decreased libido.

Interactions
Drug-drug. *Benzodiazepines, theophylline, warfarin:* May reduce clearance of these drugs. Use together cautiously (except for diazepam, which shouldn't be used with fluvoxamine). Adjust dosage as needed.
Carbamazepine, clozapine, methadone, metoprolol, propranolol, theophylline, tricyclic antidepressants: May increase levels of these drugs. Use together cautiously, and monitor patient closely for adverse reactions. Dosage adjustments may be needed.
Diltiazem: May cause bradycardia. Monitor heart rate.
Lithium, tryptophan: May enhance effects of fluvoxamine. Use together cautiously.
Pimozide, thioridazine: May increase risk of prolonged QTc interval. Avoid using together.
Sumatriptan: May cause weakness, hyperreflexia, and incoordination. Monitor pa-

tient closely. May cause serotonin syndrome (CNS irritability, shivering, and altered consciousness). Avoid using within 2 weeks of MAO inhibitor.
MAO inhibitors (phenelzine, selegiline, tranylcypromine): May cause serotonin syndrome (CNS irritability, shivering, and altered consciousness). Avoid using within 2 weeks of MAO inhibitor.
Drug-lifestyle. *Alcohol use:* May increase CNS effects. Discourage use together.
Smoking: May decrease drug's effectiveness. Urge patient to stop smoking.

Nursing considerations

- Record mood changes. Monitor patient for suicidal tendencies.
- Drug isn't approved for depression in the U.S. Don't use for the treatment of major depressive disorders in children younger than age 18. Increased risk of suicidal behavior has been reported, but the relationship to the drug hasn't been established.

!!ALERT Don't confuse Luvox with Lasix or fluvoxamine with fluoxetine.

- Patients shouldn't stop drug without first consulting prescriber; abruptly stopping drug may cause withdrawal syndrome, including headache, muscle ache, and flulike symptoms.

Patient teaching

- Warn patient to avoid hazardous activities until CNS effects of drug are known.
- Tell woman to notify prescriber about planned, suspected, or known pregnancy.
- Tell patient who develops a rash, hives, or a related allergic reaction to notify prescriber.
- Inform patient that several weeks of therapy may be needed to obtain full therapeutic effect. Once improvement occurs, advise patient not to stop drug until directed by prescriber.
- Advise patient to check with prescriber before taking OTC drugs; drug interactions can occur.
- Tell patient drug can be taken with or without food.

folic acid (vitamin B_9)
Folvite, Novo-Folacid†

Pregnancy risk category A

Indications & dosages

➲ RDA
Adults and children age 14 and older: 400 mcg.
Children ages 9 to 13: 300 mcg.
Children ages 4 to 8: 200 mcg.
Children ages 1 to 3: 150 mcg.
Infants ages 6 months to 1 year: 80 mcg.
Neonates and infants younger than age 6 months: 65 mcg.
Pregnant women: 600 mcg.
Breast-feeding women: 500 mcg.

➲ Megaloblastic or macrocytic anemia from folic acid or other nutritional deficiency, hepatic disease, alcoholism, intestinal obstruction, or excessive hemolysis
Adults and children age 4 and older: 0.4 to 1 mg P.O., I.M., or S.C. daily. After anemia caused by folic acid deficiency is corrected, proper diet and RDA supplements are needed to prevent recurrence.
Children younger than age 4: Up to 0.3 mg P.O., I.M., or S.C. daily.
Pregnant and breast-feeding women: 0.8 mg P.O., I.M., or S.C. daily.

➲ To prevent fetal neural tube defects during pregnancy
Adults: 0.4 mg P.O. daily.

➲ To prevent megaloblastic anemia during pregnancy to prevent fetal damage
Adults: Up to 1 mg P.O., I.M., or S.C. daily throughout pregnancy.

➲ Test for folic acid deficiency in patients with megaloblastic anemia without masking pernicious anemia
Adults and children: 0.1 to 0.2 mg P.O. or I.M. for 10 days while maintaining a diet low in folate and vitamin B_{12}.

➲ Tropical sprue
Adults: 3 to 15 mg P.O. daily.

Contraindications & cautions

- Contraindicated in patients with undiagnosed anemia (it may mask pernicious anemia) and in those with vitamin B_{12} deficiency.

Adverse reactions

CNS: altered sleep pattern, general malaise, difficulty concentrating, confusion, impaired judgment, irritability, hyperactivity.
GI: anorexia, nausea, flatulence, bitter taste.
Respiratory: ***bronchospasm***.
Skin: allergic reactions including rash, pruritus, and erythema.

Interactions

Drug-drug. *Aminosalicylic acid, chloramphenicol, hormonal contraceptives, methotrexate, sulfasalazine, trimethoprim:* May antagonize folic acid. Watch for decreased folic acid effect. Use together cautiously.
Phenytoin: May increase anticonvulsant metabolism, which decreases anticonvulsant level. Monitor phenytoin level closely.

Nursing considerations

- The U.S. Public Health Service recommends use of folic acid during pregnancy to decrease fetal neural tube defects. Patients with history of fetal neural tube defects in pregnancy should increase folic acid intake for 1 month before and 3 months after conception.
- Patients with small-bowel resections and intestinal malabsorption may need parenteral administration.
- Most CNS and GI adverse reactions occur at higher doses, such as 15 mg daily for 1 month.
- Don't mix with other drugs in same syringe for I.M. injections.
- Protect drug from light and heat; store at room temperature.

!!ALERT Don't confuse folic acid with folinic acid.

Patient teaching

- Teach patient about proper nutrition to prevent recurrence of anemia.
- Stress importance of follow-up visits and laboratory studies.
- Teach patient about foods that contain folic acid: liver, oranges, whole wheat, broccoli, Brussels sprouts.

fomivirsen sodium

Vitravene

Pregnancy risk category C

Indications & dosages

➲ **Local treatment of cytomegalovirus (CMV) retinitis in patients with AIDS who have intolerance or a contraindication to other treatments or who didn't respond to previous treatment**
Adults: Induction dose is 330 mcg (0.05 ml) by intravitreal injection every other week for two doses. Subsequent maintenance dose is 330 mcg (0.05 ml) by intravitreal injection once q 4 weeks after induction.

Contraindications & cautions

- Contraindicated in patients hypersensitive to drug or its components and in those who have recently (within 2 to 4 weeks) been treated with either I.V. or intravitreal cidofovir because of an increased risk of exaggerated ocular inflammation.

Adverse reactions

CNS: asthenia, headache, fever, abnormal thinking, depression, dizziness, neuropathy, pain.
CV: chest pain.
EENT: abnormal or blurred vision, anterior chamber inflammation, cataract, conjunctival hemorrhage, decreased visual acuity, desaturation of color vision, eye pain, floaters, increased intraocular pressure, photophobia, retinal detachment, retinal edema, retinal hemorrhage, retinal pigment changes, *uveitis*, *vitritis*, application site reaction, conjunctival hyperemia, conjunctivitis, corneal edema, decreased peripheral vision, eye irritation, hypotony, keratic precipitates, optic neuritis, photopsia, retinal vascular disease, visual field defect, vitreous hemorrhage, vitreous opacity, sinusitis.
GI: abdominal pain, anorexia, diarrhea, nausea, vomiting, oral candidiasis, ***pancreatitis***.
GU: catheter infection, ***renal failure***.
Hematologic: anemia, lymphoma-like reaction, ***neutropenia***, ***thrombocytopenia***.
Metabolic: dehydration, weight loss.
Musculoskeletal: back pain.

Respiratory: bronchitis, dyspnea, increased cough, pneumonia.
Skin: rash, sweating.
Other: allergic reactions, cachexia, flu syndrome, infection, ***sepsis***, systemic CMV.

Interactions

None significant.

Nursing considerations

!! ALERT Drug is for ophthalmic use by intravitreal injection only.

- Drug provides localized therapy limited to the treated eye and doesn't provide treatment for systemic CMV disease. Monitor patient for extraocular CMV disease or disease in the other eye.
- Ocular inflammation (uveitis) is more common during induction dosing.
- Monitor light perception and optic nerve head perfusion postinjection.
- Watch for intraocular pressure. This is usually transient and returns to normal without treatment or with temporary use of topical drugs.

Patient teaching

- Inform patient that drug doesn't cure CMV retinitis, and that some patients experience worsening of retinal inflammation during and after treatment.
- Tell patient that drug treats only the eye in which it has been injected and that CMV may also exist in the body. Stress importance of follow-up visits to monitor progress and to check for additional infections.
- Instruct patient to also have regular eye care follow-up examinations.
- Advise HIV-infected patient to continue taking antiretroviral therapy, as indicated.

fondaparinux sodium
Arixtra

Pregnancy risk category B

Indications & dosages

➲ To prevent DVT, which may lead to pulmonary embolism, in patients undergoing surgery for hip fracture, hip replacement, knee replacement, or abdominal surgery
Adults: 2.5 mg S.C. once daily for 5 to 9 days. Give first dose after hemostasis is established, 6 to 8 hours after surgery. Giving the dose earlier than 6 hours after surgery increases the risk of major bleeding. Patients undergoing hip fracture surgery should receive an extended prophylaxis course of up to 24 additional days; a total of 32 days (perioperative and extended prophylaxis) has been tolerated.

➲ Acute DVT (with warfarin); acute pulmonary embolism (with warfarin) when treatment is started in the hospital
Adults weighing more than 100 kg (220 lb): 10 mg S.C. daily for 5 to 9 days, and until INR level is 2 to 3. Begin warfarin therapy as soon as possible, usually within 72 hours.
Adults weighing 50 to 100 kg (110 to 220 lb): 7.5 mg S.C. daily for 5 to 9 days, and until INR level is 2 to 3. Begin warfarin therapy as soon as possible, usually within 72 hours.
Adults weighing less than 50 kg: 5 mg S.C. daily for 5 to 9 days, and until INR level is 2 to 3. Begin warfarin therapy as soon as possible, usually within 72 hours.

Contraindications & cautions

- Contraindicated in patients with creatinine clearance less than 30 ml/minute and in those who are hypersensitive to the drug or weigh less than 50 kg (110 lb).
- Contraindicated in patients with active major bleeding, bacterial endocarditis, or thrombocytopenia with a positive test result for antiplatelet antibody after taking fondaparinux.
- Use cautiously in patients being treated with platelet inhibitors; in those at increased risk for bleeding, such as congenital or acquired bleeding disorders; in those with active ulcerative and angiodysplastic GI disease; in those with hemorrhagic stroke; and in patients shortly after brain, spinal, or ophthalmologic surgery.
- Use cautiously in patients who have had epidural or spinal anesthesia or spinal puncture; they are at increased risk for developing an epidural or spinal hematoma (which may cause paralysis).
- Use cautiously in elderly patients, in patients with creatinine clearance of 30 to 50 ml/minute, and in those with a history of heparin-induced thrombocytopenia, a bleeding diathesis, uncontrolled arterial hypertension, or a history of recent GI ulceration, diabetic retinopathy, or hemorrhage.

Adverse reactions

CNS: *fever*, insomnia, dizziness, confusion, headache, pain.
CV: hypotension, edema.
GI: *nausea*, constipation, vomiting, diarrhea, dyspepsia.
GU: UTI, urine retention.
Hematologic: ***hemorrhage***, *anemia*, hematoma, ***postoperative hemorrhage, thrombocytopenia***.
Metabolic: hypokalemia.
Skin: mild local irritation (injection site bleeding, rash, pruritus); bullous eruption; purpura; rash; increased wound drainage.

Interactions

Drug-drug. *Drugs that increase risk of bleeding (NSAIDs, platelet inhibitors, anticoagulants):* May increase risk of hemorrhage. Stop these drugs before starting fondaparinux. If use together is unavoidable, monitor patient closely.

Nursing considerations

- Give by S.C. injection only, never I.M. Inspect the single-dose, prefilled syringe for particulate matter and discoloration before administration.
- Don't mix with other injections or infusions.
- Don't use interchangeably with heparin, low-molecular-weight heparins, or heparinoids.

!!ALERT To avoid loss of drug, don't expel air bubble from the syringe.

- Give the drug S.C. in fatty tissue, rotating injection sites. If the drug has been properly injected, the needle will pull back into the syringe security sleeve and the white safety indicator will appear above the blue upper body. A soft click may be heard or felt when the syringe plunger is fully released. After injection of the syringe contents, the plunger automatically rises while the needle withdraws from the skin and retracts into the security sleeve. Don't recap the needle.

!!ALERT Patients who have received epidural or spinal anesthesia are at increased risk for developing an epidural or spinal hematoma, which may result in long-term or permanent paralysis. Monitor these patients closely for neurologic impairment.

- Monitor renal function periodically and stop drug in patients who develop unstable renal function or severe renal impairment while receiving therapy.
- Routinely assess patient for signs and symptoms of bleeding, and regularly monitor CBC, platelet count, creatinine level, and stool occult blood test results. Stop use if platelet count is less than 100,000/mm^3.
- Anticoagulant effects may last for 2 to 4 days after stopping drug in patients with normal renal function.
- PT and activated PTT aren't suitable monitoring tests to measure fondaparinux activity. If coagulation parameters change unexpectedly or patient develops major bleeding, stop drug.

Patient teaching

- Tell patient to report signs and symptoms of bleeding.
- Instruct patient to avoid OTC products that contain aspirin or other salicylates.
- Teach patient the correct technique of S.C. drug administration if patient is to self-administer.

formoterol fumarate inhalation powder

Foradil Aerolizer

Pregnancy risk category C

Indications & dosages

➲ Maintenance treatment and prevention of bronchospasm in patients with reversible obstructive airway disease or nocturnal asthma, who usually require treatment with short-acting inhaled beta$_2$ agonists
Adults and children age 5 and older: One 12-mcg capsule by inhalation via Aerolizer inhaler q 12 hours. Total daily dosage shouldn't exceed 1 capsule b.i.d. (24 mcg/day). If symptoms occur between doses, use a short-acting beta$_2$ agonist for immediate relief.

➲ To prevent exercise-induced bronchospasm
Adults and children age 5 and older: One 12-mcg capsule by inhalation via Aerolizer inhaler at least 15 minutes before exercise, p.r.n. Don't give additional doses within 12 hours of first dose.

Contraindications & cautions

- Contraindicated in patients hypersensitive to drug or its components.
- Use cautiously in patients with CV disease, particularly coronary insufficiency, cardiac arrhythmias, and hypertension, and in those who are unusually responsive to sympathomimetic amines.
- Use cautiously in patients with diabetes mellitus because hyperglycemia and ketoacidosis have occurred rarely with the use of beta agonists.
- Use cautiously in patients with seizure disorders or thyrotoxicosis.

Adverse reactions

CNS: tremor, dizziness, insomnia, nervousness, headache, fatigue, malaise.
CV: chest pain, angina, hypertension, hypotension, tachycardia, ***arrhythmias***, palpitations.
EENT: dry mouth, tonsillitis, dysphonia.
GI: nausea.
Metabolic: hypokalemia, hyperglycemia, ***metabolic acidosis***.
Musculoskeletal: muscle cramps.
Respiratory: bronchitis, chest infection, dyspnea.
Skin: rash.
Other: viral infection.

Interactions

Drug-drug. *Adrenergics:* May potentiate sympathetic effects of formoterol. Use together cautiously.
Beta blockers: May antagonize effects of beta agonists, causing bronchospasm in asthmatic patients. Avoid use except when benefit outweighs risks. Use cardioselective beta blockers with caution to minimize risk of bronchospasm.
Diuretics, steroids, xanthine derivatives: May increase hypokalemic effect of formoterol. Use together cautiously.
MAO inhibitors, tricyclic antidepressants, other drugs that prolong QT interval: May increase risk of ventricular arrhythmias. Use together cautiously.
Non–potassium-sparing diuretics (such as loop or thiazide diuretics): May worsen ECG changes or hypokalemia. Use together cautiously, and monitor patient for toxicity.

Nursing considerations

- Drug isn't indicated for patients who can control asthma symptoms with just occasional use of inhaled, short-acting $beta_2$ agonists or for treatment of acute bronchospasm requiring immediate reversal with short-acting $beta_2$ agonists.
- Drug may be used along with short-acting beta agonists, inhaled corticosteroids, and theophylline therapy for asthma management.
- Patients using drug twice daily shouldn't take additional doses to prevent exercise-induced bronchospasm.
- Don't use as a substitute for short-acting $beta_2$ agonists for immediate relief of bronchospasm or as substitute for inhaled or oral corticosteroids.
- Don't begin use in patients with rapidly deteriorating or significantly worsening asthma.
- If usual dose doesn't control symptoms of bronchoconstriction, and patient's short-acting beta agonist becomes less effective, reevaluate patient and treatment regimen.
- For patients formerly using regularly scheduled short-acting $beta_2$ agonists, decrease use of the short-acting drug to an as-needed basis when starting long-acting formoterol.

!!ALERT As with all $beta_2$ agonists, formoterol may produce life-threatening paradoxical bronchospasm. If bronchospasm occurs, stop formoterol immediately and use an alternative drug.

•

!!ALERT If patient develops tachycardia, hypertension, or other CV adverse effects occur, drug may need to be stopped.

- Watch for immediate hypersensitivity reactions, such as anaphylaxis, urticaria, angioedema, rash, and bronchospasm.
- Give Foradil capsules only by oral inhalation and only with the Aerolizer inhaler. They aren't for oral ingestion. Patient shouldn't exhale into the device. Capsules should remain in the unopened blister until administration time and only be removed immediately before use.
- Don't use Foradil Aerolizer with a spacer device.
- Pierce capsules only once. In rare instances, the gelatin capsule may break into small pieces and get delivered to the mouth or throat upon inhalation. The Aerolizer

contains a screen that should catch any broken pieces before they leave the device. To minimize the possibility of shattering the capsule, strictly follow storage and use instructions.

- No overall differences in safety or efficacy have been observed in elderly patients, but increased sensitivity is possible.
- It's unknown if drug appears in breast milk. Use cautiously in breast-feeding women.

!!ALERT Don't confuse Foradil (formoterol fumarate) with Toradol (ketorolac).

Patient teaching

- Tell patient not to increase the dosage or frequency of use without medical advice.
- Warn patient not to stop or reduce other medication taken for asthma.
- Advise patient that drug isn't to be used for acute asthmatic episodes. Prescriber should give a short-acting $beta_2$ agonist for this use.
- Advise patient to report worsening symptoms, treatment that becomes less effective, or increased use of short-acting beta agonists.
- Tell patient to report nausea, vomiting, shakiness, headache, fast or irregular heartbeat, or sleeplessness.
- Warn patient not to exceed the recommended daily dosage.
- Tell patient being treated for exercise-induced bronchospasm to take drug at least 15 minutes before exercise and to wait 12 hours before taking additional doses.
- Warn patient of possible side effects, which may include palpitations, chest pain, rapid heart rate, tremor, and nervousness.
- Tell patient not to use the Foradil Aerolizer with a spacer device or to exhale or blow into the Aerolizer inhaler.
- Advise patient to avoid washing the Aerolizer and to always keep it dry. Each refill contains a new device to replace the old one.
- Tell patient to avoid exposing capsules to moisture and to handle them only with dry hands.
- Advise patient to notify prescriber if she becomes pregnant or is breast-feeding.

fosamprenavir calcium
Lexiva

Pregnancy risk category C

Indications & dosages

➲ HIV infection, with other antiretrovirals

Adults: In patients not previously treated, 1,400 mg P.O. b.i.d. (without ritonavir). Or, 1,400 mg P.O. once daily and ritonavir 200 mg P.O. once daily. Or, 700 mg P.O. b.i.d. and ritonavir 100 mg P.O. b.i.d. In patients previously treated with a protease inhibitor, 700 mg P.O. b.i.d. plus ritonavir 100 mg P.O. b.i.d.

If the patient receives efavirenz, fosamprenavir, and ritonavir once daily, give an additional 100 mg/day of ritonavir (300 mg total). If the patient has mild or moderate hepatic impairment and takes fosamprenavir without ritonavir, reduce the dosage to 700 mg P.O. b.i.d.

Contraindications & cautions

- Contraindicated in patients hypersensitive to amprenavir or its components.
- Contraindicated with dihydroergotamine, ergonovine, ergotamine, flecainide, methylergonovine, midazolam, pimozide, propafenone, and triazolam.
- Avoid use in patients with severe hepatic impairment.
- Use cautiously in patients allergic to sulfonamides and those with mild to moderate hepatic impairment.
- Use in pregnant patient only when benefit to mother justifies risk to fetus.
- Tell patient not to breast-feed during fosamprenavir therapy.

Adverse reactions

CNS: *depression, fatigue, headache, oral paresthesia.*
GI: *abdominal pain, diarrhea, nausea, vomiting.*
Metabolic: hyperglycemia.
Skin: pruritus, *rash.*

Interactions

Drug-drug. *Amitriptyline, cyclosporine, imipramine, rapamycin, tacrolimus:* May increase levels of these drugs. Monitor drug levels.

Antiarrhythmics (amiodarone, systemic lidocaine, quinidine): May increase antiarrhythmic level. Use together cautiously, and monitor antiarrhythmic levels.
Atorvastatin: May increase atorvastatin level. Give 20 mg/day or less of atorvastatin, and monitor patient carefully. Or, consider other HMG-CoA reductase inhibitors, such as fluvastatin, pravastatin, or rosuvastatin.
Benzodiazepines (alprazolam, clorazepate, diazepam, flurazepam): May increase benzodiazepine level. Decrease benzodiazepine dosage as needed.
Bepridil: May increase bepridil level, possibly leading to arrhythmias. Use together cautiously.
Calcium channel blockers (amlodipine, diltiazem, felodipine, isradipine, nifedipine, nicardipine, nimodipine, nisoldipine, verapamil): May increase calcium channel blocker level. Use together cautiously.
Carbamazepine, dexamethasone, H_2-receptor antagonists, phenobarbital, phenytoin, proton-pump inhibitors: May decrease amprenavir level. Use together cautiously.
Delavirdine: May cause loss of virologic response and resistance to delavirdine. Avoid using together.
Dihydroergotamine, ergonovine, ergotamine, flecainide, methylergonovine, midazolam, pimozide, propafenone, triazolam: May cause serious adverse reactions. Avoid using together.
Efavirenz, nevirapine, saquinavir: May decrease amprenavir level. Appropriate combination doses haven't been established.
Efavirenz with ritonavir: May decrease amprenavir level. Increase ritonavir by 100 mg/day (300 mg total) when giving efavirenz, fosamprenavir, and ritonavir once daily. No change needed in ritonavir when giving efavirenz, fosamprenavir, and ritonavir twice daily.
Ethinyl estradiol and norethindrone: May increase ethinyl estradiol and norethinrone levels. Recommend nonhormonal contraception.
Indinavir, nelfinavir: May increase amprenavir level. Appropriate combination doses haven't been established.
Ketoconazole, itraconazole: May increase ketoconazole and itraconazole levels. Reduce ketoconazole or itraconazole dosage as needed if patient receives more than 400 mg/day. (More than 200 mg/day isn't recommended).
Lopinavir with ritonavir: May decrease amprenavir and lopinavir levels. Appropriate combination doses haven't been established.
Lovastatin, simvastatin: May increase risk of myopathy, including rhabdomyolysis. Avoid using together.
Methadone: May decrease methadone level. Increase methadone dosage as needed.
Rifabutin: May increase rifabutin level. Obtain CBC weekly to watch for neutropenia, and decrease rifabutin dosage by at least half. If patient receives ritonavir, decrease dosage by at least 75% from the usual 300 mg/day. (Maximum, 150 mg every other day or three times weekly.).
Rifampin: May decrease amprenavir level and drug effect. Avoid using together.
Sildenafil, vardenafil: May increase sildenafil and vardenafil levels. Recommend cautious use of sildenafil at 25 mg every 48 hours or vardenafil at no more than 2.5 mg every 24 hours. If patient receives ritonavir, advise no more than 2.5 mg vardenafil every 72 hours, and tell patient to report adverse events.
Warfarin: May alter warfarin level. Monitor INR.
Drug-herb. *St. John's wort:* May cause loss of virologic response and resistance to fosamprenavir or its class of protease inhibitors. Discourage use together.

Nursing considerations

- Patients with hepatitis B or C or marked increase in transaminases before treatment may have increased risk of transaminase elevation. Monitor patient closely during treatment.
- Monitor triglyceride, lipase, ALT, AST, and glucose levels before starting therapy and periodically throughout treatment.
- Ask patient if he's allergic to sulfa drugs.
- Monitor patient with hemophilia for spontaneous bleeding.
- During first treatment, monitor patient for such opportunistic infections as mycobacterium avium complex, cytomegalovirus, *Pneumocystis carinii* pneumonia, and tuberculosis.
- Assess patient for redistribution or accumulation of body fat, as in central obesity, dorsocervical fat enlargement (buffalo

hump), peripheral wasting, facial wasting, breast enlargement, and a cushingoid appearance.

Patient teaching

- Tell patient that fosamprenavir doesn't reduce the risk of transmitting HIV to others.
- Inform patient that the drug may reduce the risk of progression to AIDS.
- Explain that fosamprenavir must be used with other antiretrovirals.
- Tell patient not to alter the dose or stop taking fosamprenavir without consulting prescriber.
- Because fosamprenavir interacts with many drugs, urge patient to tell prescriber about any prescription drugs, OTC drugs, or herbs he's taking (especially St. John's wort).
- Explain that body fat may redistribute or accumulate.

foscarnet sodium (phosphonoformic acid)

Foscavir

Pregnancy risk category C

Indications & dosages

➲ **CMV retinitis in patients with AIDS**

Adults: Initially, for induction, 60 mg/kg I.V. q 8 hours or 90 mg/kg I.V. q 12 hours for 2 to 3 weeks, depending on patient response. Follow with a maintenance infusion of 90 to 120 mg/kg daily.

➲ **Acyclovir-resistant herpes simplex virus infections**

Adults: 40 mg/kg I.V. over 1 hour q 8 to 12 hours for 2 to 3 weeks or until healed.

Adjust dosage when creatinine clearance is less than 1.4 ml/minute/kg. If clearance falls below 0.4 ml/minute/kg, stop drug. Consult manufacturer's package insert for specific dosage adjustments.

Contraindications & cautions

- Contraindicated in patients hypersensitive to drug.
- Use cautiously and at reduced dosage in patients with abnormal renal function. Because drug is nephrotoxic, it can worsen renal impairment. Some degree of nephrotoxicity occurs in most patients treated with drug.

Adverse reactions

CNS: cerebrovascular disorder, *headache,* ***seizures****, fatigue, malaise, asthenia, paresthesia, dizziness, hypoesthesia, neuropathy,* pain, tremor, ataxia, generalized spasms, dementia, stupor, sensory disturbances, meningitis, *fever,* aphasia, abnormal coordination, EEG abnormalities, depression, confusion, aggression, anxiety, insomnia, somnolence, nervousness, amnesia, agitation, hallucinations.
CV: *hypertension, palpitations, ECG abnormalities, sinus tachycardia, first-degree AV block, hypotension, flushing,* edema, chest pain.
EENT: visual disturbances, eye pain, conjunctivitis, sinusitis, pharyngitis, rhinitis.
GI: taste perversion, *nausea, diarrhea, vomiting, abdominal pain, anorexia,* constipation, dysphagia, rectal hemorrhage, dry mouth, dyspepsia, melena, flatulence, ulcerative stomatitis, ***pancreatitis***.
GU: *abnormal renal function,* albuminuria, dysuria, polyuria, urethral disorder, urine retention, UTI, ***acute renal failure***, candidiasis.
Hematologic: *anemia,* ***granulocytopenia, leukopenia, bone marrow suppression, thrombocytopenia***, thrombocytosis.
Hepatic: abnormal hepatic function.
Metabolic: *hypokalemia, hypomagnesemia, hypophosphatemia, hyperphosphatemia, hypocalcemia, hyponatremia.*
Musculoskeletal: leg cramps, arthralgia, myalgia, back pain.
Respiratory: *cough, dyspnea,* pneumonitis, respiratory insufficiency, pulmonary infiltration, stridor, pneumothorax, ***bronchospasm***, hemoptysis.
Skin: *rash, diaphoresis,* pruritus, skin ulceration, erythematous rash, seborrhea, skin discoloration, facial edema.
Other: lymphadenopathy, ***sepsis***, rigors, inflammation and pain at infusion site, lymphoma-like disorder, ***sarcoma***, bacterial or fungal infections, abscess, flulike symptoms.

Interactions

Drug-drug. *Nephrotoxic drugs (such as aminoglycosides, amphotericin B):* May increase risk of nephrotoxicity. Avoid using together.
Pentamidine: May increase risk of nephrotoxicity; severe hypocalcemia also has been

reported. Monitor renal function tests and electrolytes.
Zidovudine: May increase risk or severity of anemia. Monitor blood counts.

Nursing considerations

- Because drug is highly toxic and toxicity is probably dose related, always use the lowest effective maintenance dose during therapy.
- Monitor creatinine clearance frequently during therapy because of drug's adverse effects on renal function. A baseline 24-hour creatinine clearance is recommended; then regular determinations two to three times weekly during induction and at least once every 1 to 2 weeks during maintenance.
- Because drug can alter electrolyte levels, monitor levels using a schedule similar to that established for creatinine clearance. Assess patient for tetany and seizures caused by abnormal electrolyte levels.
- Monitor patient's hemoglobin level and hematocrit. Anemia occurs in up to 33% of patients treated with drug. It may be severe enough to require transfusions.
- Drug may cause a dose-related transient decrease in ionized calcium, which may not always be reflected in patient's laboratory values.

Patient teaching

- Explain the importance of adequate hydration throughout therapy.
- Advise patient to report tingling around the mouth, numbness in the arms and legs, and pins-and-needles sensations.
- Tell patient to alert nurse about discomfort at I.V. insertion site.

---

fosinopril sodium
Monopril

Pregnancy risk category C; D in 2nd and 3rd trimesters

Indications & dosages

➲ Hypertension
Adults: Initially, 10 mg P.O. daily; adjust dosage based on blood pressure response at peak and trough levels. Usual dosage is 20 to 40 mg daily; maximum is 80 mg daily. Dosage may be divided.

➲ Heart failure
Adults: Initially, 10 mg P.O. once daily. Increase dosage over several weeks to a maximum of 40 mg P.O. daily, if needed.

For patients with moderate to severe renal failure or vigorous diuresis, start with 5 mg P.O. once daily.

Contraindications & cautions

- Contraindicated in patients hypersensitive to drug or other ACE inhibitors and in breast-feeding women.
- Use cautiously in patients with impaired renal or hepatic function.

Adverse reactions

CNS: ***CVA***, headache, *dizziness*, fatigue, syncope, paresthesia, sleep disturbance.
CV: chest pain, angina pectoris, ***MI***, rhythm disturbances, palpitations, hypotension, orthostatic hypotension.
EENT: tinnitus, sinusitis.
GI: nausea, vomiting, diarrhea, ***pancreatitis***, dry mouth, abdominal distention, abdominal pain, constipation.
GU: sexual dysfunction, renal insufficiency.
Hepatic: ***hepatitis***.
Metabolic: ***hyperkalemia***.
Musculoskeletal: arthralgia, musculoskeletal pain, myalgia.
Respiratory: ***bronchospasm***; *dry, persistent, tickling, nonproductive cough.*
Skin: urticaria, rash, photosensitivity reactions, pruritus.
Other: ***angioedema***, decreased libido, gout.

Interactions

Drug-drug. *Antacids:* May impair absorption. Separate dosage times by at least 2 hours.
Azathioprine: May increase risk of anemia or leukopenia. Monitor hematologic studies if used together.
Diuretics, other antihypertensives: May cause excessive hypotension. Diuretic may need to be stopped or fosinopril dosage lowered.
Lithium: May increase lithium level and lithium toxicity. Monitor lithium level.
Nesiritide: May increase hypotensive effects. Monitor blood pressure.
NSAIDs: May decrease antihypertensive effects. Monitor blood pressure.
Potassium-sparing diuretics, potassium supplements: May cause risk of hyperkalemia. Monitor patient closely.

Drug-herb. *Capsaicin:* May cause cough. Discourage use together.
Ma huang: May decrease antihypertensive effects. Discourage use together.
Drug-food. *Salt substitutes containing potassium:* May cause hyperkalemia. Discourage use together.

Nursing considerations

- Monitor blood pressure for drug effect.
- Although ACE inhibitors reduce blood pressure in all races, they reduce it less in blacks taking the ACE inhibitor alone. Black patients should take drug with a thiazide diuretic for a more favorable response.
- ACE inhibitors appear to cause a higher risk of angioedema in black patients.
- Monitor potassium intake and potassium level. Diabetic patients, those with impaired renal function, and those receiving drugs that can increase potassium level may develop hyperkalemia.
- Other ACE inhibitors may cause agranulocytosis and neutropenia. Monitor CBC with differential counts before therapy and periodically thereafter.
- Assess renal and hepatic function before and periodically throughout therapy.

!!ALERT Don't confuse fosinopril with lisinopril.
!!ALERT Don't confuse Monopril with Monurol.

Patient teaching

- Tell patient to avoid salt substitutes; these products may contain potassium, which can cause high potassium level in patients taking drug.
- Instruct patient to contact prescriber if light-headedness or fainting occurs.
- Advise patient to report evidence of infection, such as fever and sore throat.
- Instruct patient to call prescriber if he develops easy bruising or bleeding; swelling of tongue, lips, face, eyes, mucous membranes, arms, or legs; difficulty swallowing or breathing; and hoarseness.
- Urge patient to use caution in hot weather and during exercise. Inadequate fluid intake, vomiting, diarrhea, and excessive perspiration can lead to light-headedness and fainting.
- Tell woman of childbearing age to notify prescriber if pregnancy occurs. Drug will need to be stopped.

fosphenytoin sodium
Cerebyx

Pregnancy risk category D

Indications & dosages

➲ Status epilepticus
Adults: 15 to 20 mg phenytoin sodium equivalent (PE)/kg I.V. at 100 to 150 mg PE/minute as loading dose; then 4 to 6 mg PE/kg daily I.V. as maintenance dose.
➲ To prevent and treat seizures during neurosurgery (nonemergent loading or maintenance dosing)
Adults: Loading dose of 10 to 20 mg PE/kg I.M. or I.V. at infusion rate not exceeding 150 mg PE/minute. Maintenance dose is 4 to 6 mg PE/kg daily I.V. or I.M.
➲ Short-term substitution for oral phenytoin therapy
Adults: Same total daily dose equivalent as oral phenytoin sodium therapy given as a single daily dose I.M. or I.V. at infusion rate not exceeding 150 mg PE/minute. Some patients may need more frequent dosing.
Elderly patients: Phenytoin clearance is decreased slightly in elderly patients; lower or less-frequent dosing may be required.

Contraindications & cautions

- Contraindicated in patients hypersensitive to drug or its components, phenytoin, or other hydantoins.
- Contraindicated in those with sinus bradycardia, SA block, second- or third-degree AV block, or Adams-Stokes syndrome.
- Use cautiously in patients with porphyria and in those with history of hypersensitivity to similarly structured drugs, such as barbiturates, oxazolidinediones, and succinimide.

Adverse reactions

CNS: increased or decreased reflexes, speech disorders, asthenia, ***intracranial hypertension***, thinking abnormalities, nervousness, hypesthesia, dysarthria, extrapyramidal syndrome, ***brain edema***, headache, *dizziness, somnolence, ataxia*, stupor, incoordination, paresthesia, tremor, agitation, vertigo, fever.
CV: hypertension, vasodilation, tachycardia, hypotension.

EENT: amblyopia, deafness, diplopia, tinnitus, *nystagmus.*
GI: constipation, taste perversion, dry mouth, tongue disorder, vomiting.
Metabolic: hypokalemia.
Musculoskeletal: pelvic pain, back pain, myasthenia.
Respiratory: pneumonia.
Skin: rash, ecchymoses, *pruritus*, injection site reaction and pain.
Other: accidental injury, infection, chills, facial edema.

Interactions

Drug-drug. *Amiodarone, chloramphenicol, chlordiazepoxide, cimetidine, diazepam, dicumarol, disulfiram, estrogens, ethosuximide, fluoxetine, H_2 antagonists, halothane, isoniazid, methylphenidate, phenothiazines, phenylbutazone, salicylates, succinimides, sulfonamides, tolbutamide, trazodone:* May increase phenytoin level and effect. Use together cautiously.
Carbamazepine, reserpine: May decrease phenytoin level. Monitor patient.
Corticosteroids, coumarin, digitoxin, doxycycline, estrogens, furosemide, oral contraceptives, quinidine, rifampin, theophylline, vitamin D: May decrease effects of these drugs because of increased hepatic metabolism. Monitor patient closely.
Lithium: May increase lithium toxicity. Monitor patient's neurologic status closely. Marked neurologic symptoms have been reported despite normal lithium level.
Phenobarbital, valproate sodium, valproic acid: May increase or decrease phenytoin level. May increase or decrease levels of these drugs. Monitor patient.
Tricyclic antidepressants: May lower seizure threshold and require adjustments in phenytoin dosage. Use together cautiously.
Drug-lifestyle. *Alcohol use:* Acute intoxication may increase phenytoin level and effect. Discourage use together.
Long-term alcohol use: May decrease phenytoin level. Monitor patient.

Nursing considerations

- Most significant drug interactions are those commonly seen with phenytoin.

!!ALERT Fosphenytoin should always be prescribed and dispensed in phenytoin sodium equivalent units (PE). Don't make adjustments in the recommended doses when substituting fosphenytoin for phenytoin, and vice versa.

- In status epilepticus, phenytoin may be used instead of fosphenytoin as maintenance, using the appropriate dose.
- Phosphate load provided by fosphenytoin (0.0037 mmol phosphate/mg PE fosphenytoin) must be taken into consideration when treating patients who need phosphate restriction, such as those with severe renal impairment. Monitor laboratory values.
- Stop drug and notify prescriber if patient gets exfoliative, purpuric, or bullous rash or signs and symptoms of lupus erythematosus, Stevens-Johnson syndrome, or toxic epidermal necrolysis. If rash is mild (measles-like or scarlatiniform), therapy may resume after rash disappears. If rash recurs when therapy is resumed, further fosphenytoin or phenytoin administration is contraindicated. Document that patient is allergic to drug.
- Stop drug in patients with acute hepatotoxicity.
- I.M. administration generates systemic phenytoin levels similar enough to oral phenytoin sodium to allow essentially interchangeable use.
- After administration, phenytoin levels shouldn't be monitored until conversion to phenytoin is essentially complete—about 2 hours after the end of an I.V. infusion or 4 hours after I.M. administration.
- Interpret total phenytoin levels cautiously in patients with renal or hepatic disease or hypoalbuminemia caused by an increased fraction in unbound phenytoin. It may be more useful to monitor unbound phenytoin levels in these patients. When giving drug I.V., monitor patients with renal and hepatic disease because they are at increased risk for more frequent and severe adverse reactions.
- Monitor glucose level closely in diabetic patients; drug may cause hyperglycemia.
- Abrupt withdrawal of drug may precipitate status epilepticus.
- Store drug under refrigeration. Don't store at room temperature longer than 48 hours. Discard vials that develop particulate matter.

!!ALERT Don't confuse Cerebyx with Cerezyme, Celexa, or Celebrex.

Patient teaching

- Warn patient that sensory disturbances may occur with I.V. administration.
- Instruct patient to report immediately adverse reactions, especially rash.
- Warn patient not to stop drug abruptly or adjust dosage without discussing with prescriber.
- Advise woman of childbearing age to discuss drug therapy with prescriber if she's considering pregnancy.
- Advise woman of childbearing age that breast-feeding isn't recommended during therapy.

frovatriptan succinate
Frova

Pregnancy risk category C

Indications & dosages

➲ Acute treatment of migraine attacks with or without aura

Adults: 2.5 mg P.O. taken at the first sign of migraine attack. If the headache recurs, a second tablet may be taken at least 2 hours after the first dose. The total daily dose shouldn't exceed 7.5 mg.

Contraindications & cautions

- Contraindicated in patients hypersensitive to drug or any of its components.
- Contraindicated in patients with history or symptoms of ischemic heart disease or coronary artery vasospasm, including Prinzmetal's angina; in those with cerebrovascular or peripheral vascular disease, including ischemic bowel disease; in those with uncontrolled hypertension; and in those with hemiplegic or basilar migraine.
- Contraindicated within 24 hours of another 5-HT_1 agonist, drug containing ergotamine, or ergot-type drug.
- Contraindicated in patients with risk factors for coronary artery disease (CAD) such as hypertension, hypercholesterolemia, smoking, obesity, diabetes, strong family history of CAD, postmenopausal women, or men older than age 40, unless patient is free from cardiac disease. If drug is used in such a patient, monitor patient closely and consider obtaining an ECG after the first dose. Intermittent, long-term users of 5-HT_1 agonists or those with risk factors should undergo periodic cardiac evaluation while using frovatriptan.
- Use cautiously in breast-feeding women. It's unknown if drug appears in breast milk.

Adverse reactions

CNS: dizziness, headache, fatigue, paresthesia, insomnia, anxiety, somnolence, dysesthesia, hypoesthesia, hot or cold sensation, pain.
CV: flushing, palpitations, chest pain, ***coronary artery vasospasm, transient myocardial ischemia, MI, ventricular tachycardia, ventricular fibrillation.***
EENT: abnormal vision, tinnitus, sinusitis, rhinitis.
GI: dry mouth, dyspepsia, vomiting, abdominal pain, diarrhea, nausea.
Musculoskeletal: skeletal pain.
Skin: increased sweating.

Interactions

Drug-drug. *5-HT_1 agonists:* May cause additive effects. Separate doses by 24 hours.
Ergotamine-containing or ergot-type drugs (such as dihydroergotamine or methysergide): May cause prolonged vasospastic reactions. Separate doses by 24 hours.
SSRIs (such as citalopram, fluoxetine, fluvoxamine, paroxetine, sertraline): May cause weakness, hyperreflexia, and incoordination. Monitor patient closely.

Nursing considerations

!!ALERT Serious cardiac events, including acute MI, life-threatening cardiac arrhythmias, and death, have been reported within a few hours of administration of 5-HT agonists.

- Use drug only when patient has a clear diagnosis of migraine. If a patient has no response for the first migraine attack treated with frovatriptan, reconsider the diagnosis of migraine.
- The safety of treating an average of more than four migraine headaches in a 30-day period hasn't been established.

Patient teaching

- Instruct patient to take dose at first sign of migraine headache. If headache comes back after first dose, he may take a second dose after 2 hours. Tell patient not to take more than 3 tablets in 24 hours.

• Caution patient to take extra care or avoid driving and operating machinery if dizziness or fatigue develops after taking drug.
• Stress importance of immediately reporting pain, tightness, heaviness, or pressure in chest, throat, neck, or jaw, or rash or itching after taking drug.
• Instruct the patient not to take drug within 24 hours of taking another serotonin-receptor agonist or ergot-type drug.

fulvestrant
Faslodex

Pregnancy risk category D

Indications & dosages

➲ Hormone receptor–positive metastatic breast cancer in postmenopausal women with disease progression after antiestrogen therapy
Adults: 250 mg (one 5-ml syringe or two 2.5-ml syringes) by slow I.M. injection into buttocks once monthly.

Contraindications & cautions

• Contraindicated in pregnant women and in patients allergic to drug or any of its components.
• Use cautiously in patients with moderate or severe hepatic impairment.

Adverse reactions

CNS: dizziness, *asthenia, headache,* insomnia, fever, paresthesia, depression, anxiety, *pain.*
CV: *hot flashes,* chest pain, peripheral edema.
EENT: *pharyngitis.*
GI: *nausea, vomiting, constipation, abdominal pain, diarrhea,* anorexia.
GU: UTI.
Hematologic: anemia.
Musculoskeletal: *bone pain, back pain, pelvic pain,* arthritis.
Respiratory: *dyspnea, cough.*
Skin: rash, *injection site pain,* sweating.
Other: accidental injury, flulike syndrome.

Interactions

None reported.

Nursing considerations

• Because drug is given I.M., don't use in patients with bleeding diatheses or thrombocytopenia, or in those taking anticoagulants.
• Make sure patient isn't pregnant before starting drug.
• Expel gas bubble from syringe before administration.
!!ALERT When using the 2.5-ml syringes, both must be given to obtain full dose.

Patient teaching

• Caution women of childbearing age to avoid pregnancy and to report suspected pregnancy immediately.
• Inform patient of the most common side effects, including pain at injection site, headache, GI symptoms, back pain, hot flashes, and sore throat.

furosemide (frusemide†)
Apo-Furosemide†, Furoside†, Lasix*, Novosemide†, Uritol†

Pregnancy risk category C

Indications & dosages

➲ Acute pulmonary edema
Adults: 40 mg I.V. injected slowly over 1 to 2 minutes; then 80 mg I.V. in 60 to 90 minutes if needed.
➲ Edema
Adults: 20 to 80 mg P.O. daily in the morning, with second dose in 6 to 8 hours; carefully adjusted up to 600 mg daily if needed. Or, 20 to 40 mg I.V. or I.M., increased by 20 mg q 2 hours until desired effect achieved.
Infants and children: 2 mg/kg P.O. daily, increased by 1 to 2 mg/kg in 6 to 8 hours if needed; carefully adjusted up to 6 mg/kg daily if needed.
➲ Hypertension
Adults: 40 mg P.O. b.i.d. Dosage adjusted based on response. May be used as adjunct to other antihypertensives if needed.

Contraindications & cautions

• Contraindicated in patients hypersensitive to drug and in those with anuria.
• Use cautiously in patients with hepatic cirrhosis and in those allergic to sulfonamides. Use furosemide during pregnancy only if po-

tential benefits to mother clearly outweigh risks to fetus.

Adverse reactions

CNS: vertigo, headache, dizziness, paresthesia, weakness, restlessness, fever.
CV: orthostatic hypotension, thrombophlebitis with I.V. administration.
EENT: transient deafness, blurred or yellowed vision.
GI: abdominal discomfort and pain, diarrhea, anorexia, nausea, vomiting, constipation, ***pancreatitis***.
GU: nocturia, polyuria, frequent urination, oliguria.
Hematologic: ***agranulocytosis***, ***leukopenia***, ***thrombocytopenia***, azotemia, anemia, ***aplastic anemia***.
Hepatic: hepatic dysfunction.
Metabolic: volume depletion and dehydration, asymptomatic hyperuricemia, impaired glucose tolerance, hypokalemia, hypochloremic alkalosis, hyperglycemia, dilutional hyponatremia, hypocalcemia, hypomagnesemia.
Musculoskeletal: muscle spasm.
Skin: dermatitis, purpura, photosensitivity reactions, transient pain at I.M. injection site.
Other: gout.

Interactions

Drug-drug. *Aminoglycoside antibiotics, cisplatin:* May increase ototoxicity. Use together cautiously.
Amphotericin B, corticosteroids, corticotropin, metolazone: May increase risk of hypokalemia. Monitor potassium level closely.
Antidiabetics: May decrease hypoglycemic effects. Monitor glucose level.
Antihypertensives: May increase risk of hypotension. Use together cautiously.
Cardiac glycosides, neuromuscular blockers: May increase toxicity of these drugs from furosemide-induced hypokalemia. Monitor potassium level.
Chlorothiazide, chlorthalidone, hydrochlorothiazide, indapamide, metolazone: May cause excessive diuretic response, causing serious electrolyte abnormalities or dehydration. Adjust doses carefully, and monitor patient closely for signs and symptoms of excessive diuretic response.
Ethacrynic acid: May increase risk of ototoxicity. Avoid using together.
Lithium: May decrease lithium excretion, resulting in lithium toxicity. Monitor lithium level.
NSAIDs: May inhibit diuretic response. Use together cautiously.
Phenytoin: May decrease diuretic effects of furosemide. Use together cautiously.
Propanolol: May increase propranolol level. Monitor patient closely.
Salicylates: May cause salicylate toxicity. Use together cautiously.
Sucralfate: May reduce diuretic and antihypertensive effect. Separate doses by 2 hours.
Drug-herb. *Aloe:* May increase drug effects. Discourage use together.
Dandelion: May interfere with diuretic activity. Discourage use together.
Ginseng: May decrease loop diuretic effect. Discourage use together.
Licorice: May cause unexpected rapid potassium loss. Discourage use together.
Drug-lifestyle. *Sun exposure:* May increase risk for photosensitivity reactions. Advise patient to avoid excessive sunlight exposure.

Nursing considerations

- To prevent nocturia, give P.O. and I.M. preparations in the morning. Give second dose in early afternoon.

!! ALERT Monitor weight, blood pressure, and pulse rate routinely with long-term use and during rapid diuresis. Furosemide can lead to profound water and electrolyte depletion.

- If oliguria or azotemia develops or increases, drug may need to be stopped.
- Monitor fluid intake and output and electrolyte, BUN, and carbon dioxide levels frequently.
- Watch for signs of hypokalemia, such as muscle weakness and cramps.
- Consult prescriber and dietitian about a high-potassium diet. Foods rich in potassium include citrus fruits, tomatoes, bananas, dates, and apricots.
- Monitor glucose level in diabetic patients.
- Furosemide may not be well absorbed orally in patient with severe heart failure. Drug may need to be given I.V. even if patient is taking other oral drugs.
- Monitor uric acid level, especially in patients with a history of gout.
- Monitor elderly patients, who are especially susceptible to excessive diuresis, because circulatory collapse and thromboembolic complications are possible.

• Store tablets in light-resistant container to prevent discoloration (doesn't affect potency). Refrigerate oral furosemide solution to ensure drug stability.

!!ALERT Don't confuse furosemide with torsemide or Lasix with Lonox.

Patient teaching

• Advise patient to take drug with food to prevent GI upset, and to take drug in morning to prevent need to urinate at night. If patient needs second dose, tell him to take it in early afternoon, 6 to 8 hours after morning dose.
• Inform patient of possible need for potassium or magnesium supplements.
• Instruct patient to stand slowly to prevent dizziness and to limit alcohol intake and strenuous exercise in hot weather to avoid worsening dizziness upon standing quickly.
• Advise patient to immediately report ringing in ears, severe abdominal pain, or sore throat and fever; these symptoms may indicate furosemide toxicity.

!!ALERT Discourage patient taking furosemide at home from storing different types of drugs in the same container, increasing the risk of drug errors. The most popular strengths of furosemide and digoxin are white tablets about equal in size.

• Tell patient to check with prescriber or pharmacist before taking OTC drugs.
• Teach patient to avoid direct sunlight and to use protective clothing and a sunblock because of risk of photosensitivity reactions.

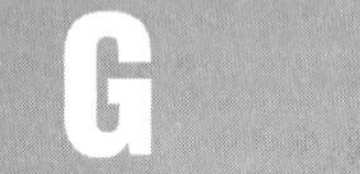

gabapentin
Neurontin

Pregnancy risk category C

Indications & dosages

➲ Adjunctive treatment of partial seizures with or without secondary generalization in adults with epilepsy
Adults: Initially, 300 mg P.O. t.i.d. Increase dosage as needed and tolerated to 1,800 mg daily in divided doses. Dosages up to 3,600 mg daily have been well tolerated.

➲ Adjunctive treatment to control partial seizures in children
Starting dosage, children ages 3 to 12: 10 to 15 mg/kg daily P.O. in three divided doses, adjusting over 3 days to reach effective dosage.
Effective dosage, children ages 5 to 12: 25 to 35 mg/kg daily P.O. in three divided doses.
Effective dosage, children ages 3 to 4: 40 mg/kg daily P.O. in three divided doses.

➲ Postherpetic neuralgia
Adults: 300 mg P.O. once daily on first day, 300 mg b.i.d. on day 2, and 300 mg t.i.d. on day 3. Adjust p.r.n. for pain to a maximum daily dose of 1,800 mg in three divided doses.

In patients age 12 and older with creatinine clearance 30 to 59 ml/minute, give 400 to 1,400 mg daily, divided into two doses. For clearance 15 to 29 ml/minute, give 200 to 700 mg daily in single dose. For clearance less than 15 ml/minute, give 100 to 300 mg daily, in single dose. Reduce daily dose in proportion to creatinine clearance (patients with a clearance of 7.5 ml/minute should receive one-half the daily dose of those with a clearance of 15 ml/minute). For patients receiving hemodialysis, maintenance dose is based on estimates of creatinine clearance. Give supplemental dose of 125 to 350 mg after each 4 hours of hemodialysis.

Contraindications & cautions

• Contraindicated in patients hypersensitive to drug.

Adverse reactions

CNS: *fatigue, somnolence, dizziness, ataxia,* nystagmus, tremor, nervousness, dysarthria, amnesia, depression, abnormal thinking, twitching, incoordination.
CV: peripheral edema, vasodilation.
EENT: diplopia, rhinitis, pharyngitis, dry throat, amblyopia.
GI: nausea, vomiting, dyspepsia, dry mouth, constipation, increased appetite.
GU: impotence.
Hematologic: ***leukopenia.***
Metabolic: weight gain.
Musculoskeletal: back pain, myalgia, fractures.
Respiratory: coughing.
Skin: pruritus, abrasion.
Other: dental abnormalities.

Interactions

Drug-drug. *Antacids:* May decrease absorption of gabapentin. Separate dosage times by at least 2 hours.
Hydrocodone: May increase gabapentin level and decrease hydrocodone level. Monitor patient for increased adverse effects or loss of clinical effect.

Nursing considerations

- Give first dose at bedtime to minimize drowsiness, dizziness, fatigue, and ataxia.
- If drug is to be stopped or an alternative drug is substituted, do so gradually over at least 1 week, to minimize risk of precipitating seizures.

!!ALERT Don't suddenly withdraw other anticonvulsants in patients starting gabapentin therapy.

- Routine monitoring of drug levels isn't necessary. Drug doesn't appear to alter levels of other anticonvulsants.

!!ALERT Don't confuse Neurontin with Noroxin.

Patient teaching

- Advise patient that drug may be taken without regard to meals.
- Instruct patient to take first dose at bedtime to minimize adverse reactions.
- Warn patient to avoid driving and operating heavy machinery until drug's CNS effects are known.
- Advise patient not to stop drug abruptly.
- Advise woman to discuss drug therapy with prescriber if she's considering pregnancy.
- Tell patient to keep oral solution refrigerated.

galantamine hydrobromide
Razadyne, Razadyne ER

Pregnancy risk category B

Indications & dosages

➲ Mild to moderate Alzheimer's dementia
Adults: Initially, 4 mg b.i.d., preferably with morning and evening meals. If dose is well tolerated after minimum of 4 weeks of therapy, increase dosage to 8 mg b.i.d. A further increase to 12 mg b.i.d. may be attempted, but only after at least 4 weeks of therapy at the previous dosage. Dosage range is 16 to 24 mg daily in two divided doses.

Or, 8 mg extended-release tablets P.O. once daily in the morning with food. Increase to 16 mg P.O. once daily after a minimum of 4 weeks. May further increase to 24 mg once daily after a minimum of 4 weeks, based upon patient response and tolerability.

For patients with Child-Pugh score of 7 to 9, dosage usually shouldn't exceed 16 mg daily. Drug isn't recommended for patients with Child-Pugh score of 10 to 15. For patients with moderate renal impairment, dosage usually shouldn't exceed 16 mg daily. For patients with creatinine clearance less than 9 ml/minute, drug isn't recommended.

Contraindications & cautions

- Contraindicated in patients hypersensitive to drug or its components.
- Use cautiously in patients with supraventricular cardiac conduction disorders and in those taking other drugs that significantly slow heart rate.
- Use cautiously during or before procedures involving anesthesia using succinylcholine-type or similar neuromuscular blockers.
- Use cautiously in patients with history of peptic ulcer disease and in those taking NSAIDs. Because of the potential for cholinomimetic effects, use cautiously in patients with bladder outflow obstruction, seizures, asthma, or COPD.

Adverse reactions

CNS: depression, dizziness, headache, tremor, insomnia, somnolence, fatigue, syncope.
CV: ***bradycardia***.
EENT: rhinitis.
GI: *nausea, vomiting,* anorexia, *diarrhea,* abdominal pain, dyspepsia, anorexia.
GU: UTI, hematuria.
Hematologic: anemia.
Metabolic: weight loss.

Interactions

Drug-drug. *Amitriptyline, fluoxetine, fluvoxamine, quinidine:* May decrease galantamine clearance. Monitor patient closely.
Anticholinergics: May antagonize anticholinergic activity. Monitor patient.

Cholinergics (such as bethanechol, succinylcholine): May have synergistic effect. Monitor patient closely. May need to avoid use before procedures using general anesthesia with succinylcholine-type neuromuscular blockers.
Cimetidine, clarithromycin, erythromycin, ketoconazole, paroxetine: May increase galantamine bioavailability. Monitor patient closely.

Nursing considerations

- Bradycardia and heart block may occur in patients with and without underlying cardiac conduction abnormalities. Consider all patients at risk for adverse effects on cardiac conduction.
- Give drug with food and antiemetics and ensure adequate fluid intake to decrease the risk of nausea and vomiting.

!!ALERT The trade name, "Reminyl," was changed to "Razadyne" because of drug errors with the antidiabetic Amaryl.

- Use proper technique when dispensing the oral solution with the pipette. Dispense measured amount in a nonalcoholic beverage and give right away.
- If drug is stopped for several days or longer, restart at the lowest dose and gradually increase, at 4-week or longer intervals, to the previous dosage level.
- Because of the risk of increased gastric acid secretion, monitor patients closely for symptoms of active or occult GI bleeding, especially those with an increased risk of developing ulcers.

Patient teaching

- Advise caregiver to give drug with morning and evening meals (for the conventional form), or only in the morning (for the extended-release form).
- Inform patient that nausea and vomiting are common adverse effects.
- Teach caregiver the proper technique when measuring the oral solution with the pipette. Place measured amount in a nonalcoholic beverage and have patient drink right away.
- Urge patient or caregiver to report slow heartbeat immediately.
- Advise patient and caregiver that although drug may improve cognitive function, it doesn't alter the underlying disease process.

ganciclovir
Cytovene

Pregnancy risk category C

Indications & dosages

➲ CMV retinitis in immunocompromised patients, including those with AIDS and normal renal function
Adults and children older than age 3 months: Induction treatment is 5 mg/kg I.V. q 12 hours for 14 to 21 days. Maintenance treatment is 5 mg/kg daily or 6 mg/ kg daily five times weekly. Or, for maintenance therapy, give 1,000 mg P.O. t.i.d. with food or 500 mg P.O. q 3 hours while awake (six times daily).
➲ To prevent CMV disease in patients with advanced HIV infection and normal renal function
Adults: 1,000 mg P.O. t.i.d. with food.
➲ To prevent CMV disease in transplant recipients with normal renal function
Adults: 5 mg/kg I.V. (given at a constant rate over 1 hour) q 12 hours for 7 to 14 days; then 5 mg/kg daily or 6 mg/kg daily five times weekly. Duration of therapy depends on degree of immunosuppression.

Adjust dosage in patients with renal impairment according to the table. If patient is receiving hemodialysis, first I.V. dosage is 1.25 mg/kg three times weekly, given shortly after hemodialysis session is complete; maintenance I.V. dosage is 0.625 mg/kg three times weekly; and P.O. dosage is 500 mg three times weekly.

Initial I.V. therapy

Creatinine clearance (ml/min)	Dose (mg/kg)	Interval
50–69	2.5	12 hr
25–49	2.5	24 hr
10–24	1.25	24 hr
< 10	1.25	3 times weekly

Maintenance I.V. therapy

Creatinine clearance (ml/min)	Dose (mg/kg)	Interval
50–69	2.5	24 hr
25–49	1.25	24 hr
10–24	0.625	24 hr
< 10	0.625	3 times weekly

P.O. therapy

Creatinine clearance (ml/min)	Dose (mg/kg)	Interval
50–69	1,500	24 hr
	500	8 hr
25–49	1,000	24 hr
	500	12 hr
10–24	500	24 hr
< 10	500	3 times weekly

Contraindications & cautions

- Contraindicated in patients hypersensitive to drug or acyclovir and in those with an absolute neutrophil count below 500/mm³ or a platelet count below 25,000/mm³.
- Use cautiously and reduce dosage in patients with renal dysfunction. Monitor renal function tests.

Adverse reactions

CNS: altered dreams, *fever*, confusion, ataxia, headache, ***seizures***, ***coma***, dizziness, somnolence, tremor, abnormal thinking, agitation, amnesia, anxiety, neuropathy, paresthesia, asthenia.
EENT: retinal detachment in CMV retinitis patients.
GI: *nausea, vomiting, diarrhea, anorexia, abdominal pain*, flatulence, dyspepsia, dry mouth.
Hematologic: ***agranulocytosis***, ***thrombocytopenia***, ***leukopenia***, *anemia.*
Respiratory: pneumonia.
Skin: *rash, sweating*, pruritus, inflammation, pain, and phlebitis at injection site.
Other: infection, chills, ***sepsis***.

Interactions

Drug-drug. *Amphotericin B, cyclosporine, other nephrotoxic drugs:* May increase risk of nephrotoxicity. Monitor renal function.
Cilastatin, imipenem: May increase seizure activity. Use together only if potential benefits outweigh risks.
Cytotoxic drugs: May increase toxic effects, especially hematologic effects and stomatitis. Monitor patient closely.
Immunosuppressants (such as azathioprine, corticosteroids, cyclosporine): May enhance immune and bone marrow suppression. Use together cautiously.
Probenecid: May increase ganciclovir level. Monitor patient closely.
Zidovudine: May increase risk of agranulocytosis. Use together cautiously; monitor hematologic function closely.

Nursing considerations

- Use caution when preparing ganciclovir solution, which is alkaline.

!!ALERT Don't give S.C. or I.M.

- Because of the frequency of agranulocytosis and thrombocytopenia, obtain neutrophil and platelet counts every 2 days during twice-daily ganciclovir doses and at least weekly thereafter.

Patient teaching

- Explain importance of drinking plenty of fluids during therapy.
- Instruct patient to report adverse reactions promptly.
- Tell patient to report discomfort at I.V. insertion site.
- Advise patient that drug causes birth defects. Instruct women to use effective birth control methods during treatment; men should use barrier contraception during and for at least 90 days after treatment with ganciclovir.

gatifloxacin (ophthalmic)

Zymar

Pregnancy risk category C

Indications & dosages

➲ Bacterial conjunctivitis
Adults and children age 1 and older: Instill 1 drop into affected eye q 2 hours while patient is awake, up to eight times daily for 2 days. Then instill 1 drop up to q.i.d. for 5 more days.

Contraindications & cautions

- Contraindicated in patients hypersensitive to drug, quinolones, or their components.
- Use cautiously in pregnant or breast-feeding women.

Adverse reactions

CNS: headache.
EENT: chemosis, conjunctival hemorrhage, *conjunctival irritation*, discharge, dry eyes, eye irritation, eyelid edema, *increased lacrimation*, *keratitis*, pain, *papillary conjunctivitis*, red eyes, reduced visual acuity.
GI: taste disturbance.

Interactions

None reported.

Nursing considerations

- Don't inject solution subconjunctivally or into the anterior chamber of the eye.
- Systemic gatifloxacin has caused serious hypersensitivity reactions. If allergic reaction occurs, stop drug and treat symptoms.
- Monitor patient for superinfection.

Patient teaching

- Urge patient to immediately stop drug and seek medical treatment if evidence of a serious allergic reaction develops, such as itching, rash, swelling of the face or throat, or difficulty breathing.
- Tell patient not to wear contact lenses during treatment.
- Warn patient to avoid touching the applicator tip to anything, including eyes and fingers.
- Teach patient that prolonged use may encourage infections with nonsusceptible bacteria.

gatifloxacin (systemic)
Tequin

Pregnancy risk category C

Indications & dosages

➲ **Acute bacterial worsening of chronic bronchitis caused by *Streptococcus pneumoniae, Haemophilus influenzae, H. parainfluenzae, Moraxella catarrhalis,* or *Staphylococcus aureus;* complicated UTI caused by *Escherichia coli, Klebsiella pneumoniae,* or *Proteus mirabilis;* acute pyelonephritis caused by *E. coli***
Adults: 400 mg I.V. or P.O. daily for 7 to 10 days for acute pyelonephritis and complicated UTIs and 5 days for chronic bronchitis.
➲ **Uncomplicated skin and skin-structure infections from *S. pyogenes* or methicillin-susceptible *S. aureus***
Adults: 400 mg I.V. or P.O. daily for 7 to 10 days.
➲ **Acute sinusitis caused by *S. pneumoniae* or *H. influenzae***
Adults: 400 mg I.V. or P.O. daily for 10 days.
➲ **Community-acquired pneumonia from *S. pneumoniae, H. influenzae, H. parainfluenzae, M. catarrhalis, S. aureus, Mycoplasma pneumoniae, Chlamydia pneumoniae,* or *Legionella pneumophila***
Adults: 400 mg I.V. or P.O. daily for 7 to 14 days.

For patients with creatinine clearance less than 40 ml/minute, those receiving hemodialysis, and those receiving continuous peritoneal dialysis, first dose is 400 mg I.V. or P.O. daily, and subsequent doses are 200 mg I.V. or P.O. daily. For patients receiving hemodialysis, give dose after hemodialysis session ends.
➲ **Uncomplicated urethral gonorrhea in men and cervical gonorrhea or acute uncomplicated rectal infections in women caused by *Neisseria gonorrhoeae***
Adults: 400 mg P.O. as single dose.
➲ **Uncomplicated UTIs caused by *E. coli, K. pneumoniae,* or *P. mirabilis***
Adults: 400 mg I.V. or P.O. as single dose, or 200 mg I.V. or P.O. daily for 3 days.

Contraindications & cautions

- Contraindicated in patients hypersensitive to fluoroquinolones.
- Don't use in patients with prolonged QTc interval or uncorrected hypokalemia.
- Use cautiously in patients with clinically significant bradycardia, acute myocardial ischemia, known or suspected CNS disorders, or renal insufficiency.

Adverse reactions

CNS: abnormal dreams, dizziness, headache, insomnia, fever, paresthesia, tremor, vertigo.
CV: palpitations, chest pain, peripheral edema.

EENT: tinnitus, abnormal vision, pharyngitis.
GI: nausea, diarrhea, abdominal pain, constipation, dyspepsia, oral candidiasis, glossitis, stomatitis, mouth ulcer, vomiting, taste perversion.
GU: dysuria, hematuria, vaginitis.
Musculoskeletal: arthralgia, myalgia, tendon rupture, back pain.
Respiratory: dyspnea.
Skin: redness at injection site, rash, sweating.
Other: hypersensitivity reaction, ***anaphylaxis***, chills.

Interactions

Drug-drug. *Aluminum hydroxide, didanosine (buffered solution, tablets, or buffered powder), aluminum-magnesium hydroxide, calcium carbonate, magnesium hydroxide, products containing zinc:* May decrease effects of gatifloxacin. Give drug at least 6 hours before or 2 hours after gatifloxacin.
Antidiabetics (glyburide, insulin): May cause symptomatic hypoglycemia or hyperglycemia. Monitor glucose level.
Antipsychotics, erythromycin, tricyclic antidepressants: May prolong QTc interval. Use together cautiously.
Class IA antiarrhythmics (procainamide, quinidine), class III antiarrhythmics (amiodarone, dofetilide, sotalol): May prolong QTc interval. Avoid using together.
Digoxin: May increase digoxin level. Watch for signs of digoxin toxicity.
NSAIDs: May increase risk of CNS stimulation and seizures. Use together cautiously.
Probenecid: May increase gatifloxacin level and prolong its half-life. Monitor patient closely.
Warfarin: May enhance effects of warfarin. Monitor PT and INR.
Drug-herb. *Dong quai, St. John's wort:* May cause photosensitivity. Advise patient to avoid excessive sunlight exposure.
Drug-lifestyle. *Sun exposure:* May cause photosensitivity. Advise patient to avoid excessive sunlight exposure.

Nursing considerations

- Monitor glucose level in patients with diabetes.
- Monitor patients also receiving digoxin for signs and symptoms of digoxin toxicity.
- Monitor kidney function in patients with renal insufficiency.
- Stop drug if patient experiences seizures, increased intracranial pressure, psychosis, or CNS stimulation leading to tremors, restlessness, light-headedness, confusion, hallucinations, paranoia, depression, nightmares, or insomnia.
- Stop drug if rash or other sign of hypersensitivity occurs.
- Stop drug if patient experiences pain, inflammation, or rupture of a tendon.
- In patients being treated for gonorrhea, test for syphilis at time of diagnosis.

Patient teaching

- Tell patient to take drug as prescribed and to finish it, even if symptoms disappear.
- Advise patient to appropriately space products containing aluminum, magnesium, zinc, or iron when taking drug.
- Advise patient to use sunscreen and protective clothing when exposed to excessive sunlight.
- Warn patient to avoid hazardous tasks until adverse effects of drug are known.
- Advise diabetic patient to monitor blood sugar levels and notify prescriber if low blood sugar occurs.
- Advise patient to immediately report palpitations; fainting spells; rash; hives; difficulty swallowing or breathing; tightness in throat; hoarseness; swelling of lips, tongue, or face; or other symptoms of allergic reaction.
- Advise patient to stop drug, refrain from exercise, and notify prescriber if pain, inflammation, or rupture of a tendon occurs.

gefitinib
Iressa

Pregnancy risk category D

Indications & dosages

➲ **Locally advanced or metastatic non-small-cell lung cancer after platinum-based and docetaxel chemotherapies have failed**
Adults: 250 mg P.O. once daily.

If patient takes a CYP3A4 enzyme inducer, gefitinib dosage may be increased to 500 mg daily.

Contraindications & cautions

- Contraindicated in patients hypersensitive to drug or its components.
- Use cautiously in patients with severe renal impairment.
- Drug may harm the fetus. Consider risks and benefits before giving drug to pregnant woman.
- Drug may harm breast-feeding infant; woman should avoid breast-feeding during treatment.
- Safety and effectiveness in children haven't been established.

Adverse reactions

CV: peripheral edema.
EENT: amblyopia, conjunctivitis.
GI: anorexia, *diarrhea*, mouth ulcers, *nausea, vomiting*, weight loss.
Respiratory: ***dyspnea, interstitial lung disease***.
Skin: *acne, dry skin*, pruritus, *rash*.

Interactions

Drug-drug. *Drugs that increase gastric pH, such as antacids, H_2 blockers, sodium bicarbonate, or ranitidine:* May reduce availability and efficacy of gefitinib. Monitor patient closely.
Drugs that induce CYP3A4, such as phenytoin and rifampin: May decrease gefitinib level. If patient has no severe adverse reactions, gefitinib dosage may be increased to 500 mg daily.
Drugs that inhibit CYP3A4, such as itraconazole and ketoconazole: May increase gefitinib level. Monitor patient closely, and adjust dosage as needed.
Warfarin: May increase INR and risk of bleeding. Monitor INR and patient closely.

Nursing considerations

!!ALERT Patients who develop acute dyspnea, cough, and a low-grade fever may have interstitial lung disease—and these effects may worsen quickly. Stop drug immediately. One-third of patients who develop this form of pulmonary toxicity die.

- Monitor liver function tests periodically during treatment.
- If patient takes warfarin, monitor PT and INR closely.
- Patients who have severe adverse GI or skin reactions may need to stop drug for up to 14 days; restart at 250 mg daily.
- Patients who develop eye pain; corneal erosion, sloughing, or ulceration; abnormal eyelash growth; ocular ischemia or hemorrhage may need to stop taking the drug.

Patient teaching

- Teach patient how to avoid dehydration.
- Tell patient to seek medical care immediately for severe or persistent diarrhea, nausea, anorexia, or vomiting; new or worsening pulmonary problems, such as shortness of breath or coughing; eye problems, such as irritation, pain, or altered vision; or a rash.
- Urge women of childbearing age to avoid becoming pregnant.
- Tell pregnant patient that drug may harm fetus.

gemcitabine hydrochloride
Gemzar

Pregnancy risk category D

Indications & dosages

➲ Locally advanced or metastatic adenocarcinoma of pancreas
Adults: 1,000 mg/m^2 I.V. over 30 minutes once weekly for up to 7 weeks, unless toxicity occurs. Monitor CBC with differential and platelet count before giving each dose.

If bone marrow suppression is detected, adjust therapy. If absolute granulocyte count (AGC) is 1,000/mm^3 or more and platelet count is 100,000/mm^3 or more, give full dose. If AGC is 500 to 999/mm^3 or platelet count is 50,000 to 99,999/mm^3, give 75% of dose. If AGC is below 500/mm^3 or platelet count is below 50,000/mm^3, withhold dose. Treatment course of 7 weeks is followed by 1 week of rest. Subsequent dosage cycles consist of one infusion weekly for 3 of 4 consecutive weeks. Dosage adjustments for subsequent cycles are based on AGC and platelet count nadirs and degree of nonhematologic toxicity.

➲ With cisplatin, first-line treatment of inoperable, locally advanced, or metastatic non–small-cell lung cancer
Adults: For 4-week schedule, 1,000 mg/m^2 I.V. over 30 minutes on days 1, 8, and 15 of each 28-day cycle. Cisplatin 100 mg/m^2 on day 1 after gemcitabine infusion.

For 3-week schedule, 1,250 mg/m² I.V. over 30 minutes on days 1 and 8 of each 21-day cycle. Cisplatin 100 mg/m² on day 1 after gemcitabine infusion.

➲ **With paclitaxel, first-line therapy for metastatic breast cancer after failure of other adjuvant chemotherapy with an anthracycline**

Adults: 1,250 mg/m² I.V. over 30 minutes on days 1 and 8 of each 21-day cycle, with 175 mg/m² paclitaxel I.V. as a 3-hour infusion given before gemcitabine dose on day 1 of the cycle. Adjust dosage based on total granulocyte and platelet counts taken on day 8 of the cycle.

If absolute granulocyte count is 1,000 to 1,199/mm³ or platelet count is 50,000 to 75,000/mm³, give 75% of dose. If absolute granulocyte count is 700 to 999/mm³ and platelet count is 50,000/mm³ or above, give 50% of dose. If absolute granulocyte count is below 700/mm³ or platelet count is below 50,000/mm³, withhold dose.

Contraindications & cautions

- Contraindicated in patients hypersensitive to drug and in pregnant or breast-feeding women.
- Use cautiously in patients with renal or hepatic impairment.

Adverse reactions

CNS: *somnolence, paresthesia, pain, fever.*
CV: *edema, peripheral edema.*
GI: *stomatitis, nausea, vomiting, constipation, diarrhea.*
GU: *proteinuria, hematuria.*
Hematologic: *anemia,* ***leukopenia, neutropenia, thrombocytopenia.***
Hepatic: ***hepatotoxicity.***
Respiratory: *dyspnea,* ***bronchospasm.***
Skin: *alopecia, rash,* pain at injection site.
Other: *flulike syndrome, infection.*

Interactions

None significant.

Nursing considerations

- Monitor patient closely. Expect dosage modification according to toxicity and degree of myelosuppression. Age, gender, and presence of renal impairment may predispose patient to toxicity.
- Carefully monitor hematologic values, especially of neutrophil and platelet counts.
- Obtain baseline and periodic renal and hepatic laboratory tests.
- Safety and effectiveness of drug in children haven't been determined.

Patient teaching

- Advise patient to watch for evidence of infection (fever, sore throat, fatigue) and bleeding (easy bruising, nosebleeds, bleeding gums, tarry stools). Tell patient to take temperature daily.
- Advise patient to promptly report flulike symptoms or breathing problems.
- Tell patient that adverse effects may continue after treatment ends.
- Caution woman of childbearing age to avoid pregnancy or breast-feeding during therapy.

gemfibrozil

Apo-Gemfibrozil†, Lopid

Pregnancy risk category C

Indications & dosages

➲ **Types IV and V hyperlipidemia unresponsive to diet and other drugs; to reduce risk of coronary heart disease in patients with type IIb hyperlipidemia who can't tolerate or who are refractory to treatment with bile-acid sequestrants or niacin**

Adults: 1,200 mg P.O. daily in two divided doses, 30 minutes before morning and evening meals.

Contraindications & cautions

- Contraindicated in patients hypersensitive to drug and in those with hepatic or severe renal dysfunction (including primary biliary cirrhosis) or gallbladder disease.

Adverse reactions

CNS: headache, fatigue, vertigo.
CV: atrial fibrillation.
GI: *abdominal and epigastric pain,* diarrhea, nausea, vomiting, *dyspepsia,* constipation, acute appendicitis.
Hematologic: anemia, ***leukopenia,*** eosinophilia, ***thrombocytopenia.***
Hepatic: bile duct obstruction.
Metabolic: hypokalemia.
Skin: rash, dermatitis, pruritus, eczema.

Interactions

Drug-drug. *Glyburide:* May increase hypoglycemic effects. Monitor glucose level, and watch for signs of hypoglycemia.
HMG-CoA reductase inhibitors: May cause myopathy with rhabdomyolysis. Avoid using together.
Oral anticoagulants: May enhance effects of oral anticoagulants. Monitor patient closely.
Repaglinide: May increase repaglinide level. Avoid using together if possible. If already taking both drugs, monitor glucose levels and adjust repaglinide dosage.

Nursing considerations

- Check CBC and test liver function periodically during the first 12 months of therapy.
- If drug has no beneficial effects after 3 months of therapy, expect prescriber to stop drug.
- Patient shouldn't take drug together with repaglinide or itraconazole.

Patient teaching

- Instruct patient to take drug 30 minutes before breakfast and dinner.
- Teach patient about proper dietary management of cholesterol and triglycerides. When appropriate, recommend weight control, exercise, and smoking cessation programs.
- Because of possible dizziness and blurred vision, advise patient to avoid driving or other potentially hazardous activities until effects of drug are known.
- Tell patient to observe bowel movements and to report evidence of excess fat in feces or other signs of bile duct obstruction.

---

gemifloxacin mesylate
Factive

Pregnancy risk category C

Indications & dosages

➲ Acute bacterial worsening of chronic bronchitis caused by *Streptococcus pneumoniae, Haemophilus influenzae, H. parainfluenzae,* or *Moraxella catarrhalis*
Adults: 320 mg P.O. once daily for 5 days.
➲ Mild to moderate community-acquired pneumonia caused by *S. pneumoniae* (including multidrug-resistant strains), *H. influenzae, M. catarrhalis, Mycoplasma pneumoniae, Chlamydia pneumoniae,* or *Klebsiella pneumoniae*
Adults: 320 mg P.O. once daily for 7 days.

If creatinine clearance is 40 ml/minute or less, or if patient receives routine hemodialysis or continuous ambulatory peritoneal dialysis, reduce dosage to 160 mg P.O. once daily.

Contraindications & cautions

- Contraindicated in patients hypersensitive to fluoroquinolones, gemifloxacin, or their components.
- Contraindicated in patients with a history of prolonged QTc interval, those with uncorrected electrolyte disorders (such as hypokalemia or hypomagnesemia), and those taking a drug that could prolong the QTc interval.
- Use cautiously in patients with a proarrhythmic condition (such as bradycardia or acute myocardial ischemia), epilepsy, or a predisposition to seizures.
- Safety and efficacy haven't been established for children younger than age 18. Don't use drug in children.

Adverse reactions

CNS: headache.
GI: diarrhea, nausea.
Musculoskeletal: ruptured tendons.
Skin: rash.
Other: hypersensitivity reactions.

Interactions

Drug-drug. *Antacids (magnesium or aluminum), didanosine (chewable tablets, buffered tablets, or pediatric powder for oral solution), ferrous sulfate, multivitamins containing metal cations (such as zinc):* May decrease gemifloxacin level. Give these drugs at least 3 hours before or 2 hours after gemifloxacin.
Antiarrhythmics of class IA (procainamide, quinidine) or class III (amiodarone, sotalol): May increase risk of prolonged QTc interval. Avoid using together.
Antipsychotics, erythromycin, tricyclic antidepressants: May increase risk of prolonged QTc interval. Use together cautiously.
Probenecid: May increase gemifloxacin level. May use with probenecid for this reason.
Sucralfate: May decrease gemifloxacin level. Use together cautiously.

Warfarin: May increase anticoagulation effect. Monitor PT and INR.

Drug-lifestyle. *Sun exposure:* May increase risk of photosensitivity. Advise patient to avoid excessive sunlight exposure.

Nursing considerations

- Use drug only for infections caused by susceptible bacteria.

!!ALERT Don't exceed recommended dosage because of increased risk of prolonging the QTc interval.

- Mild to moderate maculopapular rash may appear, usually 8 to 10 days after therapy starts. It's more likely in women younger than age 40, especially those taking hormone therapy. Stop drug if rash appears.

!!ALERT Serious, occasionally fatal, hypersensitivity reactions may occur. Stop drug immediately if hypersensitivity reaction occurs.

- Fluoroquinolones may cause tendon rupture, arthropathy, or osteochondrosis; stop drug if patient reports pain or inflammation or ruptures a tendon.
- Stop drug if patient has a photosensitivity reaction.
- Fluoroquinolones may cause CNS effects, such as tremors and anxiety. Monitor patient carefully.
- Serious diarrhea may reflect pseudomembranous colitis; drug may need to be stopped.
- Keep patient adequately hydrated to avoid concentration of urine.

Patient teaching

- Urge patient to finish full course of treatment, even if symptoms improve.
- Tell patient that drug may be taken with or without food but that it shouldn't be taken within 3 hours after or 2 hours before an antacid.
- Tell patient to stop drug and seek medical care if evidence of hypersensitivity reaction develops.
- Instruct patient to drink fluids liberally during treatment.
- Warn patient against taking OTC medications or dietary supplements with this drug without consulting his prescriber.
- Tell patient to avoid excessive exposure to sunlight or ultraviolet light.
- Urge patient to report pain, inflammation, or rupture of tendons.
- Warn patient to avoid driving or other hazardous activities until effects of drug are known.

gemtuzumab ozogamicin
Mylotarg

Pregnancy risk category D

Indications & dosages

➲ **CD33-positive acute myeloid leukemia patients who are in first relapse and aren't candidates for cytotoxic chemotherapy**
Adults age 60 and older: 9 mg/m^2 I.V. over 2 hours q 14 days for a total of two doses. Premedicate with diphenhydramine 50 mg P.O. and acetaminophen 650 to 1,000 mg P.O. 1 hour before infusion.

Contraindications & cautions

- Contraindicated in patients hypersensitive to drug or its components.
- Use cautiously in patients with hepatic impairment.

Adverse reactions

CNS: *asthenia*, depression, *dizziness, headache, insomnia, pain, fever.*
CV: *hypertension, hypotension, tachycardia, peripheral edema.*
EENT: *epistaxis, pharyngitis, rhinitis.*
GI: enlarged abdomen, *abdominal pain, anorexia, constipation, diarrhea, dyspepsia, nausea, stomatitis, vomiting.*
GU: *hematuria,* ***vaginal hemorrhage.***
Hematologic: *anemia,* HEMORRHAGE, LEUKOPENIA, NEUTROPENIA, NEUTROPENIC FEVER, THROMBOCYTOPENIA.
Hepatic: ***hepatotoxicity.***
Metabolic: hyperglycemia, *hypokalemia, hypomagnesemia.*
Musculoskeletal: arthralgia, *back pain.*
Respiratory: *cough, dyspnea,* ***hypoxia,*** *pneumonia.*
Skin: ecchymoses, local reaction, petechiae, rash.
Other: *chills,* herpes simplex, SEPSIS.

Interactions

None known.

Nursing considerations

- Use drug only under the supervision of a clinician experienced in the use of cancer chemotherapeutics.
- Premedicate with diphenhydramine and acetaminophen. Additional doses of acetaminophen 650 to 1,000 mg P.O. can be given every 4 hours, as needed.
- Monitor vital signs during infusion and for 4 hours after infusion.
- Monitor post-infusion symptom complex of chills, fever, hypotension, hypertension, hyperglycemia, hypoxia, and dyspnea that may occur during first 24 hours after administration.

!!ALERT Severe myelosuppression occurs in all patients given recommended dose of drug. Careful hematologic monitoring is required.

- Monitor electrolytes, hepatic function, CBC, and platelet counts during therapy.

!!ALERT Fatal hepatic reno-occlusive disease may occur after treatment with gemtuzumab with subsequent chemotherapy.

- Tumor lysis syndrome may occur. Provide adequate hydration and treat with allopurinol to prevent hyperuricemia.

Patient teaching

- Advise patient about postinfusion symptoms and instruct him to continue to take acetaminophen 650 to 1,000 mg every 4 hours, as needed.
- Urge patient to watch for fever, sore throat, and fatigue and for easy bruising, nosebleeds, bleeding gums, or tarry stools. Tell him to take temperature daily.
- Tell patient to avoid OTC products that contain aspirin.

gentamicin sulfate (ophthalmic)

Garamycin, Genoptic, Gentacidin, Gentak

Pregnancy risk category C

Indications & dosages

➲ **External ocular infections (conjunctivitis, keratoconjunctivitis, corneal ulcers, blepharitis, blepharoconjunctivitis, meibomianitis, and dacryocystitis) caused by susceptible organisms, especially *Pseudomonas aeruginosa, Proteus, Klebsiella pneumoniae, Escherichia coli,* and other gram-negative organisms**

Adults and children: 1 or 2 drops in eye q 4 hours. In severe infections, up to 2 drops q hour. Or, apply ointment to lower conjunctival sac b.i.d. or t.i.d.

Contraindications & cautions

- Contraindicated in patients hypersensitive to drug.
- Use cautiously in patients with history of sensitivity to aminoglycosides because cross-sensitivity may occur.

Adverse reactions

EENT: burning, stinging, or blurred vision with ointment, transient irritation from solution, conjunctival hyperemia.

Other: overgrowth of nonsusceptible organisms with long-term use.

Interactions

None significant.

Nursing considerations

- Obtain culture before giving drug. Therapy may begin before culture results are known.
- If ophthalmic gentamicin is given together with systemic gentamicin, monitor gentamicin level.
- Systemic absorption from excessive use may cause toxicities.
- Solution isn't for injection into conjunctiva or anterior chamber of eye.
- Store drug away from heat.

Patient teaching

- Tell patient to clean eye area of excessive discharge before instilling drug.
- Teach patient how to instill drops or apply ointment. Advise him to wash hands before and after applying ointment or solution and not to touch tip of dropper or tube to eye or surrounding tissue.
- Instruct patient to apply light finger pressure on lacrimal sac for 1 minute after drops are instilled.
- Instruct patient to stop drug and notify prescriber if signs and symptoms of sensitivity (itching lids, swelling, or constant burning) occur.
- Advise patient not to share drug, washcloths, or towels with family members and

to notify prescriber if anyone develops same signs or symptoms.

• Tell patient that vision may be blurred for few minutes after application of ointment.

!!ALERT Stress importance of following recommended therapy. *Pseudomonas* infections can cause complete vision loss within 24 hours if infection isn't controlled.

gentamicin sulfate (systemic)
Cidomycin†, Garamycin

Pregnancy risk category D

Indications & dosages

➲ **Serious infections caused by sensitive strains of *Pseudomonas aeruginosa, Escherichia coli, Proteus, Klebsiella,* or *Staphylococcus***

Adults: 3 mg/kg daily in three divided doses I.M. or I.V. infusion q 8 hours. For life-threatening infections, patient may receive up to 5 mg/kg daily in three to four divided doses; reduce dosage to 3 mg/kg daily as soon as patient improves.

Children: 2 to 2.5 mg/kg q 8 hours I.M. or by I.V. infusion.

Neonates older than 1 week and infants: 2.5 mg/kg q 8 hours I.M. or by I.V. infusion.

Neonates younger than 1 week and preterm infants: 2.5 mg/kg q 12 hours I.M. or by I.V. infusion.

➲ **To prevent endocarditis before GI or GU procedure or surgery**

Adults: 1.5 mg/kg I.M. or I.V. 30 minutes before procedure or surgery. Maximum dose is 80 mg. Give with ampicillin (vancomycin in penicillin-allergic patients).

Children: 2 mg/kg I.M. or I.V. 30 minutes before procedure or surgery. Maximum dose is 80 mg. Give with ampicillin (vancomycin in penicillin-allergic patients).

For adults with impaired renal function, doses and frequency are determined by gentamicin level and renal function. To maintain therapeutic blood levels, adults should receive 1 to 1.7 mg/kg I.M. or by I.V. infusion after each dialysis session, and children should receive 2 to 2.5 mg/kg I.M. or by I.V. infusion after each dialysis session.

Contraindications & cautions

• Contraindicated in patients hypersensitive to drug or other aminoglycosides.

• Use cautiously in neonates, infants, elderly patients, and patients with impaired renal function or neuromuscular disorders.

Adverse reactions

CNS: fever, headache, lethargy, ***encephalopathy***, confusion, dizziness, ***seizures***, numbness, peripheral neuropathy, vertigo, ataxia, tingling.

CV: hypotension.

EENT: *ototoxicity*, blurred vision, tinnitus.

GI: vomiting, nausea.

GU: ***nephrotoxicity***, possible increase in urinary excretion of casts.

Hematologic: anemia, eosinophilia, ***leukopenia, thrombocytopenia, agranulocytosis***.

Musculoskeletal: muscle twitching, myasthenia gravis–like syndrome.

Respiratory: ***apnea***.

Skin: rash, urticaria, pruritus, injection site pain.

Other: ***anaphylaxis***.

Interactions

Drug-drug. *Acyclovir, amphotericin B, cephalosporins, cidofovir, cisplatin, methoxyflurane, vancomycin, other aminoglycosides:* May increase ototoxicity and nephrotoxicity. Monitor hearing and renal function test results.

Atracurium, doxacurium, mivacurium, pancuronium, rocuronium, tubocurarine, vecuronium: May increase effects of nondepolarizing muscle relaxants, including prolonged respiratory depression. Use together only when necessary, and expect to reduce dosage of nondepolarizing muscle relaxant.

Dimenhydrinate: May mask ototoxicity symptoms. Monitor patient's hearing.

General anesthetics: May increase neuromuscular blockade. Monitor patient closely.

Indomethacin: May increase peak and trough levels of gentamicin. Monitor gentamicin level.

I.V. loop diuretics (such as furosemide): May increase risk of ototoxicity. Monitor patient's hearing.

Parenteral penicillins (such as ampicillin and ticarcillin): May inactivate gentamicin in vitro. Don't mix.

Nursing considerations

- Obtain specimen for culture and sensitivity tests before giving first dose. Therapy may begin while awaiting results.
- Evaluate patient's hearing before and during therapy. Notify prescriber if patient complains of tinnitus, vertigo, or hearing loss.
- Weigh patient and review renal function studies before therapy begins.

!! ALERT Use preservative-free formulations of gentamicin when intrathecal route is ordered.

- Obtain blood for peak gentamicin level 1 hour after I.M. injection or 30 minutes after I.V. infusion finishes; for trough levels, draw blood just before next dose. Don't collect blood in a heparinized tube; heparin is incompatible with aminoglycosides.
- Maintain peak levels at 4 to 12 mcg/ml and trough levels at 1 to 2 mcg/ml. The maximum peak level is usually 8 mcg/ml, except in patients with cystic fibrosis, who need increased lung penetration. Prolonged peak levels of 10 to 12 mcg/ml or prolonged trough levels greater than 2 mcg/ml may increase risk of toxicity.
- Monitor renal function: urine output, specific gravity, urinalysis, BUN and creatinine levels, and creatinine clearance. Report to prescriber evidence of declining renal function.
- Hemodialysis for 8 hours may remove up to 50% of drug from blood.
- Watch for signs and symptoms of superinfection (especially of upper respiratory tract), such as continued fever, chills, and increased pulse rate.
- Therapy usually continues for 7 to 10 days. If no response occurs in 3 to 5 days, stop therapy and obtain new specimens for culture and sensitivity testing.

Patient teaching

- Instruct patient to promptly report adverse reactions, such as dizziness, vertigo, unsteady gait, ringing in the ears, hearing loss, numbness, tingling, or muscle twitching.
- Encourage patient to drink plenty of fluids.
- Warn patient to avoid hazardous activities if adverse CNS reactions occur.

gentamicin sulfate (topical)
Garamycin, G-Myticin

Pregnancy risk category C

Indications & dosages

➲ To treat or prevent superficial infections and superficial burns of the skin caused by susceptible bacteria

Adults and children older than age 1: Rub in small amount gently t.i.d. or q.i.d., with or without gauze dressing.

Contraindications & cautions

- Contraindicated in patients hypersensitive to drug or its components and in those who may have cross-sensitivity with other aminoglycosides such as neomycin.

Adverse reactions

Skin: minor skin irritation, photosensitivity, allergic contact dermatitis.

Interactions

None significant.

Nursing considerations

!! ALERT Avoid use on large skin lesions or over a wide area because of possible systemic toxic effects.

- Restrict use of drug to selected patients; widespread use may lead to resistant organisms.
- Prolonged use may result in overgrowth of nonsusceptible organisms.

Patient teaching

- Tell patient to clean affected area and, to increase absorption, remove crusts of impetigo before applying drug.
- Tell patient to wash hands after each application.
- Instruct patient to store drug in cool place.
- Tell patient to stop using drug and notify prescriber immediately if no improvement occurs or if condition worsens.

glatiramer acetate injection
Copaxone

Pregnancy risk category B

Indications & dosages
➲ **Reduce frequency of relapse in patients with relapsing-remitting multiple sclerosis**
Adults: 20 mg S.C. daily.

Contraindications & cautions
- Contraindicated in patients hypersensitive to drug or mannitol.

Adverse reactions
CNS: abnormal dreams, fever, agitation, *anxiety, asthenia,* confusion, emotional lability, migraine, nervousness, speech disorder, stupor, tremor, vertigo, syncope.
CV: *chest pain,* hypertension, *palpitations, vasodilation,* tachycardia.
EENT: ear pain, eye disorder, laryngismus, *rhinitis,* nystagmus.
GI: anorexia, bowel urgency, *diarrhea,* gastroenteritis, GI disorder, *nausea,* oral candidiasis, salivary gland enlargement, ulcerative stomatitis, vomiting.
GU: amenorrhea, dysmenorrhea, hematuria, impotence, menorrhagia, abnormal Papanicolaou smear, *urinary urgency,* vaginal candidiasis, ***vaginal hemorrhage***.
Hematologic: ecchymosis, ***lymphadenopathy***.
Metabolic: weight gain.
Musculoskeletal: *arthralgia, back pain,* neck pain, foot drop, *hypertonia.*
Respiratory: bronchitis, *dyspnea,* hyperventilation.
Skin: eczema, erythema, *pruritus, rash, injection site reaction,* or hemorrhage, skin atrophy, nodule, *diaphoresis,* urticaria, warts.
Other: bacterial infection, herpes simplex and zoster, chills, cyst, dental caries, peripheral and facial edema, *flulike syndrome, infection, pain.*

Interactions
None significant.

Nursing considerations
- Give drug only by S.C. injection.
- Store drug in refrigerator (36° to 46° F [2° to 8° C]); allow drug to warm to room temperature for 20 minutes before use.
- Drug doesn't contain preservatives; discard if solution contains particulate matter.
- Don't try to expell the air bubble from the pre-filled syringe. This may lead to loss of drug and an incorrect dose.
- Immediate postinjection reactions have occurred in some patients with multiple sclerosis; symptoms include flushing, chest pain, palpitations, anxiety, dyspnea, constriction of the throat, and urticaria. They typically are transient and self-limiting and don't need specific treatment. Onset of postinjection reaction may occur several months after treatment starts, and patients may have more than one episode.
- Some patients have experienced at least one episode of transient chest pain, which usually begins at least 1 month after treatment starts; it isn't accompanied by other signs or symptoms and doesn't appear to be clinically important.

!! ALERT Don't confuse Copaxone with Compazine.

Patient teaching
- Instruct patient how to self-inject drug. Supervise first injection.
- Explain need for aseptic self-injection techniques and warn patient against reuse of needles and syringes. Periodically review proper disposal of needles, syringes, drug containers, and unused drug.
- Tell patient to notify prescriber about planned, suspected, or known pregnancy.
- Tell woman to notify prescriber if she is breast-feeding.
- Advise patient not to change drug or dosage schedule or to stop drug without medical approval.
- Tell patient to notify prescriber immediately if dizziness, hives, profuse sweating, chest pain, difficulty breathing, or if severe pain occurs after drug injection.

glimepiride
Amaryl

Pregnancy risk category C

Indications & dosages

➲ **Adjunct to diet and exercise to lower glucose level in patients with type 2 (non–insulin-dependent) diabetes whose hyperglycemia can't be managed by diet and exercise alone**
Adults: Initially, 1 or 2 mg P.O. once daily with first main meal of day; usual maintenance dose is 1 to 4 mg P.O. once daily. After reaching 2 mg, dosage is increased in increments not exceeding 2 mg q 1 to 2 weeks, based on patient's glucose level response. Maximum dose is 8 mg daily.

➲ **Adjunct to diet and exercise in conjunction with insulin or metformin therapy in patients with type 2 diabetes whose hyperglycemia can't be managed with the maximum dosage of glimepiride alone**
Adults: 8 mg P.O. once daily with first main meal of day; used with low-dose insulin or metformin. Increase insulin or metformin dosage weekly, p.r.n., based on patient's glucose level response.

For patients with renal or hepatic impairment, initially, 1 mg P.O. once daily with first main meal of day; then adjust to appropriate dosage, p.r.n.

Contraindications & cautions

- Contraindicated in patients hypersensitive to drug and in those with diabetic ketoacidosis, which should be treated with insulin.
- Contraindicated in pregnant or elderly patients and as sole therapy for type 1 diabetes.
- Contraindicated in breast-feeding patients because it may cause hypoglycemia in breast-fed infants.
- Use cautiously in debilitated or malnourished patients and in those with adrenal, pituitary, hepatic, or renal insufficiency; these patients are more susceptible to the hypoglycemic action of glucose-lowering drugs.
- Use cautiously in patients allergic to sulfonamides.
- Safety and effectiveness of drug in children haven't been established.

Adverse reactions

CNS: dizziness, asthenia, headache.
EENT: changes in accommodation.
GI: nausea.
Hematologic: ***leukopenia***, hemolytic anemia, ***agranulocytosis***, ***thrombocytopenia***, ***aplastic anemia***, ***pancytopenia***.
Hepatic: cholestatic jaundice.
Metabolic: ***hypoglycemia***, dilutional hyponatremia.
Skin: pruritus, erythema, urticaria, morbilliform or maculopapular eruptions, photosensitivity reactions.

Interactions

Drug-drug. *Beta blockers:* May mask symptoms of hypoglycemia. Monitor glucose level.
Drugs that tend to produce hyperglycemia (such as corticosteroids, estrogens, fosphenytoin, hormonal contraceptives, isoniazid, nicotinic acid, other diuretics, phenothiazines, phenytoin, sympathomimetic thiazides, thyroid products): May lead to loss of glucose control. Adjust dosage.
Insulin: May increase risk of hypoglycemia. Avoid using together.
NSAIDs, other drugs that are highly protein-bound (such as beta blockers, chloramphenicol, coumarin, MAO inhibitors, probenecid, salicylates, sulfonamides): May increase hypoglycemic action of sulfonylureas such as glimepiride. Monitor glucose level carefully.
Drug-herb. *Burdock, dandelion, eucalyptus, marshmallow:* May increase hypoglycemic effects. Discourage use together.
Drug-lifestyle. *Alcohol use:* May alter glycemic control, most commonly causing hypoglycemia. May also cause disulfiram-like reaction. Discourage use together.

Nursing considerations

- Glimepiride and insulin may be used together in patients who lose glucose control after first responding to therapy.
- Monitor fasting glucose level periodically to determine therapeutic response. Also monitor glycosylated hemoglobin level, usually every 3 to 6 months, to precisely assess long-term glycemic control.
- Use of oral hypoglycemics may carry higher risk of CV mortality than use of diet alone or of diet and insulin therapy.

• When changing patient from other sulfonylureas to glimepiride, a transition period isn't needed.

!!ALERT Don't confuse glimepiride with glyburide or glipizide.

Patient teaching

• Tell patient to take drug with first meal of the day.

• Make sure patient understands that therapy relieves symptoms but doesn't cure the disease. He should also understand potential risks and advantages of taking drug and of other treatment methods.

• Stress importance of adhering to diet, weight reduction, exercise, and personal hygiene programs. Explain to patient and family how and when to monitor glucose level, and teach recognition of and intervention for signs and symptoms of high and low glucose levels.

• Advise patient to wear or carry medical identification at all times.

• Advise woman to consult prescriber before planning pregnancy. Insulin may be needed during pregnancy and breast-feeding.

• Advise patient to consult prescriber before taking any OTC products.

• Teach patient to carry candy or other simple sugars to treat mild episodes of low glucose level. Patient experiencing severe episode may need hospital treatment.

• Advise patient to avoid alcohol, which lowers glucose level.

glipizide
Glucotrol, Glucotrol XL

Pregnancy risk category C

Indications & dosages

➲ Adjunct to diet to lower glucose level in patients with type 2 (non–insulin-dependent) diabetes

Immediate-release tablets

Patients older than age 65: First dose is 2.5 mg P.O. daily.

Adults: Initially, 5 mg P.O. daily 30 minutes before breakfast. Maximum once-daily dose is 15 mg. Divide doses of more than 15 mg. Maximum total daily dose is 40 mg.

Extended-release tablets

Adults: Initially, 5 mg P.O. with breakfast daily. Increase by 5 mg q 3 months, depending on level of glycemic control. Maximum daily dosage is 20 mg.

For patients with liver disease, first dose is 2.5 mg P.O. daily.

➲ To replace insulin therapy

Adults: If insulin dosage is more than 20 units daily, start patient at usual dosage in addition to 50% of insulin. If insulin dosage is less than or equal to 20 units daily, insulin may be stopped when glipizide starts.

Contraindications & cautions

• Contraindicated in patients hypersensitive to drug and in those with diabetic ketoacidosis with or without coma.

• Contraindicated in pregnant or breast-feeding women and as sole therapy in type 1 diabetes.

• Use cautiously in patients with renal or hepatic disease, in those allergic to sulfonamides, and in debilitated, malnourished, or elderly patients.

Adverse reactions

CNS: dizziness, drowsiness, headache.
GI: nausea, constipation, diarrhea.
Hematologic: ***leukopenia***, hemolytic anemia, ***agranulocytosis***, ***thrombocytopenia***, ***aplastic anemia***.
Hepatic: cholestatic jaundice.
Metabolic: ***hypoglycemia***.
Skin: rash, pruritus, photosensitivity.

Interactions

Drug-drug. *Amantadine, anabolic steroids, antifungal antibiotics (miconazole, fluconazole), chloramphenicol, clofibrate, guanethidine, MAO inhibitors, probenecid, salicylates, sulfonamides:* May increase hypoglycemic activity. Monitor glucose level.

Beta blockers: May prolong hypoglycemic effect and mask symptoms of hypoglycemia. Use together cautiously.

Corticosteroids, glucagon, phenytoin, rifampin, thiazide diuretics: May decrease hypoglycemic response. Monitor glucose level.

Oral anticoagulants: May increase hypoglycemic activity or enhanced anticoagulant effect. Monitor glucose level, PT, and INR.

Drug-herb. *Burdock, dandelion, eucalyptus, marshmallow:* May increase hypoglycemic effects. Discourage use together.
Drug-lifestyle. *Alcohol use:* May alter glycemic control, most commonly causing hypoglycemia. May cause disulfiram-like reaction. Discourage use together.

Nursing considerations

- Give immediate-release tablet about 30 minutes before meals.
- Some patients may attain effective control on a once-daily regimen, whereas others respond better with divided dosing.
- Patient may switch from immediate-release dose to extended-release tablets at the nearest equivalent total daily dose.
- Glipizide is a second-generation sulfonylurea. The frequency of adverse reactions appears to be lower than with first-generation drugs such as chlorpropamide.
- During periods of increased stress, patient may need insulin therapy. Monitor patient closely for hyperglycemia in these situations.
- Patient switching from insulin therapy to an oral antidiabetic should check glucose level at least three times a day before meals. Patient may need hospitalization during transition.

!!ALERT Don't confuse glipizide with glyburide or glimepiride.

Patient teaching

- Instruct patient about disease and importance of following therapeutic regimen, adhering to diet, losing weight, getting exercise, following personal hygiene programs, and avoiding infection. Explain how and when to monitor glucose level, and teach recognition of episodes of low and high glucose levels.
- Tell patient to carry candy or other simple sugars to treat mild low-glucose episodes. Patient experiencing severe episode may need hospital treatment.
- Instruct patient not to change drug dosage without prescriber's consent and to report abnormal blood or urine glucose test results.
- Tell patient not to take other drugs, including OTC drugs, without first checking with prescriber.
- Advise patient to wear or carry medical identification at all times.
- Advise woman planning pregnancy to first consult prescriber. Insulin may be needed during pregnancy and breast-feeding.
- Advise patient to avoid alcohol, which lowers glucose level.

glipizide and metformin hydrochloride
Metaglip

Pregnancy risk category C

Indications & dosages

➲ First-line therapy, adjunct to diet and exercise, to improve glycemic control in patients with type 2 diabetes
Adults: Initially, 2.5 mg/250 mg P.O. once daily with a meal. In patients whose fasting glucose is 280 to 320 mg/dl, start with 2.5 mg/500 mg P.O. b.i.d. Dosage may be increased in increments of one tablet per day q 2 weeks, up to a maximum of 10 mg/1,000 mg or 10 mg/2,000 mg daily in divided doses.
➲ Second-line therapy in patients with type 2 diabetes for whom diet, exercise, and initial treatment with a sulfonylurea or metformin don't provide adequate glycemic control
Adults: Initially, 2.5 mg/500 mg or 5 mg/500 mg P.O. b.i.d. with the morning and evening meals. Increase in increments of no more than 5 mg/500 mg, up to the minimum effective dose needed to adequately control glucose or to a maximum daily dose of 20 mg/2,000 mg.

Contraindications & cautions

- Contraindicated in patients hypersensitive to any components of the drug and in those with renal disease, creatinine level at least 1.5 mg/dl in men and at least 1.4 mg/dl in women, abnormal creatinine clearance, heart failure, shock, acute MI, septicemia, or acute or chronic metabolic acidosis, including diabetic ketoacidosis.
- Contraindicated after surgical procedures, in pregnant or breast-feeding patients, and in patients age 80 or older unless renal function is normal.
- Use cautiously in elderly patients and in patients with hepatic dysfunction, malnourished or debilitated patients, and those with

adrenal or pituitary insufficiency. Don't give elderly patients the maximum dose.
- Use cautiously in patients with abnormal vitamin B_{12} level or hypoglycemia and in those who consume alcohol.

Adverse reactions

CNS: *headache*, dizziness.
CV: hypertension.
GI: nausea, *diarrhea*, vomiting, abdominal pain.
GU: UTI.
Metabolic: ***hypoglycemia***, ***lactic acidosis***.
Musculoskeletal: pain.
Respiratory: *upper respiratory tract infection.*

Interactions

Drug-drug. *Azoles, beta blockers, chloramphenicol, coumarin, MAO inhibitors, NSAIDs, probenecid, salicylates, sulfonamides:* May increase the effect of sulfonylureas. Monitor closely for hypoglycemia. May increase loss of glucose control when these drugs are withdrawn.
Calcium channel blockers, corticosteroids, estrogens, highly protein-bound drugs, isoniazid, hormonal contraceptives, nicotinic acid, phenytoin, phenothiazines, sympathomimetics, thyroid products, thiazides and other diuretics: May increase risk of hyperglycemia and loss of glucose control. May increase risk of hypoglycemia when these drugs are withdrawn. Monitor glucose level.
Cationic drugs (amiloride, digoxin, morphine, procainamide, quinidine, quinine, ranitidine, triamterene, trimethoprim, vancomycin): May increase metformin level. Monitor patient carefully.
Furosemide: May increase metformin level and decrease furosemide level. Monitor patient closely.
Iodinated contrast material used in radiologic studies: May increase risk of acute renal failure. Stop the drug for 48 hours before and after such tests.
Nifedipine: May increase metformin level. Metformin dose may need to be decreased.
Drug-herb. *Juniper berries, ginseng, garlic, fenugreek, coriander, dandelion root, celery:* May increase risk of hypoglycemia. Discourage use together.
Drug-lifestyle. *Alcohol use:* May increase risk of hypoglycemia and lactic acidosis. Discourage use together.

Nursing considerations

- Temporarily stop drug in patients undergoing radiologic studies involving contrast media containing iodine or any surgical procedure.
- To reduce the risk of lactic acidosis, use the minimum effective dose and monitor renal function regularly during treatment.
- Stop drug in patients with any condition linked to hypoxemia, dehydration, or sepsis.
- Evaluate patient for ketoacidosis or lactic acidosis if laboratory abnormalities or vague, poorly defined illness occurs. Stop drug immediately if acidosis occurs.
- Periodically monitor fasting glucose level and glycosylated hemoglobin level.
- Monitor CBC and renal function annually.
- Drug shouldn't be used in pregnant patients unless the benefits outweigh the risks. If the drug is used, stop therapy at least 1 month before delivery.

Patient teaching

- Tell patient to take once daily with breakfast or twice daily with breakfast and dinner.
- Tell patient to immediately report signs of lactic acidosis—unexplained hyperventilation, myalgia, malaise, unusual drowsiness, suddenly developing a slow or irregular heartbeat, or feeling cold, dizzy, or lightheaded.
- Tell patient that GI symptoms are common during initial therapy but should resolve. Tell patient to report persistent or new onset of GI symptoms.
- Advise patient to avoid alcohol intake.
- Teach patient about diabetes and the warning signs of hypoglycemia and hyperglycemia, along with how to self-monitor glucose level. Also teach patient the importance of good hygiene to help avoid infections and of adhering to diet, exercise, and medication schedule.
- Instruct patient to wear or carry medical identification.

glucagon

GlucaGen Diagnostic Kit, Glucagon Diagnostic Kit, Glucagon Emergency Kit

Pregnancy risk category B

Indications & dosages

➲ Hypoglycemia

Adults and children weighing more than 20 kg (44 lb): 1 mg (1 unit) I.V., I.M., S.C.

Children weighing 20 kg or less: 0.5 mg (0.5 units) or 20 to 30 mcg/kg I.V., I.M., S.C.; maximum dose 1 mg. May repeat in 15 minutes, if needed. I.V. glucose must be given if patient fails to respond.

➲ Diagnostic aid for radiologic examination

Adults: 0.25 to 2 mg I.V. or I.M. before radiologic examination.

Contraindications & cautions

- Contraindicated in patients hypersensitive to drug and in those with pheochromocytoma.
- Use cautiously in patients with history of insulinoma or pheochromocytoma.

Adverse reactions

GI: nausea, vomiting.

Respiratory: ***bronchospasm, respiratory distress.***

Other: hypersensitivity reactions.

Interactions

Drug-drug. *Anticoagulants:* May enhance anticoagulant effect. Monitor prothrombin activity, and watch for signs of bleeding.

Nursing considerations

- Use drug only in emergency situations.
- Monitor glucose level before, during, and after administration.

!! ALERT Arouse patient from coma as quickly as possible and give additional carbohydrates orally to prevent secondary hypoglycemic reactions.

!! ALERT Don't confuse glucagon with Glaucon.

Patient teaching

- Instruct patient and caregivers how to give glucagon and recognize a low glucose episode.
- Explain importance of calling prescriber at once in emergencies.

glyburide (glibenclamide)

DiaBeta, Euglucon†, Glynase PresTab, Micronase

Pregnancy risk category B

Indications & dosages

➲ Adjunct to diet to lower glucose level in patients with type 2 (non-insulin-dependent) diabetes

Nonmicronized form

Adults: Initially, 2.5 to 5 mg P.O. once daily with breakfast or first main meal. Usual daily maintenance dosage is 1.25 to 20 mg, as single dose or divided doses. Maximum daily dose is 20 mg P.O.

Micronized form

Adults: Initially, 1.5 to 3 mg daily with breakfast or first main meal. Usual daily maintenance dosage is 0.75 to 12 mg. Dosages exceeding 6 mg daily may have better response with b.i.d. dosing. Maximum dose is 12 mg P.O. daily.

For patients who are more sensitive to antidiabetics and for those with adrenal or pituitary insufficiency, start with 1.25 mg daily. When using micronized tablets, patients who are more sensitive to antidiabetics should start with 0.75 mg daily.

➲ To replace insulin therapy

Adults: If insulin dosage is less than 40 units/day, patient may be switched directly to glyburide when insulin is stopped. If insulin dosage is 40 or more units/day, initially, 5-mg regular tablets or 3-mg micronized tablets can be given P.O. once daily in addition to 50% of insulin dosage.

Contraindications & cautions

- Contraindicated in patients hypersensitive to drug and in those with diabetic ketoacidosis with or without coma.
- Contraindicated as sole therapy for type 1 diabetes and in pregnant or breast-feeding women.
- Use cautiously in patients with hepatic or renal impairment; in debilitated, malnourished, or elderly patients; and in patients allergic to sulfonamides.

Adverse reactions

EENT: changes in accommodation or blurred vision.
GI: nausea, epigastric fullness, heartburn.
Hematologic: ***leukopenia***, hemolytic anemia, ***agranulocytosis***, ***thrombocytopenia***, ***aplastic anemia***.
Hepatic: cholestatic jaundice, ***hepatitis***.
Metabolic: ***hypoglycemia***.
Musculoskeletal: arthralgia, myalgia.
Skin: rash, pruritus, other allergic reactions.
Other: ***angioedema***.

Interactions

Drug-drug. *Anabolic steroids, chloramphenicol, clofibrate, guanethidine, MAO inhibitors, probenecid, phenylbutazone, salicylates, sulfonamides:* May increase hypoglycemic activity. Monitor glucose level.
Beta blockers: May prolong hypoglycemic effect and mask symptoms of hypoglycemia. Use together cautiously.
Carbamazepine, corticosteroids, glucagon, rifampin, thiazide diuretics: May decrease hypoglycemic response. Monitor glucose level.
Oral anticoagulants: May increase hypoglycemic activity or enhance anticoagulant effect. Monitor glucose level, PT, and INR.
Drug-herb. *Burdock, dandelion, eucalyptus, marshmallow:* May increase hypoglycemic effect. Discourage use together.
Drug-lifestyle. *Alcohol use:* May alter glycemic control, most commonly causing hypoglycemia. May cause disulfiram-like reaction. Discourage use together.

Nursing considerations

!!ALERT Micronized glyburide (Glynase PresTab) contains drug in a smaller particle size and isn't bioequivalent to regular glyburide tablets. Patients who have been taking Micronase or DiaBeta need dosage readjustment.
- Although most patients may take drug once daily, those taking more than 10 mg daily may achieve better results with twice-daily dosage.
- Glyburide is a second-generation sulfonylurea. Adverse effects are less common with second-generation drugs than with first-generation drugs such as chlorpropamide.
- During periods of increased stress, such as infection, fever, surgery, or trauma, patient may need insulin therapy. Monitor patient closely for hyperglycemia in these situations.
- Patient switching from insulin therapy to an oral antidiabetic should check glucose level at least three times a day before meals. Patient may need hospitalization during transition.

!!ALERT Don't confuse glyburide with glimepiride or glipizide.
- DiaBeta may contain tartrazine.

Patient teaching

- Instruct patient about nature of disease and importance of following therapeutic regimen, adhering to specific diet, losing weight, getting exercise, following personal hygiene programs, and avoiding infection. Explain how and when to monitor glucose level, and teach recognition of and intervention for low- and high-glucose episodes.
- Tell patient not to change drug dosage without prescriber's consent and to report abnormal blood or urine glucose test results.
- Teach patient to carry candy or other simple sugars to treat mild low-glucose episodes. Patient experiencing severe episode may need hospital treatment.
- Advise patient not to take other drugs, including OTC drugs, without first checking with prescriber.
- Advise patient to wear or carry medical identification at all times.

!!ALERT Instruct patient to report episodes of low glucose to prescriber immediately; severe low glucose is sometimes fatal in patients receiving as little as 2.5 to 5 mg glyburide daily.
- Advise patient to avoid alcohol, which may lower glucose level.

glyburide and metformin hydrochloride
Glucovance

Pregnancy risk category B

Indications & dosages

➲ **Adjunct to diet and exercise to improve glycemic control in patients with type 2 (non–insulin-dependent) diabetes in whom hyperglycemia can't be controlled with diet and exercise alone**
Adults: Initially, 1.25 mg glyburide/250 mg metformin hydrochloride P.O. once daily or

b.i.d. with meals. In patients with HbA_{1c} greater than 9% or a fasting glucose level greater than 200 mg/dl, start with 1.25 mg glyburide/250 mg metformin hydrochloride b.i.d. with morning and evening meals. May increase daily dose by 1.25 mg glyburide/250 mg metformin hydrochloride q 2 weeks, up to the minimum effective dose needed to achieve adequate control of glucose level. Maximum daily dose is 20 mg glyburide/2,000 mg metformin.

➲ **Second-line therapy in patients with type 2 diabetes when diet, exercise, and first-line treatment with a sulfonylurea or metformin don't adequately control glucose level**

Adults: Initially, 2.5 mg glyburide/500 mg metformin hydrochloride or 5 mg glyburide/500 mg metformin hydrochloride b.i.d. with meals. Increase by no more than 5 mg glyburide/500 mg metformin hydrochloride, up to the minimum effective dose needed to achieve adequate glucose level control. Maximum daily dose is 20 mg glyburide/2,000 mg metformin hydrochloride.

Elderly patients: First and maintenance dosages are conservative because of the potential for decreased renal function in these patients. Any dosage adjustment requires careful assessment of renal function. Don't give the maximum dosage to avoid the risk of hypoglycemia.

In debilitated or malnourished patients, don't give the maximum dosage to avoid the risk of hypoglycemia.

Contraindications & cautions

- Contraindicated in patients hypersensitive to glyburide or metformin and in those with renal disease, renal dysfunction, or metabolic acidosis (including diabetic ketoacidosis).
- Contraindicated in breast-feeding women and patients with heart failure requiring pharmacologic treatment.
- Use cautiously in elderly, hepatically impaired, debilitated, or malnourished patients and in those with adrenal or pituitary insufficiency because of increased risk of hypoglycemia.

Adverse reactions

CNS: headache, dizziness.
GI: *diarrhea*, nausea, vomiting, abdominal pain.
Metabolic: ***hypoglycemia, lactic acidosis***.
Respiratory: *upper respiratory tract infection.*

Interactions

Drug-drug. *Beta blockers, chloramphenicol, ciprofloxacin, coumarin, highly protein-bound drugs, MAO inhibitors, miconazole, NSAIDs, probenecid, salicylates, sulfonamides:* May increase hypoglycemic activity of glyburide. Monitor glucose level.
Calcium channel blockers, corticosteroids, estrogens, hormonal contraceptives, isoniazid, nicotinic acid, phenothiazines, phenytoin, sympathomimetics, thiazides and other diuretics, thyroid agents: May cause hyperglycemia. Monitor glucose level.
Cationic drugs (such as amiloride, cimetidine, digoxin, morphine, procainamide, quinidine, quinine, ranitidine, triamterene, trimethoprim, vancomycin): May increase metformin level. Monitor glucose level.
Furosemide: May increase metformin level and decrease furosemide level. Monitor patient closely.
Nifedipine: May increase metformin level. Metformin dosage may need to be decreased.
Drug-lifestyle. *Alcohol use:* May alter glycemic control, most commonly causing hypoglycemia. May cause disulfiram-like reaction with glyburide component. Discourage use together.

Nursing considerations

- In elderly patients, monitor renal function regularly.
- For patients requiring additional glycemic control, a thiazolidinedione may be added to Glucovance therapy.
- Assess glucose level before and regularly after therapy. Monitor glycosylated hemoglobin level to assess long-term therapy.

!!ALERT Obtain baseline renal function test results and don't start drug if creatinine level is 1.5 mg/dl or greater (in men) or 1.4 mg/dl or greater (in women). Monitor renal function at least once yearly while patient is on long-term therapy and more often if renal dysfunction is anticipated. If renal impairment is detected, stop drug.

- Temporarily stop drug in patients undergoing radiologic studies involving contrast media containing iodine because these products may acutely alter renal function.

• For patients previously treated with glyburide or metformin, the starting dose of drug shouldn't exceed daily dose of the glyburide (or equivalent dose of another sulfonylurea) and metformin already being taken.
• Monitor patient closely during times of increased stress, such as infection, fever, surgery, or trauma; insulin therapy may be needed. Temporarily suspend drug for any surgical procedure that requires restricted intake of food and fluids, and don't restart until patient's oral intake has resumed.
• Lactic acidosis is a rare but serious (50% fatal) metabolic complication caused by metformin accumulation. Lactic acidosis occurs primarily in diabetic patients with significant renal insufficiency; multiple medical or surgical problems; and multiple drug regimens. The risk of lactic acidosis increases with the degree of renal impairment and patient age.
• Early symptoms of lactic acidosis may include malaise, myalgias, respiratory distress, increasing somnolence, and nonspecific abdominal distress.
• GI symptoms that occur after patient is stabilized on drug are unlikely to be drug-related and could be caused by lactic acidosis or other serious disease.
• Suspect lactic acidosis in any diabetic patient with metabolic acidosis lacking evidence of ketoacidosis.
• Monitor patient's hematologic status for megaloblastic anemia. Patients with inadequate vitamin B_{12} or calcium intake or absorption seem predisposed to developing subnormal vitamin B_{12} levels when taking metformin. Check the vitamin B_{12} level in these patients every 2 to 3 years.
• Stop drug if CV collapse, acute heart failure, acute MI, or other conditions characterized by hypoxemia occur because these conditions may be linked to lactic acidosis and may cause prerenal azotemia.
• Watch for ketoacidosis or lactic acidosis in patient who develops laboratory abnormalities or clinical illness, by evaluating laboratory values, including electrolyte, ketone, glucose, pH, lactate, pyruvate, and metformin levels. Stop drug if signs or symptoms of acidosis develop.
• Obtain a baseline creatinine level that indicates normal renal function before starting therapy. Don't start therapy in patients age 80 or older, unless creatinine clearance level demonstrates normal renal function.
• Drug shouldn't usually be increased to maximum dose.

Patient teaching

• Tell patient to take once-daily dose with breakfast and twice-daily dose with breakfast and dinner.
• Teach patient about diabetes and importance of following therapeutic regimen; adhering to diet, weight reduction, regular exercise and hygiene programs; and avoiding infection. Explain how and when to self-monitor glucose level and how to differentiate between symptoms of low and high glucose levels.
• Instruct patient to stop drug and tell prescriber of unexplained hyperventilation, muscle pain, malaise, unusual sleepiness, or other symptoms of early lactic acidosis.
• Tell patient that GI symptoms are common with initial drug therapy. He should report promptly GI symptoms occurring after prolonged therapy, as they may be related to lactic acidosis or other serious disease.
• Advise patient not to drink too much alcohol.
• Advise patient not to take any other drugs, including OTC drugs, without checking with prescriber.
• Instruct patient to carry medical identification.

glycopyrrolate

Robinul, Robinul Forte

Pregnancy risk category B

Indications & dosages

➲ To block adverse cholinergic effects caused by anticholinesterases used to reverse neuromuscular blockade
Adults and children: 0.2 mg I.V. for each 1 mg of neostigmine or 5 mg of pyridostigmine. May be given I.V. without dilution or may be added to dextrose injection and given by infusion.

➲ Preoperatively to diminish secretions and block cardiac vagal reflexes
Adults and children age 2 and older: 0.0044 mg/kg I.M. 30 to 60 minutes before anesthesia.

Children younger than age 2: 0.0088 mg/kg I.M. 30 to 60 minutes before anesthesia.

➲ **Adjunctive therapy in peptic ulcerations and other GI disorders**

Adults: 1 to 2 mg P.O. t.i.d. or 0.1 to 0.2 mg I.M. or I.V. t.i.d. or q.i.d. Dosage must be individualized. Maximum oral dosage, 8 mg daily.

Contraindications & cautions

- Contraindicated in patients hypersensitive to drug, in neonates, and in those with glaucoma, obstructive uropathy, obstructive disease of the GI tract, myasthenia gravis, paralytic ileus, intestinal atony, unstable CV status in acute hemorrhage, tachycardia secondary to cardiac insufficiency or thyrotoxicosis, severe ulcerative colitis, toxic megacolon, or known or suspected GI infection.
- Use cautiously in patients with autonomic neuropathy, hyperthyroidism, coronary artery disease, arrhythmias, heart failure, hypertension, hiatal hernia, hepatic or renal disease, ulcerative colitis, and known or suspected GI infection.
- Use cautiously in patients in hot or humid environments; drug can cause heatstroke.

Adverse reactions

CNS: fever, weakness, nervousness, insomnia, drowsiness, dizziness, headache, confusion, excitement.
CV: palpitations, tachycardia.
EENT: *dilated pupils, blurred vision,* photophobia, increased intraocular pressure.
GI: *constipation, dry mouth,* nausea, loss of taste, abdominal distention, vomiting, epigastric distress.
GU: urinary hesitancy, urine retention, impotence.
Skin: urticaria, decreased sweating or anhidrosis.
Other: allergic reactions, ***anaphylaxis***.

Interactions

Drug-drug. *Amantadine, antihistamines, antiparkinsonians, disopyramide, glutethimide, meperidine, phenothiazines, procainamide, quinidine, tricyclic antidepressants:* May have additive adverse effects. Avoid using together.
Potassium chloride: May slow transit time and increase risk of potassium-induced GI lesions. Avoid wax-based potassium products.

Nursing considerations

- Give oral form 30 to 60 minutes before meals.

!!ALERT Check all dosages carefully; slight overdose can lead to toxicity.

!!ALERT Overdose may cause curarelike effects, such as respiratory paralysis. Keep emergency equipment available.

- Monitor vital signs carefully. Watch closely for adverse reactions, especially in geriatric or debilitated patients. Call prescriber promptly if reactions occur.
- Elderly patients may be more susceptible to adverse effects and typically receive smaller doses.

Patient teaching

- Tell patient to take oral drug 30 to 60 minutes before meals.
- Tell patient not to crush or chew extended-release products.
- Warn patient to avoid activities that require alertness until drug's CNS effects are known.
- Advise patient to report signs and symptoms of urinary hesitancy or urine retention.

goserelin acetate
Zoladex

Pregnancy risk category X (endometriosis and endometrial thinning); D (breast cancer)

Indications & dosages

➲ **Endometriosis, including pain relief and lesion reduction; palliative treatment of advanced prostate cancer**

Adults: 3.6 mg S.C. q 28 days into upper abdominal wall. For endometriosis, maximum duration of therapy is 6 months. For prostate cancer, 10.8 mg S.C. into upper abdominal wall q 12 weeks.

➲ **Endometrial thinning before endometrial ablation**

Adults: 3.6 mg S.C. into upper abdominal wall. Give one or two implants, 4 weeks apart.

➲ Palliative treatment of advanced breast cancer in premenopausal and perimenopausal women
Adults: 3.6 mg S.C. q 28 days into upper abdominal wall.

Contraindications & cautions

- Contraindicated in patients hypersensitive to LH-RH, LH-RH agonist analogues, or goserelin acetate.
- Contraindicated in pregnant or breast-feeding women and in patients with obstructive uropathy or vertebral metastases.
- The 10.8-mg implant is contraindicated in women because of insufficient data supporting reliable suppression of estradiol.
- Because drug may cause bone mineral density loss in women, use cautiously in patients with risk factors for osteoporosis, such as family history of osteoporosis, chronic alcohol or tobacco abuse, or use of drugs—such as corticosteroids or anticonvulsants—that affect bone density.

Adverse reactions

CNS: lethargy, pain, dizziness, *insomnia*, anxiety, *depression*, *headache*, chills, *emotional lability*, ***CVA***, *asthenia*.
CV: edema, ***heart failure***, ***arrhythmias***, *peripheral edema*, hypertension, ***MI***, peripheral vascular disorder, chest pain, *hot flashes*.
GI: nausea, vomiting, diarrhea, constipation, ulcer, anorexia, abdominal pain.
GU: *sexual dysfunction*, *impotence*, *lower urinary tract symptoms*, renal insufficiency, urinary obstruction, *vaginitis*, UTI, *amenorrhea*.
Hematologic: anemia.
Metabolic: hypercalcemia, hyperglycemia, weight increase, gout.
Musculoskeletal: back pain, osteoporosis.
Respiratory: COPD, upper respiratory tract infection.
Skin: rash, *diaphoresis*, *acne*, *seborrhea*, hirsutism.
Other: breast swelling, pain, and tenderness, *changes in breast size*, *changes in libido*, *infection*.

Interactions

None significant.

Nursing considerations

- Before giving to women, rule out pregnancy.
- Never give by I.V. injection.
- Give drug into upper abdominal wall using aseptic technique. After cleaning area with an alcohol swab and injecting a local anesthetic, stretch patient's skin with one hand while grasping barrel of syringe with the other. Insert needle into the subcutaneous fat; then change direction of needle so that it parallels the abdominal wall. Push needle in until hub touches patient's skin; withdraw about 1 cm (this creates a gap for drug to be injected) before depressing plunger completely.
- To avoid need for a new syringe and injection site, don't aspirate after inserting needle. If needle penetrates a blood vessel, blood will appear in the syringe chamber. Withdraw needle, and inject elsewhere with a new syringe.

!! ALERT Implant comes in a preloaded syringe. If package is damaged, don't use the syringe. Make sure drug is visible in the translucent chamber of the syringe.

- When drug is used for prostate cancer, LH-RH analogues such as goserelin may initially worsen symptoms because drug first increases testosterone level. Some patients may temporarily have increased bone pain. Rarely, disease may get worse (spinal cord compression or ureteral obstruction), although the relationship to therapy is uncertain.
- When drug is used for endometrial thinning, if one implant is given, surgery should be performed 4 weeks later; if two implants are given, surgery should be performed 2 to 4 weeks after patient receives second implant.

Patient teaching

- Advise patient to return every 28 days for a new implant. A delay of a couple of days is permissible.
- Tell patient that pain may worsen for first 30 days of treatment.
- Tell woman to use a nonhormonal form of contraception during treatment. Caution patient about significant risks to fetus.
- Urge woman to call prescriber if menstruation persists or if breakthrough bleeding occurs. Menstruation should stop during treatment.

• Inform woman that a delayed return of menstruation may occur after therapy ends. Persistent lack of menstruation is rare.

granisetron hydrochloride
Kytril

Pregnancy risk category B

Indications & dosages

➲ To prevent nausea and vomiting from emetogenic cancer chemotherapy
Adults and children age 2 and older: 10 mcg/kg I.V. undiluted and given by direct injection over 30 seconds, or diluted and infused over 5 minutes. Begin administration within 30 minutes before use of chemotherapy. Or, for adults, 1 mg P.O. up to 1 hour before chemotherapy and repeated 12 hours later. Or, for adults, 2 mg P.O. daily given up to 1 hour before chemotherapy.

➲ To prevent nausea and vomiting from radiation, including total body irradiation and fractionated abdominal radiation
Adults: 2 mg P.O. once daily within 1 hour of radiation.

➲ Postoperative nausea and vomiting
Adults: 1 mg I.V. undiluted and given over 30 seconds. For prevention, give before anesthesia induction or immediately before reversal.

Contraindications & cautions

• Contraindicated in patients hypersensitive to drug.

Adverse reactions

CNS: *headache, asthenia, fever,* somnolence, dizziness, anxiety, agitation, CNS stimulation, insomnia.
CV: hypertension, hypotension, ***bradycardia***.
GI: diarrhea, *constipation,* abdominal pain, *nausea, vomiting,* decreased appetite, taste disorder, flatulence, dyspepsia.
GU: UTI, oliguria.
Hematologic: ***leukopenia****, anemia,* ***thrombocytopenia, leukocytosis***.
Respiratory: cough, increased sputum.
Skin: alopecia rash dermatitis.
Other: ***hypersensitivity reactions (anaphylaxis, urticaria, dyspnea, hypotension)****, pain,* infection.

Interactions

Drug-herb. *Horehound:* May enhance serotoninergic effects. Discourage use together.

Nursing considerations

• Drug regimen is given only on days when chemotherapy is given. Treatment at other times hasn't been found useful.
!! ALERT Don't mix with other drugs; data regarding compatibility are limited.

Patient teaching

• Stress importance of taking second dose of oral drug 12 hours after the first for maximum effectiveness.
• Tell patient to report adverse reactions immediately.

guaifenesin (glyceryl guaiacolate)
Allfen Jr, Anti-Tuss ◇ *, Ganidin NR, Guiatuss ◇ *, Hytuss ◇, Hytuss 2X ◇, Mucinex ◇, Naldecon Senior EX ◇, Robitussin ◇ *, Scot-Tussin Expectorant ◇

Pregnancy risk category C

Indications & dosages

➲ Expectorant
Adults and children age 12 and older: 200 to 400 mg P.O. q 4 hours, or 600 to 1,200 mg extended-release capsules or tablets q 12 hours. Maximum, 2,400 mg daily.
Children ages 6 to 11: 100 to 200 mg P.O. q 4 hours. Maximum, 1,200 mg daily.
Children ages 2 to 5: 50 to 100 mg P.O. q 4 hours. Maximum, 600 mg daily.

Contraindications & cautions

• Contraindicated in patients hypersensitive to drug.

Adverse reactions

CNS: dizziness, headache.
GI: vomiting, nausea.
Skin: rash.

Interactions

None significant.

Nursing considerations

• Drug is used to liquefy thick, tenacious sputum. Evidence suggests that guaifenesin is effective as an expectorant, but no evidence exists to support its role as an antitussive.

- Monitor cough type and frequency.

!!ALERT Don't confuse guaifenesin with guanfacine.

Patient teaching

!!ALERT Make sure patient understands that persistent cough may indicate a serious condition and that he should contact his prescriber if cough lasts longer than 1 week, recurs frequently, or is accompanied by high fever, rash, or severe headache.

- Inform patient that drug shouldn't be used for chronic or persistent cough, such as with smoking, asthma, chronic bronchitis, or emphysema.
- Advise patient to take each dose with one glass of water; increasing fluid intake may prove beneficial.
- Encourage deep-breathing exercises.

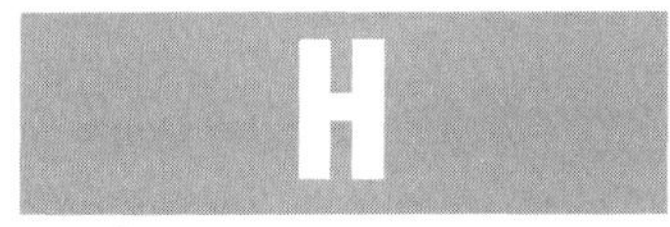

Haemophilus b conjugate vaccines

Haemophilus b conjugate vaccine, diphtheria CRM_{197} protein conjugate (HbOC)
HibTITER

Haemophilus b conjugate vaccine, diphtheria toxoid conjugate (PRP-D)
Prohibit

Haemophilus b conjugate vaccine, meningococcal protein conjugate (PRP-OMP)
Pedvaxhib

Haemophilus b conjugate, tetanus toxoid conjugate (PRP-T)
ActHIB

Pregnancy risk category C

Indications & dosages

➲ Immunization against HIB infection

Conjugate vaccine, diphtheria CRM_{197} protein conjugate

Infants: 0.5 ml I.M. at age 2 months. Repeat at 4 months and 6 months. Give booster dose at age 15 months.

Previously unvaccinated children ages 15 months to 6 years: 0.5 ml I.M. Booster dose isn't needed.

Previously unvaccinated infants ages 12 to 14 months: 0.5 ml I.M. Give booster dose at age 15 months (but no sooner than 2 months after first vaccination).

Previously unvaccinated infants ages 7 to 11 months: 0.5 ml I.M. Repeat in 2 months, for a total of two doses. Give booster dose at age 15 months (but no sooner than 2 months after last vaccination).

Previously unvaccinated infants ages 2 to 6 months: 0.5 ml I.M. Repeat in 2 months and again in 4 months for total of three doses. Give booster at age 15 months.

Conjugate vaccine, diphtheria toxoid conjugate

Previously unvaccinated children ages 15 to 71 months: 0.5 ml I.M. Booster dose isn't needed.

Conjugate vaccine, meningococcal protein conjugate

Infants: 0.5 ml I.M. at age 2 months; repeat at age 4 months. Give booster dose at age 12 months.

Previously unvaccinated children ages 15 months to 6 years: 0.5 ml I.M. Booster dose isn't needed.

Premature infants follow same schedule as full-term infants.

Previously unvaccinated infants ages 12 to 14 months: 0.5 ml I.M. Give booster dose at age 15 months (but no sooner than 2 months after first vaccination).

Previously unvaccinated infants ages 7 to 11 months: 0.5 ml I.M.; repeat in 2 months. Give booster dose at age 15 months (but no sooner than 2 months after last vaccination).

Previously unvaccinated infants ages 2 to 6 months: 0.5 ml I.M.; repeat in 2 months. Give booster dose at age 12 months.

Conjugate vaccine, tetanus toxoid conjugate

Infants: 0.5 ml I.M. at age 2 months. Repeat at ages 4 months and 6 months. Give booster doses at ages 15 to 18 months.

Previously unvaccinated infants ages 7 to 11 months: 0.5 ml I.M. Repeat in 2 months, for a total of two doses. Give booster doses at ages 15 to 18 months.

Previously unvaccinated infants ages 12 to 14 months: 0.5 ml I.M. Repeat in 2 months, for a total of two doses.

Contraindications & cautions

- Contraindicated in patients hypersensitive to vaccine or its components and in those with acute illness.

Adverse reactions

CNS: fever.
GI: diarrhea, vomiting.
Skin: *erythema, pain at injection site.*
Other: ***anaphylaxis***, crying.

Interactions

Drug-drug. *Immunosuppressants:* May suppress antibody response to HIB vaccine. Postpone immunization.

Nursing considerations

- HIB is an important cause of meningitis in infants and preschool children.
- Immunization against HIB infection is recommended for children with HIV infections. Follow usual immunization schedule.
- Vaccine and DTP may be given simultaneously. A combination product is commercially available.
- Diphtheria toxoid conjugate vaccine (Prohibit) isn't recommended in children younger than age 15 months.
- Vaccine isn't routinely given to adults or children older than age 5 unless they're at high risk for infection (including patients with chronic conditions, such as functional asplenia, splenectomy, Hodgkin's disease, or sickle cell anemia).
- ActHIB reconstituted with diphtheria and tetanus toxoids and acellular pertussis vaccine adsorbed (DTaP; Tripedia) provides a combination containing antigens to diphtheria, tetanus, pertussis, and haemophilus b (TriHIBit). This combination can be used in children ages 15 to 18 months requiring both a fourth dose of DTaP and *Haemophilus* b vaccine. Don't use this combination for the first three primary doses or in children younger than age 15 months. Refer to manufacturer's instructions to reconstitute ActHIB with Tripedia.
- Keep epinephrine 1:1,000 available to treat anaphylaxis.
- Don't give vaccine I.D. or I.V.; give it only I.M.

!!ALERT Don't give to febrile children.

- Give vaccine into anterolateral aspect of upper thigh in small children. Injections may be made into deltoid muscle of larger children if sufficient muscle is present.
- Drug may interfere with interpretation of antigen detection tests used to diagnose systemic HIB disease.

Patient teaching

- Warn patient or parents that pain may occur at injection site.
- Tell patient or parents to notify prescriber if adverse reactions persist or become severe.

halcinonide

Halog, Halog-E

Pregnancy risk category C

Indications & dosages

➲ Inflammation from dermatoses responsive to corticosteroids

Adults and children: Clean area; apply cream, ointment, or topical solution sparingly b.i.d. or t.i.d. Rub cream in gently.

Contraindications & cautions

- Contraindicated in patients hypersensitive to drug or its components.

Adverse reactions

GU: glycosuria.
Metabolic: hyperglycemia.
Skin: burning, pruritus, irritation, dryness, erythema, folliculitis, hypertrichosis, hypopigmentation, acneiform eruptions, allergic contact dermatitis, *atrophy, maceration, secondary infection, striae, miliaria with occlusive dressings.*

Other: *hypothalamic-pituitary-adrenal axis suppression*, Cushing's syndrome.

Interactions

None significant.

Nursing considerations

- Gently wash skin before applying. To prevent skin damage, rub in gently, leaving a thin coat. When treating hairy sites, part hair and apply directly to lesions.
- Avoid applying near eyes or mucous membranes or in ear canal, axillae, groin, or rectal area.
- Gently rub small amount of cream into lesion until it disappears. Reapply, leaving a thin coating on lesion, and cover with occlusive dressing, if ordered. Don't leave dressing in place for longer than 12 hours each day.
- Don't use occlusive dressings on infected or exudative lesions.
- For patients with eczematous dermatitis whose skin may be irritated by adhesive material, hold dressing in place with gauze, stockings, or stockinette.
- Stop drug and tell prescriber if skin infection, striae, or atrophy occurs.
- Good results have been obtained by applying occlusive dressings in the evening and removing them in the morning, providing 12-hour occlusion. Then reapply drug; don't apply occlusive dressings during the day.
- If an occlusive dressing has been applied and a fever develops, notify prescriber and remove dressing.
- If antifungal or antibiotic combined with corticosteroid fails to provide prompt improvement, stop corticosteroid until infection is controlled.
- Systemic absorption is especially likely with use of occlusive dressings, prolonged treatment, or extensive body surface treatment. Watch for symptoms, such as hyperglycemia, glycosuria, and hypothalamic-pituitary-adrenal axis suppression.
- Avoid using plastic pants or tight-fitting diapers on treated areas in young children. Children may absorb larger amounts of drug and be more susceptible to systemic toxicity.
- Continue treatment for a few days after lesions clear.

Patient teaching

- Teach patient how to apply drug.
- If an occlusive dressing is ordered, advise patient to leave it in place for no longer than 12 hours each day and not to use the dressing on infected or weeping lesions.
- Tell patient to stop drug and report signs of systemic absorption, skin irritation or ulceration, hypersensitivity, or infection.

haloperidol

Apo-Haloperidol†, Haldol, Novo-Peridol†, Peridol†

haloperidol decanoate

Haldol Decanoate, Haldol LA†

haloperidol lactate

Haldol, Haldol Concentrate, Haloperidol Intensol

Pregnancy risk category C

Indications & dosages

➲ Psychotic disorders

Adults and children older than age 12: Dosage varies for each patient. Initially, 0.5 to 5 mg P.O. b.i.d. or t.i.d. Or, 2 to 5 mg I.M. haldol lactate q 4 to 8 hours, although hourly administration may be needed until control is obtained. Maximum, 100 mg P.O. daily.

Children ages 3 to 12 weighing 15 to 40 kg (33 to 88 lb): Initially, 0.5 mg P.O. daily divided b.i.d. or t.i.d. May increase dose by 0.5 mg at 5- to 7-day intervals, depending on therapeutic response and patient tolerance. Maintenance dose, 0.05 mg/kg to 0.15 mg/kg P.O. daily given in two to three divided doses. Severely disturbed children may need higher doses.

➲ Chronic psychosis requiring prolonged therapy

Adults: 50 to 100 mg I.M. haloperidol decanoate q 4 weeks.

➲ Nonpsychotic behavior disorders

Children ages 3 to 12: 0.05 to 0.075 mg/kg P.O. daily, in two or three divided doses. Maximum, 6 mg daily.

➲ Tourette syndrome

Adults: 0.5 to 5 mg P.O. b.i.d., t.i.d., or p.r.n.
Children ages 3 to 12: 0.05 to 0.075 mg/kg P.O. daily, in two or three divided doses.

Elderly patients: 0.5 to 2 mg P.O. b.i.d. or t.i.d.; increase gradually, p.r.n.

For debilitated patients, initially, 0.5 to 2 mg P.O. b.i.d. or t.i.d.; increase gradually, p.r.n.

Contraindications & cautions

- Contraindicated in patients hypersensitive to drug and in those with parkinsonism, coma, or CNS depression.
- Use cautiously in elderly and debilitated patients; in patients with history of seizures or EEG abnormalities, severe CV disorders, allergies, glaucoma, or urine retention; and in those taking anticonvulsants, anticoagulants, antiparkinsonians, or lithium.

Adverse reactions

CNS: *severe extrapyramidal reactions, tardive dyskinesia,* sedation, drowsiness, lethargy, headache, insomnia, confusion, vertigo, ***seizures, neuroleptic malignant syndrome.***
CV: tachycardia, hypotension, hypertension, ECG changes, ***torsades de pointes,*** with I.V. use.
EENT: blurred vision.
GI: dry mouth, anorexia, constipation, diarrhea, nausea, vomiting, dyspepsia.
GU: urine retention, menstrual irregularities, priapism.
Hematologic: ***leukopenia,*** leukocytosis.
Hepatic: jaundice.
Skin: rash, other skin reactions, diaphoresis.
Other: gynecomastia.

Interactions

Drug-drug. *Anticholinergics:* May increase anticholinergic effects and glaucoma. Use together cautiously.
Azole antifungals, buspirone, macrolides: May increase haloperidol level. Monitor patient for increased adverse reactions; haloperidol dose may need to be adjusted.
Carbamazepine: May decrease haloperidol level. Monitor patient.
CNS depressants: May increase CNS depression. Use together cautiously.
Lithium: May cause lethargy and confusion after high doses. Monitor patient.
Methyldopa: May cause dementia. Monitor patient closely.
Rifampin: May decrease haloperidol level. Monitor patient for clinical effect.
Drug-lifestyle. *Alcohol use:* May increase CNS depression. Discourage use together.

Nursing considerations

- Protect drug from light. Slight yellowing of injection or concentrate is common and doesn't affect potency. Discard markedly discolored solutions.
- When switching from tablets to decanoate injection, give 10 to 15 times the oral dose once a month (maximum 100 mg).
- Dilute oral dose with water or a beverage, such as orange juice, apple juice, tomato juice, or cola, immediately before administration.

!!ALERT Don't give decanoate form I.V.

- Monitor patient for tardive dyskinesia, which may occur after prolonged use. It may not appear until months or years later and may disappear spontaneously or persist for life, despite ending drug.

!!ALERT Watch for signs and symptoms of neuroleptic malignant syndrome (extrapyramidal effects, hyperthermia, autonomic disturbance), which is rare but commonly fatal. It may not be related to length of drug use or type of neuroleptic; more than 60% of affected patients are men.

- Don't withdraw drug abruptly unless required by severe adverse reactions.

!!ALERT Haldol may contain tartrazine.

!!ALERT Don't confuse Haldol with Halcion or Halog.

Patient teaching

- Although drug is the least sedating of the antipsychotics, warn patient to avoid activities that require alertness and good coordination until effects of drug are known. Drowsiness and dizziness usually subside after a few weeks.
- Warn patient to avoid alcohol while taking drug.
- Tell patient to relieve dry mouth with sugarless gum or hard candy.

heparin calcium

heparin sodium

Hepalean†, Heparin Leo†, Heparin Lock Flush Solution (with Tubex), Heparin Sodium Injection, Hep-Lock, Hep-Pak

Pregnancy risk category C

Indications & dosages

➲ Full-dose continuous I.V. infusion therapy for DVT, MI, pulmonary embolism
Adults: Initially, 5,000 units by I.V. bolus; then 750 to 1,500 units/hour by I.V. infusion with pump. Titrate hourly rate based on PTT results (q 4 to 6 hours in the early stages of treatment).
Children: Initially, 50 units/kg I.V.; then 25 units/kg/hour or 20,000 units/m^2 daily by I.V. infusion pump. Titrate dosage based on PTT.

➲ Full-dose S.C. therapy for DVT, MI, pulmonary embolism
Adults: Initially, 5,000 units I.V. bolus and 10,000 to 20,000 units in a concentrated solution S.C.; then 8,000 to 10,000 units S.C. q 8 hours or 15,000 to 20,000 units in a concentrated solution q 12 hours.

➲ Full-dose intermittent I.V. therapy for DVT, MI, pulmonary embolism
Adults: Initially, 10,000 units by I.V. bolus; then titrated according to PTT, and 5,000 to 10,000 units I.V. q 4 to 6 hours.
Children: Initially, 100 units/kg by I.V. bolus; then 50 to 100 units/kg q 4 hours.

➲ Fixed low-dose therapy for venous thrombosis, pulmonary embolism, atrial fibrillation with embolism, postoperative DVT, and prevention of embolism
Adults: 5,000 units S.C. q 12 hours. In surgical patients, give first dose 1 to 2 hours before procedure; then 5,000 units S.C. q 8 to 12 hours for 5 to 7 days or until patient can walk.

➲ Consumptive coagulopathy (such as disseminated intravascular coagulation)
Adults: 50 to 100 units/kg by I.V. bolus or continuous I.V. infusion q 4 hours.
Children: 25 to 50 units/kg by I.V. bolus or continuous I.V. infusion every 4 hours. If no improvement within 4 to 8 hours, stop heparin.

➲ Open-heart surgery
Adults: For total body perfusion, 150 to 400 units/kg continuous I.V. infusion.

➲ Patency maintenance of I.V. indwelling catheters
Adults: 10 to 100 units I.V. flush. Use sufficient volume to fill device. Not intended for therapeutic use.

Contraindications & cautions

- Contraindicated in patients hypersensitive to drug. Conditionally contraindicated in patients with active bleeding, blood dyscrasia, or bleeding tendencies, such as hemophilia, thrombocytopenia, or hepatic disease with hypoprothrombinemia; suspected intracranial hemorrhage; suppurative thrombophlebitis; inaccessible ulcerative lesions (especially of GI tract) and open ulcerative wounds; extensive denudation of skin; ascorbic acid deficiency and other conditions that cause increased capillary permeability.
- Conditionally contraindicated during or after brain, eye, or spinal cord surgery; during spinal tap or spinal anesthesia; during continuous tube drainage of stomach or small intestine; and in subacute bacterial endocarditis, shock, advanced renal disease, threatened abortion, or severe hypertension.
- Use cautiously in women during menses or after childbirth and in patients with mild hepatic or renal disease, alcoholism, occupations with high risk of physical injury, or history of allergies, asthma, or GI ulcerations.

Adverse reactions

CNS: fever.
EENT: rhinitis.
Hematologic: ***hemorrhage, overly prolonged clotting time, thrombocytopenia.***
Skin: irritation, mild pain, hematoma, ulceration, cutaneous or S.C. necrosis, pruritus, urticaria.
Other: ***white clot syndrome;*** hypersensitivity reactions, including chills; ***anaphylactoid reactions.***

Interactions

Drug-drug. *Aspirin:* May increase risk of bleeding. Monitor coagulation studies and patient closely.
Oral anticoagulants: May increase additive anticoagulation. Monitor PT, INR, and PTT.

Salicylates, other antiplatelet drugs: May increase anticoagulant effect. Avoid using together.
Thrombolytics: May increase risk of hemorrhage. Monitor patient closely.
Drug-herb. *Garlic, ginkgo, motherwort, red clover, white willow:* May increase risk of bleeding. Discourage use together.

Nursing considerations

- Although heparin use is clearly hazardous in certain conditions, its risks and benefits must be evaluated.
- Draw blood to establish baseline coagulation parameters before therapy.
- When patient needs anticoagulation during pregnancy, most prescribers use heparin.
- Some commercially available heparin injections contain benzyl alcohol. Avoid using these products in neonates and pregnant women if possible.
- Drug requirements are higher in early phases of thrombogenic diseases and febrile states; they are lower when patient's condition stabilizes.
- Elderly patients should usually start at lower dosage.
- Check order and vial carefully; heparin comes in various concentrations.

!!ALERT USP units and IU aren't equivalent for heparin.
!!ALERT Heparin, low-molecular-weight heparins, and danaparoid aren't interchangeable.
!!ALERT Don't change concentrations of infusions unless absolutely necessary. This is a common source of dosage errors.

- Give low-dose injections sequentially between iliac crests in lower abdomen deep into S.C. fat. Inject drug S.C. slowly into fat pad. Leave needle in place for 10 seconds after injection; then withdraw needle. Don't massage after S.C. injection, and watch for signs of bleeding at injection site. Alternate sites every 12 hours—right for morning, left for evening.
- Draw blood for PTT 4 to 6 hours after dose given by S.C. injection.
- Avoid excessive I.M. injections of other drugs to prevent or minimize hematomas. If possible, don't give I.M. injections at all.
- Measure PTT carefully and regularly. Anticoagulation is present when PTT values are 1½ to 2 times the control values.
- Monitor platelet count regularly. When new thrombosis accompanies thrombocytopenia (white clot syndrome), stop heparin.
- Regularly inspect patient for bleeding gums, bruises on arms or legs, petechiae, nosebleeds, melena, tarry stools, hematuria, and hematemesis.
- Monitor vital signs.

!!ALERT To treat severe heparin calcium or sodium overdose, use protamine sulfate, a heparin antagonist. Dosage is based on the dose of heparin, its route of administration, and the time since it was given. Generally, 1 to 1.5 mg of protamine/100 units of heparin is given if only a few minutes have elapsed; 0.5 to 0.75 mg protamine/100 units heparin, if 30 to 60 minutes have elapsed; and 0.25 to 0.375 mg protamine/100 units heparin, if 2 hours or more have elapsed. Don't give more than 50 mg protamine in a 10-minute period.

- Abrupt withdrawal may cause increased coagulability; warfarin therapy usually overlaps heparin therapy for continuation of prophylaxis or treatment.

Patient teaching

- Instruct patient and family to watch for signs of bleeding or bruising and to notify prescriber immediately if any occur.
- Tell patient to avoid OTC drugs containing aspirin, other salicylates, or drugs that may interact with heparin unless ordered by prescriber.

hepatitis A vaccine, inactivated

Havrix, Vaqta

Pregnancy risk category C

Indications & dosages

➲ Active immunization against hepatitis A virus
Adults: 1,440 ELU Havrix or 50 units Vaqta I.M. as single dose. For booster dose, give 1,440 ELU Havrix 6 to 12 months after first dose or 50 units Vaqta I.M. 6 to 18 months after first dose. Booster is recommended for prolonged immunity.
Children ages 2 to 18: 720 ELU Havrix or 25 units Vaqta I.M. as single dose. Then, give booster dose of 720 ELU Havrix 6 to 12 months after first dose or 25 units Vaqta

I.M. 6 to 18 months after first dose. Booster is recommended for prolonged immunity.

➲ **To prevent hepatitis A in patients who are or will be at high risk of exposure to hepatitis A, or to prevent or control hepatitis A outbreaks in intermediate- to high-risk populations**

Adults: 1,440 ELU Havrix I.M. or 50 units Vaqta I.M. as single dose. For booster dose, give 1,440 ELU Havrix I.M. 6 to 12 months after first dose or 50 units Vaqta I.M. 6 to 18 months after first dose. Booster is recommended for prolonged immunity.

Children ages 2 to 18: 720 ELU Havrix or 25 units Vaqta I.M. as single dose. Then, give booster dose of 720 ELU Havrix I.M. 6 to 12 months after first dose or 25 units Vaqta I.M. 6 to 18 months after first dose. Booster is recommended for prolonged immunity.

Contraindications & cautions

- Contraindicated in patients hypersensitive to vaccine's components.
- Use cautiously in patients with thrombocytopenia or bleeding disorders and in those who are taking an anticoagulant because bleeding may occur after an I.M. injection.

Adverse reactions

CNS: hypertonia, insomnia, *fever*, vertigo, *headache*, *fatigue*, *malaise*, ***seizures***, encephalopathy, dizziness.
EENT: pharyngitis, photophobia.
GI: *anorexia*, *nausea*, abdominal pain, diarrhea, dysgeusia, vomiting.
GU: menstrual disorders.
Musculoskeletal: arthralgia, myalgia.
Respiratory: upper respiratory tract infections.
Skin: pruritus, rash, urticaria, *induration*, *redness*, *swelling*, hematoma, *injection site soreness*, jaundice.
Other: lymphadenopathy, ***anaphylaxis***.

Interactions

Drug-drug. *Anticoagulants:* May increase risk of bleeding. Give I.M. injection cautiously.
Immunosuppressants: May suppress antibody response in patients receiving immunosuppressive therapy. Monitor patient.

Nursing considerations

- As with other vaccines, postpone hepatitis A vaccination, if possible, in patient with febrile illness.
- Keep epinephrine 1:1,000 available to treat anaphylaxis.
- If vaccine is given to immunosuppressed persons or those receiving immunosuppressants, expected immune response may not occur.
- Persons who should receive vaccine include people traveling to or living in areas endemic for hepatitis A (Africa, Asia [except Japan], the Mediterranean basin, Eastern Europe, the Middle East, Central and South America, Mexico, and parts of the Caribbean), military personnel, Native Americans and Alaskans, persons engaging in high-risk sexual activity, and users of illegal injectable drugs. Certain institutional workers, employees of child day-care centers, laboratory workers who handle live hepatitis A virus, and primate handlers also may benefit.
- For I.M. use, shake vial or syringe well before withdrawal. After it has been agitated thoroughly, vaccine is an opaque white suspension. Discard if it appears otherwise. No dilution or reconstitution is needed.
- Give as I.M. injection into the deltoid region in adults. Don't give in gluteal region; such injections may result in suboptimal response. Never inject I.V., S.C., or I.D.

Patient teaching

- Inform patient that vaccine won't prevent hepatitis caused by other drugs or pathogens known to infect the liver.
- Warn patient about local adverse reactions. Tell him to report persistent or severe reactions promptly.
- Alert travelers to dangers of eating raw or undercooked shellfish or consuming food or drink in countries with poor hygienic conditions.
- Remind patient to return for second injection 6 to 12 months after the first.

hepatitis B immune globulin, human
BayHep B, Nabi-HB

Pregnancy risk category C

Indications & dosages
➲ Hepatitis B exposure in high-risk patients
Adults and children: 0.06 ml/kg (usual dose is 3 ml to 5 ml) I.M. within 7 days after exposure. Repeat dose 28 days after exposure if patient doesn't elect to receive the hepatitis B vaccine.
Neonates born to hepatitis B surface antigen (HBsAg)–positive patients: 0.5 ml I.M. within 12 hours of birth.

Contraindications & cautions
- Contraindicated in patients with history of anaphylactic reactions to immune serum.
- Give to patients with coagulation disorders or thrombocytopenia only if benefit outweighs risk.

Adverse reactions
Skin: urticaria, *pain and tenderness at injection site.*
Other: ***anaphylaxis, angioedema.***

Interactions
Drug-drug. *Live-virus vaccines:* May interfere with response to live-virus vaccines. Postpone routine immunization for 3 months.

Nursing considerations
- Obtain history of allergies and reactions to immunizations. Keep epinephrine 1:1,000 available.
- Inspect for discoloration or particulates. Make sure drug is clear, slightly amber, and moderately viscous.
- Inject into anterolateral thigh or deltoid muscle in older children and adults; inject into anterolateral thigh in neonates and children younger than age 3.
- For postexposure prophylaxis (such as after needlestick or direct contact), drug should be given with hepatitis B vaccine.

!!ALERT This immune globulin provides passive immunity; don't confuse with hepatitis B vaccine. Both drugs may be given at same time. Don't mix in the same syringe.

!!ALERT Don't confuse HyperHep with Hyperstat or Hyper-Tet.

Patient teaching
- Inform patient that pain and tenderness may occur at injection site.
- Tell patient to report signs and symptoms of hypersensitivity immediately.

hepatitis B vaccine, recombinant
Engerix-B, Recombivax HB, Recombivax HB Dialysis Formulation

Pregnancy risk category C

Indications & dosages
➲ Immunization against infection from all known subtypes of hepatitis B virus (HBV), primary preexposure prophylaxis against HBV, postexposure prophylaxis (when given with hepatitis B immune globulin)
Engerix-B
Adults age 20 and older: Initially, 20 mcg I.M.; then second dose of 20 mcg I.M. after 30 days. A third dose of 20 mcg I.M. is given 6 months after the first dose.

For adults undergoing dialysis or receiving immunosuppressants, initially, 40 mcg I.M. (divided into two 20-mcg doses and given at different sites). Then second dose of 40 mcg I.M. in 30 days, a third dose after 2 months, and final dose of 40 mcg I.M. 6 months after first dose.
Adolescents ages 11 to 19: Initially, 10 mcg (pediatric and adolescent formulation) I.M.; then second dose of 10 mcg I.M. 30 days later. Give third dose of 10 mcg I.M. 6 months after first dose. Or, 20 mcg (adult formulation) I.M.; then second dose of 20 mcg I.M. 30 days later. Give third dose of 20 mcg I.M. 6 months after first dose.
Neonates and children up to age 10: Initially, 10 mcg I.M.; then second dose of 10 mcg I.M. 30 days later. Give third dose of 10 mcg I.M. 6 months after first dose.
Recombivax HB
Adults age 20 and older: Initially, 10 mcg I.M.; then second dose of 10 mcg I.M. after 30 days. Give third dose of 10 mcg I.M. 6 months after first dose.

For adults undergoing dialysis, initially, 40 mcg I.M. (use dialysis formulation, which contains 40 mcg/ml); then second

dose of 40 mcg I.M. in 30 days, and final dose of 40 mcg I.M. 6 months after first dose. A booster or revaccination may be indicated if anti-HBs level is below 10 mIU/ml 1 to 2 months after third dose.
Infants, children, and adolescents from birth to age 19: Initially, 5 mcg I.M.; then second dose of 5 mcg I.M. after 30 days. Give third dose of 5 mcg I.M. 6 months after first dose. Or, in adolescents ages 11 to 15, give 10 mcg (1 ml adult formulation) I.M.; then second dose of 10 mcg 4 to 6 months later.
Infants born of HBsAg-positive mothers or mothers of unknown HbsAg status: Initially, 5 mcg I.M.; then second dose of 5 mcg I.M. after 30 days. Give third dose of 5 mcg I.M. 6 months after first dose.
Infants born of HBsAg-negative mothers: Initially, 5 mcg I.M.; then second dose of 5 mcg I.M. after 30 days. Give third dose of 5 mcg I.M. 6 months after first dose *Note*: If the mother is found to be HbsAg-positive within 7 days of delivery, also give the infant a dose of HBIG (0.5 ml) in the opposite anterolateral thigh.

➲ **Chronic hepatitis C infection**
Engerix-B
Adults: Initially, 20 mcg I.M.; then second dose of 20 mcg I.M. after 30 days. Give third dose of 20 mcg I.M. 6 months after first dose.

Contraindications & cautions

- Contraindicated in patients hypersensitive to yeast or components of vaccine; recombinant vaccines are derived from yeast cultures.
- Use cautiously in patients with serious, active infections or compromised cardiac or pulmonary status and in those for whom a febrile or systemic reaction could pose a risk.

Adverse reactions

CNS: headache, fever, dizziness, insomnia, paresthesia, neuropathy, transient malaise.
EENT: pharyngitis.
GI: anorexia, diarrhea, nausea, vomiting.
Musculoskeletal: myalgia, arthralgia, neck stiffness.
Skin: local inflammation, *soreness at injection site*, pruritus.
Other: ***anaphylaxis***, slight flulike syndrome.

Interactions

Drug-drug. *Immunosuppressants:* May decrease circulating antibody level. May need to increase doses of hepatitis B vaccine (recombinant).

Nursing considerations

- The American Academy of Pediatrics recommends hepatitis B vaccination for all neonates and encourages immunization for adolescents when resources allow.
- The Recombivax HB vaccine pediatric and adolescent formulation without preservatives may be used for persons for whom a thimerosal-free vaccine is recommended (such as infants up to age 6 months who may receive other vaccines containing thimerosal).
- Certain populations (neonates born to infected mothers, persons recently exposed to virus, and travelers to high-risk areas) may receive the four-dose regimen because it can induce immunity more quickly.
- Certain people are at increased risk for infection and should be considered for vaccine, including health care personnel (especially those working with dialysis patients, with high-risk patients and patient contacts who may be infected, in blood banks, in emergency medicine, or among populations in which infection is endemic [Indo-Chinese, native peoples of Alaska, and Haitian refugees]), certain military personnel, morticians and embalmers, sexually active homosexual men, prostitutes, prisoners, and users of illegal injectable drugs.
- Although anaphylaxis hasn't been reported, always keep epinephrine available when giving vaccine to counteract possible reaction.
- Thoroughly agitate vial just before giving to restore suspension.
- Inspect product for particulates or discoloration before giving. Make sure product is a slightly opaque white suspension. Discard if it appears otherwise.
- Give vaccine in deltoid muscle for adults and adolescents; give in anterolateral aspect of thigh for infants and young children. Never give I.V.
- Give S.C. in patients at risk for hemorrhage, such as hemophiliacs. Otherwise, don't use this route; it may lead to an increased occurrence or severity of local reactions.

• Recombinant hepatitis B vaccine isn't made with human plasma products.

Patient teaching

• Warn patient or parents about local adverse reactions, such as swelling or redness at injection site. Tell patient to report persistent or severe reactions promptly.
• Review immunization schedule with patient or parents; stress importance of completing series.

high–molecular-weight hyaluronan
Orthovisc

Pregnancy risk category NR

Indications & dosages

➲ To reduce pain caused by osteoarthritis of the knee in patients who haven't responded to nondrug therapy or simple analgesics
Adults: Intra-articular injection (one syringe) into affected knee once weekly for a total of three to four injections.

Contraindications & cautions

• Contraindicated in patients allergic to hyaluronate preparations, birds, eggs, feathers, and poultry. Also contraindicated in patients with infection or skin disease in area of injection site or joint.

Adverse reactions

CNS: *headache*, pain.
Musculoskeletal: *arthralgia*, back pain, bursitis.
Other: injection site pain.

Interactions

Drug-drug. *Skin preparation disinfectants that contain quaternary ammonium salts:* May cause hyaluronan to precipitate. Avoid using together.

Nursing considerations

• Drug should be given by staff trained in intra-articular administration.
• Remove joint effusion before injecting drug.
• Use an 18G to 21G needle. Using strict aseptic technique, inject contents of one syringe into one knee; if needed, use a second syringe for the second knee.
• Pain may not be relieved until after the third injection.
• Don't give less than three injections in a treatment cycle.
• Use of drug for more than one treatment cycle or in joints other than the knee haven't been studied.
• Inflammation may increase briefly in affected knee in patients with inflammatory osteoarthritis.
• Don't use drug if original package is open or damaged. Give drug immediately after opening. Store in original package at room temperature lower than 77° F (25° C); don't freeze. Discard unused drug.

Patient teaching

• Tell patient that pain and inflammation may increase briefly after the injection.
• Urge patient to avoid strenuous activity or prolonged (more than 1 hour) weight-bearing activity, such as in running or tennis, within 48 hours after the injection.
• Tell patient to report injection site reactions, such as pain, swelling, itching, heat, rash, bruising, or redness.
• Inform patient that a treatment cycle includes at least three injections and that pain may not be relieved until after the third injection.
• Caution patient to report planned or suspected pregnancy.

hydralazine hydrochloride
Apresoline, Novo-Hylazin†, Supres†

Pregnancy risk category C

Indications & dosages

➲ Essential hypertension (orally, alone, or with other antihypertensives), severe essential hypertension (parenterally, to lower blood pressure quickly)
Adults: Initially, 10 mg P.O. q.i.d.; gradually increased to 50 mg q.i.d., p.r.n. Maximum recommended dose is 200 mg daily, but some patients may need 300 to 400 mg daily.

Or, give 10 to 20 mg I.V. slowly, and repeat p.r.n.; switch to oral form as soon as possible.

Or, give 10 to 50 mg I.M., and repeat p.r.n.; switch to oral form as soon as possible.

Children: Initially, 0.75 mg/kg daily P.O. divided into four doses; gradually increased over 3 to 4 weeks to maximum of 7.5 mg/kg or 200 mg daily. Maximum first P.O. dose is 25 mg.

Or, 0.1 to 0.2 mg/kg I.V. q 4 to 6 hours, p.r.n. Maximum first parenteral dose is 20 mg.

➲ **Preeclampsia, eclampsia**

Adults: Initially, 5 to 10 mg I.V., followed by 5- to 10-mg I.V. doses (range 5 to 20 mg) q 20 to 30 minutes, p.r.n. Or, 0.5 to 10 mg/hour I.V. infusion.

➲ **Heart failure♦**

Adults: Initially, 50 to 75 mg P.O. daily. Maintenance doses range from 200 to 600 mg P.O. daily in divided doses q 6 to 12 hours.

Contraindications & cautions

- Contraindicated in patients hypersensitive to drug
- Contraindicated in those with coronary artery disease or mitral valvular rheumatic heart disease.
- Use cautiously in patients with suspected cardiac disease, CVA, or severe renal impairment and in those taking other antihypertensives.

Adverse reactions

CNS: peripheral neuritis, *headache*, dizziness.
CV: orthostatic hypotension, *tachycardia*, edema, *angina pectoris, palpitations*.
EENT: nasal congestion.
GI: *nausea, vomiting, diarrhea, anorexia*, constipation.
Hematologic: ***neutropenia*, *leukopenia*, *agranulocytopenia*, *agranulocytosis*, *thrombocytopenia with or without purpura***.
Skin: rash.
Other: *lupuslike syndrome*.

Interactions

Drug-drug. *Diazoxide, MAO inhibitors:* May cause severe hypotension. Use together cautiously.
Diuretics, other hypotensive drugs: May cause excessive hypotension. Dosage adjustment may be needed.
Indomethacin: May decrease effects of hydralazine. Monitor blood pressure.
Metoprolol, propranolol: May increase levels and effects of these beta blockers. Monitor patient closely. May need to adjust dosage of either drug.

Nursing considerations

- Monitor patient's blood pressure, pulse rate, and body weight frequently. Hydralazine may be given with diuretics and beta blockers to decrease sodium retention and tachycardia and to prevent angina attacks.
- Elderly patients may be more sensitive to drug's hypotensive effects.
- Monitor CBC, lupus erythematosus cell preparation, and antinuclear antibody titer determination before therapy and periodically during long-term therapy.

!! ALERT Monitor patient closely for signs and symptoms of lupuslike syndrome (sore throat, fever, muscle and joint aches, rash), and notify prescriber immediately if they develop.

- Improve patient compliance by giving drug b.i.d. Check with prescriber.

!! ALERT Don't confuse hydralazine with hydroxyzine or Apresoline with Apresazide.

- Apresoline may contain tartrazine.

Patient teaching

- Instruct patient to take oral form with meals to increase absorption.
- Inform patient that low blood pressure and dizziness upon standing can be minimized by rising slowly and avoiding sudden position changes.
- Tell woman of childbearing age to notify prescriber if she suspects pregnancy. Drug will need to be stopped.
- Tell patient to notify prescriber of unexplained prolonged general tiredness or fever, muscle or joint aching, or chest pain.

hydrochlorothiazide

Apo-Hydro†, Diuchlor H†, Esidrix, Ezide, HydroDIURIL, Hydro-Par, Microzide, Neo-Codema†, Novo-Hydrazide†, Oretic, Urozide†

Pregnancy risk category B

Indications & dosages

➲ Edema

Adults: 25 to 100 mg P.O. daily or intermittently; up to 200 mg initially for several days until nonedematous weight is attained.

➲ Hypertension

Adults: 12.5 to 50 mg P.O. once daily. Increase or decrease daily dose based on blood pressure.

Children ages 2 to 12: 2.2 mg/kg or 60 mg/m² daily in two divided doses. Usual dosage range is 37.5 to 100 mg daily.

Children ages 6 months to 2 years: 2.2 mg/kg or 60 mg/m² daily in two divided doses. Usual dosage range is 12.5 to 37.5 mg daily.

Children younger than age 6 months: Up to 3.3 mg/kg P.O. daily in two divided doses.

Contraindications & cautions

- Contraindicated in patients with anuria and patients hypersensitive to other thiazides or other sulfonamide derivatives.
- Use cautiously in children and in patients with severe renal disease, impaired hepatic function, or progressive hepatic disease.

Adverse reactions

CNS: dizziness, vertigo, headache, paresthesia, weakness, restlessness.

CV: orthostatic hypotension, allergic myocarditis, vasculitis.

GI: anorexia, nausea, ***pancreatitis***, epigastric distress, vomiting, abdominal pain, diarrhea, constipation.

GU: polyuria, frequent urination, ***renal failure***, interstitial nephritis.

Hematologic: ***aplastic anemia***, ***agranulocytosis***, ***leukopenia***, ***thrombocytopenia***, hemolytic anemia.

Hepatic: jaundice.

Metabolic: asymptomatic hyperuricemia, hypokalemia, hyperglycemia and impaired glucose tolerance, fluid and electrolyte imbalances, including dilutional hyponatremia and hypochloremia, metabolic alkalosis, hypercalcemia, volume depletion and dehydration.

Musculoskeletal: muscle cramps.

Respiratory: ***respiratory distress***, pneumonitis.

Skin: dermatitis, photosensitivity reactions, rash, purpura, alopecia.

Other: hypersensitivity reactions, gout, ***anaphylactic reactions***.

Interactions

Drug-drug. *Amphotericin B, corticosteroids:* May increase risk of hypokalemia. Monitor potassium level closely.

Antidiabetics: May decrease hypoglycemic effects. Dosage adjustments may be needed. Monitor glucose level.

Antihypertensives: May have additive antihypertensive effect. Use together cautiously.

Barbiturates, opioids: May increase orthostatic hypotensive effect. Monitor patient closely.

Bumetanide, ethacrynic acid, furosemide, torsemide: May cause excessive diuretic response, causing serious electrolyte abnormalities or dehydration. Adjust doses carefully, and monitor patient closely for signs and symptoms of excessive diuretic response.

Cardiac glycosides: May increase risk of digoxin toxicity from diuretic-induced hypokalemia. Monitor potassium and digoxin levels.

Cholestyramine, colestipol: May decrease intestinal absorption of thiazides. Separate doses by 2 hours.

Diazoxide: May increase antihypertensive, hyperglycemic, and hyperuricemic effects. Use together cautiously.

Lithium: May decrease lithium excretion, increasing risk of lithium toxicity. Monitor lithium level.

NSAIDs: May increase risk of renal failure. Monitor renal function closely.

Drug-herb. *Dandelion:* May interfere with diuretic activity. Discourage use together.

Licorice: May cause unexpected rapid potassium loss. Discourage use together.

Drug-lifestyle. *Alcohol use:* May increase orthostatic hypotensive effect. Discourage use together.

Nursing considerations

- To prevent nocturia, give drug in the morning.
- Monitor fluid intake and output, weight, blood pressure, and electrolyte levels.
- Watch for signs and symptoms of hypokalemia, such as muscle weakness and cramps.
- Drug may be used with potassium-sparing diuretic to prevent potassium loss.
- Consult prescriber and dietitian about a high-potassium diet. Foods rich in potassium include citrus fruits, tomatoes, bananas, dates, and apricots.
- Monitor creatinine and BUN levels regularly. Cumulative effects of drug may occur with impaired renal function.
- Monitor uric acid level, especially in patients with history of gout.
- Monitor glucose level, especially in diabetic patients.
- Monitor elderly patients, who are especially susceptible to excessive diuresis.
- Stop thiazides and thiazide-like diuretics before parathyroid function tests.
- In patients with hypertension, therapeutic response may be delayed several weeks.

Patient teaching

- Instruct patient to take drug with food to minimize GI upset.
- Advise patient to take drug in morning to avoid need to urinate at night; if patient needs second dose, have him take it in early afternoon.
- Advise patient to avoid sudden posture changes and to rise slowly to avoid dizziness upon standing quickly.
- Encourage patient to use a sunblock to prevent photosensitivity reactions.
- Tell patient to check with prescriber or pharmacist before using OTC drugs.

hydrocortisone (systemic)
Aquacort†, Cortef, Cortenema, Hydrocortone

hydrocortisone acetate
Anucort-HC, Anusol-HC, Cortifoam, Proctocort

hydrocortisone cypionate
Cortef

hydrocortisone sodium phosphate

hydrocortisone sodium succinate
A-Hydrocort, Solu-Cortef

Pregnancy risk category C

Indications & dosages

➲ Severe inflammation, adrenal insufficiency

Adults: 5 to 30 mg P.O. b.i.d., t.i.d., or q.i.d. (as much as 80 mg q.i.d. may be given in acute situations). Or, initially, 100 to 500 mg succinate I.M. or I.V.; then 50 to 100 mg I.M., as indicated. Or, 15 to 240 mg phosphate I.M., S.C., or I.V. daily in divided doses q 12 hours. Or, 5 to 75 mg acetate into joints or soft tissue repeated at 3 to 5 days for bursae and 1 to 4 weeks for joints. Dosage varies with size of joint. Local anesthetics commonly are injected with dose.

➲ Shock

Adults: Initially, 50 mg/kg succinate I.V., repeated in 4 hours. Repeat dosage q 24 hours, p.r.n. Or, 100 to 500 mg to 2 g q 2 to 6 hours, continued until patient is stabilized (usually not longer than 48 to 72 hours).

Children: Phosphate (I.M.) or succinate (I.M. or I.V.) 0.16 to 1 mg/kg or 6 to 30 mg/m^2 given once or twice daily.

➲ Adjunct treatment for ulcerative colitis and proctitis

Adults: 1 enema (100 mg) P.R. nightly for 21 days. Or, 1 applicatorful (90-mg foam) P.R. daily or b.i.d. for 14 to 21 days. Or, 25 mg rectal suppository b.i.d. for 2 weeks. For severe proctitis, 25 mg P.R. t.i.d. or 50 mg b.i.d.

Contraindications & cautions

- Contraindicated in patients hypersensitive to drug or its ingredients, in those with sys-

temic fungal infections, in those receiving immunosuppressive doses together with live-virus vaccines, and in premature infants (succinate).
- Use with caution in patient with recent MI.
- Use cautiously in patients with GI ulcer, renal disease, hypertension, osteoporosis, diabetes mellitus, hypothyroidism, cirrhosis, diverticulitis, nonspecific ulcerative colitis, active hepatitis, lactation, recent intestinal anastomoses, thromboembolic disorders, seizures, myasthenia gravis, heart failure, tuberculosis, ocular herpes simplex, emotional instability, and psychotic tendencies.

Adverse reactions

CNS: *euphoria, insomnia,* psychotic behavior, ***pseudotumor cerebri***, vertigo, headache, paresthesia, ***seizures***.
CV: ***heart failure***, hypertension, edema, ***arrhythmias***, thrombophlebitis, ***thromboembolism***.
EENT: cataracts, glaucoma.
GI: *peptic ulceration*, GI irritation, increased appetite, ***pancreatitis***, nausea, vomiting.
GU: menstrual irregularities, increased urine calcium levels.
Hematologic: easy bruising.
Metabolic: hypokalemia, hyperglycemia, carbohydrate intolerance, hypercholesterolemia, hypocalcemia.
Musculoskeletal: growth suppression in children, muscle weakness, osteoporosis.
Skin: hirsutism, delayed wound healing, acne, skin eruptions.
Other: cushingoid state, susceptibility to infections, ***acute adrenal insufficiency after increased stress or abrupt withdrawal after long-term therapy***.
After abrupt withdrawal: rebound inflammation; fatigue; weakness; arthralgia; fever; dizziness; lethargy; depression; fainting; orthostatic hypotension; dyspnea; anorexia; ***hypoglycemia. After prolonged use, sudden withdrawal may be fatal***.

Interactions

Drug-drug. *Aspirin, indomethacin, other NSAIDs:* May increase risk of GI distress and bleeding. Use together cautiously.
Barbiturates, carbamazepine, fosphenytoin, phenytoin, rifampin: May decrease corticosteroid effect. Increase corticosteroid dosage.
Cyclosporine: May increase toxicity. Monitor patient closely.
Live attenuated virus vaccines, other toxoids and vaccines: May decrease antibody response and increase risk of neurologic complications. Avoid using together.
Oral anticoagulants: May alter dosage requirements. Monitor PT and INR closely.
Potassium-depleting drugs such as thiazide diuretics: May enhance potassium-wasting effects of hydrocortisone. Monitor potassium level.
Skin-test antigens: May decrease response. Postpone skin testing until after therapy.
Drug-herb. *Echinacea:* May increase immune-stimulating effects. Discourage use together.
Ginseng: May increase immune-modulating response. Discourage use together.

Nursing considerations

- Determine whether patient is sensitive to other corticosteroids.
- Most adverse reactions to corticosteroids are dose- or duration-dependent.
- For better results and less toxicity, give a once-daily dose in morning.
- Give oral dose with food when possible. Patient may need medication to prevent GI irritation.

!!ALERT Salt formulations aren't interchangeable.
- Give I.M. injection deeply into gluteal muscle. Rotate injection sites to prevent muscle atrophy. Avoid S.C. injection because atrophy and sterile abscesses may occur.
- Injectable forms aren't used for alternate-day therapy.

!!ALERT Only hydrocortisone sodium phosphate and sodium succinate can be given I.V.
- Enema may produce same systemic effects as other forms of hydrocortisone. If enema therapy must exceed 21 days, stop gradually by reducing use to every other night for 2 to 3 weeks.
- High-dose therapy usually isn't continued beyond 48 hours.
- Always adjust to lowest effective dose.
- Monitor patient's weight, blood pressure, and electrolyte level.
- Monitor patient for cushingoid effects, including moon face, buffalo hump, central

obesity, thinning hair, hypertension, and increased susceptibility to infection.
- Unless contraindicated, give a low-sodium diet that is high in potassium and protein. Give potassium supplements.
- Drug may mask or worsen infections, including latent amebiasis.
- Stress (fever, trauma, surgery, and emotional problems) may increase adrenal insufficiency. Increase dosage.
- Watch for depression or psychotic episodes, especially during high-dose therapy.
- Inspect patient's skin for petechiae.
- Diabetic patient may need increased insulin; monitor glucose level.
- Periodic measurement of growth and development may be needed during high-dose or prolonged therapy in children.
- Elderly patients may be more susceptible to osteoporosis with prolonged use.
- Gradually reduce dosage after long-term therapy.

!!ALERT Don't confuse Solu-Cortef with Solu-Medrol (methylprednisolone sodium succinate), or hydrocortisone with hydroxychloroquine.

Patient teaching

- Tell patient not to stop drug abruptly or without prescriber's consent.
- Instruct patient to take oral form of drug with milk or food.
- Warn patient on long-term therapy about cushingoid effects (moon face, buffalo hump) and the need to notify prescriber about sudden weight gain or swelling.
- Teach patient signs and symptoms of early adrenal insufficiency: fatigue, muscle weakness, joint pain, fever, anorexia, nausea, shortness of breath, dizziness, and fainting.
- Instruct patient to carry or wear medical identification indicating his need for supplemental systemic glucocorticoids during stress. This card should contain prescriber's name and name and dosage of drug.
- Warn patient about easy bruising.
- Urge patient receiving long-term therapy to consider exercise or physical therapy. Also, tell him to ask prescriber about vitamin D or calcium supplement.
- Advise patient receiving long-term therapy to have periodic eye examinations.
- Caution patient to avoid exposure to infections (such as chickenpox or measles) and to notify prescriber if such exposure occurs.

hydrocortisone (topical)

Acticort 100, Aeroseb-HC, Ala-Cort, Ala-Scalp, Anusol-HC, Bactine Hydrocortisone ◇, Cetacort, Cort-Dome, Cortisone-5 ◇, Cortisone-10 ◇, Delcort, Dermolate Anti-Itch ◇, Dermtex HC ◇, Hi-Cor 2.5, Hycort, HydroTex, Hytone, LactiCare-HC, Penecort, Procort ◇, Proctocort ◇, Scalpicin ◇, Synacort, Tegrin-HC ◇, Texacort, T/Scalp

hydrocortisone acetate

Anu-Med HC, Anusol HC-1 ◇, Caldecort (Maximum Strength), Cortaid ◇, Cortamed†, Cortef Feminine Itch ◇, Corticaine ◇, Dermol HC, Gynecort ◇, Hemril-HC Uniserts, Lanacort-5 ◇, Lanacort 10 ◇, ProctoCream-HC, ProctoFoam-HC

hydrocortisone butyrate

Locoid

hydrocortisone valerate

Westcort

Pregnancy risk category C

Indications & dosages

➲ Inflammation and pruritus from dermatoses responsive to corticosteroids, adjunctive topical management of seborrheic dermatitis of scalp

Adults and children: Clean area; apply cream, gel, lotion, ointment, or topical solution sparingly daily to q.i.d. Spray aerosol onto affected area daily to q.i.d. until acute phase is controlled; then reduce dosage to one to three times weekly, p.r.n. Give children lowest dose that provides positive results.

➲ Inflammation from proctitis

Adults: 1 applicatorful of rectal foam P.R. daily or b.i.d. for 2 to 3 weeks; then every other day, p.r.n. Give enema once nightly for 21 days or until patient improves; may use every other night for 2 to 3 months. Insert suppository b.i.d. for 2 weeks.

Contraindications & cautions

- Contraindicated in patients hypersensitive to drug or its components.

Adverse reactions

Topical
GU: glycosuria.
Metabolic: hyperglycemia.
Skin: burning, pruritus, irritation, dryness, erythema, folliculitis, hypertrichosis, hypopigmentation, acneiform eruptions, allergic contact dermatitis, *atrophy, maceration, secondary infection, striae, miliaria with occlusive dressings.*
Other: ***hypothalamic-pituitary-adrenal axis suppression***, Cushing's syndrome.
Rectal
CNS: ***seizures, increased intracranial pressure***, vertigo, headache.
CV: hypertension.
EENT: cataracts, glaucoma.
GI: peptic ulcer, ***pancreatitis***, abdominal distention.
GU: menstrual irregularities.
Metabolic: fluid or electrolyte disturbances, decreased carbohydrate tolerance.
Musculoskeletal: muscle weakness, osteoporosis, necrosis and fractures in bone.
Skin: impaired wound healing, fragile skin, petechiae, erythema, sweating.

Interactions

None significant.

Nursing considerations

- Gently wash skin before applying. To prevent skin damage, rub in gently, leaving a thin coat. When treating hairy sites, part hair and apply directly to lesions.
- Avoid applying near eyes or mucous membranes or in ear canal; may be safely used on face, groin, and armpits and under breasts.
- If an occlusive dressing is applied and a fever develops, notify prescriber and remove dressing.
- Change dressing as prescribed. Stop drug and tell prescriber if skin infection, striae, or atrophy occurs.
- When using aerosol near the face, cover patient's eyes and warn against inhaling spray. Aerosol contains alcohol and may cause irritation or burning when used on open lesions. Don't spray longer than 3 seconds or from closer than 6 inches (15 cm) to avoid freezing tissues. If spray is applied to dry scalp after shampooing, drug need not be massaged into scalp.
- If antifungal or antibiotic combined with corticosteroid fails to provide prompt improvement, stop corticosteroid until infection is controlled.
- Systemic absorption is likely with use of occlusive dressings, prolonged treatment, or extensive body surface treatment. Watch for symptoms, such as hyperglycemia, glycosuria, and hypothalamic-pituitary-adrenal axis suppression.
- Avoid using plastic pants or tight-fitting diapers on treated areas in young children. Children may absorb larger amounts of drug and be more susceptible to systemic toxicity.
- Continue treatment for a few days after lesions clear.
- Monitor patient for fluid or electrolyte disturbances (sodium and fluid retention, potassium loss, hypokalemic alkalosis, negative nitrogen balance from catabolism of protein).
- Drug may suppress skin reaction testing.

!! ALERT Don't confuse hydrocortisone with hydroxychloroquine.

Patient teaching

- Teach patient or family member how to apply drug.
- Tell patient to wash hands after application.
- If an occlusive dressing is ordered, advise patient to leave it in place for no longer than 12 hours each day and not to use the dressing on infected or weeping lesions.
- Tell patient to stop drug and report signs of systemic absorption, skin irritation or ulceration, hypersensitivity, infection, or lack of improvement.
- Instruct patient to insert suppositories blunt end first after removing foil wrapper.
- For perianal application, instruct patient to place small amount of drug on a tissue and gently rub in.
- Tell patient to disassemble applicator or aerosol cap and clean with warm water after each use.

hydromorphone hydrochloride (dihydromorphinone hydrochloride)

Dilaudid, Dilaudid-5, Dilaudid-HP, Palladone

Pregnancy risk category C
Controlled substance schedule II

Indications & dosages

➲ Moderate to severe pain
Adults: 2 to 4 mg P.O. q 4 to 6 hours, p.r.n. Or, 1 to 4 mg I.M., S.C., or I.V. (slowly over at least 2 to 5 minutes) q 4 to 6 hours, p.r.n. Or, 3 mg P.R. suppository q 6 to 8 hours, p.r.n.

➲ Management of persistent moderate to severe pain in opioid-tolerant patients who require continuous, around-the-clock pain relief for an extended period (Palladone)
Adults: To determine an appropriate daily starting dose of hydromorphone, multiply the total daily dose of milligrams for the previous opioid used by the conversion factor below. Patient's receiving high-dose parenteral opioids require a more conservative conversion factor (50% of what's listed below). Appropriate immediate-release supplemental analgesia should be available for breakthrough or predictable pain.

Opioid	Oral conversion factor	Parenteral conversion factor
codeine	0.04	none
hydrocodone	0.22	none
hydromorphone	1	5
levorphanol	1.88	3.75
meperidine	0.02	0.1
methadone	0.38	0.75
morphine	0.12	0.75
oxycodone	0.25	none

When converting from fentanyl transdermal, give 12 mg once daily for each 50 mcg/hour of fentanyl. When converting from a fixed-combination opioid, give 12 mg once daily if patient is taking more than or equal to 45 mg oxycodone or hydrocodone, or 300 mg codeine. The nonopioid component of the combination product may be continued separately.

Adjust as needed every 2 to 3 days by 25% to 50% of the current daily dose (including supplemental analgesia).

➲ Cough
Adults and children older than age 12: 1 mg cough syrup P.O. q 3 to 4 hours, p.r.n.
Children ages 6 to 12 years: 0.5 mg cough syrup P.O. q 3 to 4 hours, p.r.n.

Contraindications & cautions

- Contraindicated in patients hypersensitive to drug; in those with intracranial lesions that cause increased intracranial pressure; and in those with depressed ventilation, such as in status asthmaticus, COPD, cor pulmonale, emphysema, and kyphoscoliosis. Palladone capsules are contraindicated for p.r.n. use.
- Use with caution in elderly or debilitated patients and in those with hepatic or renal disease, hypothyroidism, Addison's disease, prostatic hyperplasia, or urethral stricture.

Adverse reactions

CNS: sedation, somnolence, clouded sensorium, dizziness, euphoria, light-headedness.
CV: hypotension, flushing, ***bradycardia***.
EENT: blurred vision, diplopia, nystagmus.
GI: nausea, vomiting, constipation, ileus, dry mouth.
GU: urine retention.
Respiratory: ***respiratory depression***, ***bronchospasm***.
Skin: diaphoresis, pruritus.
Other: induration with repeated S.C. injections, physical dependence.

Interactions

Drug-drug. *CNS depressants, general anesthetics, hypnotics, MAO inhibitors, other opioid analgesics, sedatives, tranquilizers, tricyclic antidepressants:* May cause additive effects. Use together with caution; reduce hydromorphone dose and monitor patient response.
Drug-lifestyle. *Alcohol use:* May cause additive effects. Advise patient to use together cautiously.

Nursing considerations

- Reassess patient's level of pain at least 15 and 30 minutes after administration.

- For better analgesic effect, give drug before patient has intense pain.
- Dilaudid-HP, a highly concentrated form (10 mg/ml), may be given in smaller volumes to prevent the discomfort of large-volume I.M. or S.C. injections. Check dosage carefully.
- Rotate injection sites to avoid induration with S.C. injection.

!! **ALERT** Palladone is indicated in opioid-tolerant patients only. Use in non–opioid-tolerant patients may lead to fatal respiratory depression.

- Monitor respiratory and circulatory status and bowel function.
- Keep opioid antagonist (naloxone) available.
- Drug may worsen or mask gallbladder pain.
- Drug is a commonly abused opioid.

!! **ALERT** Cough syrup may contain tartrazine.

!! **ALERT** Don't confuse hydromorphone with morphine or oxymorphone or Dilaudid with Dilantin.

Patient teaching

- Instruct patient to request or take drug before pain becomes intense.
- Tell patient to store suppositories in refrigerator.
- Advise patient to take drug with food if GI upset occurs.
- When drug is used after surgery, encourage patient to turn, cough, and breathe deeply to avoid lung problems.
- Caution ambulatory patient about getting out of bed or walking. Warn outpatient to avoid hazardous activities that require mental alertness until drug's CNS effects are known.
- Advise patient to avoid alcohol during therapy.

hydroxychloroquine sulfate
Plaquenil Sulfate

Pregnancy risk category C

Indications & dosages

➲ **Suppressive prevention of malaria attacks caused by *Plasmodium vivax, P. malariae, P. ovale,* and susceptible strains of *P. falciparum***

Adults: 310 mg base P.O. weekly on the same day each week, beginning 1 to 2 weeks before entering malaria-endemic area and continuing for 4 weeks after leaving area. If not started before exposure, double first dose to 620 mg base in two divided doses 6 hours apart.

Children: 5 mg/kg base P.O. weekly on the same day each week, beginning 1 to 2 weeks before entering malaria-endemic area and continuing for 4 weeks after leaving area. Don't exceed adult dose. If not started before exposure, double first dose to 10 mg/kg base in two divided doses, 6 hours apart.

➲ **Acute malarial attacks**

Adults: Initially, 620 mg base P.O., followed by 310 mg base 6 to 8 hours after first dose; then 310 mg base daily for 2 days.

Children: Initially, 10 mg/kg base P.O.; then 5 mg/kg base at 6, 24, and 48 hours after the first dose.

➲ **Lupus erythematosus**

Adults: 310 mg base P.O. daily or b.i.d., continued for several weeks or months, depending on response. For prolonged maintenance dose, 155 to 310 mg base daily.

➲ **Rheumatoid arthritis**

Adults: Initially, 310 to 465 mg base P.O. daily. When good response occurs, usually in 4 to 12 weeks, cut dosage in half.

Contraindications & cautions

- Contraindicated in patients hypersensitive to drug and in those with retinal or visual field changes or porphyria.
- Contraindicated as long-term therapy for children.
- Use with caution in patients with severe GI, neurologic, or blood disorders.
- Use with caution in patients with hepatic disease or alcoholism because drug concentrates in liver.
- Use with caution in those with G6PD deficiency or psoriasis because drug may worsen these conditions.

Adverse reactions

CNS: irritability, nightmares, ataxia, ***seizures***, psychosis, vertigo, dizziness, hypoactive deep tendon reflexes, lassitude, headache.

CV: T-wave inversion or depression, widening of QRS complex.
EENT: blurred vision, difficulty in focusing, reversible corneal changes, nystagmus, typically irreversible, sometimes progressive or delayed retinal changes such as narrowing of arterioles, macular lesions, pallor of optic disk, optic atrophy.
GI: anorexia, abdominal cramps, diarrhea, nausea, vomiting.
Hematologic: ***agranulocytosis, leukopenia, thrombocytopenia, hemolysis in patients with G6PD deficiency, aplastic anemia.***
Metabolic: weight loss.
Musculoskeletal: skeletal muscle weakness.
Skin: pruritus, lichen planus eruptions, skin and mucosal pigmentary changes, pleomorphic skin eruptions, worsened psoriasis, alopecia, bleaching of hair.

Interactions

Drug-drug. *Aluminum salts (kaolin), magnesium:* May decrease GI absorption. Separate dose times.
Cimetidine: May decrease hepatic metabolism of hydroxychloroquine. Monitor patient for toxicity.
Digoxin: May increase digoxin level. Monitor drug levels; monitor patient for toxicity.

Nursing considerations

!!ALERT Drug dosage may be discussed in "mg" or "mg base"; be aware of the difference.
- Ensure that baseline and periodic ophthalmic examinations are performed. Check periodically for ocular muscle weakness after long-term use.
- Assist patient with obtaining audiometric examinations before, during, and after therapy, especially if therapy is long-term.
- Monitor CBC and liver function studies periodically during long-term therapy; if severe blood disorder not attributable to disease develops, drug may need to be stopped.

!!ALERT Monitor patient for possible overdose, which can quickly lead to toxic signs or symptoms: headache, drowsiness, visual disturbances, CV collapse, and seizures—then cardiopulmonary arrest. Children are extremely susceptible to toxicity; avoid long-term treatment.

Patient teaching

- Advise patient taking drug for prevention to take drug immediately before or after a meal on the same day each week, to improve compliance.
- Instruct patient to report adverse reactions promptly.

hydroxyurea
Droxia, Hydrea

Pregnancy risk category D

Indications & dosages

➲ Melanoma; resistant chronic myelocytic leukemia; recurrent, metastatic, or inoperable ovarian cancer; head and neck cancers
Adults: 80 mg/kg Hydrea P.O. as single dose q 3 days; or 20 to 30 mg/kg P.O. as single daily dose.
➲ To reduce frequency of painful crises and need for blood transfusions in adult patients with sickle-cell anemia with recurrent moderate to severe painful crises
Adults: 15 mg/kg Droxia P.O. once daily. If blood counts are in acceptable range, dose may be increased by 5 mg/kg daily q 12 weeks until maximum tolerated dose or 35 mg/kg daily has been reached. If blood counts are considered toxic, withhold drug until hematologic recovery occurs. Resume treatment after reducing dose by 2.5 mg/kg daily. Every 12 weeks, drug may then be adjusted up or down in 2.5-mg/kg daily increments until patient is at stable, nontoxic dose for 24 weeks.
➲ To reduce platelet count and prevent thrombosis in patients with essential thrombocythemia♦
Adults: 15 mg/kg Hydrea P.O. daily.
➲ Refractory psoriasis♦
Adults: 0.5 to 1.5 g Hydrea P.O. daily.

Contraindications & cautions

- Contraindicated in patients hypersensitive to drug and in those with fewer than 2,500/mm^3 WBCs, fewer than 100,000/mm^3 platelets, or severe anemia.
- Use cautiously in patients with renal dysfunction.

Adverse reactions

CNS: hallucinations, headache, dizziness, disorientation, ***seizures***, malaise, fever.
GI: *anorexia, nausea, vomiting, diarrhea*, stomatitis, constipation.
Hematologic: ***leukopenia, thrombocytopenia***, *anemia, megaloblastosis*, **bone marrow suppression**.
Metabolic: hyperuricemia, weight gain.
Skin: rash, itching, alopecia.
Other: chills.

Interactions

Drug-drug. *Cytotoxic drugs, radiation therapy:* May enhance toxicity of hydroxyurea. Use together cautiously.

Nursing considerations

- Routinely measure BUN, uric acid, liver enzyme, and creatinine levels; monitor blood counts every 2 weeks.
- Acceptable blood counts during dosage adjustment are neutrophil count of 2,500 cells/mm^3 or more; platelet count 95,000/mm^3 or more; hemoglobin level more than 5.3 g/dl; and reticulocyte count (if hemoglobin level is below 9 g/dl) more than 95,000/mm^3. Toxic levels are neutrophil count below 2,000 cells/mm^3, platelet count below 80,000/mm, hemoglobin level less than 4.5 g/dl, and reticulocyte count (if hemoglobin level is below 9 g/dl) below 80,000/mm^3.
- Hydroxyurea may dramatically lower the WBC count in 24 to 48 hours.
- Monitor fluid intake and output; keep patient hydrated.
- Allopurinol is used to treat or prevent tumor lysis syndrome.
- To prevent bleeding, avoid all I.M. injections when platelet count is below 50,000/mm^3.
- Anticipate need for blood transfusions because of cumulative anemia. Patient may receive injections of RBC colony–stimulating factors to promote RBC production and decrease need for blood transfusions.
- Dosage modification may be needed after chemotherapy or radiation therapy.
- Auditory and visual hallucinations and hematologic toxicity increase when renal function decreases.
- Drug crosses blood-brain barrier.
- Radiation therapy may increase risk or severity of GI distress or stomatitis.

Patient teaching

- Tell patient who can't swallow capsules that he may empty contents into water, drink immediately, and rinse mouth with water afterward. Inform patient that some inert material may not dissolve.
- Advise patient to watch for signs and symptoms of infection (fever, sore throat, fatigue) and bleeding (easy bruising, nosebleeds, bleeding gums, tarry stools). He also should take his temperature daily.
- Caution woman of childbearing age to consult prescriber before becoming pregnant.

hydroxyzine hydrochloride

Anx, Apo-Hydroxyzine†, Atarax*, Novo-Hydroxyzin†, PMS-Hydroxyzine†, Vistaril

hydroxyzine pamoate

Vistaril

Pregnancy risk category NR

Indications & dosages

➲ Anxiety
Adults: 50 to 100 mg P.O. q.i.d.
Children age 6 and older: 50 to 100 mg P.O. daily in divided doses.
Children younger than age 6: 50 mg P.O. daily in divided doses.

➲ Preoperative and postoperative adjunctive therapy for sedation
Adults: 25 to 100 mg I.M. or 50 to 100 mg P.O.
Children: 1.1 mg/kg I.M. or 0.6 mg/kg P.O.

➲ Pruritus from allergies
Adults: 25 mg P.O. t.i.d. or q.i.d.
Children age 6 and older: 50 to 100 mg P.O. daily in divided doses.
Children younger than age 6: 50 mg P.O. daily in divided doses.

➲ Psychiatric and emotional emergencies, including acute alcoholism
Adults: 50 to 100 mg I.M. q 4 to 6 hours, p.r.n.

➲ Nausea and vomiting (excluding nausea and vomiting of pregnancy)
Adults: 25 to 100 mg I.M.
Children: 1.1 mg/kg I.M.

➲ Antepartum and postpartum adjunctive therapy
Adults: 25 to 100 mg I.M.

Contraindications & cautions

- Contraindicated in patients hypersensitive to drug, patients in early pregnancy, and breast-feeding women.

Adverse reactions

CNS: *drowsiness*, involuntary motor activity.
GI: *dry mouth*, constipation.
Other: pain at I.M. injection site, hypersensitivity reactions.

Interactions

Drug-drug. *Anticholinergics:* May cause additive anticholinergic effects. Use together cautiously.
CNS depressants: May increase CNS depression. Use together cautiously; dosage adjustments may be needed.
Epinephrine: May inhibit and reverse vasopressor effect of epinephrine. Avoid using together.
Drug-lifestyle. *Alcohol use:* May increase CNS depression. Discourage use together.

Nursing considerations

- Parenteral form (hydroxyzine hydrochloride) is for I.M. use only, preferably by Z-track injection. Never give drug I.V. or S.C.
- Aspirate I.M. injection carefully to prevent inadvertent intravascular injection. Inject deeply into a large muscle.
- If patient takes other CNS drugs, observe for oversedation.

!!ALERT Don't confuse hydroxyzine with hydroxyurea or hydralazine.

Patient teaching

- Warn patient to avoid hazardous activities that require alertness and good coordination until effects of drug are known.
- Tell patient to avoid alcohol while taking drug.
- Advise patient to use sugarless hard candy or gum to relieve dry mouth.
- Warn woman of childbearing age to avoid use during pregnancy and breast-feeding.

hyoscyamine
Cystospaz

hyoscyamine sulfate
Anaspaz, Cystospaz, Cystospaz-M, Gastrosed, Levbid, Levsin*, Levsin Drops*, Levsin SL, Levsinex Timecaps, NuLev

Pregnancy risk category C

Indications & dosages

➲ **GI tract disorders caused by spasm; to diminish secretions and block cardiac vagal reflexes preoperatively; as adjunctive therapy for peptic ulcers, cystitis, renal colic; as drying agent to relieve symptoms of allergic rhinitis**
Adults and children age 12 and older: 0.125 to 0.25 mg P.O. or S.L. t.i.d. or q.i.d. before meals and h.s. Or, 0.375 to 0.75 mg extended-release form P.O. q 8 to 12 hours. Or, 0.25 to 0.5 mg or 1 or 2 ml I.M., I.V., or S.C. b.i.d. to q.i.d. Oral drug is substituted when symptoms are controlled. Maximum, 1.5 mg daily.
Children younger than age 12: Individualize dosage according to weight. Usual dose is ½ to 1 tablet P.O. q 4 hours or p.r.n. Don't exceed 6 tablets or 0.75 mg in 24 hours.

Contraindications & cautions

- Contraindicated in patients hypersensitive to anticholinergics and in those with glaucoma, obstructive uropathy, obstructive disease of the GI tract, severe ulcerative colitis, myasthenia gravis, paralytic ileus, intestinal atony, unstable CV status in acute hemorrhage, tachycardia secondary to cardiac insufficiency of thyrotoxicosis, or toxic megacolon.
- Use cautiously in patients with autonomic neuropathy, hyperthyroidism, coronary artery disease, arrhythmias, heart failure, hypertension, hiatal hernia with reflux esophagitis, hepatic or renal disease, known or suspected GI infection, and ulcerative colitis.
- Use cautiously in patients in hot or humid environments; drug can cause heatstroke.

Adverse reactions

CNS: fever, headache, insomnia, drowsiness, dizziness, *confusion or excitement in elderly patients*, nervousness, weakness.
CV: *palpitations*, tachycardia.
EENT: *blurred vision*, mydriasis, increased intraocular pressure, cycloplegia, photophobia.
GI: *dry mouth*, dysphagia, *constipation*, heartburn, loss of taste, nausea, vomiting, *paralytic ileus*.
GU: *urinary hesitancy, urine retention*, impotence.
Skin: urticaria, decreased or lack of sweating.
Other: hypersensitivity reactions.

Interactions

Drug-drug. *Amantadine, antihistamines, antiparkinsonians, disopyramide, glutethimide, MAO inhibitors, meperidine, phenothiazines, procainamide, quinidine, tricyclic antidepressants:* May have additive adverse effects. Avoid using together.
Antacids: May decrease absorption of oral anticholinergics. Separate doses by 2 or 3 hours.
Ketoconazole: May interfere with ketoconazole absorption. Separate doses by 2 or 3 hours.

Nursing considerations

- Give drug 30 minutes to 1 hour before meals and at bedtime. Bedtime dose can be larger; give at least 2 hours after last meal of day.

!!ALERT Overdose may cause curarelike effects, such as respiratory paralysis. Keep emergency equipment available.

- Monitor patient's vital signs and urine output carefully.
- Injection contains sodium metabisulfite, which may cause allergic reaction in certain people.

Patient teaching

- Urge patient to take drug as prescribed.
- Caution patient not to crush or chew extended-release tablets.
- Advise patient to avoid driving and other hazardous activities if drowsiness, dizziness, or blurred vision occurs; to drink plenty of fluids to help prevent constipation; and to report rash or other skin eruption.

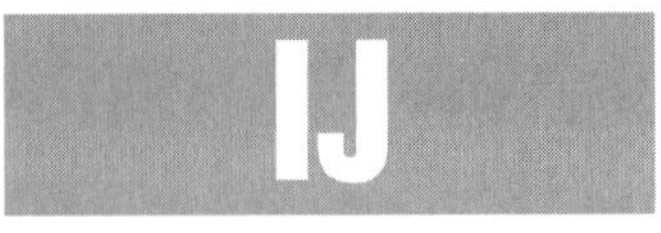

ibuprofen

Advil ◇, Apo-Ibuprofen†, Bayer Select Ibuprofen Pain Relief Formula, Children's Advil, Children's Motrin ◇, Excedrin IB ◇, Genpril ◇, Haltran ◇, Ibu-Tab ◇, Medipren ◇, Menadol, Midol IB, Motrin ◇, Novo-Profen†, Nuprin ◇, Pamprin-IB, Rufen, Saleto-200, Trendar ◇

Pregnancy risk category B; D in 3rd trimester

Indications & dosages

➲ **Rheumatoid arthritis, osteoarthritis, arthritis**
Adults: 300 to 800 mg P.O. t.i.d. or q.i.d. Maximum daily dose is 3.2 g.
➲ **Mild to moderate pain, dysmenorrhea**
Adults: 400 mg P.O. q 4 to 6 hours, p.r.n.
➲ **Fever**
Adults: 200 to 400 mg P.O. q 4 to 6 hours, for no longer than 3 days. Maximum daily dose is 1.2 g.
Children ages 6 months to 12 years: If child's temperature is below 102.5°F (39.2° C), give 5 mg/kg P.O. q 6 to 8 hours. Treat higher temperatures with 10 mg/kg q 6 to 8 hours. Maximum daily dose is 40 mg/kg.
➲ **Juvenile arthritis**
Children: 30 to 40 mg/kg daily P.O. in three or four divided doses. Maximum daily dose is 50 mg/kg.

Contraindications & cautions

- Contraindicated in patients hypersensitive to drug and in those with angioedema, syndrome of nasal polyps, or bronchospastic reaction to aspirin or other NSAIDs.
- Contraindicated in pregnant women.
- Use cautiously in patients with GI disorders, history of peptic ulcer disease, hepatic or renal disease, cardiac decompensation, hypertension, preexisting asthma, or known intrinsic coagulation defects.

Adverse reactions

CNS: headache, dizziness, nervousness, ***aseptic meningitis***.

CV: peripheral edema, fluid retention, edema.
EENT: tinnitus.
GI: epigastric distress, nausea, occult blood loss, peptic ulceration, diarrhea, constipation, abdominal pain, bloating, GI fullness, dyspepsia, flatulence, heartburn, decreased appetite.
GU: ***acute renal failure***, azotemia, cystitis, hematuria.
Hematologic: prolonged bleeding time, anemia, ***neutropenia, pancytopenia, thrombocytopenia, aplastic anemia, leukopenia, agranulocytosis***.
Metabolic: ***hypoglycemia, hyperkalemia***.
Respiratory: ***bronchospasm***.
Skin: pruritus, rash, urticaria, ***Stevens-Johnson syndrome***.

Interactions

Drug-drug. *Antihypertensives, furosemide, thiazide diuretics:* May decrease the effectiveness of diuretics or antihypertensives. Monitor patient closely.
Aspirin: May decrease ibuprofen level. Avoid using together.
Aspirin, corticosteroids: May cause adverse GI reactions. Avoid using together.
Bisphosphonates: May increase risk of gastric ulceration. Monitor patient for signs of gastric irritation or bleeding.
Cyclosporine: May increase nephrotoxicity of both drugs. Avoid using together.
Digoxin, lithium, oral anticoagulants: May increase levels or effects of these drugs. Monitor patient toxicity.
Methotrexate: May decrease methotrexate clearance and increases toxicity. Use together cautiously.
Drug-herb. *Dong quai, feverfew, garlic, ginger, ginkgo biloba, horse chestnut, red clover:* May increase risk of bleeding, based on the known effects of components. Discourage use together.
White willow: Herb and drug contain similar components. Discourage use together.
Drug-lifestyle. *Alcohol use:* May cause adverse GI reactions. Discourage use together.
Sun exposure: May cause photosensitivity reactions. Advise patient to avoid excessive sunlight exposure.

Nursing considerations

- Check renal and hepatic function periodically in patients on long-term therapy. Stop drug if abnormalities occur and notify prescriber.
- Because of their antipyretic and anti-inflammatory actions, NSAIDs may mask signs and symptoms of infection.
- Blurred or diminished vision and changes in color vision have occurred.
- It may take 1 or 2 weeks before full anti-inflammatory effects occur.
- Serious GI toxicity, including peptic ulcers and bleeding, can occur in patient taking NSAIDs, despite lack of symptoms.
- If patient consumes three or more alcoholic drinks per day, use of ibuprofen may lead to stomach bleeding.

!!ALERT Don't confuse Trendar with Trandate.

Patient teaching

- Tell patient to take with meals or milk to reduce adverse GI reactions.

!!ALERT Drug is available OTC. Instruct patient not to exceed 1.2 g daily, not to give to children younger than age 12, or not to take for extended periods (longer than 3 days for fever or longer than 10 days for pain) without consulting prescriber.

- Tell patient that full therapeutic effect for arthritis may be delayed for 2 to 4 weeks. Although pain relief occurs at low dosage levels, inflammation doesn't improve at dosages less than 400 mg q.i.d.
- Caution patient that use with aspirin, alcohol, or corticosteroids may increase risk of GI adverse reactions.
- Teach patient to watch for and report to prescriber immediately signs and symptoms of GI bleeding, including blood in vomit, urine, or stool; coffee-ground vomit; and black, tarry stool.
- Tell patient to contact prescriber before using this drug if fluid intake hasn't been adequate or if fluids have been lost as a result of vomiting or diarrhea.
- Warn patient to avoid hazardous activities that require mental alertness until effects on CNS are known.
- Advise patient to wear sunscreen to avoid hypersensitivity to sunlight.

ibutilide fumarate
Corvert

Pregnancy risk category C

Indications & dosages
➲ Rapid conversion of recent onset atrial fibrillation or atrial flutter to sinus rhythm
Adults weighing 60 kg (132 lb) or more: 1 mg I.V. over 10 minutes.
Adults weighing less than 60 kg: 0.01 mg/kg I.V. over 10 minutes.

Contraindications & cautions
- Contraindicated in patients hypersensitive to drug or its components.
- Contraindicated in patients with history of polymorphic ventricular tachycardia and in breast-feeding women.
- Use cautiously in patients with hepatic or renal dysfunction.
- Safety and effectiveness of drug haven't been established in children.

Adverse reactions
CNS: headache.
CV: ventricular extrasystoles, nonsustained ventricular tachycardia, hypotension, bundle-branch block, ***sustained polymorphic ventricular tachycardia***, ***AV block***, ***heart failure***, hypertension, prolonged QT interval, ***bradycardia***, palpitations, tachycardia.
GI: nausea.

Interactions
Drug-drug. *Class IA antiarrhythmics (disopyramide, procainamide, quinidine), other class III drugs (amiodarone, sotalol):* May increase potential for prolonged refractoriness. Don't give these drugs for at least five half-lives before and 4 hours after ibutilide dose.
Digoxin: Supraventricular arrhythmias may mask cardiotoxicity from excessive digoxin level. Use with caution in patients who may have an increased digoxin therapeutic range.
H_1-receptor antagonist antihistamines, phenothiazines, tetracyclic antidepressants, tricyclic antidepressants, other drugs that prolong QT interval: May increase risk for proarrhythmia. Monitor patient closely.

Nursing considerations
- Skilled personnel only should give drug. Cardiac monitor, intracardiac pacing, cardioverter or defibrillator, and drugs to treat sustained ventricular tachycardia must be available.
- Before therapy, correct hypokalemia and hypomagnesemia to reduce proarrhythmia potential. Patients with atrial fibrillation lasting longer than 2 to 3 days must be adequately anticoagulated, generally over at least 2 weeks.
- Monitor ECG continuously during administration and for at least 4 hours afterward or until QTc interval returns to baseline; drug can induce or worsen ventricular arrhythmias. Longer monitoring is required if ECG shows arrhythmia or patient has hepatic insufficiency.
- Don't give class IA or other class III antiarrhythmics with ibutilide infusion or for 4 hours afterward.

Patient teaching
- Tell patient to report adverse reactions promptly.
- Instruct patient to alert nurse of discomfort at injection site.

idarubicin hydrochloride
Idamycin, Idamycin PFS

Pregnancy risk category D

Indications & dosages
Dosages vary. Check treatment protocol with prescriber.
➲ Acute myeloid leukemia, including French-American-British (FAB) classifications M1 through M7, with other approved antileukemic drugs
Adults: 12 mg/m^2 daily for 3 days by slow I.V. injection (over 10 to 15 minutes) with 100 mg/m^2 daily of cytarabine for 7 days by continuous I.V. infusion. Or, as a 25-mg/m^2 bolus (cytarabine); then 200 mg/m^2 daily (cytarabine) for 5 days by continuous infusion. A second course may be given, if needed.

If patient experiences severe mucositis, delay therapy until recovery is complete and reduce dosage by 25%. Reduce dosage in patients with hepatic or renal impairment.

Don't give idarubicin if bilirubin level exceeds 5 mg/dl.

Contraindications & cautions

- Use cautiously in patients with bone marrow suppression induced by previous drug therapy or radiotherapy, impaired hepatic or renal function, previous treatment with anthracyclines or cardiotoxic drugs, or a cardiac condition.

Adverse reactions

CNS: *headache, changed mental status,* peripheral neuropathy, ***seizures****, fever.*
CV: ***heart failure***, atrial fibrillation, chest pain, ***MI***, asymptomatic decline in left ventricular ejection fraction, ***myocardial insufficiency, arrhythmias***, HEMORRHAGE, ***myocardial toxicity***.
GI: *nausea, vomiting, cramps, diarrhea, mucositis.*
GU: renal dysfunction, red urine.
Hematologic: ***myelosuppression***.
Hepatic: changes in hepatic function.
Metabolic: hyperuricemia.
Skin: *alopecia, rash, urticaria, bullous erythrodermatous rash on palms and soles,* urticaria, erythema at previously irradiated sites, tissue necrosis if extravasation occurs.
Other: INFECTION, ***hypersensitivity reactions***.

Interactions

Drug-drug. *Alkaline solutions, heparin:* These combinations are incompatible. Don't mix idarubicin with other drugs unless specific compatibility data are known.

Nursing considerations

- Cardiotoxicity is the dose-limiting toxicity of drug.
- Take preventive measures, including adequate hydration, before starting treatment. Hyperuricemia may result from rapid lysis of leukemic cells. Allopurinol may be ordered.
- Assess patient for systemic infection and ensure that it's controlled before therapy begins.
- Give antiemetics to prevent or treat nausea and vomiting.
- Drug must never be given I.M. or S.C.
- Monitor hepatic and renal function tests and CBC frequently.
- To prevent bleeding, avoid all I.M. injections when platelet count is below 50,000/mm^3.
- Anticipate need for blood transfusions to combat anemia. Patient may receive injections of RBC colony–stimulating factor to promote RBC production and decrease need for blood transfusions.
- Notify prescriber if signs or symptoms of heart failure occur.

!!ALERT Don't confuse idarubicin with daunorubicin or doxorubicin.

Patient teaching

- Teach patient to recognize signs and symptoms of leakage of drug into surrounding tissue, and tell him to report them if they occur.
- Warn patient to watch for signs and symptoms of infection (fever, sore throat, fatigue) and bleeding (easy bruising, nosebleeds, bleeding gums, tarry stools).
- Advise patient that red urine for several days is normal and doesn't indicate presence of blood.
- Caution woman of childbearing age to avoid becoming pregnant during therapy. Recommend that she consult prescriber before becoming pregnant.

ifosfamide
Ifex

Pregnancy risk category D

Indications & dosages

➲ Testicular cancer
Adults: 1.2 g/m^2 daily I.V. for 5 consecutive days. Repeat treatment q 3 weeks or after patient recovers from hematologic toxicity Don't repeat doses until WBC count exceeds 4,000/mm^3 and platelet count exceeds 100,000/mm^3.

➲ Sarcomas, small-cell lung cancer, cervical cancer, ovarian cancer, uterine cancer♦
Adults: 1.2 to 2.5 g/m^2 I.V. daily for 3 to 5 days. Repeat cycle p.r.n., based on patient response.

Contraindications & cautions

- Contraindicated in patients hypersensitive to drug and in those with severe bone marrow suppression.

• Use cautiously in patients with renal impairment or compromised bone marrow reserve as indicated by leukopenia, granulocytopenia, extensive bone marrow metastases, previous radiation therapy, or previous therapy with cytotoxic drugs.

Adverse reactions

CNS: *somnolence, confusion,* ***coma, seizures***, ataxia, hallucinations, depressive psychosis, dizziness, disorientation, cranial nerve dysfunction.
GI: *nausea, vomiting,* diarrhea.
GU: *hemorrhagic cystitis, hematuria,* ***nephrotoxicity***, Fanconi's syndrome.
Hematologic: ***leukopenia, thrombocytopenia, myelosuppression***.
Hepatic: ***hepatotoxicity***.
Metabolic: ***metabolic acidosis***.
Skin: *alopecia.*
Other: infection, phlebitis.

Interactions

Drug-drug. *Anticoagulants, aspirin, NSAIDs:* May increase risk of bleeding. Avoid using together.
Barbiturates, chloral hydrate, fosphenytoin, phenytoin: May increase ifosfamide toxicity. Monitor patient closely.
Corticosteroids: May inhibit hepatic enzymes, reducing ifosfamide's effect. Monitor patient for increased ifosfamide toxicity if corticosteroid dosage is suddenly reduced or stopped.
Cyclophosphamide: May increase risk of cardiac tamponade in patients with thalassemia. Monitor patient closely.
Myelosuppressives: May enhance hematologic toxicity. Dosage adjustment may be needed.

Nursing considerations

• Give antiemetic before drug, to reduce nausea.
• Don't give drug at bedtime; infrequent urination during the night may increase possibility of cystitis. If cystitis develops, stop drug and notify prescriber.
• Bladder irrigation with normal saline solution may be done to treat cystitis.
• Monitor CBC and renal and liver function tests.
• To prevent bleeding, avoid all I.M. injections when platelet count is less than 50,000/mm^3.
• Anticipate blood transfusions because of cumulative anemia. Patients may receive injections of RBC colony-stimulating factor to promote RBC production and decrease need for blood transfusions.
• Assess patient for mental status changes; dosage may have to be decreased.
!!ALERT Don't confuse ifosfamide with cyclophosphamide.

Patient teaching

• Remind patient to urinate frequently to minimize contact of drug and its metabolites with the lining of the bladder.
• Advise patient to watch for signs and symptoms of infection (fever, sore throat, fatigue) and bleeding (easy bruising, nosebleeds, bleeding gums, tarry stools). Tell patient to take temperature daily.
• Instruct patient to avoid OTC products that contain aspirin.
• Advise women to stop breast-feeding during therapy because of possible risk of toxicity to infant.
• Caution woman of childbearing age to avoid becoming pregnant during therapy. Recommend that she consult prescriber before becoming pregnant.

iloprost
Ventavis

Pregnancy risk category C

Indications & dosages

➲ Pulmonary arterial hypertension in patients with NYHA Class III or IV symptoms
Adults: Initially, 2.5 mcg inhaled using the Prodose AAD System. As tolerated, increase to 5 mcg inhaled six to nine times daily while patient is awake, p.r.n., but to no more than q 2 hours. Maximum, 5 mcg nine times daily.

Contraindications & cautions

• No contraindications known.Don't use in patients whose systolic blood pressure is less than 85 mm Hg.
• Use cautiously in elderly patients, patients with hepatic or renal impairment, and patients with COPD, severe asthma, or acute pulmonary infection.

Adverse reactions

CNS: *headache*, insomnia, syncope.
CV: ***chest pain, heart failure***, *hypotension*, palpitations, peripheral edema, ***supraventricular tachycardia***, *vasodilation*.
GI: tongue pain, *nausea*, vomiting.
GU: ***renal failure***.
Musculoskeletal: *trismus*, back pain, muscle cramps.
Respiratory: *cough*, dyspnea, hemoptysis, pneumonia.
Other: *flulike syndrome*.

Interactions

Drug-drug. *Antihypertensives, vasodilators:* May increase effects of these drugs. Monitor patient's blood pressure.
Anticoagulants: May increase risk of bleeding. Monitor patient closely.

Nursing considerations

- Keep drug away from skin and eyes.
- Give drug only through Prodose AAD device.
- Take care not to inhale drug while providing treatment.
- Monitor patient's vital signs carefully at start of treatment.
- Watch for syncope.
- If patient develops evidence of pulmonary edema, stop treatment immediately.

Patient teaching

- Advise patient to take drug exactly as prescribed and using Prodose AAD.
- Urge patient to follow manufacturer instructions for preparing and inhaling drug.
- Advise patient to keep a backup Prodose AAD in case the original malfunctions.
- Tell patient to keep drug away from skin and eyes and to rinse the area immediately if contact occurs.
- Caution patient not to ingest drug solution.
- Inform patient that drug may cause dizziness and fainting. Urge him to stand up slowly from a sitting or lying position and to report to prescriber worsening of symptoms.
- Tell patient to take drug before physical exertion but no more than every 2 hours.
- Discourage exposing other people—especially pregnant women and babies—to drug.
- Teach patient how to clean equipment and safely dispose of used ampules after each treatment. Caution patient not to save or use leftover solution.

imatinib mesylate
Gleevec

Pregnancy risk category D

Indications & dosages

➲ Chronic myeloid leukemia (CML) in blast crisis, in accelerated phase, or in chronic phase after failure of alfa interferon therapy; newly diagnosed Philadelphia chromosome–positive chronic phase CML
Adults: For chronic-phase CML, 400 mg P.O. daily as single dose with a meal and large glass of water. For accelerated-phase CML or blast crisis, 600 mg P.O. daily as single dose with a meal and large glass of water. Continue treatment as long as patient continues to benefit. May increase daily dose to 600 mg P.O. in chronic phase or to 800 mg P.O. (400 mg P.O. b.i.d.) in accelerated phase or blast crisis.

Consider dosage increases only if there is an absence of severe adverse reactions and absence of severe non–leukemia-related neutropenia or thrombocytopenia in the following circumstances: disease progression (at any time), failure to achieve a satisfactory hematologic response after at least 3 months of treatment, failure to achieve a cytogenetic response after 6 to 12 months of treatment, or loss of a previously achieved hematologic or cytogenetic response.

➲ Kit (CD117)-positive unresectable or metastatic malignant GI stromal tumors (GIST)
Adults: 400 or 600 mg P.O. daily.

➲ Philadelphia chromosome–positive chronic phase CML in patients whose disease has recurred after stem cell transplant or who are resistant to interferon alfa therapy
Children age 3 and older: 260 mg/m^2 daily P.O. as a single dose or divided into two doses. Have patient take with meal and large glass of water. May increase dosage to 340 mg/m^2 daily.

For severe nonhematologic adverse reactions (severe hepatotoxicity or severe fluid retention), withhold drug until event has resolved; resume treatment as appropriate based on initial severity of event. For elevations in bilirubin level more than three times the institutional upper limit of normal (IULN) or liver transaminase levels more than five times IULN, withhold drug until bilirubin level returns to less than $1\frac{1}{2}$ IULN and transaminase levels to less than $2\frac{1}{2}$ IULN. May then resume drug at reduced daily dose. (Adults' dosages can be decreased from 400 mg to 300 mg or from 600 mg to 400 mg. Children's dosages can be decreased from 260 mg/m^2 daily to 200 mg/m^2 daily or from 340 mg/m^2 daily to 260 mg/m^2 daily.)

For hematologic adverse reactions in patients with chronic-phase CML, give starting dose 400 mg in adults or 260 mg/m^2 in children; in those with GIST, give starting dose 400 mg or 600 mg. If absolute neutrophil count (ANC) less than 1 × 10^9/L or platelets less than 50 × 10^9/L, or both, follow these steps.

- Stop drug until ANC is 1.5 × 10^9/L or greater and platelets are 75 × 10^9/L or greater.
- Resume treatment at original starting dose of 400 mg or 600 mg, or 260 mg/m^2 in children.
- If recurrence of ANC less than 1 × 10^9/L, and/or platelets less than 50 × 10^9/L, repeat step 1 and resume drug at reduced dose (300 mg if starting dose was 400 mg; 400 mg if starting dose was 600 mg; or in children, 200 mg/m^2 if starting dose was 260 mg/m^2).

In patients with accelerated phase CML and blast crisis, give starting dose 600 mg; if ANC less than 0.5 × 10^9/L or platelets less than 10 × 10^9/L, or both, after at least 1 month of treatment, follow these steps.

- Check via marrow aspirate or biopsy to see if cytopenia is related to leukemia.
- If cytopenia is unrelated to leukemia, reduce dose of drug to 400 mg.
- If cytopenia persists 2 weeks, reduce further to 300 mg.
- If cytopenia persists 4 weeks and is still unrelated to leukemia, stop Gleevec until ANC is 1 × 10^9/L or greater and platelets are 20 × 10^9/L or greater and then resume treatment at 300 mg.

Contraindications & cautions

- Contraindicated in patients hypersensitive to drug or its components.
- Use cautiously in elderly patients and in those with hepatic impairment.
- Safety and effectiveness in children younger than age 3 haven't been established.

Adverse reactions

CNS: *headache*, ***CEREBRAL HEMORRHAGE***, *fatigue, weakness, pyrexia.*
CV: *edema.*
EENT: nasopharyngitis, *epistaxis.*
GI: *anorexia, nausea, diarrhea, abdominal pain, constipation, vomiting, dyspepsia,* **GI HEMORRHAGE.**
Hematologic: **HEMORRHAGE, NEUTROPENIA, THROMBOCYTOPENIA,** *anemia.*
Metabolic: *hypokalemia*, weight increase.
Musculoskeletal: *myalgia, muscle cramps, musculoskeletal pain, arthralgia.*
Respiratory: *cough, dyspnea, pneumonia.*
Skin: *rash*, pruritus, *petechiae.*
Other: *night sweats.*

Interactions

Drug-drug. *Acetaminophen:* May increase risk of hepatic toxicity. Monitor patient closely.
CYP3A4 inducers (carbamazepine, dexamethasone, phenobarbital, phenytoin, rifampin): May increase metabolism and decrease imatinib level. Use together cautiously.
CYP3A4 inhibitors (clarithromycin, erythromycin, itraconazole, ketoconazole): May decrease metabolism and increase imatinib level. Monitor patient for toxicity.
Dihydropyridine-calcium channel blockers, certain HMG-CoA reductase inhibitors (simvastatin), cyclosporine, pimozide, triazolobenzodiazepines: May increase levels of these drugs. Monitor patient for toxicity and obtain drug levels, if appropriate.
Warfarin: May alter metabolism of warfarin. Avoid using together; use standard heparin or a low-molecular-weight heparin.
Drug-herb. *St. John's wort:* May decrease imatinib effects. Discourage use together.

Nursing considerations

- Elderly patients may have an increased incidence of edema when taking this drug.

• Monitor patient closely for possibly severe fluid retention.
• Monitor weight daily. Evaluate and treat unexpected rapid weight gain.
• Monitor CBC weekly for first month; then decrease to biweekly for second month, and periodically thereafter.
• Because GI irritation is common, tell patient to take drug with food.
• For patients unable to swallow tablets, disperse the tablets in water or apple juice (50 ml for 100-mg tablet or 200 ml for 400-mg tablet). Stir and have patient drink immediately.
• Monitor liver function tests carefully because hepatotoxicity (occasionally severe) may occur; decrease dosage as needed.
• Although there are no data on long-term safety of this drug, monitor renal and liver toxicity and immunosuppression carefully.
• Consider dosage increases only if there are no severe adverse reactions or severe non–leukemia-related neutropenia or thrombocytopenia in the following circumstances: disease progression (at any time), failure to achieve a satisfactory hematologic response after at least 3 months of treatment, or loss of a previously achieved hematologic response.

Patient teaching

• Tell patient to take drug with food and a large glass of water.
• Advise patient unable to swallow tablets that the tablets can be dispersed in water or apple juice (50 ml for 100-mg tablet or 200 ml for 400-mg tablet). Stir and drink immediately.
• Advise patient to report to prescriber any adverse effects, such as fluid retention.
• Advise patient to obtain periodic liver and kidney function tests and blood work to determine blood counts.
• Tell patient to avoid or restrict the use of acetaminophen in OTC or prescription products due to potential toxic effects on the liver.

imipenem and cilastatin sodium

Primaxin I.M., Primaxin I.V.

Pregnancy risk category C

Indications & dosages

➲ **Serious lower respiratory tract, bone, intra-abdominal, gynecologic, joint, skin, and soft-tissue infections; UTIs; endocarditis; and bacterial septicemia, caused by *Acinetobacter, Enterococcus, Staphylococcus, Streptococcus, Escherichia coli, Haemophilus, Klebsiella, Morganella, Proteus, Enterobacter, Pseudomonas aeruginosa,* and *Bacteroides,* including *B. fragilis***

Adults weighing more than 70 kg (154 lb): 250 mg to 1 g by I.V. infusion q 6 to 8 hours. Maximum daily dose is 50 mg/kg/day or 4 g/day, whichever is less. Or, 500 to 750 mg I.M. q 12 hours. Maximum I.M. daily dose is 1,500 mg.

Children age 3 months and older (except for CNS infections): 15 to 25 mg/kg I.V. q 6 hours. Maximum daily dose is 2 to 4 g.

Infants ages 4 weeks to 3 months, weighing 1.5 kg (3.3 lb) or more (except for CNS infections): 25 mg/kg I.V. q 6 hours.

Neonates ages 1 to 4 weeks, weighing 1.5 kg or more (except for CNS infections): 25 mg/kg I.V. q 8 hours.

Neonates younger than age 1 week, weighing 1.5 kg or more (except for CNS infections): 25 mg/kg I.V. q 12 hours.

If creatinine clearance is less than 70 ml/minute, adjust dosage and monitor renal function test results. Consult manufacturer's package insert for specific dosage adjustments.

Contraindications & cautions

• Contraindicated in patients hypersensitive to drug, in those with a history of hypersensitivity to local anesthetics of the amide type, and in those with severe shock or heart block.
• Use cautiously in patients allergic to penicillins or cephalosporins because drug has similar properties.
• Use cautiously in patients with history of seizure disorders, especially if they also have compromised renal function.
• Use cautiously in children younger than age 3 months.

Adverse reactions

CNS: ***seizures***, dizziness, fever, somnolence.
CV: hypotension, thrombophlebitis.
GI: nausea, vomiting, diarrhea, ***pseudomembranous colitis***.
Hematologic: eosinophilia, ***thrombocytopenia***, ***leukopenia***.
Skin: rash, urticaria, pruritus, injection site pain.
Other: hypersensitivity reactions, ***anaphylaxis***.

Interactions

Drug-drug. *Beta-lactam antibiotics:* May have antagonistic effect. Avoid using together.
Ganciclovir: May cause seizures. Avoid using together.
Probenecid: May increase cilastatin level. May be used together for this effect.

Nursing considerations

!!ALERT Don't use for CNS infections in children because it increases the risk of seizures.
- Obtain specimen culture and sensitivity tests before giving first dose. Therapy may begin pending results.

!!ALERT Don't give I.M. solution by I.V. route.

!!ALERT If seizures develop and persist despite anticonvulsant therapy, stop drug and notify prescriber.
- Monitor patient for bacterial or fungal superinfections and resistant infections during and after therapy.

Patient teaching

- Instruct patient to report adverse reactions promptly.
- Tell patient to report discomfort at I.V. insertion site.
- Urge patient to notify prescriber about loose stools or diarrhea.

imipramine hydrochloride

Apo-Imipramine†, Impril†, Novopramine†, Tofranil

imipramine pamoate

Tofranil-PM

Pregnancy risk category D

Indications & dosages

➲ Depression
Adults: 75 to 100 mg P.O. daily in divided doses, increased by 25 to 50 mg. Maximum daily dose is 200 mg for outpatients and 300 mg for hospitalized patients. Give entire dose h.s.
Adolescents and elderly patients: Initially, 30 to 40 mg daily; maximum shouldn't exceed 100 mg daily.

➲ Childhood enuresis
Children age 5 and older: 25 mg P.O. 1 hour before bedtime. If patient doesn't improve within 1 week, increase dose to 50 mg if child is younger than age 12; increase dose to 75 mg for children age 12 and older. In either case, maximum daily dose is 2.5 mg/kg.

Contraindications & cautions

- Contraindicated in patients hypersensitive to drug and in those receiving MAO inhibitors; also contraindicated during acute recovery phase of MI.
- Use with extreme caution in patients at risk for suicide; in patients with history of urine retention, angle-closure glaucoma, or seizure disorders; in patients with increased intraocular pressure, CV disease, impaired hepatic function, hyperthyroidism, or impaired renal function; and in patients receiving thyroid drugs. Injectable form contains sulfites, which may cause allergic reactions in hypersensitive patients.

Adverse reactions

CNS: ***CVA***, *drowsiness*, *dizziness*, excitation, tremor, confusion, hallucinations, anxiety, ataxia, paresthesia, nervousness, EEG changes, ***seizures***, extrapyramidal reactions.
CV: *orthostatic hypotension*, *tachycardia*, *ECG changes*, hypertension, ***MI***, ***arrhythmias***, ***heart block***, precipitation of heart failure.
EENT: *blurred vision*, tinnitus, mydriasis.

GI: *dry mouth, constipation,* nausea, vomiting, anorexia, paralytic ileus, abdominal cramps.
GU: *urine retention.*
Metabolic: ***hypoglycemia***, hyperglycemia.
Skin: rash, urticaria, photosensitivity reactions, pruritus, diaphoresis.
Other: hypersensitivity reactions.

Interactions

Drug-drug. *Barbiturates, CNS depressants:* May enhance CNS depression. Avoid using together.
Cimetidine, fluoxetine, paroxetine: May increase imipramine level. Monitor patient for adverse reactions.
Clonidine: May cause potentially life-threatening elevations in blood pressure. Avoid using together.
Epinephrine, norepinephrine: May increase hypertensive effect. Use together cautiously.
MAO inhibitors: May cause hyperpyretic crisis, severe seizures, and death. Avoid using within 14 days of MAO inhibitor therapy.
Drug-herb. *Evening primrose oil:* May cause additive or synergistic effect, resulting in lower seizure threshold and increasing the risk of seizure. Discourage use together.
St. John's wort, SAM-e, yohimbe: May cause serotonin syndrome. Discourage use together.
Drug-lifestyle. *Alcohol use:* May enhance CNS depression. Discourage use together.
Smoking: May lower level of imipramine. Monitor patient for lack of effect.
Sun exposure: May increase risk of photosensitivity reactions. Advise patient to avoid excessive sunlight exposure.

Nursing considerations

- Monitor patient for nausea, headache, and malaise after abrupt withdrawal of long-term therapy; these symptoms don't indicate addiction.
- Don't withdraw drug abruptly.
- Because of hypertensive episodes during surgery in patients receiving tricyclic antidepressants, stop drug gradually several days before surgery.
- If signs or symptoms of psychosis occur or increase, expect prescriber to reduce dosage. Record mood changes. Monitor patient for suicidal tendencies, and allow only a minimum supply of drug.
- To prevent relapse in children receiving drug for enuresis, withdraw drug gradually.
- Recommend sugarless hard candy or gum to relieve dry mouth. Saliva substitutes may be useful.

!!ALERT Tofranil and Tofranil PM may contain tartrazine.
!!ALERT Don't confuse imipramine with desipramine.

Patient teaching

- Tell patient to take full dose at bedtime whenever possible, but warn him of possible morning dizziness upon standing up quickly.
- If child is an early-night bed wetter, tell parents it may be more effective to divide dose and give the first dose earlier in day.
- Tell patient to avoid alcohol while taking this drug.
- Advise patient to consult prescriber before taking other prescription or OTC drugs.
- Warn patient to avoid hazardous activities that require alertness and good coordination until effects of the drug are known. Drowsiness and dizziness usually subside after a few weeks.
- Warn patient not to stop drug suddenly.
- To prevent oversensitivity to the sun, advise patient to use sunblock, wear protective clothing, and avoid prolonged exposure to strong sunlight.

imiquimod
Aldara

Pregnancy risk category B

Indications & dosages

➲ External genital and perianal warts
Adults and adolescents age 12 and older: Apply thin layer to affected area three times weekly before normal sleeping hours and leave on skin for 6 to 10 hours. Continue treatment until genital or perianal warts clear completely or maximum of 16 weeks.
➲ Typical, nonhyperkeratotic, nonhypertrophic actinic keratoses on the face or scalp in immunocompetent adults
Adults: Wash area with mild soap and water and dry at least 10 minutes. Apply cream to face or scalp, but not both concurrently, twice weekly at bedtime and wash off after about 8 hours. Treat for 16 weeks.

Contraindications & cautions

- Drug isn't recommended for treatment of urethral, intravaginal, cervical, rectal, or intra-anal human papillomavirus disease.
- Safety of drug in breast-feeding women is unknown.

Adverse reactions

CNS: headache.
Musculoskeletal: myalgia.
Skin: local itching, burning, pain, soreness, erythema, ulceration, edema, erosion, induration, flaking, excoriation.
Other: flulike symptoms, *fungal infection.*

Interactions

None significant.

Nursing considerations

- Don't use until genital or perianal tissue is healed from previous drug or surgical treatment.
- Patient usually experiences local skin reactions at site of application or surrounding areas. Use nonocclusive dressings, such as cotton gauze, or cotton undergarments in management of skin reactions. Patient's discomfort or severity of the local skin reaction may require a rest period of several days. Resume treatment once reaction subsides.
- Drug isn't a cure; new warts may develop during therapy.

Patient teaching

- Advise patient that effect of cream on transmission of genital or perianal warts is unknown. New warts may develop during therapy; drug isn't a cure.
- Tell patient to use cream only as directed and to avoid contact with eyes.
- Tell patient to wash hands before and after applying cream.
- Advise patient to apply cream in thin layer over affected area and rub in until cream isn't visible. Advise patient to avoid excessive use of cream. Tell him not to occlude area after applying cream and to wash with mild soap and water 6 to 10 hours after application of cream.
- Advise patient that mild local skin reactions, such as redness, erosion, excoriation, flaking, and swelling at site of application or surrounding areas, are common. Tell him that most skin reactions are mild to moderate. Advise him to report severe skin reactions promptly.
- Instruct uncircumcised man being treated for warts under the foreskin to retract foreskin and clean area daily.
- Advise patient that drug can weaken condoms and vaginal diaphragms and that use together isn't recommended.
- Advise patient to avoid sexual contact while cream is on the skin.
- Tell patient to store drug at temperatures below 86° F (30° C) and to avoid freezing.

---

immune globulin intramuscular (gamma globulin, IG, IGIM)

BayGam

immune globulin intravenous (IGIV)

Carimune, Gamimune N, Gammagard S/D, Gammar-P I.V., Gamunex, Iveegam EN, Octagam, Panglobulin, Polygam S/D, Venoglobulin-S

Pregnancy risk category C

Indications & dosages

➲ **Primary immunodeficiency (IGIV)**

Carimune, Panglobulin

Adults and children: 200 mg/kg I.V. once monthly. May increase dose to maximum of 300 mg/kg once monthly or give more often to produce desired effect.

Gamimune N

Adults and children: 100 to 200 mg/kg I.V. once monthly; maximum 400 mg/kg once monthly.

Gammagard S/D

Adults and children: 200 to 400 mg/kg I.V. once monthly; minimum 100 mg/kg once monthly.

Gamunex

Adults and children: 300 to 600 mg/kg I.V. q 3 to 4 weeks.

Iveegam EN

Adults and children: 200 mg/kg I.V. once monthly. May increase dose to maximum of 800 mg/kg, or give more often to produce desired effect.

Octagam

Adults and children: 300 to 600 mg/kg I.V. q 3 to 4 weeks. Adjust dose over time to produce desired effect.

Polygam S/D
Adults and children: 200 to 400 mg/kg I.V. once monthly. Minimum dose is 100 mg/kg once monthly

➲ **Primary defective antibody synthesis such as agammaglobulinemia or hypogammaglobulinemia in patients at increased risk of infection**
Gammar-P I.V.
Adults: 200 to 400 mg/kg I.V. q 3 to 4 weeks.
Adolescents and children: 200 mg/kg I.V. q 3 to 4 weeks. Adjust dosage according to clinical effect and to maintain immunoglobulin G (IgG) at desired level.
Venoglobulin-S
Adults and children: 200 mg/kg I.V. once monthly. May increase dose to 300 to 400 mg/kg, or give more often to maintain IgG at desired level.

➲ **Idiopathic thrombocytopenic purpura (IGIV)**
Carimune, Panglobulin
Adults and children: 400 mg/kg I.V. daily for 2 to 5 consecutive days; maximum 1 g/kg/day.
Gamimune N
Adults and children: 400 mg/kg 5% or 10% solution I.V. for 2 to 5 consecutive days; or 1 g/kg 5% or 10% solution I.V. for 1 to 2 consecutive days with maintenance dose of 5% or 10% solution at 400 to 1,000 mg/kg I.V. single infusion to maintain platelet count over 30,000/mm^3.
Gammagard S/D, Polygam S/D
Adults and children: 1 g/kg I.V. Additional doses depend on response. Up to three doses may be given on alternate days, if needed.
Gamunex
Adults and children: 1 g/kg I.V. daily for 2 consecutive days. If adequate increase in platelet count occurs after first dose, second dose may be withheld. Or, 400 mg/kg I.V. daily for 5 consecutive days. Total dosage is 2 g/kg.
Venoglobulin-S
Adults and children: Maximum of 2 g/kg I.V. divided over up to 5 days. Maintenance dose is 1 g/kg I.V. p.r.n. to maintain platelet counts of 30,000/mm^3 in children and 20,000/mm^3 in adults, or to prevent bleeding episodes.

➲ **Bone marrow transplantation (IGIV)**
Gamimune N
Adults older than age 20: 500 mg/kg 5% or 10% solution I.V. on days 7 and 2 before transplantation; then weekly until 90 days after transplantation.

➲ **B-cell chronic lymphocytic leukemia (IGIV)**
Adults: 400 mg/kg Gammagard S/D or Polygam S/D I.V. q 3 to 4 weeks.

➲ **To prevent coronary artery aneurysm in patients with Kawasaki syndrome (IGIV)**
Adults and children: Combine with high-dose aspirin therapy and start within 10 days of fever.
Iveegam EN, Venoglobulin-S 5% or 10%
Adults and children: 2 g/kg I.V. over 10 to 12 hours; may give another dose.
Gammagard S/D
Adults and children: Single 1-g/kg dose Or, 400 mg/kg/day for 4 consecutive days.

➲ **Pediatric HIV infection (IGIV)**
Children: 400 mg/kg Gamimune N 5% or 10% solution I.V. q 28 days.

➲ **Hepatitis A exposure (IGIM)**
Adults and children: 0.02 ml/kg I.M. as soon as possible after exposure; may give up to 0.06 ml/kg for prolonged or intense exposure.

➲ **Measles exposure (IGIM)**
Adults and children: 0.2 to 0.25 ml/kg I.M. within 6 days after exposure.

➲ **Postexposure prophylaxis of measles (IGIM)**
Immunocompromised children age 12 months and older: 0.5 ml/kg I.M. within 6 days after exposure (maximum 15 ml).

➲ **Chickenpox exposure (IGIM)** ♦
Adults and children: 0.6 to 1.2 ml/kg I.M. as soon as exposed.

Contraindications & cautions

- Contraindicated in patients hypersensitive to drug or its components.
- IGIV administration may be linked to thrombotic events. Use IGIV cautiously in patients with a history of CV disease or thrombotic episodes.
- Use IGIV cautiously in patients with renal dysfunction or a predisposition to renal failure, including patients with pre-existing renal insufficiency, diabetes mellitus, age older than 65, volume depletion, sepsis, par-

aproteinemia, or those receiving known nephrotoxic drugs.

Adverse reactions

CNS: headache, fever, faintness, malaise, ***severe headache requiring hospitalization***.
CV: chest pain, MI, congestive cardiac failure.
GI: nausea, vomiting.
Musculoskeletal: hip pain, chest pain, chest tightness, muscle stiffness at injection site.
Respiratory: dyspnea, ***pulmonary embolism, transfusion related acute lung injury***.
Skin: urticaria, pain, erythema.
Other: ***anaphylaxis***, chills.

Interactions

Drug-drug. *Live-virus vaccines:* Length of time to wait before giving live-virus vaccinations varies with dose of immune globulin given. Refer to recommendations by American Academy of Pediatrics.

Nursing considerations

- Obtain history of allergies and reactions to immunizations. Keep epinephrine 1:1,000 available to treat anaphylaxis.
- If risk of a thrombotic event is possible, make sure infusion concentration is no more than 5% and start infusion rate no faster than 0.5 ml/kg body weight per hour. Advance rate slowly only if well tolerated, to a maximum rate of 4 ml/kg body weight per hour.
- When giving I.M., use gluteal region. Divide doses larger than 10 ml and inject into several muscle sites to reduce pain and discomfort.
- Give drug soon after reconstitution.
- Don't give immune globulin for prophylaxis against hepatitis A if 6 weeks or more have elapsed since exposure or onset of clinical illness.

Patient teaching

- Explain to patient and family how drug will be given.
- Tell patient that local reactions may occur at injection site. Instruct him to notify prescriber promptly if adverse reactions persist or become severe.
- Inform patient of possible need to have therapy more than once monthly to maintain appropriate immunoglobulin G levels.

inamrinone lactate

Pregnancy risk category C

Indications & dosages

➲ **Short-term management of heart failure**
Adults: Initially, 0.75 mg/kg I.V. bolus over 2 to 3 minutes. Then begin maintenance infusion of 5 to 10 mcg/kg/minute. May give additional bolus of 0.75 mg/kg 30 minutes after starting therapy. Don't exceed total daily dose of 10 mg/kg.

Contraindications & cautions

- Contraindicated in patients hypersensitive to inamrinone or bisulfites.
- Contraindicated in patients with severe aortic or pulmonic valvular disease in place of surgery or during acute phase of MI.
- Use cautiously in patients with hypertrophic cardiomyopathy.
- Safety and effectiveness haven't been established in children younger than age 18.

Adverse reactions

CNS: fever.
CV: ***arrhythmias***, hypotension, chest pain.
GI: nausea, vomiting, anorexia, abdominal pain.
Hematologic: ***thrombocytopenia***.
Metabolic: hypokalemia.
Skin: burning at injection site.
Other: hypersensitivity reactions.

Interactions

Drug-drug. *Cardiac glycosides:* May increase inotropic effect, which is a beneficial drug interaction. Monitor patient.
Disopyramide: May cause excessive hypotension. Monitor blood pressure.

Nursing considerations

- Inamrinone is prescribed primarily for patients who haven't responded to cardiac glycosides, diuretics, and vasodilators.
- Dosage depends on clinical response, including assessment of pulmonary wedge pressure and cardiac output.
- Anticipate that drug may be added to cardiac glycoside therapy in patients with atrial fibrillation and flutter because it slightly enhances AV conduction and increases ventricular response rate.

• Correct hypokalemia before or during therapy.
• Monitor platelet count. If it falls below 150,000/mm^3, decrease dosage.
• Monitor patient for hypersensitivity reactions, such as pericarditis, ascites, myositis vasculitis, and pleuritis.
• Monitor intake and output and daily weight.
• Patients with end-stage cardiac disease may receive home treatment with an inamrinone drip while awaiting heart transplantation.

!! ALERT Because of confusion with amiodarone, the generic name *amrinone* was changed to *inamrinone*.

Patient teaching

• Warn patient that burning may occur at injection site.
• Instruct home care patient and family on drug administration; tell them to report adverse reactions promptly.

indapamide

Lozide†, Lozol

Pregnancy risk category B

Indications & dosages

➲ Edema

Adults: Initially, 2.5 mg P.O. daily in the morning. Increased to 5 mg daily after 1 week, if needed.

➲ Hypertension

Adults: Initially, 1.25 mg P.O. daily in the morning. Increased to 2.5 mg daily after 4 weeks, if needed. Increased to 5 mg daily after 4 more weeks, if needed.

Contraindications & cautions

• Contraindicated in patients hypersensitive to other sulfonamide-derived drugs and in those with anuria.
• Use cautiously in patients with severe renal disease, impaired hepatic function, or progressive hepatic disease.

Adverse reactions

CNS: headache, nervousness, dizziness, light-headedness, weakness, vertigo, restlessness, drowsiness, fatigue, anxiety, depression, numbness of limbs, irritability, agitation.
CV: orthostatic hypotension, palpitations, PVCs, irregular heartbeat, vasculitis, flushing.
EENT: rhinorrhea.
GI: anorexia, nausea, epigastric distress, vomiting, abdominal pain, diarrhea, constipation.
GU: nocturia, polyuria, frequent urination, impotence.
Metabolic: asymptomatic hyperuricemia, fluid and electrolyte imbalances, including dilutional hyponatremia, hypochloremia, metabolic alkalosis, and hypokalemia, weight loss, volume depletion and dehydration, hyperglycemia.
Musculoskeletal: muscle cramps and spasms.
Skin: rash, pruritus, urticaria.
Other: gout.

Interactions

Drug-drug. *Amphotericin B, corticosteroids:* May increase risk of hypokalemia. Monitor potassium level closely.
Antidiabetics: May decrease hypoglycemic effect. May need to adjust dosage. Monitor glucose level.
Barbiturates, opioids: May increase orthostasis. Monitor patient closely.
Bumetanide, ethacrynic acid, furosemide, torsemide: May cause excessive diuretic response, causing serious electrolyte abnormalities or dehydration. Adjust doses carefully, and monitor patient closely for signs and symptoms of excessive diuretic response.
Cardiac glycosides: May increase risk of digoxin toxicity from indapamide-induced hypokalemia. Monitor potassium and digoxin levels.
Cholestyramine, colestipol: May decrease absorption of thiazides. Separate doses by 2 hours.
Diazoxide: May increase antihypertensive, hyperglycemic, and hyperuricemic effects. Use together cautiously.
Lithium: May decrease lithium clearance that may increase lithium toxicity. Avoid using together.
NSAIDs: May increase risk of NSAID-induced renal failure. Monitor patient for signs and symptoms of renal failure.
Drug-herb. *Dandelion:* May interfere with diuretic activity. Discourage use together.

Licorice: May cause unexpected rapid potassium loss. Discourage use together.
Drug-lifestyle. *Alcohol use:* May increase orthostatic hypotensive effect. Discourage use together.

Nursing considerations

- To prevent nocturia, give drug in the morning.
- Monitor fluid intake and output, weight, blood pressure, and electrolyte levels.
- Watch for signs of hypokalemia, such as muscle weakness and cramps. Drug may be used with potassium-sparing diuretic to prevent potassium loss.
- Consult prescriber and dietitian about a high-potassium diet. Foods rich in potassium include citrus fruits, tomatoes, bananas, dates, and apricots.
- Monitor creatinine and BUN levels regularly. Cumulative effects of drug may occur in patients with impaired renal function.
- Monitor uric acid level, especially in patients with history of gout.
- Monitor glucose level, especially in diabetic patients.
- Monitor elderly patients, who are especially susceptible to excessive diuresis.
- Stop thiazides and thiazide-like diuretics before parathyroid function tests.
- Therapeutic response may be delayed several weeks in hypertensive patients.

Patient teaching

- Instruct patient to take drug in morning to prevent need to urinate at night.
- Tell patient to take drug with food to minimize GI upset.
- Advise patient to avoid sudden posture changes and to rise slowly to avoid dizziness upon standing quickly.

indinavir sulfate

Crixivan

Pregnancy risk category C

Indications & dosages

➲ **HIV infection, with other antiretrovirals, when antiretroviral therapy is warranted**
Adults: 800 mg P.O. q 8 hours.

For patients with mild to moderate hepatic insufficiency from cirrhosis, reduce dosage to 600 mg P.O. q 8 hours.

Contraindications & cautions

- Contraindicated in patients hypersensitive to drug or its components.
- Use cautiously in patients with hepatic insufficiency from cirrhosis.
- Safety and effectiveness in children haven't been established. Don't use drug in children.

Adverse reactions

CNS: headache, insomnia, dizziness, somnolence, asthenia, malaise, fatigue.
CV: chest pain, palpitations.
EENT: blurred vision, eye pain or swelling.
GI: abdominal pain, *nausea*, diarrhea, vomiting, acid regurgitation, anorexia, dry mouth, taste perversion.
GU: nephrolithiasis, hematuria.
Hematologic: ***neutropenia, thrombocytopenia***, anemia.
Metabolic: *hyperbilirubinemia*, hyperglycemia.
Musculoskeletal: back pain.
Other: flank pain.

Interactions

Drug-drug. *Amprenavir, saquinavir:* May increase levels of these drugs. Dosage adjustments not needed.
Carbamazepine: May decrease indinavir exposure to the body. Consider an alternative drug.
Clarithromycin: May alter clarithromycin level. Dosage adjustments not needed.
Delavirdine, itraconazole, ketoconazole: May increase indinavir level. Consider reducing indinavir to 600 mg q 8 hours.
Didanosine: May alter absorption of indinavir. Separate doses by 1 hour and give on an empty stomach.
Efavirenz, nevirapine: May decrease indinavir level. Increase indinavir to 1,000 mg q 8 hours.
HMG-CoA reductase inhibitors: May increase levels of these drugs and increase risk of myopathy and rhabdomyolysis. Avoid using together.
Lopinavir and ritonavir combination: May increase indinavir level. Adjust indinavir dosage to 600 mg b.i.d.

Midazolam, triazolam: May inhibit metabolism of these drugs, which may cause serious or life-threatening events, such as arrhythmias or prolonged sedation. Avoid using together.
Nelfinavir: May increase indinavir level by 50% and nelfinavir by 80%. May need to adjust dosage to indinavir 1,200 mg b.i.d. and nelfinavir 1,250 mg b.i.d. Monitor patient closely.
Rifabutin: May increase rifabutin level and decrease indinavir level. Give indinavir 1,000 mg q 8 hours and decrease the rifabutin dose to either 150 mg daily or 300 mg two to three times a week.
Rifampin: May decrease indinavir level. Avoid using together.
Ritonavir: May increase indinavir level twofold to fivefold. Adjust dosage to indinavir 400 mg b.i.d. and ritonavir 400 mg b.i.d., or indinavir 800 mg b.i.d. and ritonavir 100 to 200 mg b.i.d.
Sildenafil: May increase sildenafil level and increase adverse effects (hypotension, visual changes, and priapism). Tell patient not to exceed 25 mg of sildenafil in 48 hours.
Drug-herb. *St. John's wort:* May reduce indinavir level by more than 50%. Discourage use together.
Drug-food. *Grapefruit and grapefruit juice:* May decrease level and therapeutic effect of indinavir. Discourage use together.

Nursing considerations

- Drug must be taken at 8-hour intervals.
- Drug may cause nephrolithiasis. If signs and symptoms of nephrolithiasis occur, prescriber may stop drug for 1 to 3 days during acute phases.
- To prevent nephrolithiasis, patient should maintain adequate hydration (at least 48 ounces or 1.5 L of fluids q 24 hours while taking indinavir).

Patient teaching

- Tell patient that drug doesn't cure HIV infection and that he may continue to develop opportunistic infections and other complications of HIV infection. Drug hasn't been shown to reduce the risk of HIV transmission.
- Advise patient to use barrier protection during sexual intercourse.
- Caution patient not to adjust dosage or stop indinavir therapy without first consulting prescriber.
- Advise patient that if a dose of indinavir is missed, he should take the next dose at the regularly scheduled time and shouldn't double the dose.
- Instruct patient to take drug on an empty stomach with water 1 hour before or 2 hours after a meal. Or, he may take it with other liquids (such as skim milk, juice, coffee, or tea) or a light meal. Inform patient that a meal high in fat, calories, and protein reduces absorption of drug.
- Instruct patient to store capsules in the original container and to keep desiccant in the bottle; capsules are sensitive to moisture.
- Tell patient to drink at least 48 ounces (1.5 L) of fluid daily.
- Advise woman to avoid breast-feeding because indinavir may appear in breast milk. Also, to prevent transmitting virus to infant, advise an HIV-positive woman not to breastfeed.
- Advise patient taking sildenafil that he may be at higher risk of sildenafil-related adverse events, including low blood pressure, visual changes, and painful erections. Tell him to promptly report any symptoms to his prescriber. Patient shouldn't take more than 25 mg of sildenafil in a 48-hour period.

indomethacin

Apo-Indomethacin†, Indocid SR†, Indocin, Indocin SR, Novo-Methacin†

indomethacin sodium trihydrate

Apo-Indomethacin†, Indocin I.V, Novo-Methacin†

Pregnancy risk category B; D in 3rd trimester

Indications & dosages

➲ **Moderate to severe rheumatoid arthritis or osteoarthritis, ankylosing spondylitis**
Adults: 25 mg P.O. or P.R. b.i.d. or t.i.d. with food or antacids; increase daily dose by 25 or 50 mg q 7 days, up to 200 mg daily. Or, 75 mg sustained-release capsules P.O. to

start, in morning or h.s., followed by 75 mg sustained-release capsules b.i.d. if needed.

➲ **Acute gouty arthritis**

Adults: 50 mg P.O. t.i.d. Reduce dose as soon as possible; then stop therapy. Don't use sustained-release form.

➲ **Acute painful shoulders (bursitis or tendinitis)**

Adults: 75 to 150 mg P.O. daily in divided doses t.i.d. or q.i.d. for 7 to 14 days.

➲ **To close a hemodynamically significant patent ductus arteriosus in premature neonates (I.V. form only)**

Neonates older than age 7 days: 0.2 mg/kg I.V.; then two doses of 0.25 mg/kg at 12- to 24-hour intervals.

Neonates ages 2 to 7 days: 0.2 mg/kg I.V.; then two doses of 0.2 mg/kg at 12- to 24-hour intervals.

Neonates younger than age 48 hours: 0.2 mg/kg I.V.; then two doses of 0.1 mg/kg at 12- to 24-hour intervals.

Contraindications & cautions

- Contraindicated in patients hypersensitive to drug and in those with a history of aspirin- or NSAID-induced asthma, rhinitis, or urticaria.
- Contraindicated in pregnant or breast-feeding women and in neonates with untreated infection, active bleeding, coagulation defects or thrombocytopenia, congenital heart disease needing patency of the ductus arteriosus, necrotizing enterocolitis, or significant renal impairment. Suppositories are contraindicated in patients with history of proctitis or recent rectal bleeding.
- Contraindicated in pregnant women.
- Use cautiously in elderly patients, those with history of GI disease, and those with epilepsy, parkinsonism, hepatic or renal disease, CV disease, infection, and mental illness or depression.

Adverse reactions

P.O. and P.R.

CNS: *headache*, dizziness, depression, drowsiness, confusion, somnolence, fatigue, peripheral neuropathy, psychic disturbances, syncope, vertigo.

CV: hypertension, edema.

EENT: hearing loss, tinnitus.

GI: nausea, anorexia, diarrhea, abdominal pain, peptic ulceration, GI bleeding, constipation, dyspepsia, ***pancreatitis***.

GU: hematuria.

Hematologic: iron deficiency anemia.

Metabolic: ***hyperkalemia***.

Skin: pruritus, urticaria, ***Stevens-Johnson syndrome***.

Other: hypersensitivity reactions.

I.V.

GU: hematuria, proteinuria, interstitial nephritis.

Interactions

Drug-drug. *Aminoglycosides, cyclosporine, methotrexate:* May enhance toxicity of these drugs. Avoid using together.

Anticoagulants: May cause bleeding. Monitor patient closely.

Antihypertensives: May decrease antihypertensive effect. Monitor patient closely.

Antihypertensives, furosemide, thiazide diuretics: May impair response to both drugs. Avoid using together, if possible.

Aspirin: May decrease level of indomethacin. Avoid using together.

Aspirin, corticosteroids: May increase risk of GI toxicity. Avoid using together.

Bisphosphonates: May increase risk of gastric ulceration. Monitor patient for symptoms of gastric irritation or GI bleeding.

Diflunisal, probenecid: May decrease indomethacin excretion. Watch for increased indomethacin adverse reactions.

Digoxin: May prolong half-life of digoxin. Use together cautiously.

Dipyridamole: May enhance fluid retention. Avoid using together.

Lithium: May increase lithium level. Monitor patient for toxicity.

Penicillamine: May increase bioavailability of penicillamine. Monitor patient closely.

Phenytoin: May increase phenytoin level. Monitor patient closely.

Triamterene: May cause nephrotoxicity. Monitor patient closely.

Drug-herb. *Dong quai, feverfew, garlic, ginger, horse chestnut, red clover:* May cause bleeding. Discourage use together.

Senna: May inhibit diarrheal effects. Discourage use together.

White willow: Herb contains components similar to those of aspirin. Discourage use together.

Drug-lifestyle. *Alcohol use:* May cause GI toxicity. Discourage use together.

Nursing considerations

- Because of the high risk of adverse effects from long-term use, indomethacin shouldn't be used routinely as an analgesic or antipyretic.
- Sustained-release capsules shouldn't be used for treatment of acute gouty arthritis.
- Give oral dose with food, milk, or antacid to decrease GI upset.
- If ductus arteriosus reopens, a second course of one to three doses may be given. If ineffective, surgery may be needed.
- Watch for bleeding in patients receiving anticoagulants, patients with coagulation defects, and neonates.
- Because NSAIDs impair synthesis of renal prostaglandins, they can decrease renal blood flow and lead to reversible renal impairment, especially in patients with renal failure, heart failure, or liver dysfunction; in elderly patients; and in those taking diuretics. Monitor these patients closely.
- Drug causes sodium retention; watch for weight gain (especially in elderly patients) and increased blood pressure in patients with hypertension.
- Monitor patient for rash and respiratory distress, which may indicate a hypersensitivity reaction.
- Because of their antipyretic and anti-inflammatory actions, NSAIDs may mask signs and symptoms of infection.
- Serious GI toxicity (including peptic ulcers and bleeding) can occur in patient taking NSAIDs, despite lack of symptoms.

Patient teaching

- Tell patient to take oral drug with food, milk, or antacid to prevent GI upset.
- Alert patient that using oral form with aspirin, alcohol, other NSAIDs, or corticosteroids may increase risk of adverse GI reactions.
- Teach patient signs and symptoms of GI bleeding, including blood in vomit, urine, or stool; coffee-ground vomit; and black, tarry stool. Tell him to notify prescriber immediately if any of these occurs.
- Warn patient to avoid hazardous activities that require mental alertness until CNS effects are known.
- Tell patient to notify prescriber immediately if visual or hearing changes occur. Monitor patient on long-term oral therapy for toxicity by conducting regular eye examinations, hearing tests, complete blood counts, and kidney function tests.

infliximab
Remicade

Pregnancy risk category B

Indications & dosages

➲ **Reduction of signs and symptoms, and induction and maintenance of clinical remission in patients with moderately to severely active Crohn's disease who have had an inadequate response to conventional therapy; reduction in the number of draining enterocutaneous and rectovaginal fistulas and maintenance of fistula closure in patients with fistulizing Crohn's disease**

Adults: 5 mg/kg I.V. infusion over 2 hours, given as an induction regimen at 0, 2, and 6 weeks, followed by a maintenance regimen of 5 mg/kg q 8 weeks thereafter. For patients who respond and then lose their response, consideration may be given to treatment with 10 mg/kg. Patients who don't respond by week 14 are unlikely to respond with continued therapy. In those patients, consider stopping infliximab.

➲ **With methotrexate to reduce signs and symptoms, and to inhibit progression of structural damage and improve physical function in patients with moderately to severely active rheumatoid arthritis**

Adults: 3 mg/kg I.V. infusion over at least 2 hours. Give additional doses of 3 mg/kg at 2 and 6 weeks after first infusion and q 8 weeks thereafter. Dose may be increased up to 10 mg/kg, or doses may be given q 4 weeks if response is inadequate.

➲ **Ankylosing spondylitis**

Adults: 5 mg/kg I.V. infusion over at least 2 hours. Give additional doses of 5 mg/kg at 2 and 6 weeks after first infusion then q 6 weeks thereafter.

➲ **Psoriatic arthritis, with or without methotrexate**

Adults: 5 mg/kg I.V. infusion over at least 2 hours. Give additional doses of 5 mg/kg at 2 and 6 weeks after first infusion then q 8 weeks thereafter.

Contraindications & cautions

- Contraindicated in patients hypersensitive to murine proteins or other components of drug and in those with congestive heart failure.
- Use cautiously in elderly patients and in patients with active infection or history of chronic or recurrent infections. In patients who have resided in regions where histoplasmosis is endemic, carefully consider the benefits and risks of infliximab therapy before starting therapy.
- Use cautiously in patients with a history of hematologic abnormalities or those with pre-existing or recent onset of CNS demyelinating or seizure disorders.

Adverse reactions

CNS: *fever, headache, fatigue*, dizziness, malaise, insomnia, depression, systemic and cutaneous vasculitis.
CV: *hypertension*, hypotension, tachycardia, chest pain, pericardial effusion, flushing.
EENT: *pharyngitis, rhinitis, sinusitis*, conjunctivitis.
GI: *nausea, abdominal pain*, vomiting, constipation, *dyspepsia, diarrhea*, flatulence, ***intestinal obstruction***, oral pain, ulcerative stomatitis.
GU: dysuria, increased urinary frequency, *UTI*.
Hematologic: anemia, hematoma, ***leukopenia, neutropenia, thrombocytopenia, pancytopenia***.
Musculoskeletal: myalgia, *arthralgia, back pain*, arthritis.
Respiratory: *upper respiratory tract infections*, bronchitis, *coughing*, dyspnea, respiratory tract allergic reaction.
Skin: *rash*, pruritus, candidiasis, acne, alopecia, eczema, erythema, erythematous rash, maculopapular rash, papular rash, dry skin, increased sweating, urticaria.
Other: toothache, flulike syndrome, ecchymosis, chills, pain, peripheral edema, hot flashes, abscess.

Interactions

Drug-drug. *Anakinra:* May increase the risk of serious infections and neutropenia. Avoid use together.
Vaccines: May affect normal immune response. Postpone live-virus vaccine until therapy stops.

Nursing considerations

!!ALERT Watch for infusion-related reactions, including fever, chills, pruritus, urticaria, dyspnea, hypotension, hypertension, and chest pain, during administration and for 2 hours afterward. If an infusion-related reaction occurs, stop drug, notify prescriber, and be prepared to give acetaminophen, antihistamines, corticosteroids, and epinephrine.
- Consider stopping treatment in patients who develop significant hematologic abnormalities or CNS adverse reactions.
- Watch for development of lymphoma and infection. Patient with chronic Crohn's disease and long-term exposure to immunosuppressants is more likely to develop lymphoma and infection.
- Drug may affect normal immune responses. Patient may develop autoimmune antibodies and lupus-like syndrome; stop drug if this happens. Symptoms can be expected to resolve.

!!ALERT Drug may cause disseminated or extrapulmonary tuberculosis and fatal opportunistic infections.
- Evaluate patient for latent tuberculosis infection with a tuberculin skin test. Treat latent tuberculosis infection before starting therapy with infliximab.

Patient teaching

- Tell patient about infusion-reaction symptoms and instruct him to report them.
- Inform patient of adverse effects that may occur after infusion, and instruct him to report them promptly.
- Advise patient to seek immediate medical attention for signs and symptoms of infection or strange or unusual bleeding or bruising
- Tell breast-feeding woman to stop breastfeeding during therapy.
- Instruct patient to tell prescriber of drug use before receiving vaccines.

insulin aspart (rDNA origin) injection
NovoLog

insulin aspart (rDNA origin) protamine suspension and insulin aspart (rDNA origin) injection
NovoLog 70/30

Pregnancy risk category C

Indications & dosages

➲ Control of hyperglycemia in patients with diabetes

NovoLog

Adults and children age 6 and older: Dosage is highly individualized. Typical daily insulin requirement is 0.5 to 1 unit/kg/day, divided in a meal-related treatment regimen. About 50% to 70% of dose is provided with NovoLog and the remainder by an intermediate- or long-acting insulin. Give 5 to 10 minutes before start of meal by S.C. injection in the abdominal wall, thigh, or upper arm. External insulin infusion pumps: initially, based on the total daily insulin dose of the previous regimen. Usually 50% of the total dose is given as meal-related boluses, and the remainder as basal infusion. Adjust dose p.r.n.

NovoLog 70/30

Adults: Dosage is individualized based on the needs of the patient. Doses are usually given twice daily within 15 minutes of meals.

Contraindications & cautions

- Contraindicated during episodes of hypoglycemia and in patients hypersensitive to NovoLog or one of its components.
- Use cautiously in patients susceptible to hypoglycemia and hypokalemia, such as those who have autonomic neuropathy or are fasting, taking potassium-lowering drugs, or taking drugs sensitive to potassium level.

Adverse reactions

Metabolic: ***hypoglycemia***, hypokalemia.
Skin: injection site reactions, lipodystrophy, pruritus, rash.
Other: ***allergic reactions***.

Interactions

Drug-drug. *ACE inhibitors, disopyramide, fibrates, fluoxetine, MAO inhibitors, oral antidiabetics, propoxyphene, salicylates, somatostatin analogue (octreotide), sulfonamide antibiotics:* May enhance the glucose-lowering effect of insulin and potentiate hypoglycemia. Monitor glucose level, and watch for signs and symptoms of hypoglycemia. May need insulin dose adjustment.
Beta blockers, clonidine: May increase or decrease the glucose-lowering effect of insulin and cause hypoglycemia or hyperglycemia. May reduce or mask symptoms of hypoglycemia. Monitor glucose level.
Corticosteroids, danazol, diuretics, estrogens, progestins (as in hormonal contraceptives), isoniazid, niacin, phenothiazine derivatives, somatropin, sympathomimetics (epinephrine, salbutamol, terbutaline), and thyroid hormones: May decrease the glucose-lowering effect of insulin and cause hyperglycemia. Monitor glucose level. May require insulin dose adjustment.
Crystalline zinc preparations: May be incompatible with NovoLog. Don't mix together.
Guanethidine, reserpine: May reduce or mask symptoms of hypoglycemia. Monitor glucose level.
Lithium salts, pentamidine: May increase or decrease glucose-lowering effect of insulin and may cause hypoglycemia or hyperglycemia. Pentamidine may cause hypoglycemia, sometimes followed by hyperglycemia. Monitor glucose level.
Drug-herb. *Burdock, dandelion, eucalyptus, marshmallow:* May increase hypoglycemic effects. Discourage use together.
Drug-lifestyle. *Alcohol use:* May increase or decrease glucose-lowering effect of insulin, causing hypoglycemia or hyperglycemia. Advise patient to monitor glucose level.
Exercise: May alter the need for insulin, requiring dose adjustment. Advise patient to report changes in physical activity.
Marijuana use: May increase glucose level. Tell patient to avoid marijuana use.
Smoking: May increase glucose level and decrease response to insulin. Monitor glucose level.

Nursing considerations

- Give NovoLog 5 to 10 minutes before the start of a meal. Give NovoLog 70/30 up to 15 minutes before the start of a meal. Because of its rapid onset of action and short duration of action, patients also may need longer-acting insulins to prevent pre-meal hyperglycemia.

- Let insulin warm to room temperature before administering to minimize discomfort. Then give by S.C. injection into the abdominal wall, thigh, or upper arm. Rotate sites to minimize lipodystrophies.
- The time course of NovoLog action may vary among people or at different times in the same person and depends on the site of injection, blood supply, temperature, and physical activity.
- Adjustments in the dose of NovoLog or of any insulin may be needed with changes in physical activity or meal routine. Insulin requirements also may be altered during emotional disturbances, illness, or other stresses.
- When giving and mixing NovoLog with NPH human insulin, draw up NovoLog into syringe first and give immediately after dose is drawn up.
- Adjust dose regularly, according to patient's glucose measurements. Monitor glucose level regularly.
- Store drug between 36° and 46° F (2° and 8° C). Don't freeze. Don't expose vials to excessive heat or sunlight. Open vials of NovoLog 70/30 and open vials and cartridges of NovoLog are stable at room temperature for 28 days. Punctured cartridges of NovoLog 70/30 may be stored at room temperature up to 14 days; don't refrigerate punctured NovoLog 70/30 cartridges.

!!ALERT Don't confuse NovoLog 70/30 with Novolin 70/30.

- Periodically monitor glycosylated hemoglobin level.
- Assess patient for rash (including pruritus) over whole body, shortness of breath, wheezing, hypotension, rapid pulse, or sweating, which may signify a generalized allergy to insulin. Severe cases, including anaphylactic reactions, may be life threatening.
- Patients with renal dysfunction and hepatic impairment may need close glucose monitoring and dose adjustments of NovoLog.
- Observe injection sites for reactions such as redness, swelling, itching, or burning. These reactions should resolve within a few days to a few weeks.

!!ALERT Don't give I.V.

- Assess patient and notify prescriber for signs and symptoms of hypoglycemia (sweating, shaking, trembling, confusion, headache, irritability, hunger, rapid pulse, nausea) and hyperglycemia (drowsiness, fruity breath odor, frequent urination, thirst).
- Symptoms of hypoglycemia may occur in patients with diabetes, regardless of glucose value.
- Patients with long duration of diabetes, diabetic nerve disease, or intensified diabetes control may have different or less-pronounced early warning symptoms of hypoglycemia; severe hypoglycemia may occur in such patients with virtually no warning.
- Inspect insulin vials before use. NovoLog is a clear, colorless solution. It should never contain particulate matter or appear cloudy, viscous, or discolored. NovoLog 70/30 should appear uniformly white and cloudy and should never contain particulate matter or be discolored.

For external pump use with NovoLog

- Monitor patient with an external insulin pump for erythematous, pruritic, or thickened skin at injection site.

!!ALERT Pump or infusion set malfunctions or insulin degradation can lead to hyperglycemia and ketosis in a short time because there is an S.C. depot of fast-acting insulin.

- Don't dilute or mix insulin aspart with any other insulin, when using an external insulin pump.
- Teach patient how to properly use the external insulin pump.
- Insulin aspart is recommended for use with Disetronic H-TRON plus V100 with Disetronic 3.15 plastic cartridges and Classic or Tender infusion sets, Polyfin or Sof-set infusion sets, and MiniMed Models 505, 506, and 507 with MiniMed 3-ml syringes.
- Replace infusion sets, insulin aspart in the reservoir, and choose a new infusion site every 48 hours or less to avoid insulin degradation and infusion set malfunction.
- Discard insulin exposed to temperatures higher than 98.6° F (37° C). The temperature of the insulin may exceed ambient temperature when the pump housing, cover, tubing, or sport case is exposed to sunlight or radiant heat.

Patient teaching

- Tell patient not to stop insulin therapy without medical approval.
- Advise patient of the warning signs of low glucose level (shaking, sweating, moodiness, irritability, confusion, or agitation). Tell patient to carry sugar (candy, sugar packets) to counteract low glucose level.
- Teach patient proper insulin injection technique and importance of timing dose to meals and adhering to meal plans.
- Tell patient to report swelling, redness, and itching at injection site, and instruct patient on the importance of rotating injection sites to avoid lipodystrophies.
- Instruct patient to use the same brand of insulin, especially if mixing insulin. Changing brands of insulin may necessitate dosage changes.
- Tell patient not to dilute or mix insulin aspart with any other insulin when using an external insulin pump.
- Instruct patient to monitor glucose level regularly.
- Advise patient to avoid vigorous exercise immediately after insulin injection, especially of the area where injection was given; it causes increased absorption and increased risk of high glucose level.
- Advise patient to store insulin at 36° to 46° F (2° to 8° C), and avoid freezing or excessive heat or sunlight.
- Advise woman to notify prescriber about planned, suspected, or known pregnancy.
- Urge patient to wear or carry medical identification at all times.
- Instruct patient about the importance of diet and exercise. Explain long-term complications of diabetes and the importance of yearly eye and foot examinations.

insulin glargine (rDNA origin) injection

Lantus

Pregnancy risk category C

Indications & dosages

➲ **To manage type 1 (insulin-dependent) diabetes in patients who need basal (long-acting) insulin to control hyperglycemia**

Adults and children age 6 and older: Individualize dosage, and give S.C. once daily at the same time each day.

➲ **To manage type 2 (non–insulin-dependent) diabetes in patients who need basal (long-acting) insulin to control hyperglycemia**

Adults: Individualize dosage, and give S.C. once daily at the same time each day.

Contraindications & cautions

- Contraindicated in patients hypersensitive to insulin glargine or its excipients.
- Contraindicated during episodes of hypoglycemia.
- Use cautiously in patients with renal or hepatic impairment.

Adverse reactions

Metabolic: ***hypoglycemia.***
Skin: lipodystrophy, pruritus, rash.
Other: allergic reactions, pain at injection site.

Interactions

Drug-drug. *ACE inhibitors, disopyramide, fibrates, fluoxetine, MAO inhibitors, octreotide, oral antidiabetics, propoxyphene, salicylates, sulfonamide antibiotics:* May cause hypoglycemia and increase insulin effect. Monitor glucose level. May need to adjust dosage of insulin glargine.
Beta blockers, clonidine: May mask signs of hypoglycemia and may either increase or reduce insulin's glucose-lowering effect. Avoid using together, if possible. If used together, monitor glucose level carefully.
Corticosteroids, danazol, diuretics, estrogens, isoniazid, phenothiazines (such as prochlorperazine, promethazine hydrochloride), progestins (such as hormonal contraceptives), somatropin, sympathomimetics (such as albuterol, epinephrine, terbutaline), thyroid hormones: May reduce the glucose-lowering effect of insulin. Monitor glucose level. May need to adjust dosage of insulin glargine.
Guanethidine, reserpine: May mask the signs of hypoglycemia. Avoid using together, if possible. Monitor glucose level carefully.
Lithium: May either increase or decrease the glucose-lowering effect of insulin. Monitor glucose level. May require dosage adjustments of insulin glargine.
Pentamidine: May cause hypoglycemia, which may be followed by hyperglycemia. Avoid using together, if possible.

Drug-herb. *Burdock, dandelion, eucalyptus, marshmallow:* May increase hypoglycemic effects. Discourage use together.
Licorice root: May increase dosage requirements of insulin. Discourage use together.
Drug-lifestyle. *Alcohol use, emotional stress:* May increase or decrease the glucose-lowering effect of insulin. Advise patient to self-monitor glucose level.

Nursing considerations

!!ALERT Drug isn't intended for I.V. use. It's only for S.C. use. Prolonged duration of activity depends on injection into S.C. space.
- Because of prolonged duration, this isn't the insulin of choice for diabetic ketoacidosis.
- Desired glucose level, as well as the doses and timing of antidiabetic medication, must be determined individually, as with any insulin. Glucose monitoring is recommended for all patients with diabetes.
- The rate of absorption, onset, and duration of action may be affected by exercise and other variables, such as illness and emotional stress.

!!ALERT Insulin glargine must not be diluted or mixed with any other insulin or solution.
- As with any insulin therapy, lipodystrophy may occur at the site of injection and may delay insulin absorption. Continuously rotate injection sites within a given area to reduce lipodystrophy.
- Hypoglycemia is the most common adverse effect of insulin. Early symptoms may be different or less pronounced in patients with long duration of diabetes, diabetic nerve disease, or intensified diabetes control. Monitor glucose level closely in these patients because severe hypoglycemia may result before the patient develops symptoms.

!!ALERT Don't confuse Lente with Lantus.

Patient teaching

- Teach proper glucose monitoring, injection techniques, and diabetes management.
- Tell patient to take dose once daily at the same time each day.

!!ALERT Educate diabetic patients about signs and symptoms of low glucose level, such as fatigue, weakness, confusion, headache, pallor, and profuse sweating.
- Urge patient to wear or carry medical identification at all times.
- Advise patient to treat mild hypoglycemia with oral glucose tablets. Encourage patient to always carry glucose tablets in case of a low-glucose episode.
- Educate patients on the importance of maintaining a diabetic diet, and explain that adjustments in drug dosage, meal patterns, and exercise may be needed to regulate glucose.

!!ALERT Advise patient not to dilute or mix any other insulin or solution with insulin glargine. If the solution is cloudy, urge patient to discard the vial. Use solution only if it is clear and colorless.

!!ALERT Make any change of insulin cautiously and only under medical supervision. Changes in insulin type, strength, manufacturer, type (such as regular, NPH, or insulin analogues), species (animal, human), or method of manufacturer (rDNA versus animal source insulin) may require a change in dosage. Oral antidiabetic treatment taken at the same time may need to be adjusted.
- Tell patient to consult prescriber before using OTC medications.
- Inform patient to avoid alcohol, which lowers glucose level.
- Advise patient to avoid vigorous exercise immediately after insulin injection, especially of the area where injection was given; it causes increased absorption and increased risk of high glucose.
- Advise woman planning pregnancy to first consult prescriber.
- Advise patient to store unopened insulin vials in the refrigerator. Opened vials may be stored at 86° F (30° C) or less and away from direct heat. Discard opened vials after 28 days whether refrigerated or not. Don't freeze.

insulin glulisine (rDNA origin) injection
Apidra

Pregnancy risk category C

Indications & dosages

➲ Diabetes mellitus
Adults: Individualize dosage. Give by S.C. injection within 15 minutes before a meal. If regimen also includes a longer-acting insulin or basal insulin analogue, give within 20 minutes after meal starts. Or, give drug

as continuous S.C. infusion using an external infusion pump.

Contraindications & cautions

- Contraindicated during periods of hypoglycemia and in patients hypersensitive to insulin glulisine or one of its ingredients.
- Use cautiously in patients with impaired renal or hepatic function and in pregnant or breast-feeding women.

Adverse reactions

Metabolic: ***hypoglycemia***.
Skin: *injection site reactions*, lipodystrophy, pruritus, rash.
Other: allergic reactions, ***anaphylaxis***, insulin antibody production.

Interactions

Drug-drug. *ACE inhibitors, disopyramide, fibrates, fluoxetine, MAO inhibitors, oral antidiabetics, pentoxifylline, propoxyphene, salicylates, sulfonamide antibiotics:* May increase glucose-lowering effects. Monitor glucose level, and watch for evidence of hypoglycemia.
Beta blockers, clonidine, lithium, pentamidine: May cause unpredictable response to insulin. Use together cautiously; monitor patient closely.
Clozapine, corticosteroids, danazol, diazoxide, diuretics, estrogens, glucagons, isoniazid, olanzapine, phenothiazines, progestogens, protease inhibitors, somatropin, sympathomimetics (such as epinephrine, albuterol, and terbutaline), thyroid hormone: May decrease glucose-lowering effects. Monitor glucose level carefully.
Drug-lifestyle. *Alcohol:* May potentiate or reduce insulin effects, resulting in either hypoglycemia or hyperglycemia. Discourage alcohol use.

Nursing considerations

- Use with a longer-acting or basal insulin analogue.

!!ALERT Insulin glulisine has a more rapid onset and shorter duration of action than regular human insulin. Give within 15 minutes before or immediately after a meal.

- Don't mix insulin glulisine in a syringe with any other insulins except NPH.
- When used in an external S.C. infusion pump, don't mix insulin glulisine with any other insulins or with a diluent.
- Changes in insulin strength, manufacturer, type, or species may cause a need for dosage adjustment.
- Changes in physical activity or usual meal plan may cause a need for dosage adjustment.
- Insulin requirements may be altered during illness, emotional disturbances, or stress.
- Early warning signs of hypoglycemia may be different or less pronounced in patients who take beta blockers, who have had an oral antidiabetic added to the regimen, or who have long-term diabetes or diabetic nerve disease.
- Monitor patient for lipodystrophy at injection site; it may delay insulin absorption.
- Redness, swelling, or itching may occur at injection site.

Patient teaching

- Tell patient to take drug within 15 minutes before starting a meal to 20 minutes after starting a meal, depending on regimen.
- Teach patient how to give S.C. insulin injections.
- Tell patient not to mix insulin glulisine in a syringe with any insulin other than NPH.
- If patient is mixing insulin glulisine with NPH, tell patient to use U-100 syringes, to draw insulin glulisine into the syringe first, followed by NPH insulin, and to inject the mixture immediately.
- Instruct patient to rotate injection sites to avoid injection site reactions.
- If patient is using an external infusion pump, teach proper use of the device. Tell patient not to mix insulin glulisine with any other insulin or diluents. Instruct patient to change the infusion set, reservoir with insulin, and infusion site at least every 48 hours.
- Teach patient the signs and symptoms of hypoglycemia (sweating, rapid pulse, trembling, confusion, headache, irritability, and nausea). Advise the patient to treat these symptoms by eating or drinking something containing sugar.
- Instruct the patient to contact a health care provider for possible dosage adjustments if hypoglycemia occurs frequently.
- Show patient how to monitor and log glucose levels to evaluate diabetes control.
- Explain the possible long-term complications of diabetes and the importance of regular preventive therapy. Urge patient to fol-

low prescribed diet and exercise regimen. To further reduce the risk of heart disease, encourage patient to stop smoking and lose weight.
- Instruct patient to wear or carry medical identification showing that patient has diabetes.
- Tell patient to store unopened vials in the refrigerator and opened vials in the refrigerator or below 77° F (25° C). Opened vials should be used within 28 days. Drug should be protected from direct heat and light.

insulins

insulin (regular)
Humulin R ◇, Humulin R Regular U-500 (concentrated), Iletin II Regular◇, Novolin R◇, Novolin R PenFill◇, Novolin R Prefilled◇, Velosulin BR◇

insulin (lispro)
Humalog

insulin lispro protamine and insulin lispro
Humalog Mix 50/50, Humalog Mix 75/25

insulin zinc suspension (lente)
Humulin L◇, Lente Iletin II◇

extended zinc insulin suspension (ultralente)
Humulin-U Ultralente◇

isophane insulin suspension (NPH)
Humulin N◇, Novolin N◇, Novolin N PenFill◇, Novolin N Prefilled◇, NPH Iletin II◇

isophane insulin suspension and insulin injection (70% isophane insulin and 30% insulin injection)
Humulin 70/30◇, Novolin 70/30◇, Novolin 70/30 PenFill◇, Novolin 70/30 Prefilled◇

isophane insulin suspension and insulin injection (50% isophane insulin and 50% insulin injection)
Humulin 50/50◇

isophane insulin suspension and insulin injection (80% isophane insulin and 20% insulin injection)

Pregnancy risk category B

Indications & dosages
➲ Moderate to severe diabetic ketoacidosis or hyperosmolar hyperglycemia
regular insulin
Adults older than age 20: Give loading dose of 0.15 units/kg I.V. by direct injection, followed by 0.1 unit/kg/hour as a continuous infusion. Decrease rate of insulin infusion to 0.05 to 0.1 unit/kg/hour when glucose level reaches 250 to 300 mg/dl. Start infusion of D_5W in half-normal saline solution separately from the insulin infusion when glucose level is 150 to 200 mg/dl in patients with diabetic ketoacidosis or 250 to 300 mg/dl in those with hyperosmolar hyperglycemia. Give dose of insulin S.C. 1 to 2 hours before stopping insulin infusion (intermediate-acting insulin is recommended).
Adults and children age 20 or younger: Loading dose isn't recommended. Begin therapy at 0.1 unit/kg/hour I.V. infusion. Once condition improves, decrease rate of insulin infusion to 0.05 unit/kg/hour. Start infusion of D_5W in half-normal saline solution separately from the insulin infusion when glucose level is 250 mg/dl.
➲ Mild diabetic ketoacidosis
regular insulin
Adults older than age 20: Give loading dose of 0.4 to 0.6 unit/kg divided in two equal parts, with half the dose given by direct I.V. injection and half given I.M. or S.C. Subsequent doses can be based on 0.1 unit/kg/hour I.M. or S.C.
➲ Newly diagnosed diabetes
regular insulin
Adults older than age 20: Individualize therapy. Initially, 0.5 to 1 unit/kg/day S.C. as part of a regimen with short-acting and long-acting insulin therapy.

Adults and children age 20 or younger: Individualize therapy. Initially, 0.1 to 0.25 unit/kg S.C. q 6 to 8 hours for 24 hours then adjust accordingly.

➲ **Control of hyperglycemia with Humalog and longer-acting insulin in patients with type 1 diabetes**

Adults: Dosage varies among patients and must be determined by prescriber familiar with patient's metabolic needs, eating habits, and other lifestyle variables. Inject S.C. within 15 minutes before or after a meal.

➲ **Control of hyperglycemia with Humalog and sulfonylureas in patients with type 2 diabetes**

Adults and children older than age 3: Dosage varies among patients and must be determined by prescriber familiar with patient's metabolic needs, eating habits, and other lifestyle variables. Inject S.C. within 15 minutes before or after a meal.

➲ **Hyperkalemia♦**

Adults: 50 ml of dextrose 50% given over 5 minutes, followed by 5 to 10 units of regular insulin by I.V. push.

Contraindications & cautions

- Contraindicated in patients with history of systemic allergic reaction to pork when porcine-derived products are used or hypersensitivity to any component of preparation.
- Contraindicated during episodes of hypoglycemia.

Adverse reactions

Metabolic: ***hypoglycemia***, hyperglycemia, hypomagnesemia, hypokalemia.
Skin: rash, urticaria, pruritus, swelling, redness, stinging, warmth at injection site.
Other: *lipoatrophy, lipohypertrophy*, hypersensitivity reactions, ***anaphylaxis***.

Interactions

Drug-drug. *ACE inhibitors, anabolic steroids, antidiabetics, beta blockers, calcium, chloroquine, clofibrate, clonidine, disopyramide, fluoxetine, guanethidine, lithium, MAO inhibitors, mebendazole, octreotide, pentamidine, propoxyphene, pyridoxine, salicylates, sulfinpyrazone, sulfonamides, tetracyclines:* May enhance hypoglycemic effects of insulin. Monitor glucose level.
Acetazolamide, adrenocorticosteroids, AIDS antivirals, albuterol, asparaginase, calcitonin, cyclophosphamide, danazol, diazoxide, diltiazem, diuretics, dobutamine, epinephrine, estrogen-containing hormonal contraceptives, estrogens, ethacrynic acid, isoniazid, lithium, morphine, niacin, nicotine, phenothiazines, phenytoin, somatropin, terbutaline, thyroid hormones: May diminish insulin response. Monitor glucose level.
Carteolol, nadolol, pindolol, propranolol, timolol: May mask symptoms of hypoglycemia as a result of beta blockade (such as tachycardia). Use together cautiously in patients with diabetes.
Rosiglitazone: May cause fluid retention that may lead to or worsen heart failure. Monitor patient closely.
Drug-herb. *Basil, bay, bee pollen, burdock, ginseng, glucomannan, horehound, marshmallow, myrrh, sage:* May affect glycemic control. Discourage use together, and monitor glucose level carefully.
Drug-food. *Unregulated diet:* May cause hyperglycemia or hypoglycemia. Urge caution, and monitor patient's diet.
Drug-lifestyle. *Alcohol use:* May cause hypoglycemic effect. Discourage use together.
Marijuana use: May increase glucose level. Tell patient to avoid marijuana.
Smoking: May increase glucose level and decrease response to insulin administration. Monitor glucose level.

Nursing considerations

!!ALERT Regular insulin is used in patients with circulatory collapse, diabetic ketoacidosis, or hyperkalemia. Don't use Humulin R (concentrated) U-500 I.V. Don't use intermediate or long-acting insulins for coma or other emergency requiring rapid drug action. Also, ketosis-prone type 1, severely ill, and newly diagnosed diabetic patients with very high glucose levels may need hospitalization and I.V. treatment with regular fast-acting insulin.

- Insulin is drug of choice to treat diabetes during pregnancy. Insulin requirements increase in pregnant diabetic women and then decline immediately postpartum. Monitor patient closely.
- Dosage is always expressed in USP units. Use only the syringes calibrated for the particular concentration of insulin given.
- Some patients may develop insulin resistance and need large insulin doses to control symptoms of diabetes. U-500 insulin is available as Humulin R (concentrated)

U-500 for such patients. Give pharmacy sufficient notice when requesting refill prescription. Never store U-500 insulin in same area with other insulin preparations because of danger of severe overdose if given accidentally to other patients.

- To mix insulin suspension, swirl vial gently or rotate between palms or between palm and thigh. Don't shake vigorously. This causes bubbling and air in syringe.
- Lente, semilente, and ultralente insulins may be mixed in any proportion. Regular insulin may be mixed with NPH or lente insulins in any proportion. When mixing regular insulin with intermediate- or long-acting insulin, always draw up regular insulin into syringe first.
- Switching from separate injections to a prepared mixture may alter patient response. When NPH or lente is mixed with regular insulin in the same syringe, give immediately to avoid loss of potency.
- Lispro insulin may be mixed with Humulin N or Humulin U; give within 15 minutes before a meal to prevent a hypoglycemic reaction.
- Don't use insulin that changes color or becomes clumped or granular in appearance.
- Check expiration date on vial before using contents.
- Usual administration route is S.C. For proper S.C. administration, pinch a fold of skin with fingers at least 3 inches (7.6 cm) apart, and insert needle at a 45- to 90-degree angle.
- Press but don't rub site after injection. Rotate injection sites to avoid overuse of one area. Diabetic patients may achieve better control if injection site is rotated within same anatomic region.
- Monitor patient for hyperglycemia (rebound, or Somogyi effect).
- Store insulin in cool area. Refrigeration is desirable but not essential, except with Humulin R (concentrated) U-500.

Patient teaching

- Make sure patient knows that drug relieves symptoms but doesn't cure disease.
- Instruct patient about nature of disease and importance of following therapeutic regimen, adhering to specific diet, losing weight, getting exercise, following personal hygiene program, and avoiding infection. Emphasize importance of timing injections with eating and of not skipping meals.
- Stress that accuracy of measurement is important, especially with concentrated regular insulin. Aids, such as magnifying sleeve or dose magnifier, may improve accuracy. Show patient and caregivers how to measure and give insulin.
- Advise patient not to change order in which insulins are mixed or model or brand of insulin, syringe, or needle. Be sure patient knows when mixing two insulins, always draw the regular into the syringe first.
- Teach patient that glucose level and urine ketone tests provide essential guides to dosage and success of therapy. It's important for patient to recognize symptoms of high and low glucose levels. Insulin-induced low glucose level is hazardous and may cause brain damage if prolonged; most adverse effects are temporary. Instruct patient on insulin peak times and their importance.
- Instruct patient on proper use of equipment for monitoring glucose level.
- Advise patient not to smoke within 30 minutes after insulin injection because smoking decreases amount of insulin absorbed by S.C. route.
- Advise patient to avoid vigorous exercise immediately after insulin injection, especially of the area where injection was given, because it increases absorption and risk of high glucose episodes.
- Inform patient that marijuana use may increase insulin requirements.
- Teach patient to avoid alcohol use because it lowers glucose level.
- Advise patient to wear or carry medical identification at all times, to carry ample insulin and syringes on trips, to keep carbohydrates (lump of sugar or candy) on hand for emergencies, and to note time zone changes for dosage schedule when traveling.
- Advise woman planning pregnancy to first consult prescriber.
- Advise patient to store insulin at 36°to 46° F (2° to 8°C). Don't freeze or expose vials to excessive heat or sunlight.

interferon alfa-2a, recombinant (rIFN-A)
Roferon-A

Pregnancy risk category C

Indications & dosages

➲ Chronic hepatitis C

Adults: 3 million IU three times a week I.M. or S.C. for 12 months (48 to 52 weeks). Or, induction dose of 6 million IU three times weekly for the first 3 months (12 weeks) followed by 3 million IU three times weekly for 9 months (36 weeks). If no response after 3 months, stop therapy. Retreatment with either 3 or 6 million IU three times weekly for 6 to 12 months may be considered for those who relapse.

➲ Hairy cell leukemia

Adults: For induction, 3 million IU I.M. or S.C. daily for 16 to 24 weeks. For maintenance, 3 million IU I.M. or S.C. three times weekly.

➲ AIDS-related Kaposi's sarcoma

Adults: For induction, 36 million IU I.M. or S.C. daily for 10 to 12 weeks. For maintenance, 36 million IU I.M. or S.C. three times weekly. Doses may begin at 3 million IU and be escalated upward every 3 days until patient is given 36 million IU daily to decrease toxicity.

➲ Philadelphia chromosome–positive chronic myelogenous leukemia

Adults: Initially, 3 million IU I.M. or S.C. daily for 3 days; then 6 million IU for 3 days; then 9 million IU for duration of treatment.
Children: 2.5 to 5 million IU/m^2 I.M. daily.

Contraindications & cautions

- Contraindicated in patients hypersensitive to drug, murine (mouse) immunoglobulin, or other drug components. Also contraindicated in patients with history of autoimmune hepatitis or history of autoimmune disease, severe visceral AIDS-related Kaposi's sarcoma, neonates (injection contains benzyl alcohol), immunocompromised transplant patients, and severe depression or suicidal behavior.
- Use cautiously in patients with severe hepatic or renal function impairment, seizure disorders, compromised CNS function, cardiac disease, or myelosuppression.

!!ALERT Neurotoxicity and cardiotoxicity are more common in elderly patients, especially those with underlying CNS or cardiac impairment.

Adverse reactions

CNS: *dizziness, confusion,* paresthesia, numbness, lethargy, *depression, decreased mental status,* forgetfulness, ***coma***, nervousness, insomnia, sedation, apathy, anxiety, irritability, fatigue, vertigo, gait disturbances, incoordination, syncope.
CV: hypotension, chest pain, ***arrhythmias***, palpitations, ***heart failure***, hypertension, edema, ***MI***, flushing.
EENT: *dryness or inflammation of the oropharynx,* rhinorrhea, sinusitis, conjunctivitis, earache, eye irritation.
GI: *anorexia, nausea, diarrhea, vomiting,* abdominal fullness, *abdominal pain,* flatulence, constipation, hypermotility, gastric distress, excessive salivation, *change in taste.*
GU: transient impotence.
Hematologic: LEUKOPENIA, THROMBOCYTOPENIA, *anemia.*
Hepatic: ***hepatitis***.
Metabolic: *weight loss,* hypercalcemia, hyperphosphatemia.
Respiratory: cyanosis, cough, dyspnea.
Skin: *rash,* dryness, pruritus, *partial alopecia,* urticaria, diaphoresis, *inflammation at injection site.*
Other: *flulike syndrome,* night sweats, hot flashes.

Interactions

Drug-drug. *Aminophylline, theophylline:* May reduce theophylline clearance. Monitor serum level.
Aspirin: May increase risk of GI bleeding. Avoid using together.
CNS depressants: May increase CNS effects. Avoid using together.
Live-virus vaccines: May increase risk of adverse reactions and may decrease antibody response. Avoid using together.
Drugs with neurotoxic, hematotoxic, cardiotoxic effects: May increase the toxic effects of these drugs. Monitor patient for increased adverse effects.
Drug-lifestyle. *Alcohol use:* May increase risk of GI bleeding. Discourage patient from use during therapy.

Nursing considerations

!!ALERT Alpha interferons cause or aggravate fatal or life-threatening neuropsychiatric, autoimmune, ischemic, and infectious disorders. Monitor patient closely with periodic clinical and laboratory evaluations. Withdraw patients with persistently severe or worsening signs or symptoms of these conditions from therapy.

- Obtain allergy history. Drug contains phenol as a preservative and albumin as a stabilizer.
- Use S.C. administration route in patients whose platelet count is below 50,000/mm^3.
- Give drug at bedtime to minimize daytime drowsiness.
- Ensure patient is well hydrated, especially during first stages of treatment.
- At beginning of therapy, assess patient for flulike signs and symptoms, which tend to diminish with continued therapy. Premedicate patient with acetaminophen to minimize signs and symptoms.
- Monitor patient for CNS adverse reactions, such as decreased mental status and dizziness, during therapy.
- Depression and suicidal behavior have been linked to treatment.
- Monitor CBC with differential, platelet count, blood chemistry and electrolyte studies, and liver function tests. If patient has cardiac disorder or advanced stages of cancer, monitor ECG.
- For patients who develop thrombocytopenia, exercise extreme care in performing invasive procedures; inspect injection site and skin frequently for bruising; limit frequency of I.M. injections; test urine, emesis fluid, stool, and secretions for occult blood.

!!ALERT Different brands of interferon may not be equivalent and may need different dosages.

- Severe adverse reactions may need dosage reduction to one-half or stoppage of drug until reactions subside.
- Use with blood dyscrasia-causing drugs, bone marrow suppressant, or radiation therapy may increase bone marrow suppression. Dosage may need to be reduced.
- Keep drug refrigerated. Don't freeze.

Patient teaching

- Advise patient that laboratory tests will be performed before and periodically during therapy.
- Teach patient proper oral hygiene during treatment because the bone marrow suppressant effects of interferon may lead to microbial infection, delayed healing, and bleeding gums. Drug also may decrease salivary flow.
- Stress need to follow prescriber's instructions about taking and recording temperature and how and when to take acetaminophen.
- Advise patient to check with prescriber for instructions after missing dose.
- Tell patient that drug may cause temporary partial hair loss; hair should return when drug is withdrawn.
- If patient will be giving drug to himself, teach him how to prepare and give it and how to dispose of used needles, syringes, containers, and unused drug.
- Instruct patient not to take aspirin or alcohol because use together increases risk of GI bleeding.
- Instruct patient not to change brands of interferon without medical consultation.
- Warn patient against performing tasks that require mental alertness.
- Advise patient to immediately report signs and symptoms of depression.

interferon alfa-2b, recombinant (IFN-alpha 2)

Intron A

Pregnancy risk category C

Indications & dosages

➲ Hairy cell leukemia

Adults: 2 million IU/m^2 I.M. or S.C., three times weekly for 6 months or more.

➲ Condylomata acuminata (genital or venereal warts)

Adults: 1 million IU for each lesion intralesionally three times weekly for 3 weeks.

➲ AIDS-related Kaposi's sarcoma

Adults: 30 million IU/m^2 S.C. or I.M. three times weekly. Maintain dose unless disease progresses rapidly or intolerance occurs.

➲ Chronic hepatitis B

Adults: 30 to 35 million IU weekly I.M. or S.C., given as 5 million IU daily or 10 million IU three times weekly for 16 weeks.
Children ages 1 to 17: 3 million IU/m^2 S.C. three times weekly for first week; then increase to 6 million IU/m^2 S.C. three times

weekly (maximum is 10 million IU three times weekly) for total of 16 to 24 weeks.

➲ **Chronic hepatitis C**

Adults: 3 million IU I.M. or S.C. three times weekly. In patients tolerating therapy with normalization of ALT at 16 weeks of therapy, continue for 18 to 24 months. In patients who haven't normalized the ALT, consider stopping therapy.

➲ **Adjunct to surgical treatment in patients with malignant melanoma who are asymptomatic after surgery but at high risk for systemic recurrence for up to 8 weeks after surgery**

Adults: Initially, 20 million IU/m^2 by I.V. infusion 5 consecutive days weekly for 4 weeks; then maintenance dose of 10 million IU/m^2 S.C. three times weekly for 48 weeks. If adverse effects occur, stop therapy until they abate; then resume therapy at 50% of the previous dose. If intolerance persists, stop therapy.

➲ **First treatment of clinically aggressive follicular non-Hodgkin's lymphoma with chemotherapy containing anthracycline**

Adults: 5 million IU S.C. three times weekly for up to 18 months.

Contraindications & cautions

- Contraindicated in patients hypersensitive to drug or its components.
- Use cautiously in patients with history of CV disease, pulmonary disease, diabetes mellitus, coagulation disorders, and severe myelosuppression.
- Depression and suicidal behavior have been linked to drug use; patients with psychotic disorders, especially depression, shouldn't continue drug treatment.

!!ALERT Neurotoxicity and cardiotoxicity are more common in elderly patients, especially those with underlying CNS or cardiac impairment.

Adverse reactions

CNS: *dizziness, confusion, paresthesia,* lethargy, *depression, difficulty in thinking or concentrating, insomnia,* anxiety, *fatigue, hypoesthesia, amnesia,* nervousness, *somnolence,* weakness, *malaise, asthenia,* ***suicidal ideation.***

CV: hypotension, *chest pain,* flushing, tachycardia, ***bradycardia,*** angina, ***arrhythmia, cardiac failure,*** hypertension, angina.

EENT: visual disturbances, hearing disorders, pharyngitis, *nasal congestion, sinusitis,* rhinitis, stye.

GI: *anorexia, nausea, diarrhea, vomiting,* abdominal pain, *dyspepsia,* constipation, loose stools, eructation, *dry mouth,* dysgeusia, stomatitis, gingivitis.

GU: transient impotence.

Hematologic: ***leukopenia, thrombocytopenia,*** anemia.

Metabolic: hypercalcemia, hyperphosphatemia.

Musculoskeletal: *arthralgia, back pain.*

Respiratory: *dyspnea, coughing,* ***pulmonary embolism.***

Skin: *rash, dryness, pruritus, alopecia,* candidiasis, dermatitis, *increased diaphoresis.*

Other: *flulike syndrome, rigors,* gynecomastia.

Interactions

Drug-drug. *Aminophylline, theophylline:* May reduce theophylline clearance. Monitor theophylline level.

CNS depressants: May increase CNS effects. Avoid using together.

Live-virus vaccines: May increase adverse reactions to vaccine or decrease antibody response. Postpone immunization.

Zidovudine: May cause synergistic adverse effects (higher risk of neutropenia). Carefully monitor WBC count.

Nursing considerations

!!ALERT Alpha interferons cause or aggravate fatal or life-threatening neuropsychiatric, autoimmune, ischemic, and infectious disorders. Monitor patients closely with periodic clinical and laboratory evaluations. Withdraw patients with persistently severe or worsening signs or symptoms of these conditions from therapy.

- Use S.C. administration route in patients whose platelet count is below 50,000/mm^3.
- Give drug at bedtime to minimize daytime drowsiness.
- When giving interferon for condylomata acuminata, use only 10 million-IU vial because dilution of other strengths needed for intralesional use results in a hypertonic solution. Don't reconstitute drug in 10 million-IU vial with more than 1 ml of diluent. Use tuberculin or similar syringe and 25G to 30G needle. Don't inject too deep beneath lesion or too superficially. As many

as five lesions can be treated at one time. To ease discomfort, give in evening with acetaminophen.

- Ensure patient is well hydrated, especially at beginning of treatment.
- At start of treatment, monitor patient for flulike signs and symptoms, which tend to diminish with continued therapy. Premedicate patient with acetaminophen to minimize these symptoms.
- Periodically check for adverse CNS reactions, such as decreased mental status and dizziness, during therapy.
- Monitor CBC with differential, platelet count, blood chemistry and electrolyte studies, and liver function tests. Monitor ECG if patient has cardiac disorder or advanced stages of cancer.
- For patients who develop thrombocytopenia, exercise extreme care in performing invasive procedures; inspect injection site and skin frequently for signs and symptoms of bruising; limit frequency of I.M. injections; test urine, emesis fluid, stool, and secretions for occult blood.
- Severe adverse reactions may need dosage reduction to one-half or stoppage of drug until reactions subside.
- Use with blood dyscrasia-causing drugs, bone marrow suppressants, or radiation therapy may increase bone marrow suppression. Dosage reduction may be needed.
- In treatment of condylomata acuminata, maximum response usually occurs 4 to 8 weeks after therapy starts. If results aren't satisfactory after 12 to 16 weeks, a second course may be started. Patients with 6 to 10 condylomata may receive a second course of treatment; patients with more than 10 condylomata may receive additional courses.

Patient teaching

- Advise patient to avoid contact with persons with viral illness; patient is at increased risk for infection during therapy.
- Advise patient that laboratory tests will be performed before and periodically during therapy.
- Teach patient proper oral hygiene during treatment because bone marrow suppressant effects of interferon may lead to microbial infection, delayed healing, and bleeding gums. Drug also may decrease salivary flow.
- Advise patient to check with prescriber for instructions after missing a dose.
- Stress need to follow prescriber's instructions about taking and recording temperature and how and when to take acetaminophen.
- If patient will give drug to himself, teach him how to prepare injection and use disposable syringe. Give him information on drug stability.
- Tell patient that drug may cause temporary partial hair loss; hair should return after drug is withdrawn.
- Advise patient to notify prescriber if signs or symptoms of depression occur.

interferon alfacon-1

Infergen

Pregnancy risk category C

Indications & dosages

➲ **Chronic hepatitis C viral infection in patients with compensated liver disease**

Adults: 9 mcg S.C. three times weekly for 24 weeks; for patients who don't respond or who relapse, 15 mcg S.C. three times weekly for up to 48 weeks.

For patients intolerant to higher doses, dose may be reduced to 7.5 mcg. Don't give doses below 7.5 mcg because decreased efficacy may result.

Contraindications & cautions

- Contraindicated in patients hypersensitive to alpha interferons, to ***Escherichia coli***–derived products, or to any component of product; and in patients with history of severe psychiatric disorders, autoimmune hepatitis, or decompensated hepatic disease.
- Use with caution in patients with history of cardiac disease and other autoimmune or endocrine disorders, in those with abnormally low peripheral blood cell counts, and in those receiving drugs that causes myelosuppression.

Adverse reactions

CNS: *headache, insomnia, dizziness, paresthesia, amnesia, nervousness, depression, anxiety, emotional lability,* confusion, agitation, ***suicidal ideation***, *malaise.*
CV: hypertension, tachycardia, palpitations.

EENT: *retinal hemorrhages,* loss of visual acuity or visual field, conjunctivitis, tinnitus, ear pain, *pharyngitis, sinusitis, rhinitis,* epistaxis.
GI: *abdominal pain, nausea, diarrhea,* taste perversion, *anorexia, dyspepsia, vomiting,* constipation, flatulence, hemorrhoids, decreased saliva.
GU: dysmenorrhea, vaginitis.
Hematologic: ***granulocytopenia, leukopenia, thrombocytopenia,*** ecchymosis, lymphadenopathy, lymphocytosis.
Metabolic: hypothyroidism.
Respiratory: *infection, cough, congestion,* dyspnea, bronchitis.
Skin: *alopecia, pruritus, rash,* dry skin, *pain, erythema at injection site.*
Other: toothache, decreased libido, ***hypersensitivity reactions,*** *body pain, flulike symptoms.*

Interactions

Drug-drug. *Drugs metabolized by cytochrome P-450:* May alter drug levels. Monitor changes in levels of these drugs.
Myelosuppressives: May cause added hematologic toxicities, use cautiously together. Monitor CBC and therapeutic or toxic level of myelosuppressive.

Nursing considerations

- Depression and suicidal behavior have been linked to drug.
- Obtain the following laboratory tests before therapy, 2 weeks after it starts, and periodically during therapy: CBC with platelets, creatinine, albumin, bilirubin, TSH, and T_4.

!!ALERT If hypersensitivity reaction occurs, stop drug immediately and treat. Premedication with acetaminophen or ibuprofen may decrease adverse effects.

- Allow at least 48 hours to elapse between doses.
- Dosages and adverse reactions vary among different subtypes of drug. Don't use different subtypes in a single treatment regimen.
- Store drug in refrigerator at 36° to 46° F (2° to 8° C); don't freeze. Injection may be allowed to reach room temperature just before use. Avoid vigorous shaking. Discard unused portion.

Patient teaching

- If drug is to be used at home, instruct patient on appropriate use, dosage, and administration. Give the patient information leaflet available from the manufacturer to the patient. Also teach patient proper disposal procedures for needles, syringes, drug containers, and unused drug.
- Instruct patient not to reuse needles or syringes or reenter vial.
- Tell patient to discard all syringes and needles in a puncture-resistant container.
- Urge patient not to use vial that is discolored or contains particulates.
- Tell patient that nonnarcotic analgesics and bedtime administration may be used to prevent or lessen flulike symptoms (headache, fever, malaise, muscle pain) related to therapy.
- Instruct patient to immediately report symptoms of depression.

interferon beta-1a

Avonex, Rebif

Pregnancy risk category C

Indications & dosages

➲ To slow accumulation of physical disability and decrease frequency of clinical worsening in patients with relapsing forms of multiple sclerosis (MS)
Adults age 18 and older: 30 mcg Avonex I.M. once weekly. Or, initially, 8.8 mcg Rebif S.C. three times weekly for 2 weeks; then increase dose to 22 mcg three times weekly for another 2 weeks. Then increase to a maintenance dose of 44 mcg S.C. three times weekly.

For Rebif, in patients with leukopenia or elevated liver function test values (ALT greater than five times upper limit of normal), reduce dosage by 20% to 50% until toxicity is resolved. Stop treatment if jaundice or other signs of hepatic injury occur.
➲ First MS attack if brain magnetic resonance imaging shows abnormalities consistent with MS
Adults: 30 mcg Avonex I.M. once weekly.

Contraindications & cautions

- Contraindicated in patients hypersensitive to natural or recombinant interferon beta,

human albumin, or other components of drug.
- Use cautiously in patients with depression, seizure disorders, or severe cardiac conditions.
- It's unknown if drug appears in breast milk; a breast-feeding woman must either stop breast-feeding or stop drug.
- Safety and effectiveness of drug in chronic progressive multiple sclerosis or in children younger than age 18 haven't been established.

Adverse reactions

CNS: *headache, sleep difficulty, dizziness, fever*, syncope, ***suicidal tendency, depression, suicidal ideation or attempt***, *fatigue*, hypertonia, abnormal coordination, ***seizures***, speech disorder, ataxia, *asthenia*, malaise.
CV: chest pain, vasodilation.
EENT: *abnormal vision*, otitis media, decreased hearing, *sinusitis*.
GI: *nausea, diarrhea, dyspepsia*, anorexia, *abdominal pain*, dry mouth.
GU: ovarian cyst, vaginitis, increased urinary frequency, urinary incontinence.
Hematologic: anemia, ***leukopenia***, *lymphadenopathy*, ***thrombocytopenia, pancytopenia***.
Hepatic: abnormal hepatic function, bilirubinemia, autoimmune hepatitis, hepatic injury, ***hepatitis***.
Metabolic: hyperthyroidism, hypothyroidism.
Musculoskeletal: *muscle ache*, muscle spasm, arthralgia, *back pain, skeletal pain*.
Respiratory: *upper respiratory tract infection*, dyspnea.
Skin: ecchymosis at injection site, *injection site reaction*, urticaria, alopecia, nevus.
Other: *flulike syndrome, pain, chills, infection*, herpes zoster, herpes simplex, neutralizing antibodies, ***hypersensitivity reactions***.

Interactions

Drug-lifestyle. *Sun exposure:* May cause photosensitivity reactions. Advise patient to take precautions against sun exposure.

Nursing considerations

- Monitor patient closely for depression and suicidal ideation. It isn't known if these symptoms are related to the underlying neurologic basis of multiple sclerosis or to the drug.
- Monitor WBC count, platelet count, and blood chemistries, including liver function tests. Rare but severe liver injury, including liver failure, may occur in patients taking Avonex.
- To reconstitute drug, inject 1.1 ml of supplied diluent (sterile water for injection) into vial and gently swirl to dissolve drug. Don't shake.
- Use drug as soon as possible but may be used within 6 hours after being reconstituted if stored at 36° to 46° F (2° to 8° C).
- Rotate sites of injection.
- After giving each dose, discard any remaining product in the syringe.
- Give analgesics or antipyretics to decrease flulike symptoms.
- Store Rebif in the refrigerator between 36° to 46° F (2° to 8° C). Don't freeze. Rebif may also be stored at or below 77° F (25° C) for up to 30 days and away from heat and light.
- Store Avonex prefilled syringes in the refrigerator at 36° to 46° F (2° to 8° C). Once removed from refrigerator, warm to room temperature (about 30 minutes) and use within 12 hours. Don't use external heat sources such as hot water to warm syringe, or expose to high temperatures. Don't freeze. Protect from light.

Patient teaching

- Teach patient and family member how to reconstitute drug and give I.M.
- Caution patient not to change dosage or schedule of administration. If a dose is missed, tell him to take it as soon as he remembers. He may then resume his regular schedule. Tell patient not to take two injections within 2 days of each other.
- Show patient how to store drug.
- Inform patient that flulike signs and symptoms, such as fever, fatigue, muscle aches, headache, chills, and joint pain, aren't uncommon at start of therapy. Acetaminophen 650 mg P.O. may be taken immediately before injection and for another 24 hours after each injection, to lessen severity of flulike signs and symptoms.
- Advise patient to report depression, suicidal thoughts, or other adverse reactions.
- Instruct patient to keep syringes and needles away from children. Also, instruct him not to reuse needles or syringes and to discard them in a syringe-disposal unit.

• Caution woman of childbearing age not to become pregnant during therapy because of the risk of spontaneous abortion. If pregnancy occurs, instruct patient to notify prescriber immediately and to stop drug.
• Advise patient to use sunscreen and avoid sun exposure while taking drug because photosensitivity may occur.
• Tell patient to store Rebif in the refrigerator between 36° to 46° F (2° to 8° C) and not to freeze. Rebif may also be stored at or below 77° F (25° C) for up to 30 days and away from heat and light.

interferon beta-1b, recombinant
Betaseron

Pregnancy risk category C

Indications & dosages
➲ **To reduce frequency of exacerbations in relapsing forms of multiple sclerosis**
Adults: 0.0625 mg S.C. every other day for weeks 1 and 2; then 0.125 mg S.C. every other day for weeks 3 and 4; then 0.1875 mg S.C. every other day for weeks 5 and 6; then 0.25 mg S.C. every other day thereafter.

Contraindications & cautions
• Contraindicated in patients hypersensitive to interferon beta, human albumin, or components of drug.
• Use cautiously in women of childbearing age. Evidence is inconclusive about teratogenic effects, but drug may be an abortifacient.

Adverse reactions
CNS: depression, anxiety, emotional lability, depersonalization, ***suicidal tendencies***, confusion, somnolence, *hypertonia, asthenia, migraine*, ***seizures***, *headache*, dizziness.
CV: palpitations, hypertension, tachycardia, peripheral vascular disorder.
EENT: laryngitis, *sinusitis, conjunctivitis*, abnormal vision.
GI: *diarrhea, constipation, abdominal pain, vomiting.*
GU: *menstrual bleeding or spotting, early or delayed menses, fewer days of menstrual flow, menorrhagia.*
Musculoskeletal: *myasthenia.*
Respiratory: dyspnea.
Skin: *inflammation, pain, necrosis at injection site, diaphoresis*, alopecia.
Other: breast pain, *flulike syndrome, pelvic pain, lymphadenopathy, pain*, generalized edema.

Interactions
None significant.

Nursing considerations
!!ALERT Serious liver damage, including hepatic failure requiring transplant, can occur. Monitor liver function at 1, 3, and 6 months after therapy starts and periodically thereafter.
• To reconstitute, inject 1.2 ml of supplied diluent (half normal saline solution for injection) into vial and gently swirl to dissolve drug. Don't shake. Reconstituted solution contains 8 million IU (0.25 mg)/ml. Discard vial that contains particulates or discolored solution.
• Inject immediately after preparation.
• Store new formulation at room temperature. After reconstitution, if not used immediately, drug may be refrigerated for up to 3 hours.
• Rotate injection sites to minimize local reactions and observe site for necrosis.
• Monitor patient for signs of depression.

Patient teaching
• Warn woman of childbearing age about dangers to fetus. If pregnancy occurs during therapy, tell her to notify prescriber and stop taking drug.
• Teach patient how to perform S.C. injections, including solution preparation, aseptic technique, injection site rotation, and equipment disposal. Periodically reevaluate patient's technique.
• Tell patient to take drug at bedtime to minimize mild flulike signs and symptoms that commonly occur.
• Advise patient to report suicidal thoughts or depression.
• Urge patient to immediately report signs or symptoms of tissue death at injection site.

interferon gamma-1b
Actimmune

Pregnancy risk category C

Indications & dosages

➲ **Chronic granulomatous disease, severe malignant osteopetrosis**

Adults with body surface area (BSA) greater than 0.5 m²: 50 mcg/m² (1 million IU/m²) S.C. three times weekly, preferably h.s., in deltoid or anterior thigh muscle.

Adults with a BSA 0.5 m² or less: 1.5 mcg/kg S.C. three times weekly.

Contraindications & cautions

- Contraindicated in patients hypersensitive to drug or to genetically engineered products derived from ***Escherichia coli.***
- Use cautiously in patients with cardiac disease, including arrhythmias, ischemia, or heart failure. The flulike syndrome commonly seen with high doses of drug can worsen these conditions.
- Use cautiously in patients with compromised CNS function or seizure disorders. CNS adverse reactions that may occur at high doses of drug can worsen these conditions.

Adverse reactions

CNS: *fatigue*, decreased mental status, gait disturbance, dizziness.
GI: *nausea, vomiting, diarrhea*, abdominal pain.
GU: proteinuria.
Hematologic: ***neutropenia, thrombocytopenia***.
Metabolic: weight loss.
Musculoskeletal: back pain.
Skin: *erythema and tenderness at injection site, rash.*
Other: *flulike syndrome.*

Interactions

Drug-drug. *Myelosuppressives:* May increase myelosuppression. Monitor patient closely.
Zidovudine: May increase zidovudine level. Adjust dosage when used together.

Nursing considerations

!!ALERT The drug's activity is expressed in international units (1 million IU/50 mcg). This is equal to what was previously expressed as units (1.5 million U/50 mcg).
- Use myelosuppressives together with caution.
- Premedicate patient with acetaminophen to minimize signs and symptoms at start of therapy; these tend to diminish with continued therapy.
- Before beginning therapy and at 3-month intervals, monitor CBC, platelets, renal and hepatic function tests, and urinalysis.
- Discard unused drug. Each vial is for single-dose use only and doesn't contain a preservative.

Patient teaching

- If patient will give drug to himself, teach him how to give it and how to dispose of used needles, syringes, containers, and unused drug.
- Instruct patient how to manage flulike signs and symptoms (fever, fatigue, muscle aches, headache, chills, joint pain) that commonly occur.
- Advise use of acetaminophen.

ipratropium bromide
Atrovent

Pregnancy risk category B

Indications & dosages

➲ **Bronchospasm in chronic bronchitis and emphysema**

Adults: Usually, 2 inhalations (36 mcg) q.i.d.; patient may take additional inhalations p.r.n. but shouldn't exceed 12 inhalations in 24 hours or 500 mcg q 6 to 8 hours via oral nebulizer.

➲ **Rhinorrhea caused by allergic and nonallergic perennial rhinitis**

Adults and children age 6 and older: Two 0.03% nasal sprays (42 mcg) per nostril b.i.d. or t.i.d.

➲ **Rhinorrhea caused by the common cold**

Adults and children age 12 and older: Two 0.06% nasal sprays (84 mcg) per nostril t.i.d. or q.i.d.

Children ages 5 to 11: Two 0.06% nasal sprays (84 mcg) per nostril t.i.d.

➲ **Rhinorrhea caused by seasonal allergic rhinitis**
Adults and children age 5 and older: Two 0.06% nasal sprays (84 mcg) per nostril q.i.d.

Contraindications & cautions

- Contraindicated in patients hypersensitive to drug, atropine, or its derivatives and in those hypersensitive to soy lecithin or related food products, such as soybeans and peanuts.
- Use cautiously in patients with angle-closure glaucoma, prostatic hyperplasia, or bladder-neck obstruction.
- Safety and efficacy of nebulization or inhaler in children younger than age 12 haven't been established.

Adverse reactions

CNS: dizziness, pain, headache, nervousness.
CV: palpitations, hypertension, chest pain.
EENT: blurred vision, rhinitis, pharyngitis, sinusitis, epistaxis.
GI: nausea, GI distress, dry mouth.
Musculoskeletal: back pain.
Respiratory: *upper respiratory tract infection, bronchitis,* cough, dyspnea, ***bronchospasm***, increased sputum.
Skin: rash.
Other: flulike symptoms, hypersensitivity reactions.

Interactions

Drug-drug. *Anticholinergics:* May increase anticholinergic effects. Avoid using together.
Drug-herb. *Jaborandi tree:* May decrease effect of ipratropium when used together. Advise patient to use together cautiously.
Pill-bearing spurge: Choline, a chemical component of the herb, may decrease effect of ipratropium. Advise patient to use together cautiously.

Nursing considerations

- If patient uses a face mask for a nebulizer, take care to prevent leakage around the mask because eye pain or temporary blurring of vision may occur.
- Safety and efficacy of use beyond 4 days in patients with a common cold haven't been established.

!!ALERT Patient with a severe peanut allergy could have an anaphylactic reaction after using Atrovent inhalation aerosol metered-dose inhaler (MDI). Get a thorough allergy history from patient before giving any drug.
!!ALERT Don't confuse Atrovent with Alupent.

Patient teaching

- Warn patient that drug isn't effective for treating acute episodes of bronchospasm when rapid response is needed.
- Teach patient to perform oral inhalation correctly. Give the following instructions for using an MDI:
  - Shake canister.
  - Clear nasal passages and throat.
  - Breathe out, expelling as much air from lungs as possible.
  - Place mouthpiece well into mouth, and inhale deeply as you release dose from inhaler. (Patient may want to close eyes.)
  - Hold breath for several seconds, remove mouthpiece, and exhale slowly.
- Inform patient that use of a spacer device with MDI may improve drug delivery to lungs.
- Warn patient to avoid accidentally spraying drug into eyes. Temporary blurring of vision may result.
- If more than 1 inhalation is prescribed, tell patient to wait at least 2 minutes before repeating procedure.
- Instruct patient to remove canister and wash inhaler in warm, soapy water at least once weekly.
- If patient is also using a corticosteroid inhaler, instruct him to use ipratropium first and then to wait about 5 minutes before using the corticosteroid. This lets the bronchodilator open air passages for maximum effectiveness of the corticosteroid.

irbesartan
Avapro

Pregnancy risk category C; D in 2nd and 3rd trimesters

Indications & dosages

➲ **Hypertension**
Adults and children age 13 and older: Initially, 150 mg P.O. daily, increased to maximum of 300 mg daily, if needed.

Children ages 6 to 12: Initially, 75 mg P.O. once daily, increased to maximum of 150 mg daily, if needed.

For volume- and salt-depleted patients, initially, 75 mg P.O. daily.

➲ **Nephropathy in patients with type 2 diabetes**

Adults: 300 mg P.O. once daily.

Contraindications & cautions

- Contraindicated in patients hypersensitive to drug or its components.
- Use cautiously in patients with impaired renal function, heart failure, and renal artery stenosis and in breast-feeding women.
- Use during pregnancy can cause injury and death to the developing fetus. When pregnancy is detected, stop drug as soon as possible.

Adverse reactions

CNS: fatigue, anxiety, dizziness, headache.
CV: chest pain, edema, tachycardia.
EENT: pharyngitis, rhinitis, sinus abnormality.
GI: diarrhea, dyspepsia, abdominal pain, nausea, vomiting.
GU: UTI.
Musculoskeletal: musculoskeletal trauma or pain.
Respiratory: upper respiratory tract infection, cough.
Skin: rash.

Interactions

Drug-herb. *Ma huang:* May decrease antihypertensive effects. Discourage use together.

Nursing considerations

- Drug may be given with a diuretic or other antihypertensive, if needed, for control of hypertension.
- Symptomatic hypotension may occur in volume- or salt-depleted patients (vigorous diuretic use or dialysis). Correct the cause of volume depletion before administration or before a lower dose is used.
- If hypotension occurs, place patient in a supine position and give an I.V. infusion of normal saline solution, if needed. Once blood pressure has stabilized after a transient hypotensive episode, drug may be continued.
- Dizziness and orthostatic hypotension may occur more frequently in patients with type 2 diabetes and renal disease.

Patient teaching

- Warn woman of childbearing age of consequences of drug exposure to fetus. Tell her to call prescriber immediately if pregnancy is suspected.
- Tell patient that drug may be taken once daily without regard to food.

irinotecan hydrochloride
Camptosar

Pregnancy risk category D

Indications & dosages

➲ **Metastatic carcinoma of the colon or rectum that has recurred or progressed after fluorouracil (5-FU) therapy**

Adults: Initially, 125 mg/m^2 by I.V. infusion over 90 minutes once weekly for 4 weeks; then 2-week rest period. Thereafter, additional courses of treatment may be repeated q 6 weeks with 4 weeks on and 2 weeks off. Subsequent doses may be adjusted to low of 50 mg/m^2 or maximum of 150 mg/m^2 in 25 to 50-mg/m^2 increments based on patient's tolerance. Or, 350 mg/m^2 by I.V. infusion over 90 minutes once q 3 weeks. Additional courses may continue indefinitely in patients who respond favorably and in those whose disease remains stable, provided intolerable toxicity doesn't occur.

Consider reducing starting dose in patients age 65 and older, patients who have received pelvic or abdominal radiation, or who have a performance status of 2 or increased bilirubin level. Give 300 mg/m^2 by I.V. infusion over 90 minutes once q 3 weeks. Or, give 100 mg/m^2 by I.V. infusion over 90 minutes once weekly.

➲ **First-line therapy for metastatic colorectal cancer with 5-fluorouracil (5-FU) and leucovorin**

Regimen 1

Adults: 125 mg/m^2 I.V. over 90 minutes on days 1, 8, 15, and 22; then leucovorin 20 mg/m^2 I.V. bolus on days 1, 8, 15, and 22 and 5-FU 500 mg/m^2 I.V. bolus on days 1, 8, 15, and 22. Courses are repeated q 6 weeks.

Regimen 2

Adults: 180 mg/m^2 I.V. over 90 minutes on days 1, 15, and 29; then leucovorin 200 mg/m^2 I.V. over 2 hours on days 1, 2, 15, 16, 29, and 30; then 5-FU 400 mg/m^2 I.V. bolus on days 1, 2, 15, 16, 29, and 30 and 5-FU 600 mg/m^2 I.V. infusion over 22 hours on days 1, 2, 15, 16, 29, and 30.

See manufacturer's package insert for details on dosage adjustment.

Contraindications & cautions

- Contraindicated in patients hypersensitive to drug.
- Safety and effectiveness of drug in children haven't been established.
- Use cautiously in elderly patients.

Adverse reactions

CNS: *insomnia, dizziness, asthenia, headache*, akathisia, *fever, pain.*
CV: *vasodilation, edema*, orthostatic hypotension.
EENT: *rhinitis.*
GI: ***diarrhea***, *nausea, vomiting, anorexia, stomatitis, constipation, flatulence, dyspepsia, abdominal cramping, pain, and enlargement.*
Hematologic: ***leukopenia***, *anemia*, ***neutropenia, thrombocytopenia***.
Metabolic: *weight loss, dehydration.*
Musculoskeletal: *back pain.*
Respiratory: *dyspnea, increased cough.*
Skin: *alopecia, sweating, rash.*
Other: *chills, infection.*

Interactions

Drug-drug. *Dexamethasone:* May increase risk of irinotecan-induced lymphocytopenia. Monitor patient closely.
Diuretics: May increase risk of dehydration and electrolyte imbalance. Consider stopping diuretic during active periods of nausea and vomiting.
Laxative use: May increase risk of diarrhea. Avoid using together.
Prochlorperazine: May increase risk of akathisia. Monitor patient closely.
Other antineoplastics: May cause additive adverse effects, such as myelosuppression and diarrhea. Monitor patient closely.
Drug-herb. *St. John's wort:* May decrease blood levels of irinotecan by about 40%. Discourage use together.

Nursing considerations

- Pelvic or abdominal irradiation may increase risk of severe myelosuppression. Avoid use of drug in patients undergoing irradiation.
- Diuretic may be withheld during therapy and periods of active vomiting or diarrhea to decrease risk of dehydration.
- Drug can induce severe diarrhea. Diarrhea occurring within 24 hours of administration may be preceded by diaphoresis and abdominal cramping and may be relieved by 0.25 to 1 mg atropine I.V., unless contraindicated. Diarrhea occurring more than 24 hours after drug administration may be prolonged, leading to dehydration and electrolyte imbalances; it may be life-threatening.
- Treat late diarrhea (more than 24 hours after irinotecan administration) promptly with loperamide. Monitor patient for dehydration, electrolyte imbalance, or sepsis, and treat appropriately.
- Delay subsequent irinotecan treatments until normal bowel function returns for at least 24 hours without antidiarrhea medication. If grade 2, 3, or 4 late diarrhea occurs, decrease subsequent doses of irinotecan within the current cycle.
- Temporarily stop therapy if neutropenic fever occurs or if absolute neutrophil count drops below 500/mm^3. Reduce dosage, especially if WBC count is below 2,000/mm^3, neutrophil count is below 1,000/mm^3, hemoglobin level is below 8 g/dl, or platelet count is below 100,000/mm^3.
- Routine administration of a colony-stimulating factor isn't needed but may be helpful in patients with significant neutropenia.
- Monitor WBC count with differential, hemoglobin level, and platelet count before each dose of irinotecan.

Patient teaching

- Inform patient about risk of diarrhea and methods to treat it; tell him to avoid laxatives.
- Instruct patient to contact prescriber if any of the following occur: diarrhea for the first time during treatment; black or bloody stools; symptoms of dehydration such as light-headedness, dizziness, or faintness; inability to drink fluids due to nausea or vomiting; inability to control diarrhea within 24 hours; or fever or infection.

• Warn patient that hair loss may occur.
• Caution woman of childbearing age to avoid pregnancy or breast-feeding during therapy.

iron dextran
DexFerrum, InFeD

Pregnancy risk category C

Indications & dosages

➲ Iron deficiency anemia

Adults and children: I.V. or I.M. test dose is needed before administration. Total dose is calculated using the following formula:

$$\text{Dose (ml)} = 0.0442\ (\text{desired Hb} - \text{observed Hb}) \times \text{Weight in kg} + (0.26 \times \text{Weight in kg})$$

I.V.

Inject 0.5-ml test dose over 30 seconds. If no reaction occurs in 1 hour, give remainder of therapeutic I.V. dose. Repeat therapeutic I.V. dose daily. Single daily dose shouldn't exceed 100 mg. Give slowly (1 ml/minute).

I.M. (by Z-track method)

Inject 0.5-ml test dose. If no reaction occurs in 1 hour, give remainder of dose. Daily dose should ordinarily not exceed 0.5 ml (25 mg) for infants weighing less than 5 kg (11 lb); 1 ml (50 mg) for those weighing less than 10 kg (22 lb); and 2 ml (100 mg) for heavier children and adults. Don't give iron dextran in the first 4 months of life.

Contraindications & cautions

• Contraindicated in patients hypersensitive to drug, in those with acute infectious renal disease, and in those with any anemia except iron deficiency anemia.
• Use cautiously in patients who have serious hepatic impairment, rheumatoid arthritis, or other inflammatory diseases because these patients may be at higher risk for certain delays and reactions.
• Use cautiously in patients with history of significant allergies or asthma.

Adverse reactions

CNS: headache, transitory paresthesia, dizziness, malaise, fever, chills.
CV: chest pain, tachycardia, ***bradycardia***, *hypotensive reaction, peripheral vascular flushing.*
GI: nausea, anorexia.
Musculoskeletal: arthralgia, myalgia.
Respiratory: ***bronchospasm***, dyspnea.
Skin: rash, urticaria, *soreness, inflammation, brown skin discoloration at I.M. injection site, local phlebitis at I.V. injection site,* sterile abscess, necrosis, atrophy.
Other: fibrosis, ***anaphylaxis***, ***delayed sensitivity reactions***.

Interactions

None significant.

Nursing considerations

• Have epinephrine immediately available in event of acute hypersensitivity reaction.
• Don't give iron dextran with oral iron preparations.
• I.V. or I.M. injections of iron are advisable only for patients in whom oral administration is impossible or ineffective.
• For I.M. route, inject deep into upper outer quadrant of buttock—never into arm or other exposed area—with a 2- to 3-inch 19G or 20G needle. Use Z-track method to avoid leakage into subcutaneous tissue and staining of skin. After drawing up drug, use a new sterile needle to give injection.
• Monitor hemoglobin level, hematocrit, and reticulocyte count.

Patient teaching

• Teach patient signs and symptoms of hypersensitivity and iron toxicity, and tell him to report them to prescriber.
• Inform patient that drug may stain skin.

iron sucrose injection
Venofer

Pregnancy risk category B

Indications & dosages

➲ Iron deficiency anemia in patients undergoing long-term hemodialysis who are receiving supplemental erythropoietin therapy

Adults: 100 mg (5 ml) of elemental iron I.V. directly in the dialysis line, either by slow injection at a rate of 1 ml/minute or by infusion over 15 minutes during the dialysis session one to three times a week to a total of 1,000 mg in 10 doses; repeat p.r.n.

Contraindications & cautions

- Contraindicated in patients with hypersensitivity to drug or its components, evidence of iron overload, or anemia not caused by iron deficiency.
- Use cautiously in breast-feeding women.

Adverse reactions

CNS: headache, asthenia, malaise, dizziness, fever.
CV: ***heart failure***, *hypotension*, chest pain, hypertension, fluid retention.
GI: nausea, vomiting, diarrhea, abdominal pain, taste perversion.
Musculoskeletal: *leg cramps*, bone and muscle pain.
Respiratory: dyspnea, wheezing, pneumonia, cough.
Skin: rash, pruritus, application site reaction.
Other: accidental injury, pain, ***sepsis***, ***hypersensitivity reactions***.

Interactions

Drug-drug. *Oral iron preparations:* May reduce absorption of oral iron preparations. Avoid using together.

Nursing considerations

!!ALERT Rare but fatal hypersensitivity reactions characterized by anaphylactic shock, loss of consciousness, collapse, hypotension, dyspnea, or seizures may occur. Have epinephrine readily available.
- Mild to moderate hypersensitivity reactions, with wheezing, dyspnea, hypotension, rash, or pruritus, may occur.
- Giving drug by infusion may reduce the risk of hypotension.
- Transferrin saturation level increases rapidly after I.V. administration of iron sucrose. Obtain iron level 48 hours after I.V. administration.
- Monitor ferritin, transferrin saturation, and hemoglobin levels, and hematocrit.
- Withhold dose in patient with signs and symptoms of iron overload.
- Keep dose selection in elderly patients conservative because of decreased hepatic, renal, or cardiac function; other disease; and other drug therapy.

Patient teaching

- Instruct patient to notify prescriber if symptoms of overdose (headache, nausea, dizziness, joint aches, tingling, or abdominal and muscle pain) or of allergic reaction (labored breathing, collapse, or loss of consciousness) occur.

isoniazid (INH, isonicotinic acid hydrazide)

Isotamine†, Nydrazid, PMS-Isoniazid†

Pregnancy risk category C

Indications & dosages

➲ Actively growing tubercle bacilli
Adults and children age 15 and older: 5 mg/kg daily P.O. or I.M. in a single dose, up to 300 mg/day, with other drugs, continued for 6 months to 2 years. For intermittent multiple-drug regimen, 15 mg/kg (up to 900 mg) P.O. or I.M. once, twice, or three times weekly.
Infants and children: 10 to 20 mg/kg daily P.O. or I.M. in a single dose, up to 500 mg/day, continued long enough to prevent relapse. Give with at least one other antituberculotic. For intermittent multiple-drug regimen, 20 to 30 mg/kg (up to 900 mg) P.O. or I.M. twice weekly.
➲ To prevent tubercle bacilli in those exposed to tuberculosis (TB) or those with positive skin test results whose chest X-rays and bacteriologic study results indicate nonprogressive TB
Adults: 300 mg daily P.O. in a single dose, continued for 6 months to 1 year.
Infants and children: 10 mg/kg daily P.O. in a single dose, up to 300 mg/day, continued for up to 1 year.

Contraindications & cautions

- Contraindicated in patients with acute hepatic disease or isoniazid-related liver damage.
- Use cautiously in elderly patients, in those with chronic non–isoniazid-related liver disease or chronic alcoholism, in those with seizure disorders (especially if taking phenytoin), and in those with severe renal impairment.

Adverse reactions

CNS: *peripheral neuropathy*, ***seizures***, ***toxic encephalopathy***, memory impairment, toxic psychosis.
EENT: optic neuritis and atrophy.
GI: nausea, vomiting, epigastric distress.
Hematologic: ***agranulocytosis***, hemolytic anemia, ***aplastic anemia***, eosinophilia, ***thrombocytopenia***, sideroblastic anemia.
Hepatic: ***hepatitis***, jaundice, bilirubinemia.
Metabolic: hyperglycemia, metabolic acidosis, hypocalcemia, hypophosphatemia.
Skin: irritation at injection site.
Other: rheumatic and lupuslike syndromes, hypersensitivity reactions, pyridoxine deficiency, gynecomastia.

Interactions

Drug-drug. *Antacids and laxatives containing aluminum:* May decrease isoniazid absorption. Give isoniazid at least 1 hour before antacid or laxative.
Benzodiazepines, such as diazepam, triazolam: May inhibit metabolic clearance of benzodiazepines that undergo oxidative metabolism, possibly increasing benzodiazepine activity. Monitor patient for adverse reactions.
Carbamazepine, phenytoin: May increase levels of these drugs. Monitor drug levels closely.
Cycloserine: May increase CNS adverse reactions. Use safety precautions.
Disulfiram: May cause neurologic symptoms, including changes in behavior and coordination. Avoid using together.
Enflurane: In rapid acetylators of isoniazid, may cause high-output renal failure because of nephrotoxic inorganic fluoride level. Monitor renal function.
Ketoconazole: May decrease ketoconazole level. Monitor patient for lack of efficacy.
Meperidine: May increase CNS adverse reactions and hypotension. Use safety precautions.
Oral anticoagulants: May enhance anticoagulant activity. Monitor PT and INR.
Phenytoin: May inhibit phenytoin metabolism and increase phenytoin level. Monitor patient for phenytoin toxicity.
Drug-food. *Foods containing tyramine (such as aged cheese, beer, and chocolate):* May cause hypertensive crisis. Tell patient to avoid such foods or eat in small quantities.
Drug-lifestyle. *Alcohol use:* May increase risk of isoniazid-related hepatitis. Discourage use of alcohol.

Nursing considerations

- Always give isoniazid with other antituberculotics to prevent development of resistant organisms.
- Isoniazid pharmacokinetics may vary among patients because drug is metabolized in the liver by genetically controlled acetylation. Fast acetylators metabolize drug up to five times as fast as slow acetylators. About 50% of blacks and whites are slow acetylators; more than 80% of Chinese, Japanese, and Inuits are fast acetylators.
- Peripheral neuropathy is more common in patients who are slow acetylators or who are malnourished, alcoholic, or diabetic.
- Monitor hepatic function closely for changes. Elevated liver function study results occur in about 15% of patients; most abnormalities are mild and transient, but some may persist throughout treatment.

!!ALERT Severe and sometimes fatal hepatitis may develop, even after many months of treatment. Risk increases with age. Monitor liver study results closely.

- Give pyridoxine to prevent peripheral neuropathy, especially in malnourished patients.

Patient teaching

- Instruct patient to take drug exactly as prescribed; warn against stopping drug without prescriber's consent.
- Advise patient to take drug 1 hour before or 2 hours after meals.
- Tell patient to notify prescriber immediately if signs and symptoms of liver impairment occur, such as appetite loss, fatigue, malaise, yellow skin or eye discoloration, and dark urine.
- Advise patient to avoid alcoholic beverages while taking drug. Also tell him to avoid certain foods (fish such as skipjack and tuna and products containing tyramine, such as aged cheese, beer, and chocolate), because drug has some MAO inhibitor activity.
- Encourage patient to comply fully with treatment, which may take months or years.

isoproterenol hydrochloride
Isuprel

Pregnancy risk category C

Indications & dosages

➲ Bronchospasm during anesthesia
Adults: Dilute 1 ml of a 1:5,000 solution with 10 ml of normal saline or D_5W. Give 0.01 to 0.02 mg I.V. and repeat as necessary. Or, give 1:50,000 solution undiluted using same dose.

➲ Heart block, ventricular arrhythmias
Adults: Initially, 0.02 to 0.06 mg I.V.; then 0.01 to 0.2 mg I.V. or 5 mcg/minute I.V. Or, initially, 0.2 mg I.M.; then 0.02 to 1 mg I.M., p.r.n.
Children: Initial I.V. infusion of 0.1 mcg/kg/minute. Adjust dosage based on patient's response. Usual dosage range is 0.1 to 1 mcg/kg/minute.

➲ Shock
Adults and children: 0.5 to 5 mcg/minute isoproterenol hydrochloride by continuous I.V. infusion. Usual concentration is 1 mg or 5 ml in 500 ml D_5W. Titrate infusion rate according to heart rate, central venous pressure, blood pressure, and urine flow.

➲ Postoperative cardiac patients with bradycardia♦
Children: I.V. infusion of 0.029 mcg/kg/minute.

➲ As an aid in diagnosing the cause of mitral regurgitation♦
Adults: 4 mcg/minute I.V. infusion.

➲ As an aid in diagnosing coronary artery disease or lesions♦
Adults: 1 to 3 mcg/minute I.V. infusion.

Contraindications & cautions

- Contraindicated in patients with tachycardia or AV block caused by digoxin intoxication, arrhythmias (other than those that may respond to treatment with isoproterenol), angina pectoris, or angle-closure glaucoma.
- Contraindicated when used with general anesthetics with halogenated drugs or cyclopropane.
- Use cautiously in elderly patients and in those with renal or CV disease, coronary insufficiency, diabetes, hyperthyroidism, or history of sensitivity to sympathomimetic amines.

Adverse reactions

CNS: headache, mild tremor, weakness, dizziness, nervousness, insomnia, anxiety.
CV: *palpitations, tachycardia, angina,* ***arrhythmias, cardiac arrest****, rapid rise and fall in blood pressure.*
GI: nausea, vomiting.
Metabolic: hyperglycemia.
Skin: diaphoresis.
Other: swelling of parotid glands with prolonged use.

Interactions

Drug-drug. *Epinephrine, other sympathomimetics:* May increase risk of arrhythmias. Use together cautiously. If used together, give at least 4 hours apart.
Halogenated general anesthetics or cyclopropane: May increase risk of arrhythmias. Avoid using together.
Propranolol, other beta blockers: May block bronchodilating effect of isoproterenol. Monitor patient carefully.

Nursing considerations

- Drug isn't a substitute for blood or fluid volume deficit. Correct volume deficit before giving vasopressors.
- Don't use solution if it's discolored or contains precipitate.

!!ALERT Notify prescriber if heart rate exceeds 110 beats/minute with I.V. infusion. Doses sufficient to increase the heart rate to more than 130 beats/minute may induce ventricular arrhythmias.

- Isoproterenol may cause a slight increase in systolic blood pressure and a slight-to-marked decrease in diastolic blood pressure.
- Monitor patient for adverse reactions.

!!ALERT Don't confuse Isuprel with Isordil.

Patient teaching

- Tell patient to report chest pain, fluttering in chest, or other adverse reactions.
- Remind patient to report pain at the I.V. injection site.

isosorbide dinitrate

Apo-ISDN†, Cedocard SR†, Dilatrate-SR, Isordil, Isordil Tembids, Isordil Titradose

isosorbide mononitrate

Imdur, ISMO, Isotrate ER, Monoket

Pregnancy risk category C

Indications & dosages

➲ Acute anginal attacks (S.L. isosorbide dinitrate only); to prevent situations that may cause anginal attacks

Adults: 2.5 to 5 mg S.L. tablets for prompt relief of angina, repeated q 5 to 10 minutes (maximum of three doses for each 30-minute period). For prevention, 2.5 to 10 mg q 2 to 3 hours.

Or, 5 to 40 mg isosorbide dinitrate P.O. b.i.d. or t.i.d. for prevention only (use smallest effective dose).

Or, 30 to 60 mg isosorbide mononitrate using Imdur P.O. once daily on arising; increased to 120 mg once daily after several days, if needed.

Or, 20 mg isosorbide mononitrate using ISMO or Monoket b.i.d. with the two doses given 7 hours apart.

Contraindications & cautions

- Contraindicated in patients with hypersensitivity or idiosyncrasy to nitrates and in those with severe hypotension, angle-closure glaucoma, increased intracranial pressure, shock, or acute MI with low left ventricular filling pressure.
- Use cautiously in patients with blood volume depletion (such as from diuretic therapy) or mild hypotension.

Adverse reactions

CNS: *headache*, dizziness, weakness.
CV: *orthostatic hypotension*, *tachycardia*, *palpitations*, *ankle edema*, fainting, *flushing*.
EENT: S.L. burning.
GI: nausea, vomiting.
Skin: cutaneous vasodilation, rash.

Interactions

Drug-drug. *Antihypertensives:* May increase hypotensive effects. Monitor patient closely during initial therapy.
Sildenafil, tadalafil, vardenafil: May cause severe hypotension. Use of nitrates in any form with these drugs is contraindicated.
Drug-lifestyle. *Alcohol use:* May increase hypotension. Discourage use together.

Nursing considerations

- To prevent tolerance, a nitrate-free interval of 8 to 12 hours per day is recommended. The regimen for isosorbide mononitrate (1 tablet on awakening with the second dose in 7 hours, or 1 extended-release tablet daily) is intended to minimize nitrate tolerance by providing a substantial nitrate-free interval.
- Monitor blood pressure and intensity and duration of drug response.
- Drug may cause headaches, especially at beginning of therapy. Dosage may be reduced temporarily, but tolerance usually develops. Treat headache with aspirin or acetaminophen.
- Methemoglobinemia has been seen with nitrates. Symptoms are those of impaired oxygen delivery despite adequate cardiac output and adequate arterial partial pressure of oxygen.

!! ALERT Don't confuse Isordil with Isuprel or Inderal.

Patient teaching

- Caution patient to take drug regularly, as prescribed, and to keep it accessible at all times.

!! ALERT Advise patient that stopping drug abruptly may cause spasm of the coronary arteries with increased angina symptoms and potential risk of heart attack.

- Tell patient to take S.L. tablet at first sign of attack. He should wet tablet with saliva and place under his tongue until absorbed; he should sit down and rest. Dose may be repeated every 10 to 15 minutes for a maximum of three doses. If drug doesn't provide relief, tell patient to seek medical help promptly.
- Advise patient who complains of tingling sensation with S.L. drug to try holding tablet in cheek.
- Warn patient not to confuse S.L. with P.O. form.
- Advise patient taking P.O. form of isosorbide dinitrate to take oral tablet on an empty stomach either 30 minutes before or 1 to 2

hours after meals and to swallow oral tablets whole.

- Tell patient to minimize dizziness upon standing up by changing to upright position slowly. Advise him to go up and down stairs carefully and to lie down at first sign of dizziness.
- Caution patient to avoid alcohol because it may worsen low blood pressure effects.
- Advise patient that use of sildenafil, tadalafil, or vardenafil with any nitrate may cause severe low blood pressure. Patient should talk to his prescriber before using these drugs together.
- Instruct patient to store drug in a cool place, in a tightly closed container, and away from light.

isotretinoin

Accutane, Amnesteem, Claravis, Sotret

Pregnancy risk category X

Indications & dosages

➲ **Severe recalcitrant nodular acne unresponsive to conventional therapy**
Adults and adolescents: 0.5 to 2 mg/kg P.O. daily in two divided doses with food for 15 to 20 weeks.

Contraindications & cautions

- Contraindicated in patients hypersensitive to parabens (used as preservatives), vitamin A, or other retinoids.
- Contraindicated in woman of childbearing potential, unless patient has had two negative pregnancy test results before beginning therapy, will begin drug therapy on second or third day of next menstrual period, and will comply with stringent contraceptive measures for 1 month before therapy, during therapy, and for at least 1 month after therapy.
- Use cautiously in patients with a history of mental illness or a family history of psychiatric disorders, asthma, liver disease, diabetes, heart disease, osteoporosis, genetic predisposition for age-related osteoporosis, history of childhood osteoporosis, weak bones, anorexia nervosa, osteomalacia, or other disorders of bone metabolism.

Adverse reactions

CNS: ***depression, psychosis, suicidal ideation or attempts, suicide, aggressive and violent behavior***, emotional instability, headache, fatigue, *pseudotumor cerebri.*
EENT: *conjunctivitis,* corneal deposits, dry eyes, visual disturbances, *epistaxis, drying of mucous membranes, dry nose,* hearing impairment (sometimes irreversible), decreased night vision.
GI: nonspecific GI symptoms, *nausea, vomiting,* anorexia, *abdominal pain, dry mouth,* gum bleeding and inflammation, ***acute pancreatitis***, inflammatory bowel disease.
Hematologic: anemia, thrombocytosis, *increased erythrocyte sedimentation rate.*
Hepatic: ***hepatitis***.
Metabolic: *hypertriglyceridemia,* hyperglycemia.
Musculoskeletal: skeletal hyperostosis, tendon and ligament calcification, premature epiphyseal closure, decreased bone mineral density and other bone abnormalities, back pain, arthralgia, arthritis, tendinitis, ***rhabdomyolysis***.
Skin: *cheilosis, rash, dry skin, facial skin desquamation,* peeling of palms and toes, *petechiae, nail brittleness,* thinning of hair, skin infection, photosensitivity reaction, *cheilitis, pruritus, fragility.*

Interactions

Drug-drug. *Corticosteroids:* May increase risk of osteoporosis. Use together cautiously.
Medicated soaps, cleansers, and coverups, topical resorcinol peeling agents (benzoyl peroxide), alcohol-containing preparations: May have cumulative drying effect. Use together cautiously.
Micro-dosed progesterone oral contraceptives ("minipills") that don't contain estrogen: May decrease effectiveness of contraceptive. Advise patient to use different contraceptive method.
Phenytoin: May increase risk of osteomalacia. Use together cautiously.
Tetracyclines: May increase risk of pseudotumor cerebri. Avoid using together.
Vitamin A, products containing vitamin A: May increase toxic effects of isotretinoin. Avoid using together.
Drug-food. *Any food:* May increase absorption of drug. Advise patient to take drug with milk, a meal, or shortly after a meal.

Drug-lifestyle. *Alcohol use:* May increase risk of hypertriglyceridemia. Discourage use together.
Sun exposure: May increase photosensitivity reaction. Advise patient to avoid excessive sunlight exposure.

Nursing considerations

- Before use, have patient read patient information and sign accompanying consent form.
- Patient must have negative results from two urine or serum pregnancy tests; one is performed in the office when the patient is qualified for therapy, the second during the first 5 days of the next normal menstrual period immediately preceding the beginning of therapy. For patients with amenorrhea, the second test should be done at least 11 days after the last unprotected act of sexual intercourse. A pregnancy test must be repeated every month before the patient receives the prescription.
- Monitor baseline lipid studies, liver function tests, and pregnancy tests before therapy and at monthly intervals.
- Regularly monitor glucose level and CK levels in patients who participate in vigorous physical activity.
- Most adverse reactions occur at doses exceeding 1 mg/kg daily. Reactions are generally reversible when therapy is stopped or dosage is reduced.

!!ALERT Screen for papilledema if patient experiences headache, nausea and vomiting, or visual disturbances. Signs and symptoms of pseudotumor cerebri require immediate discontinuation of drug and prompt neurologic intervention.

!!ALERT Severe fetal abnormalities may occur if this drug is used during pregnancy.

- The FDA and drug manufacturer designed the program System to Manage Accutane Related Teratogenicity (S.M.A.R.T.) to encourage the safe and appropriate use of drug, which can cause birth defects and fetal death if taken by a pregnant woman.
- If patient becomes pregnant during treatment, prescribers are encouraged to call Roche Medical Services at 1-800-526-6367 or FDA (MedWatch) at 1-800-FDA-1088.
- A second course of therapy may begin 8 weeks after completion of the first course, if necessary. Improvements may continue after first course is complete.
- Patients may be at increased risk of bone fractures or injury when participating in sports with repetitive impact.
- Spontaneous reports of osteoporosis, osteopenia, bone fractures, and delayed healing of bone fractures have occurred in patients taking drug. To decrease this risk, don't exceed recommended doses and duration.

Patient teaching

- Advise patient to take drug with or shortly after meals to facilitate absorption.
- Tell patient to immediately report visual disturbances and bone, muscle, or joint pain.
- Warn patient that contact lenses may feel uncomfortable during therapy.
- Warn patient against using abrasives, medicated soaps and cleansers, acne preparations containing peeling drugs, and topical products containing alcohol (including cosmetics, aftershave, cologne) because they may cause cumulative irritation or excessive drying of skin.
- Tell patient to avoid prolonged sun exposure and to use sunblock. Drug may have additive effect if used with other drugs that cause photosensitivity reaction.
- Advise patient of childbearing age to either abstain from sex or use two reliable forms of contraception simultaneously for 1 month before, during, and for 1 month after treatment.
- Tell women that manufacturer will supply urine pregnancy tests for monthly testing during therapy.
- Warn patient that transient exacerbations may occur during therapy.
- Warn patient not to donate blood during therapy and for 1 month after stopping drug because drug could harm fetus of a pregnant recipient.
- Tell patient to report adverse reactions immediately, especially depression, suicidal thoughts, persistent headaches, and persistent GI pain.

itraconazole
Sporanox

Pregnancy risk category C

Indications & dosages

➲ **Pulmonary and extrapulmonary blastomycosis, nonmeningeal histoplasmosis**
Adults: 200 mg P.O. daily; increase as needed and tolerated by 100 mg to maximum of 400 mg daily. Give dosages exceeding 200 mg P.O. daily in two divided doses. Or, give 200 mg I.V. b.i.d. over 1 hour for four doses, followed by 200 mg I.V. daily for up to 14 days; then change to P.O. form. Continue treatment for at least 3 months. In life-threatening illness, give a loading dose of 200 mg P.O. t.i.d. for 3 days.

➲ **Aspergillosis**
Adults: 200 to 400 mg P.O. daily. Or, 200 mg I.V. b.i.d. over 1 hour for four doses, followed by 200 mg I.V. daily for up to 14 days; then change to P.O. form.

➲ **Onychomycosis of the toenail (with or without fingernail involvement)**
Adults: 200 mg P.O. b.i.d. for 1 week, followed by 3 weeks drug free. Repeat cycle twice, for a total of three cycles.

➲ **Onychomycosis of the fingernail**
Adults: 200 mg P.O. b.i.d. for 1 week, followed by 3 weeks drug free. Repeat dosage.

➲ **Oropharyngeal candidiasis**
Adults: 200 mg oral solution swished in mouth vigorously and swallowed daily, for 1 to 2 weeks.

➲ **Oropharyngeal candidiasis in patients unresponsive to fluconazole tablets**
Adults: 100 mg oral solution swished in mouth vigorously and swallowed b.i.d., for 2 to 4 weeks.

➲ **Esophageal candidiasis**
Adults: 100 to 200 mg oral solution swished in mouth vigorously and swallowed daily, for at least 3 weeks. Treatment should continue for 2 weeks after symptoms resolve.

Contraindications & cautions

- Contraindicated in patients hypersensitive to drug or those receiving alprazolam, triazolam, midazolam, pimozide, quinidine, dofetilide, lovastatin, or simvastatin; in those with ventricular dysfunction or a history of heart failure; and in those who are breast-feeding. If signs and symptoms of heart failure occur, stop itraconazole.
- Use cautiously in patients with hypochlorhydria; they may not absorb drug readily.
- Use cautiously in HIV-infected patients because hypochlorhydria can accompany HIV infection.
- Use cautiously in patients receiving other highly bound drugs.

Adverse reactions

CNS: fever, *headache*, dizziness, somnolence, fatigue, malaise, asthenia, pain, tremor, abnormal dreams, anxiety, depression.
CV: hypertension, edema, orthostatic hypotension, ***heart failure***.
EENT: rhinitis, sinusitis, pharyngitis.
GI: *nausea*, vomiting, diarrhea, abdominal pain, anorexia, dyspepsia, flatulence, increased appetite, constipation, gastritis, gastroenteritis, ulcerative stomatitis, gingivitis.
GU: albuminuria, impotence, cystitis, UTI.
Hematologic: ***neutropenia***.
Hepatic: impaired hepatic function, ***hepatotoxicity***, ***liver failure***.
Metabolic: hypokalemia, hypertriglyceridemia.
Musculoskeletal: myalgia.
Respiratory: upper respiratory tract infection, ***pulmonary edema***.
Skin: rash, pruritus.
Other: decreased libido, injury, herpes zoster, ***hypersensitivity reactions (urticaria, angioedema, Stevens-Johnson syndrome)***.

Interactions

Drug-drug. *Alprazolam, midazolam, triazolam:* May increase and prolong drug levels, CNS depression, and psychomotor impairment. Avoid using together.
Antacids, carbamazepine, H_2-receptor antagonists, isoniazid, phenobarbital, phenytoin, rifabutin, rifampin: May decrease itraconazole level. Avoid using together.
Chlordiazepoxide, clonazepam, clorazepate, diazepam, estazolam, flurazepam, quazepam: May increase and prolong drug levels, CNS depression, and psychomotor impairment. Avoid using together.
Clarithromycin, erythromycin: May increase itraconazole levels. Monitor patient for signs of itraconazole toxicity.

Cyclosporine, digoxin, tacrolimus: May increase levels of these drugs. Monitor drug levels.
Dofetilide, pimozide, quinidine: May increase levels of these drugs by cytochrome P-450 metabolism, causing serious CV events, including torsades de pointes, QT interval prolongation, ventricular tachycardia, cardiac arrest, and sudden death. Avoid using together.
HMG-CoA reductase inhibitors (atorvastatin, fluvastatin, lovastatin, pravastatin, simvastatin): May increase levels and adverse effects of these drugs. Avoid using together, or reduce dose of HMG-CoA reductase inhibitor. Don't use itraconazole with lovastatin or simvastatin.
Indinavir, ritonavir, saquinavir: May increase levels of these drugs; indinavir and ritonavir may increase itraconazole levels. Monitor patient for toxicity.
Oral anticoagulants: May enhance anticoagulant effect. Monitor PT and INR.
Oral antidiabetics: May cause hypoglycemia, similar to effect of other antifungals. Monitor glucose level. Avoid using together.
Drug-food. *Grapefruit and orange juice:* May decrease itraconazole level and therapeutic effect. Give with liquid other than grapefruit or orange juice.

Nursing considerations

!!ALERT Capsules and oral solution aren't interchangeable.

- Confirm the diagnosis of onychomycosis before starting therapy, by having nail specimens undergo appropriate laboratory testing.
- Perform baseline liver function tests, and monitor results periodically. Unless the patient's condition is life-threatening, avoid therapy in patients with baseline hepatic impairment. If liver dysfunction occurs during therapy, notify prescriber immediately.

Patient teaching

- Teach patient to recognize and report signs and symptoms of liver disease (anorexia, dark urine, pale stools, unusual fatigue, and jaundice).
- Instruct patient not to use oral solution interchangeably with capsules.
- Tell patient to use 10 ml of the oral solution at a time.
- Advise patient to take solution without food and to take capsules with a full meal.
- Urge patient to tell prescriber about all drugs he's taking to avoid potential drug interactions.
- Advise women of childbearing potential that an effective form of contraception must be used during therapy and for two menstrual cycles (2 months) after stopping therapy with itraconazole capsules.

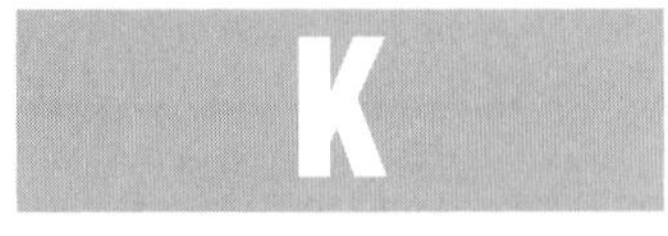

ketoconazole (systemic)
Nizoral

Pregnancy risk category C

Indications & dosages

➲ **Systemic candidiasis, chronic mucocandidiasis, oral candidiasis, candiduria, coccidioidomycosis, blastomycosis, histoplasmosis, chromomycosis, and paracoccidioidomycosis; severe cutaneous dermatophyte infections that are resistant to therapy with topical or oral griseofulvin**
Adults and children weighing more than 40 kg (88 lb): Initially, 200 mg P.O. daily in a single dose. Dosage may be increased to 400 mg once daily in patients who don't respond.
Children age 2 and older: 3.3 to 6.6 mg/kg P.O. daily in a single dose.
➲ **Onychomycosis (caused by *Trichophyton* and *Candida* species); pityriasis versicolor (tinea versicolor); tinea pedis, tinea corporis, and tinea cruris♦**
Adults: 200 to 400 mg P.O. daily.
➲ **Tinea capitis♦**
Adults: 3.3 to 6.6 mg/kg P.O. daily.

Contraindications & cautions

- Contraindicated in patients hypersensitive to drug and in those taking alprazolam or oral triazolam.
- Use cautiously in patients with hepatic disease and in those taking other hepatotoxic drugs.

Adverse reactions

CNS: fever, headache, nervousness, dizziness, somnolence, ***suicidal tendencies***, severe depression.
EENT: photophobia.
GI: *nausea, vomiting,* abdominal pain, diarrhea.
GU: impotence.
Hematologic: ***thrombocytopenia***, hemolytic anemia, ***leukopenia***.
Hepatic: ***fatal hepatotoxicity***.
Metabolic: hyperlipidemia.
Skin: pruritus.
Other: gynecomastia with tenderness, chills.

Interactions

Drug-drug. *Alprazolam, triazolam:* May increase and prolong levels of these drugs. May cause CNS depression and psychomotor impairment. Avoid using together.
Antacids, anticholinergics, H_2-receptor antagonists: May decrease absorption of ketoconazole. Wait at least 2 hours after ketoconazole dose before giving these drugs.
Chlordiazepoxide, clonazepam, clorazepate, diazepam, estazolam, flurazepam, midazolam, quazepam: May increase and prolong levels of these drugs. May cause CNS depression and psychomotor impairment. Avoid using together.
Cyclosporine, methylprednisolone, tacrolimus: May increase drug levels. Monitor drug levels, if appropriate.
Digoxin: May increase digoxin level. Monitor digoxin level.
Isoniazid, rifampin: May increase ketoconazole metabolism. Monitor patient for decreased antifungal effect.
HMG-CoA reductase inhibitors (atorvastatin, fluvastatin, lovastatin, pravastatin, simvastatin): May increase levels and adverse effects of these drugs. Avoid using together, or reduce dose of HMG-CoA reductase inhibitor.
Oral antidiabetics: May cause hypoglycemia. Monitor glucose level.
Paclitaxel: May inhibit metabolism. Use together cautiously.
Phenytoin: May alter the metabolism of one or both drugs. Monitor patient for adverse effects.
Rifampin, isoniazid: May decrease ketoconazole level. Avoid using together.
Theophylline: May decrease theophylline level. Monitor theophylline level.
Warfarin: May enhance effects of anticoagulant. Monitor INR, PT, and PTT and adjust dosage, as needed.
Drug-herb. *Yew:* May inhibit ketoconazole metabolism. Discourage use together.

Nursing considerations

!!ALERT Because of potential for hepatotoxicity, ketoconazole shouldn't be used for less serious conditions, such as fungal infections of skin or nails.

- Monitor patient for signs and symptoms of hepatotoxicity, including elevated liver enzyme levels, nausea that doesn't subside, and unusual fatigue, jaundice, dark urine, or pale stool.
- Doses up to 800 mg/day can be used to treat fungal meningitis and intracerebral fungal lesions.

!!ALERT Ketoconazole is a potent inhibitor of the cytochrome P-450 enzyme system. Giving this drug with drugs metabolized by the cytochrome P-450 3A4 enzyme system may lead to increased drug levels, which could increase or prolong therapeutic and adverse effects.

Patient teaching

- Instruct patient with achlorhydria to dissolve each tablet in 4 ml aqueous solution of 0.2 N hydrochloric acid, sip mixture through a glass or plastic straw, and then drink a glass of water because ketoconazole needs gastric acidity for dissolution and absorption.
- Instruct patient to wait at least 2 hours after dose before taking antacids.
- Make sure patient understands that treatment should continue until all tests indicate that active fungal infection has subsided. If drug is stopped too soon, infection will recur. Minimum treatment for candidiasis is 7 to 14 days; for other systemic fungal infections, 6 months; for resistant dermatophyte infections, at least 4 weeks.
- Reassure patient that nausea, which is common early in therapy, will subside. To minimize nausea, instruct patient to divide daily amount into two doses or take drug with meals.
- Review signs and symptoms of hepatotoxicity with patient; instruct him to stop medication and notify prescriber if they occur.

- Advise patient to discuss any new medications or herbal supplements with prescriber.

ketoconazole

Nizoral, Nizoral A-D ◇

Pregnancy risk category C

Indications & dosages

➲ Tinea corporis, tinea cruris, tinea pedis, tinea versicolor from susceptible organisms; seborrheic dermatitis; cutaneous candidiasis

Adults: Cover affected and immediate surrounding areas daily for at least 2 weeks. For seborrheic dermatitis, apply b.i.d. for 4 weeks. Patients with tinea pedis need 6 weeks of treatment.

➲ Scaling caused by dandruff

Adults: Using shampoo, wet hair, lather, and massage for 1 minute. Leave drug on scalp for 3 minutes; then rinse and repeat. Shampoo twice weekly for 4 weeks, with at least 3 days between shampoos and then intermittently, p.r.n., to maintain control.

Contraindications & cautions

- Contraindicated in patients hypersensitive to drug or its components.
- Use cautiously in breast-feeding women.

Adverse reactions

Skin: severe irritation, pruritus, and stinging with cream; increase in normal hair loss; irritation; abnormal hair texture; scalp pustules; pruritus, oiliness, or dryness of hair and scalp with shampoo use.

Interactions

Drug-drug. *Topical corticosteroids:* May cause increased absorption of corticosteroid. Avoid using together.

Nursing considerations

- Most patients show improvement soon after treatment begins.
- Treatment of tinea corporis or tinea cruris should continue for at least 2 weeks to reduce possibility of recurrence.

!!ALERT Product contains sodium sulfite anhydrous, which may cause severe or life-threatening allergic reactions, including anaphylaxis, in patients with asthma.

Patient teaching

- Tell patient to stop drug and notify prescriber if hypersensitivity reaction occurs.
- Advise patient to check with prescriber if condition worsens; drug may have to be stopped and diagnosis reevaluated.
- Tell patient to avoid using shampoo on scalp if skin is broken or inflamed.
- Warn patient that shampoo applied to permanent-waved hair removes curl.
- Warn patient to avoid drug contact with eyes.
- Tell patient to continue drug for intended duration of therapy, even if signs and symptoms improve soon after starting treatment.
- Tell patient not to store drug above room temperature (77° F [25° C]) and to protect from light.

ketoprofen

Actron, Apo-Keto†, Apo-Keto-E†, Novo-Keto-EC†, Orudis, Orudis E†, Orudis KT ◇, Oruvail, Rhodis†, Rhodis-EC†

Pregnancy risk category B; D in 3rd trimester

Indications & dosages

➲ Rheumatoid arthritis, osteoarthritis

Adults: 75 mg t.i.d. or 50 mg q.i.d., or 200 mg as an extended-release tablet once daily. Maximum dose is 300 mg daily, or 200 mg daily for extended-release capsules. Or, 50 or 100 mg P.R. b.i.d.; or one suppository h.s. (with oral ketoprofen during the day).

Adults older than age 75: 75 to 150 mg P.O. daily. Adjust dose according to patient's response and tolerance.

➲ Mild to moderate pain, dysmenorrhea

Adults: 25 to 50 mg P.O. q 6 to 8 hours, p.r.n. Maximum dose is 300 mg daily.

➲ Minor aches and pain or fever

Adults: 12.5 mg q 4 to 6 hours. Don't exceed 25 mg in 4 to 6 hours or 75 mg in 24 hours.

For elderly patients and those with impaired renal function, reduce first dose to between one-third and one-half normal first dose.

Contraindications & cautions

- Contraindicated in patients hypersensitive to drug and in those with history of aspirin- or NSAID-induced asthma, urticaria, or other allergic reactions.
- Avoid use during last trimester of pregnancy.
- Drug isn't recommended for children or breast-feeding women.
- Use cautiously in patients with history of peptic ulcer disease, renal dysfunction, hypertension, heart failure, or fluid retention.

Adverse reactions

CNS: headache, dizziness, CNS excitation (which includes insomnia, and nervousness, and dreams) or CNS depression (which includes somnolence and malaise).
CV: peripheral edema.
EENT: tinnitus, visual disturbances.
GI: nausea, abdominal pain, diarrhea, constipation, flatulence, peptic ulceration, *dyspepsia*, anorexia, vomiting, stomatitis.
GU: ***nephrotoxicity***.
Hematologic: prolonged bleeding time.
Respiratory: dyspnea.
Skin: rash, photosensitivity reactions.

Interactions

Drug-drug. *Aspirin, corticosteroids:* May increase risk of adverse GI reactions. Avoid using together.
Aspirin, probenecid: May increase ketoprofen level. Avoid using together.
Cyclosporine: May increase nephrotoxicity. Avoid using together.
Hydrochlorothiazide, other diuretics: May decrease diuretic effectiveness. Monitor patient for lack of effect.
Lithium, methotrexate, phenytoin: May increase levels of these drugs, leading to toxicity. Monitor patient closely.
Warfarin: May increase risk of bleeding. Monitor patient closely.
Drug-herb. *Dong quai, feverfew, garlic, ginger, horse chestnut, red clover:* May cause bleeding based on the known effects of components. Discourage use together.
White willow: Herb and drug contain similar components. Discourage use together.
Drug-lifestyle. *Alcohol use:* May cause GI toxicity. Discourage use together.
Sun exposure: May cause photosensitivity reactions. Advise patient to avoid excessive sunlight exposure.

Nursing considerations

- Sustained-release form isn't recommended for patients in acute pain.
- Because NSAIDs impair synthesis of renal prostaglandins, they can decrease renal blood flow and lead to reversible renal impairment, especially in patients with renal or heart failure or liver dysfunction, in elderly patients, and in those taking diuretics. Monitor these patients closely.
- Check renal and hepatic function every 6 months or as indicated.
- Drug decreases platelet adhesion and aggregation, and can prolong bleeding time about 3 to 4 minutes from baseline.
- NSAIDs may mask signs and symptoms of infection because of their antipyretic and anti-inflammatory actions.
- Serious GI toxicity, including peptic ulcers and bleeding, can occur in patient taking NSAIDs, despite lack of symptoms.

Patient teaching

!!ALERT Drug is available without prescription. Instruct patient not to exceed 75 mg daily.

- Tell patient to take drug 30 minutes before or 2 hours after meals with a full glass of water. If adverse GI reactions occur, patient may take drug with milk or meals.
- Tell patient not to crush delayed-release or extended-release tablets.
- Tell patient that full therapeutic effect may be delayed for 2 to 4 weeks.
- Teach patient signs and symptoms of GI bleeding, including blood in vomit, urine, or stool; coffee-ground vomit; and black, tarry stool. Tell him to notify prescriber immediately if any of these occurs.
- Alert patient that using with aspirin, alcohol, other NSAIDs, or corticosteroids may increase risk of adverse GI reactions.
- Warn patient to avoid hazardous activities that require mental alertness until CNS effects are known.
- Because of possibility of sensitivity to the sun, advise patient to use a sunblock, wear protective clothing, and avoid prolonged exposure to sunlight.
- Instruct patient to report problems with vision or hearing immediately.
- Tell patient to protect drug from direct light and excessive heat and humidity.

ketorolac tromethamine
Acular, Acular LS

Pregnancy risk category C

Indications & dosages

➲ **Relief from ocular itching caused by seasonal allergic conjunctivitis**

Adults: 1 drop into conjunctival sac in each eye q.i.d.

➲ **Postoperative inflammation in patients who have had cataract extraction**

Adults: 1 drop to affected eye q.i.d. beginning 24 hours after cataract surgery and continuing through first 2 weeks of postoperative period.

➲ **Reduce ocular pain, burning, and stinging after corneal refractive surgery (Acular LS)**

Adults and children age 3 and older: 1 drop q.i.d. to affected eye, p.r.n., for up to 4 days after surgery.

Contraindications & cautions

- Contraindicated in patients hypersensitive to components of drug and in those wearing soft contact lenses.
- Use cautiously in patients with bleeding disorders or those hypersensitive to other NSAIDs or aspirin. Use cautiously in breast-feeding women.

Adverse reactions

CNS: headache (Acular LS).

EENT: *transient stinging and burning on instillation*, superficial keratitis, superficial ocular infections, ocular irritation, ocular pain, corneal edema, iritis, ocular inflammation (Acular), conjunctival hyperemia, corneal infiltrates, ocular edema and ocular pain (Acular LS).

Other: hypersensitivity reactions.

Interactions

None significant.

Nursing considerations

- Store drug away from heat in a dark, tightly closed container and protect from freezing.

!!ALERT Don't confuse Acular with Acthar.

Patient teaching

- Teach patient how to instill drops. Advise him to wash hands before and after instilling solution, and warn him not to touch tip of dropper to eye or surrounding tissue.
- Advise patient to apply light finger pressure on lacrimal sac for 1 minute after instillation.
- Stress importance of compliance with recommended therapy.
- Tell patient not to instill drops while wearing contact lenses.
- Advise patient to report excessive bleeding or bruising to prescriber.
- Remind patient to discard drug when it's no longer needed.

ketorolac tromethamine
Toradol

Pregnancy risk category C; D in 3rd trimester

Indications & dosages

➲ **Short-term management of moderately severe, acute pain for single-dose treatment**

Adults: For patients younger than age 65, 60 mg I.M. or 30 mg I.V.

Children ages 2 to 16: 1 mg/kg I.M. (maximum dose 30 mg) or 0.5 mg/kg I.V. (maximum dose 15 mg).

Elderly patients: In patients age 65 and older, 30 mg I.M. or 15 mg I.V.

For renally impaired patients or those weighing less than 50 kg (110 lb), 30 mg I.M. or 15 mg I.V.

➲ **Short-term management of moderately severe, acute pain for multiple-dose treatment**

Adults: In patients younger than age 65, 30 mg I.M. or I.V. q 6 hours for maximum of 5 days. Maximum daily dose is 120 mg.

Elderly patients: In patients age 65 and older, 15 mg I.M. or I.V. q 6 hours for maximum of 5 days. Maximum daily dose is 60 mg.

For renally impaired patients or those weighing less than 50 kg, 15 mg I.M. or I.V. q 6 hours. Maximum daily dose is 60 mg.

➲ **Short-term management of moderately severe, acute pain when switching from parenteral to oral administration (oral therapy is indicated only as continuation**

of parenterally given drug and should never be given without patient first having received parenteral therapy)
Adults: For patients younger than age 65, 20 mg P.O. as single dose; then 10 mg P.O. q 4 to 6 hours for maximum of 5 days. Maximum daily dose is 40 mg.
Elderly patients: For patients age 65 and older, 10 mg P.O. as single dose; then 10 mg P.O. q 4 to 6 hours for maximum of 5 days. Maximum daily dose is 40 mg.

For renally impaired patients or those weighing less than 50 kg, 10 mg P.O. as single dose; then 10 mg P.O. q 4 to 6 hours. Maximum daily dose is 40 mg.

Contraindications & cautions

- Contraindicated in patients hypersensitive to drug and in those with active peptic ulcer disease, recent GI bleeding or perforation, advanced renal impairment, cerebrovascular bleeding, hemorrhagic diathesis, or incomplete hemostasis, and those at risk for renal impairment from volume depletion or at risk of bleeding.
- Contraindicated in children younger than age 2 and in patients with history of peptic ulcer disease or GI bleeding, past allergic reactions to aspirin or other NSAIDs, and during labor and delivery or breast-feeding.
- Contraindicated as prophylactic analgesic before major surgery or intraoperatively when hemostasis is critical; and in patients currently receiving aspirin, an NSAID, or probenecid.
- Use cautiously in patients who are elderly or have hepatic or renal impairment or cardiac decompensation.

Adverse reactions

CNS: drowsiness, sedation, dizziness, *headache.*
CV: edema, hypertension, palpitations, ***arrhythmias.***
GI: *nausea, dyspepsia, GI pain,* diarrhea, peptic ulceration, vomiting, constipation, flatulence, stomatitis.
Hematologic: decreased platelet adhesion, purpura, prolonged bleeding time.
Skin: pruritus, rash, diaphoresis.
Other: pain at injection site.

Interactions

Drug-drug. *ACE inhibitors:* May cause renal impairment, particularly in volume-depleted patients. Avoid using together in volume-depleted patients.
Anticoagulants, salicylates: May increase salicylate or anticoagulant levels in the blood. Use together with extreme caution and monitor patient closely.
Antihypertensives, diuretics: May decrease effectiveness. Monitor patient closely.
Lithium: May increase lithium level. Monitor patient closely.
Methotrexate: May decrease methotrexate clearance and increased toxicity. Avoid using together.
Drug-herb. *Dong quai, feverfew, garlic, ginger, horse chestnut, red clover:* May cause bleeding. Discourage use together.
White willow: Herb and drug contain similar components. Discourage use together.

Nursing considerations

- Correct hypovolemia before giving ketorolac.

!!ALERT The maximum combined duration of parenteral and oral therapy is 5 days.

- When appropriate, give by deep I.M. injection. Patient may feel pain at injection site. Put pressure on site for 15 to 30 seconds after injection to minimize local effects.
- Use in children age 2 and older is for a single dose only.
- Don't give drug epidurally or intrathecally because of alcohol content.
- Carefully observe patients with coagulopathies and those taking anticoagulants. Drug inhibits platelet aggregation and can prolong bleeding time. This effect disappears within 48 hours of stopping drug and doesn't alter platelet count, INR, PTT, or PT.
- NSAIDs may mask signs and symptoms of infection because of their antipyretic and anti-inflammatory actions.
- Serious GI toxicity, including peptic ulcers and bleeding, can occur in patient taking NSAIDs, despite lack of symptoms.

!!ALERT Don't confuse Toradol with Tegretol or Foradil.

Patient teaching

- Warn patient receiving drug I.M. that pain may occur at injection site.
- Teach patient signs and symptoms of GI bleeding, including blood in vomit, urine, or stool; coffee-ground vomit; and black, tarry

stool. Tell him to notify prescriber immediately if any of these occurs.

ketotifen fumarate
Zaditor

Pregnancy risk category C

Indications & dosages
➲ To temporarily prevent eye itching from allergic conjunctivitis
Adults and children age 4 and older: Instill 1 drop in affected eye q 8 to 12 hours.

Contraindications & cautions
- Contraindicated in patients hypersensitive to components of drug.
- Contraindicated for irritation related to contact lenses.

Adverse reactions
CNS: *headache.*
EENT: *conjunctival infection, rhinitis,* ocular allergic reactions, burning or stinging of eyes, conjunctivitis, eye discharge, dry eyes, eye pain, eyelid disorder, itching of eyes, keratitis, lacrimation disorder, mydriasis, photophobia, ocular rash, pharyngitis.
Other: flulike syndrome.

Interactions
None significant.

Nursing considerations
- Drug is for ophthalmic use only. Don't inject or give orally.
- Drug isn't indicated for irritation related to contact lenses.
- Soft contact lenses may absorb the preservative benzalkonium. Contact lenses shouldn't be inserted until 10 minutes after drug is instilled.
- To prevent contaminating dropper tip and solution, don't touch eyelids or surrounding areas with dropper tip of bottle.

Patient teaching
- Teach patient the proper technique for instilling drops.
- Advise patient not to wear contact lens if eye is red. Warn him not to use drug to treat contact lens–related irritation.
- Instruct patient who wears soft contact lenses and whose eyes aren't red to wait at least 10 minutes after instilling drug before inserting contact lenses.
- Advise patient to report adverse reactions.
- Advise patient to keep bottle tightly closed when not in use.

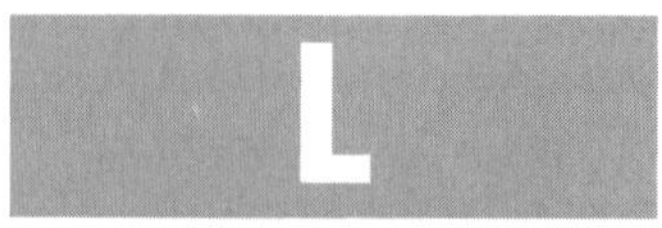

labetalol hydrochloride
Normodyne, Trandate

Pregnancy risk category C

Indications & dosages
➲ Hypertension
Adults: 100 mg P.O. b.i.d. with or without a diuretic. If needed, dosage is increased to 200 mg b.i.d. after 2 days. Further increases may be made q 2 to 3 days until optimum response is reached. Usual maintenance dosage is 200 to 400 mg b.i.d.
➲ Severe hypertension, hypertensive emergency
Adults: 200 mg diluted in 160 ml of D_5W, infused at 2 mg/minute until satisfactory response is obtained; then infusion is stopped. May be repeated q 6 to 12 hours.

Or, give by repeated I.V. injection: initially, 20 mg I.V. slowly over 2 minutes. Repeat injections of 40 to 80 mg q 10 minutes until maximum dose of 300 mg is reached, p.r.n.

Contraindications & cautions
- Contraindicated in patients hypersensitive to drug and in those with bronchial asthma, overt cardiac failure, greater than first-degree heart block, cardiogenic shock, severe bradycardia, and other conditions that may cause severe and prolonged hypotension.
- Use cautiously in patients with heart failure, hepatic failure, chronic bronchitis, emphysema, peripheral vascular disease, and pheochromocytoma.

Adverse reactions
CNS: vivid dreams, fatigue, headache, paresthesia, transient scalp tingling, *dizziness,* syncope.

CV: *orthostatic hypotension,* ***ventricular arrhythmias.***
EENT: nasal congestion.
GI: nausea, vomiting.
GU: sexual dysfunction, urine retention.
Respiratory: dyspnea, ***bronchospasm.***
Skin: rash.

Interactions

Drug-drug. *Beta agonists:* May blunt bronchodilator effect of these drugs in patients with bronchospasm. May need to increase dosages of these drugs.
Cimetidine: May enhance labetalol's effect. Use together cautiously.
Halothane: May increase hypotensive effect. Monitor blood pressure closely.
Insulin, oral antidiabetics: May alter dosage requirements in previously stabilized diabetic patient. Monitor patient closely.
NSAIDs: May decrease antihypertensive effects. Monitor blood pressure.
Drug-herb. *Ma huang:* May decrease antihypertensive effects. Discourage use together.

Nursing considerations

- Monitor blood pressure frequently. Drug masks common signs and symptoms of shock.
- If dizziness occurs, ask prescriber if patient may take a dose at bedtime or take smaller doses t.i.d. to help minimize this adverse reaction.
- When switching from I.V. to P.O. form, begin P.O. regimen at 200 mg after blood pressure begins to rise; repeat dose with 200 to 400 mg in 6 to 12 hours. Adjust dosage according to blood pressure response.
- Monitor glucose level in diabetic patients closely because beta blockers may mask certain signs and symptoms of hypoglycemia.

!!ALERT Don't confuse Trandate with Trental or Tridrate.

!!ALERT Sodium bicarbonate injection is incompatible with I.V. labetalol.

Patient teaching

!!ALERT Tell patient that stopping drug abruptly can worsen chest pain and trigger an MI.

- Advise patient that dizziness is the most troublesome adverse reaction and tends to occur in the early stages of treatment, in patients also receiving diuretics, and in those receiving higher dosages. Inform patient that dizziness can be minimized by rising slowly and avoiding sudden position changes.
- Warn patient that occasional harmless scalp tingling may occur, especially when therapy begins.

lactulose

Cephulac, Cholac, Chronulac, Constilac, Constulose, Duphalac, Enulose, Kristalose, Lactulax†

Pregnancy risk category B

Indications & dosages

➲ Constipation
Adults: 10 to 20 g or 15 to 30 ml P.O. daily, increased to 60 ml/day, if needed.

➲ To prevent and treat hepatic encephalopathy, including hepatic precoma and coma in patients with severe hepatic disease
Adults: Initially, 20 to 30 g or 30 to 45 ml P.O. t.i.d. or q.i.d., until two or three soft stools are produced daily. Usual dose is 60 to 100 g daily in divided doses. Or, 200 g or 300 ml diluted with 700 ml of water or normal saline solution and given as retention enema P.R. q 4 to 6 hours, p.r.n.

Contraindications & cautions

- Contraindicated in patients on a low galactose diet.
- Use cautiously in patients with diabetes mellitus.

Adverse reactions

GI: *abdominal cramps, belching, diarrhea, gaseous distention, flatulence,* nausea, vomiting.

Interactions

Drug-drug. *Antacids, antibiotics, oral neomycin:* May decrease lactulose effectiveness. Avoid using together.

Nursing considerations

- To minimize sweet taste, dilute with water or fruit juice or give with food.
- Prepare enema (not commercially available) by adding 200 g (300 ml) to 700 ml of water or normal saline solution. The diluted

solution is given as retention enema for 30 to 60 minutes. Use a rectal balloon.
- If enema isn't retained for at least 30 minutes, be prepared to repeat dose.
- Monitor sodium level for hypernatremia, especially when giving in higher doses to treat hepatic encephalopathy.
- Monitor mental status and potassium levels when giving to patients with hepatic encephalopathy.
- Be prepared to replace fluid loss.

!!ALERT Don't confuse lactulose with lactose.

Patient teaching

- Show home care patient how to mix and use drug.
- Inform patient about adverse reactions and tell him to notify prescriber if reactions become bothersome or if diarrhea occurs.
- Instruct patient not to take other laxatives during lactulose therapy.

lamivudine

Epivir, Epivir-HBV

Pregnancy risk category C

Indications & dosages

➲ HIV infection, with other antiretrovirals

Adults and children older than age 16: 300 mg Epivir P.O. once daily or 150 mg P.O. b.i.d.

Children ages 3 months to 16 years: 4 mg/kg Epivir P.O. b.i.d. Maximum dose is 150 mg b.i.d.

Neonates age 30 days and younger♦: 2 mg/kg Epivir P.O. b.i.d.

For patients with creatinine clearance of 30 to 49 ml/minute, give 150 mg Epivir P.O. daily. If clearance is 15 to 29 ml/minute, give 150 mg P.O. on day 1 and then 100 mg daily; if it's 5 to 14 ml/minute, give 150 mg on day 1 and then 50 mg daily; if it's less than 5 ml/minute, give 50 mg on day 1 and then 25 mg daily.

➲ Chronic hepatitis B with evidence of hepatitis B viral replication and active liver inflammation

Adults: 100 mg Epivir-HBV P.O. once daily.

Children ages 2 to 17: 3 mg/kg Epivir-HBV P.O. once daily, up to a maximum dose of 100 mg daily. Optimum duration of treatment isn't known; safety and efficacy of treatment beyond 1 year haven't been established.

For adult patients with creatinine clearance of 30 to 49 ml/minute, give first dose of 100 mg Epivir-HBV; then give 50 mg P.O. once daily. If clearance is 15 to 29 ml/minute, give first dose of 100 mg; then give 25 mg P.O. once daily. If clearance is 5 to 14 ml/minute, give first dose of 35 mg; then give 15 mg P.O. once daily. If clearance is less than 5 ml/minute, give first dose of 35 mg; then give 10 mg P.O. once daily.

Contraindications & cautions

- Contraindicated in patients hypersensitive to drug.
- Use cautiously in patients with renal impairment.

!!ALERT Use drug cautiously, if at all, in children with history of pancreatitis or other significant risk factors for development of pancreatitis.
- An Antiretroviral Pregnancy Registry monitors maternal-fetal outcomes of pregnant women exposed to lamivudine. To register a pregnant patient, the prescriber can call the Antiretroviral Pregnancy Registry at 1-800-258-4263.

Adverse reactions

Adverse reactions pertain to the combination therapy of lamivudine and zidovudine.

CNS: *headache, fatigue, fever, neuropathy, malaise, dizziness, insomnia and other sleep disorders*, depressive disorders.

EENT: *nasal symptoms.*

GI: *nausea, diarrhea, vomiting, anorexia,* abdominal pain, abdominal cramps, dyspepsia, ***pancreatitis***.

Hematologic: ***neutropenia***, anemia, ***thrombocytopenia***.

Hepatic: ***hepatotoxicity***.

Metabolic: ***lactic acidosis***.

Musculoskeletal: *musculoskeletal pain*, myalgia, arthralgia.

Respiratory: *cough.*

Skin: rash.

Other: *chills.*

Interactions

Drug-drug. *Trimethoprim and sulfamethoxazole:* May increase lamivudine level because of decreased clearance of drug. Monitor patient for toxicity.

Zalcitabine: May inhibit activation of both drugs. Avoid using together.
Zidovudine: May increase zidovudine level. Monitor patient closely for adverse reactions.

Nursing considerations

!!ALERT Stop lamivudine treatment immediately and notify prescriber if signs, symptoms, or laboratory abnormalities suggest pancreatitis. Monitor amylase level.
!!ALERT Lactic acidosis and hepatotoxicity have been reported. Notify prescriber if signs of lactic acidosis or hepatotoxicity occurs.

- Hepatitis may recur in some patients with chronic hepatitis B virus when they stop taking drug.
- Safety and effectiveness of treatment with Epivir-HBV for longer than 1 year haven't been established; optimum duration of treatment isn't known. Test patients for HIV before starting treatment and during therapy because formulation and dosage of lamivudine in Epivir-HBV aren't appropriate for those infected with both hepatitis B virus and HIV. If lamivudine is given to patients with hepatitis B virus and HIV, use the higher dosage indicated for HIV therapy as part of an appropriate combination regimen.
- Because of a high rate of early virologic resistance, don't use triple antiretroviral therapy with abacavir, lamivudine, and tenofovir as new treatment regimen for naive or pretreated patients. Monitor patients currently controlled with this combination and those who use this combination in addition to other antiretrovirals, and consider modification of therapy.
- Because of a high rate of early virologic failure and emergence of resistance, therapy with tenofovir in combination with didanosine and lamivudine isn't recommended as a new treatment regimen for therapy-naive or experienced patients with HIV infection. Patients on this regimen should be considered for treatment modification.
- Monitor patient's CBC, platelet count, and renal and liver function studies. Report abnormalities.

Patient teaching

- Inform patient that long-term effects of lamivudine are unknown.
- Stress importance of taking lamivudine exactly as prescribed.
- Inform patient that drug doesn't cure HIV infection, that opportunistic infections and other complications of HIV infection may still occur, and that transmission of HIV to others through sexual contact or blood contamination is still possible.
- Teach parents or guardians the signs and symptoms of inflammation of the pancreas (pancreatitis). Advise them to report signs and symptoms immediately.

lamivudine and zidovudine

Combivir

Pregnancy risk category C

Indications & dosages

➲ HIV infection
Adults and children age 12 and older, weighing more than 50 kg (110 lb): 1 tablet P.O. b.i.d.

Contraindications & cautions

- Contraindicated in patients hypersensitive to drug or its components and in those who are younger than age 12, who weigh less than 50 kg, or who have creatinine clearance below 50 ml/minute. Also contraindicated in patients experiencing dose-limiting adverse effects.
- Use combination cautiously in patients with bone marrow suppression as evidenced by granulocyte count less than 1,000 cells/mm or hemoglobin level below 9.5 g/dl.
- An Antiretroviral Pregnancy Registry monitors maternal-fetal outcomes of pregnant women exposed to Combivir. To register a pregnant patient, prescriber can call the Antiretroviral Pregnancy Registry at 1-800-258-4263.

Adverse reactions

CNS: *headache, malaise, fatigue, insomnia, dizziness, neuropathy,* depression, *fever.*
EENT: *nasal signs and symptoms.*
GI: *nausea, diarrhea, vomiting, anorexia,* abdominal pain, abdominal cramps, dyspepsia.
Hematologic: ***neutropenia***, anemia.
Musculoskeletal: *musculoskeletal pain,* myalgia, arthralgia.

Respiratory: *cough.*
Skin: rash.
Other: *chills.*

Interactions

Drug-drug. *Atovaquone, fluconazole, methadone, probenecid, valproic acid:* May increase bioavailability of zidovudine. Dosage modification isn't needed.
Co-trimoxazole, nelfinavir: May increase bioavailability of lamivudine. Dosage modification isn't needed.
Doxorubicin, ribavirin, stavudine: May have antagonistic effects when used with zidovudine. Avoid using together.
Ganciclovir, interferon alfa, and other bone marrow suppressive or cytotoxic drugs: May increase hematologic toxicity of zidovudine. Use together cautiously.
Nelfinavir, ritonavir: May decrease bioavailability of zidovudine. Dosage modification isn't needed.
Zalcitabine: Zalcitabine and lamivudine may inhibit intracellular phosphorylation of one another. Use together isn't recommended.

Nursing considerations

- Some patients with chronic hepatitis B virus (HBV) may experience recurrence of hepatitis if lamivudine is stopped. Patients with liver disease may have more severe consequences. Patients with liver disease and HBV should have periodic monitoring of both liver function tests and markers of HBV replication.
- Safety and efficacy of lamivudine haven't been established for treatment of HBV in patients infected with both HIV and HBV. Emergence of lamivudine-resistant HBV variants has been reported in patients with HBV and HIV who have received antiretroviral regimens containing lamivudine.
- Lactic acidosis and severe hepatomegaly with steatosis have been reported in patients receiving lamivudine and zidovudine, either alone or as adjunctive therapy. Notify prescriber if signs and symptoms of lactic acidosis or hepatotoxicity (abdominal pain, jaundice) develop.

!!ALERT Monitor patient for bone marrow toxicity with frequent blood counts, particularly in patients with advanced HIV infection. Monitor patients for signs and symptoms of lactic acidosis and hepatotoxicity.

- Assess patient's fine motor skills and peripheral sensation for evidence of peripheral neuropathies. Assess patient for myopathy and myositis.

!!ALERT Don't confuse Combivir with Combivent.

Patient teaching

- Tell patient that the lamivudine-zidovudine combination therapy doesn't cure HIV infection and that he may continue to experience illness, including opportunistic infections.
- Warn patient that HIV transmission can still occur with drug therapy.
- Educate patient about using condoms when engaging in sexual activities to prevent disease transmission.
- Teach patient signs and symptoms of a drop in WBC count and hemoglobin (fever, chills, infection, fatigue), and instruct him to report such occurrences.
- Tell patient to have blood counts followed closely while taking drug, especially if he has advanced disease.
- Advise patient to consult prescriber before taking other drugs.
- Warn patient to report abdominal pain immediately.
- Instruct patient to report signs and symptoms of muscle disease (myopathy or myositis), including muscle inflammation, pain, weakness, decrease in muscle size.
- Stress importance of taking combination therapy exactly as prescribed to reduce the development of resistance.
- Tell patient he may take drug combination with or without food.
- Inform woman that breast-feeding is contraindicated in HIV infection and during drug therapy.

lamotrigine
Lamictal

Pregnancy risk category C

Indications & dosages

➲ **Adjunct treatment of partial seizures caused by epilepsy or generalized seizures of Lennox-Gastaut syndrome**
Adults and children older than age 12 taking other enzyme-inducing anticonvulsants with valproic acid: 25 mg P.O. every other day for 2 weeks; then 25 mg P.O. daily for 2 weeks. Continue to increase, p.r.n., by 25 to 50 mg daily q 1 to 2 weeks until an effective maintenance dosage of 100 to 400 mg daily given in one or two divided doses is reached. When added to valproic acid alone, the usual daily maintenance dose is 100 to 200 mg.
Adults and children older than age 12 taking other enzyme-inducing anticonvulsants but not valproic acid: 50 mg P.O. daily for 2 weeks; then 100 mg P.O. daily in two divided doses for 2 weeks. Increase, p.r.n., by 100 mg daily q 1 to 2 weeks. Usual maintenance dosage is 300 to 500 mg P.O. daily in two divided doses.
Children ages 2 to 12 weighing 6.7 to 40 kg (15 to 88 lb) taking other enzyme-inducing anticonvulsants with valproic acid: 0.15 mg/kg P.O. daily in one or two divided doses (rounded down to nearest whole tablet) for 2 weeks, followed by 0.3 mg/kg daily in one or two divided doses for another 2 weeks. Thereafter, usual maintenance dosage is 1 to 5 mg/kg daily (maximum, 200 mg daily in one to two divided doses).
Children ages 2 to 12 weighing 6.7 to 40 kg (15 to 88 lb) taking other enzyme-inducing anticonvulsants but not valproic acid: 0.6 mg/kg P.O. daily in two divided doses (rounded down to nearest whole tablet) for 2 weeks; then 1.2 mg/kg daily in two divided doses for another 2 weeks. Usual maintenance dosage is 5 to 15 mg/kg P.O. daily (maximum 400 mg daily in two divided doses).
➲ **To convert patients from therapy with a hepatic enzyme-inducing anticonvulsant alone to lamotrigine therapy**
Adults and children age 16 and older: Add lamotrigine 50 mg P.O. once daily to current drug regimen for 2 weeks, followed by 100 mg P.O. daily in two divided doses for 2 weeks. Then increase daily dosage by 100 mg q 1 to 2 weeks until maintenance dose of 500 mg daily in two divided doses is reached. The concomitant hepatic enzyme-inducing anticonvulsant can then be gradually reduced by 20% decrements weekly for 4 weeks.

For patients with severe renal impairment, use lower maintenance dosage.
➲ **To convert patients with partial seizures from adjunctive therapy with valproate to therapy with lamotrigine alone**
Adults and children age 16 and older : Add lamotrigine until 200 mg daily is achieved; then gradually decrease valproate to 500 mg daily by decrements of no more than 500 mg daily per week. Maintain these dosages for 1 week, then increase lamotrigine to 300 mg daily while decreasing valproate to 250 mg daily. Maintain these dosages for 1 week, then stop valproate completely while increasing lamotrigine by 100 mg daily q week until a dose of 500 mg daily is reached.
➲ **Bipolar disorder**
Adults: Initially, 25 mg P.O. once daily for 2 weeks; then 50 mg P.O. once daily for 2 weeks. Dosage may then be doubled at weekly intervals, to maintenance dosage of 200 mg daily.
Adults taking carbamazepine or other hepatic enzyme-inducing drugs without valproic acid: Initially, 50 mg P.O. once daily for 2 weeks; then 100 mg daily in two divided doses for 2 weeks. Dosage is then increased by 100 mg weekly to maintenance dosage of 400 mg daily, given in two divided doses.
Adults taking valproic acid: Initially, 25 mg P.O. every other day for 2 weeks; then 25 mg P.O. once daily for 2 weeks. Dosage may then be doubled at weekly intervals to maintenance dosage of 100 mg daily.

Contraindications & cautions

- Contraindicated in patients hypersensitive to drug or its components.
- Safety and efficacy of drug in children younger than age 16 (other than those with Lennox-Gastaut syndrome) haven't been established. Don't give drug to children younger than age 16. Don't give drug to children weighing less than 17 kg (37 lb) because therapy can't be started using dosing

guidelines and currently available tablet strength.
• Use cautiously in patients with renal, hepatic, or cardiac impairment.

Adverse reactions

CNS: *dizziness, headache, ataxia, somnolence,* fever, incoordination, insomnia, tremor, depression, anxiety, ***seizures***, irritability, speech disorder, decreased memory, aggravated reaction, concentration disturbance, sleep disorder, emotional lability, vertigo, mind racing, dysarthria, malaise.
CV: palpitations.
EENT: *diplopia, blurred vision,* vision abnormality, nystagmus, *rhinitis,* pharyngitis.
GI: *nausea, vomiting,* diarrhea, dyspepsia, abdominal pain, constipation, anorexia, dry mouth.
GU: dysmenorrhea, vaginitis, amenorrhea.
Musculoskeletal: muscle spasm, neck pain.
Respiratory: cough, dyspnea.
Skin: *rash,* ***Stevens-Johnson syndrome, toxic epidermal necrolysis***, pruritus, hot flashes, alopecia, acne.
Other: flulike syndrome, infection, chills, tooth disorder.

Interactions

Drug-drug. *Acetaminophen:* May decrease therapeutic effects of lamotrigine. Monitor patient.
Carbamazepine, ethosuximide, oral contraceptives, oxcarbazepine, phenobarbital, phenytoin, primidone: May decrease lamotrigine level. Monitor patient closely.
Folate inhibitors, such as co-trimoxazole and methotrexate: May have additive effect because lamotrigine inhibits dihydrofolate reductase, an enzyme involved in folic acid synthesis. Monitor patient.
Valproic acid: May decrease clearance of lamotrigine, which increases lamotrigine level; also decreases valproic acid level. Monitor patient for toxicity.
Drug-lifestyle. *Sun exposure:* May cause photosensitivity reactions. Advise patient to avoid excessive sun exposure.

Nursing considerations

• Don't stop drug abruptly because this may increase seizure frequency. Instead, taper drug over at least 2 weeks.
!!ALERT Stop drug at first sign of rash, unless rash is clearly not drug related.
• Reduce lamotrigine dose if drug is added to a multidrug regimen that includes valproic acid.
• Chewable dispersible tablets may be swallowed whole, chewed, or dispersed in water or diluted fruit juice. If tablets are chewed, give a small amount of water or diluted fruit juice to aid in swallowing.
• Evaluate patients for changes in seizure activity. Check adjunct anticonvulsant level.
!!ALERT Don't confuse lamotrigine with lamivudine or Lamictal with Lamisil, Ludiomil, labetalol, or Lomotil.

Patient teaching

• Inform patient that drug may cause rash. Combination therapy of valproic acid and lamotrigine may cause a serious rash. Tell patient to report rash or signs or symptoms of hypersensitivity promptly to prescriber because they may warrant drug discontinuation.
• Warn patient not to engage in hazardous activity until drug's CNS effects are known.
• Warn patient that the drug may trigger sensitivity to the sun and to take precautions until tolerance is determined.
• Warn patient not to stop drug abruptly.
• Advise woman of childbearing age to discuss drug therapy with prescriber if she's considering pregnancy.
• Advise woman of childbearing age that breast-feeding isn't recommended during therapy.

lansoprazole

Prevacid, Prevacid I.V., Prevacid SoluTab

Pregnancy risk category B

Indications & dosages

➲ Short-term treatment of active duodenal ulcer
Adults: 15 mg P.O. daily before eating for 4 weeks.
➲ Maintenance of healed duodenal ulcers
Adults: 15 mg P.O. daily.
➲ Short-term treatment of active benign gastric ulcer
Adults: 30 mg P.O. once daily for up to 8 weeks.

➲ Short-term I.V. therapy for erosive esophagitis when patient can't take P.O. drug
Adults: 30 mg I.V. daily over 30 minutes for up to 7 days. As soon as patient can take drug orally, switch to P.O. form and continue for 6 to 8 weeks.
➲ Short-term treatment of erosive esophagitis
Adults: 30 mg P.O. daily before eating for up to 8 weeks. If healing doesn't occur, 8 more weeks of therapy may be given. Maintenance dosage for healing is 15 mg P.O. daily.
Children ages 12 to 17: 30 mg P.O. once daily for up to 8 weeks.
Children ages 1 to 11, weighing more than 30 kg (66 lb): 30 mg P.O. once daily for up to 12 weeks. Increase dosage up to 30 mg b.i.d. in patients who remain symptomatic after 2 weeks.
Children ages 1 to 11, weighing 30 kg or less: 15 mg P.O. once daily for up to 12 weeks. Increase dosage up to 30 mg b.i.d. in patients who remain symptomatic after 2 weeks.
➲ Long-term therapy for pathologic hypersecretory conditions, including Zollinger-Ellison syndrome
Adults: Initially, 60 mg P.O. once daily. Increase dosage, p.r.n. Give daily amounts above 120 mg in evenly divided doses.
➲ *Helicobacter pylori* eradication to reduce risk of duodenal ulcer recurrence
Adults: For patients receiving dual therapy, 30 mg P.O. lansoprazole with 1 g P.O. amoxicillin, each given t.i.d. for 14 days. For patients receiving triple therapy, 30 mg P.O. lansoprazole with 1 g P.O. amoxicillin and 500 mg P.O. clarithromycin, all given b.i.d. for 10 to 14 days.
➲ Short-term treatment of symptomatic gastroesophageal reflux disease (GERD)
Adults: 15 mg P.O. once daily for up to 8 weeks.
➲ Short-term treatment of symptomatic GERD; short-term treatment of erosive esophagitis
Children ages 12 to 17: 15 mg P.O. once daily for up to 8 weeks.
Children ages 1 to 11, weighing more than 30 kg: 30 mg P.O. once daily for up to 12 weeks. Dosage can be increased up to 30 mg b.i.d. in patients who remain symptomatic after 2 weeks.
Children ages 1 to 11, weighing 30 kg (66 lb) or less: 15 mg P.O. once daily for up to 12 weeks. Dosage can be increased up to 30 mg b.i.d in patients who remain symptomatic after 2 weeks.
➲ NSAID-related ulcer in patients who take NSAIDs
Adults: 30 mg P.O. daily for 8 weeks.
➲ To reduce risk of NSAID-related ulcer in patients with history of gastric ulcer who need NSAIDs
Adults: 15 mg P.O. daily for up to 12 weeks.

Contraindications & cautions

- Contraindicated in patients hypersensitive to drug.

Adverse reactions

GI: diarrhea, nausea, abdominal pain.

Interactions

Drug-drug. *Ampicillin esters, digoxin, iron salts, ketoconazole:* May inhibit absorption of these drugs. Monitor patient closely.
Sucralfate: May cause delayed lansoprazole absorption. Give lansoprazole at least 30 minutes before sucralfate.
Theophylline: May mildly increase theophylline clearance. Dosage adjustment of theophylline may be needed when lansoprazole is started or stopped. Use together cautiously.
Drug-herb. *Male fern:* May cause alkaline environment, in which herb is inactivated. Discourage use together.
St. John's wort: May increase risk of sun sensitivity. Advise patient to avoid excessive sunlight exposure.
Drug-food. *Food:* May decrease rate and extent of GI absorption. Advise patient to take before meals.

Nursing considerations

- Patients with severe liver disease may need dosage adjustment, but don't adjust dosage for elderly patients or those with renal insufficiency.
- The contents of capsule can be mixed with 40 ml of apple juice in a syringe and given within 3 to 5 minutes via a nasogastric tube. Flush with additional apple juice to give entire dose and maintain patency of the tube.
- To give orally disintegrating tablets using an oral syringe, dissolve a 15-mg tablet in 4 ml water or a 30-mg tablet in 10 ml water

and give within 15 minutes. Refill the syringe with about 2 ml (15-mg tablet) or 5 ml (30-mg tablet) of water, shake gently, and give any remaining contents.
- To give orally disintegrating tablets through a nasogastric tube 8 French or larger, dissolve a 15-mg tablet in 4 ml water or a 30-mg tablet in 10 ml water and give within 15 minutes. Refill the syringe with about 5 ml of water, shake gently, and flush the nasogastric tube.
- Orally disintegrating tablets contain 2.5 mg phenylalanine/15-mg tablet and 5.1 mg phenylalanine/30-mg tablet.
- A symptomatic response to lansoprazole therapy doesn't preclude presence of gastric malignancy.
- It's unknown if lansoprazole appears in breast milk. Breast-feeding women should either stop breast-feeding or stop drug.

Patient teaching

- For best effect, instruct patient to take drug no more than 30 minutes before eating.
- Tell patient he may mix the capsule's contents with a small amount (about 2 ounces) of apple, cranberry, grape, orange, pineapple, prune, tomato, or vegetable juice. The patient must drink the mixture within 30 minutes. To ensure complete delivery of the dose, the patient should fill the glass two or more times with juice and swallow the contents immediately.
- Contents of capsule can be mixed with 1 tablespoon of applesauce, Ensure pudding, cottage cheese, yogurt, or strained pears and swallowed immediately. The granules shouldn't be chewed or crushed.
- For the oral suspension, instruct patient to empty packet contents into 30 ml of water, stir well, and drink immediately. Tell him not to crush or chew the granules and not to take with other liquids or food. If any material remains after drinking, tell him to add more water, stir, and drink immediately.
- Tell patient taking orally disintegrating tablets to allow tablet to dissolve on tongue until all particles can be swallowed.

lanthanum carbonate
Fosrenol

Pregnancy risk category C

Indications & dosages

To reduce phosphate level in patients with end-stage renal disease (ESRD)
Adults: Initially, 250 to 500 mg P.O. t.i.d. with meals. Adjust q 2 to 3 weeks by 750 mg daily until reaching desired phosphate level. Reducing phosphate level to less than 6 mg/dl usually requires 1,500 to 3,000 mg daily.

Contraindications & cautions

- No known contraindications.
- Use cautiously in breast-feeding women and patients with acute peptic ulcer, ulcerative colitis, Crohn's disease, or bowel obstruction.

Adverse reactions

CNS: headache.
CV: *hypotension.*
EENT: rhinitis.
GI: abdominal pain, *constipation, diarrhea, nausea, vomiting.*
Metabolic: hypercalcemia.
Respiratory: bronchitis.
Other: *dialysis graft complication, dialysis graft occlusion.*

Interactions

None reported.

Nursing considerations

- Give drug with or just after a meal.
- Monitor patient for bone pain and skeletal deformities.
- Check serum phosphate levels during dosage adjustment and regularly as needed throughout treatment.
- Drug isn't recommended for children because it's deposited in developing bone, including the growth plate.

Patient teaching

- Urge patient to follow a low-phosphorus diet. Assist with meal planning as needed.
- Tell patient to take drug with or immediately after meals.

!!ALERT Remind patient to chew tablets completely before swallowing them.

• Instruct patient to avoid taking lanthanum within 2 hours of oral drugs known to interact with antacids.
• Explain that the most common side effects are nausea and vomiting and that they tend to subside over time.

latanoprost
Xalatan

Pregnancy risk category C

Indications & dosages

➲ **First-line treatment of increased intraocular pressure (IOP) in patients with ocular hypertension or open-angle glaucoma**
Adults: Instill 1 drop in conjunctival sac of affected eyes once daily h.s.

Contraindications & cautions

• Contraindicated in patients hypersensitive to drug, benzalkonium chloride, or other components of drug.
• Use cautiously in patients with impaired renal or hepatic function.
• Use cautiously in breast-feeding women; it's unknown if drug appears in breast milk.
• Safety and efficacy of drug in children haven't been established.

Adverse reactions

CV: angina pectoris.
EENT: *blurred vision, burning, stinging,* conjunctival hyperemia, *foreign body sensation, itching, increased brown pigmentation of the iris,* dry eye, punctate epithelial keratopathy, lid crusting or edema, lid discomfort, excessive tearing, eye pain, photophobia, eyelash changes.
Musculoskeletal: muscle, joint, or back pain.
Respiratory: upper respiratory tract infection.
Skin: rash, allergic skin reaction.
Other: cold, flulike syndrome.

Interactions

Drug-drug. *Eyedrops that contain thimerosal:* May cause precipitation of eyedrops. Give at least 5 minutes apart.

Nursing considerations

• Don't give drug while patient is wearing contact lenses.
• Giving drug more frequently than recommended may decrease its IOP-lowering effects.
• Drug may gradually change eye color, increasing amount of brown pigment in iris. This change in iris color occurs slowly and may not be noticeable for months or years. Increased pigmentation may be permanent.
• To avoid ocular infections, don't allow tip of dispenser to contact eye or surrounding tissue. Serious damage to eye and subsequent vision loss may be caused by contaminated solutions.

Patient teaching

• Inform patient of risk that iris color may change in treated eye.
• Teach patient how to instill drops, and advise him to wash hands before and after instilling solution. Warn him not to touch tip of dropper to eye or surrounding tissue.
• Advise patient to apply light finger pressure on lacrimal sac for 1 minute after instillation to minimize systemic absorption.
• Instruct patient to report reactions in the eye, especially eye inflammation and lid reactions.
• Tell patient who wears contact lenses to remove them before instilling solution and not to reinsert the lenses until 15 minutes have elapsed.
• If patient is using more than one topical ophthalmic drug, tell him to apply them at least 5 minutes apart.
• If patient develops another eye condition (such as trauma or infection) or needs eye surgery, advise him to contact prescriber about continued use of multidose container.
• Stress importance of compliance with recommended therapy.

leflunomide
Arava

Pregnancy risk category X

Indications & dosages

➲ **To reduce signs and symptoms of active rheumatoid arthritis; to slow structural damage as shown by erosions and joint space narrowing seen on X-ray; to improve physical function**
Adults: 100 mg P.O. q 24 hours for 3 days; then 20 mg (maximum daily dose) P.O. q 24

hours. Dose may be decreased to 10 mg daily if higher dose isn't well tolerated.

Contraindications & cautions

- Contraindicated in patients hypersensitive to drug or its components and in women who are or may become pregnant or who are breast-feeding.
- Drug isn't recommended for patients with significant hepatic impairment, evidence of infection with hepatitis B or C viruses, severe immunodeficiency, bone marrow dysplasia, or severe uncontrolled infections; in patients younger than age 18; or in men attempting to father a child.
- Use cautiously in patients with renal insufficiency.

Adverse reactions

CNS: asthenia, dizziness, fever, headache, paresthesia, malaise, migraine, sleep disorder, vertigo, neuritis, anxiety, depression, insomnia, neuralgia.
CV: angina pectoris, *hypertension*, chest pain, palpitations, tachycardia, vasculitis, vasodilation, varicose veins, peripheral edema.
EENT: pharyngitis, rhinitis, sinusitis, epistaxis, blurred vision, cataracts, conjunctivitis, eye disorder.
GI: mouth ulcer, oral candidiasis, gingivitis, enlarged salivary glands, stomatitis, dry mouth, taste perversion, anorexia, *diarrhea*, dyspepsia, gastroenteritis, nausea, abdominal pain, vomiting, cholelithiasis, colitis, constipation, esophagitis, flatulence, gastritis, melena.
GU: UTI, albuminuria, cystitis, dysuria, hematuria, menstrual disorder, pelvic pain, vaginal candidiasis, prostate disorder, urinary frequency.
Hematologic: anemia.
Hepatic: ***hepatotoxicity***.
Metabolic: diabetes mellitus, hyperglycemia, hyperthyroidism, hypokalemia, hyperlipidemia, weight loss.
Musculoskeletal: arthralgia, arthrosis, back pain, bursitis, muscle cramps, myalgia, bone necrosis, bone pain, leg cramps, joint disorder, neck pain, synovitis, tendon rupture, tenosynovitis.
Respiratory: bronchitis, increased cough, pneumonia, *respiratory infection*, asthma, dyspnea, lung disorder.
Skin: *alopecia*, eczema, pruritus, *rash*, dry skin, acne, contact dermatitis, fungal dermatitis, hair discoloration, hematoma, nail disorder, skin nodule, subcutaneous nodule, maculopapular rash, skin disorder, skin discoloration, skin ulcer.
Other: tooth disorder, allergic reaction, flu-like syndrome, injury or accident, pain, abscess, cyst, hernia, increased sweating, ecchymoses, herpes simplex, herpes zoster.

Interactions

Drug-drug. *Charcoal, cholestyramine:* May decrease leflunomide level. Sometimes used for this effect in overdose.
Methotrexate, other hepatotoxic drugs: May increase risk of hepatotoxicity. Monitor liver enzymes.
NSAIDs (diclofenac, ibuprofen): May increase NSAID level. Monitor patient.
Rifampin: May increase active leflunomide metabolite level. Use together cautiously.
Tolbutamide: May increase tolbutamide level. Monitor patient.

Nursing considerations

- Vaccination with live vaccines isn't recommended. Consider the long half-life of drug when contemplating giving a live vaccine after stopping drug treatment.

!!ALERT Men planning to father a child should stop drug therapy and follow recommended leflunomide removal protocol (cholestyramine 8 g, P.O. t.i.d. for 11 days). In addition to cholestyramine, verify drug levels are less than 0.02 mg/L by two separate tests at least 14 days apart. If level is greater than 0.02 mg/L, consider additional cholestyramine treatment.

- Risk of malignancy, particularly lymphoproliferative disorders, is increased with use of some immunosuppressants, including leflunomide.

!!ALERT Monitor ALT levels, platelet and WBC counts, and hemoglobin level or hematocrit at baseline and monthly for 6 months after starting therapy and every 6 to 8 weeks thereafter.

!!ALERT Monitor AST, ALT, and serum albumin levels monthly if treatment includes methotrexate or other potential immunosuppressives.

- Stop drug and start cholestyramine or charcoal therapy if bone marrow suppression occurs.

• Watch for overlapping hematologic toxicity when switching to another antirheumatic.

!!ALERT Rare cases of severe liver injury, including cases with fatal outcome, have occurred during leflunomide therapy. Most cases occur within 6 months of therapy and in a setting of multiple risk factors for hepatotoxicity (liver disease, other hepatotoxins).

• For confirmed ALT elevations between two and three times the upper limit of normal (ULN), reduce dose to 10 mg/day; if elevations persist despite dose reduction or if ALT elevations of greater than three times ULN are present, stop drug and give cholestyramine or charcoal.

• Carefully monitor patient after dose reduction. Because the active metabolite of leflunomide has a prolonged half-life, it may take several weeks for levels to decline.

Patient teaching

• Explain need for and frequency of required blood tests and monitoring.

• Instruct patient to use birth control during course of treatment and until it's been determined that drug is no longer active.

• Warn patient to immediately notify prescriber if signs or symptoms of pregnancy occur (such as late menstrual periods or breast tenderness).

• Advise breast-feeding woman to stop breast-feeding during therapy.

• Inform patient he may continue taking aspirin, other NSAIDs, and low-dose corticosteroids during treatment.

letrozole
Femara

Pregnancy risk category D

Indications & dosages

➲ **Metastatic breast cancer in postmenopausal women with disease progression after antiestrogen therapy (such as tamoxifen)**
Adults: 2.5 mg P.O. as single daily dose.

➲ **First-line treatment of hormone receptor–positive or hormone receptor–unknown, locally advanced, or metastatic breast cancer in postmenopausal women**
Adults: 2.5 mg P.O. once daily until tumor progression is evident.

Contraindications & cautions

• Contraindicated in patients hypersensitive to drug or its components.

• Use cautiously in patients with severe liver impairment; dosage adjustment isn't needed in those with mild to moderate liver dysfunction.

Adverse reactions

CNS: headache, somnolence, dizziness, fatigue, mood changes.
CV: hypertension, ***thromboembolism***, chest pain, edema, *hot flashes*, ***MI***.
GI: *nausea*, vomiting, constipation, diarrhea, abdominal pain, anorexia.
Metabolic: hypercholesterolemia, weight gain.
Musculoskeletal: *bone pain, limb pain, back pain*, arthralgia.
Respiratory: dyspnea, cough.
Skin: rash, pruritus.
Other: viral infections, breast pain, alopecia, diaphoresis.

Interactions

None significant.

Nursing considerations

• Dosage adjustment isn't needed in patients with creatinine clearance of 10 ml/minute or more.

• Food doesn't affect drug absorption.

!!ALERT Don't confuse Femara (letrozole) with FemHRT (ethinyl estradiol and norethindrone acetate).

Patient teaching

• Instruct patient to take drug exactly as prescribed.

• Tell patient to take drug with or without food.

• Inform patient about potential adverse reactions.

leucovorin calcium (citrovorum factor, folinic acid)

Pregnancy risk category C

Indications & dosages

➲ Overdose of folic acid antagonist (methotrexate, trimethoprim, or pyrimethamine)
Adults and children: I.M. or I.V. dose equivalent to weight of antagonist given. For methotrexate overdose, up to 75 mg I.V. infusion within 12 hours, followed by 12 mg I.M. q 6 hours for four doses. For adverse effects after average doses of methotrexate, 6 to 12 mg I.M. q 6 hours for four doses.

➲ Leucovorin rescue after high methotrexate dose in treatment of malignant disease
Adults and children: 10 mg/m^2 P.O., I.M., or I.V. q 6 hours until methotrexate level falls below 5×10^{-8} M.

➲ Megaloblastic anemia from congenital enzyme deficiency
Adults and children: 3 to 6 mg I.M. daily.

➲ Folate-deficient megaloblastic anemia
Adults and children: Up to 1 mg I.M. daily. Duration of treatment depends on hematologic response.

➲ To prevent hematologic toxicity from pyrimethamine or trimethoprim therapy
Adults and children: 400 mcg to 5 mg I.M. with each dose of folic acid antagonist. Oral dosages of 10 to 35 mg once daily or 25 mg once weekly may also be used.

➲ Hematologic toxicity from pyrimethamine or trimethoprim therapy
Adults and children: 5 to 15 mg I.M. daily.

➲ Palliative treatment of advanced colorectal cancer
Adults: 20 mg/m^2 I.V.; then fluorouracil 425 mg/m^2 I.V. or 200 mg/m^2 I.V. (over 3 minutes or longer) followed by fluorouracil 370 mg/m^2 daily for 5 consecutive days. Repeat at 4-week intervals for two additional courses; then at intervals of 4 to 5 weeks, if tolerated.

Contraindications & cautions

- Contraindicated in patients with pernicious anemia and other megaloblastic anemias secondary to lack of vitamin B. Don't give leucovorin calcium intrathecally.
- In elderly or debilitated patients, use combined leucovorin and fluorouracil therapy cautiously because of increased risk of severe GI toxicity.

Adverse reactions

Skin: urticaria.
Other: hypersensitivity reactions, ***anaphylactoid reactions***.

Interactions

Drug-drug. *Anticonvulsants:* May decrease effectiveness of these drugs. Monitor for seizure activity.
Fluorouracil: May increase fluorouracil toxicity. Fluorouracil dose may need to be reduced.
Methotrexate: High doses of leucovorin may decrease efficacy of intrathecal methotrexate. Monitor effects.

Nursing considerations

- I.V. route is preferred in patients with GI toxicity when doses exceed 25 mg.
- Drug may mask diagnosis of pernicious anemia.
- Follow leucovorin rescue schedule and protocol closely.
- Don't give leucovorin with systemic methotrexate.

!!ALERT Don't confuse leucovorin (folinic acid) with folic acid.

Patient teaching

- Explain need for drug to patient and family, and answer any questions or concerns.
- Tell patient to report symptoms of hypersensitivity promptly.

levetiracetam
Keppra

Pregnancy risk category C

Indications & dosages

➲ Adjunctive treatment for partial seizures
Adults: Initially, 500 mg b.i.d. Dosage can be increased by 500 mg b.i.d., p.r.n., for seizure control at 2-week intervals to maximum of 1,500 mg b.i.d.

For patients with renal impairment, if creatinine clearance is more than 80 ml/minute, give 500 to 1,500 mg q 12 hours; if clearance is 50 to 80 ml/minute, give 500 to 1,000 mg q 12 hours; if clearance is 30 to 50 ml/minute, give 250 to 750 mg q 12 hours; if clearance is less than 30 ml/minute, give 250 to 500 mg q 12 hours. For dialysis patients, give 500 to 1,000 mg q 24 hours. Give a 250- to 500-mg dose after dialysis.

Contraindications & cautions

- Contraindicated in patients hypersensitive to drug.
- Leukopenia and neutropenia have been reported with drug use. Use cautiously in immunocompromised patients, such as those with cancer or HIV infection.
- Patients with poor renal function need dosage adjustment.

Adverse reactions

CNS: *asthenia, headache, somnolence,* dizziness, depression, vertigo, paresthesia, nervousness, hostility, emotional lability, ataxia, amnesia, anxiety.
EENT: diplopia, pharyngitis, rhinitis, sinusitis.
GI: anorexia.
Hematologic: ***leukopenia, neutropenia.***
Musculoskeletal: pain.
Respiratory: cough, infection.

Interactions

Drug-drug. *Antihistamines, benzodiazepines, opioids, other drugs that cause drowsiness, tricyclic antidepressants:* May lead to severe sedation. Avoid using together.
Drug-lifestyle. *Alcohol use:* May lead to severe sedation. Discourage use together.

Nursing considerations

!!ALERT Don't confuse Keppra (levetiracetam) with Kaletra (lopinavir and ritonavir).
- Drug can be taken with or without food.
- Use drug only with other anticonvulsants; it's not recommended for monotherapy.
- Seizures can occur if drug is stopped abruptly. Tapering is recommended.
- Monitor patients closely for such adverse reactions as dizziness, which may lead to falls.

Patient teaching

- Warn patient to use extra care when sitting or standing to avoid falling.
- Advise patient to call prescriber and not to stop drug suddenly if adverse reactions occur.
- Tell patient to take with other prescribed seizure drugs.
- Inform patient that drug can be taken with or without food.

levobunolol hydrochloride
AKBeta, Betagan

Pregnancy risk category C

Indications & dosages

➲ Chronic open-angle glaucoma, ocular hypertension
Adults: 1 or 2 drops once daily (0.5%) or b.i.d. (0.25%).

Contraindications & cautions

- Contraindicated in patients hypersensitive to drug and in those with bronchial asthma, sinus bradycardia, second- or third-degree AV block, cardiac failure, cardiogenic shock, or history of bronchial asthma or severe COPD.
- Use cautiously in patients with chronic bronchitis, emphysema, diabetes mellitus, hyperthyroidism, or myasthenia gravis.
- Safe use in pregnant or breast-feeding women hasn't been established.

Adverse reactions

CNS: headache, depression, insomnia, *syncope.*
CV: slight reduction in resting heart rate, *hypotension,* ***bradycardia, heart failure.***
EENT: *transient eye stinging and burning,* tearing, erythema, itching, keratitis, corneal punctate staining, photophobia, decreased corneal sensitivity, blepharoconjunctivitis.
GI: nausea.
Respiratory: ***bronchospasm.***
Skin: urticaria.

Interactions

Drug-drug. *Dipivefrin, epinephrine, systemically administered carbonic anhydrase inhibitors, topical miotics:* May further reduce intraocular pressure (IOP). Use together cautiously.
Metoprolol, propranolol, other oral beta blockers: May increase ocular and systemic effects. Use together cautiously.

Reserpine, other catecholamine-depleting drugs: May increase hypotensive and bradycardiac effects. Monitor blood pressure and heart rate closely.

Drug-lifestyle. *Sun exposure:* May cause photophobia. Advise patient to wear sunglasses.

Nursing considerations

- Don't let tip of dropper touch patient's eye or surrounding tissue.

Patient teaching

- Teach patient how to instill drug. Advise him to wash hands before and after instillation and to apply light finger pressure on lacrimal sac for 1 minute after drops are instilled.
- Warn patient not to touch tip of dropper to eye or surrounding tissue.
- Advise elderly patient to report shortness of breath, chest pain, or heart irregularities to prescriber. Drug may be absorbed systemically and produce signs and symptoms of beta blockade.
- Advise patient to wear or carry medical identification at all times during therapy.

levodopa
Larodopa

Pregnancy risk category NR

Indications & dosages

➲ Idiopathic parkinsonism, postencephalitic parkinsonism, and symptomatic parkinsonism after carbon monoxide or manganese intoxication or with cerebral arteriosclerosis

Adults and children age 12 or older: Initially, 0.5 to 1 g P.O. daily, divided in two or more doses with food; increase by no more than 0.75 g daily q 3 to 7 days until maximum response is achieved. Don't exceed 8 g daily. Adjust dosage to patient requirements, tolerance, and response. Higher dosage needs close supervision.

Contraindications & cautions

- Contraindicated in patients hypersensitive to drug and in those with acute angle-closure glaucoma, melanoma, or undiagnosed skin lesions; also contraindicated within 14 days of MAO inhibitor therapy.
- Use cautiously in patients with severe CV, renal, hepatic, and pulmonary disorders; peptic ulcer; psychiatric illness; MI with residual arrhythmias; bronchial asthma; emphysema; and endocrine disease.

Adverse reactions

CNS: *aggressive behavior, involuntary grimacing, head movements, myoclonic body jerks,* ***seizures****, ataxia, tremor, muscle twitching, bradykinetic episodes, psychiatric disturbances, mood changes, nervousness, anxiety, disturbing dreams, euphoria, malaise, fatigue, severe depression,* ***suicidal tendencies****, dementia, delirium, hallucinations, choreiform, dystonic, and dyskinetic movements.*

CV: *orthostatic hypotension*, phlebitis, cardiac irregularities.

EENT: blepharospasm, blurred vision, diplopia, mydriasis or miosis, activation of latent Horner's syndrome, oculogyric crises.

GI: dry mouth, bitter taste, *nausea, vomiting, anorexia*, constipation, flatulence, diarrhea, abdominal pain, excessive salivation.

GU: urinary frequency, urine retention, incontinence, darkened urine, priapism.

Hematologic: ***leukopenia***, hemolytic anemia, ***agranulocytosis***.

Hepatic: ***hepatotoxicity***.

Metabolic: weight loss.

Respiratory: hiccups, hyperventilation.

Skin: dark perspiration.

Interactions

Drug-drug. *Antacids:* May increase absorption of levodopa. Give antacids 1 hour after levodopa.

Furazolidone, MAO inhibitors, phenelzine, procarbazine, tranylcypromine: May cause severe hypertension. Avoid using together.

Inhaled anesthetics, sympathomimetics: May increase risk of arrhythmias. Monitor patient closely.

Iron salts: May reduce bioavailability of levodopa. Separate dosage times.

Metoclopramide: May accelerate gastric emptying of levodopa. Give metoclopramide 1 hour after levodopa.

Papaverine, phenothiazines, other antipsychotics, phenytoin, rauwolfia alkaloids: May decrease levodopa effect. Avoid using together.

Pyridoxine (vitamin B_6): May decrease the effectiveness of levodopa; has little to no effect on the combination drug levodopa and carbidopa. Avoid using pyridoxine with levodopa.
Drug-herb. *Kava:* May increase parkinsonism symptoms. Discourage kava use altogether.
Drug-food. *Foods high in protein:* May decrease levodopa absorption. Discourage use together.
Drug-lifestyle. *Cocaine use:* May increase risk of arrhythmias. Inform patient of this interaction.

Nursing considerations

- Capsules may contain tartrazine.
- Patients who need surgery should continue levodopa therapy as long as oral intake is permitted, usually until 6 to 24 hours before surgery. Resume therapy as soon as patient can take drug orally.

!!ALERT Because of risk of triggering a symptom complex resembling neuroleptic malignant syndrome, observe patient closely if levodopa dosage is reduced abruptly or stopped.

- Giving levodopa and carbidopa together typically decreases amount of levodopa needed by 75%, reducing risk of adverse reactions.
- Monitor vital signs, especially while adjusting dosage. Report changes.

!!ALERT Watch for muscle twitching and blepharospasm, which may be early signs of drug overdose; report immediately.

!!ALERT Hallucinations may require reduction or withdrawal of drug.

- An accurate measure for urine glucose can be obtained if paper strip is partially immersed in the urine sample. Urine migrates up the strip, as with an ascending chromatographic system. Read only the top of the strip.
- Test patients receiving long-term therapy regularly for diabetes and acromegaly; also periodically monitor renal, hepatic, and hematopoietic function.

Patient teaching

- Tell patient to take drug with food to minimize GI upset, but tell him high-protein meals can impair absorption and reduce effectiveness.
- If patient has trouble swallowing pills, tell him or caregiver to crush tablets and mix with applesauce or pureed fruit.
- Warn patient or caregiver not to increase dosage unless ordered. Daily dosage shouldn't exceed 8 g.
- Tell patient to protect drug from heat, light, and moisture. If preparation darkens, it has lost potency; tell him to discard it.
- Warn patient about possible dizziness upon standing quickly, especially at start of therapy. Tell him to change positions slowly and dangle legs before rising. Elastic stockings may control these adverse reactions.
- Advise patient and caregivers that multivitamin preparations, fortified cereals, and certain OTC drugs may contain pyridoxine (vitamin B_6), which can block the effects of levodopa by enhancing its peripheral metabolism.

levodopa and carbidopa

Sinemet, Sinemet CR

Pregnancy risk category C

Indications & dosages

➲ **Idiopathic Parkinson's disease, postencephalitic parkinsonism, and symptomatic parkinsonism resulting from carbon monoxide or manganese intoxication**
Adults: 1 tablet of 100 mg levodopa with 25 mg carbidopa P.O. t.i.d.; then increased by 1 tablet daily or every other day, p.r.n., to maximum daily dosage of 8 tablets. May use 250 mg levodopa with 25 mg carbidopa or 100 mg levodopa with 10 mg carbidopa tablets, as directed, to obtain maximum response. Optimum daily dose must be determined by careful adjustment for each patient.

Patients given conventional tablets may receive extended-release tablets; dosage is calculated on current levodopa intake. Extended-release tablets should provide 10% more levodopa daily, increased p.r.n. and as tolerated to 30% more levodopa daily. Give in divided doses at intervals of 4 to 8 hours.

Contraindications & cautions

- Contraindicated in patients hypersensitive to drug and in those with angle-closure

glaucoma, melanoma, or undiagnosed skin lesions.
- Contraindicated within 14 days of MAO inhibitor therapy.
- Use cautiously in patients with severe CV, renal, hepatic, endocrine, or pulmonary disorders; history of peptic ulcer; psychiatric illness; MI with residual arrhythmias; bronchial asthma; emphysema; or well-controlled, chronic open-angle glaucoma.

Adverse reactions

CNS: *choreiform, dystonic, dyskinetic movements, involuntary grimacing, head movements, myoclonic body jerks, ataxia,* tremor, muscle twitching, bradykinetic episodes, psychiatric disturbances, anxiety, disturbing dreams, euphoria, malaise, fatigue, severe depression, ***suicidal tendencies***, dementia, delirium, hallucinations, confusion, insomnia, agitation.
CV: *orthostatic hypotension*, cardiac irregularities, phlebitis.
EENT: blepharospasm, blurred vision, diplopia, mydriasis or miosis, oculogyric crises, excessive salivation.
GI: *dry mouth*, bitter taste, *nausea, vomiting, anorexia*, constipation, flatulence, diarrhea, abdominal pain.
GU: urinary frequency, urine retention, urinary incontinence, darkened urine, priapism.
Hematologic: hemolytic anemia, ***thrombocytopenia, leukopenia, agranulocytosis***.
Hepatic: ***hepatotoxicity***.
Metabolic: weight loss.
Respiratory: hiccups, hyperventilation.
Skin: dark perspiration.

Interactions

Drug-drug. *Antihypertensives:* May cause additive hypotensive effects. Use together cautiously.
Iron salts: May reduce bioavailability of levodopa and carbidopa. Give iron 1 hour before or 2 hours after Sinemet.
MAO inhibitors: May cause risk of severe hypertension. Avoid using together.
Papaverine, phenytoin: May antagonize antiparkinsonian actions. Avoid using together.
Phenothiazines, other antipsychotics: May antagonize antiparkinsonian actions. Use together cautiously.
Drug-herb. *Kava:* May decrease action of drug. Discourage kava use altogether.
Octacosanol: May worsen dyskinesias. Discourage use together.
Drug-food. *Foods high in protein:* May decrease levodopa absorption. Don't give levodopa with high-protein foods.

Nursing considerations

- If patient takes levodopa, stop drug at least 8 hours before starting levodopa-carbidopa.
- Giving levodopa and carbidopa together typically decreases amount of levodopa needed by 75%, reducing risk of adverse reactions.
- Therapeutic and adverse reactions occur more rapidly with levodopa and carbidopa than with levodopa alone. Observe patient and monitor vital signs, especially while adjusting dosage. Report significant changes.

!! ALERT Because of risk of precipitating a symptom complex resembling neuroleptic malignant syndrome, observe patient closely if levodopa dosage is reduced abruptly or stopped.
- Hallucinations may require reduction or withdrawal of drug.

!! ALERT Muscle twitching and blepharospasm may be early signs of drug overdose; report immediately.
- Test patients receiving long-term therapy regularly for diabetes and acromegaly, and periodically for hepatic, renal, and hematopoietic function.

Patient teaching

- Tell patient to take drug with food to minimize GI upset; however, high-protein meals can impair absorption and reduce effectiveness.
- Tell patient not to chew or crush extended-release form.
- Warn patient and caregivers not to increase dosage without prescriber's orders.
- Caution patient about possible dizziness when standing up quickly, especially at start of therapy. Tell him to change positions slowly and dangle his legs before getting out of bed. Elastic stockings may control these adverse reactions in some patients.
- Instruct patient to report adverse reactions and therapeutic effects.
- Inform patient that pyridoxine (vitamin B_6) doesn't reverse beneficial effects of levodopa and carbidopa. Multivitamins can be taken without reversing levodopa's effects.

levodopa, carbidopa, and entacapone
Stalevo

Pregnancy risk category C

Indications & dosages

➲ Idiopathic Parkinson's disease, to replace (with equivalent strengths) levodopa, carbidopa, and entacapone given individually or to replace immediate-release levodopa and carbidopa for a patient with end-of-dose "wearing off" taking a total daily levodopa dose of 600 mg or less and no dyskinesia
Adults: 1 tablet P.O.; determine dose and interval by therapeutic response. Maximum, 8 tablets daily.

Contraindications & cautions

- Contraindicated in patients hypersensitive to drug or its ingredients.
- Contraindicated in patients with angle-closure glaucoma, suspicious undiagnosed skin lesions, or a history of melanoma.
- Contraindicated within 2 weeks of MAO inhibitor therapy.
- Use cautiously in patients with past or current psychosis and in patients with severe cardiovascular or pulmonary disease, bronchial asthma, biliary obstruction, or renal, hepatic, or endocrine disease.
- Use cautiously in patients with chronic open-angle glaucoma or a history of MI and residual atrial, nodal, or ventricular arrhythmias.

Adverse reactions

levodopa and carbidopa
CNS: agitation, asthenia, confusion, delusions, dementia, depression, dizziness, dyskinesia, hallucinations, headache, increased libido, insomnia, ***neuroleptic malignant syndrome***, nightmares, paranoid ideation, paresthesias, psychosis, somnolence, syncope.
CV: cardiac irregularities, chest pain, hypertension, hypotension, orthostatic hypotension, palpitations, phlebitis.
GI: anorexia, constipation, dark saliva, diarrhea, dry mouth, duodenal ulcer, dyspepsia, GI bleeding, nausea, taste alterations, vomiting.
GU: dark urine, urinary frequency, UTI.
Hematologic: ***agranulocytosis***, anemia, ***leukopenia, thrombocytopenia***.
Musculoskeletal: back pain, muscle cramps, shoulder pain.
Respiratory: dyspnea, upper respiratory infection.
Skin: alopecia, bullous lesions, dark sweat, Henoch-Schönlein purpura, increased sweating, pruritus, rash, urticaria.
Other: ***angioedema***.
entacapone
CNS: agitation, anxiety, asthenia, dizziness, *dyskinesia*, fatigue, *hyperkinesia*, hypokinesia, somnolence.
GI: abdominal pain, constipation, *diarrhea*, dry mouth, dyspepsia, flatulence, gastritis, *nausea*, taste perversion, vomiting.
GU: *urine discoloration*.
Musculoskeletal: back pain.
Respiratory: dyspnea.
Skin: increased sweating, purpura.
Other: bacterial infection.

Interactions

Drug-drug. *Ampicillin, chloramphenicol, cholestyramine, erythromycin, probenecid, rifampicin:* May interfere with entacapone excretion. Use together cautiously.
Antihypertensives: May cause orthostatic hypotension. Adjust antihypertensive dosage as needed.
CNS depressants: Additive effects. Use together cautiously.
Dopamine (D2) receptor antagonists such as butyrophenones, iron salts, isoniazid, metoclopramide, papaverine, phenothiazines, phenytoin, and risperidone: May decrease levodopa, carbidopa, and entacapone effects. Monitor patient for effectiveness.
Drugs metabolized by COMT, such as alpha-methyldopa, apomorphine, bitolterol, dobutamine, dopamine, epinephrine, isoproterenol, isoetharine, and norepinephrine: May increase heart rate, arrhythmias, and excessive blood pressure changes. Use together cautiously.
Metoclopramide: May increase availability of levodopa and carbidopa by increasing gastric emptying. Monitor patient for adverse effects.
Nonselective MAO inhibitor: May disrupt catecholamine metabolism. Avoid using together.

Selegiline: May cause severe hypotension. Use together cautiously, and monitor blood pressure.
Tricyclic antidepressants: May increase risk of hypertension and dyskinesia. Monitor patient closely.

Nursing considerations

- Certain CNS effects, such as dyskinesia, may occur at lower dosages and sooner with levodopa, carbidopa, and entacapone than with levodopa alone. Dyskinesia may require a reduced dosage.
- During the first adjustment period, monitor a patient with CV disease carefully and in a facility equipped to provide intensive cardiac care.
- Neuroleptic malignant syndrome may develop when levodopa and carbidopa are reduced or stopped, especially in patients taking antipsychotic drugs. Watch patient carefully for fever, hyperthermia, muscle rigidity, involuntary movements, altered consciousness, mental status changes, and autonomic dysfunction.
- During extended therapy, periodically monitor hepatic, hematopoietic, CV, and renal function.
- Diarrhea is common; it usually develops 4 to 12 weeks after treatment starts but may appear as early as the first week or as late as many months after treatment starts.
- Monitor patient for hallucinations, depression, and suicidal tendencies.

Patient teaching

- Advise patient to take drug exactly as prescribed.
- Tell patient to report a "wearing-off" effect, which may occur at the end of the dosing interval.
- Tell patient that urine, sweat, and saliva may turn dark (red, brown, or black) during treatment.
- Advise patient to notify the prescriber if problems making voluntary movements increase.
- Tell patient that diarrhea is common with this treatment.
- Inform patient that hallucinations may occur.
- Urge patient to immediately report depression or suicidal thoughts.
- Explain that he may become dizzy if he rises quickly. Urge patient to use caution when rising.
- Tell patient that a high-protein diet, excessive acidity, and iron salts may reduce the drug's effectiveness.
- Urge patient to avoid hazardous activities until the CNS effects of the drug are known.
- Advise patient to notify prescriber if she becomes pregnant.

levofloxacin

Levaquin

Pregnancy risk category C

Indications & dosages

➲ **Acute maxillary sinusitis caused by susceptible strains of *Streptococcus pneumoniae, Moraxella catarrhalis,* or *Haemophilus influenzae***
Adults: 500 mg P.O. or I.V. daily for 10 to 14 days.

➲ **Mild to moderate skin and skin-structure infections caused by *Staphylococcus aureus* or *S. pyogenes***
Adults: 500 mg P.O. or I.V. q 24 hours for 7 to 10 days.

➲ **Acute bacterial worsening of chronic bronchitis caused by *S. aureus, S. pneumoniae, M. catarrhalis, H. influenzae,* or *H. parainfluenzae***
Adults: 500 mg P.O. or I.V. over 60 minutes q 24 hours for 7 days.

➲ **Community-acquired pneumonia from multidrug-resistant *S. pneumoniae* (resistance to two or more of the following antibiotics: penicillin, second-generation cephalosporins, macrolides, trimethoprim-sulfamethoxazole, tetracyclines), *S. aureus, M. catarrhalis, H. influenzae, H. parainfluenzae, Klebsiella pneumoniae, Chlamydia pneumoniae, Legionella pneumophila,* or *Mycoplasma pneumoniae***
Adults: 500 mg P.O. or I.V. infusion over 60 minutes q 24 hours for 7 to 14 days.

➲ **Prevention of inhalation anthrax following confirmed or suspected exposure to *Bacillus anthracis***
Adults: 500 mg I.V. or P.O. q 24 hours for 60 days.

➲ **Chronic bacterial prostatitis caused by *Escherichia coli, Enterococcus faecalis,* or *Staphylococcus epidermidis***
Adults: 500 mg P.O. or I.V. over 60 minutes q 24 hours for 28 days.

In patients with a creatinine clearance of 20 to 49 ml/minute, give first dose of 500 mg and then 250 mg daily. If clearance is 10 to 19 ml/minute, give first dose of 500 mg and then 250 mg q 48 hours. For patients receiving dialysis or chronic ambulatory peritoneal dialysis, give first dose of 500 mg and then 250 mg q 48 hours.

➲ **Community-acquired pneumonia from *S. pneumoniae* (excluding multidrug-resistant strains), *H. influenzae, H. parainfluenzae, M. pneumoniae,* and *C. pneumoniae***
Adults: 750 mg P.O. or I.V. over 90 minutes q 24 hours for 5 days.

➲ **Complicated skin and skin-structure infections caused by methicillin-sensitive *S. aureus, E. faecalis, S. pyogenes,* or *Proteus mirabilis***
Adults: 750 mg P.O. or I.V. infusion over 90 minutes q 24 hours for 7 to 14 days.

➲ **Nosocomial pneumonia caused by methicillin-susceptible *S. aureus, Pseudomonas aeruginosa, Serratia marcescens, E. coli, K. pneumoniae, H. influenzae,* or *S. pneumoniae***
Adults: 750 mg P.O. or I.V. infusion over 90 minutes q 24 hours for 7 to 14 days.

If creatinine clearance is 20 to 49 ml/minute, give 750 mg initially and then 750 mg q 48 hours; if clearance is 10 to 19 ml/minute, or patient is receiving hemodialysis or chronic ambulatory peritoneal dialysis, give 750 mg initially and then 500 mg q 48 hours.

➲ **Mild to moderate UTI caused by *E. faecalis, Enterobacter cloacae, E. coli, K. pneumoniae, P. mirabilis,* or *P. aeruginosa;* mild to moderate acute pyelonephritis caused by *E. coli***
Adults: 250 mg P.O. or I.V. over 60 minutes q 24 hours for 10 days.

If creatinine clearance is 10 to 19 ml/minute, increase dosage interval to q 48 hours.

➲ **Mild to moderate uncomplicated UTI caused by *E. coli, K. pneumoniae,* or *S. saprophyticus***
Adults: 250 mg P.O. daily for 3 days.

➲ **Traveler's diarrhea♦**
Adults: 500 mg P.O. daily for up to 3 days.

➲ **To prevent traveler's diarrhea♦**
Adults: 500 mg P.O. once daily during period of risk, for up to 3 weeks.

➲ **Uncomplicated cervical, urethral, or rectal gonorrhea♦**
Adults: 250 mg P.O. as a single dose.

➲ **Disseminated gonococcal infection♦**
Adults: 250 mg I.V. once daily and continued for 24 to 48 hours after patient starts to improve. Therapy may be switched to 500 mg P.O. daily to complete at least 1 week of therapy.

➲ **Nongonococcal urethritis; urogenital chlamydial infections♦**
Adults: 500 mg P.O. once daily for 7 days.

➲ **Acute pelvic inflammatory disease♦**
Adults: 500 mg I.V. once daily with or without metronidazole 500 mg q 8 hours. Stop parenteral therapy 24 hours after patient improves; then begin doxycycline 100 mg P.O. b.i.d. to complete 14 days of treatment. Or, 500 mg P.O. once daily for 14 days with or without metronidazole 500 mg b.i.d. for 14 days.

Contraindications & cautions

- Contraindicated in patients hypersensitive to drug, its components, or other fluoroquinolones.
- Use cautiously in patients with history of seizure disorders or other CNS diseases, such as cerebral arteriosclerosis.
- Use cautiously and with dosage adjustment in patients with renal impairment.
- Safety and efficacy of drug in children younger than age 18 and in pregnant and breast-feeding women haven't been established.

Adverse reactions

CNS: headache, insomnia, pain, dizziness, ***encephalopathy***, paresthesia, ***seizures***.
CV: chest pain, palpitations, vasodilation.
GI: nausea, diarrhea, constipation, vomiting, abdominal pain, dyspepsia, flatulence, ***pseudomembranous colitis***.
GU: vaginitis.
Hematologic: eosinophilia, hemolytic anemia, ***lymphopenia***.
Metabolic: ***hypoglycemia***.
Musculoskeletal: back pain, tendon rupture.
Respiratory: allergic pneumonitis.

Skin: rash, photosensitivity, pruritus, ***erythema multiforme, Stevens-Johnson syndrome***.
Other: hypersensitivity reactions, ***anaphylaxis, multisystem organ failure***.

Interactions

Drug-drug. *Aluminum hydroxide, aluminum–magnesium hydroxide, calcium carbonate, didanosine, magnesium hydroxide, products containing zinc, sucralfate:* May interfere with GI absorption of levofloxacin. Give levofloxacin 2 hours before or 6 hours after these products.
Antidiabetics: May alter glucose level. Monitor glucose level closely.
Iron salts: May decrease absorption of levofloxacin, reducing anti-infective response. Separate doses by at least 2 hours.
NSAIDs: May increase CNS stimulation. Monitor patient for seizure activity.
Theophylline: May decrease clearance of theophylline. Monitor theophylline level.
Warfarin and derivatives: May increase effect of oral anticoagulant. Monitor PT and INR.
Drug-herb. *Dong quai, St. John's wort:* May cause photosensitivity reactions. Advise patient to avoid excessive sunlight exposure.
Drug-lifestyle. *Sun exposure:* May cause photosensitivity reactions. Advise patient to avoid excessive sunlight exposure.

Nursing considerations

- If patient experiences symptoms of excessive CNS stimulation (restlessness, tremor, confusion, hallucinations), stop drug and notify prescriber. Begin seizure precautions.
- Patients with acute hypersensitivity reactions may need treatment with epinephrine, oxygen, I.V. fluids, antihistamines, corticosteroids, pressor amines, and airway management.
- Most antibacterial drugs can cause pseudomembranous colitis. Notify prescriber if diarrhea occurs. Drug may be stopped.
- Drug may cause an abnormal ECG.
- Obtain specimen for culture and sensitivity tests before starting therapy and as needed to determine if bacterial resistance has occurred.

!!ALERT If *P. aeruginosa* is a confirmed or suspected pathogen, use combination therapy with a beta-lactam.

- Monitor glucose level and renal, hepatic, and hematopoietic blood studies.

Patient teaching

- Tell patient to take drug as prescribed, even if signs and symptoms disappear.
- Advise patient to take drug with plenty of fluids and to appropriately space antacids, sucralfate, and products containing iron or zinc after each dose of levofloxacin.
- Tell patient to take oral solution one hour before or two hours after eating.
- Warn patient to avoid hazardous tasks until adverse effects of drug are known.
- Advise patient to avoid excessive sunlight, use sunscreen, and wear protective clothing when outdoors.
- Instruct patient to stop drug and notify prescriber if rash or other signs or symptoms of hypersensitivity develop.
- Tell patient that tendon rupture may occur with drug and to notify prescriber if he experiences pain or inflammation.
- Instruct diabetic patient to monitor glucose level and notify prescriber about low-glucose reaction.
- Instruct patient to notify prescriber if he has loose stools or diarrhea.

levothyroxine sodium
(T_4 L-thyroxine sodium)
Eltroxin†, Levo-T, Levotec†, Levothroid, Levoxine, Levoxyl, Novothyrox, Synthroid, Thyro-Tabs, Unithroid

Pregnancy risk category A

Indications & dosages

➲ Myxedema coma
Adults: 300 to 500 mcg I.V., followed by parenteral maintenance dose of 75 to 100 mcg I.V. daily. Switch patient to oral maintenance as soon as possible.

➲ Thyroid hormone replacement
Adults: Initially, 25 to 50 mcg P.O. daily; increase by 25 mcg P.O. q 4 to 8 weeks until desired response occurs. Maintenance dosage is 75 to 200 mcg P.O. daily.
Children older than age 12: More than 150 mcg or 2 to 3 mcg/kg P.O. daily.
Children ages 6 to 12: 100 to 150 mcg or 4 to 5 mcg/kg P.O. daily.

Children ages 1 to 5: 75 to 100 mcg or 5 to 6 mcg/kg P.O. daily.
Children ages 6 months to 1 year: 50 to 75 mcg or 6 to 8 mcg/kg P.O. daily.
Children younger than age 6 months: 25 to 50 mcg or 8 to 10 mcg/kg P.O. daily.
Patients older than age 65: 12.5 to 50 mcg P.O. daily; increase by 12.5 to 25 mcg q 6 to 8 weeks, depending on response.

Contraindications & cautions

- Contraindicated in patients hypersensitive to drug and in those with acute MI uncomplicated by hypothyroidism, untreated thyrotoxicosis, or uncorrected adrenal insufficiency.
- Use cautiously in elderly patients and in those with angina pectoris, hypertension, other CV disorders, renal insufficiency, or ischemia.
- Use cautiously in patients with diabetes mellitus, diabetes insipidus, or myxedema and during rapid replacement in those with arteriosclerosis.

Adverse reactions

CNS: *nervousness, insomnia, tremor,* headache, fever.
CV: *tachycardia, palpitations,* ***arrhythmias****, angina pectoris,* ***cardiac arrest****.*
GI: diarrhea, vomiting.
GU: menstrual irregularities.
Metabolic: weight loss.
Musculoskeletal: decreased bone density.
Skin: allergic skin reactions, diaphoresis.
Other: heat intolerance.

Interactions

Drug-drug. *Beta blockers:* May reduce beta blocker effects. Monitor patient.
Cholestyramine, colestipol: May impair levothyroxine absorption. Separate doses by 4 to 5 hours.
Digoxin: May decrease glycoside effects. Monitor patient for clinical effect.
Estrogens: May decrease free levothyroxines. Monitor patient for decreased effectiveness of thyroid hormone.
Fosphenytoin, phenytoin: May release free thyroid hormone. Monitor patient for tachycardia.
Insulin, oral antidiabetics: May alter glucose level. Monitor glucose level. Dosage adjustments may be needed.
Oral anticoagulants: May alter PT. Monitor PT and INR. Dosage adjustments may be needed.
Sympathomimetics such as epinephrine: May increase risk of coronary insufficiency. Monitor patient closely.
Theophylline: May decrease theophylline clearance in hypothyroidism; clearance may return to normal when euthyroid state is achieved. Monitor theophylline level.
Drug-herb. *Horseradish:* May cause abnormal thyroid function. Discourage use in patients undergoing thyroid function tests.
Lemon balm: May have antithyroid effects; may inhibit thyroid-stimulating hormone. Discourage use together.

Nursing considerations

!!ALERT Drug may be given I.V. or I.M. when P.O. ingestion is precluded for long periods. However, dosage adjustment is needed.

- Patients with diabetes mellitus may need increased antidiabetic doses when starting thyroid hormone replacement.
- Watch for angina, coronary occlusion, or CVA in patients with arteriosclerosis who are receiving rapid replacement.
- In patients with coronary artery disease who must receive thyroid hormone, observe carefully for possible coronary insufficiency.
- Thyroid hormone replacement requirements are about 25% lower in patients older than age 60 than in young adults.
- Patients with adult hypothyroidism are unusually sensitive to thyroid hormone. Start at lowest dosage and adjust to higher dosages according to patient's symptoms and laboratory data until euthyroid state is reached.
- When changing from levothyroxine to liothyronine, stop levothyroxine and begin liothyronine. Increase dosage in small increments after residual effects of levothyroxine have disappeared. When changing from liothyronine to levothyroxine, start levothyroxine several days before withdrawing liothyronine to avoid relapse. Drugs aren't interchangeable.
- Long-term therapy causes bone loss in premenopausal and postmenopausal women. Consider a basal bone density measurement and monitor patient closely for osteoporosis.

- Patients taking levothyroxine who need to have ^{131}I uptake studies performed must stop drug 4 weeks before test.
- Patients taking anticoagulants may need their dosage modified; they require careful monitoring of coagulation status.
- Dosage may need to be increased in pregnant patients.

!! ALERT Don't confuse levothyroxine with liothyronine or liotrix.

- Synthroid may contain tartrazine.

Patient teaching

- Teach patient the importance of compliance. Tell him to take thyroid hormones at same time each day, preferably ½ to 1 hour before breakfast, to maintain constant hormone levels and help prevent insomnia.
- Make sure patient understands that replacement therapy is usually for a lifetime. The drug should never be stopped unless directed by prescriber.
- Warn patient (especially elderly patient) to notify prescriber at once about chest pain, palpitations, sweating, nervousness, shortness of breath, or other signals of overdose or aggravated CV disease.
- Tell caregiver of infant or child who can't swallow tablets to crush tablet and suspend in small amount of formula (except soy formula, which may decrease the absorption), breast milk, or water, and give by spoon or dropper. Crushed tablet can be sprinkled over food, except foods containing large amounts of soybean, fiber, or iron.
- Tell patient to take pill with plenty of water to avoid choking, gagging, or getting the pill stuck in his throat.
- Advise patient who has achieved stable response not to change brands.
- Tell patient to report unusual bleeding and bruising.
- Advise patient not to take OTC or other prescription medications without first consulting prescriber.
- Advise patient to report pregnancy to prescriber, because dosage may need adjustment.

lidocaine hydrochloride (lignocaine hydrochloride)

LidoPen Auto-Injector, Xylocaine

Pregnancy risk category B

Indications & dosages

➲ Ventricular arrhythmias caused by MI, cardiac manipulation, or cardiac glycosides

Adults: 50 to 100 mg (1 to 1.5 mg/kg) by I.V. bolus at 25 to 50 mg/minute. Bolus dose is repeated q 3 to 5 minutes until arrhythmias subside or adverse reactions develop. Don't exceed 300-mg total bolus during a 1-hour period. Simultaneously, constant infusion of 20 to 50 mcg/kg/minute (1 to 4 mg/minute) is begun. If single bolus has been given, smaller bolus dose may be repeated 15 to 20 minutes after start of infusion to maintain therapeutic level. Or, 200 to 300 mg I.M.; then second I.M. dose 60 to 90 minutes later, if needed.

Children: 1 mg/kg by I.V. or intraosseous bolus. If no response, start infusion of 20 to 50 mcg/kg/minute. Give an additional bolus dose of 0.5 to 1 mg/kg if delay of greater than 15 minutes between initial bolus and starting the infusion. Bolus doses shouldn't exceed 3 to 5 mg/kg.

Elderly patients: Reduce dosage and rate of infusion by 50%.

For patients with heart failure, with renal or liver disease, or who weigh less than 50 kg (110 lb), reduce dosage.

Contraindications & cautions

- Contraindicated in patients hypersensitive to the amide-type local anesthetics.
- Contraindicated in those with Adams-Stokes syndrome, Wolff-Parkinson-White syndrome, and severe degrees of SA, AV, or intraventricular block in the absence of an artificial pacemaker.
- Use cautiously and at reduced dosages in patients with complete or second-degree heart block or sinus bradycardia, in elderly patients, in those with heart failure or renal or hepatic disease, and in those weighing less than 50 kg (110 lb).

Adverse reactions

CNS: *confusion, tremor,* lethargy, somnolence, *stupor, restlessness,* anxiety, halluci-

nations, nervousness, *light-headedness*, paresthesia, muscle twitching, ***seizures***.
CV: *hypotension*, ***bradycardia, new or worsened arrhythmias, cardiac arrest***.
EENT: *tinnitus, blurred or double vision*.
GI: vomiting.
Respiratory: ***respiratory depression and arrest***.
Skin: soreness at injection site.
Other: ***anaphylaxis***, sensation of cold.

Interactions

Drug-drug. *Atenolol, metoprolol, nadolol, pindolol, propranolol:* May reduce hepatic metabolism of lidocaine, increasing the risk of toxicity. Give bolus doses of lidocaine at a slower rate, and monitor lidocaine level closely.
Cimetidine: May decrease clearance of lidocaine increasing the risk of toxicity. Consider using a different H_2 receptor antagonist if possible. Monitor lidocaine level closely.
Mexiletine, tocainide: May increase pharmacologic effects. Avoid using together.
Phenytoin, procainamide, propranolol, quinidine: May increase cardiac depressant effects. Monitor patient closely.
Succinylcholine: May prolong neuromuscular blockade. Monitor patient closely.
Drug-herb. *Pareira:* May increase the effects of neuromuscular blockade. Discourage use together.
Drug-lifestyle. *Smoking:* May increase metabolism of lidocaine. Monitor patient closely.

Nursing considerations

- Give I.M. injections in the deltoid muscle only.
- Monitor isoenzymes when using I.M. drug for suspected MI. A patient who has received I.M. lidocaine will show a sevenfold increase in CK level. Such an increase originates in the skeletal muscle, not the heart.
- Monitor drug level. Therapeutic levels are 2 to 5 mcg/ml.

!! ALERT Monitor patient for toxicity. In many severely ill patients, seizures may be the first sign of toxicity, but severe reactions are usually preceded by somnolence, confusion, tremors, and paresthesia.

- If signs of toxicity such as dizziness occur, stop drug at once and notify prescriber. Continuing could lead to seizures and coma. Give oxygen through a nasal cannula if not contraindicated. Keep oxygen and cardiopulmonary resuscitation equipment available.
- Monitor patient's response, especially blood pressure and electrolytes, BUN, and creatinine levels. Notify prescriber promptly if abnormalities develop.
- Stop infusion and notify prescriber if arrhythmias worsen or ECG changes, such as widening QRS complex or substantially prolonged PR interval, appear.

Patient teaching

- Tell patient receiving lidocaine I.M. that drug may cause soreness at injection site. Tell him to report discomfort at the site.
- Tell patient to report adverse reactions promptly because toxicity can occur.

linezolid
Zyvox

Pregnancy risk category C

Indications & dosages

➲ **Vancomycin-resistant *Enterococcus faecium* infections, including those with concurrent bacteremia**
Adults and children age 12 and older: 600 mg I.V. or P.O. q 12 hours for 14 to 28 days.
Neonates age 7 days or older and infants and children through age 11: 10 mg/kg I.V. or P.O. q 8 hours for 14 to 28 days.
Neonates younger than age 7 days: 10 mg/kg I.V. or P.O. q 12 hours for 14 to 28 days. Increase to 10 mg/kg q 8 hours when patient is 7 days old. Consider this dosage increase if neonate has inadequate response.
➲ **Nosocomial pneumonia caused by *Staphylococcus aureus* (methicillin-susceptible [MSSA] and methicillin-resistant [MRSA] strains) or *Streptococcus pneumoniae* (including multidrug-resistant strains [MDRSP]); complicated skin and skin-structure infections, including diabetic foot infections without osteomyelitis caused by *S. aureus* (MSSA and MRSA), *S. pyogenes, or S. agalactiae*; community-acquired pneumonia caused by *S. pneumoniae* (including MDRSP), in-**

cluding those with concurrent bacteremia, or *S. aureus* (MSSA only)
Adults and children age 12 and older: 600 mg I.V. or P.O. q 12 hours for 10 to 14 days.
Neonates 7 days or older, infants and children through 11 years: 10 mg/kg I.V. or P.O. q 8 hours for 10 to 14 days.
Neonates younger than age 7 days: 10 mg/kg I.V. or P.O. q 12 hours for 10 to 14 days. Increase to 10 mg/kg q 8 hours when patient is 7 days old. Consider this dosage increase if neonate has inadequate response.

➲ **Uncomplicated skin and skin-structure infections caused by *S. aureus* (MSSA only) or *S. pyogenes***
Adults: 400 mg P.O. q 12 hours for 10 to 14 days.
Children ages 12 to 18: 600 mg P.O. q 12 hours for 10 to 14 days.
Children ages 5 to 11: 10 mg/kg P.O. q 12 hours for 10 to 14 days.
Neonates age 7 days or older and infants and children younger than age 5: 10 mg/kg P.O. q 8 hours for 10 to 14 days.
Neonates younger than age 7 days: 10 mg/kg P.O. q 12 hours for 10 to 14 days. Increase to 10 mg/kg q 8 hours when patient is 7 days old. Consider this dosage increase if neonate has inadequate response.

Contraindications & cautions

- Contraindicated in patients hypersensitive to drug or its components.

Adverse reactions

CNS: fever, *headache*, insomnia, dizziness.
GI: *diarrhea*, *nausea*, vomiting, constipation, altered taste, tongue discoloration, oral candidiasis, ***pseudomembranous colitis***.
GU: vaginal candidiasis.
Hematologic: anemia, ***leukopenia***, ***neutropenia***, ***myelosuppression***, ***thrombocytopenia***.
Skin: rash.
Other: fungal infection.

Interactions

Drug-drug. *Adrenergic drugs (such as dopamine, epinephrine, pseudoephedrine):* May cause hypertension. Monitor blood pressure and heart rate; start continuous infusions of dopamine and epinephrine at lower doses and titrate to response.
Serotoninergic drugs: May cause serotonin syndrome, including confusion, delirium, restlessness, tremors, blushing, diaphoresis, and hyperpyrexia. If you note signs and symptoms of serotonin syndrome, notify prescriber immediately.
Drug-food. *Foods and beverages high in tyramine (such as aged cheeses, air-dried meats, red wines, sauerkraut, soy sauce, tap beers):* May increase blood pressure when linezolid is used with high-tyramine diet. Advise patient that tyramine content of meals shouldn't exceed 100 mg.

Nursing considerations

- Obtain specimen for culture and sensitivity tests before linezolid therapy. Use sensitivity results to guide subsequent therapy.
- No dosage adjustment is needed when switching from I.V. to P.O. forms.
- Reconstitute oral suspension according to manufacturer's instructions. Store reconstituted suspension at room temperature and use within 21 days.

!!ALERT Don't confuse Zyvox (linezolid) with Zovirax (acyclovir). Both come in a 400-mg strength.

- Drug may cause thrombocytopenia. Monitor platelet count in patients at increased risk for bleeding, in those with existing thrombocytopenia, in those taking other drugs that may cause thrombocytopenia, and in those receiving linezolid for longer than 14 days.
- Drug may lead to myelosuppression. Monitor CBC weekly in patients receiving linezolid.

!!ALERT Pseudomembranous colitis or superinfection may occur. Consider these diagnoses and take appropriate measures in patients with persistent diarrhea or secondary infections.

- Inappropriate use of antibiotics may lead to development of resistant organisms; carefully consider alternative drugs before instituting linezolid therapy, especially in outpatient setting.

!!ALERT Safety and efficacy of drug for longer than 28 days haven't been studied.

Patient teaching

- Tell patient that tablets and oral suspension may be taken with or without meals.

• Stress importance of completing entire course of therapy, even if patient feels better.
• Tell patient to alert prescriber if he has high blood pressure, is taking cough or cold preparations, or is being treated with SSRIs or other antidepressants.
• Advise patient to avoid large quantities of tyramine-containing foods (such as aged cheeses, soy sauce, tap beers, red wine) while taking linezolid.
• Inform patient with phenylketonuria that each 5 ml of linezolid oral suspension contains 20 mg of phenylalanine. Linezolid tablets and injection don't contain phenylalanine.

liothyronine sodium (T_3)
Cytomel, Triostat

Pregnancy risk category A

Indications & dosages

➲ Congenital hypothyroidism
Children: 5 mcg P.O. daily; increase by 5 mcg q 3 to 4 days until desired response is achieved.

➲ Myxedema
Adults: Initially, 2.5 to 5 mcg P.O. daily; increase by 5 to 10 mcg q 1 to 2 weeks until daily dose reaches 25 mcg. Then, increase by 12.5 to 25 mcg daily q 1 to 2 weeks. Maintenance dosage is 50 to 100 mcg daily.

➲ Myxedema coma, premyxedema coma
Adults: Initially, 10 to 20 mcg I.V. for patients with CV disease; 25 to 50 mcg I.V. for patients who don't have CV disease. Adjust dosage based on patient's condition and response. Switch patient to oral therapy as soon as possible.

➲ Simple (nontoxic) goiter
Adults: Initially, 5 mcg P.O. daily; may increase by 5 to 10 mcg daily q 1 to 2 weeks, until daily dose reaches 25 mcg. Then, increase by 12.5 to 25 mcg daily q 1 to 2 weeks. Usual maintenance dosage is 75 mcg daily.

➲ Thyroid hormone replacement
Adults: Initially, 25 mcg P.O. daily; increase by 12.5 to 25 mcg q 1 to 2 weeks until satisfactory response occurs. Usual maintenance dosage is 25 to 50 mcg daily.
Patients older than age 65 and children: 5 mcg daily; increase by 5 mcg daily q 1 to 2 weeks.

➲ T_3 suppression test to differentiate hyperthyroidism from euthyroidism
Adults: 75 to 100 mcg P.O. daily for 7 days.

Contraindications & cautions

• Contraindicated in patients hypersensitive to drug and in those with acute MI uncomplicated by hypothyroidism, untreated thyrotoxicosis, or uncorrected adrenal insufficiency. Also contraindicated with artificial rewarming of patients.
• Use cautiously in elderly patients and in those with angina pectoris, hypertension, other CV disorders, renal insufficiency, or ischemia.
• Use cautiously in patients with diabetes mellitus, diabetes insipidus, or myxedema and during rapid replacement in those with arteriosclerosis.

Adverse reactions

CNS: *nervousness*, *insomnia*, *tremor*, headache.
CV: *tachycardia*, ***arrhythmias***, angina, ***cardiac decompensation and collapse***.
GI: diarrhea, vomiting.
GU: menstrual irregularities.
Metabolic: weight loss.
Musculoskeletal: accelerated bone maturation in infants and children.
Skin: skin reactions, diaphoresis.
Other: heat intolerance.

Interactions

Drug-drug. *Beta blockers:* May reduce beta-blocker effect. Monitor patient for clinical effect.
Cholestyramine, colestipol: May impair liothyronine absorption. Separate doses by 4 to 5 hours.
Digoxin: May decrease glycoside effect. Monitor patient for clinical effect.
Insulin, oral antidiabetics: First thyroid replacement therapy may increase insulin or oral hypoglycemic requirements. Monitor glucose level. Dosage adjustments may be needed.
Oral anticoagulants: May alter PT. Monitor PT and INR. Dosage adjustments may be needed.

Sympathomimetics such as epinephrine: May increase risk of coronary insufficiency. Monitor patient closely.
Theophylline: May decrease theophylline clearance in hypothyroidism; clearance may return to normal when euthyroid state is achieved. Monitor theophylline level.
Drug-herb. *Lemon balm:* May have antithyroid effects; may inhibit thyroid-stimulating hormone. Discourage use together.

Nursing considerations

- Watch for angina, coronary occlusion, or CVA in patients with arteriosclerosis who are receiving rapid replacement. In patients with coronary artery disease who must receive thyroid hormones, watch for possible coronary insufficiency.

!!ALERT Levothyroxine is usually the preferred drug for thyroid hormone replacement therapy. Liothyronine may be used when a rapid-onset or a rapidly reversible drug is desirable, or in patients with impaired peripheral conversion of levothyroxine to liothyronine.

- Long-term therapy causes bone loss in premenopausal and postmenopausal women. Consider a basal bone density measurement, and monitor patient closely for osteoporosis.
- Regulation of liothyronine dosage is difficult.
- Thyroid hormone replacement requirements are about 25% lower in patients older than age 60 than in young adults.
- Monitor pulse and blood pressure.
- When changing from levothyroxine to liothyronine, stop levothyroxine and start liothyronine at a low dosage. Increase dosage in small increments after residual effects of levothyroxine have disappeared. When changing from liothyronine to levothyroxine, start levothyroxine several days before stopping liothyronine to avoid relapse.
- When switching from I.V. to P.O. therapy, gradually increase I.V. dose while starting P.O. dose.
- Patients taking liothyronine who need ^{131}I uptake studies done must stop drug 7 to 10 days before test.
- Dosage may need to be increased in pregnant patients.

!!ALERT Don't confuse levothyroxine with liothyronine or liotrix. Don't confuse Cytomel with Cytotec.

!!ALERT Don't give injection I.M. or S.C.

Patient teaching

- Teach patient importance of compliance. Tell him to take thyroid hormones at same time each day, preferably before breakfast, to maintain constant hormone levels and help prevent insomnia.
- Make sure patient understands that replacement therapy is usually for a lifetime. Drug should never be stopped unless directed by prescriber.
- Advise patient who has achieved a stable response not to change brands.
- Warn patient (especially elderly patient) to notify prescriber at once about chest pain, palpitations, sweating, nervousness, or other signals of overdose or aggravated CV disease.
- Tell patient to report unusual bleeding and bruising.
- Advise diabetic patients to monitor blood glucose closely.
- Tell patient not to take OTC or other prescription medications without first consulting his prescriber.
- Advise patient to report pregnancy to prescriber, because dosage may need adjustment.

liotrix

Thyrolar†

Pregnancy risk category A

Indications & dosages

Dosages are expressed in thyroid equivalents and must be individualized to approximate the deficit in patient's thyroid secretion.

➲ Hypothyroidism
Adults: Initially, a single daily dose of Thyrolar-1/4 or Thyrolar-1/2. Adjust dosage at 2-week intervals.

Contraindications & cautions

- Contraindicated in patients hypersensitive to drug and in those with acute MI uncomplicated by hypothyroidism, untreated thyrotoxicosis, or uncorrected adrenal insufficiency.
- Use cautiously in elderly patients and in those with angina pectoris, hypertension,

other CV disorders, renal insufficiency, or ischemia.
- Use cautiously in patients with diabetes mellitus, diabetes insipidus, or myxedema and during rapid replacement in those with arteriosclerosis.

Adverse reactions

CNS: *nervousness, insomnia, tremor,* headache.
CV: *tachycardia,* ***arrhythmias,*** angina pectoris, ***cardiac decompensation and collapse.***
GI: diarrhea, vomiting.
GU: menstrual irregularities.
Metabolic: weight loss.
Musculoskeletal: accelerated rate of bone maturation in infants and children.
Skin: allergic skin reactions, diaphoresis.
Other: heat intolerance.

Interactions

Drug-drug. *Beta blockers:* May reduce beta-blocker effect. Monitor patient for clinical effect.
Cholestyramine, colestipol: May impair liotrix absorption. Separate doses by 4 to 5 hours.
Digoxin: May decrease glycoside effect. Monitor patient for clinical effect.
Fosphenytoin, phenytoin: May release free thyroid hormone. Monitor patient for tachycardia.
Insulin, oral antidiabetics: May alter glucose level. Monitor glucose level. Dosage adjustments may be needed.
Oral anticoagulants: May alter PT. Monitor PT and INR. Dosage adjustments may be needed.
Sympathomimetics such as epinephrine: May increase risk of coronary insufficiency. Monitor patient closely.
Theophylline: May decrease theophylline clearance in hypothyroidism; clearance may return to normal when euthyroid state is achieved. Monitor theophylline level.
Drug-herb. *Lemon balm:* May have antithyroid effects; may inhibit thyroid-stimulating hormone. Discourage use together.

Nursing considerations

- Watch for angina, coronary occlusion, or CVA in patients with arteriosclerosis who are receiving rapid replacement.
- In patients with coronary artery disease who must receive thyroid hormones, monitor patient for possible coronary insufficiency. Also watch carefully during surgery because arrhythmias may arise.
- Thyroid hormone replacement requirements are about 25% lower in patients older than age 60 than in young adults.
- Dosage may need to be increased in pregnant patients.
- Monitor pulse and blood pressure.
- Long-term therapy causes bone loss in premenopausal and postmenopausal women. Consider a basal bone density measurement and monitor patient closely for osteoporosis.
- Patients taking liotrix must stop drug 7 to 10 days before undergoing ^{131}I uptake studies.

!!ALERT Don't confuse Thyrolar with thyroid or Synthroid; don't confuse liotrix with levothyroxine or liothyronine.

Patient teaching

- Teach patient importance of compliance. He should take thyroid hormones at same time each day, preferably before breakfast, to maintain constant hormone levels and help prevent insomnia.
- Tell patient that drug should never be stopped unless directed by prescriber.
- Warn patient (especially elderly patient) to notify prescriber at once about chest pain, palpitations, sweating, nervousness, or other signs of overdose or aggravated CV disease.
- Tell patient to report unusual bleeding and bruising.
- Advise patient not to take OTC or other prescription medications without first consulting his prescriber.
- Advise patient to report pregnancy to prescriber because dosage may need adjustment.

lisinopril
Prinivil, Zestril

Pregnancy risk category C; D in 2nd and 3rd trimesters

Indications & dosages

➲ Hypertension
Adults: Initially, 10 mg P.O. daily for patients not taking a diuretic. Most patients are well controlled on 20 to 40 mg daily as a single

dose. For patients taking a diuretic, initially, 5 mg P.O. daily.

If creatinine clearance is 10 to 30 ml/minute, give 5 mg P.O. daily; if clearance is less than 10 ml/minute, give 2.5 mg P.O. daily.

➲ Adjunct treatment (with diuretics and cardiac glycosides) for heart failure
Adults: Initially, 5 mg P.O. daily; increased p.r.n. to maximum of 20 mg P.O. daily.

If sodium level is less than 130 mEq/L or creatinine clearance less than 30 ml/minute, start treatment at 2.5 mg daily.

➲ Hemodynamically stable patients within 24 hours of acute MI to improve survival
Adults: Initially, 5 mg P.O.; then 5 mg after 24 hours, 10 mg after 48 hours, followed by 10 mg once daily for 6 weeks.

For patients with systolic blood pressure 120 mm Hg or less when treatment is started or during first 3 days after an infarct, decrease dosage to 2.5 mg P.O. If systolic blood pressure drops to 100 mm Hg or less, reduce daily maintenance dose of 5 mg to 2.5 mg, if needed. If prolonged systolic blood pressure stays under 90 mm Hg for longer than 1 hour, withdraw drug.

➲ Hypertension in children
Children ages 6 to 16: Initially, 0.07 mg/kg P.O. once daily (up to 5 mg total). Adjust dosage according to blood pressure response. Doses above 0.61 mg/kg (or above 40 mg) haven't been studied in children.

Contraindications & cautions

- Contraindicated in patients hypersensitive to ACE inhibitors and in those with a history of angioedema related to previous treatment with ACE inhibitor.
- Use cautiously in patients with impaired renal function; adjust dosage.
- Use cautiously in patients at risk for hyperkalemia and in those with aortic stenosis or hypertrophic cardiomyopathy.

Adverse reactions

CNS: *dizziness*, headache, fatigue, paresthesia.
CV: hypotension, *orthostatic hypotension*, chest pain.
EENT: *nasal congestion*.
GI: *diarrhea*, nausea, dyspepsia.
GU: impaired renal function, impotence.
Metabolic: ***hyperkalemia***.
Respiratory: dyspnea; dry, persistent, tickling, nonproductive cough.
Skin: rash.

Interactions

Drug-drug. *Allopurinol:* May cause hypersensitivity reaction. Use together cautiously.
Azathioprine: May increase risk of anemia or leukopenia. Monitor hematologic studies if used together.
Diuretics, thiazide diuretics: May cause excessive hypotension with diuretics. Monitor blood pressure closely.
Indomethacin, NSAIDs: May reduce hypotensive effects of drug. Adjust dose as needed.
Insulin, oral antidiabetics: May cause hypoglycemia, especially at start of lisinopril therapy. Monitor glucose level.
Phenothiazines: May increase hypotensive effects. Monitor blood pressure closely.
Potassium-sparing diuretics, potassium supplements: May cause hyperkalemia. Monitor laboratory values.
Tizanidine: May cause severe hypotension. Monitor patient.
Drug-herb. *Capsaicin:* May cause ACE inhibitor–induced cough. Discourage use together.
Ma huang: May decrease antihypertensive effects. Discourage use together.
Drug-food. *Potassium-containing salt substitutes:* May cause hyperkalemia. Monitor laboratory values.

Nursing considerations

- When using drug in acute MI, give patient the appropriate and standard recommended treatment, such as thrombolytics, aspirin, and beta blockers.
- The safety and efficacy of lisinopril on blood pressure in pediatric patients younger than age 6 or in pediatric patients with glomerular filtration rate less than 30 ml/minute hasn't been established.
- Although ACE inhibitors reduce blood pressure in all races, they reduce it less in blacks taking the ACE inhibitor alone. Black patients should take drug with a thiazide diuretic for a more favorable response.
- ACE inhibitors appear to increase risk of angioedema in black patients.

- Monitor blood pressure frequently. If drug doesn't adequately control blood pressure, diuretics may be added.
- Monitor WBC with differential counts before therapy, every 2 weeks for first 3 months of therapy, and periodically thereafter.

!!ALERT Don't confuse lisinopril with fosinopril or Lioresal.

!!ALERT Don't confuse Zestril with Zostrix, Zetia, Zebeta, or Zyrtec.

!!ALERT Don't confuse Prinivil with Proventil or Prilosec.

Patient teaching

!!ALERT Rarely, facial and throat swelling (including swelling of the larynx) may occur, especially after first dose. Advise patient to report signs or symptoms of breathing problems or swelling of face, eyes, lips, or tongue.

- Inform patient that light-headedness can occur, especially during first few days of therapy. Tell him to rise slowly to minimize this effect and to report symptoms to prescriber. If he faints, advise patient to stop taking drug and call prescriber immediately.
- If unpleasant adverse reactions occur, tell patient not to stop drug suddenly but to notify prescriber.
- Advise patient to report signs and symptoms of infection, such as fever and sore throat.
- Tell woman of childbearing age to notify prescriber if pregnancy occurs. Drug will need to be stopped.
- Instruct patient not to use salt substitutes that contain potassium without first consulting prescriber.

lithium carbonate

Carbolith†, Duralith†, Eskalith, Eskalith CR, Lithane, Lithizine†, Lithobid, Lithonate, Lithotabs

lithium citrate

Cibalith-S*

Pregnancy risk category D

Indications & dosages

➲ To prevent or control mania

Adults: 300 to 600 mg P.O. up to q.i.d. Or, 900-mg controlled-release tablets P.O. q 12 hours. Increase dosage based on blood levels to achieve optimal dosage. Recommended therapeutic lithium levels are 1 to 1.5 mEq/L for acute mania and 0.6 to 1.2 mEq/L for maintenance therapy.

Contraindications & cautions

- Contraindicated if therapy can't be closely monitored.
- Avoid using in pregnant patient unless benefits outweigh risks.
- Use with caution in patients receiving neuromuscular blockers and diuretics; in elderly or debilitated patients; and in patients with thyroid disease, seizure disorder, infection, renal or CV disease, severe debilitation or dehydration, or sodium depletion.

Adverse reactions

CNS: tremors, drowsiness, headache, confusion, restlessness, dizziness, psychomotor retardation, *lethargy*, ***coma***, blackouts, ***epileptiform seizures***, EEG changes, worsened organic mental syndrome, impaired speech, ataxia, incoordination, *fatigue*.

CV: reversible ECG changes, ***arrhythmias***, hypotension, ***bradycardia***.

EENT: tinnitus, blurred vision.

GI: dry mouth, metallic taste, nausea, *vomiting*, *anorexia*, *diarrhea*, *thirst*, abdominal pain, flatulence, indigestion.

GU: *polyuria*, glycosuria, decreased creatinine clearance, albuminuria, ***renal toxicity***, with long-term use.

Hematologic: *leukocytosis with leukocyte count of 14,000 to 18,000/mm^3.*

Metabolic: transient hyperglycemia, goiter, hypothyroidism, hyponatremia.

Musculoskeletal: *muscle weakness*.

Skin: pruritus, rash, diminished or absent sensation, drying and thinning of hair, psoriasis, acne, alopecia.

Other: ankle and wrist edema.

Interactions

Drug-drug. *ACE inhibitors:* May increase lithium level. Monitor lithium level; adjust lithium dosage, as needed.

Aminophylline, sodium bicarbonate, urine alkalinizers: May increase lithium excretion. Avoid excessive salt, and monitor lithium levels.

Calcium channel blockers (verapamil): May decrease lithium levels and may increase

risk of neurotoxicity. Use together cautiously.
Carbamazepine, fluoxetine, methyldopa, NSAIDs, probenecid: May increase effect of lithium. Monitor patient for lithium toxicity.
Neuromuscular blockers: May cause prolonged paralysis or weakness. Monitor patient closely.
Thiazide diuretics: May increase reabsorption of lithium by kidneys, with possible toxic effect. Use with caution, and monitor lithium and electrolyte levels (especially sodium).
Drug-food. *Caffeine:* May decrease lithium level and drug effect. Advise patient who ingests large amounts of caffeine to tell prescriber before stopping caffeine. Adjust lithium dosage, as needed.

Nursing considerations

- Lithane may contain tartrazine.

!!ALERT Determination of lithium level is crucial to safe use of drug. Don't use drug in patients who can't have regular tests. Monitor lithium level 8 to 12 hours after first dose, the morning before second dose is given, two or three times weekly for the first month, and then weekly to monthly during maintenance therapy.

- When lithium level is less than 1.5 mEq/L, adverse reactions are usually mild.
- Monitor baseline ECG, thyroid studies, renal studies, and electrolyte levels.
- Check fluid intake and output, especially when surgery is scheduled.
- Weigh patient daily; check for edema or sudden weight gain.
- Adjust fluid and salt ingestion to compensate if excessive loss occurs from protracted diaphoresis or diarrhea. Under normal conditions, patient fluid intake should be 2½ to 3 L daily and he should follow a balanced diet with adequate salt intake.
- Check urine specific gravity and report level below 1.005, which may indicate diabetes insipidus.
- Drug alters glucose tolerance in diabetics. Monitor glucose level closely.
- Perform outpatient follow-up of thyroid and renal functions every 6 to 12 months. Palpate thyroid to check for enlargement.

!!ALERT Don't confuse Lithobid with Levbid, Lithonate with Lithostat, or Lithotabs with Lithobid or Lithostat.

Patient teaching

- Tell patient to take drug with plenty of water and after meals to minimize GI upset.
- Explain that lithium has a narrow therapeutic margin of safety. A level that's even slightly high can be dangerous.
- Warn patient and caregivers to expect transient nausea, large amounts of urine, thirst, and discomfort during first few days of therapy and to watch for evidence of toxicity (diarrhea, vomiting, tremor, drowsiness, muscle weakness, incoordination).
- Instruct patient to withhold one dose and call prescriber if signs and symptoms of toxicity appear, but not to stop drug abruptly.
- Warn patient to avoid hazardous activities that require alertness and good psychomotor coordination until CNS effects of drug are known.
- Tell patient not to switch brands of lithium or take other prescription or OTC drugs without prescriber's guidance.
- Tell patient to wear or carry medical identification at all times.

lomustine (CCNU)

CeeNU

Pregnancy risk category D

Indications & dosages

➲ **Brain tumor, Hodgkin's disease**
Adults and children: 100 to 130 mg/m^2 P.O. as single dose q 6 weeks. Repeat doses shouldn't be given until WBC count exceeds 4,000/mm^3 and platelet count is greater than 100,000/mm^3.

Reduce dosage according to degree of bone marrow suppression or when used with other myelosuppressive drugs. Reduce dosage by 30% for WBC count nadir 2,000 to 2,999/mm^3 and platelet count nadir 25,000 to 74,999/mm^3; by 50% for WBC count nadir less than 2,000/mm^3 and platelet count nadir less than 25,000/mm^3.

Contraindications & cautions

- Contraindicated in patients hypersensitive to drug.
- Use cautiously in patients with decreased platelet, WBC, or RBC counts and in those receiving other myelosuppressives.

Adverse reactions

CNS: disorientation, lethargy, ataxia.
GI: *nausea, vomiting*, stomatitis.
GU: ***nephrotoxicity***, progressive azotemia, ***renal failure***, amenorrhea, azoospermia.
Hematologic: *anemia*, ***leukopenia, thrombocytopenia, bone marrow suppression***.
Hepatic: ***hepatotoxicity***.
Respiratory: ***pulmonary fibrosis***.
Skin: alopecia.
Other: ***secondary malignant disease***.

Interactions

Drug-drug. *Anticoagulants, aspirin, NSAIDs:* May increase risk of bleeding. Avoid using together.
Myelosuppressives: May increase myelosuppression. Monitor patient.

Nursing considerations

- Give antiemetic before drug, to reduce nausea.
- Give 2 to 4 hours after meals; drug will be more completely absorbed if taken when stomach is empty.
- Monitor CBC weekly. Usually not given more often than every 6 weeks; bone marrow toxicity is cumulative and delayed, usually occurring 4 to 6 weeks after drug administration.
- Periodically monitor liver function test results.
- To prevent bleeding, avoid all I.M. injections when platelet count is less than 50,000/mm^3.
- Anticipate blood transfusions because of cumulative anemia. Patients may receive RBC colony-stimulating factor to promote RBC production and decrease need for blood transfusions.
- Therapeutic effects are commonly accompanied by toxicity.
- Store capsules at room temperature. Avoid exposure to moisture, and protect from temperatures greater than 104° F (40° C).

Patient teaching

- Advise patient to take capsules on an empty stomach, if possible.
- Advise patient to watch for signs and symptoms of infection (fever, sore throat, fatigue) and bleeding (easy bruising, nosebleeds, bleeding gums, tarry stools). Tell patient to take temperature daily.
- Instruct patient to avoid OTC products that contain aspirin or NSAIDs.
- Advise women to stop breast-feeding during therapy because of possible risk of toxicity to infant.
- Caution woman of childbearing age to avoid becoming pregnant during therapy. Recommend that she consult prescriber before becoming pregnant.

loperamide

Imodium, Imodium A-D ◇, Kaopectate II Caplets ◇, Maalox Anti-Diarrheal Caplets ◇, Pepto Diarrhea Control ◇

Pregnancy risk category B

Indications & dosages

➲ Acute, nonspecific diarrhea
Adults and children older than age 12: Initially, 4 mg P.O.; then 2 mg after each unformed stool. Maximum, 8 mg daily, unless otherwise directed.
Children ages 8 to 12: 2 mg P.O. t.i.d. on first day. Subsequent dosages of 5 ml or 0.1 mg/kg of body weight may be given after each unformed stool. Maximum, 6 mg daily.
Children ages 6 to 8: 2 mg P.O. b.i.d. on first day. If diarrhea persists, contact prescriber. Maximum, 4 mg daily.
Children ages 2 to 5: 1 mg P.O. t.i.d. on first day. If diarrhea persists, contact prescriber.
➲ Chronic diarrhea
Adults: Initially, 4 mg P.O.; then 2 mg after each unformed stool until diarrhea subsides. Adjust dosage to individual response.

Contraindications & cautions

- Contraindicated in patients hypersensitive to drug and in those who must avoid constipation.
- Contraindicated in patients with bloody diarrhea or diarrhea with fever greater than 101° F (38° C), in breast-feeding women, and in children younger than age 2.
- Use cautiously in patients with hepatic disease.

Adverse reactions

CNS: drowsiness, fatigue, dizziness.

GI: dry mouth, abdominal pain, distention, or discomfort, *constipation*, nausea, vomiting.
Skin: rash, hypersensitivity reactions.

Interactions

Drug-drug. *Saquinavir:* May increase loperamide levels and decrease saquinavir levels. Avoid use together.

Nursing considerations

- If clinical symptoms don't improve within 48 hours, stop therapy and consider other alternatives.
- Drug produces antidiarrheal action similar to that of diphenoxylate but without as many adverse CNS effects.

!!ALERT Monitor children closely for CNS effects; children may be more sensitive to these effects than adults.
!!ALERT Don't confuse Imodium with Ionamin.

Patient teaching

- Advise patient not to exceed recommended dosage.
- Tell patient with acute diarrhea to stop drug and seek medical attention if no improvement occurs within 48 hours. In chronic diarrhea, tell patient to notify prescriber and to stop drug if no improvement occurs after taking 16 mg daily for at least 10 days.
- Advise patient with acute colitis to stop drug immediately and notify prescriber about abdominal distention.
- Warn patient to avoid activities that require mental alertness until CNS effects of drug are known.
- Tell patient to report nausea, abdominal pain, or abdominal discomfort.
- Advise patient to relieve dry mouth with ice chips or sugarless gum.
- Advise breast-feeding patients to avoid use.

lopinavir and ritonavir
Kaletra

Pregnancy risk category C

Indications & dosages

➲ Once-daily dosing for HIV infection, with other antiretrovirals in treatment-naive adults
Adults: 800 mg lopinavir and 200 mg ritonavir (6 capsules or 10 ml) P.O. once daily with food.

➲ HIV infection, with other antiretrovirals
Adults and children older than age 12: 400 mg lopinavir and 100 mg ritonavir (3 capsules or 5 ml) P.O. b.i.d. with food.

In treatment-experienced patient also taking efavirenz or nevirapine, when reduced susceptibility to lopinavir is suspected, consider dosage of 533 mg lopinavir and 133 mg ritonavir (4 capsules or 6.5 ml) P.O. b.i.d. with food.

Children ages 6 months to 12 years, weighing 15 to 40 kg (33 to 88 lb): 10 mg/kg (lopinavir content) P.O. b.i.d. with food up to a maximum of 400 mg lopinavir and 100 mg ritonavir in children weighing more than 40 kg.

In treatment-experienced patient also taking efavirenz or nevirapine who weighs 15 to 50 kg (33 to 110 lb), when reduced susceptibility to lopinavir is suspected, consider dosage of 11 mg/kg (lopinavir content) P.O. b.i.d. Treatment-experienced children weighing more than 50 kg can receive adult dosage.

Children ages 6 months to 12 years, weighing 7 to 15 kg (15 to 33 lb): 12 mg/kg (lopinavir content) P.O. b.i.d. with food.

In treatment-experienced patient also taking efavirenz or nevirapine, when reduced susceptibility to lopinavir is suspected, consider dosage of 13 mg/kg (lopinavir content) P.O. b.i.d. with food.

Contraindications & cautions

- Contraindicated in patients hypersensitive to drug or any of its components.
- Use cautiously in patients with a history of pancreatitis or with hepatic impairment, hepatitis B or C, marked elevations in liver enzyme levels, or hemophilia.
- Use cautiously in elderly patients.

• The Antiretroviral Pregnancy Registry monitors maternal-fetal outcomes of pregnant women exposed to lopinavir-ritonavir combination. Health care providers are encouraged to enroll patients by calling 1-800-258-4263.

Adverse reactions

CNS: asthenia, headache, pain, insomnia, malaise, fever, abnormal dreams, agitation, amnesia, anxiety, ataxia, confusion, depression, dizziness, dyskinesia, emotional lability, ***encephalopathy***, hypertonia, nervousness, neuropathy, paresthesia, peripheral neuritis, somnolence, abnormal thinking, tremors.
CV: chest pain, deep vein thrombosis, hypertension, palpitations, thrombophlebitis, vasculitis, edema.
EENT: sinusitis, abnormal vision, eye disorder, otitis media, tinnitus.
GI: abdominal pain, abnormal stools, *diarrhea*, *nausea*, vomiting, anorexia, cholecystitis, constipation, dry mouth, dyspepsia, dysphagia, enterocolitis, eructation, esophagitis, fecal incontinence, flatulence, gastritis, gastroenteritis, GI disorder, ***hemorrhagic colitis***, increased appetite, ***pancreatitis***, inflammation of the salivary glands, stomatitis, ulcerative stomatitis, taste perversion.
GU: abnormal ejaculation, hypogonadism, renal calculus, urine abnormality.
Hematologic: anemia, ***leukopenia***, ***neutropenia***, ***thrombocytopenia in children***.
Hepatic: hyperbilirubinemia in children.
Metabolic: Cushing's syndrome, hypothyroidism, dehydration, decreased glucose tolerance, lactic acidosis, weight loss, hyperglycemia, hyperuricemia, hyponatremia in children.
Musculoskeletal: back pain, arthralgia, arthrosis, myalgia.
Respiratory: bronchitis, dyspnea, lung edema.
Skin: rash, acne, alopecia, dry skin, exfoliative dermatitis, furunculosis, nail disorder, pruritus, benign skin neoplasm, skin discoloration, sweating.
Other: gynecomastia, chills, facial edema, flu syndrome, viral infection, lymphadenopathy, peripheral edema, decreased libido.

Interactions

Drug-drug. *Amiodarone, bepridil, lidocaine, quinidine:* May increase antiarrhythmic level. Use together cautiously. Monitor levels of these drugs, if possible.
Amprenavir, indinavir, saquinavir: May increase levels of these drugs. Avoid using together.
Antiarrhythmics (flecainide, propafenone), pimozide: May increase risk of cardiac arrhythmias. Avoid using together.
Atorvastatin: May increase level of this drug. Use lowest possible dose and monitor patient carefully.
Atovaquone, methadone: May decrease levels of these drugs. Consider increasing doses of these drugs.
Carbamazepine, dexamethasone, phenobarbital, phenytoin: May decrease lopinavir level. Use together cautiously.
Clarithromycin: May increase clarithromycin level in patients with renal impairment. Adjust clarithromycin dosage.
Cyclosporine, rapamycin, tacrolimus: May increase levels of these drugs. Monitor therapeutic levels.
Delavirdine: May increase lopinavir level. Avoid using together.
Didanosine: May decrease absorption of didanosine because lopinavir-ritonavir combination is taken with food. Give didanosine 1 hour before or 2 hours after lopinavir-ritonavir combination.
Dihydroergotamine, ergonovine, ergotamine, methylergonovine: May increase risk of ergot toxicity characterized by peripheral vasospasm and ischemia. Avoid using together.
Disulfiram, metronidazole: May cause disulfiram-like reaction. Avoid using together.
Efavirenz, nevirapine: May decrease lopinavir level. Consider increasing dose of lopinavir-ritonavir combination.
Felodipine, nicardipine, nifedipine: May increase levels of these drugs. Use together cautiously.
Hormonal contraceptives (ethinyl estradiol): May decrease effectiveness of contraceptives. Recommend alternative contraception measures.
Itraconazole, ketoconazole: May increase levels of these drugs. Don't give more than 200 mg/day of these drugs.
Lovastatin, simvastatin: May increase risk of adverse reactions, such as myopathy, rhabdomyolysis. Avoid using together.

Midazolam, triazolam: May cause prolonged or increased sedation or respiratory depression. Avoid using together.
Rifabutin: May increase rifabutin level. Decrease rifabutin dose by 75%. Monitor patient for adverse effects.
Rifampin: May decrease effectiveness of lopinavir-ritonavir combination. Avoid using together.
Sildenafil: May increase sildenafil level and adverse effects, such as hypotension and priapism. Warn patient not to take more than 25 mg of sildenafil in 48 hours.
Warfarin: May affect warfarin level. Monitor PT and INR.
Drug-herb. *St. John's wort:* Loss of virologic response and possible resistance to lopinavir and ritonavir. Discourage use together.
Drug-food. *Any food:* May increase absorption of drug. Tell patient to take with food.

Nursing considerations

!!ALERT Many drug interactions are possible. Review all drugs patient is taking.
- Give drug with food.
- Refrigerated drug remains stable until expiration date on package. If stored at room temperature, use drug within 2 months.
- Monitor patient for signs of fat redistribution, including central obesity, buffalo hump, peripheral wasting, breast enlargement, and cushingoid appearance.
- Monitor total cholesterol and triglycerides before starting therapy and periodically thereafter.
- Monitor patient for signs and symptoms of pancreatitis (nausea, vomiting, abdominal pain, or increased lipase and amylase values).
- Monitor patient for signs and symptoms of bleeding (hypotension, rapid heart rate).

!!ALERT Don't confuse Kaletra with Keppra.

Patient teaching

- Tell patient to take drug with food.
- Tell patient also taking didanosine to take it 1 hour before or 2 hours after lopinavir-ritonavir combination.
- Advise patient to report side effects to prescriber.
- Tell patient to immediately report severe nausea, vomiting, or abdominal pain.
- Inform patient that drug doesn't cure HIV infection, that opportunistic infections and other complications of HIV infection may still occur, and that transmission of HIV to others through sexual contact or blood contamination remains possible.
- Advise patient taking sildenafil of an increased risk of sildenafil-related adverse events, including low blood pressure, visual changes, and painful erections, and to promptly report any symptoms to his prescriber. Tell him not to take more than 25 mg of sildenafil in 48 hours.
- Warn patient to tell prescriber about any other prescription or nonprescription medicine that he's taking, including herbal supplements.

loratadine

Alavert ◇, Claritin ◇, Claritin Reditabs ◇, Claritin Syrup ◇, Tavist ND Allergy ◇

Pregnancy risk category B

Indications & dosages

➲ **Hay fever or other upper respiratory allergies; chronic idiopathic urticaria**
Adults and children age 6 and older: 10 mg P.O. daily.
Children ages 2 to 5 years: 5 mg P.O. daily.

In adults and children age 6 and older with hepatic failure or creatinine clearance less than 30 ml/minute, give 10 mg every other day. In children ages 2 to 5 years with hepatic failure or renal insufficiency, give 5 mg every other day.

Contraindications & cautions

- Contraindicated in patients hypersensitive to drug.
- Use cautiously in patients with hepatic or renal impairment and in breast-feeding patients.

Adverse reactions

CNS: *headache*, drowsiness, fatigue, insomnia, nervousness.
GI: dry mouth.

Interactions

Drug-drug. *Cimetidine, ketoconazole, macrolide antibiotics (clarithromycin, erythromycin, troleandomycin):* May increase plasma loratadine levels. Monitor patient closely.

Drug-lifestyle. *Alcohol use:* May increase CNS depression. Discourage use together.

Nursing considerations

- Stop drug 4 days before patient undergoes diagnostic skin tests because drug can prevent, reduce, or mask positive skin test response.

Patient teaching

- Make sure patient understands to take drug once daily. If symptoms persist or worsen, tell him to contact prescriber.
- Tell patient taking Claritin Reditabs to use tablet immediately after opening individual blister.
- Advise patient taking Claritin Reditabs to place tablet on the tongue, where it disintegrates within a few seconds. It can be swallowed with or without water.
- Warn patient to avoid alcohol and hazardous activities that require alertness until CNS effects of drug are known.
- Tell patient that dry mouth can be relieved with sugarless gum, hard candy, or ice chips.

lorazepam

Apo-Lorazepam†, Ativan, Lorazepam Intensol, Novo-Lorazem†, Nu-Loraz† ◇

Pregnancy risk category D
Controlled substance schedule IV

Indications & dosages

➲ **Anxiety**
Adults: 2 to 6 mg P.O. daily in divided doses. Maximum, 10 mg daily.
Elderly patients: 1 to 2 mg P.O. daily in divided doses. Maximum, 10 mg daily.
➲ **Insomnia from anxiety**
Adults: 2 to 4 mg P.O. h.s.
➲ **Preoperative sedation**
Adults: 0.05 mg/kg I.M. 2 hours before procedure. Total dose shouldn't exceed 4 mg. Or, 2 mg I.V. total or 0.044 mg/kg I.V., whichever is smaller. Larger doses up to 0.05 mg/kg I.V., to total of 4 mg, may be needed.
➲ **Status epilepticus♦**
Adults and children: 0.05 to 0.1 mg/kg. Repeat dose q 10 to 15 minutes, p.r.n. Or, give adults 4 to 8 mg I.V.
➲ **Nausea and vomiting caused by emetogenic cancer chemotherapy♦**
Adults: 2.5 mg P.O. the evening before and just after starting chemotherapy. Or, 1.5 mg/m^2 (usually up to a maximum dose of 3 mg) I.V. (over 5 minutes) 45 minutes before starting chemotherapy.

Contraindications & cautions

- Contraindicated in patients hypersensitive to drug, other benzodiazepines, or the vehicle used in parenteral dosage form; in patients with acute angle-closure glaucoma; and in pregnant women, especially in the first trimester.
- Use cautiously in patients with pulmonary, renal, or hepatic impairment.
- Use cautiously in elderly, acutely ill, or debilitated patients.

Adverse reactions

CNS: *drowsiness,* amnesia, insomnia, agitation, *sedation*, dizziness, weakness, unsteadiness, disorientation, depression, headache.
CV: hypotension.
EENT: visual disturbances.
GI: abdominal discomfort, nausea, change in appetite.

Interactions

Drug-drug. *CNS depressants:* May increase CNS depression. Use together cautiously.
Digoxin: May increase digoxin level and risk of toxicity. Monitor patient and digoxin level closely.
Drug-herb. *Kava:* May increase sedation. Discourage use together.
Drug-lifestyle. *Alcohol use:* May cause additive CNS effects. Discourage use together.
Smoking: May decrease benzodiazepine effectiveness. Monitor patient closely.

Nursing considerations

- For I.M. administration, inject deeply into a muscle. Don't dilute.
- Refrigerate parenteral form to prolong shelf life.
- Monitor hepatic, renal, and hematopoietic function periodically in patients receiving repeated or prolonged therapy.

!!ALERT Use of this drug may lead to abuse and addiction. Don't stop drug abruptly after long-term use because withdrawal symptoms may occur.

!!ALERT Don't confuse lorazepam with alprazolam.

Patient teaching

- When used as a drug before surgery, lorazepam causes substantial preoperative amnesia. Patient teaching requires extra care to ensure adequate recall. Provide written materials or inform a family member, if possible.
- Warn patient to avoid hazardous activities that require alertness or good coordination until effects of drug are known.
- Tell patient to avoid alcohol while taking drug.
- Notify patient that smoking may decrease drug's effectiveness.
- Warn patient not to stop drug abruptly because withdrawal symptoms may occur.
- Warn woman of childbearing age to avoid use during pregnancy.

losartan potassium
Cozaar

Pregnancy risk category C; D in 2nd and 3rd trimesters

Indications & dosages

➲ Hypertension

Adults: Initially, 25 to 50 mg P.O. daily. Maximum daily dose is 100 mg in one or two divided doses.

For patients who are hepatically impaired or intravascularly volume-depleted (such as those taking diuretics), initially, 25 mg.

➲ Nephropathy in type 2 diabetic patients

Adults: 50 mg P.O. once daily. Increase dosage to 100 mg once daily based on blood pressure response.

➲ To reduce risk of CVA in patients with hypertension and left ventricular hypertrophy

Adults: Initially, 50 mg losartan P.O. once daily. Adjust dosage based on blood pressure response, adding hydrochlorothiazide 12.5 mg once daily, increasing losartan to 100 mg daily, or both. If further adjustments are required, may increase the daily dosage of hydrochlorothiazide to 25 mg.

Contraindications & cautions

- Contraindicated in patients hypersensitive to drug. Breast-feeding isn't recommended during losartan therapy.
- Use cautiously in patients with impaired renal or hepatic function.
- Drugs that act directly on the renin-angiotensin system (such as losartan) can cause fetal and neonatal morbidity and death when given to women in the second or third trimester of pregnancy. These problems haven't been detected when exposure was limited to the first trimester. If pregnancy is suspected, notify prescriber because drug should be stopped.

Adverse reactions

Patients with hypertension or left ventricular hypertrophy

CNS: dizziness, asthenia, fatigue, headache, insomnia.

CV: edema, chest pain.

EENT: nasal congestion, sinusitis, pharyngitis, sinus disorder.

GI: abdominal pain, nausea, diarrhea, dyspepsia.

Musculoskeletal: muscle cramps, myalgia, back or leg pain.

Respiratory: cough, upper respiratory infection.

Other: ***angioedema***.

Patients with nephropathy

CNS: *asthenia*, *fatigue*, fever, hypesthesia.

CV: *chest pain*, hypotension, orthostatic hypotension.

EENT: sinusitis, cataract.

GI: *diarrhea*, dyspepsia, gastritis.

GU: *UTI*.

Hematologic: *anemia*.

Metabolic: ***hyperkalemia***, ***hypoglycemia***, weight gain.

Musculoskeletal: *back pain*, leg or knee pain, muscle weakness.

Respiratory: *cough*, *bronchitis*.

Skin: cellulitis.

Other: infection, *flulike syndrome*, trauma, diabetic neuropathy, ***diabetic vascular disease***, ***angioedema***.

Interactions

Drug-drug. *Lithium:* May increase lithium level. Monitor lithium level and patient for toxicity.

NSAIDs: May decrease antihypertensive effects. Monitor blood pressure.

Potassium-sparing diuretics, potassium supplements: May cause hyperkalemia. Monitor patient closely.
Drug-herb. *Ma huang:* May decrease antihypertensive effects. Discourage use together.
Drug-food. *Salt substitutes containing potassium:* May cause hyperkalemia. Monitor patient closely.

Nursing considerations

- Drug can be used alone or with other antihypertensives.
- If antihypertensive effect is inadequate using once-daily doses, a twice daily regimen using the same or increased total daily dose may give a more satisfactory response.
- Monitor patient's blood pressure closely to evaluate effectiveness of therapy. When used alone, drug has less of an effect on blood pressure in black patients than in patients of other races.
- Monitor patients who are also taking diuretics for symptomatic hypotension.
- Regularly assess the patient's renal function (via creatinine and BUN levels).
- Patients with severe heart failure whose renal function depends on the angiotensin-aldosterone system have experienced acute renal failure during ACE inhibitor therapy. Losartan's manufacturer states that drug would be expected to have the same effect. Closely monitor patient, especially during first few weeks of therapy.

!!ALERT Don't confuse Cozaar with Zocor.

Patient teaching

- Tell patient to avoid salt substitutes; these products may contain potassium, which can cause high potassium level in patients taking losartan.
- Inform woman of childbearing age about consequences of second and third trimester exposure to drug. Prescriber should be notified immediately if pregnancy is suspected.
- Advise patient to immediately report swelling of face, eyes, lips, or tongue or any breathing difficulty.

lovastatin (mevinolin)
Altoprev, Mevacor

Pregnancy risk category X

Indications & dosages

➲ To prevent and treat coronary heart disease; hyperlipidemia
Adults: Initially, 20 mg P.O. once daily with evening meal. Recommended range is 10 to 80 mg as a single dose or in two divided doses; maximum daily recommended dose is 80 mg.

Or, 20 to 60 mg extended-release tablets P.O. h.s. Starting dose of 10 mg can be used for patients requiring smaller reductions; usual dosage range is 10 to 60 mg daily.

➲ Heterozygous familial hypercholesterolemia in adolescents
Adolescents ages 10 to 17: 10 to 40 mg daily P.O. with evening meal. Patients requiring reductions in LDL cholesterol level of 20% or more should start with 20 mg daily.

For patients also taking cyclosporine, give 10 mg P.O. daily, not to exceed 20 mg daily. Avoid use of lovastatin with fibrates or niacin; if combined with either, the dosage of lovastatin shouldn't exceed 20 mg daily. For patient with creatinine clearance less than 30 ml/minute, carefully consider dosage increase greater than 20 mg daily and implement cautiously if necessary.

Contraindications & cautions

- Contraindicated in patients hypersensitive to drug and in those with active liver disease or unexplained persistently increased transaminase level.
- Contraindicated in pregnant and breast-feeding women and in women of childbearing age.
- Use cautiously in patients who consume substantial quantities of alcohol or have a history of liver disease.

Adverse reactions

CNS: *headache*, dizziness, peripheral neuropathy, insomnia.
CV: chest pain.
EENT: blurred vision.
GI: constipation, diarrhea, dyspepsia, flatulence, abdominal pain or cramps, heartburn, nausea, vomiting.

Musculoskeletal: muscle cramps, myalgia, myositis, ***rhabdomyolysis***.
Skin: rash, pruritus, alopecia.

Interactions

Drug-drug. *Amiodarone, verapamil:* May cause myopathy and rhabdomyolysis. Don't exceed 40 mg lovastatin daily.
Azole antifungals, clarithromycin, erythromycin, HIV protease inhibitors, nefazodone: May cause myopathy and rhabdomyolysis. Avoid using together.
Cyclosporine, gemfibrozil or other fibrates, niacin: May cause myopathy and rhabdomyolysis. Don't exceed 20 mg lovastatin daily.
Oral anticoagulants: May increase oral anticoagulant effect. Monitor patient closely.
Drug-herb. *Eucalyptus, jin bu huan, kava:* May increase risk of hepatotoxicity. Discourage use together.
Pectin: May decrease lovastatin effect. Discourage use together.
Red yeast rice: May increase risk of adverse reactions because herb contains compounds similar to those of statin drugs. Discourage use together.
Drug-food. *Grapefruit juice:* May increase drug level, increasing risk of side effects. Discourage use together.
Drug-lifestyle. *Alcohol use:* May increase risk of hepatotoxicity. Discourage use together.

Nursing considerations

- Use only after diet and other nondrug therapies prove ineffective. Have patient follow a standard low-cholesterol diet during therapy.
- Obtain liver function test results at the start of therapy, at 6 and 12 weeks after the start of therapy, and when increasing dose; then monitor results periodically.
- Heterozygous familial hypercholesterolemia can be diagnosed in adolescent boys and in girls who are at least 1 year postmenarche and are 10 to 17 years old; if after an adequate trial of diet therapy LDL cholesterol level remains over 189 mg/dl or LDL cholesterol over 160 mg/dl and patient has a positive family history of premature CV disease or two or more other CV disease risk factors.

!!ALERT Don't confuse lovastatin with Lotensin, Leustatin, or Livostin.
!!ALERT Don't confuse Mevacor with Mivacron.

Patient teaching

- Instruct patient to take drug with the evening meal, which improves absorption and cholesterol biosynthesis.
- Teach patient about proper dietary management of cholesterol and triglycerides. When appropriate, recommend weight control, exercise, and smoking cessation programs.
- Advise patient to have periodic eye examinations; related compounds cause cataracts.
- Instruct patient to store tablets at room temperature in a light-resistant container.
- Advise patient to promptly report unexplained muscle pain, tenderness, or weakness, particularly when accompanied by malaise or fever.

!!ALERT Tell woman to stop drug and notify prescriber immediately if she is or may be pregnant or if she's breast-feeding.
!!ALERT Advise patient not to crush or chew extended-release tablets.

loxapine succinate
Loxitane

Pregnancy risk category NR

Indications & dosages

➲ Psychotic disorders
Adults: 10 mg P.O. b.i.d. to q.i.d., rapidly increasing to 60 to 100 mg P.O. daily for most patients; dosage varies.
Elderly patients: Initially, 5 mg P.O. b.i.d. Adjust dosage as needed and as tolerated.

Contraindications & cautions

- Contraindicated in patients hypersensitive to dibenzapines, in those in a coma, and in those with severe CNS depression or drug-induced depressed states.
- Use with caution in patients with seizure disorder, CV disorder, glaucoma, or history of urine retention.

Adverse reactions

CNS: *extrapyramidal reactions, sedation,* drowsiness, ***seizures***, numbness, confusion, syncope, *tardive dyskinesia,* pseudoparkin-

sonism, EEG changes, dizziness, ***neuroleptic malignant syndrome***.
CV: orthostatic hypotension, tachycardia, ECG changes, hypertension.
EENT: *blurred vision*, nasal congestion.
GI: *dry mouth, constipation*, nausea, vomiting, paralytic ileus.
GU: *urine retention*, menstrual irregularities.
Hematologic: ***leukopenia, agranulocytosis, thrombocytopenia***.
Hepatic: jaundice.
Metabolic: weight gain.
Skin: allergic reactions, rash, pruritus.
Other: gynecomastia, galactorrhea.

Interactions

Drug-drug. *Anticholinergics:* May increase anticholinergic effect. Use together cautiously.
CNS depressants: May increase CNS depression. Use together cautiously.
Epinephrine: May inhibit vasopressor effect of epinephrine. Avoid using together.
Drug-lifestyle. *Alcohol use:* May increase CNS depression. Discourage use together.

Nursing considerations

- Obtain baseline blood pressure measurements before starting therapy and monitor pressure regularly.
- Monitor patient for tardive dyskinesia, which may occur after prolonged use. It may not appear until months or years later and may disappear spontaneously or persist for life, despite ending drug.

!!ALERT Watch for evidence of neuroleptic malignant syndrome (extrapyramidal effects, hyperthermia, autonomic disturbance), which is rare but commonly fatal. It may not be related to length of drug use or type of neuroleptic; more than 60% of affected patients are men.

Patient teaching

- Warn patient to avoid activities that require alertness and good coordination until effects of drug are known. Drowsiness and dizziness usually subside after first few weeks.
- Advise patient to report bruising, fever, or sore throat immediately.
- Tell patient to avoid alcohol while taking drug.
- Advise patient to get up slowly to avoid dizziness upon standing quickly.
- Tell patient to relieve dry mouth with sugarless gum or hard candy.
- Recommend periodic eye examinations.

lymphocyte immune globulin (antithymocyte globulin [equine], ATG, LIG)
Atgam

Pregnancy risk category C

Indications & dosages

➲ To prevent acute renal allograft rejection
Adults and children: 15 mg/kg I.V. daily for 14 days; then alternate-day therapy for 14 days. Give first dose within 24 hours of transplantation.
➲ Acute renal allograft rejection
Adults and children: 10 to 15 mg/kg I.V. daily for 14 days. Additional alternate-day therapy to total of 21 doses can be given. Start therapy when rejection is diagnosed.
➲ Aplastic anemia
Adults: 10 to 20 mg/kg I.V. daily for 8 to 14 days. Additional alternate-day therapy to total of 21 doses can be given.

Contraindications & cautions

- Contraindicated in patients hypersensitive to drug.
- Use cautiously in patients receiving additional immunosuppressive therapy (such as corticosteroids or azathioprine) because of increased risk of infection.

Adverse reactions

CNS: malaise, ***seizures***, headache.
CV: *hypotension, chest pain*, thrombophlebitis, tachycardia, edema, iliac vein obstruction.
EENT: ***laryngospasm***.
GI: *nausea, vomiting, diarrhea*, hiccups, epigastric pain, abdominal distention, stomatitis.
GU: renal artery stenosis.
Hematologic: LEUKOPENIA, THROMBOCYTOPENIA, hemolysis, ***aplastic anemia***.
Metabolic: hyperglycemia.
Musculoskeletal: *arthralgia, myalgia*.

Respiratory: *dyspnea, **pulmonary edema**.*
Skin: *rash, pruritus, urticaria.*
Other: febrile reactions, hypersensitivity reactions, serum sickness, ***anaphylaxis***, infections, night sweats, lymphadenopathy, chills.

Interactions
None significant.

Nursing considerations
!!ALERT An intradermal skin test is recommended at least 1 hour before first dose. Give an intradermal dose of 0.1 ml of a 1:1,000 lymphocyte immune globulin along with a contralateral normal saline control. Marked local swelling or erythema larger than 10 mm indicates increased risk of severe systemic reaction such as anaphylaxis. Severe reactions to skin test, such as hypotension, tachycardia, dyspnea, generalized rash, or anaphylaxis, usually preclude further use of drug. Anaphylaxis has occurred in patients with negative skin tests.
- Monitor patient for hypotension, respiratory distress, and chest, flank, or back pain, which may indicate anaphylaxis or hemolysis.
- Keep airway adjuncts and anaphylaxis drugs at bedside during administration.
- Watch for signs and symptoms of infection, such as fever, sore throat, malaise.

Patient teaching
- Instruct patient to report adverse drug reactions promptly, especially signs and symptoms of infection (fever, sore throat, fatigue).
- Tell patient to immediately report discomfort at I.V. insertion site because drug can cause a chemical phlebitis.
- Advise woman of childbearing age to avoid pregnancy during therapy.

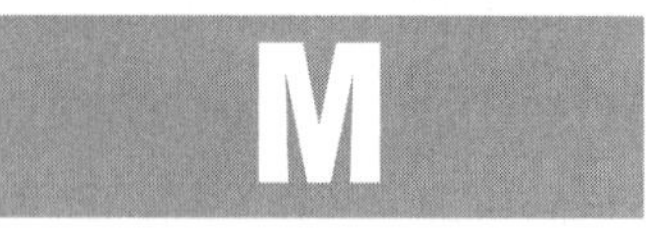

magnesium chloride
Slow-Mag ◇

magnesium sulfate

Pregnancy risk category D

Indications & dosages
➲ Mild hypomagnesemia
Adults: 1 g I.V. by piggyback or I.M. q 6 hours for four doses, depending on magnesium level. Or, 3 g P.O. q 6 hours for four doses.
➲ Symptomatic severe hypomagnesemia, with magnesium 0.8 mEq/L or less
Adults: 2 to 5 g I.V. in 1 L of solution over 3 hours. Base subsequent doses on magnesium level.
➲ Magnesium supplementation
Adults: 64 mg (one tablet) P.O. t.i.d.
➲ Magnesium supplementation in total parenteral nutrition (TPN)
Adults and children: 4 to 24 mEq I.V. daily added to TPN solution.
Infants: 2 to 10 mEq I.V. daily added to TPN solution. Each 2 ml of 50% solution contains 1 g, or 8.12 mEq, magnesium sulfate.
➲ Seizures
Adults: 4 to 5 g magnesium sulfate 50% solution I.M. q 4 hours, p.r.n. Or 4 g of 10% to 20% magnesium sulfate solution I.V. at no more than 1.5 ml/minute of 10% solution. Or, for I.V. infusion, 4 to 5 g in 250 ml of D_5W or sodium chloride, not exceeding 3 ml/minute.
Children: 20 to 40 mg/kg I.M. in a 20% solution. Repeat p.r.n.

Contraindications & cautions
- Contraindicated in patients with myocardial damage or heart block and in pregnant women in actively progressing labor.
- Use parenteral magnesium with caution in patients with impaired renal function.

Adverse reactions
CNS: toxicity, *weak or absent deep tendon reflexes*, flaccid paralysis, drowsiness, stupor.

CV: slow, weak pulse, ***arrhythmias***, *hypotension*, ***circulatory collapse***, flushing.
GI: diarrhea.
Metabolic: hypocalcemia.
Respiratory: ***respiratory paralysis***.
Skin: diaphoresis.
Other: hypothermia.

Interactions

Drug-drug. *Alendronate, fluoroquinolones, nitrofurantoin, penicillamine, sodium polystyrene sulfonate, tetracyclines:* May decrease bioavailability with oral magnesium supplements. Separate doses by 2 to 3 hours.
Cardiac glycosides: May cause serious cardiac conduction changes. Use together with caution.
CNS depressants: May have additive effect. Use together cautiously.
Neuromuscular blockers: May cause increased neuromuscular blockage. Use together cautiously.

Nursing considerations

- Undiluted 50% solutions may be given by deep I.M. injection to adults. Dilute solutions to 20% or less for use in children.
- Keep I.V. calcium available to reverse magnesium intoxication.
- Test knee-jerk and patellar reflexes before each additional dose. If absent, notify prescriber and give no more magnesium until reflexes return; otherwise, patient may develop temporary respiratory failure and need cardiopulmonary resuscitation or I.V. administration of calcium.
- Check magnesium level after repeated doses.
- Monitor fluid intake and output. Output should be 100 ml or more during 4-hour period before dose.
- Monitor renal function.
- After giving to toxemic pregnant woman within 24 hours before delivery, watch neonate for signs and symptoms of magnesium toxicity, including neuromuscular and respiratory depression.

Patient teaching

- Explain use and administration of drug to patient and family.
- Tell patient to report adverse effects.

magnesium citrate (citrate of magnesia)

Citroma ◇, Citro-Mag†

magnesium hydroxide (milk of magnesia)

Milk of Magnesia ◇, Milk of Magnesia-Concentrated ◇, Phillips' Milk of Magnesia ◇

magnesium sulfate ◇ (epsom salts ◇)

Pregnancy risk category B

Indications & dosages

➲ Constipation, to evacuate bowel before surgery
Adults and children age 12 and older: 11 to 25 g magnesium citrate P.O. daily as a single or divided dose. Or, 2.4 to 4.8 g or 30 to 60 ml magnesium hydroxide P.O. (2 to 4 tablespoons at bedtime or upon arising, followed by 8 ounces of liquid) daily as a single dose or divided. Or, 10 to 30 g magnesium sulfate P.O. daily as a single or divided dose.
Children ages 6 to 11: 5.5 to 12.5 g magnesium citrate P.O. daily as a single or divided dose. Or, 1.2 to 2.4 g or 15 to 30 ml magnesium hydroxide P.O. (1 to 2 tablespoons, followed by 8 ounces of liquid) daily as a single or divided dose. Or, 5 to 10 g magnesium sulfate P.O. daily as a single or divided dose. Don't use dosage cup.
Children ages 2 to 5: 2.7 to 6.25 g magnesium citrate P.O. daily as a single or divided dose. Or, 0.4 to 1.2 g or 5 to 15 ml magnesium hydroxide P.O. (1 to 3 tsp, followed by 8 ounces of liquid) daily as a single or divided dose. Or, 2.5 to 5 g magnesium sulfate P.O. daily as a single or divided dose. Don't use dosage cup.
➲ Acid indigestion
Adults and children age 12 and older: 1 to 3 tsp with a little water, up to four times a day, or as directed. Don't use dosage cup.

Contraindications & cautions

- Contraindicated in pregnant patients about to deliver and in patients with myocardial damage, heart block, fecal impaction, rectal fissures, intestinal obstruction or perfo-

ration, renal disease, or signs and symptoms of appendicitis or acute surgical abdomen, such as abdominal pain, nausea, or vomiting.
- Use cautiously in patients with rectal bleeding.

Adverse reactions
GI: *abdominal cramping, nausea, diarrhea.*
Metabolic: fluid and electrolyte disturbances with daily use.
Other: laxative dependence with long-term or excessive use.

Interactions
Drug-drug. *Oral drugs:* May impair absorption. Separate doses.

Nursing considerations
- Give drug at times that don't interfere with scheduled activities or sleep. Drug produces watery stools in 3 to 6 hours.
- Before giving drug for constipation, determine whether patient has adequate fluid intake, exercise, and diet.
- Chill magnesium citrate before use to improve its palatability.
- Shake suspension well; give with a large amount of water when used as laxative. When giving by nasogastric tube, make sure tube is placed properly and is patent. After instilling drug, flush tube with water to ensure passage to stomach and maintain tube patency.

!! ALERT Monitor electrolyte levels during prolonged use. Magnesium may accumulate if patient has renal insufficiency.
- Drug is recommended for short-term use only.
- Magnesium sulfate is more potent than other saline laxatives.

Patient teaching
- Teach patient how to use drug.
- Teach patient about dietary sources of bulk, including bran and other cereals, fresh fruit, and vegetables.
- Warn patient that frequent or prolonged use as a laxative may cause dependence.

magnesium oxide
Mag-Ox 400 ◇, Maox ◇, Uro-Mag ◇

Pregnancy risk category B

Indications & dosages
➲ Acid indigestion
Adults: 140 mg P.O. with water or milk after meals and h.s.
➲ Oral replacement therapy in mild hypomagnesemia
Adults: 400 to 840 mg P.O. daily. Monitor magnesium level.

Contraindications & cautions
- Contraindicated in patients with severe renal disease.
- Use cautiously in patients with mild renal impairment.

Adverse reactions
GI: *diarrhea*, nausea, abdominal pain.
Metabolic: hypermagnesemia.

Interactions
Drug-drug. *Allopurinol, antibiotics, digoxin, iron salts, penicillamine, phenothiazines:* May decrease effects of these drugs because may impair absorption. Separate doses by 1 to 2 hours.
Enteric-coated drugs: May be released prematurely in stomach. Separate doses by at least 1 hour.

Nursing considerations
!! ALERT Monitor magnesium level. With prolonged use and renal impairment, watch for evidence of hypermagnesemia (hypotension, nausea, vomiting, depressed reflexes, respiratory depression, and coma).
- If diarrhea occurs, be prepared to suggest alternative preparation.

Patient teaching
- Advise patient not to take magnesium oxide indiscriminately or to switch antacids without prescriber's advice.
- Urge patient to report signs of GI bleeding, such as tarry stools, or coffee-ground vomitus.

magnesium sulfate

Pregnancy risk category A

Indications & dosages

➲ To prevent or control seizures in preeclampsia or eclampsia

Women: Initially, 4 g I.V. in 250 ml D_5W or normal saline and 4 to 5 g deep I.M. into each buttock; then 4 to 5 g deep I.M. into alternate buttock q 4 hours, p.r.n. Or, 4 g I.V. loading dose; then 1 to 3 g hourly as I.V. infusion. Total dose shouldn't exceed 30 or 40 g daily.

➲ Hypomagnesemia

Adults: For mild deficiency, 1 g I.M. q 6 hours for four doses; for severe deficiency, 5 g in 1,000 ml D_5W or normal saline solution infused over 3 hours.

➲ Seizures, hypertension, and encephalopathy with acute nephritis in children

Children: 0.2 ml/kg of 50% solution I.M. q 4 to 6 hours, p.r.n. For severe symptoms, 100 to 200 mg/kg as a 1% to 3% solution I.V. slowly over 1 hour with 50% of dose given in first 15 to 20 minutes. Adjust dosage according to magnesium level and seizure response.

➲ To manage paroxysmal atrial tachycardia

Adults: 3 to 4 g I.V. over 30 seconds, with extreme caution.

➲ To manage life-threatening ventricular arrhythmias, such as sustained ventricular tachycardia or torsades de pointes♦

Adults: 1 to 6 g I.V. over several minutes; then continuous I.V. infusion of 3 to 20 mg/minute for 5 to 48 hours. Base dosage and duration of therapy on patient response and magnesium level.

➲ To manage preterm labor♦

Adults: 4 to 6 g I.V. over 20 minutes, followed by 2 to 4 g/hr I.V. infusion for 12 to 24 hours, as tolerated, after contractions have ceased.

Contraindications & cautions

- Parenteral administration contraindicated in patients with heart block or myocardial damage.
- Contraindicated in patients with toxemia of pregnancy during 2 hours preceding delivery.
- Use cautiously in patients with impaired renal function.
- Use cautiously in pregnant women during labor.

Adverse reactions

CNS: drowsiness, *depressed reflexes*, flaccid paralysis, hypothermia.
CV: *hypotension*, *flushing*, ***bradycardia***, ***circulatory collapse***, depressed cardiac function.
EENT: diplopia.
Metabolic: hypocalcemia.
Respiratory: ***respiratory paralysis***.
Skin: diaphoresis.

Interactions

Drug-drug. *Anesthetics, CNS depressants:* May cause additive CNS depression. Use together cautiously.
Cardiac glycosides: May worsen arrhythmias. Use together cautiously.
Neuromuscular blockers: May cause increased neuromuscular blockade. Use together cautiously.

Nursing considerations

- If used to treat seizures, take appropriate seizure precautions.

!!ALERT Watch for respiratory depression and signs and symptoms of heart block.

- Keep I.V. calcium gluconate available to reverse magnesium intoxication, but use cautiously in digitalized patients because of danger of arrhythmias.
- Check magnesium level after repeated doses. Disappearance of knee-jerk and patellar reflexes is sign of impending magnesium toxicity.
- Signs of hypermagnesemia begin to appear at levels of 4 mEq/L.
- Effective anticonvulsant level ranges from 2.5 to 7.5 mEq/L.
- Monitor fluid intake and output. Make sure urine output is 100 ml or more in 4-hour period before each dose.
- Observe neonates for signs of magnesium toxicity, including neuromuscular or respiratory depression, when giving I.V. form of drug to toxemic mothers within 24 hours before delivery.

!!ALERT Don't confuse magnesium sulfate with manganese sulfate.

Patient teaching

- Inform patient of short-term need for drug and answer any questions and address concerns.
- Review potential adverse reactions and instruct patient to promptly report any occurrences. Reassure patient that, although adverse reactions can occur, vital signs, reflexes, and drug level will be monitored frequently to ensure safety.

mannitol

Osmitrol

Pregnancy risk category C

Indications & dosages

➲ **Test dose for marked oliguria or suspected inadequate renal function**
Adults and children older than age 12: 200 mg/kg or 12.5 g as a 15% to 20% I.V. solution over 3 to 5 minutes. Response is adequate if 30 to 50 ml of urine/hour is excreted over 2 to 3 hours; if response is inadequate, a second test dose is given. If still no response after second dose, stop drug.

➲ **Oliguria**
Adults and children older than age 12: 50 to 100 g I.V. as a 15% to 25% solution over 90 minutes to several hours.

➲ **To prevent oliguria or acute renal failure**
Adults and children older than age 12: 50 to 100 g I.V. of a 5% to 25% solution. Determine exact concentration by fluid requirements.

➲ **To reduce intraocular or intracranial pressure**
Adults and children older than age 12: 1.5 to 2 g/kg as a 15% to 20% I.V. solution over 30 to 60 minutes. For maximum intraocular pressure reduction before surgery, give 60 to 90 minutes preoperatively.

➲ **Diuresis in drug intoxication**
Adults and children older than age 12: 5% to 10% solution continuously up to 200 g I.V., while maintaining 100 to 500 ml urine output/hour and a positive fluid balance.

➲ **Irrigating solution during transurethral resection of prostate gland**
Adults: 2.5% to 5% solution, p.r.n.

Contraindications & cautions

- Contraindicated in patients hypersensitive to drug.
- Contraindicated in patients with anuria, severe pulmonary congestion, frank pulmonary edema, severe heart failure, severe dehydration, metabolic edema, progressive renal disease or dysfunction, or active intracranial bleeding (except during craniotomy).

Adverse reactions

CNS: ***seizures***, dizziness, headache, fever.
CV: edema, thrombophlebitis, hypotension, hypertension, ***heart failure***, tachycardia, angina-like chest pain, vascular overload.
EENT: blurred vision, rhinitis.
GI: thirst, dry mouth, nausea, vomiting, *diarrhea.*
GU: urine retention.
Metabolic: dehydration.
Skin: local pain, urticaria.
Other: chills.

Interactions

Drug-drug. *Lithium:* May increase urinary excretion of lithium. Monitor lithium level closely.

Nursing considerations

- Monitor vital signs, including central venous pressure and fluid intake and output hourly. Report increasing oliguria. Check weight, renal function, fluid balance, and serum and urine sodium and potassium levels daily.
- Use urinary catheter in comatose or incontinent patient because therapy is based on strict evaluation of fluid intake and output. If patient has urinary catheter, use an hourly urometer collection bag to evaluate output accurately and easily.
- Drug can be used to measure glomerular filtration rate.
- To relieve thirst, give frequent mouth care or fluids.
- Drug is commonly used in chemotherapy regimens to enhance diuresis of renally toxic drugs.
- Don't give electrolyte-free mannitol solutions with blood. If blood is given simultaneously, add at least 20 mEq of sodium chloride to each liter of mannitol solution to avoid pseudoagglutination.

Patient teaching

- Tell patient that he may feel thirsty or have a dry mouth, and emphasize importance of drinking only the amount of fluids ordered.
- Instruct patient to promptly report adverse reactions and discomfort at I.V. site.

measles and rubella virus vaccine, live attenuated

M-R-Vax II

Pregnancy risk category C

Indications & dosages

➲ Immunization

Adults and children age 15 months and older: 0.5 ml (1,000 units) S.C.

Contraindications & cautions

- Contraindicated in immunosuppressed patients; in those with cancer, blood dyscrasia, gamma globulin disorders, fever, active untreated tuberculosis, or anaphylactic or anaphylactoid reactions to eggs or neomycin; in those receiving corticosteroid or radiation therapy; and in pregnant women.

Adverse reactions

CNS: fever.
Musculoskeletal: arthralgia.
Skin: rash, *burning and stinging at injection site.*
Other: lymphadenopathy, ***anaphylaxis***.

Interactions

Drug-drug. *Immune serum globulin, plasma, whole blood:* Antibodies in serum may interfere with immune response. Don't use vaccine within 3 months of transfusion.
Immunosuppressants: May reduce immune response to vaccine. Postpone immunization until immunosuppressant is stopped.

Nursing considerations

- Obtain history of allergies, especially anaphylactic reactions to antibiotics.
- Keep epinephrine 1:1,000 available to treat anaphylaxis.
- If skin test is needed, give it either before or simultaneously with vaccine.
- Use only diluent supplied. Discard vaccine 8 hours after reconstituting.
- Inject into outer upper arm. Don't inject I.V.
- Store in refrigerator and protect from light. Make sure reconstituted solution is clear yellow.

!!ALERT Don't give vaccine within 1 month of other live-virus vaccines. Postpone immunization in patients with acute illness.

- Allow at least 3 weeks between BCG and rubella vaccines.

Patient teaching

- Warn patient or parents about adverse reactions linked to vaccine.
- Caution woman of childbearing age to avoid pregnancy until 3 months after immunization.
- Advise use of fever-reducing drugs to control fever.

measles virus vaccine, live attenuated

Attenuvax

Pregnancy risk category C

Indications & dosages

➲ Immunization

Adults and children age 15 months and older: 0.5 ml (1,000 units) S.C. A two-dose schedule is recommended, with first dose given at 15 months (12 months in high-risk areas) and second dose given at ages 4 to 6 or 11 to 12.

➲ Measles outbreak control

Adults: Revaccinate school personnel born in or after 1957 if they lack evidence of measles immunity. If outbreak is in a medical facility, revaccinate all workers born in or after 1957 if they lack evidence of immunity.
Children: If cases occur in children younger than age 1, vaccinate children as young as age 6 months. Revaccinate all students and siblings if they lack documentation of measles immunity.

Contraindications & cautions

- Contraindicated in pregnant women; in immunosuppressed patients; in patients with cancer, blood dyscrasia, gamma globulin disorders, fever, active untreated tuberculosis, or anaphylactic or anaphylactoid reactions to neomycin or eggs; and in patients receiving corticosteroid or radiation therapy.

• Don't give vaccine within 3 months of receiving blood or plasma transfusion or human immune serum globulin.

Adverse reactions

CNS: ***febrile seizures in susceptible children***, fever.
GI: anorexia.
Hematologic: *leukopenia, thrombocytopenia*.
Skin: rash, erythema, swelling, tenderness at injection site.
Other: lymphadenopathy, ***anaphylaxis***.

Interactions

Drug-drug. *Immune serum globulin, plasma, whole blood:* Antibodies in serum may interfere with immune response. Don't use vaccine for at least 3 months after giving these products.

Nursing considerations

• Obtain history of allergies, especially anaphylactic reactions to antibiotics, or reaction to immunization. Postpone immunization in patients with acute illness or after giving blood or plasma.
• Keep epinephrine 1:1,000 available to treat anaphylaxis.
• If skin test is needed, give it either before or simultaneously with vaccine.
• Use only diluent supplied. Discard vaccine 8 hours after reconstituting.
• Don't give vaccine I.V.
• The Immunization Practices Advisory Committee recommends that colleges, other post-high school educational institutions, and medical institutions obtain documentation of receipt of two doses of vaccine after age 1 (or other evidence of immunity, such as infection, documented by prescriber). Combined measles, mumps, and rubella vaccine is preferred.

!!ALERT The Centers for Disease Control and Prevention recommends that during a health care facility measles outbreak, susceptible personnel exposed to the measles virus (whether they received measles vaccine or immune globulin) avoid patient contact for days 5 through 21 after exposure. If personnel become ill, they should avoid patient contact for at least 7 days after developing rash.

• Attenuated measles vaccine given immediately after exposure to the disease may provide some protection. This level of protection is significantly increased if vaccine is given even a few days before exposure.

Patient teaching

• Warn patient or parents about adverse reactions linked to vaccine.
• Review immunization schedule with patient or parents and stress importance of receiving second injection at appropriate time.
• Stress importance of avoiding pregnancy for 3 months after vaccination. Provide contraception information, if needed.

measles, mumps, and rubella virus vaccine, live

M-M-R II

Pregnancy risk category C

Indications & dosages

➲ Routine immunization
Adults: 0.5 ml S.C. Patients born after 1957 should receive two doses at least 1 month apart.
Children: 0.5 ml S.C. A two-dose schedule is recommended, with first dose given at 15 months (12 months in high-risk areas) and second dose given either at ages 4 to 6 or 11 to 12.

Contraindications & cautions

• Contraindicated in immunosuppressed patients; in those with cancer, blood dyscrasia, gamma globulin disorders, fever, active untreated tuberculosis, or anaphylactic or anaphylactoid reactions to neomycin or eggs; in those receiving corticosteroid or radiation therapy; and in pregnant women.

Adverse reactions

GI: diarrhea.
Musculoskeletal: arthritis, arthralgia.
Skin: rash, erythema at injection site, urticaria.
Other: regional lymphadenopathy, ***anaphylaxis***.

Interactions

Drug-drug. *Immune serum globulin, plasma, whole blood:* Antibodies in serum may interfere with immune response. Don't use vaccine within 3 to 11 months of these

products, depending on dose of antibody or blood given.
Immunosuppressants: May decrease immune response to vaccine. Postpone immunization until immunosuppressant is stopped.

Nursing considerations

- Obtain history of allergies, especially anaphylactic reactions to antibiotics, or reaction to immunization.
- Keep epinephrine 1:1,000 available to treat anaphylaxis.
- If skin test is needed, give it either before or simultaneously with vaccine.
- Use only diluent supplied. Discard vaccine 8 hours after reconstituting.
- Inject into outer aspect of upper arm with a 25G 5/8 -inch needle. Don't give I.V.
- Refrigerate vaccine; protect from light. Solution may be used if red, pink, or yellow but must be clear.
- Risk of adverse effects is low (0.5% to 4%).
- Treat fever with antipyretics such as acetaminophen.
- Presence of maternal antibodies may prevent response in children younger than age 12 months.
- The Immunization Practices Advisory Committee recommends that colleges, other post-high school educational institutions, and medical institutions obtain documentation of receipt of two doses of vaccine after age 1 (or other evidence of immunity, such as infection, documented by prescriber). Combined measles, mumps, and rubella vaccine is preferred.

!!ALERT The Centers for Disease Control and Prevention recommend that, during a measles outbreak in a health care facility, susceptible personnel exposed to measles virus (whether they received measles vaccine or immunoglobulin) avoid patient contact for days 5 through 21 after such exposure. If personnel become ill, they should avoid patient contact for at least 7 days after developing rash.

Patient teaching

- Warn patient or parents about adverse reactions linked to vaccine.
- Review immunization schedule with parents, and stress importance of receiving second injection at the appropriate time to maintain immunization.
- Tell woman of childbearing age to use contraceptive measures until 3 months after immunization.
- Febrile seizures have rarely occurred in children after vaccination. Tell parents to treat and promptly report fever, especially in patient with family history of seizures.

mebendazole
Vermox

Pregnancy risk category C

Indications & dosages

➲ Pinworm
Adults and children older than age 2: 100 mg P.O. as a single dose; repeat if infestation persists 2 to 3 weeks later.
➲ Roundworm, whipworm, and hookworm
Adults and children older than age 2: 100 mg P.O. b.i.d. for 3 days; repeat if infestation persists 3 weeks later.
➲ Trichinosis♦
Adults: 200 to 400 mg P.O. t.i.d. for 3 days; then 400 to 500 mg t.i.d. for 10 days.
➲ Capillariasis♦
Adults and children: 200 mg P.O. b.i.d. for 20 days.
➲ Dracunculiasis♦
Adults: 400 to 800 mg P.O. daily for 6 days.

Contraindications & cautions

- Contraindicated in patients hypersensitive to drug.
- Safe use in children younger than age 2 hasn't been established.

Adverse reactions

CNS: ***seizures***, fever.
GI: transient abdominal pain and diarrhea in massive infestation and during expulsion of worms.
Skin: urticaria.

Interactions

Drug-drug. *Carbamazepine, hydantoin:* May decrease plasma mebendazole level, which may decrease drug's effect. Monitor patient for drug effectiveness.

Cimetidine: May increase plasma mebendazole level. Monitor patient for increased adverse effects if used together.

Nursing considerations

- Tablets may be chewed, swallowed whole, or crushed and mixed with food.
- Give drug to all family members to decrease risk of spreading the infestation.
- No dietary restrictions, laxatives, or enemas are needed.

Patient teaching

- Teach patient about personal hygiene, especially good hand-washing technique. Advise him to refrain from preparing food for others.
- To avoid reinfestation, teach patient to wash perianal area daily, change undergarments and bedclothes daily, and wash hands and clean fingernails before meals and after bowel movements.

mechlorethamine hydrochloride (nitrogen mustard)

Mustargen

Pregnancy risk category D

Indications & dosages

Dosage is based on patient response and degree of toxicity.

➲ Hodgkin's disease

Adults and children: 6 mg/m^2 daily on days 1 and 8 of 28-day cycle with other antineoplastics, such as mechlorethamine-vincristine-procarbazine-prednisone (MOPP) regimen. Repeat dosage for six cycles.

Subsequent doses reduced by 50% in MOPP regimen when WBC count is 3,000 to 3,999/mm^3 and by 75% when WBC count is 1,000 to 2,999/mm^3 or platelet count is 50,000 to 100,000/mm^3.

➲ Polycythemia vera, chronic lymphocytic leukemia, chronic myelocytic leukemia, bronchogenic cancer

Adults and children: 0.4 mg/kg as single dose or 0.1 to 0.2 mg/kg divided in two or four successive daily doses during each course of therapy.

➲ Malignant effusions (pericardial, peritoneal, pleural)

Adults: 0.4 mg/kg intracavitarily, although 0.2 mg/kg (10 to 20 mg) has been used intrapericardially.

Contraindications & cautions

- Contraindicated in patients hypersensitive to drug and in those with infectious diseases.
- Use cautiously in patients with severe anemia or depressed neutrophil or platelet count and in those who have recently undergone radiation therapy or chemotherapy.

Adverse reactions

CNS: weakness, vertigo, neurotoxicity.
CV: *thrombophlebitis.*
EENT: tinnitus, deafness with high doses.
GI: *nausea, vomiting, anorexia,* diarrhea, metallic taste.
GU: menstrual irregularities, impaired spermatogenesis.
Hematologic: ***thrombocytopenia,*** lymphocytopenia, ***agranulocytosis,*** mild anemia beginning in 2 to 3 weeks.
Hepatic: jaundice.
Metabolic: hyperuricemia.
Skin: *alopecia,* rash, sloughing, severe skin irritation with extravasation or contact.
Other: precipitation of herpes zoster, ***anaphylaxis, secondary malignant disease.***

Interactions

Drug-drug. *Anticoagulants, aspirin, NSAIDs:* May increase risk of bleeding. Avoid using together.
Myelosuppressives: May increase myelosuppression. Monitor patient.

Nursing considerations

- When given intracavitarily for sclerosing effect, dilute using up to 100 ml of normal saline solution for injection. Turn patient from side to side every 5 to 10 minutes for 1 hour to distribute drug.
- Monitor uric acid level. To prevent hyperuricemia with resulting uric acid or nephropathy, mechlorethamine may be used with adequate hydration.
- Therapeutic effects are commonly accompanied by toxicity.
- Neurotoxicity increases with dosage and patient age.

- To prevent bleeding, avoid all I.M. injections when platelet count is less than $50,000/mm^3$.
- Monitor patient closely for bone marrow suppression (nadir of myelosuppression occurring between days 4 and 10 and lasting 10 to 21 days).
- Anticipate need for blood transfusions because of cumulative anemia. Patients may receive RBC colony–stimulating factor to promote RBC cell production and decrease need for blood transfusions.

Patient teaching

- Advise patient to report any pain or burning at site of injection during or after administration.
- Advise patient to watch for signs and symptoms of infection (fever, sore throat, fatigue) and bleeding (easy bruising, nosebleeds, bleeding gums, tarry stools). Tell patient to take temperature daily.
- Tell patient that severe nausea and vomiting can occur.
- Instruct patient to avoid OTC products that contain aspirin or NSAIDs.
- Advise women to stop breast-feeding during therapy because of risk of toxicity to infant.
- Advise women of childbearing age to consult prescriber before becoming pregnant.
- Tell patient about the risk of sterility.

meclizine hydrochloride (meclozine hydrochloride)

Antivert, Antivert/25 ◇, Antivert/50, Bonamine†, Bonine ◇, Dramamine Less Drowsy Formula

Pregnancy risk category B

Indications & dosages

➲ Vertigo
Adults: 25 to 100 mg P.O. daily in divided doses. Dosage varies with response.

➲ Motion sickness
Adults and children age 12 and older: 25 to 50 mg P.O. 1 hour before travel; then daily for duration of trip.

Contraindications & cautions

- Contraindicated in patients hypersensitive to drug.
- Use cautiously in patients with asthma, glaucoma, or prostatic hyperplasia.

Adverse reactions

CNS: *drowsiness*, restlessness, excitation, nervousness, auditory and visual hallucinations.
CV: hypotension, palpitations, tachycardia.
EENT: blurred vision, diplopia, tinnitus, dry nose and throat.
GI: dry mouth, constipation, anorexia, nausea, vomiting, diarrhea.
GU: urine retention, urinary frequency.
Skin: urticaria, rash.

Interactions

Drug-drug. *CNS depressants:* May increase drowsiness. Use together cautiously.

Nursing considerations

- Stop drug 4 days before diagnostic skin tests to avoid interference with test response.
- Drug may mask signs and symptoms of ototoxicity, brain tumor, or intestinal obstruction.

!!ALERT Don't confuse Antivert (meclizine) with Axert (almotriptan).

Patient teaching

- Advise patient to avoid hazardous activities that require alertness until CNS effects of drug are known.
- Urge patient to report persistent or serious adverse reactions promptly.

medroxyprogesterone acetate

Amen, Cycrin, Depo-Provera†, Provera

Pregnancy risk category X

Indications & dosages

➲ Abnormal uterine bleeding caused by hormonal imbalance
Women: 5 to 10 mg P.O. daily for 5 to 10 days beginning on day 16 of menstrual cycle. If patient also has received estrogen, give 10 mg P.O. daily for 10 days beginning on day 16 or 21 of cycle.

➲ Secondary amenorrhea
Women: 5 to 10 mg P.O. daily for 5 to 10 days. Start at any time during menstrual cycle (usually during latter half of cycle).

➲ Endometrial or renal cancer
Adults: 400 to 1,000 mg I.M. weekly. Dosage may be decreased to 400 mg/month when disease has stabilized.
➲ Contraception
Women: 150 mg I.M. once q 3 months.

Contraindications & cautions

- Contraindicated in patients hypersensitive to drug and in those with active thromboembolic disorders or history of thromboembolic disorders, cerebrovascular disease, apoplexy, breast cancer, undiagnosed abnormal vaginal bleeding, missed abortion, or hepatic dysfunction; also contraindicated during pregnancy. Tablets are contraindicated in patients with liver dysfunction or known or suspected malignant disease of genital organs.
- Use cautiously in patients with diabetes, seizures, migraine, cardiac or renal disease, asthma, or depression.

Adverse reactions

CNS: depression, ***CVA***, pain.
CV: thrombophlebitis, ***pulmonary embolism***, edema, ***thromboembolism***.
EENT: exophthalmos, diplopia.
GI: *bloating, abdominal pain.*
GU: *breakthrough bleeding*, dysmenorrhea, *amenorrhea*, cervical erosion, abnormal secretions.
Hepatic: cholestatic jaundice.
Metabolic: weight changes.
Skin: rash, induration, sterile abscesses, acne, pruritus, melasma, alopecia, hirsutism.
Other: breast tenderness, enlargement, or secretion.

Interactions

Drug-drug. *Aminoglutethimide, carbamazepine, fosphenytoin, phenobarbital, phenytoin, rifampin:* May decrease progestin effects. Monitor patient for diminished therapeutic response. Tell patient to use a nonhormonal contraceptive during therapy with these drugs.
Drug-food. *Caffeine:* May increase caffeine level. Advise caution.
Drug-lifestyle. *Smoking:* May increase risk of adverse CV effects. If smoking continues, may need alternative therapy.

Nursing considerations

- Drug shouldn't be used as test for pregnancy; it may cause birth defects and masculinization of female fetus.
- I.M. injection may be painful. Monitor sites for evidence of sterile abscess. Rotate injection sites to prevent muscle atrophy.
- Monitor patient for pain, swelling, warmth, or redness in calves; sudden, severe headaches; visual disturbances; numbness in extremities; signs of depression; signs of liver dysfunction (abdominal pain, dark urine, jaundice).

Patient teaching

- According to FDA regulations, patient must read package insert explaining possible adverse effects of progestins before receiving first dose. Also, give patient verbal explanation.
- Advise patient to take medication with food if GI upset occurs.

!!ALERT Tell patient to report unusual symptoms immediately and to stop drug and notify prescriber about visual disturbances or migraine.

- Teach woman how to perform routine breast self-examination.
- Advise patient to immediately report to prescriber any breast abnormalities, vaginal bleeding, swelling, yellowed skin or eyes, dark urine, clay-colored stools, shortness of breath, chest pain, or pregnancy.
- Advise patient that injection must be given every 3 months to maintain adequate contraceptive effects.
- Tell patient to immediately report to prescriber a suspected pregnancy.

mefloquine hydrochloride
Lariam

Pregnancy risk category C

Indications & dosages

➲ Acute malaria infections caused by mefloquine-sensitive strains of *Plasmodium falciparum* or *P. vivax*
Adults: 1,250 mg (5 tablets) P.O. as a single dose with food and at least 8 ounces of water. Patients with *P. vivax* infections should receive subsequent therapy with primaquine or other 8-aminoquinolines to avoid relapse after treatment of the initial infection.

Children: 20 to 25 mg/kg P.O. as a single dose with food and at least 8 ounces of water. Maximum dose 1,250 mg. Dosage may be divided into two doses given 6 to 8 hours apart to reduce the incidence and severity of adverse effects. Patients with *P. vivax* infections should receive subsequent therapy with primaquine or other 8-aminoquinolines to avoid relapse after treatment of the initial infection.

➲ To prevent malaria

Adults and children weighing more than 45 kg (99 lb): 250 mg P.O. once weekly. Prevention therapy should start 1 week before entering endemic area and continue for 4 weeks after returning. If patient returns to an area without malaria after a prolonged stay in an endemic area, prevention therapy should end after three doses.

Children weighing 31 to 45 kg (68 to 99 lb): 187.5 mg (3/4 of a 250-mg tablet) P.O. once weekly.

Children weighing 20 to 30 kg (44 to 66 lb): 125 mg (1/2 of a 250-mg tablet) P.O. once weekly.

Children weighing 15 to 19 kg (33 to 42 lb): 62.5 mg (1/4 of a 250-mg tablet) P.O. once weekly.

Children weighing less than 15 kg (33 lb): 5 mg/kg P.O. once weekly.

Contraindications & cautions

- Contraindicated in patients hypersensitive to mefloquine or related compounds.
- Contraindicated for prevention of malaria in patients with a history of seizures or an active or recent history of depression, generalized anxiety disorder, psychosis, schizophrenia, or other major psychiatric disorders.
- Use cautiously as treatment for patients with cardiac disease or seizure disorders.

Adverse reactions

CNS: fever, dizziness, syncope, headache, psychotic changes, hallucinations, confusion, anxiety, fatigue, vertigo, depression, ***seizures***, tremor, ataxia, mood changes, panic attacks, ***suicide***.

CV: chest pain, edema.

EENT: tinnitus, visual disturbances.

GI: anorexia, vomiting, *nausea*, loose stools, diarrhea, abdominal discomfort or pain, dyspepsia.

Hematologic: ***leukopenia, thrombocytopenia.***

Musculoskeletal: myalgia.

Skin: rash.

Other: chills.

Interactions

Drug-drug. *Beta blockers, quinidine, quinine:* May cause ECG abnormalities and cardiac arrest. Avoid using together.

Carbamazepine, phenobarbital, phenytoin, valproic acid: May decrease drug levels and loss of seizure control at start of mefloquine therapy. Monitor anticonvulsant level.

Chloroquine, quinine: May increase risk of seizures and ECG abnormalities. Give mefloquine at least 12 hours after last dose.

Valproic acid: May decrease valproic acid level and loss of seizure control at start of mefloquine therapy. Monitor anticonvulsant level.

Nursing considerations

- Because giving quinine and mefloquine together poses a health risk, give mefloquine no sooner than 12 hours after the last dose of quinine or quinidine.
- Patients with *P. vivax* infections are at high risk for relapse because drug doesn't eliminate the hepatic-phase exoerythrocytic parasites. Follow-up therapy with primaquine is advisable.
- Monitor liver function test results periodically.
- If overdose is suspected, induce vomiting or perform gastric lavage as appropriate because of potential for cardiotoxicity. Mefloquine has produced cardiac actions similar to quinidine and quinine.

!! ALERT When drug is used preventatively, psychiatric symptoms (acute anxiety, depression, restlessness, confusion) that occur may precede onset of a more serious event. Replace drug with alternate therapy.

Patient teaching

- Advise patient taking drug for prevention to take dose immediately before or after a meal on the same day each week, to improve compliance.
- Tell patient not to take drug on an empty stomach and always to take it with at least 8 ounces of water.
- Advise patient to use caution when performing activities that require alertness and

coordination because dizziness, disturbed sense of balance, and neuropsychiatric reactions may occur.
- Instruct patient taking drug for prevention to stop drug and notify prescriber if signs or symptoms of impending toxicity occur, such as unexplained anxiety, depression, confusion, or restlessness.
- Advise patient undergoing long-term therapy to have periodic ophthalmic examinations because drug may cause ocular lesions.
- Advise women of childbearing age to use reliable contraception during treatment.

megestrol acetate
Megace, Megace OS†

Pregnancy risk category D

Indications & dosages
➲ Breast cancer
Adults: 40 mg P.O. q.i.d.
➲ Endometrial cancer
Adults: 40 to 320 mg P.O. daily in divided doses.
➲ Anorexia, cachexia, or unexplained significant weight loss in patients with AIDS
Adults: 800 mg P.O. (oral suspension) daily.
➲ Anorexia or cachexia in patients with cancer♦
Adults: 480 to 600 mg P.O. daily.

Contraindications & cautions
- Contraindicated in patients hypersensitive to drug.
- Contraindicated as a diagnostic test for pregnancy.
- Use cautiously in patients with history of thrombophlebitis or thromboembolism.

Adverse reactions
CV: thrombophlebitis, ***heart failure***, hypertension, ***thromboembolism***.
GI: nausea, vomiting, diarrhea, flatulence, constipation, dry mouth, increased appetite.
GU: breakthrough menstrual bleeding, impotence, vaginal bleeding or discharge, UTI.
Metabolic: hyperglycemia, *weight gain*.
Musculoskeletal: carpal tunnel syndrome.
Respiratory: ***pulmonary embolism***, dyspnea.
Skin: alopecia, rash.
Other: gynecomastia, tumor flare.

Interactions
None significant.

Nursing considerations
- Glucose level may increase in diabetic patients.
- Drug is relatively nontoxic with a low risk of adverse effects.
- Two months is an adequate trial period in patients with cancer.

Patient teaching
- Inform patient that therapeutic response isn't immediate.
- Advise breast-feeding woman to stop breast-feeding during therapy because of risk of toxicity to infant.
- Advise woman of childbearing age to use an effective form of contraception while receiving drug.

meloxicam
Mobic

Pregnancy risk category C; D in 3rd trimester

Indications & dosages
➲ Relief from signs and symptoms of osteoarthritis
Adults: 7.5 mg P.O. once daily. May increase p.r.n. to maximum dose of 15 mg daily.
➲ Relief from signs and symptoms of rheumatoid arthritis
Adults: 7.5 mg P.O. once daily. May increase p.r.n. to maximum dose of 15 mg daily.

Contraindications & cautions
- Contraindicated in patients hypersensitive to drug and in those who have experienced asthma, urticaria, or allergic reactions after taking aspirin or other NSAIDs.
- Contraindicated in patients late in pregnancy.
- Use with caution in patients with history of ulcers, GI bleeding, or preexisting asthma. Use cautiously in patients with dehydration, anemia, hepatic disease, renal disease, hypertension, fluid retention, heart failure, or asthma. Also use cautiously in elderly and

debilitated patients because of increased risk of fatal GI bleeding.

Adverse reactions

CNS: dizziness, headache, insomnia, fatigue, ***seizures***, paresthesia, tremor, vertigo, anxiety, confusion, depression, nervousness, somnolence, malaise, syncope, fever.
CV: ***arrhythmias***, palpitations, tachycardia, angina pectoris, ***heart failure***, hypertension, hypotension, ***MI***, edema.
EENT: pharyngitis, abnormal vision, conjunctivitis, tinnitus, taste perversion.
GI: abdominal pain, diarrhea, dyspepsia, flatulence, nausea, constipation, colitis, dry mouth, duodenal ulcer, esophagitis, gastric ulcer, gastritis, gastroesophageal reflux, ***hemorrhage***, ***pancreatitis***, vomiting, increased appetite.
GU: albuminuria, hematuria, urinary frequency, ***renal failure***, UTI.
Hematologic: anemia, ***leukopenia***, purpura, ***thrombocytopenia***.
Hepatic: ***hepatitis***.
Metabolic: dehydration, weight increase or decrease.
Musculoskeletal: arthralgia, back pain.
Respiratory: upper respiratory tract infection, ***asthma***, ***bronchospasm***, dyspnea, coughing.
Skin: rash, pruritus, alopecia, bullous eruption, photosensitivity reactions, sweating, urticaria.
Other: accidental injury, allergic reaction, ***angioedema***, flulike symptoms.

Interactions

Drug-drug. *ACE inhibitors:* May decrease antihypertensive effects. Monitor blood pressure.
Aspirin: May cause adverse effects. Avoid using together.
Furosemide, thiazide diuretics: May reduce sodium excretion caused by diuretics, leading to sodium retention. Monitor patient for edema and increased blood pressure.
Lithium: May increase lithium level. Monitor lithium level closely.
Warfarin: May increase PT and INR and increases risk of bleeding complications. Monitor PT and INR, and check for signs and symptoms of bleeding.
Drug-lifestyle. *Alcohol use:* May cause GI irritation and bleeding. Discourage use together.
Smoking: May cause GI irritation and bleeding. Discourage use together.

Nursing considerations

!!ALERT Patient may be allergic to meloxicam, and the drug can produce allergic reactions in those hypersensitive to aspirin and other NSAIDs.
- Rehydrate dehydrated patients before starting drug. Patient with a history of ulcers or GI bleeding is at higher risk for GI bleeding while taking NSAIDs. Other risk factors for GI bleeding include treatment with corticosteroids or anticoagulants, longer duration of NSAID treatment, smoking, alcoholism, older age, and poor overall health.
- Watch for signs and symptoms of overt and occult bleeding.
- NSAIDs can cause fluid retention; closely monitor patients who have hypertension, edema, or heart failure.
- Drug may be hepatotoxic. Watch for elevated ALT and AST levels. If signs and symptoms of liver disease develop or if systemic signs and symptoms such as eosinophilia rash occur, stop drug and call prescriber.
- Monitor hemoglobin level and hematocrit in patients on long-term therapy.

Patient teaching

- Tell patient to report history of allergic reactions to aspirin or other NSAIDs before starting therapy.
- Tell patient drug can be taken without regard to meals.
- Advise patient to report signs and symptoms of GI ulcers and bleeding, such as blood in vomit or stool and black, tarry stools, and to contact prescriber if they occur.
- Instruct patient to report any skin rash, weight gain, or swelling.
- Advise patient to report warning signs of liver damage, such as nausea, fatigue, lethargy, itching, yellowed skin or eyes, right upper quadrant tenderness, and flulike symptoms.
- Warn patient with history of asthma that drug may trigger an asthma attack. Tell him to stop drug and contact prescriber if he has an asthma attack.
- Tell woman of childbearing age to notify prescriber if she becomes pregnant or is

planning to become pregnant while taking drug.
- Inform patient that it may take several days to achieve consistent pain relief.
- Advise patient that use of OTC NSAIDs in combination with meloxicam may increase the risk of GI toxicity.

melphalan (L-phenylalanine mustard)
Alkeran

melphalan hydrochloride
Alkeran

Pregnancy risk category D

Indications & dosages

➲ Multiple myeloma

Adults: Initially, 6 mg P.O. daily for 2 to 3 weeks; then stop drug for up to 4 weeks or until WBC and platelet counts stop dropping and begin to rise again; maintenance dose is 2 mg daily. Or, 0.15 mg/kg P.O. daily for 7 days, or 0.25 mg/kg for 4 days; repeat q 4 to 6 weeks.

Or, give I.V. to patients who can't tolerate oral therapy, 16 mg/m^2 given by infusion over 15 to 20 minutes at 2-week intervals for four doses. After patient has recovered from toxicity, give drug at 4-week intervals.

For patients with renal insufficiency, reduce dosage by up to 50%.

➲ Nonresectable advanced ovarian cancer

Adults: 0.2 mg/kg P.O. daily for 5 days. Repeat q 4 to 6 weeks, depending on bone marrow recovery.

Contraindications & cautions

- Contraindicated in patients hypersensitive to drug and in those whose disease is resistant to drug. Patients hypersensitive to chlorambucil may have cross-sensitivity to melphalan.
- Contraindicated in patients with severe leukopenia, thrombocytopenia, or anemia and in those with chronic lymphocytic leukemia.
- Use cautiously in patients receiving radiation and chemotherapy.
- Safe use in children hasn't been established.

Adverse reactions

CV: hypotension, tachycardia, edema.
GI: nausea, vomiting, diarrhea, oral ulceration, stomatitis.
Hematologic: ***thrombocytopenia, leukopenia, bone marrow suppression***, hemolytic anemia.
Hepatic: ***hepatotoxicity***.
Metabolic: hyperuricemia.
Respiratory: ***pneumonitis, pulmonary fibrosis***, dyspnea, ***bronchospasm***.
Skin: pruritus, alopecia, urticaria, ulceration at injection site.
Other: ***anaphylaxis***, hypersensitivity reactions.

Interactions

Drug-drug (I.V. melphalan only). *Anticoagulants, aspirin, NSAIDs:* May increase risk of bleeding. Avoid using together.
Carmustine: May decrease threshold for pulmonary toxicity. Use together cautiously.
Cimetidine: May decrease melphalan level. Monitor patient closely.
Cisplatin: May increase renal impairment, decreasing melphalan clearance. Monitor patient closely.
Cyclosporine: May cause severe renal impairment. Monitor renal function closely.
Interferon alfa: May increase melphalan elimination. Monitor patient closely.
Myelosuppressives: May increase myelosuppression. Monitor patient.
Vaccines: May decrease effectiveness of killed-virus vaccines and increase risk of toxicity from live-virus vaccines. Postpone routine immunization for at least 3 months after last dose of melphalan.
Drug-food. *Any food:* May decrease oral drug absorption. Advise patient to take drug on empty stomach.

Nursing considerations

- Dosage may need to be reduced in patients with renal impairment.
- Melphalan is drug of choice with prednisone in patients with multiple myeloma.
- Give oral form on empty stomach because food decreases drug absorption.
- Monitor uric acid level and CBC.
- To prevent bleeding, avoid all I.M. injections when platelet count is less than 50,000/mm^3.
- Anticipate need for blood transfusions because of cumulative anemia. Patients may

receive RBC colony-stimulating factor to promote RBC production and decrease need for blood transfusions.
- Anaphylaxis may occur. Keep antihistamines and steroids readily available to give if needed.

!! ALERT Don't confuse melphalan with Mephyton.

Patient teaching
- Advise patient to take tablets on empty stomach.
- Advise patient to watch for signs and symptoms of infection (fever, sore throat, fatigue) and bleeding (easy bruising, nosebleeds, bleeding gums, tarry stools). Tell patient to take temperature daily.
- Instruct patient to avoid OTC products that contain aspirin or NSAIDs.
- Advise women to stop breast-feeding during therapy because of risk of toxicity to infant.
- Advise women of childbearing age to consult prescriber before becoming pregnant.

memantine hydrochloride
Namenda

Pregnancy risk category B

Indications & dosages
➲ Moderate to severe dementia of the Alzheimer's type

Adults: Initially, 5 mg P.O. once daily. Increase by 5 mg/day q week until target dose is reached. Maximum, 10 mg P.O. b.i.d. Doses greater than 5 mg should be divided b.i.d.

Reduce dosage in patients with moderate renal impairment.

Contraindications & cautions
- Contraindicated in patients allergic to drug or its components.
- Not recommended for patients with severe renal impairment.
- Use cautiously in patients with seizures, hepatic impairment, or moderate renal impairment.
- Use cautiously in patients who may have an increased urine pH (from drugs, diet, renal tubular acidosis, or severe UTI, for example).

Adverse reactions
CNS: aggressiveness, agitation, anxiety, ataxia, confusion, ***CVA***, depression, dizziness, fatigue, hallucinations, headache, hypokinesia, insomnia, pain, somnolence, syncope, transient ischemic attack, vertigo.
CV: edema, ***heart failure***, hypertension.
EENT: cataracts, conjunctivitis.
GI: anorexia, constipation, diarrhea, nausea, vomiting.
GU: incontinence, urinary frequency, UTI.
Hematologic: anemia.
Metabolic: weight loss.
Musculoskeletal: arthralgia, back pain.
Respiratory: bronchitis, coughing, dyspnea, flulike symptoms, pneumonia, upper respiratory tract infection.
Skin: rash.
Other: abnormal gait, falls, injury.

Interactions
Drug-drug. *Cimetidine, hydrochlorothiazide, quinidine, ranitidine, triamterene:* May alter levels of both drugs. Monitor patient.
NMDA antagonists (amantadine, dextromethorphan, ketamine): Combined use unknown. Use together cautiously.
Urine alkalinizers (carbonic anhydrase inhibitors, sodium bicarbonate): May decrease memantine clearance. Monitor patient for adverse effects.
Drug-herb. *Herbs that alkalinize urine:* May increase drug level and adverse effects. Use together cautiously.
Drug-food. *Foods that alkalinize urine:* May increase drug level and adverse effects. Use together cautiously.
Drug-lifestyle. *Alcohol use:* May alter drug adherence, decrease its effectiveness, or increase adverse effects. Discourage use together.
Nicotine: May alter levels of drug and nicotine. Discourage use together.

Nursing considerations
- Memantine isn't indicated for mild Alzheimer's disease or other types of dementia.
- In elderly patients, even those with a normal creatinine level, use of this drug may impair renal function. Estimate creatinine clearance; reduce dosage in patients with moderate renal impairment. Don't give drug to patients with severe renal impairment.

Patient teaching

- Explain that memantine doesn't cure Alzheimer's disease but may improve the symptoms.
- Tell patient to report adverse effects.
- Urge patient to avoid alcohol during treatment.
- To avoid possible interactions, advise patient not to take herbal or OTC products without consulting prescriber.

meningococcal polysaccharide vaccine

Menomune-A/C/Y/W-135

Pregnancy risk category C

Indications & dosages

➲ To prevent meningococcal meningitis

Adults and children age 2 and older: 0.5 ml S.C.

Contraindications & cautions

- Contraindicated in patients hypersensitive to thimerosal or other vaccine components; also contraindicated in pregnant women. Postpone vaccination in patients with acute illness.
- Don't give vaccine within 3 months of receiving blood or plasma transfusion or human immune serum globulin administration.

Adverse reactions

CNS: headache, fever, malaise.
Musculoskeletal: muscle cramps.
Skin: *pain, tenderness, erythema, induration at injection site.*
Other: chills, ***anaphylaxis***, mild lymphadenopathy.

Interactions

Drug-drug. *Immunosuppressants:* May reduce immune response to vaccine. Postpone immunization until 3 months after immunosuppressant therapy is stopped.

Nursing considerations

- Obtain history of allergies and reaction to immunization.
- Keep epinephrine 1:1,000 available to treat anaphylaxis.
- Don't give I.V., I.M., or I.D.
- Vaccine may be given with other immunizations and to immunocompromised patients.
- Routine vaccination isn't recommended. Reserve vaccine for persons at risk, such as those who live in or are traveling to epidemic or highly endemic areas, household or institutional contacts of meningococcal disease as an adjunct to appropriate antibiotic chemoprophylaxis, medical and laboratory personnel at risk for exposure to meningococcal disease, patients with terminal complement component deficiency, and those with anatomic or functional asplenia.
- Reconstitute vaccine only with supplied diluent.
- Some prescribers revaccinate children if they are at high risk and if they previously received vaccine before age 4.

Patient teaching

- Warn patient or parents about adverse reactions linked to vaccine.
- Stress importance of avoiding pregnancy for 3 months after vaccination. Provide contraception information, if needed.
- Instruct patient to take correct acetaminophen dose to control fever.

menotropins

Pergonal, Repronex

Pregnancy risk category X

Indications & dosages

➲ Anovulation

Women: 75 IU each of FSH and LH I.M. daily for 7 to 12 days; then 5,000 to 10,000 units of human chorionic gonadotropin (hCG) I.M. 1 day after last dose of menotropins. Don't exceed 12 days of menotropins. Repeat for one to three menstrual cycles, until ovulation occurs.

➲ Infertility with ovulation

Women: 75 IU each of FSH and LH I.M. daily for 7 to 12 days; then 10,000 units hCG I.M. 1 day after last dose of menotropins. Repeat for two menstrual cycles. Then 150 IU each of FSH and LH daily for 7 to 12 days, followed by 10,000 units hCG I.M. 1 day after last dose of menotropins. Repeat for two menstrual cycles.

➲ Infertility in men
Men: Initially, 5,000 units hCG three times a week for 4 to 6 months; then 75 IU each of FSH and LH I.M. three times a week (given with 2,000 units hCG twice a week) for at least 4 months. If spermatogenesis doesn't improve, increase to 150 IU each of FSH and LH three times a week (no change in hCG dose).

Contraindications & cautions

- Contraindicated in patients hypersensitive to drug and in those with primary ovarian failure, uncontrolled thyroid or adrenal dysfunction, pituitary tumor, abnormal uterine bleeding, uterine fibromas, ovarian cysts or enlargement, or any cause of infertility other than anovulation.
- Contraindicated in pregnant women and in men with normal pituitary function, primary testicular failure, or infertility disorders other than hypogonadotropic hypogonadism.

Adverse reactions

CNS: headache, malaise, fever, dizziness, ***CVA***.
CV: tachycardia, venous thrombophlebitis, ***arterial occlusion, pulmonary embolism***.
GI: nausea, vomiting, diarrhea, abdominal cramps, bloating.
GU: *ovarian enlargement with pain and abdominal distention*, multiple births, ovarian hyperstimulation syndrome, ovarian cysts, ectopic pregnancy.
Musculoskeletal: aches, joint pains.
Respiratory: atelectasis, ***acute respiratory distress syndrome***, ***pulmonary infarction***, dyspnea, tachypnea.
Skin: rash.
Other: *gynecomastia*, hypersensitivity reactions, ***anaphylaxis***, chills.

Interactions

None significant.

Nursing considerations

- Prescriber should be experienced in fertility treatment.
- Monitor patient closely to ensure adequate ovarian stimulation without hyperstimulation.

!! ALERT Watch for ovarian hyperstimulation syndrome, which may progress rapidly to a serious medical event characterized by dramatic increase in vascular permeability, which causes rapid accumulation of fluid in the peritoneal cavity, thorax, and pericardium. Signs and symptoms are hypovolemia, hemoconcentration, electrolyte imbalance, ascites, hemoperitoneum, pleural effusion, hydrothorax, and thromboembolism. Condition is common and severe if patient becomes pregnant.

- Refrigerate powder or store at room temperature.
- Reconstitute with 1 to 2 ml of sterile normal saline solution for injection. Use immediately.
- Rotate injection sites.

Patient teaching

- Tell patient about possibility of multiple births. (It occurs about 20% of the time.)
- In women being treated for infertility, encourage daily intercourse from day before hCG is given until ovulation occurs.
- Instruct patient to immediately report severe abdominal pain, bloating, swelling of hands or feet, nausea, vomiting, diarrhea, substantial weight gain, or shortness of breath.

meperidine hydrochloride (pethidine hydrochloride)
Demerol

Pregnancy risk category B; D if used for prolonged periods or in high doses at term
Controlled substance schedule II

Indications & dosages

➲ Moderate to severe pain
Adults: 50 to 150 mg P.O., I.M., or S.C. q 3 to 4 hours, p.r.n.
Children: 1.1 to 1.8 mg/kg P.O., I.M., or S.C. q 3 to 4 hours. Maximum, 100 mg q 4 hours, p.r.n.

➲ Preoperative analgesia
Adults: 50 to 100 mg I.M. or S.C. 30 to 90 minutes before surgery.
Children: 1 to 2.2 mg/kg I.M. or S.C. up to the adult dose 30 to 90 minutes before surgery.

➲ Adjunct to anesthesia
Adults: Repeated slow I.V. injections of fractional doses (10 mg/ml). Or, continuous I.V. infusion of a more dilute solution (1 mg/ml) titrated to patient's needs.

➲ Obstetric analgesia
Adults: 50 to 100 mg I.M. or S.C. when pain becomes regular; repeated at 1- to 3-hour intervals.

Contraindications & cautions

- Contraindicated in patients hypersensitive to drug and in those who have received MAO inhibitors within past 14 days.
- Avoid use in patients with end-stage renal disease.
- Use with caution in elderly or debilitated patients and in those with increased intracranial pressure, head injury, asthma and other respiratory conditions, supraventricular tachycardias, seizures, acute abdominal conditions, hepatic or renal disease, hypothyroidism, Addison's disease, urethral stricture, and prostatic hyperplasia.

Adverse reactions

CNS: physical dependence, *sedation, somnolence, clouded sensorium, euphoria,* paradoxical anxiety, tremor, *dizziness,* ***seizures,*** headache, hallucinations, syncope, *lightheadedness.*
CV: hypotension, ***bradycardia,*** tachycardia, ***cardiac arrest, shock.***
GI: constipation, ileus, dry mouth, *nausea, vomiting,* biliary tract spasms.
GU: urine retention.
Musculoskeletal: muscle twitching.
Respiratory: ***respiratory depression, respiratory arrest.***
Skin: pruritus, urticaria, *diaphoresis.*
Other: phlebitis after I.V. delivery, pain at injection site, local tissue irritation, induration.

Interactions

Drug-drug. *Aminophylline, barbiturates, heparin, methicillin, morphine sulfate, phenytoin, sodium bicarbonate, sulfonamides:* Incompatible when mixed in same I.V. container. Avoid using together.
Cimetidine: May increase respiratory and CNS depression. Monitor patient closely.
Chlorpromazine: May cause excessive sedation and hypotension. Avoid using together.
CNS depressants, general anesthetics, hypnotics, other opioid analgesics, phenothiazines, sedatives, tricyclic antidepressants: May cause respiratory depression, hypotension, profound sedation, or coma. Use together with caution; reduce meperidine dosage.
MAO inhibitors: May increase CNS excitation or depression that can be severe or fatal. Avoid using together.
Phenytoin: May decrease meperidine level. Watch for decreased analgesia.
Protease inhibitors: May increase respiratory and CNS depression. Avoid using together.
Drug-lifestyle. *Alcohol use:* May cause additive effects. Discourage use together.

Nursing considerations

- Active metabolite of meperidine may accumulate in patients with renal dysfunction, causing increased adverse CNS reactions.
- Drug may be used in some patients who are allergic to morphine.
- Reassess patient's level of pain at least 15 and 30 minutes after administration.
- S.C. injection isn't recommended because it's very painful, but it may be suitable for occasional use. Monitor patient for pain at injection site, local tissue irritation, and induration after S.C. injection.

!!ALERT Oral dose is less than half as effective as parenteral dose. Give I.M., if possible. When changing from parenteral to oral route, increase dosage.

- Syrup has local anesthetic effect. Give with full glass of water.
- Drug and its active metabolite, normeperidine, accumulate in the body. Watch for increased toxic effect, especially in patients with impaired renal function.
- Because drug toxicity frequently appears after several days of treatment, drug isn't recommended for treatment of chronic pain.
- Monitor respirations of neonates exposed to drug during labor. Have resuscitation equipment and naloxone available.
- Monitor respiratory and CV status carefully. Don't give if respirations are below 12 breaths/minute, if respiratory rate or depth is decreased, or if change in pupils is noted.
- Watch for withdrawal symptoms if drug is stopped abruptly after long-term use.
- Monitor bladder function in postoperative patients.
- Monitor bowel function. Patient may need a laxative or stool softener.

!!ALERT Don't confuse Demerol with Demulen.

Patient teaching

- When drug is used postoperatively, encourage patient to turn, cough, and deep-breathe and to use an incentive spirometer to prevent lung problems.
- Caution ambulatory patient about getting out of bed or walking. Warn outpatient to avoid driving and other potentially hazardous activities that require mental alertness until drug's CNS effects are known.
- Advise patient to avoid alcohol during therapy.

mercaptopurine (6-mercaptopurine, 6-MP)

Purinethol

Pregnancy risk category D

Indications & dosages

➲ **Acute lymphoblastic leukemia, acute myeloblastic leukemia**

Adults and children: 2.5 mg/kg P.O. once daily (rounded to nearest 25 mg). May increase to 5 mg/kg daily after 4 weeks if no improvement.

After remission is attained, usual maintenance dose for adults and children is 1.5 to 2.5 mg/kg once daily.

Contraindications & cautions

- Contraindicated in patients resistant or hypersensitive to drug.

Adverse reactions

GI: nausea, vomiting, anorexia, painful oral ulcers, diarrhea, ***pancreatitis***, GI ulceration.
Hematologic: ***leukopenia, thrombocytopenia***, *anemia*.
Hepatic: *jaundice*, ***hepatotoxicity***.
Metabolic: hyperuricemia.
Skin: rash, hyperpigmentation.

Interactions

Drug-drug. *Allopurinol:* Slows inactivation of mercaptopurine. Decrease mercaptopurine to 25% or 33% of normal dose.
Co-trimoxazole: May enhance bone marrow suppression. Monitor CBC with differential carefully.
Hepatotoxic drugs: May enhance hepatotoxicity of mercaptopurine. Monitor patient for hepatotoxicity.
Nondepolarizing neuromuscular blockers: May antagonize muscle relaxant effect. Notify anesthesiologist that patient is receiving mercaptopurine.
Warfarin: May decrease or increase anticoagulant effect. Monitor PT and INR.

Nursing considerations

- Consider modifying dosage after chemotherapy or radiation therapy in patients who have depressed neutrophil or platelet counts or impaired hepatic or renal function.

!!ALERT Drug may be ordered as "6-mercaptopurine" or as "6-MP." The numeral 6 is part of drug name and doesn't refer to dosage.

- Monitor CBC and transaminase, alkaline phosphatase, and bilirubin levels weekly during induction and monthly during maintenance.
- Leukopenia, thrombocytopenia, or anemia may persist for several days after drug is stopped.
- Watch for signs of bleeding and infection.
- Monitor fluid intake and output. Encourage 3 L fluid intake daily.

!!ALERT Watch for jaundice, clay-colored stools, and frothy, dark urine. Hepatic dysfunction is reversible when drug is stopped. If right-sided abdominal tenderness occurs, stop drug and notify prescriber.

- Monitor uric acid level. Use allopurinol cautiously.
- To prevent bleeding, avoid all I.M. injections when platelet count is below 100,000/mm^3.
- Anticipate need for blood transfusions because of cumulative anemia. Patient may receive injections of RBC colony-stimulating factors to promote RBC production and decrease need for blood transfusions.
- GI adverse reactions are less common in children than in adults.

Patient teaching

- Instruct patient to watch for signs and symptoms of infection (fever, sore throat, fatigue) and bleeding (easy bruising, nosebleeds, bleeding gums, tarry stools). Tell patient to take temperature daily.
- Caution woman of childbearing age to consult prescriber before becoming pregnant.

• Advise woman to stop breast-feeding during therapy because of risk of toxicity to infant.

meropenem
Merrem IV

Pregnancy risk category B

Indications & dosages

➲ **Complicated skin and skin-structure infections from *Staphylococcus aureus* (beta-lactamase or non-beta-lactamase producing, methicillin-susceptible isolates only), *Streptococcus pyogenes, S. agalactiae,* viridans group streptococci, *Enterococcus faecalis* (excluding vancomycin-resistant isolates), *Pseudomonas aeruginosa, Escherichia coli, Proteus mirabilis, Bacteroides fragilis* and *Peptostreptococcus species.***
Adults and children who weigh more than 50 kg (110 lb): 500 mg I.V. q 8 hours over 15 to 30 minutes as I.V. infusion.
Children ages 3 months and older who weigh 50 kg or less: 10 mg/kg I.V. q 8 hours over 15 to 30 minutes as I.V. infusion or over 3 to 5 minutes as I.V. bolus injection (5 to 20 ml); maximum dose is 500 mg I.V. q 8 hours.

➲ **Complicated appendicitis and peritonitis from viridans group streptococci, *Escherichia coli, Klebsiella pneumoniae, Pseudomonas aeruginosa, Bacteroides fragilis, B. thetaiotaomicron,* and *Peptostreptococcus species***
Adults and children who weigh more than 50 kg: 1 g I.V. q 8 hours over 15 to 30 minutes as I.V. infusion or over 3 to 5 minutes as I.V. bolus injection (5 to 20 ml).
Children ages 3 months and older, who weigh 50 kg or less: 20 mg/kg I.V. q 8 hours over 15 to 30 minutes as I.V. infusion or over 3 to 5 minutes as I.V. bolus injection (5 to 20 ml); maximum dose is 1 g I.V. q 8 hours.

For adults with creatinine clearance of 26 to 50 ml/minute, give usual dose q 12 hours. If clearance is 10 to 25 ml/minute, give half usual dose q 12 hours; if clearance is less than 10 ml/minute, give half usual dose q 24 hours

➲ **Bacterial meningitis from *Streptococcus pneumoniae, Haemophilus influenzae,* and *Neisseria meningitidis***
Children who weigh more than 50 kg: 2 g I.V. q 8 hours.
Children ages 3 months and older, who weigh 50 kg or less: 40 mg/kg I.V. q 8 hours; maximum dose, 2 g I.V. q 8 hours.

Contraindications & cautions

• Contraindicated in patients hypersensitive to components of drug or other drugs in same class and in patients who have had anaphylactic reactions to beta-lactams.
• Use cautiously in elderly patients and in those with a history of seizure disorders or impaired renal function.
• Safety and effectiveness of drug haven't been established for patients younger than age 3 months. Don't use drug in these patients.
• Use drug cautiously in breast-feeding women; it's unknown if drug appears in breast milk.
• Drug isn't used to treat methicillin-resistant staphylococci.

Adverse reactions

CNS: ***seizures***, headache.
CV: phlebitis, thrombophlebitis.
GI: diarrhea, nausea, vomiting, constipation, ***pseudomembranous colitis***, oral candidiasis, glossitis.
GU: presence of RBCs in urine.
Respiratory: ***apnea***, dyspnea.
Skin: rash, pruritus, injection site inflammation.
Other: hypersensitivity reactions, ***anaphylaxis***, inflammation.

Interactions

Drug-drug. *Probenecid:* May decrease renal excretion of meropenem; probenecid competes with meropenem for active tubular secretion, which significantly increases elimination half-life of meropenem and extent of systemic exposure. Avoid using together.

Nursing considerations

• Obtain specimen for culture and sensitivity tests before giving first dose. Therapy may begin pending test results.
!! ALERT Serious and occasionally fatal hypersensitivity reactions may occur in pa-

tients receiving beta-lactams. Before therapy begins, determine if patient has had previous hypersensitivity reactions to penicillins, cephalosporins, other beta-lactams, or other allergens.
- Stop drug and notify prescriber if an allergic reaction occurs. Serious anaphylactic reactions require immediate emergency treatment.
- Drug may cause seizures and other CNS adverse reactions in patients with CNS disorders, bacterial meningitis, and compromised renal function.
- If seizures occur during drug therapy, stop infusion and notify prescriber. Dosage adjustment may be needed.
- Monitor patient for signs and symptoms of superinfection. Drug may cause overgrowth of nonsusceptible bacteria or fungi.
- Periodic assessment of organ system functions, including renal, hepatic, and hematopoietic function, is recommended during prolonged therapy.
- Monitor patient's fluid balance and weight carefully.

Patient teaching
- Advise breast-feeding woman to use another way to feed the baby during therapy.
- Instruct patient to report adverse reactions or signs and symptoms of superinfection.
- Advise patient to report loose stools to prescriber.

mesalamine
Asacol, Canasa, Mesasal, Pentasa, Rowasa, Salofalk

Pregnancy risk category B

Indications & dosages
➲ **Active mild to moderate distal ulcerative colitis, proctitis, or proctosigmoiditis**
Adults: 800 mg P.O. (tablets) t.i.d. for total dose of 2.4 g/day for 6 weeks; or 1 g P.O. (capsules) q.i.d. for total dose of 4 g up to 8 weeks; or 500 mg P.R. (suppository) retained in the rectum for 1 to 3 hours or longer, b.i.d., increased to t.i.d. after 2 weeks; or 4 g as retention enema once daily (preferably h.s.). Patient should retain rectal dosage form overnight (for about 8 hours). Usual course of therapy for rectal form is 3 to 6 weeks.

Contraindications & cautions
- Contraindicated in children and in patients allergic to mesalamine, sulfites (including sulfasalazine), any salicylates, or any component of the preparation.
- Use cautiously in renally impaired, elderly, pregnant, and breast-feeding patients.

Adverse reactions
CNS: *headache*, dizziness, fever, fatigue, malaise, asthenia.
CV: chest pain.
EENT: *pharyngitis*.
GI: abdominal pain, cramps, discomfort, flatulence, diarrhea, rectal pain, bloating, nausea, *pancolitis*, vomiting, constipation, eructation.
GU: interstitial nephritis, nephropathy, ***nephrotoxicity***.
Musculoskeletal: arthralgia, myalgia, back pain, hypertonia.
Respiratory: wheezing.
Skin: itching, rash, urticaria, hair loss.
Other: chills, acne.

Interactions
Drug-drug. *Lactulose:* May impair release of delayed or extended-release products. Monitor patient closely.
Omeprazole: May increase absorption of mesalamine. Monitor patient closely.

Nursing considerations
- Shake suspension well before each use and remove sheath before inserting into rectum.
- Intact or partially intact tablets may be seen in stool. Notify prescriber if this occurs repeatedly.
- Monitor periodic renal function studies in patients on long-term therapy.
- Because the mesalamine rectal suspension contains potassium metabisulfite, it may cause hypersensitivity reactions in patients sensitive to sulfites.
- Absorption of drug may be nephrotoxic.

!! **ALERT** Don't confuse Asacol with Os-Cal.

Patient teaching
- Instruct patient to carefully follow instructions supplied with drug and to swallow tablets whole without crushing or chewing.
- Advise patient to stop drug if fever or rash occurs. Patient intolerant of sulfasalazine may also be hypersensitive to mesalamine.

• Tell patient to remove foil wrapper from suppositories before inserting into rectum.
• Teach patient about proper use of retention enema.
• Tell patient that enema solution may stain bedsheets and clothing. Patient should use protective underpads and linens.

mesna
Mesnex

Pregnancy risk category B

Indications & dosages

➲ To prevent hemorrhagic cystitis in patients receiving ifosfamide
Adults: Dosage varies with amount of ifosfamide given; calculated as 20% of ifosfamide dose at time of ifosfamide administration. Usual dose is 240 mg/m^2 as an I.V. bolus with administration of ifosfamide; repeated at 4 and 8 hours after administration of ifosfamide. Or, calculate daily dose as 100% of the ifosfamide dose. Give as a single bolus injection (20%), followed by two oral doses (40% each). Protocols that use 1.2 g/m^2 ifosfamide would use 240 mg/m^2 I.V. mesna at 0 hours, and then 480 mg/m^2 P.O. at 2 and 6 hours.

Contraindications & cautions

• Contraindicated in patients hypersensitive to mesna or compounds containing thiol.

Adverse reactions

CNS: *fatigue, fever, asthenia,* dizziness, headache, somnolence, anxiety, confusion, insomnia.
CV: chest pain, edema, hypotension, tachycardia, flushing.
GI: *nausea, vomiting,* diarrhea, *constipation, anorexia, abdominal pain,* dyspepsia.
GU: hematuria.
Hematologic: ***leukopenia, thrombocytopenia, anemia, granulocytopenia.***
Metabolic: hypokalemia, dehydration.
Musculoskeletal: back pain.
Respiratory: dyspnea, coughing, pneumonia.
Skin: alopecia, increased sweating, injection site reaction, pallor.
Other: allergy, pain.

Interactions

None significant.

Nursing considerations

• Mesna isn't effective in preventing hematuria from other causes (such as thrombocytopenia).
• Because mesna is used with ifosfamide and other chemotherapeutic drugs, it's difficult to determine adverse reactions attributable solely to mesna.
• Although formulated to prevent hemorrhagic cystitis from ifosfamide, drug won't protect against other toxicities from drug therapy.
• Patients who vomit within 2 hours of taking P.O. mesna should repeat the dose or receive I.V. mesna.
• Monitor urine samples for hematuria daily. Monitor BUN and creatinine levels and intake and output.
• Drug contains benzyl alcohol, which has been linked to fatal gasping syndrome in premature infants.

Patient teaching

• Explain to patient and family or other caregiver why drug is needed and how it's given.
• Instruct patient to report persistent or severe adverse reactions.
• Advise patient to promptly report blood in urine.

metformin hydrochloride
Fortamet, Glucophage, Glucophage XR, Glumetza, Riomet

Pregnancy risk category B

Indications & dosages

➲ Adjunct to diet to lower glucose level in patients with type 2 (non–insulin-dependent) diabetes
Adults: If using regular-release tablets or oral solution, initially 500 mg P.O. b.i.d. given with morning and evening meals, or 850 mg P.O. once daily given with morning meal. When 500-mg dose of regular-release form is used, increase dosage by 500 mg weekly to maximum dose of 2,500 mg P.O. daily in divided doses, p.r.n. When 850-mg dose of regular-release form is used, increase dosage by 850 mg every other week to maxi-

mum dose of 2,550 mg P.O. daily in divided doses, p.r.n. If using extended-release formulation, start therapy at 500 mg P.O. once daily with the evening meal. May increase dose weekly in increments of 500 mg daily, up to a maximum dose of 2,000 mg once daily. If higher doses are required, consider using the regular-release formulation up to its maximum dose.
Children ages 10 to 16: 500 mg P.O. b.i.d. using the regular-release formulation only. Increase dosage in increments of 500 mg weekly up to a maximum of 2,000 mg daily in divided doses.
Elderly patients: Dosage should be conservative because of potential decrease in renal function.

For debilitated patients, dosage should be conservative because of potential decrease in renal function.

➲ **Adjunct to diet and exercise in type 2 diabetes as monotherapy or with a sulfonylurea or insulin (Fortamet)**
Adults age 17 and older: Initially, 500 to 1,000 mg P.O. with evening meal. Increase dosage based on glucose level in increments of 500 mg weekly to a maximum of 2,500 mg daily. When used with a sulfonylurea or insulin, base dosage on glucose level and adjust slowly until desired therapeutic effect occurs. Decrease insulin dose by 10% to 25% when fasting blood glucose level is less than 120 mg/dl.
Elderly patients: Use conservative initial and maintenance dosage because of potential decrease in renal function. Adjust dosage carefully. Don't adjust to maximum dosage.

➲ **Adjunct to diet and exercise in type 2 diabetes as monotherapy or with a sulfonylurea or insulin (Glumetza)**
Adults: Initially, 1,000 mg P.O. once daily in the evening with food. Increase as needed in weekly increments of 500 mg, to a maximum of 2,000 mg daily. If glycemic control not attained at this dose, give 1,000 mg b.i.d.

When used with insulin or a sulfonylurea, base dosage on glucose level and adjust slowly until desired therapeutic effect occurs. Decrease insulin dose by 10% to 25% when fasting glucose level is less than 120 mg/dl.

For malnourished or debilitated patients, don't adjust to maximum dosage.

Contraindications & cautions

- Contraindicated in patients hypersensitive to drug and in those with renal disease, hepatic disease, or metabolic acidosis.
- Contraindicated in patients with heart failure requiring pharmacologic intervention and patients with conditions predisposing to renal dysfunction, CV collapse, MI, hypoxia, and septicemia. Temporarily withhold from patients having radiologic studies involving use of contrast media containing iodine.
- Use caution when giving drug to elderly, debilitated, or malnourished patients and to those with adrenal or pituitary insufficiency because of increased risk of hypoglycemia.

Adverse reactions

GI: *diarrhea, nausea, vomiting,* abdominal bloating, flatulence, anorexia, taste perversion.
Hematologic: megaloblastic anemia.
Metabolic: ***lactic acidosis***, **HYPOGLYCEMIA**.

Interactions

Drug-drug. *Calcium channel blockers, corticosteroids, estrogens, fosphenytoin, hormonal contraceptives, isoniazid, nicotinic acid, phenothiazines, phenytoin, sympathomimetics, thiazide and other diuretics, thyroid drugs:* May produce hyperglycemia. Monitor patient's glycemic control. Metformin dosage may need to be increased.
Cationic drugs (such as amiloride, cimetidine, digoxin, morphine, procainamide, quinidine, quinine, ranitidine, triamterene, trimethoprim, vancomycin): May compete for common renal tubular transport systems, which may increase metformin level. Monitor glucose level.
Nifedipine: May increase metformin level. Monitor patient closely. Metformin dosage may need to be decreased.
Radiologic contrast dye: May cause acute renal failure. Withhold metformin for 24 hours before procedure.
Drug-herb. *Guar gum:* May decrease hypoglycemic effect. Discourage use together.
Drug-lifestyle. *Alcohol use:* May increase drug effects. Discourage use together.

Nursing considerations

- Before therapy begins and at least annually thereafter, assess patient's renal function. If renal impairment is detected, expect prescriber to switch patient to a different antidiabetic. This is particularly important in elderly patients.

- Give with meals. Maximum doses may be better tolerated if total dose is divided into t.i.d. dosing and given with meals.
- When switching patients from standard oral hypoglycemics (except chlorpropamide) to metformin, no transition period is usually needed. When switching patients from chlorpropamide to metformin, take care during the first 2 weeks of metformin therapy because the prolonged retention of chlorpropamide increases the risk of hypoglycemia during this time.
- Monitor patient's glucose level regularly to evaluate effectiveness of therapy. Notify prescriber if glucose level increases despite therapy.
- If patient hasn't responded to 4 weeks of therapy with maximum dosage, prescriber may add an oral sulfonylurea while keeping metformin at maximum dosage. If patient still doesn't respond after several months of therapy with both drugs at maximum dosage, prescriber may stop both and start insulin therapy.
- Monitor patient closely during times of increased stress, such as infection, fever, surgery, or trauma. Insulin therapy may be needed in these situations.
- Risk of drug-induced lactic acidosis is very low. Reported cases have occurred primarily in diabetic patients with significant renal insufficiency; in those with other medical or surgical problems; and in those with other drug regimens. Risk increases with degree of renal impairment and patient age.

!!ALERT Stop drug immediately and notify prescriber if patient develops a condition related to hypoxemia or dehydration because of risk of lactic acidosis.

- Expect drug therapy to be temporarily suspended for surgical procedures (except minor procedures that don't restrict intake of food and fluids) and for patients undergoing radiologic studies involving use of contrast media containing iodine. Therapy shouldn't be restarted until patient's oral intake has resumed and renal function has been deemed normal by prescriber.
- Monitor patient's hematologic status for evidence of megaloblastic anemia. Patients with inadequate vitamin B_{12} or calcium intake or absorption appear to be predisposed to developing subnormal vitamin B_{12} level. These patients should have routine vitamin B_{12} level determinations every 2 to 3 years.

!!ALERT Don't confuse Glucophage with Glucovance.

Patient teaching

- Instruct patient about nature of diabetes and importance of following therapeutic regimen, adhering to specific diet, losing weight, getting exercise, following personal hygiene programs, and avoiding infection. Explain how and when to monitor glucose level. Teach evidence of low and high glucose levels. Explain emergency measures.

!!ALERT Instruct patient to stop drug and immediately notify prescriber about unexplained hyperventilation, muscle pain, malaise, unusual sleepiness, or other nonspecific symptoms of early lactic acidosis.

- Warn patient not to consume excessive alcohol while taking drug.
- Tell patient not to change drug dosage without prescriber's consent. Encourage patient to report abnormal glucose level test results.

!!ALERT Advise patient not to cut, crush, or chew extended-release tablets; instead, he should swallow them whole.

- Advise patient not to take other drugs, including OTC drugs, without first checking with prescriber.
- Instruct patient to wear or carry medical identification at all times.

methadone hydrochloride

Dolophine, Methadose

Pregnancy risk category C
Controlled substance schedule II

Indications & dosages

➲ Severe pain
Adults: 2.5 to 10 mg P.O., I.M., or S.C. q 3 to 4 hours, p.r.n.

➲ Severe chronic pain
Adults: 5 to 20 mg P.O. q. 6 to 8 hours, p.r.n.

➲ Opioid withdrawal syndrome
Adults: 15 to 20 mg P.O. daily often suppresses withdrawal symptoms (highly individualized; some patients may require a higher dose). Maintenance dose is 20 to 120 mg P.O. daily. Dosage adjusted, p.r.n.

Contraindications & cautions

- Contraindicated in patients hypersensitive to drug.
- Use with caution in elderly or debilitated patients and in those with acute abdominal conditions, severe hepatic or renal impairment, hypothyroidism, Addison's disease, prostatic hyperplasia, urethral stricture, head injury, increased intracranial pressure, asthma, and other respiratory conditions.

Adverse reactions

CNS: *sedation, somnolence, clouded sensorium*, euphoria, *dizziness*, choreic movements, ***seizures***, headache, insomnia, agitation, *light-headedness*, syncope.
CV: hypotension, ***arrhythmias, bradycardia, shock, cardiac arrest***, palpitations, edema.
EENT: visual disturbances.
GI: *nausea, vomiting*, constipation, ileus, dry mouth, anorexia, biliary tract spasm.
GU: urine retention.
Respiratory: ***respiratory depression, respiratory arrest.***
Skin: diaphoresis, pruritus, urticaria.
Other: physical dependence, pain at injection site, tissue irritation, induration, decreased libido.

Interactions

Drug-drug. *Ammonium chloride, other urine acidifiers, phenytoin:* May reduce methadone effect. Watch for decreased pain control.
CNS depressants, general anesthetics, hypnotics, MAO inhibitors, sedatives, tranquilizers, tricyclic antidepressants: May cause respiratory depression, hypotension, profound sedation, or coma. Use together with caution. Monitor patient response.
Protease inhibitors, cimetidine, fluvoxamine: May increase respiratory and CNS depression. Monitor patient closely.
Rifampin: May cause withdrawal symptoms; reduces level of methadone. Use together cautiously.
Drug-lifestyle. *Alcohol use:* May cause additive effects. Discourage use together.

Nursing considerations

- Reassess patient's level of pain at least 15 and 30 minutes after parenteral administration and 30 minutes after oral administration.
- When used in opioid withdrawal syndrome, daily doses of more than 120 mg require special state and federal approval.
- Oral liquid form legally required in maintenance programs. Completely dissolve tablets in 1/2 cup of orange juice or powdered citrus drink.
- For parenteral use, I.M. injection is preferred. Rotate injection sites.
- Monitor patient for pain at injection site, tissue irritation, and induration after S.C. injection.
- Oral dose is one-half as potent as injected dose.
- An around-the-clock regimen is needed to manage severe, chronic pain.
- Patient treated for opioid withdrawal syndrome usually needs an additional analgesic if pain control is needed.
- Monitor patient closely because drug has cumulative effect; marked sedation can occur after repeated doses.
- Monitor circulatory and respiratory status and bladder and bowel function. Patient may need a stool softener or laxative.
- When used as an adjunct in the treatment of opioid addiction (maintenance), withdrawal is usually delayed and mild.

!! ALERT High doses of methadone may cause or contribute to QT interval prolongation and torsades de point.

Patient teaching

- Caution ambulatory patient about getting out of bed or walking. Warn outpatient to avoid hazardous activities that require mental alertness until drug's CNS effects are known.
- Instruct patient to increase fluid and fiber in diet, if not contraindicated, to combat constipation.
- Advise patient to avoid alcohol during therapy.

methimazole

Tapazole

Pregnancy risk category D

Indications & dosages

➲ Hyperthyroidism
Adults: If mild, 15 mg P.O. daily. If moderately severe, 30 to 40 mg daily. If severe, 60 mg daily. Daily amount is divided into

three equal doses and given at 8-hour intervals. Maintenance dosage is 5 to 30 mg daily.
Children: 0.4 mg/kg P.O. in three divided doses daily. Maintenance dosage is 0.2 mg/kg in divided doses daily.

Contraindications & cautions

- Contraindicated in patients hypersensitive to drug and in breast-feeding women.
- Use cautiously in pregnant patients.

Adverse reactions

CNS: headache, drowsiness, vertigo, paresthesia, neuritis, neuropathies, CNS stimulation, depression, fever.
GI: diarrhea, nausea, vomiting, salivary gland enlargement, loss of taste, epigastric distress.
GU: nephritis.
Hematologic: ***agranulocytosis, leukopenia, thrombocytopenia, aplastic anemia.***
Hepatic: jaundice, hepatic dysfunction, ***hepatitis.***
Metabolic: hypothyroidism.
Musculoskeletal: arthralgia, myalgia.
Skin: rash, urticaria, discoloration, pruritus, erythema nodosum, exfoliative dermatitis, lupuslike syndrome, abnormal hair loss.
Other: lymphadenopathy.

Interactions

Drug-drug. *Aminophylline, oxtriphylline, theophylline:* May decrease clearance of these drugs. Dosage may need to be adjusted.
Anticoagulants: May alter dosage requirements. Monitor PT, PTT, and INR.
Beta blockers: Hyperthyroidism may increase beta-blocker clearance. May need to reduce dosage of beta blocker when patient becomes euthyroid.
Cardiac glycosides: May increase cardiac glycoside level. Cardiac glycoside dosage may need to be reduced.
Potassium iodide: May decrease response to drug. Methimazole dosage may need to be increased.

Nursing considerations

- Pregnant women may need less drug as pregnancy progresses. Monitor thyroid function studies closely. Thyroid hormone may be added to regimen. Drug may be stopped during last few weeks of pregnancy.
- Monitor CBC periodically to detect impending leukopenia, thrombocytopenia, and agranulocytosis; also monitor hepatic function.

!!ALERT Doses higher than 30 mg daily increase risk of agranulocytosis.
!!ALERT Patients older than age 40 may have an increased risk of drug-induced agranulocytosis.

- Watch for evidence of hypothyroidism (mental depression; cold intolerance; hard, nonpitting edema); notify prescriber because patient may need dosage adjustment.

!!ALERT Stop drug and notify prescriber if severe rash or enlarged cervical lymph nodes develop.
!!ALERT Don't confuse methimazole with mebendazole or methazolamide.

Patient teaching

- Tell patient to take drug with meals to reduce adverse GI reactions.
- Warn patient to report fever, sore throat, mouth sores, skin eruptions, anorexia, itching, right upper quadrant pain, yellow skin or eyes.
- Tell patient to ask prescriber about using iodized salt and eating shellfish because the iodine in these products may make the drug less effective.
- Warn patient that drug may cause drowsiness; advise patient to use caution when operating machinery or a vehicle.
- Instruct patient to store drug in light-resistant container.
- Teach patient to watch for evidence of hypothyroidism (unexplained weight gain, fatigue, cold intolerance) and to notify prescriber if it arises.
- Tell woman not to use drug while breast-feeding.

methotrexate (amethopterin, MTX)

methotrexate sodium

Methotrexate LPF, Rheumatrex, Trexall

Pregnancy risk category X

Indications & dosages

➲ Trophoblastic tumors (choriocarcinoma, hydatidiform mole)
Adults: 15 to 30 mg P.O. or I.M. daily for 5 days. Repeat after 1 or more weeks, based on response or toxicity. Number of courses is three to maximum of five.

➲ Acute lymphocytic leukemia
Adults and children: 3.3 mg/m^2 daily P.O., I.V., or I.M. with 40 to 60 mg/m^2 prednisone daily for 4 to 6 weeks or until remission occurs; then 20 to 30 mg/m^2 P.O. or I.M. weekly in two divided doses or 2.5 mg/kg I.V. q 14 days.

➲ Meningeal leukemia
Adults and children: 12 mg/m^2 or less (maximum 15 mg) intrathecally q 2 to 5 days until CSF is normal; then one additional dose. Or, for children, use dosages based on age.
Children age 3 and older: 12 mg intrathecally q 2 to 5 days.
Children ages 2 to 3: 10 mg intrathecally q 2 to 5 days.
Children ages 1 to 2: 8 mg intrathecally q 2 to 5 days.
Children younger than age 1: 6 mg intrathecally q 2 to 5 days.

➲ Burkitt's lymphoma (stage I, II, or III)
Adults: 10 to 25 mg P.O. daily for 4 to 8 days, with 1-week rest intervals.

➲ Lymphosarcoma (stage III)
Adults: 0.625 to 2.5 mg/kg daily P.O., I.M., or I.V.

➲ Osteosarcoma
Adults: Initially, 12 g/m^2 I.V. as 4-hour infusion. Give subsequent doses 15 g/m^2 I.V. as 4-hour I.V. infusion at postoperative weeks 4, 5, 6, 7, 11, 12, 15, 16, 29, 30, 44, and 45. Give with leucovorin, 15 mg P.O. q 6 hours for 10 doses, beginning 24 hours after start of methotrexate infusion.

➲ Breast cancer
Adults: 40 mg/m^2 I.V. on days 1 and 8 of each cycle, combined with cyclophosphamide and fluorouracil.

In patients older than age 60, give 30 mg/m^2.

➲ Mycosis fungoides
Adults: 2.5 to 10 mg P.O. daily; or 50 mg I.M. weekly; or 25 mg I.M. twice weekly.

➲ Psoriasis
Adults: 10 to 25 mg P.O., I.M., or I.V. as single weekly dose; or 2.5 to 5 mg P.O. q 12 hours for three doses weekly. Dosage shouldn't exceed 30 mg per week.

➲ Rheumatoid arthritis
Adults: Initially, 7.5 mg P.O. weekly, either in single dose or divided as 2.5 mg P.O. q 12 hours for three doses once weekly. Dosage may be gradually increased to maximum of 20 mg weekly.

Contraindications & cautions

- Contraindicated in patients hypersensitive to drug and in those with psoriasis or rheumatoid arthritis who also have alcoholism, alcoholic liver, chronic liver disease, immunodeficiency syndromes, or blood dyscrasias.
- Contraindicated in pregnant or breast-feeding women.
- Use cautiously and at modified dosage in patients with impaired hepatic or renal function, bone marrow suppression, aplasia, leukopenia, thrombocytopenia, or anemia.
- Use cautiously in very young, elderly, or debilitated patients and in those with infection, peptic ulceration, or ulcerative colitis.

Adverse reactions

CNS: ***arachnoiditis within hours of intrathecal use***, subacute neurotoxicity possibly beginning a few weeks later, ***leukoencephalopathy***, demyelination, malaise, fatigue, dizziness, headache, aphasia, hemiparesis, fever, drowsiness, ***seizures***.
EENT: pharyngitis, blurred vision.
GI: gingivitis, *stomatitis, diarrhea*, abdominal distress, anorexia, GI ulceration and bleeding, enteritis, *nausea, vomiting*.
GU: nephropathy, *tubular necrosis*, ***renal failure***, hematuria, menstrual dysfunction, defective spermatogenesis, infertility, abortion, cystitis.
Hematologic: *anemia*, ***leukopenia***, ***thrombocytopenia***.
Hepatic: ***acute toxicity***, ***chronic toxicity***, including cirrhosis and, ***hepatic fibrosis***.
Metabolic: diabetes, hyperuricemia.

Musculoskeletal: arthralgia, myalgia, osteoporosis in children on long-term therapy.
Respiratory: ***pulmonary fibrosis***; ***pulmonary interstitial infiltrates***; pneumonitis; dry, nonproductive cough.
Skin: *urticaria*, pruritus, hyperpigmentation, erythematous rashes, ecchymoses, rash, photosensitivity, alopecia, acne, psoriatic lesions aggravated by exposure to sun.
Other: chills, reduced resistance to infection, septicemia, ***sudden death***.

Interactions

Drug-drug. *Acyclovir:* Use with intrathecal methotrexate may cause neurologic abnormalities. Monitor patient closely.
Digoxin: May decrease digoxin level. Monitor digoxin level closely.
Folic acid derivatives: Antagonizes methotrexate effect. Avoid using together, except for leucovorin rescue with high-dose methotrexate therapy.
Fosphenytoin, phenytoin: May decrease phenytoin and fosphenytoin levels. Monitor drug levels closely.
Hepatotoxic drugs: May increase risk of hepatotoxicity. Monitor patient closely.
NSAIDs, phenylbutazone, salicylates, sulfonamides: May increase methotrexate toxicity. Avoid using together.
Oral antibiotics: May decrease absorption of methotrexate. Monitor patient closely.
Penicillins, sulfonamides: May increase methotrexate level. Monitor patient for methotrexate toxicity.
Probenecid: May impair excretion of methotrexate, causing increased level, effect, and toxicity of methotrexate. Monitor methotrexate level closely and adjust dosage accordingly.
Procarbazine: May increase risk of nephrotoxicity. Monitor patient closely.
Theophylline: May increase theophylline level. Monitor theophylline level closely.
Thiopurines: May increase thiopurine level. Monitor patient closely.
Vaccines: May make immunizations ineffective; may cause risk of disseminated infection with live virus vaccines. Postpone immunization, if possible.
Drug-food. *Any food:* May delay absorption and reduce peak level of methotrexate. Instruct patient to take drug on an empty stomach.
Drug-lifestyle. *Alcohol use:* May increase hepatotoxicity. Discourage alcohol use.
Sun exposure: May cause photosensitivity reactions. Advise patient to avoid excessive sunlight exposure.

Nursing considerations

!!ALERT Methotrexate may be given daily or once weekly, depending on the disease. To avoid administration errors, be aware of which disease the patient has.

- Monitor pulmonary function tests periodically and fluid intake and output daily. Encourage fluid intake of 2 to 3 L daily.
- Monitor uric acid level.
- Methotrexate distributes readily into pleural effusions and other third-space compartments, such as ascites, leading to prolonged systemic level and potential for toxicity. Use drug cautiously in these patients.
- Methotrexate tablets may contain lactose. May give OTC lactose enzyme supplement.

!!ALERT Alkalinize urine by giving sodium bicarbonate tablets or I.V. fluids containing sodium bicarbonate to prevent precipitation of drug, especially at high doses. Maintain urine pH above 7. Reduce dosage if BUN level is 20 to 30 mg/dl or creatinine level is 1.2 to 2 mg/dl. Stop drug and notify prescriber if BUN level exceeds 30 mg/dl or creatinine level is higher than 2 mg/dl.

- Use preservative-free formulation for intrathecal administration.
- Watch for increases in AST, ALT, and alkaline phosphatase levels, which may signal hepatic dysfunction.
- Watch for signs and symptoms of bleeding (especially GI) and infection.
- To prevent bleeding, avoid all I.M. injections when platelet count is below 50,000/mm^3.
- Anticipate blood transfusions because of cumulative anemia. Patient may receive injections of RBC colony–stimulating factors to promote RBC production and decrease need for blood transfusions.
- Leucovorin rescue is needed with doses over 100 mg and starts 24 hours after methotrexate therapy is begun. Leucovorin is continued until methotrexate level falls below 5×10^{-8} M. Consult specialized references for specific recommendations for leucovorin dosage.
- Monitor methotrexate level and adjust leucovorin dose.

• The WBC and platelet count nadirs usually occur on day 7.

Patient teaching

• Advise patient to watch for signs and symptoms of infection (fever, sore throat, fatigue) and bleeding (easy bruising, nosebleeds, bleeding gums, tarry stools). Tell patient to take temperature daily.
• Teach and encourage diligent mouth care to reduce risk of superinfection in the mouth.
• Instruct patient how to take leucovorin. Stress the importance of taking medication as prescribed until instructed by prescriber to stop medication.
• Tell patient to use highly protective sunblock when exposed to sunlight.
• Warn patient to avoid conception during and immediately after therapy because of possible abortion or birth defects or problems.
• Advise breast-feeding woman to stop breast-feeding during therapy because of risk of toxicity to infant.

methyldopa

Aldomet, Apo-Methyldopa†, Dopamet†, Novo-Medopa†, Nu-Medopa†

methyldopate hydrochloride

Aldomet

Pregnancy risk category B for P.O.; C for I.V.

Indications & dosages

➲ Hypertension, hypertensive crisis
Adults: Initially, 250 mg P.O. b.i.d. to t.i.d. in first 48 hours. Increase p.r.n. q 2 days. May give entire daily dose in evening or at bedtime. Adjust dosages if other antihypertensives are added to or deleted from therapy. Maintenance dosage is 500 mg to 2 g daily in two to four divided doses. Maximum recommended daily dose is 3 g. Or, 250 to 500 mg I.V. q 6 hours. Maximum dosage is 1 g q 6 hours. Switch to oral antihypertensives as soon as possible.
Children: Initially, 10 mg/kg P.O. daily in two to four divided doses; or, 20 to 40 mg/kg I.V. daily in four divided doses. Increase dose daily until desired response occurs. Maximum daily dose is 65 mg/kg or 3 g, whichever is less.

Contraindications & cautions

• Contraindicated in patients hypersensitive to drug and in those with active hepatic disease (such as acute hepatitis) or active cirrhosis.
• Contraindicated in those whose previous methyldopa therapy caused liver problems and in those taking MAO inhibitors.
• Use cautiously in patients with history of impaired hepatic function or sulfite sensitivity and in breast-feeding women.

Adverse reactions

CNS: *sedation, headache,* weakness, dizziness, *decreased mental acuity,* paresthesia, parkinsonism, involuntary choreoathetoid movements, psychic disturbances, depression, nightmares.
CV: ***bradycardia****, orthostatic hypotension,* aggravated angina, ***myocarditis****, edema.*
EENT: *nasal congestion.*
GI: nausea, vomiting, diarrhea, ***pancreatitis****, dry mouth,* constipation.
GU: galactorrhea.
Hematologic: hemolytic anemia, ***thrombocytopenia, leukopenia, bone marrow depression.***
Hepatic: ***hepatic necrosis, hepatitis.***
Musculoskeletal: arthralgia.
Skin: rash.
Other: drug-induced fever, gynecomastia.

Interactions

Drug-drug. *Amphetamines, nonselective beta blockers, norepinephrine, phenothiazines, tricyclic antidepressants:* May cause hypertensive effects. Monitor patient closely.
Anesthetics: May need lower doses of anesthetics. Use together cautiously.
Barbiturates: May decrease actions of methyldopa. Monitor patient closely.
Haloperidol: May cause psychomotor retardation, impaired memory, and difficulty concentrating in nonschizophrenic patients; increases sedation. Use together cautiously.
Levodopa: May increase hypotensive effects, which may increase adverse CNS reactions. Monitor patient closely.
Lithium: May increase lithium level. Watch for increased lithium level and signs and symptoms of toxicity.

MAO inhibitors: May cause excessive sympathetic stimulation. Avoid using together.
Tolbutamide: May impair metabolism of tolbutamide. Monitor patient for hypoglycemic effect.
Drug-herb. *Capsicum:* May reduce antihypertensive effectiveness. Discourage use together.

Nursing considerations

- Monitor patient's blood pressure regularly. Elderly patients are more likely to experience hypotension and sedation.
- Occasionally tolerance may occur, usually between the second and third months of therapy. The addition of a diuretic or a dosage adjustment may be needed. Notify prescriber if patient response changes significantly.
- After dialysis, monitor patient for hypertension and notify prescriber, if needed. Patient may need an extra dose of methyldopa.
- Monitor CBC with differential counts before therapy and periodically thereafter.
- Patients who need blood transfusions should have direct and indirect Coombs' tests to prevent crossmatching problems.
- Monitor patient's Coombs' test results. In patients who have received drug for several months, positive reaction to direct Coombs' test indicates hemolytic anemia.
- Observe for and report involuntary choreoathetoid movements. Drug may have to be stopped.

!!ALERT Don't confuse Aldomet with Aldoril or Anzemet.

Patient teaching

- Tell patient not to suddenly stop taking drug, but to notify prescriber if unpleasant adverse reactions occur.
- Instruct patient to report signs and symptoms of infection.
- Tell patient to check his weight daily and to notify prescriber if he gains more than 5 lb. Sodium and water retention may occur but can be relieved with diuretics.
- Warn patient that drug may impair ability to perform tasks that require mental alertness, particularly at start of therapy. A once-daily dose at bedtime minimizes daytime drowsiness.
- Inform patient that low blood pressure and dizziness on standing can be minimized by rising slowly and avoiding sudden position changes. Dry mouth can be relieved by chewing gum or sucking on hard candy or ice chips.
- Tell patient that urine may turn dark if left standing in toilet bowl or if toilet bowl has been treated with bleach.

methylphenidate hydrochloride

Concerta, Metadate CD, Metadate ER, Methylin, Methylin ER, Ritalin, Ritalin LA, Ritalin-SR

Pregnancy risk category NR; C (for Concerta, Metadate CD, Ritalin LA)
Controlled substance schedule II

Indications & dosages

➲ Attention deficit hyperactivity disorder (ADHD)

Children age 6 and older: Initially, 5 mg P.O. b.i.d. immediate-release form before breakfast and lunch, increasing by 5 to 10 mg at weekly intervals, p.r.n., until an optimum daily dosage of 2 mg/kg is reached, not to exceed 60 mg/day. To use Ritalin-SR, Metadate ER, and Methylin ER tablets in place of immediate-release methylphenidate tablets, calculate methylphenidate dosage in 8-hour intervals.

Concerta

Adolescents age 13 to 17 not currently taking methylphenidate, or for patients taking other stimulants: 18 mg P.O. extended-release Concerta once daily in the morning. Adjust dosage by 18 mg at weekly intervals to a maximum of 72 mg P.O. (not to exceed 2 mg/kg) once daily in the morning.

Children age 6 to 12 not currently taking methylphenidate or patients taking stimulants other than methylphenidate: 18 mg P.O. (extended-release) once daily q morning. Adjust dosage by 18 mg at weekly intervals to a maximum of 54 mg daily q morning.

Adolescents and children age 6 and older currently taking methylphenidate: If previous methylphenidate dosage was 5 mg b.i.d. or t.i.d. or 20 mg sustained-release, give 18 mg P.O. q morning. If previous dosage was 10 mg b.i.d. or t.i.d. or 40 mg sustained-release, give 36 mg P.O. q morning. If previous dosage was 15 mg b.i.d. or t.i.d. or 60 mg sustained-release, give 54 mg P.O. q morning. Maximum conversion daily dosage is 54 mg. Once conversion complete, adjust adolescents age 13 to 17 to maximum dose of 72 mg once daily (not to exceed 2 mg/kg).

Metadate CD

Children age 6 and older: Initially, 20 mg P.O. daily before breakfast, increasing by 20 mg at weekly intervals to a maximum of 60 mg daily.

Ritalin LA

Children age 6 and older: 20 mg P.O. once daily. Increase by 10 mg at weekly intervals to a maximum of 60 mg daily. If previous methylphenidate dosage was 10 mg b.i.d. or 20 mg sustained-release, give 20 mg P.O. once daily. If previous methylphenidate dosage was 15 mg b.i.d., give 30 mg P.O. once daily. If previous methylphenidate dosage was 20 mg b.i.d. or 40 mg sustained-release, give 40 mg P.O. once daily. If previous methylphenidate dosage was 30 mg b.i.d. or 60 mg sustained-release, give 60 mg P.O. once daily.

➲ Narcolepsy

Adults: 10 mg P.O. b.i.d. or t.i.d. immediate-release, 30 to 45 minutes before meals. Dosage varies; average is 40 to 60 mg/day. To use Ritalin-SR, Metadate ER, or Methylin ER tablets in place of immediate-release methylphenidate tablets, calculate the dose of methylphenidate in 8-hour intervals.

Contraindications & cautions

- Contraindicated in patients hypersensitive to drug and in those with glaucoma, motor tics, family history or diagnosis of Tourette syndrome, or history of marked anxiety, tension, or agitation.
- Because it doesn't dissolve, Concerta isn't recommended in patients with a history of peritonitis or with severe GI narrowing (such as small bowel inflammatory disease, short-gut syndrome caused by adhesions or decreased transit time, cystic fibrosis, chronic intestinal pseudo-obstruction, or Meckel's diverticulum).
- Ritalin, Ritalin-SR, and Ritalin LA are contraindicated within 14 days of MAO inhibitor therapy.
- Use cautiously in patients with a history of seizures, EEG abnormalities, or hypertension, and in patients whose underlying medical conditions might be compromised by increases in blood pressure or heart rate, such as those with preexisting hypertension, heart failure, recent MI, or hyperthyroidism.
- Use cautiously in patients who are emotionally unstable or who have a history of drug dependence or alcoholism.

Adverse reactions

CNS: *nervousness, insomnia,* tics, dizziness, *headache,* akathisia, dyskinesia, ***seizures,*** drowsiness.
CV: *palpitations, tachycardia,* hypertension, ***arrhythmias.***
EENT: pharyngitis, sinusitis.
GI: nausea, abdominal pain, anorexia, vomiting.
Hematologic: ***thrombocytopenia, thrombocytopenic purpura, leukopenia,*** anemia.
Metabolic: weight loss.
Respiratory: cough, upper respiratory tract infection.
Skin: rash, urticaria, *exfoliative dermatitis,* ***erythema multiforme.***

Interactions

Drug-drug. *Centrally acting alpha$_2$ agonists, clonidine:* May cause serious adverse events. Avoid using together.
Centrally acting antihypertensives: May decrease antihypertensive effect. Monitor blood pressure.
MAO inhibitors: May cause severe hypertension or hypertensive crisis. Avoid using within 14 days of MAO inhibitor therapy.
Tricyclic antidepressants: May increase levels of these drugs. Monitor patient for adverse reactions.
Drug-food. *Caffeine:* May increase amphetamine and related amine effects. Discourage use together.

Nursing considerations

- Don't use drug to prevent fatigue or treat severe depression.
- Drug may trigger Tourette syndrome in children. Monitor patient, especially at start of therapy.
- Observe patient for signs of excessive stimulation. Monitor blood pressure.
- Monitor results of periodic CBC, differential, and platelet counts with long-term use.
- Monitor height and weight in children on long-term therapy. Drug may delay growth spurt, but children will attain normal height when drug is stopped.

- Monitor patient for tolerance or psychological dependence.
- Chewable tablets contain phenylalanine.

!!ALERT Don't confuse Ritalin with Rifadin.

Patient teaching

- Tell patient or caregiver to give last daily dose at least 6 hours before bedtime to prevent insomnia and after meals to reduce appetite-suppressant effects.
- Warn patient against chewing sustained-release tablets.
- Metadate CD may be swallowed whole, or the contents of the capsule may be sprinkled onto a small amount of applesauce and taken immediately.

!!ALERT Warn patient to take chewable tablet with at least 8-oz of water. Not using enough water to swallow tablet may cause the tablet to swell and block the throat, causing choking.

- Caution patient to avoid activities that require alertness or good psychomotor coordination until CNS effects of drug are known.
- Warn patient with seizure disorder that drug may decrease seizure threshold. Urge him to notify prescriber if seizure occurs.
- Advise patient to avoid beverages containing caffeine while taking drug.

methylprednisolone
Medrol

methylprednisolone acetate
depMedalone 40, depMedalone 80, Depo-Medrol, Depopred-40, Depopred-80

methylprednisolone sodium succinate
A-Methapred, Solu-Medrol

Pregnancy risk category C

Indications & dosages

➲ Severe inflammation or immunosuppression

Adults: 2 to 60 mg base P.O. usually in four divided doses, 10 to 80 mg acetate I.M. daily, or 10 to 250 mg succinate I.M. or I.V. up to six times daily. Or, 4 to 40 mg acetate into smaller joints or 20 to 80 mg acetate into larger joints. Intralesional use is usually 20 to 60 mg acetate. Intralesional and intra-articular injections may be repeated q 1 to 5 weeks.

Children: 0.03 to 0.2 mg/kg or 1 to 6.25 mg/m^2 succinate I.M. once daily or b.i.d.

➲ Shock

Adults: 100 to 250 mg succinate I.V. at 2- to 6-hour intervals. Or, 30 mg/kg I.V. initially, repeated q 4 to 6 hours, p.r.n. Give over 3 to 15 minutes. Continue therapy for 2 to 3 days or until patient is stable.

Contraindications & cautions

- Contraindicated in patients hypersensitive to drug or its ingredients, in those with systemic fungal infections, in premature infants (acetate and succinate), and in patients receiving immunosuppressive doses together with live virus vaccines.
- Use cautiously in patients with GI ulceration or renal disease, hypertension, osteoporosis, diabetes mellitus, hypothyroidism, cirrhosis, diverticulitis, nonspecific ulcerative colitis, recent intestinal anastomoses, thromboembolic disorders, seizures, active hepatitis, lactation, myasthenia gravis, heart failure, tuberculosis, ocular herpes simplex, emotional instability, and psychotic tendencies.

Adverse reactions

CNS: *euphoria, insomnia*, psychotic behavior, ***pseudotumor cerebri***, vertigo, headache, paresthesia, ***seizures***.
CV: ***heart failure***, hypertension, edema, ***arrhythmias***, thrombophlebitis, ***thromboembolism, cardiac arrest, circulatory collapse***, after rapid use of large I.V. doses.
EENT: cataracts, glaucoma.
GI: *peptic ulceration*, GI irritation, increased appetite, ***pancreatitis***, nausea, vomiting.
GU: menstrual irregularities, increased urine calcium levels.
Metabolic: hypokalemia, hyperglycemia, carbohydrate intolerance, hypercholesterolemia, hypocalcemia.
Musculoskeletal: growth suppression in children, muscle weakness, osteoporosis.
Skin: hirsutism, delayed wound healing, acne, various skin eruptions.
Other: cushingoid state, susceptibility to infections, ***acute adrenal insufficiency after increased stress or abrupt withdrawal after long-term therapy***.

After abrupt withdrawal: rebound inflammation, fatigue, weakness, arthralgia, fever, dizziness, lethargy, depression, fainting, orthostatic hypotension, dyspnea, anorexia, hypoglycemia. After prolonged use, sudden withdrawal may be fatal.

Interactions

Drug-drug. *Aspirin, indomethacin, other NSAIDs:* May increase risk of GI distress and bleeding. Use together cautiously.
Barbiturates, carbamazepine, phenytoin, rifampin: May decrease corticosteroid effect. Increase corticosteroid dosage.
Cyclosporine: May increase toxicity. Monitor patient closely.
Ketoconazole and macrolide antibiotics: May decrease methylprednisolone clearance. Decreased dose may be required.
Oral anticoagulants: May alter dosage requirements. Monitor PT and INR closely.
Potassium-depleting drugs such as thiazide diuretics: May enhance potassium-wasting effects of methylprednisolone. Monitor potassium level.
Salicylates: May decrease salicylate levels. Monitor patient for lack of salicylate effectiveness.
Skin-test antigens: May decrease response. Postpone skin testing until after therapy.
Toxoids, vaccines: May decrease antibody response and may increase risk of neurologic complications. Avoid using together.
Drug-herb. *Echinacea:* May increase immune-stimulating effects. Discourage use together.
Ginseng: May increase immune-modulating response. Discourage use together.

Nursing considerations

- Determine whether patient is sensitive to other corticosteroids.
- Medrol may contain tartrazine.
- Drug may be used for alternate-day therapy.
- Most adverse reactions to corticosteroids are dose- or duration-dependent.
- For better results and less toxicity, give a once-daily dose in the morning.
- Give oral dose with food when possible. Critically ill patients may need to take drug together with antacid or H_2-receptor antagonist.

!!ALERT Salt formulations aren't interchangeable.

!!ALERT Don't give Solu-Medrol intrathecally because severe adverse reactions may occur.

- Give I.M. injection deeply into gluteal muscle. Avoid S.C. injection because atrophy and sterile abscesses may occur.
- Dermal atrophy may occur with large doses of acetate salt. Use several small injections rather than a single large dose, and rotate injection sites.
- Don't use acetate if immediate onset of action is needed.
- Discard reconstituted solution after 48 hours.
- Always adjust to lowest effective dose.
- Monitor patient's weight, blood pressure, electrolyte level, and sleep patterns. Euphoria may initially interfere with sleep, but patients typically adjust to therapy in 1 to 3 weeks.
- Monitor patient for cushingoid effects, including moon face, buffalo hump, central obesity, thinning hair, hypertension, and increased susceptibility to infection.
- Drug may mask or worsen infections, including latent amebiasis.
- Watch for depression or psychotic episodes, especially in high-dose therapy.
- Diabetic patient may need increased insulin; monitor glucose level.
- Watch for an enhanced response to drug in patients with hypothyroidism or cirrhosis.
- Watch for allergic reaction to tartrazine in patients with sensitivity to aspirin.
- Unless contraindicated, give low-sodium diet that's high in potassium and protein. Give potassium supplements, as needed.
- Elderly patients may be more susceptible to osteoporosis with prolonged use.
- Gradually reduce dosage after long-term therapy.

!!ALERT Don't confuse Solu-Medrol with Solu-Cortef (hydrocortisone sodium succinate) or methylprednisolone with medroxyprogesterone.

Patient teaching

- Tell patient not to stop drug abruptly or without prescriber's consent.
- Instruct patient to take oral form of drug with milk or food.
- Teach patient signs and symptoms of early adrenal insufficiency: fatigue, muscle weakness, joint pain, fever, anorexia, nausea,

shortness of breath, dizziness, and fainting.
- Instruct patient to carry or wear medical identification indicating his need for supplemental systemic glucocorticoids during stress. This card should contain prescriber's name, name of drug, and dosage taken.
- Warn patient on long-term therapy about cushingoid effects (moon face, buffalo hump) and the need to notify prescriber about sudden weight gain or swelling.
- Advise patient receiving long-term therapy to consider exercise or physical therapy. Also, tell patient to ask prescriber about vitamin D or calcium supplement.
- Instruct patient to avoid exposure to infections (such as chickenpox or measles) and to contact prescriber if such exposure occurs.

methyltestosterone
Android, Metandren†, Methitest, Testred, Virilon

Pregnancy risk category X
Controlled substance schedule III

Indications & dosages
➲ **Breast cancer in women 1 to 5 years postmenopausal**
Women: 50 to 200 mg P.O. daily or 25 to 100 mg buccally daily.
➲ **Male hypogonadism**
Men: 10 to 50 mg P.O. daily or 5 to 25 mg buccally daily.
➲ **Postpubertal cryptorchidism**
Men: 30 mg P.O. daily or 15 mg buccally daily.

Contraindications & cautions
- Contraindicated in pregnant or breast-feeding women and in men with breast or prostate cancer.
- Contraindicated in patients with cardiac, hepatic, or renal disease.
- Use cautiously in elderly patients; patients with cardiac, renal, or hepatic disease; and healthy males with delayed puberty.

Adverse reactions
CNS: headache, anxiety, depression, paresthesia.
CV: edema.
GI: irritation of oral mucosa with buccal administration, nausea.
Hematologic: ***suppression of clotting factors***, polycythemia.
Hepatic: reversible jaundice, ***cholestatic hepatitis***.
Metabolic: hypernatremia, hyperkalemia, hyperphosphatemia, hypercholesterolemia, hypercalcemia.
Musculoskeletal: muscle cramps or spasms.
Skin: hypersensitivity reactions.
Other: androgenic effects in women, altered libido, *hypoestrogenic effects in women*, excessive hormonal effects in men.

Interactions
Drug-drug. *Hepatotoxic drugs:* May increase risk of hepatotoxicity. Monitor liver function closely.
Imipramine: May cause dramatic paranoid response. Monitor patient closely.
Insulin, oral antidiabetics: May decrease glucose level; may alter dosage requirements. Monitor glucose level in diabetic patients.
Oral anticoagulants: May increase sensitivity to oral anticoagulants; may alter dosage requirements. Monitor PT and INR.

Nursing considerations
- Don't give to woman of childbearing age until pregnancy is ruled out.
- In children, obtain X-rays of wrist bones before therapy begins to establish bone maturation level. During treatment, bones may mature more rapidly than they grow in length. Periodically review X-rays to monitor bone maturation.
- Buccal tablets are twice as potent as oral tablets.
- Drug is typically used only for intermittent therapy. Because of potential hepatotoxicity, watch closely for jaundice.
- Promptly report evidence of virilization in women, such as deepening of the voice, increased hair growth, acne, or baldness.
- Watch for hypoestrogenic effects in women (flushing, diaphoresis, vaginal bleeding, nervousness, emotional lability, menstrual irregularities, and vaginitis, including itching, dryness, and burning).
- Watch for excessive hormonal effects in men. If patient is prepubertal, watch for premature epiphyseal closure, acne, priapism, growth of body and facial hair, and phallic

enlargement. If he's postpubertal, watch for testicular atrophy, oligospermia, decreased ejaculatory volume, impotence, gynecomastia, and epididymitis.
- Unless contraindicated, use with high-calorie, high-protein diet. Give small, frequent meals.
- Periodically check cholesterol, calcium, and hemoglobin levels, hematocrit, and cardiac and liver function test results.
- Check weight regularly. Control edema with sodium restriction or diuretics.

!!ALERT Therapeutic response in breast cancer usually occurs within 3 months. Drug should be stopped if signs of disease progression appear.
- Report signs of hypercalcemia. In metastatic breast cancer, hypercalcemia may indicate progression of bone metastases.
- Evaluate semen every 3 to 4 months, especially in adolescent boys.

!!ALERT Don't use to enhance athletic performance or physique.

!!ALERT Testosterone and methyltestosterone aren't interchangeable. Don't confuse methyltestosterone with medroxyprogesterone.

Patient teaching

- Make sure patient understands importance of using effective contraception during therapy.
- Tell woman of childbearing age to report menstrual irregularities and to stop drug while awaiting examination.
- Instruct patient to stop drug immediately and notify prescriber if pregnancy is suspected.
- Tell patient to place buccal tablet in upper or lower buccal pouch between cheek and gum; tablet needs 30 to 60 minutes to dissolve. Tell patient not to eat, drink, chew, or smoke while buccal tablet is in place and not to swallow tablet.
- Instruct patient to change buccal tablet absorption site with each dose to minimize risk of irritation. Advise patient to rinse mouth after using buccal tablet.
- Tell woman to immediately report evidence of virilization, such as acne, swelling, weight gain, increased hair growth, hoarseness, clitoral enlargement, decreased breast size, deepening of voice, changes in libido, male-pattern baldness, and oily skin or hair.
- Teach patient signs and symptoms of low blood glucose (hypoglycemia) and method for checking glucose level; drug enhances hypoglycemia. Instruct patient to report signs or symptoms of hypoglycemia immediately.
- Advise woman to wear cotton underwear and to wash after intercourse to decrease risk of vaginitis.

metoclopramide hydrochloride
Apo-Metoclop†, Clopra, Maxeran†, Octamide PFS, Reglan

Pregnancy risk category B

Indications & dosages

➲ To prevent or reduce nausea and vomiting from emetogenic cancer chemotherapy

Adults: 1 to 2 mg/kg I.V. 30 minutes before chemotherapy; repeat q 2 hours for two doses, then q 3 hours for three doses.

➲ To prevent or reduce postoperative nausea and vomiting

Adults: 10 to 20 mg I.M. near end of surgical procedure; repeat q 4 to 6 hours, p.r.n.

➲ To facilitate small-bowel intubation, to aid in radiologic examinations

Adults and children older than age 14: 10 mg or 2 ml I.V. as a single dose over 1 to 2 minutes.

Children ages 6 to 14: 2.5 to 5 mg or 0.5 to 1 ml I.V.

Children younger than age 6: 0.1 mg/kg I.V.

➲ Delayed gastric emptying secondary to diabetic gastroparesis

Adults: 10 mg P.O. 30 minutes before each meal and h.s. for mild symptoms. Give by slow I.V. infusion over 1 to 2 minutes 30 minutes before each meal and h.s. for up to 10 days for severe symptoms; then P.O. dose may be started and continued for 2 to 8 weeks.

➲ Gastroesophageal reflux disease

Adults: 10 to 15 mg P.O. q.i.d., p.r.n., 30 minutes before meals and h.s.

For patients with creatinine clearance below 40 ml/minute, decrease dosage by half.

➲ Emesis during pregnancy♦

Adults: 5 to 10 mg P.O. or 5 to 20 mg I.V. or I.M. t.i.d.

Contraindications & cautions

- Contraindicated in patients hypersensitive to drug and in those with pheochromocytoma or seizure disorders.
- Contraindicated in patients for whom stimulation of GI motility might be dangerous (those with hemorrhage, obstruction, or perforation).
- Use cautiously in patients with history of depression, Parkinson's disease, or hypertension.

Adverse reactions

CNS: *restlessness, anxiety, drowsiness, fatigue, lassitude,* fever, depression, akathisia, insomnia, confusion, ***suicide ideation, seizures, neuroleptic malignant syndrome,*** hallucinations, headache, dizziness, extrapyramidal symptoms, tardive dyskinesia, *dystonic reactions.*
CV: transient hypertension, hypotension, ***supraventricular tachycardia, bradycardia.***
GI: nausea, bowel disorders, diarrhea.
GU: urinary frequency, incontinence.
Hematologic: ***neutropenia, agranulocytosis.***
Skin: rash, urticaria.
Other: prolactin secretion, loss of libido.

Interactions

Drug-drug. *Anticholinergics, opioid analgesics:* May antagonize GI motility effects of metoclopramide. Use together cautiously.
CNS depressants: May cause additive CNS effects. Avoid using together.
Levodopa: Levodopa and metoclopramide have opposite effects on dopamine receptors. Avoid using together.
MAO inhibitors: May increase release of catecholamines in patients with hypertension. Use together cautiously.
Phenothiazines: May increase risk of extrapyramidal effects. Monitor patient closely.
Drug-lifestyle. *Alcohol use:* May cause additive CNS effects. Discourage use together.

Nursing considerations

- Monitor bowel sounds.
- Safety and effectiveness of drug haven't been established for therapy lasting longer than 12 weeks.
- When oral solution is used (10 mg/ml) dilute in pudding, applesauce, juice, or water just before using.

!!ALERT Use diphenhydramine 25 mg I.V. to counteract extrapyramidal adverse effects from high metoclopramide doses.

Patient teaching

- Tell patient to avoid activities that require alertness for 2 hours after doses.
- Urge patient to report persistent or serious adverse reactions promptly.
- Advise patient to avoid alcohol ingestion during therapy.

metolazone
Zaroxolyn

Pregnancy risk category B

Indications & dosages

➲ **Edema in heart failure or renal disease**
Adults: 5 to 20 mg P.O. daily.
➲ **Hypertension**
Adults: 2.5 to 5 mg P.O. daily. Base maintenance dosage on blood pressure.

Contraindications & cautions

- Contraindicated in patients hypersensitive to thiazides or other sulfonamide-derived drugs and in those with anuria, hepatic coma, or precoma.
- Use cautiously in patients with impaired renal or hepatic function.

Adverse reactions

CNS: *dizziness,* headache, fatigue, vertigo, paresthesia, weakness, restlessness, drowsiness, anxiety, depression, nervousness, blurred vision.
CV: orthostatic hypotension, palpitations, vasculitis.
GI: anorexia, nausea, ***pancreatitis,*** epigastric distress, vomiting, abdominal pain, diarrhea, constipation, dry mouth.
GU: nocturia, polyuria, impotence.
Hematologic: ***aplastic anemia, agranulocytosis, leukopenia,*** purpura.
Hepatic: jaundice, ***hepatitis.***
Metabolic: hyperglycemia and impaired glucose tolerance, fluid and electrolyte imbalances, including hypokalemia, hypomagnesemia, dilutional hyponatremia and hypochloremia, metabolic alkalosis, and hypercalcemia, volume depletion and dehydration.
Musculoskeletal: muscle cramps.

Skin: dermatitis, photosensitivity reactions, rash, pruritus, urticaria.

Interactions

Drug-drug. *Amphotericin B, corticosteroids:* May increase risk of hypokalemia. Monitor potassium level closely.
Anticoagulants: May affect hypoprothrombinemic response. Monitor PT and INR.
Antidiabetics: May alter glucose level requiring dosage adjustment of antidiabetics. Monitor glucose level.
Barbiturates, opioids: May increase orthostatic hypotensive effect. Monitor patient closely.
Bumetanide, ethacrynic acid, furosemide, torsemide: May cause excessive diuretic response, causing serious electrolyte abnormalities or dehydration. Adjust doses carefully, and monitor patient closely for signs and symptoms of excessive diuretic response.
Cardiac glycosides: May increase risk of digoxin toxicity from metolazone-induced hypokalemia. Monitor potassium and digoxin levels.
Cholestyramine, colestipol: May decrease intestinal absorption of thiazides. Separate doses.
Diazoxide: May increase antihypertensive, hyperglycemic, and hyperuricemic effects. Use together cautiously.
Lithium: May decrease lithium clearance, increasing risk of lithium toxicity. Monitor lithium level.
NSAIDs: May increase risk of NSAID-induced renal failure. Monitor patient for signs of renal failure.
Other antihypertensives: May have additive effects. Use together cautiously.
Drug-herb. *Dandelion:* May interfere with diuretic activity. Discourage use together.
Licorice: May cause unexpected rapid potassium loss. Discourage use together.
Drug-lifestyle. *Alcohol use:* May increase orthostatic hypotensive effect. Discourage use together.
Sun exposure: May increase risk for photosensitivity reaction. Advise patient to avoid excessive sunlight exposure.

Nursing considerations

- To prevent nocturia, give drug in the morning.
- Monitor fluid intake and output, weight, blood pressure, and electrolyte levels.
- Watch for signs and symptoms of hypokalemia, such as muscle weakness and cramps. Drug may be used with potassium-sparing diuretic to prevent potassium loss.
- Consult prescriber and dietitian about a high-potassium diet. Foods rich in potassium include citrus fruits, tomatoes, bananas, dates, and apricots.
- Monitor glucose level, especially in diabetic patients.
- Monitor uric acid level, especially in patients with history of gout.
- Monitor elderly patients, who are especially susceptible to excessive diuresis.
- In hypertensive patients, therapeutic response may be delayed several weeks.
- Monitor blood pressure. If response is inadequate, another antihypertensive may be added.
- Metolazone and furosemide may be used together to enhance diuretic effect.
- Unlike thiazide diuretics, metolazone is effective in patients with decreased renal function.
- Stop thiazides and thiazide-like diuretics before parathyroid function tests.

!!ALERT Don't confuse Zaroxolyn with Zarontin.

Patient teaching

- Tell patient to take drug in morning to prevent need to urinate at night.
- Advise patient to avoid sudden posture changes and to rise slowly to avoid effects of dizziness upon standing quickly.
- Instruct patient to use a sunblock to prevent photosensitivity reactions.

metoprolol succinate
Toprol-XL

metoprolol tartrate
Apo-Metoprolol†, Apo-Metoprolol (Type L)†, Betaloc Durules†, Lopresor†, Lopresor SR†, Lopressor, Novo-Metoprol†, Nu-Metop†

Pregnancy risk category C

Indications & dosages

➲ Hypertension
Adults: Initially, 50 mg P.O. b.i.d. or 100 mg P.O. once daily; then up to 100 to 450 mg daily in two or three divided doses. Or, 50 to 100 mg of extended-release tablets (tartrate equivalent) once daily. Adjust dosage as needed and tolerated at intervals of not less than 1 week to maximum of 400 mg daily.

➲ Early intervention in acute MI
Adults: 5 mg metoprolol tartrate I.V. bolus q 2 minutes for three doses. Then, 15 minutes after the last I.V. dose, give 25 to 50 mg P.O. q 6 hours for 48 hours. Maintenance dosage is 100 mg P.O. b.i.d.

➲ Angina pectoris
Adults: Initially, 100 mg P.O. daily as a single dose or in two equally divided doses; increased at weekly intervals until an adequate response or a pronounced decrease in heart rate is seen. Effects of daily dose beyond 400 mg aren't known. Or, give 100 mg of extended-release tablets (tartrate equivalent) once daily. Adjust dosage as needed and tolerated at intervals of not less than 1 week to maximum of 400 mg daily.

➲ Stable symptomatic heart failure (New York Heart Association class II) resulting from ischemia, hypertension, or cardiomyopathy
Adults: 25 mg Toprol-XL P.O. once daily for 2 weeks. Double the dose q 2 weeks, as tolerated, to a maximum of 200 mg daily.

In patients with more severe heart failure, start with 12.5 mg Toprol-XL P.O. once daily for 2 weeks.

Contraindications & cautions

- Contraindicated in patients hypersensitive to drug or other beta blockers.
- Contraindicated in patients with sinus bradycardia, greater than first-degree heart block, cardiogenic shock, or overt cardiac failure when used to treat hypertension or angina. When used to treat MI, drug is contraindicated in patients with heart rate less than 45 beats/minute, greater than first-degree heart block, PR interval of 0.24 second or longer with first-degree heart block, systolic blood pressure less than 100 mm Hg, or moderate to severe cardiac failure.
- Use cautiously in patients with heart failure, diabetes, or respiratory or hepatic disease.

Adverse reactions

CNS: *fatigue, dizziness,* depression.
CV: ***bradycardia***, *hypotension*, ***heart failure, AV block***.
GI: nausea, diarrhea.
Respiratory: dyspnea.
Skin: rash.

Interactions

Drug-drug. *Amobarbital, aprobarbital, butabarbital, butalbital, mephobarbital, pentobarbital, phenobarbital, primidone, secobarbital:* May reduce metoprolol effect. May need to increase beta-blocker dose.
Cardiac glycosides, diltiazem: May cause excessive bradycardia and increased depressant effect on myocardium. Use together cautiously.
Catecholamine-depleting drugs, such as MAO inhibitors, reserpine: May have additive effect. Monitor patient for hypotension and bradycardia.
Chlorpromazine: May decrease hepatic clearance. Watch for greater beta-blocking effect.
Cimetidine: May increase beta-blocker effects. Consider another H_2 agonist or decrease dose of beta blocker.
Hydralazine: May increase levels and effects of both drugs. Monitor patient closely. May need to adjust dosage.
Indomethacin, NSAIDs: May decrease antihypertensive effect. Monitor blood pressure and adjust dosage.
Insulin, oral antidiabetics: May alter dosage requirements in previously stabilized diabetic patients. Monitor patient closely.
I.V. lidocaine: May reduce hepatic metabolism of lidocaine, increasing risk of toxicity. Give bolus doses of lidocaine at a slower rate, and monitor lidocaine level closely.

Prazosin: May increase risk of orthostatic hypotension in the early phases of use together. Assist patient to stand slowly until effects are known.
Propafenone: May increase metoprolol level. Monitor vital signs.
Rifampin: May increase metoprolol metabolism. Watch for decreased effect.
Terbutaline: May antagonize bronchodilatory effects of terbutaline. Monitor patient.
Verapamil: May increase effects of both drugs. Monitor cardiac function closely, and decrease dosages as needed.
Drug-herb. *Ma huang:* May decrease antihypertensive effects. Discourage use together.
Drug-food. *Any food:* May increase absorption. Encourage patient to take drug with food.

Nursing considerations

- Always check patient's apical pulse rate before giving drug. If it's slower than 60 beats/minute, withhold drug and call prescriber immediately.
- Monitor glucose level closely in diabetic patients because drug masks common signs and symptoms of hypoglycemia.
- Monitor blood pressure frequently; metoprolol masks common signs and symptoms of shock.
- Beta blockers may mask tachycardia caused by hyperthyroidism. In patients with suspected thyrotoxicosis, withdraw beta blocker gradually to avoid thyroid storm.
- When therapy is stopped, reduce dose gradually over 1 to 2 weeks.
- Store drug at room temperature and protect from light. Discard solution if it's discolored or contains particles.
- Beta selectivity is lost at higher doses. Watch for peripheral side effects.

!!ALERT Don't confuse metoprolol with metaproterenol or metolazone.
!!ALERT Don't confuse Toprol with Topamax.

Patient teaching

- Instruct patient to take drug exactly as prescribed and to take it with meals.
- Caution patient to avoid driving and other tasks requiring mental alertness until response to therapy has been established.
- Advise patient to inform dentist or prescriber about use of this drug before procedures or surgery.
- Tell patient to alert prescriber if shortness of breath occurs.
- Instruct patient not to stop drug suddenly but to notify prescriber about unpleasant adverse reactions. Inform him that drug must be withdrawn gradually over 1 or 2 weeks.
- Inform patient that metoprolol isn't advised in breast-feeding women.

metronidazole (systemic)

Apo-Metronidazole†, Flagyl, Flagyl 375, Flagyl ER, Novo-Nidazol†, Protostat, Trikacide†

metronidazole hydrochloride

Flagyl IV RTU, Novo-Nidazol†

Pregnancy risk category B

Indications & dosages

➲ Amebic liver abscess
Adults: 500 to 750 mg P.O. t.i.d. for 5 to 10 days; or 2.4 g P.O. once daily for 1 to 2 days. Or, 500 mg I.V. q 6 hours for 10 days if patient can't tolerate P.O. route.
Children: 30 to 50 mg/kg daily in three divided doses for 10 days. Maximum, 750 mg/dose.

➲ Intestinal amebiasis
Adults: 750 mg P.O. t.i.d. for 5 to 10 days; then treat with a luminal amebicide, such as iodoquinol or paromomycin.
Children: 30 to 50 mg/kg daily in three divided doses for 10 days; then treat with a luminal amebicide, such as iodoquinol or paromomycin.

➲ Trichomoniasis
Adults: 250 mg P.O. t.i.d. for 7 days, or 500 mg P.O. b.i.d. for 7 days, or 2 g P.O. in single dose (may give the 2-g dose in two 1-g doses, both on the same day); 4 to 6 weeks should elapse before repeat courses of therapy are given.
Children: 5 mg/kg P.O. t.i.d. for 7 days.

➲ Refractory trichomoniasis
Adults: 250 mg P.O. b.i.d. for 10 days. Or, 500 mg P.O. b.i.d. for 7 days.

➲ Bacterial infections caused by anaerobic microorganisms
Adults: Loading dose is 15 mg/kg I.V. infused over 1 hour. Maintenance dose is 7.5 mg/kg I.V. or P.O. q 6 hours. Give first maintenance dose 6 hours after loading

dose. Maximum dose shouldn't exceed 4 g daily.

➲ **To prevent postoperative infection in contaminated or potentially contaminated colorectal surgery**
Adults: 15 mg/kg I.V. infused over 30 to 60 minutes and completed about 1 hour before surgery. Then, 7.5 mg/kg I.V. infused over 30 to 60 minutes at 6 and 12 hours after first dose.

➲ **Bacterial vaginosis (Flagyl ER only)**
Adults: 750 mg (extended-release) P.O. daily for 7 days.

➲ ***Clostridium difficile*–associated diarrhea and colitis♦**
Adults: Usually 250 mg P.O. q.i.d. or 500 mg P.O. t.i.d. for 10 days. Or, 500 mg to 750 mg I.V. q 6 to 8 hours when P.O. route isn't practical.
Children: 30 to 50 mg/kg/day P.O. given in three to four equally divided doses for 7 to 10 days. Don't exceed adult dose.

➲ **Pelvic inflammatory disease (PID)♦**
Adults: 500 mg I.V. q 8 hours with ofloxacin or with I.V. levofloxacin. For ambulatory patients, 500 mg P.O. b.i.d. with ofloxacin for 14 days.

➲ **Bacterial vaginosis♦**
Nonpregnant women: 250 mg P.O. t.i.d. or 500 mg P.O. b.i.d. for 7 days. Or, 2 g P.O. as a single dose.
Pregnant women: 250 mg P.O. t.i.d. for 7 days or 2 g P.O. as a single dose.

Contraindications & cautions

- Contraindicated in patients hypersensitive to drug or other nitroimidazole derivatives and in patients in first trimester of pregnancy.

‼ALERT Although contraindicated in the first trimester of pregnancy, if drug must be taken by a pregnant patient to treat trichomoniasis, the 7-day regimen is preferred over the 2-g, single-dose regimen because the 2-g dose produces a high serum level that's more likely to reach the fetal circulation.

- Use cautiously in patients with history of blood dyscrasia, CNS disorder, or retinal or visual field changes.
- Use cautiously in patients who take hepatotoxic drugs or have hepatic disease or alcoholism.

Adverse reactions

CNS: fever, vertigo, *headache*, ataxia, dizziness, syncope, incoordination, confusion, irritability, depression, weakness, insomnia, ***seizures***, peripheral neuropathy.
CV: flattened T wave, edema, flushing, thrombophlebitis after I.V. infusion.
EENT: rhinitis, sinusitis, pharyngitis.
GI: abdominal cramping or pain, stomatitis, epigastric distress, *nausea*, vomiting, anorexia, diarrhea, constipation, proctitis, dry mouth, metallic taste.
GU: darkened urine, polyuria, dysuria, cystitis, dyspareunia, dryness of vagina and vulva, vaginal candidiasis, *vaginitis*, genital pruritus.
Hematologic: ***transient leukopenia***, ***neutropenia***.
Musculoskeletal: fleeting joint pains.
Respiratory: upper respiratory tract infection.
Skin: rash.
Other: decreased libido, overgrowth of nonsusceptible organisms, especially ***Candida*** .

Interactions

Drug-drug. *Cimetidine:* May increase risk of metronidazole toxicity because of inhibited hepatic metabolism. Monitor patient for toxicity.
Disulfiram: May cause acute psychosis and confusion. Avoid giving metronidazole within 2 weeks of disulfiram.
Lithium: May increase lithium level, which may cause toxicity. Monitor lithium level.
Oral anticoagulants: May increase anticoagulant effects. Monitor PT and INR periodically.
Phenobarbital, phenytoin: May decrease metronidazole effectiveness; may reduce total phenytoin clearance. Monitor patient.
Drug-lifestyle. *Alcohol use:* May cause disulfiram-like reaction, including nausea, vomiting, headache, cramps, and flushing. Warn patient to avoid alcohol during and for 3 days after completing drug therapy.

Nursing considerations

- Monitor liver function test results carefully in elderly patients.
- Give oral form with meals.
- Observe patient for edema, especially if he's receiving corticosteroids; Flagyl IV RTU may cause sodium retention.

• Record number and character of stools when drug is used to treat amebiasis. Give metronidazole only after *Trichomonas vaginalis* infection is confirmed by wet smear or culture or *Entameba histolytica* is identified.
• Symptomatic and asymptomatic sexual partners of patients being treated for *T. vaginalis* infection must be treated simultaneously to avoid reinfection.

Patient teaching

• Instruct patient to take extended-release tablets from at least 1 hour before or 2 hours after meals but to take all other oral forms with food to minimize GI upset.
• Inform patient of need for sexual partners to be treated simultaneously to avoid reinfection.
• Instruct patient in proper hygiene.
• Tell patient to avoid alcohol and alcohol-containing drugs during and for at least 3 days after treatment course.
• Tell patient he may experience a metallic taste and have dark or red-brown urine.
• Tell patient to report to prescriber symptoms of candidal overgrowth.
• Tell patient to report to prescriber immediately any neurologic symptoms (seizures, peripheral neuropathy).

metronidazole (topical)

MetroCream, MetroGel, MetroGel Vaginal, MetroLotion, Noritate

Pregnancy risk category B

Indications & dosages

➲ Inflammatory papules and pustules of acne rosacea

Adults: Apply thin film to affected area b.i.d., morning and evening. Frequency and duration of therapy are adjusted after response is seen. Results are usually noticed within 3 weeks.

➲ Bacterial vaginosis

Adults: 1 applicatorful intravaginally daily or b.i.d. for 5 days. For once-daily use, give h.s.

Contraindications & cautions

• Contraindicated in patients hypersensitive to drug or its ingredients, such as parabens, and other nitroimidazole derivatives.
• Use cautiously in patients with history or evidence of blood dyscrasia and in those with severe hepatic disease.
• Use vaginal gel cautiously in patients with history of CNS diseases. Oral form may cause seizures and peripheral neuropathy.

Adverse reactions

Topical forms

EENT: lacrimation if applied around eyes.
Skin: rash, *transient redness, dryness, mild burning, stinging.*

Vaginal form

GI: cramps, pain, nausea, metallic or bad taste in mouth.
GU: *cervicitis, vaginitis,* perineal and vulvovaginal itching.
Skin: *transient redness, dryness, mild burning, stinging.*
Other: overgrowth of nonsusceptible organisms.

Interactions

Drug-drug. *Disulfiram:* May cause disulfiram-like reaction when used with vaginal form. Avoid using together and wait 2 weeks after stopping disulfiram before starting metronidazole vaginal therapy.
Lithium: May increase lithium level. Monitor lithium level.
Oral anticoagulants: May increase anticoagulant effect. Monitor patient for adverse reactions.
Drug-lifestyle. *Alcohol use:* May cause disulfiram-like reaction when used with vaginal form. Discourage use together.

Nursing considerations

• Topical therapy hasn't been linked to adverse effects observed with parenteral or oral therapy, but some drug may be absorbed after topical use.
• Don't use vaginal gel in patients who have taken disulfiram within past 2 weeks.

Patient teaching

• Instruct patient to avoid use of topical gel around eyes.
• Advise patient to clean area thoroughly before use and to wait 15 to 20 minutes after cleaning skin before applying drug to minimize risk of local irritation. Cosmetics may be used after applying drug.

• If local reactions occur, advise patient to apply drug less frequently or stop using it and notify prescriber.
• Advise patient to avoid sexual intercourse while using vaginal preparation.
• Caution patient to avoid alcohol while being treated with vaginal preparation.

mexiletine hydrochloride
Mexitil

Pregnancy risk category C

Indications & dosages

➲ Life-threatening ventricular arrhythmias, including ventricular tachycardia and PVCs
Adults: Initially, 200 mg P.O. q 8 hours. If satisfactory control isn't obtained at this dosage, increase dosage by 50 to 100 mg q 2 to 3 days up to maximum of 400 mg q 8 hours. If rapid control of ventricular rate is desired, give a loading dose of 400 mg P.O., followed by 200 mg 8 hours later. Patients controlled on 300 mg or less q 8 hours can receive the total daily dose in evenly divided doses q 12 hours.

Contraindications & cautions

• Contraindicated in patients with cardiogenic shock or second- or third-degree AV block in the absence of an artificial pacemaker.
• Use cautiously in patients with first-degree heart block, a ventricular pacemaker, sinus node dysfunction, intraventricular conduction disturbances, hypotension, severe heart failure, or seizure disorder.

Adverse reactions

CNS: *tremor, dizziness,* confusion, *lightheadedness, incoordination,* changes in sleep habits, paresthesia, weakness, fatigue, speech difficulties, depression, *nervousness,* headache.
CV: NEW OR WORSENED ARRHYTHMIAS, palpitations, chest pain, nonspecific edema, angina.
EENT: blurred vision, diplopia, tinnitus.
GI: *nausea, vomiting, upper GI distress, heartburn,* diarrhea, constipation, dry mouth, changes in appetite, abdominal pain.
Skin: rash.

Interactions

Drug-drug. *Antacids, atropine, narcotics:* May slow mexiletine absorption. Monitor patient for effectiveness.
Cimetidine: May alter mexiletine level. Monitor patient.
Methylxanthines (such as caffeine, theophylline): May reduce methylxanthine clearance, which may cause toxicity. Monitor drug level.
Metoclopramide: May speed up mexiletine absorption. Monitor patient for toxicity.
Phenobarbital, phenytoin, rifampin, urine acidifiers: May decrease mexiletine level. Monitor patient for effectiveness.
Urine alkalinizers: May increase mexiletine level. Monitor patient for adverse reactions.

Nursing considerations

• When changing from lidocaine to mexiletine, stop the lidocaine infusion when the first mexiletine dose is given. But keep the infusion line open until the arrhythmia is satisfactorily controlled.
• Give oral dose with meals or antacids to lessen GI distress.
• If patient may be a good candidate for every-12-hour therapy, notify prescriber. Twice-daily dosage enhances compliance.
• Monitor therapeutic drug level, which may range from 0.5 to 2 mcg/ml.
• An early sign of mexiletine toxicity is tremor, usually a fine tremor of the hands, progressing to dizziness and then to ataxia and nystagmus as drug level in the blood increases. Watch for and ask patients about these symptoms.
• Monitor blood pressure and heart rate and rhythm frequently. Notify prescriber of significant change.

Patient teaching

• Tell patient to take drug exactly as prescribed and to take with food or antacids if GI reactions occur.
• Instruct patient to report adverse reactions promptly.
• Advise patient to notify prescriber if he develops jaundice, fever, or general tiredness; these symptoms may indicate liver damage.

micafungin sodium
Mycamine

Pregnancy risk category C

Indications & dosages

➲ Esophageal candidiasis
Adults: 150 mg I.V. daily for 10 to 30 days.

➲ To prevent candidal infection in hematopoietic stem cell transplant recipients
Adults: 50 mg I.V. daily for 6 to 51 days.

Contraindications & cautions

- Contraindicated in patients hypersensitive to drug.
- Use cautiously in patients with severe hepatic disease.

Adverse reactions

CNS: headache.
GI: abdominal pain, diarrhea, nausea, vomiting.
Hematologic: anemia, ***leukopenia***, ***neutropenia***, ***thrombocytopenia***.
Metabolic: hypocalcemia, hypokalemia, hypomagnesemia, hypophosphatemia.
Skin: infusion site inflammation, phlebitis, pruritus, rash.
Other: pyrexia, rigors.

Interactions

Drug-drug. *Nifedipine:* May increase nifedipine level. Monitor blood pressure, and decrease nifedipine dose if needed.
Sirolimus: May increase sirolimus level. Monitor patient for evidence of toxicity, and decrease sirolimus dose if needed.

Nursing considerations

- Injection site reactions occur more often in patients receiving drug by peripheral I.V.
- To reduce the risk of histamine-mediated reactions, infuse drug over at least 1 hour.

!!ALERT If patient develops signs of serious hypersensitivity reaction, including shock, stop infusion and notify prescriber.

- Monitor hepatic and renal function during therapy.
- Monitor patient for hemolysis and hemolytic anemia.
- Use drug in pregnant women only if clearly needed.
- It's unknown whether drug appears in breast milk. Use cautiously in breast-feeding women.

Patient teaching

- Advise patient to report pain or redness at infusion site.
- Tell patient to expect laboratory tests to monitor his hematologic, renal, and hepatic function.

midazolam hydrochloride
Versed, Versed Syrup

Pregnancy risk category D
Controlled substance schedule IV

Indications & dosages

➲ Preoperative sedation (to induce sleepiness or drowsiness and relieve apprehension)
Adults: 0.07 to 0.08 mg/kg I.M. about 1 hour before surgery.

➲ Conscious sedation before short diagnostic or endoscopic procedures
Adults younger than age 60: Initially, small dose not to exceed 2.5 mg I.V. given slowly; repeat in 2 minutes, if needed, in small increments of first dose over at least 2 minutes to achieve desired effect. Total dose of up to 5 mg may be used. Additional doses to maintain desired level of sedation may be given by slow titration in increments of 25% of dose used to first reach the sedative end point.
Patients age 60 or older and debilitated patients: 0.5 to 1.5 mg I.V. over at least 2 minutes. Incremental doses shouldn't exceed 1 mg. A total dose of up to 3.5 mg is usually sufficient.

➲ To induce sleepiness and amnesia and to relieve apprehension before anesthesia or before and during procedures in children
P.O.
Children ages 6 to 16 and cooperative patients: 0.25 to 0.5 mg/kg P.O. as a single dose, up to 20 mg.
Infants and children ages 6 months to 5 years and less-cooperative patients: 0.25 to 1 mg/kg P.O. as a single dose, up to 20 mg.
I.V.
Children ages 12 to 16: Initially, no more than 2.5 mg I.V. given slowly; repeat in 2

minutes, if needed, in small increments of first dose over at least 2 minutes to achieve desired effect. Total dose of up to 10 mg may be used. Additional doses to maintain desired level of sedation may be given by slow titration in increments of 25% of dose used to first reach the sedative end point.
Children ages 6 to 12: 0.025 to 0.05 mg/kg I.V. over 2 to 3 minutes. Additional doses may be given in small increments after 2 to 3 minutes. Total dose of up to 0.4 mg/kg, not to exceed 10 mg, may be used.
Children ages 6 months to 5 years: 0.05 to 0.1 mg/kg I.V. over 2 to 3 minutes. Additional doses may be given in small increments after 2 to 3 minutes. Total dose of up to 0.6 mg/kg, not to exceed 6 mg, may be used.
I.M.
Children: 0.1 to 0.15 mg/kg I.M. Use up to 0.5 mg/kg in more anxious patients.

For obese children, base dose on ideal body weight; high-risk or debilitated children and children receiving other sedatives need lower doses.

➲ To induce general anesthesia
Adults older than age 55: 0.3 mg/kg I.V. over 20 to 30 seconds if patient hasn't received premedication, or 0.2 mg/kg I.V. over 20 to 30 seconds if patient has received a sedative or opioid premedication. Additional increments of 25% of first dose may be needed to complete induction.
Adults younger than age 55: 0.3 to 0.35 mg/kg I.V. over 20 to 30 seconds if patient hasn't received premedication, or 0.25 mg/kg I.V. over 20 to 30 seconds if patient has received a sedative or opioid premedication. Additional increments of 25% of first dose may be needed to complete induction.

For debilitated patients, initially, 0.2 to 0.25 mg/kg. As little as 0.15 mg/kg may be needed.

➲ As continuous infusion to sedate intubated patients in critical care unit
Adults: Initially, 0.01 to 0.05 mg/kg may be given I.V. over several minutes, repeated at 10- to 15-minute intervals until adequate sedation is achieved. To maintain sedation, usual initial infusion rate is 0.02 to 0.1 mg/kg/hour. Higher loading dose or infusion rates may be needed in some patients. Use the lowest effective rate.
Children: Initially, 0.05 to 0.2 mg/kg may be given I.V. over 2 to 3 minutes or longer; then continuous infusion at rate of 0.06 to 0.12 mg/kg/hour. Increase or decrease infusion to maintain desired effect.
Neonates more than 32 weeks' gestational age: Initially, 0.06 mg/kg/hour. Adjust rate, p.r.n., using lowest possible rate.
Neonates less than 32 weeks' gestational age: Initially, 0.03 mg/kg/hour. Adjust rate, p.r.n., using lowest possible rate.

Contraindications & cautions

- Contraindicated in patients hypersensitive to drug and in those with acute angle-closure glaucoma, shock, coma, or acute alcohol intoxication.
- Use cautiously in patients with uncompensated acute illness and in elderly or debilitated patients.

Adverse reactions

CNS: headache, *oversedation, drowsiness,* amnesia, involuntary movements, nystagmus, paradoxical behavior or excitement.
CV: variations in blood pressure and pulse rate.
GI: *nausea,* vomiting.
Respiratory: *decreased respiratory rate,* APNEA, *hiccups.*
Other: *pain at injection site.*

Interactions

Drug-drug. *CNS depressants:* May cause apnea. Use together cautiously. Prepare to adjust dosage of midazolam if used with opiates or other CNS depressants.
Diltiazem: May increase CNS depression and prolonged effects of midazolam. Use lower dose of midazolam.
Erythromycin: May alter metabolism of midazolam. Use together cautiously.
Fluconazole, itraconazole, ketoconazole, miconazole: May increase and prolong midazolam level, CNS depression, and psychomotor impairment. Avoid using together.
Hormonal contraceptives: May prolong half-life of midazolam. Use together cautiously.
Rifampin: May decrease midazolam level. Monitor for midazolam effectiveness.
Theophylline: May antagonize sedative effect of midazolam. Use together cautiously.
Verapamil: May increase midazolam level. Monitor patient closely.

Drug-herb. *St. John's wort:* May decrease midazolam level. Discourage use together.
Drug-food. *Grapefruit juice:* May increase bioavailability of oral midazolam. Discourage use together.
Drug-lifestyle. *Alcohol use:* May cause additive CNS effects. Discourage use together.

Nursing considerations

!!**ALERT** Before giving drug, have oxygen and resuscitation equipment available in case of severe respiratory depression. Excessive amounts and rapid infusion have been linked to respiratory arrest. Continuously monitor patients who have received midazolam, including children who have received midazolam syrup, to detect potentially life-threatening respiratory depression.
- When injecting I.M., give deeply into a large muscle.
- Monitor blood pressure, heart rate and rhythm, respirations, airway integrity, and arterial oxygen saturation during procedure.

!!**ALERT** Don't confuse Versed with VePesid.

Patient teaching

- Because drug's beneficial amnesic effect diminishes patient's recall of events around the time of surgery, provide written information, family member instruction, and follow-up contact to make sure patient has adequate information.
- Warn patient to avoid hazardous activities that require alertness or good coordination until effects of drug are known.
- Tell patient to avoid alcohol while taking drug.
- Tell patient not to take oral form with grapefruit juice.

miglitol
Glyset

Pregnancy risk category B

Indications & dosages

➲ **Adjunct to diet as monotherapy to improve glycemic control in patients with type 2 (non–insulin-dependent) diabetes whose hyperglycemia can't be managed with diet alone or with a sulfonylurea when diet plus either miglitol or sulfonylurea doesn't adequately control glucose level**
Adults: 25 mg P.O. t.i.d. with first bite of each main meal. May start with 25 mg P.O. daily and increase gradually to t.i.d. to minimize GI upset; dosage may be increased after 4 to 8 weeks to 50 mg P.O. t.i.d. Dosage may then be further increased after 3 months, based on glycosylated hemoglobin level, to maximum of 100 mg P.O. t.i.d.

Contraindications & cautions

- Contraindicated in patients hypersensitive to drug or its components and in those with diabetic ketoacidosis, inflammatory bowel disease, colonic ulceration, partial intestinal obstruction, chronic intestinal diseases with marked disorders of digestion or absorption, or conditions that may deteriorate because of increased gas formation in the intestine.
- Contraindicated in those predisposed to intestinal obstruction and in those with creatinine level greater than 2 mg/dl.
- Use cautiously in patients also receiving insulin or oral sulfonylureas because drug may increase hypoglycemic potential of insulin or sulfonylureas.

Adverse reactions

GI: *abdominal pain, diarrhea, flatulence.*
Skin: rash.

Interactions

Drug-drug. *Digoxin, propranolol, ranitidine:* May decrease bioavailability of these drugs. Watch for loss of efficacy of these drugs and adjust dosage.
Intestinal absorbents (such as charcoal), digestive enzyme preparations (such as amylase, pancreatin): May reduce effectiveness of miglitol. Discourage use together.

Nursing considerations

- In patients also taking insulin or oral sulfonylureas, dosages of these drugs may be needed. Monitor patient for increased frequency of hypoglycemia.
- Management of type 2 diabetes should include diet control, exercise program, and regular testing of urine and glucose level.
- Monitor glucose level regularly, especially during situations of increased stress, such as infection, fever, surgery, or trauma.

• Besides checking glucose level regularly, monitor glycosylated hemoglobin level every 3 months to evaluate long-term glycemic control.
• Treat mild to moderate hypoglycemia with a form of dextrose, such as glucose tablets or gel. Severe hypoglycemia may necessitate I.V. glucose or glucagon.
• Give drug with the first bite of each main meal.
• Monitor patient for adverse GI effects.

Patient teaching

• Stress importance of adhering to diet, weight reduction, and exercise instructions. Urge patient to have glucose and glycosylated hemoglobin levels tested regularly.
• Inform patient that drug treatment relieves symptoms but doesn't cure diabetes.
• Teach patient how to recognize high and low glucose levels.
• Instruct patient to have a source of glucose readily available to treat hypoglycemia when miglitol is taken with a sulfonylurea or with insulin.
• Advise patient to seek medical advice promptly during periods of stress, such as fever, trauma, infection, or surgery, because dosage may have to be adjusted.
• Instruct patient to take drug three times daily with first bite of each main meal.
• Show patient how and when to monitor glucose level.
• Advise patient that sucrose (table sugar, cane sugar) or fruit juices shouldn't be used to treat low glucose reactions with miglitol. Oral glucose (dextrose) or glucagon is necessary to increase glucose.
• Advise patient that adverse GI effects are most common during first few weeks of therapy and should improve over time.
• Urge patient to wear or carry medical identification at all times.

milrinone lactate

Primacor

Pregnancy risk category C

Indications & dosages

➲ Short-term treatment of heart failure
Adults: Give first loading dose of 50 mcg/kg I.V. slowly over 10 minutes; then give continuous I.V. infusion of 0.375 to 0.75 mcg/kg/minute. Titrate infusion dose based on clinical and hemodynamic responses. Don't exceed 1.13 mg/kg/day.

If creatinine clearance is 50 ml/minute, infusion rate is 0.43 mcg/kg/minute; if 40 ml/minute, infusion rate is 0.38 mcg/kg/minute; if 30 ml/minute, infusion rate is 0.33 mcg/kg/minute; if 20 ml/minute, infusion rate is 0.28 mcg/kg/minute; if 10 ml/minute, infusion rate is 0.23 mcg/kg/minute; and if 5 ml/minute, infusion rate is 0.2 mcg/kg/minute. Don't exceed 1.13 mg/kg/day.

Contraindications & cautions

• Contraindicated in patients hypersensitive to drug.
• Contraindicated for use in patients with severe aortic or pulmonic valvular disease in place of surgery and during acute phase of MI.
• Use cautiously in patients with atrial flutter or fibrillation because drug slightly shortens AV node conduction time and may increase ventricular response rate.

Adverse reactions

CNS: headache.
CV: VENTRICULAR ARRHYTHMIAS, *ventricular ectopic activity*, nonsustained ventricular tachycardia, ***sustained ventricular tachycardia, ventricular fibrillation***.

Interactions

None significant.

Nursing considerations

• Give a cardiac glycoside, if ordered, before beginning milrinone therapy.
• Drug is typically given with digoxin and diuretics.
• Improved cardiac output may increase urine output. Expect dosage reduction in patient's diuretic therapy as heart failure improves. Potassium loss may predispose patient to digitalis toxicity.
• Monitor fluid and electrolyte status, blood pressure, heart rate, and renal function during therapy. Excessive decrease in blood pressure requires stopping or slowing rate of infusion. Correct hypoxemia if it occurs during treatment.

Patient teaching

- Instruct patient to promptly report adverse reactions to prescriber promptly, especially angina.
- Tell patient that drug may cause headache, which can be treated with analgesics.
- Tell patient to report discomfort at I.V. insertion site.

minocycline hydrochloride

Alti-Minocycline†, Apo-Minocycline†, Dynacin, Minocin, Novo-Minocycline†, PMS-Minocycline†

Pregnancy risk category D

Indications & dosages

➲ Infections caused by susceptible gram-negative and gram-positive organisms (including *Haemophilus ducreyi, Yersinia pestis,* and *Campylobacter fetus*), *Rickettsiae* species, *Mycoplasma pneumoniae,* and *Chlamydia trachomatis;* psittacosis; granuloma inguinale

Adults: Initially, 200 mg I.V.; then 100 mg I.V. q 12 hours. Don't exceed 400 mg/day. Or, 200 mg P.O. initially; then 100 mg P.O. q 12 hours. May use 100 or 200 mg P.O. initially; then 50 mg q.i.d.

Children older than age 8: Initially, 4 mg/kg P.O. or I.V.; then 2 mg/kg q 12 hours.

Give I.V. in 500- to 1,000-ml solution without calcium, over 6 hours.

➲ Gonorrhea in patients allergic to penicillin

Adults: Initially, 200 mg P.O.; then 100 mg q 12 hours for at least 4 days. Obtain samples for follow-up cultures within 2 to 3 days after treatment is finished.

➲ Syphilis in patients allergic to penicillin

Adults: Initially, 200 mg P.O.; then 100 mg q 12 hours for 10 to 15 days.

➲ Meningococcal carrier state

Adults: 100 mg P.O. q 12 hours for 5 days.

➲ Uncomplicated urethral, endocervical, or rectal infection caused by *C. trachomatis* or *Ureaplasma urealyticum*

Adults: 100 mg P.O. b.i.d. for at least 7 days.

➲ Uncomplicated gonococcal urethritis in men

Adults: 100 mg P.O. b.i.d. for 5 days.

Contraindications & cautions

- Contraindicated in patients hypersensitive to drug or other tetracyclines.
- Use cautiously in patients with impaired renal or hepatic function. Use of these drugs during last half of pregnancy and in children younger than age 8 may cause permanent discoloration of teeth, enamel defects, and bone growth retardation.

Adverse reactions

CNS: headache, ***intracranial hypertension***, light-headedness, dizziness, vertigo.
CV: pericarditis, *thrombophlebitis*.
GI: *anorexia*, dysphagia, glossitis, epigastric distress, oral candidiasis, *nausea*, vomiting, *diarrhea*, enterocolitis, inflammatory lesions in anogenital region.
Hematologic: ***neutropenia***, eosinophilia, ***thrombocytopenia***, hemolytic anemia.
Musculoskeletal: bone growth retardation in children younger than age 8.
Skin: *maculopapular and erythematous rashes, photosensitivity, increased pigmentation, urticaria.*
Other: hypersensitivity reactions, ***anaphylaxis***, superinfection, permanent discoloration of teeth, enamel defects.

Interactions

Drug-drug. *Antacids (including sodium bicarbonate) and laxatives containing aluminum, magnesium, or calcium; antidiarrheals:* May decrease antibiotic absorption. Give antibiotic 1 hour before or 2 hours after any of these drugs.
Ferrous sulfate and other iron products, zinc: May decrease antibiotic absorption. Give drug 2 hours before or 3 hours after iron.
Hormonal contraceptives: May decrease contraceptive effectiveness and increase risk of breakthrough bleeding. Advise patient to use nonhormonal contraceptive.
Methoxyflurane: May cause nephrotoxicity when given with tetracyclines. Avoid using together.
Oral anticoagulants: May increase anticoagulant effect. Monitor PT and INR, and adjust dosage.
Penicillins: May disrupt bactericidal action of penicillins. Avoid using together.
Drug-lifestyle. *Sun exposure:* May cause photosensitivity reactions. Advise patient to avoid excessive sunlight exposure.

Nursing considerations

- Monitor renal and liver function test results.
- Obtain specimen for culture and sensitivity tests before first dose. Therapy may begin while awaiting test results.

!!ALERT Check expiration date. Outdated or deteriorated tetracyclines may cause reversible nephrotoxicity (Fanconi's syndrome).

- Don't expose drug to light or heat. Keep cap tightly closed.
- If large doses are given, therapy is prolonged, or patient is at high risk, monitor patient for signs and symptoms of superinfection.
- Check patient's tongue for signs of candidal infection. Stress good oral hygiene.
- Drug may discolor teeth in young adults. Watch for brown pigmentation, and notify prescriber if it occurs.
- Don't use drug to treat neurosyphilis.
- Photosensitivity reactions may occur within a few minutes to several hours after exposure. Photosensitivity lasts after therapy ends.

!!ALERT Don't confuse Minocin, niacin, and Mithracin.

Patient teaching

- Tell patient to take entire amount of drug exactly as prescribed, even after he feels better.
- Instruct patient to take oral form of drug with a full glass of water. Drug may be taken with food. Tell patient not to take within 1 hour of bedtime, to avoid esophageal irritation or ulceration.
- Warn patient to avoid driving or other hazardous tasks because of possible adverse CNS effects.
- Caution patient to avoid direct sunlight and ultraviolet light, wear protective clothing, and use sunscreen.

mirtazapine

Remeron, Remeron Soltab

Pregnancy risk category C

Indications & dosages

➲ Depression

Adults: Initially, 15 mg P.O. h.s. Maintenance dose ranges from 15 to 45 mg daily. Adjust dosage at intervals of at least 1 week.

Contraindications & cautions

- Contraindicated in patients hypersensitive to drug and within 14 days of MAO inhibitor therapy.
- Use cautiously in patients with CV or cerebrovascular disease, seizure disorders, suicidal thoughts, hepatic or renal impairment, or history of mania or hypomania.
- Use cautiously in patients with conditions that predispose them to hypotension, such as dehydration, hypovolemia, or antihypertensive therapy.
- Give drug cautiously to elderly patients; decreased clearance has occurred in this age group.

Adverse reactions

CNS: *somnolence,* dizziness, asthenia, abnormal dreams, abnormal thinking, tremors, confusion, ***suicidal behavior***.
CV: edema, peripheral edema.
GI: nausea, *increased appetite, dry mouth, constipation.*
GU: urinary frequency.
Metabolic: *weight gain.*
Musculoskeletal: back pain, myalgia.
Respiratory: dyspnea.
Other: flulike syndrome.

Interactions

Drug-drug. *Diazepam, other CNS depressants:* May cause additive CNS effects. Avoid using together.
MAO inhibitors: May sometimes cause fatal reactions. Avoid using within 14 days of MAO inhibitor therapy.
Drug-lifestyle. *Alcohol use:* May cause additive CNS effects. Discourage use together.

Nursing considerations

- Don't use within 14 days of MAO inhibitor therapy.
- Record mood changes. Watch for suicidal tendencies.
- Although agranulocytosis occurs rarely, stop drug and monitor patient closely if he develops a sore throat, fever, stomatitis, or other signs and symptoms of infection with a low WBC count.
- Lower dosages tend to be more sedating than higher dosages.

Patient teaching

- Caution patient not to perform hazardous activities if he gets too sleepy.

• Tell patient to report signs and symptoms of infection, such as fever, chills, sore throat, mucous membrane irritation, or flulike syndrome.
• Instruct patient not to use alcohol or other CNS depressants while taking drug.
• Stress importance of following prescriber's orders.
• Instruct patient not to take other drugs without prescriber's approval.
• Tell woman of childbearing age to report suspected pregnancy immediately and to notify prescriber if she is breast-feeding.
• Instruct patient to remove orally disintegrating tablets from blister pack and place immediately on tongue.
• Advise patient not to break or split tablet.

misoprostol
Cytotec

Pregnancy risk category X

Indications & dosages

➲ To prevent NSAID-induced gastric ulcer in elderly or debilitated patients at high risk for complications from gastric ulcer and in patients with history of NSAID-induced ulcer
Adults: 200 mcg P.O. q.i.d. with food; if not tolerated, decrease to 100 mcg P.O. q.i.d. Give dosage for duration of NSAID therapy. Give last dose h.s.

Contraindications & cautions

• Contraindicated in those allergic to prostaglandins. Drug shouldn't be taken by pregnant women to reduce the risk of NSAID-induced ulcers.
• Use with caution in patients with inflammatory bowel disease.

Adverse reactions

CNS: headache.
GI: *diarrhea, abdominal pain,* nausea, flatulence, dyspepsia, vomiting, constipation.
GU: hypermenorrhea, dysmenorrhea, spotting, cramps, menstrual disorders, postmenopausal vaginal bleeding.

Interactions

Drug-food. *Any food:* May decrease absorption rate of drug. However, manufacturer recommends that patient take drug with food.

Nursing considerations

!!ALERT Take special precautions to prevent use of drug during pregnancy. Uterine rupture is linked to certain risk factors, including later trimester pregnancies, higher doses of the drug, prior cesarean delivery or uterine surgery, or five or more previous pregnancies. Make sure patient understands dangers of drug to herself and her fetus and that she receives both oral and written warnings about these dangers. Also, make sure she can comply with effective contraception and that the result of a serum pregnancy test performed within 2 weeks of starting therapy is negative. Patient shouldn't breast-feed during therapy.
• Drug causes modest decrease in basal pepsin secretion.
!!ALERT Don't confuse misoprostol (Cytotec) with mifepristone (Mifeprex).

Patient teaching

• Instruct patient not to share misoprostol.
• Remind pregnant patient that drug may cause miscarriage, often with potentially life-threatening bleeding.
• Advise woman not to begin therapy until second or third day of next normal menstrual period.
• Advise patient to take drug as prescribed for duration of NSAID therapy.
• Tell patient that diarrhea usually occurs early in the course of therapy and is usually self-limiting. Taking drug with food helps minimize the diarrhea.

mitomycin (mitomycin-C)
Mutamycin

Pregnancy risk category NR

Indications & dosages

Dosage and indications vary. Check treatment protocol with prescriber.

➲ Disseminated adenocarcinoma of stomach or pancreas
Adults: 20 mg/m^2 as an I.V. single dose. Repeat cycle after 6 to 8 weeks when WBC and platelet counts have returned to normal.

For patients with myelosuppression, if leukocytes are 2,000 to 2,999/mm^3 and platelets are 25,000 to 74,999/mm³, give 70% of initial dose. If leukocytes are less than 2,000/mm³ and platelets are less than 25,000/mm³, give 50% of initial dose.

➲ Bladder cancer♦

Adults: 20 to 60 mg intravesically once weekly for 8 weeks.

Contraindications & cautions

- Contraindicated in patients hypersensitive to drug and in those with thrombocytopenia, coagulation disorders, or an increased bleeding tendency from other causes.

Adverse reactions

CNS: headache, neurologic abnormalities, confusion, drowsiness, fatigue, *fever.*
EENT: blurred vision.
GI: mucositis, *nausea, vomiting, anorexia, diarrhea, stomatitis.*
GU: ***renal toxicity, hemolytic uremic syndrome.***
Hematologic: THROMBOCYTOPENIA, LEUKOPENIA, ***microangiopathic hemolytic anemia.***
Respiratory: ***interstitial pneumonitis,*** pulmonary edema, dyspnea, nonproductive cough, ***adult respiratory distress syndrome.***
Skin: cellulitis, induration, desquamation, pruritus, *pain at injection site, reversible alopecia,* purple bands on nails, rash, sloughing with extravasation.
Other: ***septicemia,*** ulceration, pain.

Interactions

Drug-drug. *Vinca alkaloids:* May cause acute respiratory distress when given together. Monitor patient closely.

Nursing considerations

- Never give drug I.M. or S.C.
- Continue CBC and blood studies at least 8 weeks after therapy stops. Leukopenia and thrombocytopenia are cumulative. If WBC count falls below 2,000/mm³ or granulocyte count falls below 1,000/mm³, follow institutional policy for infection control in immunocompromised patients.
- To prevent bleeding, avoid all I.M. injections when platelet count is less than 100,000/mm³.
- Anticipate need for blood transfusions to combat anemia. Patients may receive injections of RBC colony-stimulating factor to promote RBC production and decrease need for blood transfusions.
- Monitor patient for dyspnea with nonproductive cough; chest X-ray may show infiltrates.
- Monitor renal function tests.
- Leukopenia may occur up to 8 weeks after therapy and may be cumulative with successive doses.
- Hemolytic uremic syndrome is characterized by microangiopathic hemolytic anemia, thrombocytopenia, and renal failure.

!!ALERT Don't confuse mitomycin with mithramycin.

Patient teaching

- Advise patient to report any pain or burning at site of injection during or after administration.
- Warn patient to watch for signs and symptoms of infection (fever, sore throat, fatigue) and bleeding (easy bruising, nosebleeds, bleeding gums, tarry stools). Tell patient to take temperature daily.
- Inform patient that hair loss may occur, but that it's usually reversible.

mitoxantrone hydrochloride

Novantrone

Pregnancy risk category D

Indications & dosages

➲ Combination initial therapy for acute nonlymphocytic leukemia

Adults: Induction begins with 12 mg/m² I.V. daily on days 1 to 3, with 100 mg/m² daily of cytarabine on days 1 to 7. A second induction may be given if response isn't adequate. Maintenance therapy is 12 mg/m² on days 1 and 2, with cytarabine 100 mg/m² on days 1 to 5.

➲ To reduce neurologic disability and frequency of relapse in chronic progressive, progressive relapsing, or worsening relapsing-remitting multiple sclerosis

Adults: 12 mg/m² I.V. over 5 to 15 minutes q 3 months.

➲ Advanced hormone-refractory prostate cancer

Adults: 12 to 14 mg/m² as a short I.V. infusion q 21 days. Drug is given as an adjunct to corticosteroid therapy.

Contraindications & cautions

- Contraindicated in patients hypersensitive to drug.
- Use cautiously in patients with previous exposure to anthracyclines or other cardiotoxic drugs, previous radiation therapy to mediastinal area, or heart disease.

Adverse reactions

CNS: ***seizures***, *headache, fever.*
CV: ***arrhythmias***, tachycardia, ECG abnormalities.
EENT: conjunctivitis, sinusitis.
GI: *bleeding, abdominal pain, diarrhea, nausea, mucositis, vomiting, stomatitis, constipation.*
GU: ***renal failure***, *menstrual disorder, amenorrhea, UTI.*
Hematologic: ***myelosuppression***, anemia.
Hepatic: jaundice.
Metabolic: hyperuricemia.
Musculoskeletal: back pain.
Respiratory: *dyspnea, cough, upper respiratory tract infection*, pneumonia.
Skin: *alopecia*, petechiae, ecchymoses, local irritation or phlebitis.
Other: *fungal infections*, ***sepsis***.

Interactions

None significant.

Nursing considerations

- Patients with significant myelosuppression shouldn't receive drug unless benefits outweigh risks.
- Give allopurinol. Avoid uric acid nephropathy by hydrating patient before and during therapy.
- Closely monitor hematologic and laboratory chemistry parameters.
- To prevent bleeding, avoid all I.M. injections if platelet count falls below 50,000/mm^3.
- Anticipate need for blood transfusion to combat anemia. Patients may receive injections of RBC colony–stimulating factors to promote RBC production and decrease need for blood transfusions.
- Monitor left ventricular ejection fraction; cardiotoxicity incidence increases with a cumulative dose of 140 mg/m^2, although toxicities also have occurred at lower cumulative doses.
- Treat infections with antibiotics. Patients may receive injections of WBC colony–stimulating factors to promote cell growth and decrease risk of infection.
- If severe nonhematologic toxicity occurs during first course, delay second course until patient recovers.

Patient teaching

- Advise patient to report any pain or burning at site of injection during or after administration.
- Tell patient that urine may appear blue-green within 24 hours after administration, and that some bluish discoloration of the whites of the eyes may occur. These effects aren't harmful and may persist during therapy.
- Advise patient to watch for signs and symptoms of bleeding and infection.
- Caution woman of childbearing age to avoid pregnancy during therapy. Recommend that she consult prescriber before becoming pregnant.

modafinil
Provigil

Pregnancy risk category C
Controlled substance schedule IV

Indications & dosages

➲ **To improve wakefulness in patients with excessive daytime sleepiness caused by narcolepsy, obstructive sleep apnea-hypoapnea syndrome, and shift-work sleep disorder**
Adults: 200 mg P.O. daily, as single dose in the morning. Patients with shift-work sleep disorder should take dose about 1 hour before the start of their shift.

In patients with severe hepatic impairment, give 100 mg P.O. daily, as single dose in the morning.

Contraindications & cautions

- Contraindicated in patients hypersensitive to drug and in those with a history of left ventricular hypertrophy or ischemic ECG changes, chest pain, arrhythmias, or other evidence of mitral valve prolapse linked to CNS stimulant use.
- Use cautiously in patients with recent MI or unstable angina and in those with history of psychosis.

- Use cautiously and give reduced dosage to patients with severe hepatic impairment, with or without cirrhosis.
- Use cautiously in patients taking MAO inhibitors.
- Safety and efficacy in patients with severe renal impairment haven't been determined.

Adverse reactions

CNS: *headache, nervousness, dizziness,* fever, depression, anxiety, cataplexy, *insomnia,* paresthesia, dyskinesia, hypertonia, confusion, syncope, amnesia, emotional lability, ataxia, tremor.
CV: hypotension, hypertension, vasodilation, ***arrhythmias,*** chest pain.
EENT: *rhinitis,* pharyngitis, epistaxis, amblyopia, abnormal vision.
GI: *nausea,* diarrhea, dry mouth, anorexia, vomiting, mouth ulcer, gingivitis, thirst.
GU: abnormal urine, urine retention, abnormal ejaculation, albuminuria.
Hematologic: eosinophilia.
Metabolic: hyperglycemia.
Musculoskeletal: joint disorder, neck pain, neck rigidity.
Respiratory: asthma, lung disorder, dyspnea.
Skin: sweating.
Other: herpes simplex, chills.

Interactions

Drug-drug. *Carbamazepine, phenobarbital, rifampin, and other inducers of CYP3A4:* May alter modafinil level. Monitor patient closely.
Cyclosporine, theophylline: May reduce levels of these drugs. Use together cautiously.
Diazepam, phenytoin, propranolol, other drugs metabolized by CYP2C19: May inhibit CYP2C19 and lead to higher levels of drugs metabolized by this enzyme. Use together cautiously; adjust dosage as needed.
Hormonal contraceptives: May reduce contraceptive effectiveness. Advise patient to use alternative or additional method of contraception during modafinil therapy and for 1 month after drug is stopped.
Itraconazole, ketoconazole, other inhibitors of CYP3A4: May alter modafinil level. Monitor patient closely.
Methylphenidate: May cause 1-hour delay if modafinil absorption. Separate dosage times.
Phenytoin, warfarin: May inhibit CYP2C9 and increase phenytoin and warfarin levels. Monitor patient closely for toxicity.
Tricyclic antidepressants (such as clomipramine, desipramine): May increase tricyclic antidepressant level. Reduce dosage of these drugs.

Nursing considerations

- Monitor hypertensive patients closely.
- Although single daily 400-mg doses have been well tolerated, the larger dose is no more beneficial than the 200-mg dose.
- Food has no effect on overall bioavailability but may delay absorption of drug by 1 hour.

Patient teaching

- Advise woman to notify prescriber about planned, suspected, or known pregnancy, or if she's breast-feeding.
- Caution patient that use of hormonal contraceptives (including depot or implantable contraceptives) together with modafinil tablets may reduce contraceptive effectiveness. Recommend an alternative method of contraception during modafinil therapy and for 1 month after drug is stopped.
- Instruct patient to confer with prescriber before taking prescription or OTC drugs to avoid drug interactions.
- Tell patient to avoid alcohol while taking drug.
- Warn patient to avoid activities that require alertness or good coordination until CNS effects of drug are known.

mometasone furoate

Asmanex Twisthaler

Pregnancy risk category C

Indications & dosages

➲ **Maintenance therapy for asthma; asthma in patients who take an oral corticosteroid**
Adults and children age 12 and older who use a bronchodilator or inhale a corticosteroid: Initially, 220 mcg by oral inhalation q day in the evening. Maximum, 440 mcg/day.
Adults and children age 12 and older who take an oral corticosteroid: 440 mcg b.i.d. by oral inhalation. Maximum, 880 mcg/day.

Reduce oral corticosteroid dosage by no more than 2.5 mg/day at weekly intervals, beginning at least 1 week after starting mometasone. After stopping oral corticosteroid, reduce mometasone dose to lowest effective amount.

Contraindications & cautions

- Contraindicated in patients hypersensitive to drug or its ingredients and in those with status asthmaticus or other acute forms of asthma or bronchospasm (as primary treatment).
- Use cautiously in patients at high risk for decreased bone mineral content (those with a family history of osteoporosis, prolonged immobilization, long-term use of drugs that reduce bone mass), patients switching from a systemic to an inhaled corticosteroid, and patients with active or dormant tuberculosis, untreated systemic infections, ocular herpes simplex, or immunosuppression.
- Use cautiously in breast-feeding women.

Adverse reactions

CNS: depression, fatigue, *headache*, insomnia.
EENT: *allergic rhinitis*, dry throat, dysphonia, earache, epistaxis, nasal irritation, *pharyngitis*, sinus congestion, sinusitis.
GI: abdominal pain, anorexia, dyspepsia, flatulence, gastroenteritis, nausea, oral candidiasis, vomiting.
GU: dysmenorrhea, menstrual disorder, UTI.
Musculoskeletal: arthralgia, back pain, myalgia, pain.
Respiratory: respiratory disorder, *upper respiratory tract infection.*
Other: accidental injury, flulike symptoms, infection.

Interactions

Drug-drug. *Ketoconazole:* May increase mometasone level. Use together cautiously.

Nursing considerations

!!ALERT Don't use for acute bronchospasm.
- Wean patient slowly from a systemic corticosteroid after he switches to mometasone. Monitor lung function tests, beta-agonist use, and asthma symptoms.

!!ALERT If patient is switching from an oral corticosteroid to an inhaled form, watch closely for evidence of adrenal insufficiency, such as fatigue, lethargy, weakness, nausea, vomiting, and hypotension.
- After an oral corticosteroid is withdrawn, hypothalamic-pituitary-adrenal (HPA) function may not recover for months. If patient has trauma, stress, infection, or surgery during this HPA recovery period, he is particularly vulnerable to adrenal insufficiency or adrenal crisis.
- Because an inhaled corticosteroid can be systemically absorbed, watch for cushingoid effects.
- Assess patient for bone loss during long-term use.
- Watch for evidence of localized mouth infections, glaucoma, and immunosuppression.
- Use drug only if benefits to mother justify risks to fetus. If a woman takes a corticosteroid during pregnancy, monitor newborn for hypoadrenalism.
- Monitor elderly patients for increased sensitivity to drug effects.

Patient teaching

- Tell patient to use drug regularly and at the same time each day. If he uses it only once daily, tell him to do so in the evening.
- Caution patient not to use drug for immediate relief of an asthma attack or bronchospasm.
- Inform patient that maximum benefits might not occur for 1 to 2 weeks or longer after therapy starts; instruct him to notify his prescriber if his condition fails to improve or worsens.
- Tell patient that if he has bronchospasm after taking drug, he should immediately use a fast-acting bronchodilator. Urge him to contact prescriber immediately if bronchospasm doesn't respond to the fast-acting bronchodilator.

!!ALERT If patient has been weaned from an oral corticosteroid, urge him to contact prescriber immediately if an asthma attack occurs or if he is experiencing a period of stress. The oral corticosteriod may need to be resumed.
- Warn patient to avoid exposure to chickenpox or measles and to notify prescriber if such contact occurs.
- Long-term use of an inhaled corticosteroid may increase the risk of cataracts or glaucoma; tell patient to report vision changes.

• Advise patient to write the date on a new inhaler on the day he opens it and to discard the inhaler after 45 days or when the dose counter reads "00."
• Instruct patient on proper use and routine care of the inhaler.

montelukast sodium
Singulair

Pregnancy risk category B

Indications & dosages
➲ Asthma, seasonal allergic rhinitis
Adults and children age 15 and older: 10 mg P.O. once daily in evening.
Children ages 6 to 14: 5 mg (chewable tablet) P.O. once daily in evening.
Children ages 2 to 5: 4 mg chewable tablet or 1 packet of oral granules P.O. once daily in the evening.
Children ages 12 to 23 months (asthma only): 1 packet of oral granules P.O. once daily in the evening.

Contraindications & cautions
• Contraindicated in patients hypersensitive to drug or its ingredients.
• Use cautiously and with appropriate monitoring in patients whose dosages of systemic corticosteroids are reduced.

Adverse reactions
CNS: fever, *headache*, dizziness, fatigue, asthenia.
EENT: nasal congestion, dental pain.
GI: dyspepsia, infectious gastroenteritis, abdominal pain.
GU: pyuria.
Respiratory: cough.
Skin: rash.
Other: trauma, influenza, ***systemic eosinophilia***.

Interactions
Drug-drug. *Phenobarbital, rifampin:* May decrease bioavailability of montelukast because of hepatic metabolism induction. Monitor patient for effectiveness.

Nursing considerations
• Assess patient's underlying condition, and monitor patient for effectiveness.

!! ALERT Don't abruptly substitute drug for inhaled or oral corticosteroids. Dose of inhaled corticosteroids may be reduced gradually.
• Drug isn't indicated for use in patients with acute asthmatic attacks, status asthmaticus, or as monotherapy for management of exercise-induced bronchospasm. Continue appropriate rescue drug for acute worsening.
• Give oral granules either directly in the mouth or mixed with a teaspoonful of cold or room-temperature applesauce, carrots, rice, or ice cream. Don't open packet until ready to use. After opening packet, give full dose within 15 minutes. If mixed with food, don't store excess for future use; discard any unused portion.
• Don't dissolve oral granules in liquid; let the patient take a drink after receiving the granules.
• Oral granules may be given without regard to meals.

Patient teaching
• Teach patient how to mix granules with applesauce, carrots, rice, or ice cream.
• Tell patient to discard any unused portion.
• Advise patient to take drug daily, even if asymptomatic, and to contact his prescriber if asthma isn't well controlled.
• Warn patient not to reduce or stop taking other prescribed antasthmatics without prescriber's approval.
• Advise patient to seek medical attention if short-acting inhaled bronchodilators are needed more often than usual during drug therapy.
• Warn patient that drug isn't beneficial in acute asthma attacks or in exercise-induced bronchospasm, and advise him to keep appropriate rescue drugs available.
• Advise patient with known aspirin sensitivity to continue to avoid using aspirin and NSAIDs during drug therapy.
• Advise patient with phenylketonuria that chewable tablet contains phenylalanine.

moricizine hydrochloride
Ethmozine

Pregnancy risk category B

Indications & dosages

➲ Life-threatening ventricular arrhythmias

Adults: Individualized dosage is based on patient response and tolerance. Begin therapy in the hospital. Most patients respond to 600 to 900 mg P.O. daily in divided doses q 8 hours. Increase daily dose by 150 mg q 3 days until desired effect occurs.

For patients with hepatic or renal impairment, 600 mg or less P.O. daily.

Contraindications & cautions

- Contraindicated in patients hypersensitive to drug, cardiogenic shock, or second- or third-degree AV block or right bundle-branch block with left hemiblock (bifascicular block), unless an artificial pacemaker is present.
- Use with caution in patients with sick sinus syndrome because drug may cause sinus bradycardia or sinus arrest.
- Use with caution in patients with coronary artery disease and left ventricular dysfunction because these patients may be at risk for sudden death when treated with the drug.
- Use with caution in patients with hepatic or renal dysfunction and in breast-feeding patients.

Adverse reactions

CNS: *dizziness*, headache, fatigue, hyperesthesia, anxiety, asthenia, depression, nervousness, paresthesia, sleep disorders.
CV: ***ventricular tachycardia***; ***PVCs***; ***supraventricular arrhythmias***; *ECG abnormalities, including conduction defects, sinus pause, junctional rhythm, and AV block*; ***heart failure***; palpitations; thrombophlebitis; chest pain; ***cardiac death***; hypotension; hypertension; vasodilation; cerebrovascular events.
EENT: blurred vision.
GI: nausea, vomiting, abdominal pain, dyspepsia, diarrhea, dry mouth.
GU: urine retention, urinary frequency, dysuria.
Musculoskeletal: musculoskeletal pain.
Respiratory: dyspnea.
Skin: rash, diaphoresis.
Other: drug-induced fever.

Interactions

Drug-drug. *Cimetidine:* May increase level and decrease clearance of moricizine. Begin moricizine at no more than 600 mg daily, and monitor drug level and therapeutic effect closely.
Digoxin, propranolol: May increase PR interval prolongation. Monitor patient closely.
Theophylline: May increase clearance and reduces level of theophylline. Monitor drug level and therapeutic response; adjust theophylline dosage, as needed.

Nursing considerations

- Monitor patients with heart failure carefully for worsening of heart failure.
- When substituting moricizine for another antiarrhythmic, withdraw previous drug for one to two of the drug's half-lives before starting moricizine. During withdrawal and adjustment to moricizine, hospitalize patients who developed life-threatening arrhythmias after withdrawal of previous antiarrhythmic. Guidelines for when to start moricizine therapy are as follows: disopyramide, 6 to 12 hours after last dose; flecainide, 12 to 24 hours after last dose; mexiletine, 8 to 12 hours after last dose; procainamide, 3 to 6 hours after last dose; propafenone, 8 to 12 hours after last dose; quinidine, 6 to 12 hours after last dose; and tocainide, 8 to 12 hours after last dose.
- Determine electrolyte status and correct imbalances before therapy, as prescribed. Hypokalemia, hyperkalemia, and hypomagnesemia may alter drug's effects.
- Because drug appears in breast milk, the decision to stop breast-feeding or stop taking the drug depends on importance of drug to the mother.

!!ALERT Don't confuse Ethmozine with Erythrocin.

Patient teaching

- Inform patient that he'll need to be hospitalized for start of therapy.
- Instruct patient to take drug exactly as prescribed and not to abruptly stop use.
- Tell patient to avoid hazardous activities if adverse CNS reactions or blurred vision occurs.

• Instruct patient to report persistent or serious adverse reactions promptly.

morphine hydrochloride
Morphitec†, M.O.S.†, M.O.S.-S.R.†

morphine sulfate
Astramorph PF, Avinza, DepoDur, Duramorph, Epimorph†, Infumorph, Infumorph 500, Kadian, M-Eslon†, Morphine H.P.†, MS Contin, MSIR, MS/L, OMS Concentrate, Oramorph SR, RMS Uniserts, Roxanol, Roxanol 100, Roxanol Rescudose, Roxanol UD, Statex

morphine tartrate

Pregnancy risk category C
Controlled substance schedule II

Indications & dosages
➲ Severe pain
Adults: 5 to 20 mg S.C. or I.M. or 2.5 to 15 mg I.V. q 4 hours, p.r.n. Or, 5 to 30 mg P.O. or 10 to 20 mg P.R. q 4 hours, p.r.n.

For continuous I.V. infusion, give loading dose of 15 mg I.V.; then continuous infusion of 0.8 to 10 mg/hour.

For extended-release tablet, give 15 or 30 mg P.O,. q 8 to 12 hours.

For sustained-release Kadian capsules used as a first opioid, give 20 mg P.O. q 12 hours or 40 mg P.O. once daily; increase consservatively in opioid-naive patients.

For epidural injection, give 5 mg by epidural catheter; then, if pain isn't relieved adequately in 1 hour, give supplementary doses of 1 to 2 mg at intervals sufficient to assess efficacy. Maximum total epidural dose shouldn't exceed 10 mg/24 hours.

For intrathecal injection, a single dose of 0.2 to 1 mg may provide pain relef for 24 hours (only in the lumbar area). Don't repeat injections.

Children: 0.1 to 0.2 mg/kg S.C. or I.M. q 4 hours. Maximum single dose, 15 mg.

➲ Moderate to severe pain requiring continuous, around-the-clock opioid
Adults: Individualize dosage of Avinza. For patients with no tolerance to opioids, begin with 30 mg Avinza P.O. daily; adjust dosage by no more than 30 mg q 4 days. When converting from another oral morphine formulation, individualize the dosing schedule according to patient's previous drug dosing schedule.

➲ Single-dose, epidural extended pain relief after major surgery
Adults: Inject 10 to 15 mg (maximum 20 mg) DepoDur via lumbar epidural administration before surgery or after clamping of umbilical cord during cesarean section. May be injected undiluted or may be diluted up to 5 ml total volume with preservative-free normal saline solution.

Contraindications & cautions
• Contraindicated in patients hypersensitive to drug and in those with conditions that would preclude administration of opioids by I.V. route (acute bronchial asthma or upper airway obstruction).
• Contraindicated in patients with GI obstruction.
• Use with caution in elderly or debilitated patients and in those with head injury, increased intracranial pressure, seizures, chronic pulmonary disease, prostatic hyperplasia, severe hepatic or renal disease, acute abdominal conditions, hypothyroidism, Addison's disease, and urethral stricture.
• Use with caution in patients with circulatory shock, biliary tract disease, CNS depression, toxic psychosis, acute alcoholism, delirium tremens, and seizure disorders.

Adverse reactions
CNS: *sedation, somnolence, clouded sensorium, euphoria,* ***seizures****, dizziness, nightmares,* physical dependence, *lightheadedness,* hallucinations, nervousness, depression, syncope.
CV: hypotension, ***bradycardia, shock, cardiac arrest***, tachycardia, hypertension.
GI: *nausea, vomiting, constipation,* ileus, dry mouth, biliary tract spasms, anorexia.
GU: urine retention.
Hematologic: ***thrombocytopenia***.
Respiratory: ***respiratory depression, apnea, respiratory arrest***.
Skin: pruritus and skin flushing, diaphoresis, edema.
Other: decreased libido.

Interactions
Drug-drug. *Cimetidine:* May increase respiratory and CNS depression when given

with morphine sulfate. Monitor patient closely.
CNS depressants, general anesthetics, hypnotics, MAO inhibitors, other opioid analgesics, sedatives, tranquilizers, tricyclic antidepressants: May cause respiratory depression, hypotension, profound sedation, or coma. Use together with caution, reduce morphine dose, and monitor patient response.
Drug-lifestyle. *Alcohol use:* May cause additive effects. Advise patient to use together cautiously.

Nursing considerations

- Reassess patient's level of pain at least 15 and 30 minutes after giving parenterally and 30 minutes after giving orally.
- Keep opioid antagonist (naloxone) and resuscitation equipment available.
- Oral solutions of various concentrations and an intensified oral solution (20 mg/ml) are available. Carefully note the strength given.

!!ALERT Don't crush, break, or chew extended-release tablets or sustained-release capsules.

- Oral capsules may be carefully opened and the entire bead contents poured into cool, soft foods, such as water, orange juice, applesauce, or pudding; patient should consume mixture immediately.
- S.L. administration may be ordered. Measure oral solution with tuberculin syringe. Give dose a few drops at a time to allow maximal S.L. absorption and minimize swallowing.
- Refrigeration of rectal suppository isn't needed. In some patients, rectal and oral absorption may not be equivalent.
- Preservative-free preparations are available for epidural and intrathecal administration.
- When drug has been given epidurally, monitor patient closely for respiratory depression up to 24 hours after the injection. Check respiratory rate and depth every 30 to 60 minutes for 24 hours.
- When drug has been given epidurally, watch for pruritus and skin flushing.
- Morphine is drug of choice in relieving MI pain; may cause transient decrease in blood pressure.
- An around-the-clock regimen best manages severe, chronic pain.
- Morphine may worsen or mask gallbladder pain.
- Monitor circulatory, respiratory, bladder, and bowel functions carefully. Drug may cause respiratory depression, hypotension, urine retention, nausea, vomiting, ileus, or altered level of consciousness regardless of the route used. Withhold dose and notify prescriber if respirations are below 12 breaths/minute.
- Constipation is commonly severe with maintenance dose. Ensure that stool softener or other laxative is ordered.
- Give morphine sulfate without regard to food.
- Taper morphine sulfate therapy gradually when stopping therapy.
- Morphine sulfate is not intended for use as a p.r.n. analgesic.

!!ALERT Don't confuse morphine with hydromorphone or Avinza with Invanz.

Patient teaching

- When drug is used after surgery, encourage patient to turn, cough, and deep-breathe and to use incentive spirometer to prevent lung problems.
- Caution ambulatory patient about getting out of bed or walking. Warn outpatient to avoid driving and other potentially hazardous activities that require mental alertness until drug's adverse CNS effects are known.
- Advise patient to avoid alcohol during therapy.
- Tell patient to swallow morphine sulfate whole or to open capsule and sprinkle beads on a small amount of applesauce immediately before ingestion.
- Teach patient that due to the risk of acute overdose, extended-release beads can't be crushed, chewed, or dissolved.

moxifloxacin hydrochloride (ophthalmic)

Vigamox

Pregnancy risk category C

Indications & dosages

➲ Bacterial conjunctivitis
Adults and children age 1 and older: 1 drop into affected eye t.i.d. for 7 days.

Contraindications & cautions

- Contraindicated in patients hypersensitive to moxifloxacin, fluoroquinolones, or their components.
- Use cautiously in pregnant or breast-feeding women.

Adverse reactions

CNS: fever.
EENT: conjunctivitis, dry eyes, increased lacrimation, keratitis, ocular discomfort, pain, and pruritus, otitis media, pharyngitis, reduced visual acuity, rhinitis, subconjunctival hemorrhage.
Respiratory: increased cough.
Skin: rash.
Other: infection.

Interactions

None reported.

Nursing considerations

- Don't inject solution subconjunctivally or into anterior chamber of the eye.
- Systemic moxifloxacin has caused serious hypersensitivity reactions. If allergic reaction occurs, stop drug and treat symptoms.
- Monitor patient for superinfection.

Patient teaching

- Tell patient to stop drug and seek medical treatment immediately if evidence of hypersensitivity reaction develops, such as itching, rash, swelling of the face or throat, or difficulty breathing.
- Tell patient not to wear contact lenses during treatment.
- Instruct patient not to touch dropper tip to anything, including eyes and fingers.

moxifloxacin hydrochloride (systemic)

Avelox, Avelox I.V.

Pregnancy risk category C

Indications & dosages

➲ **Acute bacterial sinusitis caused by *Streptococcus pneumoniae, Haemophilus influenzae,* or *Moraxella catarrhalis***
Adults: 400 mg P.O. or I.V. q 24 hours for 10 days.

➲ **Community-acquired pneumonia from multidrug-resistant *S. pneumoniae* (resistance to two or more of the following antibiotics: penicillin, second-generation cephalosporins, macrolides, trimethoprim-sulfamethoxazole, tetracyclines,), *S. aureus, M. catarrhalis, H. influenzae, H. parainfluenzae, Klebsiella pneumoniae, Chlamydia pneumoniae, Legionella pneumophila,* or *Mycoplasma pneumoniae***
Adults: 400 mg P.O. or I.V. q 24 hours for 7 to 14 days.

➲ **Acute bacterial worsening of chronic bronchitis caused by *S. pneumoniae, H. influenzae, H. parainfluenzae, K. pneumoniae, S. aureus,* or *M. catarrhalis***
Adults: 400 mg P.O. or I.V. q 24 hours for 5 days.

➲ **Uncomplicated skin-structure and skin infections caused by *S. aureus* or *S. pyogenes***
Adults: 400 mg P.O. or I.V. q 24 hours for 7 days.

Contraindications & cautions

- Contraindicated in patients hypersensitive to drug or other fluoroquinolones and in those with prolonged QT interval or uncorrected hypokalemia.
- Use cautiously in patients with ongoing proarrhythmic conditions, such as clinically significant bradycardia or acute myocardial ischemia.
- Use cautiously in patients who may have CNS disorders and in those with other risk factors that may lower the seizure threshold or predispose them to seizures.
- Safety and efficacy in children, adolescents younger than age 18, and pregnant or breast-feeding women haven't been established.

Adverse reactions

CNS: dizziness, headache, asthenia, pain, malaise, insomnia, nervousness, anxiety, confusion, somnolence, tremor, vertigo, paresthesia.
CV: ***prolongation of QT interval***, chest pain, palpitations, tachycardia, hypertension, peripheral edema.
GI: ***pseudomembranous colitis***, nausea, diarrhea, abdominal pain, vomiting, dyspepsia, dry mouth, constipation, oral candidiasis, anorexia, stomatitis, glossitis, flatulence, GI disorder, taste perversion.
GU: vaginitis, vaginal candidiasis.

Hematologic: ***thrombocytosis, thrombocytopenia, leukopenia***, eosinophilia.
Hepatic: abnormal liver function, cholestatic jaundice.
Musculoskeletal: leg pain, back pain, arthralgia, myalgia, tendon rupture.
Respiratory: dyspnea.
Skin: injection site reaction, rash (maculopapular, purpuric, pustular), pruritus, sweating.
Other: candidiasis, allergic reaction.

Interactions

Drug-drug. *Aluminum hydroxide, aluminum-magnesium hydroxide, calcium carbonate, didanosine, magnesium hydroxide, multivitamins, products containing zinc:* May interfere with GI absorption of moxifloxacin. Give moxifloxacin 4 hours before or 8 hours after these products.
Class IA antiarrhythmics (such as procainamide, quinidine), class III antiarrhythmics (such as amiodarone, sotalol): May increase risk of cardiac arrhythmias. Avoid using together.
Drugs that prolong QT interval, such as antipsychotics, erythromycin, tricyclic antidepressants: May have additive effect. Avoid using together.
NSAIDs: May increase risk of CNS stimulation and seizures. Avoid using together.
Sucralfate: May decrease absorption of moxifloxacin, reducing anti-infective response. If use together can't be avoided, give at least 6 hours apart.
Warfarin: May increase anticoagulant effects. Monitor PT and INR closely.
Drug-lifestyle. *Sun exposure:* May cause photosensitivity reactions. Advise patient to avoid excessive sunlight exposure.

Nursing considerations

- Drug may be given without regard to meals. Give at same time each day.

!!ALERT Monitor patient for adverse CNS effects, including seizures, dizziness, confusion, tremors, hallucinations, depression, and suicidal thoughts or acts. If these effects occur, stop drug and institute appropriate measures.

- Serious hypersensitivity reactions, including anaphylaxis, have occurred in patients receiving fluoroquinolones. Stop drug and institute supportive measures, as indicated.
- Consider the possibility of pseudomembranous colitis if diarrhea develops after therapy begins.
- Rupture of the Achilles and other tendons has been linked to fluoroquinolones. If pain, inflammation, or rupture of a tendon occurs, stop drug.
- Store drug at controlled room temperature.

Patient teaching

- Instruct patient to take drug once daily, at the same time each day, without regard to meals.
- Tell patient to finish entire course of therapy, even if symptoms are relieved.
- Advise patient to drink plenty of fluids.
- Tell patient to appropriately space antacids, sucralfate, multivitamins, and products containing aluminum, magnesium, iron, and zinc to avoid decreasing drug's therapeutic effects.
- Instruct patient to contact prescriber and stop drug if he experiences allergic reaction, rash, heart palpitations, fainting, or persistent diarrhea.
- Direct patient to contact prescriber, stop drug, rest, and refrain from exercise if he experiences pain, inflammation, or rupture of a tendon.
- Warn patient that drug may cause dizziness and light-headedness. Tell patient to avoid hazardous activities, such as driving or operating machinery, until effects of drug are known.
- Instruct patient to avoid excessive sunlight exposure and ultraviolet light and to report photosensitivity reactions to prescriber.

mumps virus vaccine, live

Mumpsvax

Pregnancy risk category C

Indications & dosages

➲ Immunization
Adults and children age 1 and older: 0.5 ml (20,000 units) S.C.
Not recommended in children younger than age 12 months; revaccinate children vaccinated before age 12 months.

Contraindications & cautions

- Contraindicated in immunosuppressed patients; in those with cancer, blood dyscrasia, gamma globulin disorders, fever, untreated active tuberculosis, or anaphylactic or anaphylactoid reactions to neomycin or eggs; in those receiving corticosteroid or radiation therapy; and in pregnant women.
- Vaccine isn't recommended for infants younger than age 12 months because retained maternal mumps antibodies may interfere with immune response.
- Postpone use in patients with acute or febrile illness and for at least 3 months after transfusions or treatment with immune serum globulin.
- Don't give vaccine less than 1 month before or after immunization with other live-virus vaccines.

Adverse reactions

CNS: *slight fever*, malaise.
GI: diarrhea.
Skin: rash, injection site reaction.
Other: ***anaphylaxis***, mild allergic reactions, mild lymphadenopathy.

Interactions

Drug-drug. *Immune serum globulin, plasma, whole blood:* Antibodies in serum may interfere with immune response. Don't use vaccine for at least 3 months after giving these products.

Nursing considerations

- Obtain history of allergies, especially anaphylactic reactions to antibiotics, and reaction to immunization.
- Keep epinephrine 1:1,000 available to treat anaphylaxis.
- If skin test is needed, give it either before or simultaneously with vaccine.
- Use only diluent supplied. Discard vaccine 8 hours after reconstituting.
- Use a 25G 5/8 -inch needle to inject.
- Don't give vaccine I.V.
- Refrigerate and protect from light. Reconstituted solution is clear yellow; don't use if discolored.
- Give to asymptomatic HIV-infected children.
- Don't use for delayed hypersensitivity (allergy) skin testing. Use mumps skin-test antigen, a killed viral product.

Patient teaching

- Warn patient or parents about adverse reactions linked to vaccine.
- Stress importance of avoiding pregnancy for 3 months after vaccination. Provide contraception information, if needed.
- Tell patient to treat fever with fever-reducing drugs.

mycophenolate mofetil
CellCept

mycophenolate mofetil hydrochloride
CellCept Intravenous

Pregnancy risk category C

Indications & dosages

➲ **To prevent organ rejection in patients receiving allogenic renal transplants**
Adults: 1 g P.O. or I.V. b.i.d. with corticosteroids and cyclosporine.

For patients with severe chronic renal impairment outside of immediate posttransplant period, avoid doses above 1 g b.i.d. If neutropenia develops, interrupt or reduce dosage.

➲ **To prevent organ rejection in patients receiving allogenic cardiac transplant**
Adults: 1.5 g P.O. or I.V. b.i.d. with cyclosporine and corticosteroids.

➲ **To prevent organ rejection in patients receiving allogenic hepatic transplants**
Adults: 1 g I.V. b.i.d. over no less than 2 hours or 1.5 g P.O. b.i.d. with cyclosporine and corticosteroids.

If neutropenia develops, interrupt or reduce dosage.

Contraindications & cautions

- Contraindicated in patients hypersensitive to drug, its ingredients, or mycophenolic acid and in patients sensitive to polysorbate 80.
- Drug isn't recommended for use in pregnant women (unless benefits to mother outweigh risks to fetus) or in breast-feeding women.
- Safety and effectiveness of drug in children haven't been established.
- Use cautiously in patients with GI disorders.

Adverse reactions

CNS: *tremor*, insomnia, *fever*, dizziness, *headache, asthenia.*
CV: *chest pain, hypertension, edema.*
EENT: pharyngitis.
GI: *diarrhea, constipation, nausea, dyspepsia, vomiting, oral candidiasis, abdominal pain,* ***hemorrhage****.*
GU: *UTI, hematuria,* renal tubular necrosis.
Hematologic: *anemia,* LEUKOPENIA, THROMBOCYTOPENIA, hypochromic anemia, leukocytosis.
Metabolic: *hypercholesterolemia, hypophosphatemia, hypokalemia, hyperkalemia, hyperglycemia.*
Musculoskeletal: *back pain.*
Respiratory: *dyspnea, cough, infection,* bronchitis, pneumonia.
Skin: *acne,* rash.
Other: *pain, infection,* ***sepsis****, peripheral edema.*

Interactions

Drug-drug. *Acyclovir, ganciclovir, other drugs that undergo renal tubular secretion:* May increase risk of toxicity for both drugs. Monitor patient closely.
Antacids with magnesium and aluminum hydroxides: May decrease mycophenolate absorption. Separate dosing times.
Cholestyramine: May interfere with enterohepatic recirculation, reducing mycophenolate bioavailability. Avoid using together.
Phenytoin, theophylline: May increase both drug levels. Monitor drug levels closely.
Probenecid, salicylates: May increase mycophenolate level. Monitor patient closely.

Nursing considerations

- Start drug therapy within 24 hours after transplantation. Use I.V. form in patients unable to take oral forms.
- I.V. form can be given for up to 14 days; switch patient to capsules or tablets as soon as oral drugs can be tolerated.
- Avoid doses above 1 g b.i.d. after immediate posttransplant period in patients with severe chronic renal impairment.
- Because of potential teratogenic effects, don't open or crush capsule. Avoid inhaling powder in capsule or having it contact skin or mucous membranes. If such contact occurs, wash thoroughly with soap and water, and rinse eyes with water.

Patient teaching

- Warn patient not to open or crush capsules, but to swallow them whole on an empty stomach.
- Stress importance of not interrupting or stopping therapy without first consulting prescriber.
- Tell woman to have a pregnancy test 1 week before therapy begins.
- Instruct woman of childbearing age to use two forms of contraception during therapy and for 6 weeks afterward, even with a history of infertility, unless a hysterectomy has been performed or abstinence is the chosen method. Tell her to notify prescriber immediately if she suspects pregnancy.
- Warn patient of the increased risk of lymphoma and other malignancies.

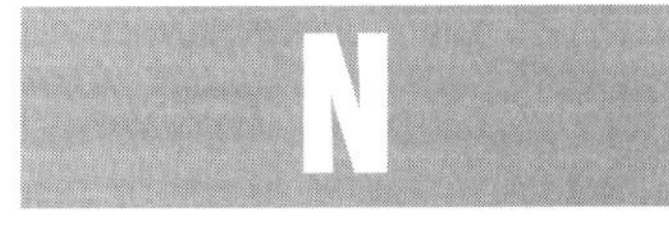

nadolol
Corgard

Pregnancy risk category C

Indications & dosages

➲ Angina pectoris
Adults: 40 mg P.O. once daily. Increase in 40- to 80-mg increments at 3- to 7-day intervals until optimum response occurs. Usual maintenance dose is 40 to 80 mg once daily; up to 240 mg once daily may be needed.

➲ Hypertension
Adults: 40 mg P.O. once daily. Increase in 40- to 80-mg increments until optimum response occurs. Usual maintenance dose is 40 to 80 mg once daily. Doses of 320 mg may be needed.

If creatinine clearance is 31 to 50 ml/minute, q 24 to 36 hours; if clearance is 10 to 30 ml/minute, q 24 to 48 hours; and if clearance is less than 10 ml/minute, q 40 to 60 hours.

Contraindications & cautions

- Contraindicated in patients with bronchial asthma, sinus bradycardia and greater than first-degree heart block, cardiogenic shock, and overt heart failure.

• Use cautiously in patients with heart failure, chronic bronchitis, emphysema, or renal or hepatic impairment and in patients undergoing major surgery involving general anesthesia.
• Use cautiously in diabetic patients because beta blockers may mask certain signs and symptoms of hypoglycemia.

Adverse reactions

CNS: fatigue, dizziness, fever.
CV: BRADYCARDIA, *hypotension*, HEART FAILURE, peripheral vascular disease, rhythm and conduction disturbances.
GI: nausea, vomiting, diarrhea, abdominal pain, constipation, anorexia.
Respiratory: *increased airway resistance.*
Skin: rash.

Interactions

Drug-drug. *Antihypertensives:* May increase antihypertensive effect. Monitor blood pressure closely.
Cardiac glycosides: May cause excessive bradycardia and additive effects on AV conduction. Use together cautiously.
Epinephrine: May decrease the patient response to epinephrine for treatment of an allergic reaction. Monitor patient closely for decreased clinical effect.
General anesthetics: May increase hypotensive effects. Consider stopping nadolol before surgery.
Insulin: May mask symptoms of hypoglycemia, as a result of beta blockade (such as tachycardia). Use with caution in patients with diabetes.
I.V. lidocaine: May reduce hepatic metabolism of lidocaine, increasing the risk of toxicity. Give bolus doses of lidocaine at a slower rate and monitor lidocaine level closely.
NSAIDs: May decrease antihypertensive effect. Monitor blood pressure and adjust dosage.
Oral antidiabetics: May alter dosage requirements in previously stabilized diabetic patients. Monitor glucose closely.
Phenothiazines: May increase hypotensive effects. Monitor blood pressure.
Prazosin: May increase risk of orthostatic hypotension in the early phases of use together. Assist patient to stand slowly until effects are known.
Reserpine: May increase hypotension or bradycardia. Monitor patient for adverse effects such as dizziness, syncope, and postural hypotension.
Verapamil: May increase effects of both drugs. Monitor cardiac function closely and decrease dosages as necessary.

Nursing considerations

• Check apical pulse before giving drug. If slower than 60 beats/minute, withhold drug and call prescriber.
• Monitor blood pressure frequently. If patient develops severe hypotension, give a vasopressor, as prescribed.
!!ALERT Abrupt stoppage can worsen angina and cause an MI. Reduce dosage gradually over 1 to 2 weeks.
• Drug masks signs and symptoms of shock and hyperthyroidism.

Patient teaching

• Explain importance of taking drug as prescribed, even when patient is feeling well.
• Teach patient how to check pulse rate and tell him to check it before each dose. If pulse rate is below 60 beats/minute, tell patient to notify prescriber.
• Warn patient not to stop drug suddenly.

nafcillin sodium

Pregnancy risk category B

Indications & dosages

➲ **Systemic infections caused by susceptible organisms (methicillin-sensitive *Staphylococcus aureus*)**
Adults: 500 mg to 1 g I.V. q 4 hours, depending on severity of infection.
Infants and children older than age 1 month: 50 to 200 mg/kg I.V. daily in divided doses q 4 to 6 hours, depending on severity of infection.
Neonates older than 7 days weighing more than 2 kg (4.4 lb): 25 mg/kg I.V. q 6 hours.
Neonates older than 7 days weighing 2 kg or less: 25 mg/kg I.V. q 8 hours.
Neonates age 7 days or younger weighing more than 2 kg: 25 mg/kg I.V. q 8 hours.
Neonates age 7 days or younger weighing 2 kg or less: 25 mg/kg I.V. q 12 hours.

➲ **Meningitis**
Adults: 100 to 200 mg/kg/day I.V. in divided doses q 4 to 6 hours.
Neonates older than 7 days weighing 2 kg (4.4 lb) or more: 50 mg/kg I.V. q 6 hours.
Neonates older than 7 days weighing less than 2 kg: 50 mg/kg I.V. q 8 hours.
Neonates age 7 days or younger weighing 2 kg or more: 50 mg/kg I.V. q 8 hours.
Neonates age 7 days or younger weighing less than 2 kg: 25 to 50 mg/kg I.V. q 12 hours.
➲ **Acute or chronic osteomyelitis caused by susceptible organism**
Adults: 1 to 2 g I.V. q 4 hours for 4 to 8 weeks.
Children older than age 1 month: 100 to 200 mg/kg/day in equally divided doses q 4 to 6 hours for 4 to 8 weeks.
➲ **Native valve endocarditis caused by susceptible organism**
Adults: 2 g I.V. q 4 hours for 4 to 6 weeks, combined with gentamicin.
Children older than age 1 month: 100 to 200 mg/kg/day in equally divided doses q 4 to 6 hours for 4 to 8 weeks in combination with gentamicin.

Contraindications & cautions

- Contraindicated in patients hypersensitive to drug or other penicillins.
- Use cautiously in patients with GI distress and in those with other drug allergies (especially to cephalosporins) because of possible cross-sensitivity.

Adverse reactions

CV: thrombophlebitis, vein irritation.
GI: *nausea*, vomiting, diarrhea, ***pseudomembranous colitis***.
Hematologic: ***neutropenia***, ***leukopenia***, eosinophilia, anemia, ***agranulocytosis***, ***thrombocytopenia***.
Other: hypersensitivity reactions, ***anaphylaxis***.

Interactions

Drug-drug. *Aminoglycosides:* May have synergistic effect; drugs are chemically and physically incompatible. Don't combine in same I.V. solution.
Hormonal contraceptives: May decrease hormonal contraceptive effectiveness. Advise use of additional form of contraception during penicillin therapy.
Probenecid: May increase nafcillin level. Probenecid may be used for this purpose.
Rifampin: May cause dose-dependent antagonism. Monitor patient closely.
Warfarin: May decrease effects of warfarin when used with nafcillin. Monitor PT and INR closely.

Nursing considerations

- Before giving drug, ask patient about allergic reactions to penicillin.
- Obtain specimen for culture and sensitivity tests before giving first dose. Therapy may begin pending results.
- If large doses are given or if therapy is prolonged, bacterial or fungal superinfection may occur, especially in elderly, debilitated, or immunosuppressed patients.
- Monitor sodium level because each gram of nafcillin contains 2.9 mEq of sodium.
- Monitor WBC counts twice weekly in patients receiving nafcillin for longer than 2 weeks. Neutropenia commonly occurs in the third week.
- An abnormal urinalysis result may indicate drug-induced interstitial nephritis.

Patient teaching

- Tell patient to report burning or irritation at the I.V. site.
- Advise patient to notify prescriber if a rash develops or if signs and symptoms of superinfection appear, such as recurring fever, chills, and malaise.

nalbuphine hydrochloride
Nubain

Pregnancy risk category B

Indications & dosages

➲ **Moderate to severe pain**
Adults: For a patient of about 70 kg [154 lb]), 10 to 20 mg S.C., I.M., or I.V. q 3 to 6 hours, p.r.n. Maximum, 160 mg daily.
➲ **Adjunct to balanced anesthesia**
Adults: 0.3 mg/kg to 3.0 mg/kg I.V. over 10 to 15 minutes; then maintenance doses of 0.25 to 0.50 mg/kg in single I.V. dose, p.r.n.

In patients with renal or hepatic impairment, decrease dosage.

Contraindications & cautions

- Contraindicated in patients hypersensitive to drug.
- Use cautiously in patients with history of drug abuse and in those with emotional instability, head injury, increased intracranial pressure, impaired ventilation, MI accompanied by nausea and vomiting, upcoming biliary surgery, and hepatic or renal disease.

!!ALERT Certain commercial preparations contain sodium metabisulfite.

Adverse reactions

CNS: *headache, sedation, dizziness, vertigo,* nervousness, depression, restlessness, crying, euphoria, hostility, confusion, unusual dreams, hallucinations, speech disorders, delusions.
CV: hypertension, hypotension, tachycardia, ***bradycardia***.
EENT: blurred vision, dry mouth.
GI: cramps, dyspepsia, bitter taste, nausea, vomiting, constipation, biliary tract spasms.
GU: urinary urgency.
Respiratory: ***respiratory depression***, dyspnea, asthma, pulmonary edema.
Skin: pruritus, burning, urticaria, clamminess, diaphoresis.

Interactions

Drug-drug. *CNS depressants, general anesthetics, hypnotics, MAO inhibitors, sedatives, tranquilizers, tricyclic antidepressants:* May cause respiratory depression, hypertension, profound sedation, or coma. Use together with caution, and monitor patient response.
Opioid analgesics: May decrease analgesic effect. Avoid using together.
Drug-lifestyle. *Alcohol use:* May cause additive effects. Discourage use together.

Nursing considerations

- Reassess patient's level of pain at least 15 and 30 minutes after parenteral administration.
- Drug acts as an opioid antagonist and may cause withdrawal syndrome. For patients who have received long-term opioids, give 25% of the usual dose initially. Watch for signs of withdrawal.

!!ALERT Drug causes respiratory depression, which at 10 mg is equal to respiratory depression produced by 10 mg of morphine.

- Monitor circulatory and respiratory status and bladder and bowel function. Withhold dose and notify prescriber if respirations are shallow or rate is below 12 breaths/minute.
- Constipation is often severe with maintenance therapy. Make sure stool softener or other laxative is ordered.
- Psychological and physical dependence may occur with prolonged use.

!!ALERT Don't confuse Nubain with Navane.

Patient teaching

- Caution ambulatory patient about getting out of bed or walking. Warn outpatient to avoid driving and other hazardous activities that require mental alertness until drug's CNS effects are known.
- Teach patient how to manage troublesome adverse effects such as constipation.

naloxone hydrochloride
Narcan

Pregnancy risk category B

Indications & dosages

➲ Known or suspected opioid-induced respiratory depression, including that caused by pentazocine and propoxyphene
Adults: 0.4 to 2 mg I.V., I.M., or S.C. Repeat dose q 2 to 3 minutes, p.r.n. If patient doesn't respond after 10 mg have been given, question diagnosis of opioid-induced toxicity.
Children: 0.01 mg/kg I.V.; then, second dose of 0.1 mg/kg I.V., if needed. If I.V. route isn't available, drug may be given I.M. or S.C. in divided doses.
Neonates: 0.01 mg/kg I.V., I.M., or S.C. Repeat dose q 2 to 3 minutes, p.r.n.
➲ Postoperative opioid depression
Adults: 0.1 to 0.2 mg I.V. q 2 to 3 minutes, p.r.n. Repeat dose within 1 to 2 hours, if needed.
Children: 0.005 to 0.01 mg I.V. repeated q 2 to 3 minutes, p.r.n.
Neonates (asphyxia neonatorum): 0.01 mg/kg I.V. into umbilical vein. May be repeated q 2 to 3 minutes.

Contraindications & cautions

- Contraindicated in patients hypersensitive to drug.

• Use cautiously in patients with cardiac irritability or opioid addiction. Abrupt reversal of opioid-induced CNS depression may result in nausea, vomiting, diaphoresis, tachycardia, CNS excitement, and increased blood pressure.

Adverse reactions

CNS: tremors, ***seizures***.
CV: tachycardia, hypertension with higher-than-recommended doses, hypotension, ***ventricular fibrillation***.
GI: nausea, vomiting.
Respiratory: pulmonary edema.
Skin: diaphoresis.
Other: withdrawal symptoms in opioid-dependent patients with higher-than-recommended doses.

Interactions

None significant.

Nursing considerations

• Duration of action of the opioid may exceed that of naloxone, and patients may relapse into respiratory depression.
• Respiratory rate increases within 1 to 2 minutes.
!!ALERT Drug is effective only in reversing respiratory depression caused by opioids, not against other drug-induced respiratory depression, including that caused by benzodiazepines.
• Patients who receive naloxone to reverse opioid-induced respiratory depression may exhibit tachypnea.
• Monitor respiratory depth and rate. Be prepared to provide oxygen, ventilation, and other resuscitation measures.
!!ALERT Don't confuse naloxone with naltrexone.

Patient teaching

• Inform family about use and administration of drug.
• Reassure family that patient will be monitored closely until effects of opioid resolve.

naltrexone hydrochloride
Depade, ReVia

Pregnancy risk category C

Indications & dosages

➲ Adjunct for maintenance of opioid-free state in detoxified persons
Adults: Initially, 25 mg P.O. If no withdrawal signs occur within 1 hour, an additional 25 mg is given. Once patient has been started on 50 mg q 24 hours, flexible maintenance schedule may be used. From 50 to 150 mg may be given daily, depending on schedule prescribed.
➲ Alcohol dependence
Adults: 50 mg P.O. once daily.

Contraindications & cautions

• Contraindicated in patients hypersensitive to drug, in those receiving opioid analgesics, in opioid-dependent patients, in patients in acute opioid withdrawal, and in those with positive urine screen for opioids or acute hepatitis or liver failure.
• Use cautiously in patients with mild hepatic disease or history of recent hepatic disease.

Adverse reactions

CNS: *insomnia, anxiety, nervousness, headache,* depression, dizziness, fatigue, somnolence, ***suicidal ideation***.
GI: *nausea, vomiting,* anorexia, *abdominal pain,* constipation, increased thirst.
GU: delayed ejaculation, decreased potency.
Hepatic: ***hepatotoxicity***.
Musculoskeletal: *muscle and joint pain.*
Skin: rash.
Other: chills.

Interactions

Drug-drug. *Opioid-containing products:* May decrease effect of opioid. Avoid using together.
Thioridazine: May increase somnolence and lethargy. Monitor patient closely.

Nursing considerations

• Treatment for opioid dependence shouldn't begin until patient receives naloxone challenge, a provocative test of opioid dependence. If signs and symptoms of opioid withdrawal persist after naloxone challenge, don't give drug.

- Patient must be completely free from opioids before taking drug or severe withdrawal symptoms may occur. Patients who have been addicted to short-acting opioids, such as heroin and meperidine, must wait at least 7 days after last opioid dose before starting drug. Patients who have been addicted to longer-acting opioids such as methadone should wait at least 10 days.
- In an emergency, anticipate that patient receiving naltrexone may be given an opioid analgesic, but dose must be higher than usual to surmount naltrexone's effect. Watch for respiratory depression from the opioid; it may be longer and deeper.
- For patients expected to be noncompliant because of history of opioid dependence, be prepared to try a flexible maintenance dose regimen of 100 mg on Monday and Wednesday and 150 mg on Friday.
- Use drug only as part of a comprehensive rehabilitation program.

!!ALERT Don't confuse naltrexone with naloxone.

Patient teaching

- Advise patient to wear or carry medical identification and to tell medical personnel that he takes naltrexone.
- Give patient names of nonopioid drugs that he can continue to take for pain, diarrhea, or cough.
- Tell patient to report adverse effects to prescriber immediately.

nandrolone decanoate
Deca-Durabolin

Pregnancy risk category X
Controlled substance schedule III

Indications & dosages

➲ Severe debility or disease states, refractory anemias

Adults and children older than age 13: 50 to 100 mg I.M. at 1- to 4-week intervals for women; 50 to 200 mg I.M. at 1- to 4-week intervals for men. Therapy should be intermittent and should be stopped if patient doesn't improve in 6 months.

Children ages 2 to 13: 25 to 50 mg I.M. q 3 to 4 weeks.

Contraindications & cautions

- Contraindicated in patients hypersensitive to anabolic steroids, patients with nephrosis or the nephrotic phase of nephritis, men with breast cancer or known or suspected prostate cancer, women with breast cancer and hypercalcemia, pregnant or breastfeeding women, and those who want to enhance their physical appearance or athletic performance.
- Use cautiously in patients with diabetes; cardiac, renal, or hepatic disease; epilepsy; or migraine or other conditions that may be aggravated by fluid retention.

Adverse reactions

CNS: excitation, insomnia, habituation, depression.
CV: edema.
GI: nausea, vomiting, diarrhea.
GU: bladder irritability.
Hematologic: ***suppression of clotting factors***.
Hepatic: reversible jaundice, ***peliosis hepatis, liver cell tumors***.
Metabolic: hypernatremia, hyperkalemia, hypercalcemia, hyperphosphatemia, hypercholesterolemia.
Skin: pain, induration at injection site, acne.
Other: *hypoestrogenic effects in women*, excessive hormonal effects in men, androgenic effects in women.

Interactions

Drug-drug. *Hepatotoxic drugs:* May increase risk of hepatotoxicity. Monitor liver function closely.
Insulin, oral antidiabetics: May alter dosage requirements. Monitor glucose level in diabetic patients.
Oral anticoagulants: May alter dosage requirements. Monitor PT and INR.

Nursing considerations

- Don't give drug to woman of childbearing age until pregnancy is ruled out.
- Make sure patient understands importance of using an effective nonhormonal contraceptive during therapy.
- Instruct patient to stop drug immediately and notify prescriber if pregnancy is suspected.
- In children, obtain X-rays of wrist bones before therapy begins to establish bone maturation level. During treatment, bones may

mature more rapidly than they grow in length. Periodically review X-ray results to monitor bone maturation.
• Inject I.M. drug deeply, preferably into upper outer quadrant of gluteal muscle in adults. Rotate injection sites to prevent muscle atrophy.
• Unless contraindicated, use with high-calorie, high-protein diet. Give small, frequent meals.
• Watch for signs of virilization, which may be irreversible even if drug is stopped. Androgenic effects in women include acne, edema, weight gain, increased hair growth, hoarseness, clitoral enlargement, decreased breast size, changes in libido, male-pattern baldness, and oily skin or hair.
• Watch for hypoestrogenic effects in women, such as flushing, diaphoresis, vaginal bleeding, nervousness, emotional lability, menstrual irregularities, and vaginitis, including itching, dryness, and burning.
• Watch for excessive hormonal effects in male patients. If patient is prepubertal, watch for premature epiphyseal closure, acne, priapism, growth of body and facial hair, and phallic enlargement. If he's postpubertal, watch for testicular atrophy, oligospermia, decreased ejaculatory volume, impotence, gynecomastia, and epididymitis.
• Closely observe boys younger than age 7 for precocious development of male sexual characteristics.
• Evaluate semen every 3 to 4 months, especially in adolescent boys.
!! ALERT Periodically evaluate hepatic function. Watch for jaundice; dosage adjustment may reverse condition. If liver function test results are abnormal, therapy should be stopped.
• Check weight regularly. Edema usually can be controlled with sodium restriction or diuretics.
• Watch for evidence of hypoglycemia in diabetic patients. Check glucose levels and adjust dosage of antidiabetic.
• Check quantitative urine and serum calcium levels. Hypercalcemia is most likely to occur in patients with breast cancer.
• When used to promote erythropoiesis in patient with refractory anemia, make sure he has adequate daily iron intake.
• Anabolic steroids may alter results of laboratory studies performed during therapy and for 2 to 3 weeks after therapy ends.

Patient teaching

• Make sure patient understands importance of using an effective nonhormonal contraceptive during therapy.
• Review signs and symptoms of virilization with woman, and instruct her to notify prescriber immediately if they occur.
• Advise woman to wear cotton underwear and to wash after intercourse to decrease risk of vaginitis.
• Warn diabetic patient to be alert for hypoglycemia, and tell him to notify prescriber if it occurs.
• Tell patient to report sudden weight gain to prescriber.
• Tell woman of childbearing age to report menstrual irregularities and to stop drug while awaiting examination.

naproxen

Apo-Naproxen†, EC-Naprosyn, Naprosyn, Naprosyn-E†, Naprosyn-SR, Naxen†, Novo-Naprox†, Nu-Naprox†

naproxen sodium

Aleve ◇, Anaprox, Anaprox DS, Apo-Napro-Na† ◇, Naprelan, Novo-Naprox Sodium†, Synflex†

Pregnancy risk category B; D in 3rd trimester

Indications & dosages

➲ Rheumatoid arthritis, osteoarthritis, ankylosing spondylitis, pain, dysmenorrhea, tendinitis, bursitis
Adults: 250 to 500 mg naproxen b.i.d.; maximum, 1.5 g daily for a limited time. Or, 375 to 500 mg delayed-release EC Naprosyn b.i.d. Or, 750 to 1,000 mg controlled-release Naprelan daily. Or, 275 to 550 mg naproxen sodium b.i.d.
➲ Juvenile arthritis
Children: 10 mg/kg P.O. in two divided doses.
➲ Acute gout
Adults: 750 mg naproxen P.O.; then 250 mg q 8 hours until attack subsides. Or, 825 mg naproxen sodium; then 275 mg q 8 hours until attack subsides. Or, 1,000 to 1,500 mg

daily controlled-release Naprelan on first day; then 1,000 mg daily until attack subsides.

➲ **Mild to moderate pain, primary dysmenorrhea**

Adults: 500 mg naproxen P.O.; then 250 mg q 6 to 8 hours up to 1.25 g daily. Or, 550 mg naproxen sodium; then 275 mg q 6 to 8 hours up to 1,375 mg daily. Or, 1,000 mg controlled-release Naprelan once daily.
Elderly patients: In patients older than age 65, don't exceed 400 mg daily.

Contraindications & cautions

- Contraindicated in patients hypersensitive to drug and in those with the syndrome of asthma, rhinitis, and nasal polyps.
- Patient should avoid drug during last trimester of pregnancy.
- Use cautiously in elderly patients and in patients with renal disease, CV disease, GI disorders, hepatic disease, or history of peptic ulcer disease.

Adverse reactions

CNS: headache, drowsiness, dizziness, vertigo.
CV: edema, palpitations.
EENT: visual disturbances, *tinnitus*, auditory disturbances.
GI: epigastric pain, occult blood loss, abdominal pain, nausea, peptic ulceration, constipation, dyspepsia, heartburn, diarrhea, stomatitis, thirst.
Hematologic: increased bleeding time, ecchymoses.
Metabolic: ***hyperkalemia***.
Respiratory: dyspnea.
Skin: pruritus, rash, urticaria, diaphoresis, purpura.

Interactions

Drug-drug. *ACE inhibitors:* May cause renal impairment. Use together cautiously.
Antihypertensives, diuretics: May decrease effect of these drugs. Monitor patient closely.
Aspirin, corticosteroids: May cause adverse GI reactions. Avoid using together.
Lithium: May increase lithium level. Observe patient for toxicity and monitor level. Adjustment of lithium dosage may be required.
Methotrexate: May cause toxicity. Monitor patient closely.
Oral anticoagulants, other sulfonylureas, highly protein-bound drugs: May cause toxicity. Monitor patient closely.
Probenecid: May decrease elimination of naproxen. Monitor patient for toxicity.
Drug-herb. *Dong quai, feverfew, garlic, ginger, horse chestnut, red clover:* May cause bleeding, based on the known effects of components. Discourage use together.
White willow: Herb contains components similar to those of aspirin. Discourage use together.
Drug-lifestyle. *Alcohol use:* May cause adverse GI reactions. Discourage use together.

Nursing considerations

- Because NSAIDs impair synthesis of renal prostaglandins, they can decrease renal blood flow and lead to reversible renal impairment, especially in patients with renal failure, heart failure, or liver dysfunction; in elderly patients; and in those taking diuretics. Monitor these patients closely.
- Monitor CBC and renal and hepatic function every 4 to 6 months during long-term therapy.
- Serious GI toxicity, including peptic ulcers and bleeding, can occur in patient taking NSAIDs, despite lack of symptoms.
- Because of their antipyretic and anti-inflammatory actions, NSAIDs may mask signs and symptoms of infection.
- Naproxen may have a heart benefit, similar to aspirin, in preventing blood clotting.

Patient teaching

!!ALERT Drug is available without prescription (naproxen sodium, 200 mg). Instruct patient not to take more than 600 mg in 24 hours. Dosage in patient older than age 65 shouldn't exceed 400 mg daily.

- Advise patient to take drug with food or milk to minimize GI upset. Tell him to take a full glass of water or other liquid with each dose.
- Tell patient taking prescription doses of naproxen for arthritis that full therapeutic effect may be delayed 2 to 4 weeks.
- Warn patient against taking naproxen and naproxen sodium at the same time.
- Teach patient signs and symptoms of GI bleeding, including blood in vomit, urine, or stool; coffee-ground vomit; and black, tarry stool. Tell him to notify prescriber immediately if any of these occurs.

• Caution patient that use with aspirin, alcohol, other NSAIDs, or corticosteroids may increase risk of adverse GI reactions.
• Warn patient against hazardous activities that require mental alertness until CNS effects are known.

naratriptan hydrochloride
Amerge

Pregnancy risk category C

Indications & dosages
➲ Acute migraine attacks with or without aura
Adults: 1 or 2.5 mg P.O. as a single dosage. If headache returns or responds only partially, dose may be repeated after 4 hours. Maximum, 5 mg in 24 hours.

For patients with mild to moderate renal or hepatic impairment, reduce dosage. Maximum, 2.5 mg in 24 hours.

Contraindications & cautions
• Contraindicated in patients hypersensitive to drug or its components, in those with prior or current cardiac ischemia, in those with cerebrovascular or peripheral vascular syndromes, and in those with uncontrolled hypertension.
• Contraindicated in elderly patients, patients with creatinine clearance below 15 ml/minute, patients with Child-Pugh grade C, and patients who have used ergot-containing, ergot-type, or other 5-HT_1 agonists within 24 hours.
• Use cautiously in patients with risk factors for coronary artery disease (CAD), such as hypertension, hypercholesterolemia, obesity, diabetes, smoking, strong family history of CAD, postmenopausal women, and men older than age 40, unless patient is free from cardiac disease. Monitor patient closely after first dose.
• Use cautiously in patients with renal or hepatic impairment.

Adverse reactions
CNS: paresthesia, dizziness, drowsiness, malaise, fatigue, vertigo, syncope.
CV: palpitations, increased blood pressure, ***tachyarrhythmias, abnormal ECG changes, coronary artery vasospasm, transient myocardial ischemia, MI, ventricular tachycardia, ventricular fibrillation.***
EENT: ear, nose, and throat infections, photophobia.
GI: nausea, hyposalivation, vomiting.
Other: sensations of warmth, cold, pressure, tightness, or heaviness.

Interactions
Drug-drug. *Ergot-containing or ergot-type drugs (dihydroergotamine, methysergide), other 5-HT_1 agonists:* May prolong vasospastic reactions. Avoid using within 24 hours of naratriptan.
Hormonal contraceptives: May slightly increase naratriptan level. Monitor patient.
SSRIs (fluoxetine, fluvoxamine, paroxetine, sertraline): May cause weakness, hyperreflexia, and incoordination. Monitor patient.
Drug-herb. *St. John's wort:* May increase serotonergic effect. Discourage use together.
Drug-lifestyle. *Smoking:* May increase naratriptan clearance. Discourage smoking.

Nursing considerations
• Assess cardiac status in patients who develop risk factors for CAD.
!! ALERT Drug can cause coronary artery vasospasm and increased risk of cerebrovascular events.
• Drug isn't intended to prevent migraines or manage hemiplegic or basilar migraine.
• Safety and effectiveness of treating cluster headaches or more than four headaches in a 30-day period haven't been established.
• Use drug only when patient has a clear diagnosis of migraine.

Patient teaching
• Instruct patient to take drug only as prescribed and to read the accompanying patient instruction leaflet before using drug.
• Tell patient that drug is intended to relieve, not prevent, migraines.
• Instruct patient to take dose soon after headache starts. If no response occurs with first tablet, tell him to seek medical approval before taking second tablet. Tell patient that if more relief is needed after first tablet (if a partial response occurs or headache returns), and prescriber has approved a second dose, he may take a second tablet (but not sooner than 4 hours after first tablet). Tell him not to exceed 2 tablets within 24 hours.

• Advise patient to increase fluid intake.
• Advise patient not to use drug if she suspects or knows that she's pregnant.
• Tell patient to alert prescriber about bothersome adverse effects.

nateglinide

Starlix

Pregnancy risk category C

Indications & dosages

➲ As monotherapy, or with metformin or a thiazolidinedione, to lower glucose level in patients with type 2 (non–insulin-dependent) diabetes whose hyperglycemia isn't adequately controlled by diet and exercise and who haven't had long-term treatment with other antidiabetics
Adults: 120 mg P.O. t.i.d. taken 1 to 30 minutes before meals. Patients near goal HbA_{1c} when treatment is started may receive 60 mg P.O. t.i.d.

Contraindications & cautions

• Contraindicated in patients hypersensitive to drug, in those with type 1 diabetes or diabetic ketoacidosis, and in breast-feeding patients.
• Use cautiously in patients with moderate to severe liver dysfunction or adrenal or pituitary insufficiency, and in elderly and malnourished patients.

Adverse reactions

CNS: dizziness.
GI: diarrhea.
Metabolic: ***hypoglycemia***.
Musculoskeletal: back pain, arthropathy.
Respiratory: *upper respiratory tract infection*, bronchitis, coughing.
Other: flulike symptoms, accidental trauma.

Interactions

Drug-drug. *Corticosteroids, sympathomimetics, thiazides, thyroid products:* May reduce hypoglycemic action of nateglinide. Monitor glucose level closely.
MAO inhibitors, nonselective beta blockers, NSAIDs, salicylates: May increase hypoglycemic action of nateglinide. Monitor glucose level closely.

Nursing considerations

• Don't use with or as a substitute for glyburide or other oral antidiabetics; may use with metformin or a thiazolidinedione.
• Give drug 1 to 30 minutes before a meal. If patient misses a meal, skip the scheduled dose.
• Monitor glucose level regularly to evaluate drug's efficacy.
• Observe patient for signs and symptoms of hypoglycemia (sweating, rapid pulse, trembling, confusion, headache, irritability, and nausea). To minimize risk of hypoglycemia, make sure that patient has a meal immediately after dose. If hypoglycemia occurs and patient remains conscious, give him an oral form of glucose. If he's unconscious, treat with I.V. glucose.
• Risk of hypoglycemia increases with strenuous exercise, alcohol ingestion, or insufficient caloric intake.
• Symptoms of hypoglycemia may be masked in patients with autonomic neuropathy and in those who use beta blockers.
• Insulin therapy may be needed for glycemic control in patients with fever, infection, or trauma and in those undergoing surgery.
• Monitor glucose level closely when other drugs are started or stopped, to detect possible drug interactions.
• Periodically monitor HbA_{1c} level.
• Drug's effectiveness may decrease over time.
• No special dosage adjustments are usually necessary in elderly patients, but some elderly patients may have greater sensitivity to glucose-lowering effect.

Patient teaching

• Tell patient to take drug 1 to 30 minutes before a meal.
• Advise patient to skip the scheduled dose if he skips a meal, to reduce risk of low glucose level.
• Instruct patient on risk of low glucose level, its signs and symptoms (sweating, rapid pulse, trembling, confusion, headache, irritability, and nausea), and ways to treat these symptoms by eating or drinking something containing sugar.
• Teach patient how to monitor and log glucose levels to evaluate diabetes control.
• Advise patient to notify prescriber for persistent low or high glucose level.

- Instruct patient to adhere to prescribed diet and exercise regimen.
- Explain possible long-term complications of diabetes and importance of regular preventive therapy.
- Encourage patient to wear a medical identification bracelet.

nefazodone hydrochloride

Pregnancy risk category C

Indications & dosages

➲ Depression

Adults: Initially, 200 mg daily P.O. in two divided doses. Dosage may be increased by 100 to 200 mg daily at intervals of at least 1 week, p.r.n. Usual dosage range is 300 to 600 mg daily.

Elderly patients: Initially, 100 mg daily P.O. in two divided doses.

For debilitated patients, initially, 100 mg daily P.O. in two divided doses.

Contraindications & cautions

- Contraindicated in patients hypersensitive to drug or other phenylpiperazine antidepressants; also contraindicated within 14 days of MAO inhibitor therapy.
- Contraindicated in patients who stopped using nefazodone because of liver injury.
- Use cautiously in patients with CV or cerebrovascular disease that could be worsened by hypotension (such as history of MI, angina, or CVA) and conditions that would predispose patients to hypotension (such as dehydration, hypovolemia, and antihypertensive therapy).
- Use cautiously in patients with a history of mania.

Adverse reactions

CNS: fever, *headache, somnolence, dizziness, asthenia, insomnia, light-headedness, confusion,* memory impairment, paresthesia, vasodilation, abnormal dreams, impaired concentration, ataxia, incoordination, psychomotor retardation, tremor, hypertonia, ***suicidal behavior***.

CV: orthostatic hypotension, hypotension, peripheral edema.

EENT: blurred vision, abnormal vision, tinnitus, visual field defect, pharyngitis.

GI: *dry mouth, nausea, constipation,* taste perversion, dyspepsia, diarrhea, increased appetite, vomiting.

GU: urinary frequency, UTI, urine retention, vaginitis.

Hepatic: ***liver failure***.

Musculoskeletal: neck rigidity, arthralgia.

Respiratory: cough.

Skin: pruritus, rash.

Other: infection, flulike syndrome, chills, breast tenderness, thirst.

Interactions

Drug-drug. *Alprazolam, triazolam:* May potentiate effects of these drugs. Avoid using together; if use together is unavoidable, greatly reduce doses of alprazolam and triazolam.

CNS drugs: May alter CNS activity. Avoid using together.

Cyclosporine: May cause cyclosporine toxicity. Monitor cyclosporine level.

Digoxin: May increase digoxin level. Use together cautiously and monitor digoxin level.

Haloperidol: May increase haloperidol level. Monitor patient for increased adverse reactions.

HMG-CoA reductase inhibitors: May increase atorvastatin, lovastatin, and simvastatin levels. Monitor patient for increased adverse effects.

MAO inhibitors (phenelzine, selegiline, tranylcypromine): May cause serotonin syndrome. Avoid using within 14 days of MAO inhibitor therapy.

Other highly protein-bound drugs: May increase risk and severity of adverse reactions. Monitor patient closely.

Drug-herb. *St. John's wort:* May cause additive effects and serotonin syndrome. Discourage use together.

Drug-lifestyle. *Alcohol use:* May enhance CNS depression. Discourage use together.

Nursing considerations

!!ALERT Drug may cause hepatic failure. Don't start drug in patients with active liver disease or with elevated baseline transaminase level. Although preexisting hepatic disease doesn't increase the likelihood of developing hepatic failure, baseline abnormalities can complicate patient monitoring. Stop drug if clinical signs and symptoms of hepatic dysfunction appear, such as increased AST or ALT level exceeding three times the

upper limit of normal. Don't restart therapy.
- Don't use within 14 days of MAO inhibitor therapy.

!!ALERT A thorough risk-versus-benefit assessment should be considered before using nefazodone to treat depression, taking into account the risk for hepatic failure and emergence of suicidal thoughts and attempts.

Patient teaching

- Warn patient not to engage in hazardous activity until effects of drug are known.

!!ALERT Instruct men who experience prolonged or inappropriate erections to stop drug immediately and notify prescriber.
- Instruct woman of childbearing age to notify prescriber if she becomes pregnant or is planning pregnancy during therapy, or if she's breastfeeding.

!!ALERT Teach patient the signs and symptoms of liver problems, including yellowed skin or eyes, appetite loss, GI complaints, and malaise. Tell patient to report these adverse events to prescriber immediately.

!!ALERT Inform family members to be particularly vigilant for suicidal tendencies during therapy with nefazodone.
- Tell patient to notify prescriber if rash, hives, or related allergic reactions occur.
- Instruct patient to avoid alcohol during therapy.
- Tell patient to notify prescriber before taking OTC drugs.
- Inform patient that several weeks of therapy may be needed to obtain full antidepressant effect. Once improvement occurs, advise him not to stop drug until directed by prescriber.

nelfinavir mesylate
Viracept

Pregnancy risk category B

Indications & dosages

➲ HIV infection, when antiretroviral therapy is warranted
Adults: 1,250 mg b.i.d. or 750 mg P.O. t.i.d. with meals or light snack.
Children ages 2 to 13: 20 to 30 mg/kg dose P.O. t.i.d. with meals or light snack; don't exceed 750 mg t.i.d.

➲ To prevent infection after occupational exposure to HIV♦
Adults: 750 mg P.O. t.i.d. with two other antiretrovirals (zidovudine and lamivudine, lamivudine and stavudine, or didanosine and stavudine) for 4 weeks.

Contraindications & cautions

- Contraindicated in patients hypersensitive to drug or its components. Drug is also contraindicated in patients receiving amiodarone, ergot derivatives, lovastatin, midazolam, pimozide, quinidine, simvastatin, or triazolam.
- Use cautiously in patients with hepatic dysfunction or hemophilia types A or B. Monitor liver function test results.
- It's not known if drug appears in breast milk. Because safety hasn't been established, advise HIV-infected women not to breast-feed, to avoid transmitting virus to the infant.

Adverse reactions

CNS: ***seizures, suicidal ideation.***
GI: nausea, *diarrhea*, flatulence, ***pancreatitis.***
Hematologic: ***leukopenia, thrombocytopenia.***
Hepatic: ***hepatitis.***
Metabolic: dehydration, diabetes mellitus, hyperlipidemia, hyperuricemia, ***hypoglycemia.***
Skin: rash.
Other: redistribution or accumulation of body fat.

Interactions

Drug-drug. *Amiodarone, ergot derivatives, lovastatin, midazolam, pimozide, quinidine, simvastatin, triazolam:* May increase levels of these drugs, causing increased risk of serious or life-threatening adverse events. Avoid using together.
Atorvastatin: May increase atorvastatin level. Use lowest possible dose or consider using pravastatin or fluvastatin instead.
Azithromycin: May increase azithromycin level. Monitor patient for liver impairment.
Carbamazepine, phenobarbital: May reduce the effectiveness of nelfinavir. Use together cautiously.
Cyclosporine, sirolimus, tacrolimus: May increase levels of these immunosuppressants. Use cautiously together.

Delavirdine, HIV protease inhibitors (indinavir, saquinavir), nevirapine: May increase levels of protease inhibitors. Use together cautiously.
Didanosine: May decrease didanosine absorption. Take nelfinavir with food at least 2 hours before or 1 hour after didanosine.
Ethinyl estradiol: May decrease contraceptive level and effectiveness. Advise patient to use alternative contraceptive measures during therapy.
Methadone, phenytoin: May decrease levels of these drugs. Adjust dosage of these drugs accordingly.
Rifabutin: May increase rifabutin level and decrease nelfinavir level. Reduce dosage of rifabutin to half the usual dose and increase nelfinavir to 1,250 mg b.i.d.
Sildenafil: May increase adverse effects of sildenafil. Caution patient not to exceed 25 mg of sildenafil in a 48-hour period.
Drug-herb. *St. John's wort:* May decrease nelfinavir level. Discourage use together.

Nursing considerations

- Drug dosage is the same whether used alone or with other antiretrovirals.
- Give oral powder to children unable to take tablets. May mix oral powder with small amount of water, milk, formula, soy formula, soy milk, or dietary supplements. Patient should consume entire contents.
- Don't reconstitute with water in the original container.
- Use reconstituted powder within 6 hours.
- Mixing with acidic foods or juice isn't recommended because of bitter taste.

!!ALERT Don't confuse nelfinavir with nevirapine.

Patient teaching

- Advise patient to take drug with food.
- Inform patient that drug doesn't cure HIV infection.
- Tell patient that long-term effects of drug are unknown and that there are no data stating that nelfinavir reduces risk of HIV transmission.
- Advise patient to take drug daily as prescribed and not to alter dose or stop drug without medical approval.
- If patient misses a dose, tell him to take it as soon as possible and then return to his normal schedule. Advise patient not to double the dose.
- Tell patient that diarrhea is the most common adverse effect and that it can be controlled with loperamide, if needed.
- Instruct patient taking hormonal contraceptives to use alternative or additional contraceptive measures while taking nelfinavir.
- Advise patient taking sildenafil about an increased risk of sildenafil-related adverse events including low blood pressure, visual changes, and painful erections. Tell him to promptly report any symptoms. Tell him not to exceed 25 mg of sildenafil in a 48-hour period.
- Warn patient with phenylketonuria that powder contains 11.2 mg phenylalanine/g.
- Advise patient to report use of other prescribed or OTC drugs because of possible drug interactions.

neomycin sulfate

Mycifradin†, Neo-fradin, Neo-Tabs

Pregnancy risk category D

Indications & dosages

➲ **Infectious diarrhea caused by enteropathogenic *Escherichia coli***
Adults: 50 mg/kg daily P.O. in four divided doses for 2 to 3 days; maximum of 3 g/day.
Children: 50 to 100 mg/kg daily P.O. in divided doses q 4 to 6 hours for 2 to 3 days.

➲ **To suppress intestinal bacteria before surgery**
Adults: After saline cathartic, 1 g P.O. q hour for four doses; then 1 g q 4 hours for the balance of the 24 hours. Or, 88 mg/kg in six equally divided doses q 4 hours. Or, 1 g neomycin with 1 g erythromycin base at 1 p.m., 2 p.m., and 11 p.m. on day before 8 a.m. surgery.
Children: After saline cathartic, 40 to 100 mg/kg daily P.O. in divided doses q 4 to 6 hours. Or, 88 mg/kg in six equally divided doses q 4 hours.

➲ **Adjunctive treatment for hepatic coma**
Adults: 1 to 3 g P.O. q.i.d. for 5 to 6 days; or 200 ml of 1% solution or 100 ml of 2% solution as enema retained for 20 to 60 minutes q 6 hours. For patients with chronic hepatic insufficiency, 4 g/day indefinitely may be needed.
Children: 50 to 100 mg/kg/day P.O. in divided doses for 5 to 6 days.

Contraindications & cautions

- Contraindicated in patients hypersensitive to other aminoglycosides and in those with intestinal obstruction.
- Use cautiously in elderly patients and in those with impaired renal function, neuromuscular disorders, or ulcerative bowel lesions.

Adverse reactions

EENT: *ototoxicity.*
GI: nausea, vomiting, diarrhea, malabsorption syndrome, ***Clostridium difficile*-related** colitis.
GU: ***nephrotoxicity***, possible increase in urinary excretion of casts.

Interactions

Drug-drug. *Acyclovir, amphotericin B, cephalosporins, cidofovir, cisplatin, methoxyflurane, vancomycin, other aminoglycosides:* May increase nephrotoxicity. Monitor renal function test results.
Atracurium, doxacurium, mivacurium, pancuronium, rocuronium, tubocurarine, vecuronium: May increase effects of nondepolarizing muscle relaxants, including prolonged respiratory depression. Use together only when necessary, and expect to reduce dosage of nondepolarizing muscle relaxants.
Digoxin: May decrease digoxin absorption. Monitor digoxin level.
I.V. loop diuretics (such as furosemide): May increase ototoxicity. Monitor patient's hearing.
Oral anticoagulants: May inhibit vitamin K–producing bacteria; may increase anticoagulant effect. Monitor PT and INR.

Nursing considerations

- Monitor renal function: urine output, specific gravity, urinalysis, BUN and creatinine levels, and creatinine clearance. Report to prescriber evidence of declining renal function.
- Evaluate patient's hearing before and during prolonged therapy. Notify prescriber if patient has tinnitus, vertigo, or hearing loss. Deafness may start several weeks after drug is stopped.
- Watch for signs and symptoms of superinfection, such as fever, chills, and increased pulse rate.
- When using drug as adjunctive treatment for hepatic coma, decrease patient's dietary protein and assess neurologic status frequently during therapy.
- When using drug for preoperative disinfection, provide a low-residue diet and a cathartic immediately before therapy.
- The ototoxic and nephrotoxic properties of neomycin limit its usefulness.

Patient teaching

- Instruct patient to report adverse reactions promptly.
- Encourage patient to maintain adequate fluid intake.

neostigmine bromide
Prostigmin

neostigmine methylsulfate
Prostigmin

Pregnancy risk category C

Indications & dosages

➲ To control myasthenia gravis symptoms
Adults: Initially, 15 mg P.O. t.i.d.; increase gradually, p.r.n. Range is 15 to 375 mg/day. Average dosage is 150 mg/day with intervals individualized. Or, 0.5 mg S.C. or I.M.; base subsequent parenteral doses on patient's response.
Children: 2 mg/kg/day P.O. divided q 3 to 4 hours, or 0.01 to 0.04 mg/kg/dose I.M. or S.C. q 2 to 3 hours, p.r.n.

➲ To prevent and treat postoperative distention and urinary retention
Adults: For prevention, 0.25 mg I.M. or S.C. as soon as possible after surgery; then q 4 to 6 hours for 2 to 3 days. For treatment, 0.5 mg I.M. or S.C. If urination hasn't occurred in 1 hour, catheterize. Continue 0.5-mg injections q 3 hours for at least 5 doses.

➲ Antidote for nondepolarizing neuromuscular blockers
Adults: 0.5 to 2 mg I.V. slowly. Repeat, p.r.n., to total of 5 mg. Before antidote dose, give 0.6 to 1.2 mg atropine sulfate I.V. if patient is bradycardic.

Contraindications & cautions

- Contraindicated in patients hypersensitive to cholinergics or bromides and in those with peritonitis or mechanical obstruction of the intestinal or urinary tract.
- Use cautiously in patients with bronchial asthma, bradycardia, seizure disorders, recent coronary occlusion, vagotonia, hyperthyroidism, arrhythmias, and peptic ulcer.

Adverse reactions

CNS: dizziness, headache, muscle weakness, loss of consciousness, drowsiness, syncope, ***seizures***.
CV: ***bradycardia***, hypotension, tachycardia, ***AV block***, flushing, ***cardiac arrest***.
EENT: blurred vision, lacrimation, miosis.
GI: *nausea, vomiting, diarrhea, abdominal cramps*, excessive salivation, flatulence, increased peristalsis.
GU: urinary frequency.
Musculoskeletal: *muscle cramps*, muscle fasciculations, arthralgia.
Respiratory: ***bronchospasm***, dyspnea, ***respiratory depression, respiratory arrest***, increased secretions, ***laryngospasm, paralysis of respiratory muscles, central respiratory paralysis***.
Skin: rash, urticaria, diaphoresis.
Other: hypersensitivity reactions, ***anaphylaxis***.

Interactions

Drug-drug. *Aminoglycosides, anticholinergics, atropine, corticosteroids, local and general anesthetics, magnesium sulfate, procainamide, quinidine:* May reverse cholinergic effects; watch for lack of drug effect. Stop all other cholinergics before giving this drug.
Succinylcholine: May worsen blockade produced by succinylcholine when used to reverse the effects of nondepolarizing neuromuscular blockers in surgical patients. Monitor patient.

Nursing considerations

- Dosage for the treatment of myasthenia gravis must be highly individualized, depending on response and tolerance of adverse effects. Therapy may be needed day and night.
- In myasthenia gravis, schedule doses before periods of fatigue. For example, if patient has difficulty swallowing, schedule dose 30 minutes before each meal.

!!ALERT Monitor vital signs frequently, especially respirations. Keep atropine injection available, and be prepared to provide respiratory support, as needed.
!!ALERT Don't confuse neostigmine with etomidate (Amidate) vials, which may look alike.

- Monitor and document patient's response after each dose. Optimum dosage is difficult to judge. Watch closely for improvement in strength, vision, and ptosis, 45 to 60 minutes after each dose.
- When drug is used to prevent abdominal distention and GI distress, insertion of a rectal tube may help passage of gas.
- When drug is given for postoperative abdominal distention and bladder atony, rule out mechanical obstruction before dose is given. If no response within 1 hour after first dose, catheterize patient.
- Patients sometimes develop resistance to neostigmine.
- If appropriate, obtain order for hospitalized patient to have bedside supply of tablets. Many patients with long-standing disease insist on self-administration.

Patient teaching

- Tell patient to take drug with food or milk to reduce adverse GI reactions.
- When giving drug for myasthenia gravis, explain that it will relieve ptosis, double vision, chewing and swallowing problems, and trunk and limb weakness. Stress the importance of taking drug exactly as prescribed, including nighttime doses. Explain that patient may need to take drug for life.
- Teach patient how to observe and record variations in muscle strength.
- Advise patient to wear or carry medical identification of myasthenia gravis condition.

nesiritide
Natrecor

Pregnancy risk category C

Indications & dosages

➲ Acutely decompensated heart failure in patients with dyspnea at rest or with minimal activity
Adults: 2 mcg/kg by I.V. bolus over 60 seconds, followed by continuous infusion of 0.01 mcg/kg/minute.

If hypotension develops during administration, reduce dosage or stop drug. Restart drug at dosage reduced by 30% with no bolus doses.

Contraindications & cautions

- Contraindicated in patients hypersensitive to drug or its components.
- Contraindicated in patients with cardiogenic shock, systolic blood pressure below 90 mm Hg, low cardiac filling pressures, conditions in which cardiac output depends on venous return, or conditions that make vasodilators inappropriate, such as valvular stenosis, restrictive or obstructive cardiomyopathy, constrictive pericarditis, and pericardial tamponade.

Adverse reactions

CNS: headache, confusion, somnolence, insomnia, dizziness, anxiety, paresthesia, tremor, fever.
CV: *hypotension*, ***ventricular tachycardia***, ventricular extrasystoles, angina, ***bradycardia***, atrial fibrillation, AV node conduction abnormalities.
GI: nausea, vomiting, abdominal pain.
Hematologic: anemia.
Musculoskeletal: back pain, leg cramps.
Respiratory: ***apnea***, cough.
Skin: injection site reactions, pain at the site, rash, sweating, pruritus.

Interactions

Drug-drug. *ACE inhibitors:* May increase hypotension symptoms. Monitor blood pressure closely.

Nursing considerations

- Don't start drug at higher-than-recommended dosage because this may cause hypotension and may increase creatinine level.

!!ALERT This drug may cause hypotension. Monitor patient's blood pressure closely, particularly if he also takes an ACE inhibitor.

!!ALERT Natrecor binds heparin and could bind the heparin lining of a heparin-coated catheter, decreasing the amount of nesiritide delivered. Don't give nesiritide through a central heparin-coated catheter.

!!ALERT Drug is incompatible with injectable forms of bumetanide, enalaprilat, ethacrynate sodium, furosemide, heparin, hydralazine, and insulin. Don't give these drugs through the same line as nesiritide.

!!ALERT The preservative sodium metabisulfite is incompatible with nesiritide. Don't give injectable drugs with this preservative through the same line as nesiritide.

- Nesiritide may affect renal function in some people. In patients with severe heart failure whose renal function depends on the renin-angiotensin-aldosterone system, treatment may lead to azotemia.
- Results of giving this drug for longer than 48 hours are unknown.

Patient teaching

- Tell patient to report discomfort at I.V. site.
- Urge patient to report to prescriber symptoms of hypotension, such as dizziness, lightheadedness, blurred vision, or sweating.
- Tell patient to report to prescriber other adverse effects promptly.

nevirapine
Viramune

Pregnancy risk category C

Indications & dosages

➲ Adjunct treatment in patients with HIV-1 infection who have experienced clinical or immunologic deterioration
Adults: 200 mg P.O. daily for the first 14 days; then 200 mg P.O. b.i.d. Used with nucleoside analogue antiretrovirals.

➲ Adjunct treatment in children infected with HIV-1
Children age 8 and older: 4 mg/kg P.O. once daily for first 14 days; then 4 mg/kg P.O.

b.i.d. thereafter. Maximum daily dose is 400 mg.
Children ages 2 months to 8 years: 4 mg/kg P.O. once daily for first 14 days; then 7 mg/kg P.O. b.i.d. thereafter. Maximum daily dose is 400 mg.

Contraindications & cautions

- Contraindicated in patients hypersensitive to drug.
- Nevirapine shouldn't be given to patients with severe hepatic impairment from drug accumulation.
- Use cautiously in patients with impaired renal and hepatic function; pharmacokinetics haven't been evaluated in those patients.
- Safety and effectiveness in children haven't been established. Don't use drug in children.
- Nevirapine appears in breast milk. Don't use drug in breast-feeding patients.

Adverse reactions

CNS: headache, *fever,* paresthesia.
GI: *nausea,* diarrhea, abdominal pain, ulcerative stomatitis.
Hematologic: ***neutropenia***.
Hepatic: ***hepatitis***.
Musculoskeletal: myalgia.
Skin: *rash, blistering,* ***Stevens-Johnson syndrome***.

Interactions

Drug-drug. *Drugs extensively metabolized by cytochrome P-450 3A:* May lower levels of these drugs. Dosage adjustment of these drugs may be needed.
Ketoconazole: May decrease ketoconazole level. Avoid using together.
Protease inhibitors or hormonal contraceptives: May decrease levels of these drugs. Use together cautiously.
Rifabutin, rifampin: Dosage adjustment may be needed. Monitor patient closely.
Drug-herb. *St. John's wort:* May decrease nevirapine level. Discourage use together.

Nursing considerations

- Perform clinical chemistry tests, including renal function tests, before starting drug therapy and regularly throughout therapy.
- Use drug with at least one other antiretroviral.

!!ALERT Severe, life-threatening, and in some cases fatal hepatotoxicity, including fulminant and cholestatic hepatitis, hepatic necrosis, and hepatic failure, have been reported in patients treated with nevirapine, including patients receiving drug for post-exposure prophylaxis, an unapproved use.
- Increased AST or ALT levels or coinfection with hepatitis B or C at the start of antiretroviral therapy suggest a greater risk of hepatic adverse events.
- In some cases, nonspecific prodromal signs or symptoms of hepatitis are present and patient progresses to hepatic failure. These events are often linked with rash and fever. Women and patients with higher CD4 cell counts are at increased risk of these hepatic events. Women with CD4 cell counts greater than 250 cells/mm^3, including pregnant women receiving long-term treatment for HIV infection, are at considerably higher risk of these events.
- Monitor patient for signs and symptoms of hepatitis, including rash. Closely monitor liver function tests at baseline and during the first 18 weeks of treatment; then monitor frequently thereafter.
- Perform liver function tests immediately if hepatitis or hypersensitivity reactions are suspected.

!!ALERT Monitor patient for blistering, oral lesions, conjunctivitis, muscle or joint aches, or general malaise. Be especially alert for a severe rash or rash accompanied by fever. Report such signs and symptoms to prescriber. Patients who experience a rash during the first 14 days of therapy shouldn't have the dosage increased until the rash has resolved. Most rashes occur within the first 6 weeks of therapy.

!!ALERT If clinical hepatitis occurs, permanently stop drug and don't restart after recovery. In some cases, hepatic injury progresses despite stopping treatment.
- Patients who have nevirapine therapy interrupted for longer than 7 days should restart therapy as if receiving drug for the first time.
- Antiretroviral therapy may be changed if disease progresses while patient is receiving nevirapine.

!!ALERT Don't confuse nevirapine with nelfinavir.

Patient teaching

- Inform patient that nevirapine doesn't cure HIV and that illnesses associated with ad-

vanced HIV-1 infection still may occur. Explain that drug doesn't reduce risk of HIV-1 transmission.
- Instruct patient to report rash immediately and to stop drug until told to resume.
- Tell patient with signs or symptoms of hepatitis (such as fatigue, malaise, anorexia, nausea, jaundice, liver tenderness or hepatomegaly, with or without initially abnormal serum transaminase levels) to stop nevirapine and seek medical evaluation immediately.
- Stress importance of taking drug exactly as prescribed. If a dose is missed, tell patient to take the next dose as soon as possible. Patient shouldn't double next dose.
- Tell patient not to use other drugs unless approved by prescriber.
- Advise woman of childbearing age that hormonal contraceptives and other hormonal methods of birth control shouldn't be used with nevirapine.
- Advise woman to avoid breast-feeding during drug therapy to reduce risk of postnatal HIV transmission.

niacin (nicotinic acid, vitamin B_3)

Nia-Bid ◇, Niacor ◇, Niaspan, Nicobid ◇, Nicotinex, Slo-Niacin ◇

niacinamide ◇ (nicotinamid ◇)

Pregnancy risk category A; C if dose exceeds RDA

Indications & dosages

➲ RDA
Adult men and boys ages 14 to 18: 16 mg.
Adult women and girls ages 14 to 18: 14 mg.
Children ages 9 to 13: 12 mg.
Children ages 4 to 8: 8 mg.
Children ages 1 to 3: 6 mg.
Infants ages 6 months to 1 year: 4 mg.
Neonates and infants younger than age 6 months: 2 mg.
Pregnant women: 18 mg.
Breast-feeding women: 17 mg.

➲ Pellagra
Adults: 300 to 500 mg P.O. daily in divided doses.
Children: 100 to 300 mg P.O. daily in divided doses.

➲ Hartnup disease
Adults: 50 to 200 mg P.O. daily.

➲ Niacin deficiency
Adults: Up to 100 mg P.O. daily.

➲ Hyperlipidemias, especially with hypercholesterolemia
Adults: 250 mg P.O. daily h.s. Increase at 4- to 7-day intervals up to 1.5 to 2 g P.O. daily divided b.i.d. to t.i.d. Maximum 6 g daily. Or, 1 to 2 g extended-release tablets P.O. daily h.s.

Contraindications & cautions

- Contraindicated in patients hypersensitive to drug and in those with hepatic dysfunction, active peptic ulcers, severe hypotension, or arterial hemorrhage.
- Use cautiously in patients with gallbladder disease, diabetes mellitus, or unstable angina and in patients with history of liver disease, peptic ulcer, allergy, gout, or significant alcohol intake.

Adverse reactions

CV: *excessive peripheral vasodilation, especially with niacin*, hypotension, atrial fibrillation, ***arrhythmias***, *flushing*.
EENT: toxic amblyopia.
GI: *nausea, vomiting, diarrhea*, possible activation of peptic ulceration, epigastric or substernal pain.
Hepatic: ***hepatic dysfunction***.
Metabolic: hyperglycemia, hyperuricemia.
Skin: pruritus, dryness, tingling, rash, hyperpigmentation.

Interactions

Drug-drug. *Antihypertensives (ganglionic or sympathetic blockers):* May increase vasodilating effect, causing orthostatic hypotension. Use together cautiously and warn patient about orthostatic hypotension.
Cholestyramine, colestipol: May decrease bioavailability of extended-release products. Separate doses by 4 to 6 hours.
Lovastatin (statin class): May lead to rhabdomyolysis. Use together cautiously.
Sulfinpyrazone: May decrease uricosuric effects. Avoid using together.
Drug-food. *Hot drinks:* May increase flushing and pruritus. Urge patient not to take with hot liquids.
Drug-lifestyle. *Alcohol use:* May increase flushing and pruritus. Discourage use together.

Nursing considerations

- After symptoms of niacin deficiency subside, advise adequate nutrition and RDA supplements to prevent recurrence.
- Most reactions are dose-dependent.
- Drug may cause dose-related increase in glucose intolerance; carefully monitor glucose level in diabetic patients. Glycosuria may occur.
- Give niacin with meals to minimize adverse GI effects.
- Give 325 mg of aspirin P.O. 30 minutes before niacin dose, to help reduce flushing response to niacin.
- Extended-release niacin or niacinamide may prevent excessive flushing that occurs with large doses. However, extended-release niacin is linked to hepatic dysfunction, even at very low doses.
- Monitor hepatic function and glucose level early in therapy.

!!ALERT Don't confuse Nicobid and Nicotinex with nicotine (NicoDerm, Nicotrol, Nicorette).

Patient teaching

- Stress that niacin is a potent drug, not just a vitamin, and may cause serious adverse effects. Explain importance of adhering to therapy.
- Explain that flushing syndrome is harmless. Tell patient that flushing and warmth may subside with continued use and that concurrent use of alcohol may increase flushing.
- Tell patient to take with food to minimize stomach upset.

nifedipine

Adalat, Adalat CC, Adalat PA†, Adalat XL†, Apo-Nifed†, Nifedical XL, Novo-Nifedin†, Nu-Nifed†, Procardia, Procardia XL

Pregnancy risk category C

Indications & dosages

➲ Vasospastic angina (Prinzmetal's or variant angina), classic chronic stable angina pectoris

Adults: Initially, 10 mg (short-acting capsules) P.O. t.i.d. Usual effective dosage range is 10 to 20 mg t.i.d. Some patients may require up to 30 mg q.i.d. Maximum daily dose is 180 mg. Adjust dosage over 7 to 14 days to evaluate response. Or, 30 to 60 mg (extended-release tablets, except Adalat CC) P.O. once daily. Maximum daily dose is 120 mg. Adjust dosage over 7 to 14 days to evaluate response.

➲ Hypertension

Adults: 30 or 60 mg P.O. (extended-release) once daily. Adjusted over 7 to 14 days. Doses larger than 90 mg (Adalat CC) and 120 mg (Procardia XL) aren't recommended.

Contraindications & cautions

- Contraindicated in patients hypersensitive to drug.
- Use cautiously in patients with heart failure or hypotension and in elderly patients. Use extended-release tablets cautiously in patients with severe GI narrowing.

Adverse reactions

CNS: *dizziness, light-headedness,* somnolence, *headache, weakness,* syncope, nervousness.
CV: *peripheral edema,* hypotension, palpitations, ***heart failure, MI,*** *flushing.*
EENT: nasal congestion.
GI: *nausea,* diarrhea, constipation, abdominal discomfort.
Musculoskeletal: muscle cramps.
Respiratory: dyspnea, pulmonary edema, cough.
Skin: rash, pruritus.

Interactions

Drug-drug. *Cimetidine, ranitidine:* May decrease nifedipine metabolism. May need to adjust dosage.
Digoxin: May cause elevated digoxin level. Monitor digoxin level.
Fentanyl: May cause severe hypotension. Monitor blood pressure.
Phenytoin: May reduce phenytoin metabolism. Monitor phenytoin level.
Propranolol, other beta blockers: May cause hypotension and heart failure. Use together cautiously.
Drug-herb. *Dong quai:* May increase antihypertensive effect. Discourage use together.
Ginkgo: May increase effects of nifedipine. Discourage use together.
Ginseng: May increase nifedipine levels; possible toxicity. Discourage use together.
Melatonin: May interfere with antihypertensive effect. Discourage use together.

Drug-food. *Grapefruit juice:* May increase bioavailability of nifedipine. Discourage use together.

Nursing considerations

- Don't give immediate-release form within 1 week of acute MI or in acute coronary syndrome.

!!ALERT Despite the previously widespread S.L. use of nifedipine capsules (or the "bite and swallow" method), avoid this route of administration. Excessive hypotension, MI, and death may result.

- Monitor blood pressure regularly, especially in patients who take beta blockers or antihypertensives.
- Watch for symptoms of heart failure.
- Although rebound effect hasn't been observed when drug is stopped, reduce dosage slowly under prescriber's supervision.

!!ALERT Don't confuse nifedipine with nimodipine or nicardipine.

Patient teaching

- If patient is kept on nitrate therapy while nifedipine dosage is being adjusted, urge continued compliance. Patient may take S.L. nitroglycerin, as needed, for acute chest pain.
- Tell patient that chest pain may worsen briefly when beginning drug or when dosage is increased.
- Instruct patient to swallow extended-release tablets without breaking, crushing, or chewing them.
- Advise patient to avoid taking drug with grapefruit juice.
- Reassure patient taking the extended-release form that a wax-matrix "ghost" from the tablet may be passed in the stools. Drug is completely absorbed before this occurs.
- Tell patient to protect capsules from direct light and moisture and to store at room temperature.

nisoldipine
Sular

Pregnancy risk category C

Indications & dosages

➲ Hypertension

Adults: Initially, 20 mg P.O. once daily; increased by 10 mg/week or at longer intervals, p.r.n. Usual maintenance dose is 20 to 40 mg daily. Doses of more than 60 mg daily aren't recommended.

Patients older than age 65: Initially, 10 mg P.O. once daily; dosage is adjusted as for adults.

For patients with impaired liver function, initially, 10 mg P.O. once daily; dosage is adjusted as for adults.

Contraindications & cautions

- Contraindicated in patients hypersensitive to dihydropyridine calcium channel blockers.
- Contraindicated in breast-feeding women.
- Use cautiously in patients with heart failure or compromised ventricular function, particularly those receiving beta blockers and those with severe hepatic dysfunction.

Adverse reactions

CNS: *headache,* dizziness.

CV: vasodilation, palpitations, chest pain, *peripheral edema.*

EENT: sinusitis, pharyngitis.

GI: nausea.

Skin: rash.

Interactions

Drug-drug. *Cimetidine:* May increase bioavailability and peak nisoldipine level. Monitor blood pressure closely.

CYP3A4 inducers such as phenytoin: May decrease nisoldipine level. Avoid using together; consider alternative antihypertensive therapy.

Quinidine: May decrease bioavailability of nisoldipine. Adjust dosage accordingly.

Drug-herb. *Ma huang:* May decrease antihypertensive effects. Discourage use together.

Peppermint oil: May decrease effect of nisoldipine. Discourage use together.

Drug-food. *Grapefruit, grapefruit juice:* May increase drug level, increasing adverse reactions. Discourage use together.

High-fat foods: May increase peak drug level. Discourage use together.

Nursing considerations

- Monitor patient carefully. Some patients, especially those with severe obstructive coronary artery disease, have developed increased frequency, duration, or severity of angina or even acute MI after starting calcium channel blocker therapy or at time of dosage increase.

- Monitor blood pressure regularly, especially when starting therapy and during dosage adjustment.

Patient teaching

- Tell patient to take drug as prescribed, even if he feels better.
- Advise patient to swallow tablet whole and not to chew, divide, or crush it.
- Remind patient not to take drug with a high-fat meal or with grapefruit juice. Both may increase drug level in the body beyond intended amount.

nitazoxanide

Alinia

Pregnancy risk category B

Indications & dosages

➲ Diarrhea caused by *Cryptosporidium parvum* or *Giardia lamblia*

Children ages 4 to 11: 10 ml (200 mg) P.O. with food q 12 hours for 3 days.

Children ages 1 to 3: 5 ml (100 mg) P.O. with food q 12 hours for 3 days.

➲ Diarrhea caused by *G. lamblia*

Adults and children age 12 and older: 500 mg P.O. (tablet or suspension) with food q 12 hours for 3 days.

Contraindications & cautions

- Contraindicated in patients hypersensitive to nitazoxanide.
- Use cautiously in patients with renal or hepatic dysfunction. Safety and efficacy haven't been established in HIV-positive patients, immunodeficient patients, children younger than age 1, or those age 12 and older being treated for diarrhea caused by ***C. parvum***.

Adverse reactions

CNS: headache.

GI: abdominal pain, diarrhea, nausea, vomiting.

Interactions

Drug-drug. *Drugs that are highly protein-bound:* May compete for binding sites. Use together cautiously.

Nursing considerations

- Give drug with food.

!!ALERT A single nitazoxanide tablet contains more of the drug than is recommended for pediatric doses and shouldn't be used in pediatric patients age 11 or younger.

- Monitor glucose level in patients with diabetes who are taking the suspension.
- Store tablets, suspension, and powder at 77° F (25° C).

Patient teaching

- Tell caregiver or patient to give drug with food.
- Instruct caregiver or patient to keep container tightly closed and to shake it well before each use.
- Advise caregiver or patient that reconstituted suspension or tablets may be stored at room temperature.
- Advise caregiver or patient to discard suspension after 7 days.
- Inform diabetic patient or his caregiver that the suspension contains 1.48 g of sucrose per 5 ml.

nitrofurantoin macrocrystals

Macrobid, Macrodantin

nitrofurantoin microcrystals

Apo-Nitrofurantoin†, Furadantin, Novo-Furantoin†

Pregnancy risk category B

Indications & dosages

➲ UTIs caused by susceptible *Escherichia coli, Staphylococcus aureus, enterococci;* or certain strains of *Klebsiella* and *Enterobacter* species

Adults and children older than age 12: 50 to 100 mg P.O. q.i.d. with meals and h.s. Or, 100 mg Macrobid P.O. q 12 hours for 7 days.

Children ages 1 month to 12 years: 5 to 7 mg/kg P.O. daily, divided q.i.d.

➲ Long-term suppression therapy

Adults: 50 to 100 mg P.O. daily h.s.

Children: 1 mg/kg P.O. daily in a single dose h.s. or divided into two doses given q 12 hours.

Contraindications & cautions

- Contraindicated in infants age 1 month and younger and in patients with anuria, ol-

iguria, or creatinine clearance less than 60 ml/minute. Also contraindicated in pregnant patients at 38 to 42 weeks' gestation and during labor and delivery.
- Use cautiously in patients with renal impairment, asthma, anemia, diabetes mellitus, electrolyte abnormalities, vitamin B deficiency, debilitating disease, and G6PD deficiency.

Adverse reactions

CNS: peripheral neuropathy, headache, dizziness, drowsiness, *ascending polyneuropathy with high doses or renal impairment.*
GI: *anorexia, nausea, vomiting,* abdominal pain, *diarrhea.*
GU: overgrowth of nonsusceptible organisms in urinary tract.
Hematologic: ***hemolysis in patients with G6PD deficiency, agranulocytosis, thrombocytopenia.***
Hepatic: ***hepatitis, hepatic necrosis.***
Metabolic: ***hypoglycemia.***
Respiratory: ***pulmonary sensitivity reactions, asthmatic attacks.***
Skin: maculopapular, erythematous, or eczematous eruption, transient alopecia, pruritus, urticaria, exfoliative dermatitis, ***Stevens-Johnson syndrome.***
Other: hypersensitivity reactions, ***anaphylaxis,*** drug fever.

Interactions

Drug-drug. *Antacids containing magnesium:* May decrease nitrofurantoin absorption. Separate dosage times by 1 hour.
Probenecid, sulfinpyrazone: May inhibit excretion of nitrofurantoin, increasing drug levels and risk of toxicity. The resulting decreased urinary levels could lessen antibacterial effects. Avoid using together.
Drug-food. *Any food:* May increase absorption. Advise patient to take drug with food or milk.

Nursing considerations

- Obtain urine specimen for culture and sensitivity tests before giving first dose. Repeat as needed. Therapy may begin pending results.
- Give drug with food or milk to minimize GI distress and improve absorption.
- Drug may cause an asthma attack in patients with a history of asthma.
- Monitor fluid intake and output carefully. May turn urine brown or dark yellow.
- Monitor CBC and pulmonary status regularly.

!! ALERT Monitor patient for signs and symptoms of superinfection. Use of nitrofurantoin may result in growth of nonsusceptible organisms, especially *Pseudomonas* species.
- Monitor patient for pulmonary sensitivity reactions, including cough, chest pain, fever, chills, dyspnea, and pulmonary infiltration with consolidation or effusions.

!! ALERT Hypersensitivity may develop when drug is used for long-term therapy.
- Some patients may experience fewer adverse GI effects with nitrofurantoin macrocrystals.
- Dual-release capsules (25 mg nitrofurantoin macrocrystals combined with 75 mg nitrofurantoin monohydrate) enable patients to take drug only twice daily.
- Continue treatment for 3 days after sterile urine specimens have been obtained.
- Store drug in amber container. Keep away from metals other than stainless steel or aluminum to avoid precipitate formation.

Patient teaching

- Instruct patient to take drug for as long as prescribed, exactly as directed, even after he feels better.
- Tell patient to take drug with food or milk to minimize stomach upset.
- Instruct patient to report adverse reactions, especially peripheral neuropathy, which can become severe or irreversible.
- Alert patient that drug may turn urine dark yellow or brown.
- Warn patient not to store drug in container made of metal other than stainless steel or aluminum.

nitroglycerin (glyceryl trinitrate)
Deponit, Minitran, Nitrek, Nitro-Bid, Nitro-Bid IV, Nitrodisc, Nitro-Dur, Nitrogard, Nitroglyn, Nitrolingual, Nitrong, NitroQuick, Nitrostat, NitroTab, Nitro-Time, NTS, Transderm-Nitro, Tridil

Pregnancy risk category C

Indications & dosages

➲ To prevent chronic anginal attacks
Adults: 2.5 or 2.6 mg sustained-release capsule or tablet q 8 to 12 hours, adjusted upward to an effective dose in 2.5- or 2.6-mg increments b.i.d. to q.i.d. Or, use 2% ointment: Start dosage with 1/2 -inch ointment, increasing by 1/2 -inch increments until desired results are achieved. Range of dosage with ointment is 1/2 to 5 inches. Usual dose is 1 to 2 inches q 6 to 8 hours. Or, transdermal disc or pad (Nitrodisc, Nitro-Dur, or Transderm-Nitro) 0.2 to 0.4 mg/hour once daily.

➲ Acute angina pectoris; to prevent or minimize anginal attacks before stressful events
Adults: 1 S.L. tablet (1/400 grain, 1/200 grain, 1/150 grain, 1/100 grain) dissolved under the tongue or in the buccal pouch as soon as angina begins. Repeat q 5 minutes, if needed, for 15 minutes. Or, using Nitrolingual spray, one or two sprays into mouth, preferably onto or under the tongue. Repeat q 3 to 5 minutes, if needed, to a maximum of three doses within a 15-minute period. Or, 1 to 3 mg transmucosally q 3 to 5 hours while awake.

➲ Hypertension from surgery, heart failure after MI, angina pectoris in acute situations, to produce controlled hypotension during surgery (by I.V. infusion)
Adults: Initially, infuse at 5 mcg/minute, increasing p.r.n. by 5 mcg/minute q 3 to 5 minutes until response occurs. If a 20-mcg/minute rate doesn't produce a response, increase dosage by as much as 20 mcg/minute q 3 to 5 minutes. Up to 100 mcg/minute may be needed.

Contraindications & cautions

- Contraindicated in patients with early MI (oral and sublingual), severe anemia, increased intracranial pressure, angle-closure glaucoma, orthostatic hypotension, allergy to adhesives (transdermal), or hypersensitivity to nitrates. I.V. nitroglycerin is contraindicated in patients hypersensitive to I.V. form, cardiac tamponade, restrictive cardiomyopathy, or constrictive pericarditis.
- Use cautiously in patients with hypotension or volume depletion.

Adverse reactions

CNS: *headache, dizziness,* weakness.
CV: *orthostatic hypotension, tachycardia, flushing, palpitations,* fainting.
EENT: S.L. burning.
GI: nausea, vomiting.
Skin: cutaneous vasodilation, contact dermatitis, rash.
Other: hypersensitivity reactions.

Interactions

Drug-drug. *Alteplase:* May decrease tPA antigen level. Avoid using together; if unavoidable, use lowest effective dose of nitroglycerin.
Antihypertensives: May increase hypotensive effect. Monitor blood pressure closely.
Heparin: I.V. nitroglycerin may interfere with anticoagulant effect of heparin. Monitor PTT.
Sildenafil, tadalafil, vardenafil: May cause severe hypotension. Use of nitrates in any form with these drugs is contraindicated.
Drug-lifestyle. *Alcohol use:* May increase hypotension. Discourage use together.

Nursing considerations

- Closely monitor vital signs during infusion, particularly blood pressure, especially in a patient with an MI. Excessive hypotension may worsen the MI.
- To apply ointment, measure the prescribed amount on the application paper; then place the paper on any nonhairy area. Don't rub in. Cover with plastic film to aid absorption and to protect clothing. Remove all excess ointment from previous site before applying the next dose. Avoid getting ointment on fingers.
- Transdermal dosage forms can be applied to any nonhairy part of the skin except distal parts of the arms or legs (absorption won't be maximal at distal sites). Patch may cause contact dermatitis.
- Remove transdermal patch before defibrillation. Because of the aluminum backing on

the patch, the electric current may cause arcing that can damage the paddles and burn the patient.

- When stopping transdermal treatment of angina, gradually reduce the dosage and frequency of application over 4 to 6 weeks.
- Monitor blood pressure and intensity and duration of drug response.
- Drug may cause headaches, especially at beginning of therapy. Dosage may be reduced temporarily, but tolerance usually develops. Treat headache with aspirin or acetaminophen.
- Tolerance to drug can be minimized with a 10- to 12-hour nitrate-free interval. To achieve this, remove the transdermal system in the early evening and apply a new system the next morning or omit the last daily dose of a buccal, sustained-release, or ointment form. Check with the prescriber for alterations in dosage regimen if tolerance is suspected.

!!ALERT Don't confuse Nitro-Bid with Nicobid or nitroglycerin with nitroprusside.

Patient teaching

- Caution patient to take nitroglycerin regularly, as prescribed, and to have it accessible at all times.

!!ALERT Advise patient that stopping drug abruptly causes spasm of the coronary arteries.

- Teach patient how to give the prescribed form of nitroglycerin.
- Tell patient to take S.L. tablet at first sign of attack. Patient should wet the tablet with saliva and place under the tongue until absorbed; he should sit down and rest. Dose may be repeated every 5 minutes for a maximum of three doses. If drug doesn't provide relief, he should obtain medical help promptly.
- Advise patient who complains of a tingling sensation with S.L. drug to try holding tablet in cheek.
- Tell patient to take oral tablets on an empty stomach either 30 minutes before or 1 to 2 hours after meals, to swallow oral tablets whole, and not to chew tablets.
- Remind patient using translingual aerosol form that he shouldn't inhale the spray, but should release it onto or under the tongue. Tell him to wait about 10 seconds or so before swallowing.
- Tell patient to place the buccal tablet between the lip and gum above the incisors or between the cheek and gum. Tablets shouldn't be swallowed or chewed.
- Tell patient to take an additional dose before anticipated stress or at bedtime if chest pain occurs at night.
- Urge patient using skin patches to dispose of them carefully because enough medication remains after normal use to be hazardous to children and pets.
- Advise patient to avoid alcohol.
- To minimize dizziness when standing up, tell patient to rise slowly. Advise him to go up and down stairs carefully and to lie down at the first sign of dizziness.
- Advise patient that use of sildenafil, tadalafil, or vardenafil with any nitrate may cause severe low blood pressure. The patient should talk to his prescriber before considering use of these drugs together.
- Tell patient to store drug in cool, dark place in a tightly closed container. Tell him to remove cotton from container because it absorbs drug.
- Tell patient to store S.L. tablets in original container or other container specifically approved for this use and to carry the container in a jacket pocket or purse, not in a pocket close to the body.

nitroprusside sodium

Nipride†, Nitropress

Pregnancy risk category C

Indications & dosages

➲ To lower blood pressure quickly in hypertensive emergencies, to produce controlled hypotension during anesthesia, to reduce preload and afterload in cardiac pump failure or cardiogenic shock (may be used with or without dopamine)

Adults and children: Begin infusion at 0.25 to 0.3 mcg/kg/minute I.V. and gradually titrate q few minutes to a maximum infusion rate of 10 mcg/kg/minute.

Patients taking other antihypertensives with nitroprusside are extremely sensitive to nitroprusside. Titrate dosage accordingly. Use with caution in patients with renal failure; reduce dosage as much as possible.

Contraindications & cautions

- Contraindicated in patients hypersensitive to drug.
- Contraindicated in those with compensatory hypertension (such as in arteriovenous shunt or coarctation of the aorta), inadequate cerebral circulation, acute heart failure with reduced peripheral vascular resistance, congenital optic atrophy, or tobacco-induced amblyopia.
- Use with extreme caution in patients with increased intracranial pressure.
- Use cautiously in patients with hypothyroidism, hepatic or renal disease, hyponatremia, or low vitamin B level.

Adverse reactions

CNS: *headache, dizziness,* loss of consciousness, apprehension, ***increased ICP***, restlessness.
CV: ***bradycardia***, hypotension, tachycardia, palpitations, ECG changes, flushing.
GI: *nausea, abdominal pain,* ileus.
Hematologic: ***methemoglobinemia***.
Metabolic: acidosis, hypothyroidism.
Musculoskeletal: *muscle twitching.*
Skin: pink color, rash, *diaphoresis.*
Other: ***thiocyanate toxicity, cyanide toxicity***, venous streaking, irritation at infusion site.

Interactions

Drug-drug. *Antihypertensives:* May cause sensitivity to nitroprusside. Adjust dosage.
Ganglionic blocking drugs, general anesthetics, negative inotropic drugs, other antihypertensives: May cause additive effects. Monitor blood pressure closely.
Sildenafil, vardenafil: May increase hypotensive effects. Monitor blood pressure.

Nursing considerations

- Obtain baseline vital signs before giving drug; find out parameters prescriber wants to achieve.
- Keep patient in the supine position when starting therapy or titrating drug.

!!ALERT Don't confuse nitroprusside with nitroglycerin.

Patient teaching

- Instruct patient to report adverse reactions promptly.
- Tell patient to alert nurse if discomfort occurs at I.V. insertion site.

norelgestromin and ethinyl estradiol transdermal system

Ortho Evra

Pregnancy risk category X

Indications & dosages

➲ Contraception
Women: Apply 1 patch weekly for 3 weeks. Apply each new patch on the same day of the week. Week 4 is patch free. On the day after week 4 ends, apply a new patch to start a new 4-week cycle. The patch-free interval between cycles should never be longer than 7 days.

Contraindications & cautions

- Contraindicated in patients hypersensitive to any component of this drug and in those with past history of deep vein thrombosis or related disorder; current or past history of cerebrovascular or coronary artery disease; past or current known or suspected breast cancer, endometrial cancer or other known or suspected estrogen-dependent neoplasia; or hepatic adenoma or cancer; and in those who are or may be pregnant.
- Contraindicated in patients with thrombophlebitis, thromboembolic disorders, valvular heart disease with complications, severe hypertension, diabetes with vascular involvement, headaches with focal neurologic symptoms, major surgery with prolonged immobilization, undiagnosed abnormal genital bleeding, cholestatic jaundice of pregnancy or jaundice with previous hormonal contraceptive use, or acute or chronic hepatocellular disease with abnormal liver function.
- Use cautiously in patients with CV disease risk factors, with conditions that might be aggravated by fluid retention, or with a history of depression.

Adverse reactions

CNS: *headache,* emotional lability.
CV: ***thromboembolic events, MI***, hypertension, edema, ***cerebral hemorrhage***.
EENT: contact lens intolerance.
GI: *nausea, abdominal pain,* vomiting, gallbladder disease.
GU: *menstrual cramps,* changes in menstrual flow, vaginal candidiasis.

Hepatic: ***hepatic adenomas***, benign liver tumors.
Metabolic: weight changes.
Respiratory: *upper respiratory tract infection.*
Skin: *application site reaction.*
Other: *breast tenderness, enlargement, or secretion.*

Interactions

Drug-drug. *Acetaminophen, clofibric acid, morphine, salicylic acid, temazepam:* May decrease levels or increase clearance of these drugs. Monitor patient for lack of effect.
Ampicillin, barbiturates, carbamazepine, felbamate, griseofulvin, oxcarbazepine, phenylbutazone, phenytoin, rifampin, topiramate: May reduce contraceptive effectiveness, resulting in unintended pregnancy or breakthrough bleeding. Encourage backup method of contraception if used together.
Ascorbic acid, atorvastatin, itraconazole, ketoconazole: May increase hormone levels. Use together cautiously.
Cyclosporine, prednisolone, theophylline: May increase levels of these drugs. Monitor patient for adverse reactions.
HIV protease inhibitors: May affect contraceptive effectiveness and safety. Use together cautiously.
Drug-herb. *St. John's wort:* May reduce effectiveness of contraceptive and cause breakthrough bleeding. Discourage use together.
Drug-lifestyle. *Smoking:* May increase risk of CV adverse effects of hormonal contraceptive use, related to age and smoking 15 or more cigarettes daily. Urge patient not to smoke.

Nursing considerations

!!ALERT Patients taking combination hormonal contraceptives may be at increased risk for thrombophlebitis, venous thrombosis with or without embolism, pulmonary embolism, MI, cerebral hemorrhage, cerebral thrombosis, hypertension, gallbladder disease, hepatic adenomas, benign liver tumors, mesenteric thrombosis, and retinal thrombosis.

- Increased risk of MI occurs primarily in smokers and women with hypertension, hypercholesterolemia, morbid obesity, and diabetes.
- Encourage women with a history of hypertension or renal disease to use a different method of contraception. If Ortho Evra is used, monitor blood pressure closely and stop use if hypertension occurs.
- Drug may be less effective in women weighing 198 lb (90 kg) or more.
- Cigarette smoking increases the risk of serious adverse cardiac effects. The risk increases with age and in those who smoke 15 or more cigarettes daily.
- The risk of thromboembolic disease increases if therapy is used postpartum or postabortion.
- Rule out pregnancy if withdrawal bleeding fails to occur for two consecutive cycles.
- If skin becomes irritated, the patch may be removed and a new patch applied at a different site.
- Stop drug and notify prescriber at least 4 weeks before and for 2 weeks after an elective surgery that increases the risk of thromboembolism, and during and after prolonged immobilization.
- Stop drug and notify prescriber if patient has headaches, vision loss, proptosis, diplopia, papilledema, retinal vascular lesions, jaundice, or depression.

Patient teaching

- Emphasize the importance of having regular annual physical examinations to check for adverse effects or developing contraindications.
- Tell patient that drug doesn't protect against HIV and other sexually transmitted diseases.
- Advise patient to immediately apply a new patch once the used patch is removed, on the same day of the week every 7 days for 3 weeks. Week 4 is patch free. Bleeding is expected to occur during this time.
- Tell patient to apply each patch to a clean, dry area of the skin on the buttocks, abdomen, upper outer arm, or upper torso. Tell patient not to apply to the breasts or to skin that is red, irritated, or cut.
- Tell patient to carefully fold the used patch in half so that it sticks to itself, before discarding.
- Tell patient to immediately stop use if pregnancy is confirmed.

• Tell patient who wears contact lenses to report visual changes or changes in lens tolerance.
• Advise patient not to smoke while using the patch.
• Stress that if patient isn't sure what to do about mistakes with patch use, she should use a backup method of birth control and contact her health care provider.

norepinephrine bitartrate (levarterenol bitartrate, noradrenaline acid tartrate)
Levophed

Pregnancy risk category C

Indications & dosages

➲ To restore blood pressure in acute hypotensive states
Adults: Initially, 8 to 12 mcg/minute by I.V. infusion; then titrated to maintain normal blood pressure. Average maintenance dose is 2 to 4 mcg/minute.
Children: 2 mcg/minute or 2 mcg/m^2/minute by I.V. infusion; adjust dosage based on patient response.
➲ Severe hypotension during cardiac arrest
Children: Initially, 0.1 mcg/kg/minute I.V. infusion. Titrate infusion rate based on patient response, up to 2 mcg/kg/minute.

Contraindications & cautions

• Contraindicated in patients with mesenteric or peripheral vascular thrombosis, profound hypoxia, hypercarbia, or hypotension resulting from blood volume deficit.
• Contraindicated during cyclopropane and halothane anesthesia.
• Use cautiously in patients taking MAO inhibitors or triptyline- or imipramine-type antidepressants.
• Use cautiously in patients with sulfite sensitivity.

Adverse reactions

CNS: *headache*, anxiety, weakness, dizziness, tremor, restlessness, insomnia.
CV: ***bradycardia***, ***severe hypertension***, ***arrhythmias***.
Respiratory: respiratory difficulties, ***asthma attacks***.
Skin: irritation with extravasation, necrosis and gangrene secondary to extravasation.
Other: ***anaphylaxis***.

Interactions

Drug-drug. *Alpha blockers:* May antagonize drug effects. Avoid using together.
Antihistamines, ergot alkaloids, guanethidine, MAO inhibitors, methyldopa, oxytocics: When given with sympathomimetics, may cause severe hypertension (hypertensive crisis). Avoid using together.
Inhaled anesthetics: May increase risk of arrhythmias. Monitor ECG.
Tricyclic antidepressants: May potentiate the pressor response and cause arrhythmias. Use together cautiously.

Nursing considerations

• Drug isn't a substitute for blood or fluid replacement therapy. If patient has volume deficit, replace fluids before giving vasopressors.
!!ALERT Never leave patient unattended during infusion. Check blood pressure every 2 minutes until stabilized; then check every 5 minutes. In previously hypertensive patients, maintain systolic blood pressure at 30 to 40 mm Hg below usual level.
• During infusion, frequently monitor ECG, cardiac output, central venous pressure, pulmonary artery wedge pressure, pulse rate, urine output, and color and temperature of limbs. Titrate infusion rate based on findings and prescriber guidelines.
• Keep emergency drugs on hand to reverse effects of norepinephrine: atropine for reflex bradycardia, phentolamine to decrease vasopressor effects, and propranolol for arrhythmias.
• Notify prescriber immediately of decreased urine output.
• When stopping drug, gradually slow infusion rate. Continue monitoring vital signs, watching for possible severe drop in blood pressure.
!!ALERT Don't confuse norepinephrine with epinephrine.

Patient teaching

• Tell patient to report adverse reactions promptly.
• Advise patient to report discomfort at I.V. insertion site.

norethindrone
Camila, Errin, Jolivette, Micronor, Nora-BE, Nor-QD

norethindrone acetate
Aygestin

Pregnancy risk category X

Indications & dosages

➲ Amenorrhea, abnormal uterine bleeding
Women: 2.5 to 10 mg norethindrone acetate P.O. daily on days 5 to 25 of menstrual cycle.

➲ Endometriosis
Women: 5 mg norethindrone acetate P.O. daily for 14 days; then increased by 2.5 mg daily q 2 weeks, up to 15 mg daily.

➲ Contraception
Women: Initially, 0.35 mg norethindrone P.O. on first day of menstruation; then 0.35 mg daily.

Contraindications & cautions

- Contraindicated in pregnant patients, patients hypersensitive to drug, and patients with breast cancer, undiagnosed abnormal vaginal bleeding, severe hepatic disease, missed abortion, or current or previous thromboembolic disorders.
- Use cautiously in patients with diabetes, seizures, migraines, cardiac or renal disease, asthma, and depression.

Adverse reactions

CNS: depression, ***CVA***.
CV: thrombophlebitis, ***pulmonary embolism***, edema, ***thromboembolism***.
EENT: exophthalmos, diplopia.
GI: *bloating, abdominal pain or cramping.*
GU: *breakthrough bleeding*, dysmenorrhea, *amenorrhea*, cervical erosion, abnormal secretions.
Hepatic: cholestatic jaundice.
Metabolic: weight changes.
Skin: melasma, rash, acne, pruritus.
Other: breast tenderness, enlargement, or secretion.

Interactions

Drug-drug. *Barbiturates, carbamazepine, fosphenytoin, phenytoin, rifampin:* May decrease progestin effects. Monitor patient for diminished therapeutic response.
Drug-food. *Caffeine:* May increase caffeine level. Urge caution.
Drug-lifestyle. *Smoking:* May increase risk of adverse CV effects. If smoking continues, may need alternative therapy.

Nursing considerations

- If switching from combined oral contraceptives to progestin-only pills (POPs), take the first POP the day after the last active combined pill.
- If switching from POPs to combined pills, take the first active combined pill on the first day of menstruation, even if the POP pack isn't finished.
- Norethindrone acetate is twice as potent as norethindrone. Norethindrone acetate shouldn't be used for contraception.
- Patients with menstrual disorders usually need preliminary estrogen treatment.
- Watch patient closely for signs of edema.
- Monitor blood pressure.

!!ALERT Don't confuse Micronor with Micro K or Micronase.

Patient teaching

- According to FDA regulations, patient must read package insert explaining possible adverse effects of progestins before receiving first dose. Also, give patient verbal explanation.
- Tell patient to take drug at the same time every day when used as a contraceptive. If she is more than 3 hours late taking the pill or if she has missed a pill, she should take the pill as soon as she remembers, and then continue the normal schedule. Also tell her to use a backup method of contraception for the next 48 hours.

!!ALERT Tell patient to report unusual symptoms immediately and to stop drug and notify prescriber about visual disturbances or migraine.

- Teach woman how to perform routine breast self-examination.
- Tell patient to report suspected pregnancy to prescriber.
- Encourage patient to stop or reduce smoking because of the risk of CV complications.

norfloxacin
Noroxin

Pregnancy risk category C

Indications & dosages

➲ **Complicated or uncomplicated UTI from susceptible strains of *Enterococcus faecalis, Escherichia coli, E. cloacae, Klebsiella pneumoniae, Enterobacter aerogenes, Proteus mirabilis, P. vulgaris, Pseudomonas aeruginosa, Citrobacter freundii, Staphylococcus agalactiae, S. aureus, S. epidermidis, S. saprophyticus,* or *Serratia marcescens***

Adults: 400 mg P.O. q 12 hours for 7 to 10 days (uncomplicated infection). Or, 400 mg P.O. q 12 hours for 10 to 21 days (complicated infection).

➲ **Prostatitis**

Adults: 400 mg P.O. q 12 hours for 28 days.

➲ **Cystitis caused by *E. coli, K. pneumoniae,* or *P. mirabilis***

Adults: 400 mg P.O. q 12 hours for 3 days.

For adult patients with creatinine clearance of 30 ml/minute or less, give 400 mg once daily for above indications.

➲ **Acute, uncomplicated urethral and cervical gonorrhea**

Adults: 800 mg P.O. as a single dose, then doxycycline therapy to treat any coexisting chlamydial infection.

Contraindications & cautions

- Contraindicated in patients hypersensitive to drug or other fluoroquinolones.
- Use cautiously in patients with conditions such as cerebral arteriosclerosis that may predispose them to seizure disorders.
- Use cautiously and monitor renal function in those with renal impairment.
- Safety in children younger than age 18 hasn't been established.

Adverse reactions

CNS: fatigue, somnolence, headache, dizziness, ***seizures***, depression, insomnia, fever.
GI: anorexia, nausea, constipation, flatulence, heartburn, dry mouth, abdominal pain, diarrhea, vomiting, ***pseudomembranous colitis***.
GU: crystalluria.
Hematologic: eosinophilia, ***neutropenia, leukopenia, thrombocytopenia***.
Musculoskeletal: back pain.
Skin: rash, photosensitivity, hyperhidrosis.
Other: hypersensitivity reactions, ***anaphylaxis***.

Interactions

Drug-drug. *Aluminum hydroxide, calcium carbonate, aluminum–magnesium hydroxide, magnesium hydroxide:* May decrease norfloxacin level. Give antacid at least 6 hours before or 2 hours after norfloxacin.
Iron salts: May decrease absorption of norfloxacin, reducing anti-infective response. Give at least 2 hours apart.
Cyclosporine: May increase cyclosporine level. Monitor cyclosporine level.
Nitrofurantoin: May antagonize norfloxacin effect. Monitor patient closely.
Oral anticoagulants: May increase anticoagulant effect. Monitor PT and INR.
Probenecid: May increase norfloxacin level by decreasing its excretion. May give probenecid for this reason, but monitor high-risk patient for toxicity.
Sucralfate: May decrease absorption of norfloxacin, reducing anti-infective response. If use together can't be avoided, give at least 6 hours apart.
Theophylline: May impair theophylline metabolism, increasing drug level and risk of toxicity. Monitor patient closely.
Drug-herb. *Dong quai, St. John's wort:* May cause photosensitivity reactions. Advise patient to avoid excessive sunlight exposure.

Nursing considerations

- Obtain specimen for culture and sensitivity testing before starting therapy.
- Tendon rupture may occur in patients receiving quinolones. Stop drug if pain or inflammation occurs or patient ruptures a tendon.
- Monitor patient for adverse CNS effects, including dizziness, headache, seizures, or depression. Stop drug and notify prescriber if these effects occur.
- Monitor patient for hypersensitivity reactions. Stop drug and initiate supportive therapy as indicated.

!!ALERT Don't confuse Noroxin (norfloxacin) with Neurontin (gabapentin) or Floxin (ofloxacin).

Patient teaching

- Tell patient to take drug as prescribed, even after he feels better.
- Advise patient to take drug 1 hour before or 2 hours after meals because food may hinder absorption.
- Advise patient to appropriately space iron products and antacids when taking norfloxacin.
- Warn patient not to exceed the recommended dosages and to drink several glasses of water throughout the day to maintain hydration and adequate urine output.
- Warn patient to avoid hazardous tasks that require alertness until effects of drug are known.
- Instruct patient to avoid exposure to sunlight, wear protective clothing, and use sunscreen while outdoors.
- Tell patient to report pain, inflammation, or tendon rupture, and to refrain from exercise until diagnosis of rupture or tendinitis is excluded.

nortriptyline hydrochloride

Aventyl, Pamelor*

Pregnancy risk category D

Indications & dosages

➲ Depression

Adults: 25 mg P.O. t.i.d. or q.i.d., gradually increased to maximum of 150 mg daily. Give entire dose h.s. Monitor level when doses above 100 mg daily are given.

Adolescents and elderly patients: 30 to 50 mg daily given once or in divided doses.

Contraindications & cautions

- Contraindicated in patients hypersensitive to drug and during acute recovery phase of MI; also contraindicated within 14 days of MAO therapy.
- Use with extreme caution in patients with glaucoma, suicidal tendency, history of urine retention or seizures, CV disease, or hyperthyroidism and in those receiving thyroid drugs.

Adverse reactions

CNS: *drowsiness, dizziness,* ***seizures***, tremor, weakness, confusion, headache, nervousness, EEG changes, ***CVA***, extrapyramidal syndrome, insomnia, nightmares, hallucinations, paresthesia, ataxia, agitation.
CV: ECG changes, *tachycardia*, hypertension, hypotension, ***MI***, ***heart block***.
EENT: *blurred vision*, tinnitus, mydriasis.
GI: dry mouth, *constipation*, nausea, vomiting, anorexia, paralytic ileus.
GU: *urine retention*.
Hematologic: bone marrow depression, ***agranulocytosis***, eosinophilia, ***thrombocytopenia***.
Metabolic: ***hypoglycemia***, hyperglycemia.
Skin: rash, urticaria, photosensitivity reactions, diaphoresis.
Other: hypersensitivity reactions.

Interactions

Drug-drug. *Barbiturates, CNS depressants:* May enhance CNS depression. Avoid using together.
Cimetidine, fluoxetine, paroxetine: May increase nortriptyline level. Watch for adverse reactions.
Clonidine: May cause life-threatening blood pressure elevations. Avoid using together.
Epinephrine, norepinephrine: May increase hypertensive effect. Use together cautiously.
MAO inhibitors: May cause severe excitation, hyperpyrexia, or seizures, usually with high doses. Avoid using within 14 days of MAO inhibitor therapy.
Drug-herb. *Evening primrose oil:* May cause additive or synergistic effect, resulting in lower seizure threshold and increasing the risk of seizure. Discourage use together.
St. John's wort, SAM-e, yohimbe: May cause serotonin syndrome and reduce drug level. Discourage use together.
Drug-lifestyle. *Alcohol use:* May enhance CNS depression. Discourage use together.
Smoking: May decrease nortriptyline level. Monitor patient for lack of effect.
Sun exposure: May increase risk of photosensitivity reactions. Advise patient to avoid excessive sunlight exposure.

Nursing considerations

- Monitor patient for nausea, headache, and malaise after abrupt withdrawal of long-term therapy; these symptoms don't indicate addiction.
- Because patients using tricyclic antidepressants may suffer hypertensive episodes during surgery, stop drug gradually several days before surgery.

• If signs or symptoms of psychosis occur or increase, expect to reduce dosage. Record mood changes. Monitor patient for suicidal tendencies and allow him only a minimum supply of drug.
!!ALERT Don't confuse nortriptyline with amitriptyline.

Patient teaching
• Advise patient to take full dose at bedtime whenever possible, to reduce risk of dizziness upon standing quickly.
• Warn patient to avoid activities that require alertness and good coordination until effects of drug are known. Drowsiness and dizziness usually subside after a few weeks.
• Recommend use of sugarless hard candy or gum to relieve dry mouth. Saliva substitutes may be needed.
• Tell patient to consult prescriber before taking other prescription or OTC drugs.
• Warn patient not to stop drug suddenly.
• To prevent oversensitivity to the sun, advise patient to use sunblock, wear protective clothing, and avoid prolonged exposure to strong sunlight.

nystatin (systemic)
Mycostatin*, Nadostine†, Nilstat, Nystex

Pregnancy risk category C

Indications & dosages
Intestinal candidiasis
Adults: 500,000 to 1 million units P.O. as tablets t.i.d.
Oral candidiasis (thrush)
Adults and children: 400,000 to 600,000 units P.O. as oral suspension q.i.d. or 200,000 to 400,000 units P.O. as lozenges four to five times daily for up to 14 days.
Infants: 200,000 units P.O. as oral suspension q.i.d.
Neonates and premature infants: 100,000 units P.O. oral suspension q.i.d.
Vaginal candidiasis
Adults: 100,000 units, as vaginal tablets, inserted high into vagina, daily at h.s. or b.i.d. for 14 days.

Contraindications & cautions
• Contraindicated in patients hypersensitive to drug.

Adverse reactions
GI: transient nausea, vomiting, diarrhea.
GU: irritation, sensitization, vulvovaginal burning (vaginal form).
Skin: rash.

Interactions
None significant.

Nursing considerations
• Nystatin isn't effective against systemic infections.
• Vaginal tablets can be used by pregnant patients up to 6 weeks before term to treat maternal infection that may cause oral candidiasis in neonates.
• To treat oral candidiasis, after the patient's mouth is clean of food debris, have him hold suspension in mouth for several minutes before swallowing. When treating infants, swab medication on oral mucosa. Prescriber may instruct immunosuppressed patients to suck on vaginal tablets (100,000 units) because this provides prolonged contact with oral mucosa.

Patient teaching
• Instruct patient not to chew or swallow lozenge but to allow it to dissolve slowly in mouth.
• Advise patient to continue taking drug for at least 2 days after signs and symptoms disappear. Consult prescriber for exact length of therapy.
• Instruct patient to continue therapy during menstruation.
• Explain that factors predisposing patient to vaginal infection include use of antibiotics, oral contraceptives, and corticosteroids; diabetes; reinfection by sexual partner; and tight-fitting pantyhose. Encourage patient to use cotton underwear.
• Instruct women in careful hygiene for affected areas, including cleaning perineal area from front to back.
• Advise patient to report redness, swelling, or irritation.
• Tell patient, especially an older patient, that overusing mouthwash or wearing poorly fitting dentures may promote infection.

nystatin (topical)
Mycostatin, Nilstat, Nystex, Pedi-Dri

Pregnancy risk category NR

Indications & dosages

➲ **Cutaneous and mucocutaneous infections caused by *Candida albicans***
Adults and children: Apply to affected area up to several times daily until healing is complete. Apply cream or ointment b.i.d. or as indicated; powder, b.i.d. or t.i.d.; lozenges, 1 or 2 four to five times daily until 48 hours after oral symptoms subside, but not longer than 14 days; suspension, 4 to 6 ml q.i.d. (one-half of dose in each side of mouth); retain dose as long as possible before swallowing.

➲ **Vulvovaginal candidiasis**
Adults: 1 vaginal tablet daily for 14 days.

Contraindications & cautions

- Contraindicated in patients hypersensitive to drug or its components.

Adverse reactions

Skin: occasional contact dermatitis from preservatives in some forms.

Interactions

None significant.

Nursing considerations

- Don't use occlusive dressings.
- Preparation doesn't stain skin or mucous membranes.
- Cream is recommended for skinfolds; powder, for moist areas; ointment, for dry areas.

!!ALERT Don't confuse nystatin with Nitrostat.

Patient teaching

- Show patient how to use vaginal tablets and tell her to continue using them during menstrual period.
- Tell patient to insert drug high in vagina (except during pregnancy) and to refrain from sexual intercourse during vaginal treatment.
- Instruct patient to refrigerate tablets.
- Tell patient to use drug for full prescribed period even if condition improves and to continue use for at least 2 days after symptoms subside (for oral therapy). Immunosuppressed patients may use drug on long-term basis.
- Warn patient to keep drug away from eyes.
- Instruct patient not to use occlusive dressings with skin application.
- Tell patient to dissolve oral lozenges slowly in mouth.
- Demonstrate and stress importance of proper oral hygiene, especially for denture wearers.

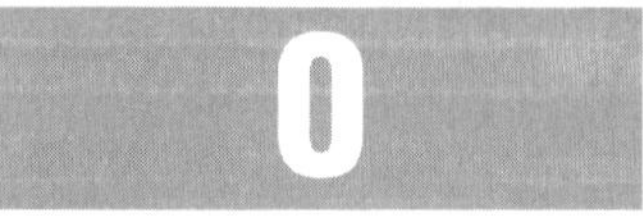

octreotide acetate
Sandostatin, Sandostatin LAR

Pregnancy risk category B

Indications & dosages

➲ **Flushing and diarrhea from carcinoid tumors**
Adults: 0.1 to 0.6 mg daily S.C. in two to four divided doses for first 2 weeks of therapy. Usual daily dosage is 0.3 mg. Base subsequent dosage on individual response.

➲ **Watery diarrhea from vasoactive intestinal polypeptide-secreting tumors (VIPomas)**
Adults: 0.2 to 0.3 mg daily S.C. in two to four divided doses for first 2 weeks of therapy. Base subsequent dosage on individual response; usually shouldn't exceed 0.45 mg daily.

➲ **Acromegaly**
Adults: Initially, 50 mcg S.C. t.i.d.; then adjust based on somatomedin C levels q 2 weeks. If Sandostatin LAR is used, give 20 mg I.M. (intragluteally) at 4-week intervals.

➲ **GI fistula♦**
Adults: 50 to 200 mcg S.C. q 8 hours.

➲ **Variceal bleeding♦**
Adults: 25 to 50 mcg/hour via continuous I.V. infusion, over 18 hours to 5 days.

➲ **AIDS-related diarrhea♦**
Adults: 100 to 500 mcg S.C. t.i.d.

➲ **Short-bowel syndrome♦**
Adults: I.V. infusion of 25 mcg/hour or 50 mcg S.C. b.i.d.

➲ Diarrhea caused by chemotherapy or radiation therapy ♦
Adults: 50 to 100 mcg S.C. t.i.d. for 1 to 3 days.
➲ Pancreatic fistula ♦
Adults: 50 to 200 mcg q 8 hours.
➲ Irritable bowel syndrome ♦
Adults: Initially, 100 mcg S.C. as single dose; maximum, 125 mcg S.C. b.i.d.

Contraindications & cautions

- Contraindicated in patients hypersensitive to drug or its components.

Adverse reactions

CNS: dizziness, light-headedness, fatigue, headache.
CV: ***bradycardia***, edema, conduction abnormalities, ***arrhythmias***.
EENT: blurred vision.
GI: *nausea, diarrhea, abdominal pain or discomfort, loose stools*, vomiting, fat malabsorption, *gallbladder abnormalities*, flatulence, constipation, ***pancreatitis***.
GU: pollakiuria, UTI.
Metabolic: hyperglycemia, ***hypoglycemia***, hypothyroidism, suppressed secretion of growth hormone and of the gastroenterohepatic peptides gastrin, vasoactive intestinal polypeptide, insulin, glucagon, secretin, motilin, and pancreatic polypeptide.
Musculoskeletal: backache, joint pain.
Skin: flushing, wheal, erythema or pain at injection site, alopecia.
Other: pain or burning at S.C. injection site, cold symptoms, flulike symptoms.

Interactions

Drug-drug. *Cyclosporine:* May decrease cyclosporine level. Monitor patient closely.

Nursing considerations

- Monitor baseline thyroid function tests.
- Monitor IGF-I (somatomedin C) levels every 2 weeks. Dosage adjustments are based on this level.
- Periodically monitor laboratory tests such as thyroid function, glucose, urine 5-hydroxyindoleacetic acid, plasma serotonin, and plasma substance P (for carcinoid tumors).
- Monitor patient regularly for gallbladder disease. Octreotide therapy may be related to the development of cholelithiasis because of its effect on gallbladder motility or fat absorption.
- Monitor patient closely for signs and symptoms of glucose imbalance. Patients with type 1 diabetes mellitus and patients receiving oral antidiabetics or oral diazoxide may need dosage adjustments during therapy. Monitor glucose level.
- Octreotide therapy may alter fluid and electrolyte balance and may cause need for adjustment of other drugs used to control symptoms of the disease, such as beta blockers.
- Half-life may be altered in patients with end-stage renal failure who are receiving dialysis.

!!ALERT Don't confuse Sandostatin with Sandimmune or Sandoglobulin.

Patient teaching

- Urge patient to report signs and symptoms of abdominal discomfort immediately.
- Stress importance of the need for periodic laboratory testing during octreotide therapy.

ofloxacin

Floxin, Floxin I.V.

Pregnancy risk category C

Indications & dosages

➲ Acute bacterial worsening of chronic bronchitis, uncomplicated skin and skin-structure infections, and community-acquired pneumonia
Adults: 400 mg P.O. or I.V. q 12 hours for 10 days.
➲ Sexually transmitted diseases, such as acute uncomplicated urethral and cervical gonorrhea, nongonococcal urethritis and cervicitis, and mixed infections of urethra and cervix
Adults: For acute uncomplicated gonorrhea, 400 mg P.O. or I.V. once as a single dose; for cervicitis and urethritis, 300 mg P.O. or I.V. q 12 hours for 7 days.
➲ Cystitis from *Escherichia coli, Klebsiella pneumoniae,* or other organisms
Adults: 200 mg P.O. or I.V. q 12 hours for 3 days (*E. coli* or *K. pneumoniae*), 200 mg P.O. or I.V. q 12 hours for 7 days (other organisms).

➲ **Complicated UTI**
Adults: 200 mg P.O. or I.V. q 12 hours for 10 days.

➲ **Prostatitis**
Adults: 300 mg P.O. or I.V. q 12 hours for 6 weeks. Switch from I.V. to P.O. after 10 days.

➲ **Pelvic inflammatory disease**
Adults: 400 mg P.O. or I.V. q 12 hours with metronidazole for 10 to 14 days.

➲ **To prevent inhalation anthrax♦**
Adults: 400 mg P.O. or I.V. b.i.d. Give first doses I.V. if signs and symptoms of disease exist. Switch to P.O. after patient's condition improves. Continue therapy for 60 days if no vaccine is available. If vaccine is available, continue for 28 to 45 days and until three doses of the vaccine have been given.

➲ **Traveler's diarrhea**
Adults: 300 mg P.O. b.i.d. for 3 days.

For patients with creatinine clearance less than 20 ml/minute, give first dose as recommended; then give subsequent doses at 50% of recommended dose q 24 hours. For patients with hepatic impairment, don't exceed 400 mg/day.

Contraindications & cautions

- Contraindicated in patients hypersensitive to drug or other fluoroquinolones.
- Use cautiously in pregnant patients and in those with seizure disorders, CNS diseases such as cerebral arteriosclerosis, hepatic disorders, or renal impairment.
- Ofloxacin appears in breast milk in levels similar to those found in plasma. Safety hasn't been established in breast-feeding women.
- Safety and efficacy in children younger than age 18 haven't been established.

Adverse reactions

CNS: dizziness, headache, fever, fatigue, lethargy, malaise, drowsiness, sleep disorders, nervousness, insomnia, visual disturbances, ***seizures***.
CV: phlebitis, chest pain.
GI: *nausea*, ***pseudomembranous colitis***, anorexia, abdominal pain or discomfort, diarrhea, vomiting, constipation, dry mouth, flatulence, dysgeusia.
GU: hematuria, glucosuria, proteinuria, vaginitis, vaginal discharge, genital pruritus.
Hematologic: eosinophilia, ***leukopenia***, ***neutropenia***, anemia, leukocytosis.
Metabolic: hyperglycemia, ***hypoglycemia***.
Musculoskeletal: body pain, tendon rupture.
Skin: rash, pruritus, photosensitivity.
Other: hypersensitivity reactions, ***anaphylactoid reaction***.

Interactions

Drug-drug. *Aluminum hydroxide, calcium carbonate, aluminum–magnesium hydroxide, magnesium hydroxide:* May decrease effects of ofloxacin. Give antacid at least 6 hours before or 2 hours after ofloxacin.
Antidiabetics: May affect glucose level, causing hypoglycemia or hyperglycemia. Monitor patient closely.
Didanosine (chewable or buffered tablets or pediatric powder for oral solution): May interfere with GI absorption of ofloxacin. Separate doses by 2 hours.
Iron salts: May decrease absorption of ofloxacin, reducing anti-infective response. Separate doses by at least 2 hours.
Sucralfate: May decrease absorption of ofloxacin, reducing anti-infective response. If use together can't be avoided, separate doses by at least 6 hours.
Theophylline: May increase theophylline level. Monitor patient closely and adjust theophylline dosage as needed.
Warfarin: May prolong PT and INR. Monitor PT and INR.
Drug-lifestyle. *Sun exposure:* May cause photosensitivity reactions. Advise patient to avoid excessive sunlight exposure.

Nursing considerations

- Give drug I.V. for no longer than 10 days; after 10 days, change I.V. to P.O.

!!ALERT Patients treated for gonorrhea should have a serologic test for syphilis. Drug isn't effective against syphilis, and treatment of gonorrhea may mask or delay symptoms of syphilis.

- Periodically assess organ system functions during prolonged therapy.
- Monitor patient for overgrowth of nonsusceptible organisms.
- Monitor renal and hepatic studies and CBC in prolonged therapy.
- Monitor patient for adverse CNS effects, including dizziness, headache, seizures, or depression. Stop drug and notify prescriber if these effects occur.

- Monitor patient for hypersensitivity reactions. Stop drug and initiate supportive therapy, as indicated.

Patient teaching

- Tell patient to drink plenty of fluids during drug therapy and to finish the entire prescription even if he starts feeling better.
- Tell patient drug may be taken without regard to meals, but he shouldn't take antacids and vitamins at the same time as ofloxacin.
- Warn patient that dizziness and lightheadedness may occur. Advise caution when driving or operating hazardous machinery until effects of drug are known.
- Warn patient that hypersensitivity reactions may follow first dose; he should stop drug at first sign of rash or other allergic reaction and call prescriber immediately.
- Advise patient to avoid prolonged exposure to direct sunlight and to use a sunscreen when outdoors.

ofloxacin 0.3%
Ocuflox

Pregnancy risk category C

Indications & dosages

➲ **Conjunctivitis caused by *Staphylococcus aureus, Staphylococcus epidermidis, Streptococcus pneumoniae, Enterobacter cloacae, Haemophilus influenzae, Proteus mirabilis,* and *Pseudomonas aeruginosa***

Adults and children older than age 1: 1 or 2 drops in conjunctival sac q 2 to 4 hours daily while patient is awake, for first 2 days; then q.i.d. for up to 5 additional days.

➲ **Bacterial corneal ulcer caused by *S. aureus, S. epidermidis, S. pneumoniae, P. aeruginosa, Serratia marcescens,* and *Propionibacterium acnes***

Adults and children older than age 1: 1 or 2 drops q 30 minutes while patient is awake and 1 or 2 drops 4 to 6 hours after he goes to bed on days 1 and 2. Days 3 to 7, 1 or 2 drops hourly while patient is awake. Days 7 to 9, 1 or 2 drops q.i.d.

Contraindications & cautions

- Contraindicated in patients hypersensitive to ofloxacin, other fluoroquinolones, or other components of drug and in breast-feeding women.

Adverse reactions

EENT: *transient ocular burning or discomfort,* stinging, redness, itching, photophobia, lacrimation, eye dryness, eye pain, chemical conjunctivitis or keratitis, periocular or facial edema.

Interactions

None significant.

Nursing considerations

!!ALERT Don't inject drug into conjunctiva or introduce directly into anterior chamber of eye.

- Stop drug if improvement doesn't occur within 7 days. Prolonged use may result in overgrowth of nonsusceptible organisms, including fungi.

!!ALERT Don't confuse Ocuflox with Ocufen.

Patient teaching

- If an allergic reaction occurs, tell patient to stop drug and notify prescriber. Serious acute hypersensitivity reactions may need emergency treatment.
- Tell patient to clean excessive discharge from eye area before application.
- Teach patient how to instill drops. Advise him to wash hands before and after instilling solution, and warn him not to touch tip of dropper to eye or surrounding tissue.
- Advise patient to apply light finger pressure on lacrimal sac for 1 minute after drug instillation.
- Tell patient not to share drug, washcloths, or towels with family members and to notify prescriber if anyone develops same signs or symptoms.
- Stress importance of compliance with recommended therapy.
- Warn patient not to use leftover drug for new eye infection.
- Remind patient to discard drug when it's no longer needed.

olanzapine
Zyprexa, Zyprexa Zydis

Pregnancy risk category C

Indications & dosages

➲ **Schizophrenia**

Adults: Initially, 5 to 10 mg P.O. once daily with the goal to be at 10 mg daily within several days of starting therapy. Adjust dose in 5-mg increments at intervals 1 week or more. Most patients respond to 10 to 15 mg daily. Safety of dosages greater than 20 mg daily hasn't been established.

➲ **Short-term treatment of acute manic episodes linked to bipolar I disorder**

Adults: Initially, 10 to 15 mg P.O. daily. Adjust dosage p.r.n. in 5-mg daily increments at intervals of 24 hours or more. Maximum, 20 mg P.O. daily. Duration of treatment is 3 to 4 weeks.

➲ **Short-term treatment, with lithium or valproate, of acute manic episodes linked to bipolar I disorder**

Adults: 10 mg P.O. once daily. Dosage range is 5 to 20 mg daily. Duration of treatment is 6 weeks.

➲ **Long-term treatment of bipolar I disorder**

Adults: 5 to 20 mg P.O. daily.

➲ **Adjunct to lithium or valproate to treat bipolar mania**

Adults: 10 mg P.O. daily. Usual range 5 to 20 mg daily.

In elderly or debilitated patients, those predisposed to hypotensive reactions, patients who may metabolize olanzapine more slowly than usual (nonsmoking women older than age 65) or may be more pharmacodynamically sensitive to olanzapine, initially, 5 mg P.O. Increase dose cautiously.

➲ **Agitation caused by schizophrenia and bipolar I mania**

Adults: 10 mg I.M. (range 2.5 to 10 mg). Subsequent doses of up to 10 mg may be given 2 hours after the first dose or 4 hours after the second dose, up to 30 mg I.M. daily. If maintenance therapy is required, convert patient to 5 to 20 mg P.O. daily.

In elderly patients, give 5 mg I.M. In debilitated patients, in those predisposed to hypotension, and in patients sensitive to effects of olanzapine, give 2.5 mg I.M.

Contraindications & cautions

- Contraindicated in patients hypersensitive to drug.
- Use cautiously in patients with heart disease, cerebrovascular disease, conditions that predispose patient to hypotension, history of seizures or conditions that might lower the seizure threshold, and hepatic impairment.
- Use cautiously in elderly patients, those with a history of paralytic ileus, and those at risk for aspiration pneumonia, prostatic hyperplasia, or angle-closure glaucoma.

Adverse reactions

CNS: *somnolence*, asthenia, abnormal gait, *insomnia, parkinsonism, dizziness*, personality disorder, akathisia, tremor, articulation impairment, ***suicide attempt***, tardive dyskinesia, ***neuroleptic malignant syndrome***, fever, asthenia, somnolence, dizziness, tremor, parkinsonism, akathisia, extrapyramidal events (I.M.).
CV: orthostatic hypotension, tachycardia, chest pain, hypertension, ecchymosis, peripheral edema, hypotension (I.M.).
EENT: amblyopia, rhinitis, pharyngitis, conjunctivitis.
GI: *constipation, dry mouth, dyspepsia*, increased appetite, increased salivation, vomiting, thirst.
GU: hematuria, metrorrhagia, urinary incontinence, urinary tract infection, amenorrhea, vaginitis.
Hematologic: ***leukopenia***.
Metabolic: weight gain, *hyperglycemia*.
Musculoskeletal: joint pain, extremity pain, back pain, neck rigidity, twitching, hypertonia.
Respiratory: increased cough, dyspnea.
Skin: sweating, injection site pain (I.M.).
Other: flulike syndrome, injury.

Interactions

Drug-drug. *Antihypertensives:* May potentiate hypotensive effects. Monitor blood pressure closely.
Carbamazepine, omeprazole, rifampin: May increase clearance of olanzapine. Monitor patient.
Ciprofloxacin: May increase olanzapine level. Monitor patient for increased adverse effects.
Diazepam: May increase CNS effects. Monitor patient.

Dopamine agonists, levodopa: May cause antagonized activity of these drugs. Monitor patient.
Fluoxetine: May increase olanzapine level. Use together cautiously.
Fluvoxamine: May increase olanzapine level. May need to reduce olanzapine dose.
Drug-herb. *St. John's wort:* May decrease olanzapine level. Discourage use together.
Drug-lifestyle. *Alcohol use:* May increase CNS effects. Discourage use together.
Smoking: May increase olanzapine clearance. Urge patient to quit smoking.

Nursing considerations

- Inspect I.M. solution for particulate matter and discoloration before administration.
- To reconstitute I.M. injection, dissolve contents of one vial with 2.1 ml of sterile water for injection to yield a clear yellow 5 mg/ml solution. Store at room temperature and give within 1 hour of reconstitution. Discard any unused solution.
- Monitor patient for abnormal body temperature regulation, especially if he exercises, is exposed to extreme heat, takes anticholinergics, or is dehydrated.
- Obtain baseline and periodic liver function test results.
- Monitor patient for weight gain.

!!ALERT Watch for evidence of neuroleptic malignant syndrome (hyperpyrexia, muscle rigidity, altered mental status, autonomic instability), which is rare but commonly fatal. Stop drug immediately; monitor and treat patient as needed.

!!ALERT Drug may cause hyperglycemia. Monitor patients with diabetes regularly. In patients with risk factors for diabetes, obtain fasting blood glucose test results at baseline and periodically.

- Monitor patient for tardive dyskinesia, which may occur after prolonged use. It may not appear until months or years later and may disappear spontaneously or persist for life, despite stopping drug.
- Periodically reevaluate the long-term usefulness of olanzapine.
- Drug may increase risk of stroke and death in elderly patients with dementia. Olanzapine isn't approved to treat patients with dementia-related psychosis.
- A patient who feels dizzy or drowsy after an I.M. injection should remain recumbent until he can be assessed for orthostatic hypotension and bradycardia. He should rest until the feeling passes.

!!ALERT Don't confuse olanzapine with olsalazine or Zyprexa with Zyrtec.

Patient teaching

- Warn patient to avoid hazardous tasks until full effects of drug are known.
- Warn patient against exposure to extreme heat; drug may impair body's ability to reduce temperature.
- Inform patient that he might gain weight.
- Advise patient to avoid alcohol.
- Tell patient to rise slowly to avoid dizziness upon standing up quickly.
- Inform patient that orally disintegrating tablets contain phenylalanine.
- Drug may be taken without regard to food.
- Urge woman of childbearing age to notify prescriber if she becomes pregnant or plans or suspects pregnancy. Tell her not to breastfeed during therapy.

olmesartan medoxomil
Benicar

Pregnancy risk category C; D in 2nd and 3rd trimesters

Indications & dosages

➲ Hypertension
Adults: 20 mg P.O. once daily if patient has no volume depletion. May increase dosage to 40 mg P.O. once daily if blood pressure isn't reduced after 2 weeks of therapy.

In patients with possible depletion of intravascular volume (those with impaired renal function who are taking diuretics), consider using lower starting dose.

Contraindications & cautions

- Contraindicated in patients hypersensitive to the drug or any of its components and in patients who are pregnant.
- Use cautiously in patients who are volume- or salt-depleted, those whose renal function depends on the renin-angiotensin-aldosterone system (such as patients with severe heart failure), and those with unilateral and bilateral renal artery stenosis.
- It's unknown if drug appears in breast milk. Patient should stop either breastfeeding or drug.

• Safety and efficacy in children haven't been established. Don't give drug to children.

Adverse reactions

CNS: headache.
EENT: pharyngitis, rhinitis, sinusitis.
GI: diarrhea.
GU: hematuria.
Metabolic: hyperglycemia, hypertriglyceridemia.
Musculoskeletal: back pain.
Respiratory: bronchitis, upper respiratory tract infection.
Other: flulike symptoms, accidental injury.

Interactions

Drug-herb. *Ma huang:* May decrease antihypertensive effects. Discourage use together.

Nursing considerations

• Symptomatic hypotension may occur in patients who are volume- or salt-depleted, especially those being treated with high doses of a diuretic. If hypotension occurs, place patient supine and treat supportively. Treatment may continue once blood pressure is stabilized.
• If blood pressure isn't adequately controlled, a diuretic or other antihypertensive drugs also may be prescribed.
• Overdose may cause hypotension and tachycardia, along with bradycardia from parasympathetic (vagal) stimulation. Treatment should be supportive.
• Closely monitor patients with heart failure for oliguria, azotemia, and acute renal failure.
• Monitor BUN and creatinine level in patients with unilateral or bilateral renal artery stenosis.
• Drugs that act on the renin-angiotensin system may cause fetal and neonatal complications and death when given to pregnant women after the first trimester. If patient taking drug becomes pregnant, stop drug immediately.

Patient teaching

• Tell patient to take drug exactly as prescribed and not to stop taking it even if he feels better.
• Tell patient that drug may be taken without regard to meals.
• Tell patient to report to health care provider any adverse reactions promptly, especially light-headedness and fainting.
• Advise woman of childbearing age to immediately report pregnancy to health care provider.
• Inform diabetic patients that glucose readings may rise and that the dosage of their diabetes drugs may need adjustment.
• Warn patients that inadequate fluid intake, excessive perspiration, diarrhea, or vomiting may lead to an excessive drop in blood pressure, light-headedness, and possibly fainting.
• Instruct patients that other antihypertensives can have additive effects. Patient should inform his prescriber of all medications he's taking, including OTC drugs.

olsalazine sodium
Dipentum

Pregnancy risk category C

Indications & dosages

➲ **Maintenance of remission of ulcerative colitis in patients intolerant of sulfasalazine**
Adults: 500 mg P.O. b.i.d. with meals.

Contraindications & cautions

• Contraindicated in patients hypersensitive to salicylates.
• Use cautiously in patients with renal disease.

Adverse reactions

CNS: headache, depression, vertigo, dizziness, fatigue.
GI: *diarrhea*, nausea, *abdominal pain*, dyspepsia, bloating, anorexia.
Musculoskeletal: arthralgia.
Skin: rash, itching.

Interactions

Drug-drug. *Anticoagulants, coumarin derivatives:* May prolong PT or INR. Monitor bleeding study results.
Drug-food. *Any food:* May decrease GI irritation. Advise patient to take drug with food.

Nursing considerations

- Regularly monitor BUN and creatinine levels and urinalysis in patients with renal disease.
- Absorption of drug or its metabolites may cause renal tubular damage.
- Diarrhea sometimes occurs during therapy. Although diarrhea appears to be dose-related, it's difficult to distinguish from worsening of disease symptoms.
- Similar drugs have caused worsening of disease.

!!ALERT Don't confuse olsalazine with olanzapine.

Patient teaching

- Teach patient to take drug in evenly divided doses and with food to minimize adverse GI reactions.
- Instruct patient to report persistent or severe adverse reactions promptly.

omalizumab
Xolair

Pregnancy risk category B

Indications & dosages

➲ Moderate to severe persistent asthma in patients with positive skin test or in vitro reactivity to a perennial aeroallergen and whose symptoms aren't adequately controlled by inhaled corticosteroids

Adults and adolescents age 12 and older: 150 to 375 mg S.C. q 2 or 4 weeks. Dose and frequency vary with pretreatment immunoglobulin E (IgE) level (IU/ml) and patient. Divide doses larger than 150 mg among more than one injection site.

Contraindications & cautions

- Contraindicated in patients severely hypersensitive to omalizumab.
- Safety and effectiveness haven't been established in children younger than age 12.

Adverse reactions

CNS: dizziness, fatigue, *headache*, pain.
EENT: earache, *pharyngitis*, *sinusitis*.
Musculoskeletal: arm pain, arthralgia, fracture, leg pain.
Respiratory: *upper respiratory tract infection.*
Skin: dermatitis, *injection site reaction*, pruritus.
Other: *viral infections.*

Interactions

None reported.

Nursing considerations

!!ALERT Don't use this drug to treat acute bronchospasm or status asthmaticus.

- Don't abruptly stop systemic or inhaled corticosteroid when omalizumab therapy starts; taper the dose gradually and under supervision.
- Because the solution is slightly viscous, it may take 5 to 10 seconds to give.
- Injection site reactions may occur, such as bruising, redness, warmth, burning, stinging, itching, hives, pain, induration, and inflammation. Most occur within 1 hour after the injection, last fewer than 8 days, and decrease in frequency with subsequent injections.

!!ALERT Observe patient after the injection, and keep drugs available to respond to anaphylactic reactions. If the patient has a severe hypersensitivity reaction, stop treatment.

- Drug increases IgE level, so it can't be used to determine appropriate dosage during therapy or for 1 year after therapy ends.

Patient teaching

- Tell patients not to stop or reduce the dosage of any other asthma drugs unless directed by the prescriber.
- Explain that patient may not notice an immediate improvement in asthma after omalizumab therapy starts.

omega-3–acid ethyl esters
Omacor

Pregnancy risk category C

Indications & dosages

➲ Adjunct to diet to reduce triglyceride levels 500 mg/dl or higher

Adults: 4 g P.O. once daily or divided as 2 g b.i.d.

Contraindications & cautions

- Contraindicated in patients hypersensitive to drug or its components.

- Use cautiously in patients sensitive to fish.

Adverse reactions

CNS: pain.
CV: angina pectoris.
GI: altered taste, belching, dyspepsia.
Musculoskeletal: back pain.
Skin: rash.
Other: flulike syndrome, infection.

Interactions

Drug-drug. *Anticoagulants:* May prolong bleeding time. Monitor patient.

Nursing considerations

- Assess patient for conditions that contribute to increased triglycerides, such as diabetes and hypothyroidism, before treatment.
- Evaluate patient's current drug regimen for any drugs known to sharply increase triglyceride levels, including estrogen therapy, thiazide diuretics, and beta blockers. Stopping these drugs, if appropriate, may negate the need for Omacor.
- Start therapy only after diet and lifestyle modifications have proven unsuccessful.
- Obtain baseline triglyceride levels to confirm that they're consistently abnormal before therapy; then recheck periodically during treatment. If patient has an inadequate response after 2 months, stop drug.
- Monitor LDL level to make sure it doesn't increase excessively during treatment.

Patient teaching

- Explain that taking Omacor doesn't reduce the importance of following the recommended diet and exercise plan.
- Remind patient of the need for follow-up blood work to evaluate progress.
- Advise patient to notify prescriber about bothersome side effects.
- Tell patient to report planned or suspected pregnancy.

omeprazole
Prilosec, Zegerid

omeprazole magnesium
Prilosec OTC ◇

Pregnancy risk category C

Indications & dosages

➲ **Symptomatic gastroesophageal reflux disease (GERD) without esophageal lesions**
Adults: 20 mg P.O., as delayed-release or oral suspension, daily for 4 weeks for patients who respond poorly to customary medical treatment, usually including an adequate course of H_2-receptor antagonists.

➲ **Erosive esophagitis and accompanying symptoms caused by GERD**
Adults: 20 mg P.O. daily for 4 to 8 weeks.

➲ **Maintenance of healing erosive esophagitis**
Adults: 20 mg P.O., as delayed-release or oral suspension, daily.

➲ **Pathologic hypersecretory conditions (such as Zollinger-Ellison syndrome)**
Adults: Initially, 60 mg P.O. daily; adjust dosage based on patient response. If daily dose exceeds 80 mg, give in divided doses. Doses up to 120 mg t.i.d. have been given. Continue therapy as long as clinically indicated.

➲ **Duodenal ulcer (short-term treatment)**
Adults: 20 mg P.O., as delayed-release or oral suspension, daily for 4 to 8 weeks.

➲ ***Helicobacter pylori* infection and duodenal ulcer disease, to eradicate *H. pylori* with clarithromycin (dual therapy)**
Adults: 40 mg P.O. q morning with clarithromycin 500 mg P.O. t.i.d. for 14 days. For patients with an ulcer at start of therapy, give another 14 days of omeprazole 20 mg P.O. once daily.

➲ ***H. pylori* infection and duodenal ulcer disease, to eradicate *H. pylori* with clarithromycin and amoxicillin (triple therapy)**
Adults: 20 mg P.O. with clarithromycin 500 mg P.O. and amoxicillin 1,000 mg P.O., each given b.i.d. for 10 days. For patients with an ulcer at start of therapy, give another 18 days of omeprazole 20 mg P.O. once daily.

➲ **Short-term treatment of active benign gastric ulcer**
Adults: 40 mg P.O. once daily for 4 to 8 weeks.
➲ **Frequent heartburn (2 or more days a week)**
Adults: 20 mg P.O. Prilosec OTC once daily before breakfast for 14 days. May repeat the 14-day course q 4 months.

Contraindications & cautions

- Contraindicated in patients hypersensitive to drug or its components.
- Zegerid is contraindicated in patients with metabolic alkalosis and hypocalcemia.
- Use cautiously in patients with Bartter's syndrome, hypokalemia, and respiratory alkalosis.
- Long-term administration of bicarbonate with calcium or milk can cause milk-alkali syndrome.

Adverse reactions

CNS: headache, dizziness, asthenia.
GI: diarrhea, abdominal pain, nausea, vomiting, constipation, flatulence.
Musculoskeletal: back pain.
Respiratory: cough, upper respiratory tract infection.
Skin: rash.

Interactions

Drug-drug. *Ampicillin esters, iron derivatives, ketoconazole:* May cause poor bioavailability of these drugs because they need a low gastric pH for optimal absorption. Avoid using together.
Diazepam, fosphenytoin, phenytoin, warfarin: May decrease hepatic clearance, possibly leading to increased levels of these drugs. Monitor drug levels.
Drug-herb. *Male fern:* May cause alkaline environment in which herb is inactivated. Discourage use together.
Pennyroyal: May change rate at which toxic pennyroyal metabolites form. Ask patient about the use of herbal remedies, and discourage use together.
St. John's wort: May increase risk of sun sensitivity. Advise patient to avoid excessive sunlight exposure.

Nursing considerations

- Dosage adjustments may be necessary in Asian patients and patients with hepatic impairment.
- Omeprazole increases its own bioavailability with repeated doses. Drug is labile in gastric acid; less drug is lost to hydrolysis because drug increases gastric pH.
- Zegerid contains 460 mg sodium per dose in the form of sodium bicarbonate.

!!ALERT Don't confuse Prilosec with Prozac, Prilocaine, or Prinivil.

- Gastrin level rises in most patients during the first 2 weeks of therapy.

Patient teaching

- Tell patient to swallow tablets or capsules whole and not to open, crush, or chew them.
- Warn patients that Zegerid contains 460 mg sodium bicarbonate per dose. Those following a sodium-restricted diet should be cautious.
- Tell patient to empty contents of Zegerid packet into a small cup containing 2 tablespoons of water. Instruct him not to use other liquids or foods. Stir contents and drink immediately. Refill cup with water and drink.
- Instruct patient to take drug 30 minutes before meals. Zegerid powder for oral suspension should be taken on an empty stomach at least 1 hour before a meal.
- Caution patient to avoid hazardous activities if he gets dizzy.
- Advise patient that Prilosec OTC isn't intended to treat infrequent heartburn (one episode of heartburn a week or less), or for those who want immediate relief of heartburn.
- Inform patient that Prilosec OTC may take 1 to 4 days for full effect, although some patients may get complete relief of symptoms within 24 hours.

ondansetron hydrochloride
Zofran, Zofran ODT

Pregnancy risk category B

Indications & dosages

➲ To prevent nausea and vomiting from emetogenic chemotherapy

Adults and children age 12 and older: 8 mg P.O. 30 minutes before chemotherapy. Then, 8 mg P.O. 8 hours after first dose. Then, 8 mg q 12 hours for 1 to 2 days. Or, a single dose of 32 mg by I.V. infusion over 15 minutes beginning 30 minutes before chemotherapy. Or, three divided doses of 0.15 mg/kg I.V. Give first dose 30 minutes before chemotherapy and subsequent doses 4 and 8 hours after first dose. Infuse drug over 15 minutes.

Children ages 4 to 12: 4 mg P.O. 30 minutes before chemotherapy. Then, 4 mg P.O. 4 and 8 hours after first dose. Then, 4 mg q 8 hours for 1 to 2 days.

Infants and children ages 6 months to 12 years: Three doses of 0.15 mg/kg I.V. Give first dose 30 minutes before chemotherapy; give subsequent doses 4 and 8 hours after first dose. Infuse drug over 15 minutes.

➲ To prevent postoperative nausea and vomiting

Adults: 4 mg I.V. undiluted over 2 to 5 minutes. Or, 16 mg P.O. 1 hour before induction of anesthesia.

Children ages 1 month to 12 years weighing more than 40 kg (88 lb): 4 mg I.V. as a single dose.

Children ages 1 month to 12 years weighing 40 kg or less: 0.1 mg/kg I.V. as a single dose.

➲ To prevent nausea and vomiting from radiotherapy in patients receiving total body irradiation, single high-dose fraction to abdomen, or daily fractions to abdomen

Adults: 8 mg P.O. t.i.d.

For patients with severe hepatic impairment, total daily dose shouldn't exceed 8 mg.

Contraindications & cautions

- Contraindicated in patients hypersensitive to drug.
- Use cautiously in patients with hepatic impairment.

Adverse reactions

CNS: *headache, malaise, fatigue, dizziness,* fever, *sedation,* extrapyramidal syndrome.
CV: chest pain, ***arrhythmias***.
GI: *diarrhea, constipation,* abdominal pain, xerostomia, decreased appetite.
GU: urine retention, gynecologic disorders.
Musculoskeletal: *pain.*
Respiratory: hypoxia.
Skin: rash, pruritus.
Other: chills, injection site reaction.

Interactions

Drug-drug. *Drugs that alter hepatic drug-metabolizing enzymes, such as cimetidine, phenobarbital, rifampin:* May change pharmacokinetics of ondansetron. No need to adjust dosage.

Drug-herb. *Horehound:* May enhance serotoninergic effects. Discourage use together.

Nursing considerations

!!ALERT Don't confuse Zofran with Zosyn, Zantac, or Zoloft.

- Monitor liver function test results. Don't exceed 8 mg in patients with hepatic impairment.

Patient teaching

- Instruct patient to immediately report difficulty breathing after drug administration.
- Tell patient receiving drug I.V. to report discomfort at insertion site.
- Instruct patient, when using disintegrating tablets, to open blister just before use by peeling backing off and not by pushing through foil blister. Using with a liquid isn't necessary.

oprelvekin
Neumega

Pregnancy risk category C

Indications & dosages

➲ To prevent severe thrombocytopenia and reduce need for platelet transfusions after myelosuppressive chemotherapy with nonmyeloid malignancies

Adults: 50 mcg/kg as single daily S.C. injection until post-nadir platelet count is at least 50,000 cells/mm^3. Treatment beyond 21 days per course isn't recommended.

Contraindications & cautions

- Contraindicated in patients hypersensitive to drug or its components.
- Use drug cautiously in patients with heart failure because of fluid retention.

Adverse reactions

CNS: *asthenia, headache, insomnia, dizziness,* paresthesia, *syncope.*
CV: *tachycardia, palpitations,* **ATRIAL FLUTTER OR FIBRILLATION,** *edema.*
EENT: blurred vision, *conjunctival injection,* eye hemorrhage, pharyngitis.
GI: *oral candidiasis, nausea, vomiting, diarrhea.*
Hematologic: anemia.
Metabolic: dehydration, hypocalcemia.
Respiratory: dyspnea, cough, pleural effusions.
Skin: *rash,* skin discoloration, exfoliative dermatitis.

Interactions

Drug-drug. *Diuretics, ifosfamide:* May cause severe hypokalemia resulting in death. Avoid using together.

Nursing considerations

- Give S.C. in the abdomen, thigh, hip, or upper arm. Don't inject I.D. or intravascularly.
- Dosing should begin 6 to 24 hours after completion of chemotherapy and end at least 2 days before starting next planned cycle of chemotherapy.
- Reconstitute each single-dose vial with 1 ml of supplied diluent. Avoid excessive or vigorous agitation. Discard unused portions.
- Use reconstituted drug within 3 hours.
- Store drug and diluent in refrigerator until ready to use. Don't freeze.
- Closely monitor fluid and electrolyte status in patients receiving long-term diuretic therapy.
- Obtain a CBC before chemotherapy and at regular intervals during drug therapy.
- Fluid retention can be severe; monitor patient closely.

Patient teaching

- Instruct patient about appropriate preparation and administration of drug if he is to self-administer at home.
- Warn patient about potential adverse reactions. Tell him to report any occurrence.
- Tell patient to keep drug refrigerated and not to reconstitute until just before use.
- Urge patient to call prescriber immediately if swelling, rapid heart beat, or difficulty breathing occurs.
- Tell patient to report signs and symptoms of increased bleeding or bruising.

orlistat
Xenical

Pregnancy risk category B

Indications & dosages

➲ **To manage obesity, including weight loss and weight maintenance with a reduced-calorie diet; to reduce risk of weight gain after previous weight loss**
Adults and children ages 12 to 16: 120 mg P.O. t.i.d. with or up to 1 hour after each main meal containing fat.

Contraindications & cautions

- Contraindicated in patients hypersensitive to drug or its components and in those with chronic malabsorption syndrome or cholestasis.
- Use cautiously in patients with history of hyperoxaluria or calcium oxalate nephrolithiasis or those at risk for anorexia nervosa or bulimia.
- Use cautiously in patients receiving cyclosporine therapy because of potential changes in cyclosporine absorption related to variations in dietary intake.

Adverse reactions

CNS: *headache,* dizziness, fatigue, sleep disorder, anxiety, depression.
CV: pedal edema.
EENT: otitis.
GI: *flatus with discharge, fecal urgency, fatty or oily stool, oily spotting, increased defecation, abdominal pain,* fecal incontinence, nausea, infectious diarrhea, rectal pain, vomiting.
GU: menstrual irregularity, vaginitis, UTI.
Musculoskeletal: *back pain, leg pain,* arthritis, myalgia, joint disorder, tendinitis.
Respiratory: *influenza, upper respiratory tract infection,* lower respiratory tract infection.
Skin: rash, dry skin.
Other: tooth and gingival disorders.

Interactions

Drug-drug. *Cyclosporine:* May alter cyclosporine absorption with variations in dietary intake. Monitor patient's cyclosporine levels if used together.
Fat-soluble vitamins (such as vitamins A and E and beta-carotene): May decrease absorption of vitamins. Separate doses by 2 hours.
Pravastatin: May slightly increase pravastatin levels and lipid-lowering effects of drug. Monitor patient.
Warfarin: May change coagulation values. Monitor INR.

Nursing considerations

- Exclude organic causes of obesity, such as hypothyroidism, before starting drug therapy.
- Drug is recommended for use in patients with an initial body mass index (BMI) of 30 kg/m^2 or more or those with a BMI of 27 kg/m^2 or more and other risk factors (such as hypertension, diabetes, or dyslipidemia).
- In diabetic patients, dosage of oral antidiabetic or insulin may need to be reduced because improved metabolic control may accompany weight loss.
- As with other weight-loss drugs, potential for misuse exists in certain patients (such as those with anorexia nervosa or bulimia).

!!ALERT Don't confuse Xenical with Xeloda.

Patient teaching

- Advise patient to follow a nutritionally balanced, reduced-calorie diet that derives only 30% of its calories from fat. Tell him to distribute daily intake of fat, carbohydrate, and protein over three main meals. If a meal is occasionally missed or contains no fat, tell patient that dose of drug can be omitted.
- Advise patient to adhere to dietary guidelines. GI effects may increase when patient takes drug with high-fat foods, specifically when more than 30% of total daily calories come from fat.
- Drug reduces absorption of some fat- soluble vitamins and beta-carotene.
- Tell patient with diabetes that weight loss may improve his glycemic control, so dosage of his oral antidiabetic (such as a sulfonylurea or metformin) or insulin may need to be reduced during drug therapy.
- Tell woman of childbearing age to inform prescriber if pregnancy or breast-feeding is planned during therapy.

oseltamivir phosphate

Tamiflu

Pregnancy risk category C

Indications & dosages

➲ Uncomplicated, acute illness caused by influenza infection in patients who have had symptoms for 2 days or less
Adults: 75 mg P.O. b.i.d. for 5 days.

For patients with creatinine clearance of 10 to 30 ml/minute, reduce dosage to 75 mg P.O. once daily for 5 days.

➲ To prevent influenza after close contact with infected person
Adults and adolescents age 13 and older: 75 mg P.O. once daily, beginning within 2 days of exposure, for at least 7 days.

➲ To prevent influenza during a community outbreak
Adults and adolescents age 13 and older: 75 mg P.O. once daily for up to 6 weeks.

➲ Influenza in children age 1 and older
Children age 1 and older, weighing more than 40 kg (88 lb): 75 mg oral suspension P.O. b.i.d.
Children age 1 and older, weighing 23 to 40 kg (51 to 88 lb): 60 mg oral suspension P.O. b.i.d.
Children age 1 and older, weighing 15 to 23 kg (33 to 51 lb): 45 mg oral suspension P.O. b.i.d.
Children age 1 and older, weighing 15 kg (33 lb) or less: 30 mg oral suspension P.O. b.i.d.

Contraindications & cautions

- Contraindicated in patients hypersensitive to drug or its components.
- Use cautiously in patients with chronic cardiac or respiratory diseases, or any medical condition that may require imminent hospitalization. Also use cautiously in patients with renal failure.
- It's unknown if drug or its metabolite appears in breast milk. Use only if benefits to patient outweigh risks to infant.

Adverse reactions

CNS: dizziness, insomnia, headache, vertigo, fatigue.
GI: abdominal pain, diarrhea, nausea, vomiting.
Respiratory: bronchitis, cough.

Interactions

None significant.

Nursing considerations

- No evidence supports drug use to treat viral infections other than influenza virus types A and B.
- Drug must be given within 2 days of onset of symptoms.
- Drug isn't a replacement for the annual influenza vaccination. Patients for whom vaccine is indicated should continue to receive the vaccine each fall.
- Safety and efficacy of repeated treatment courses haven't been established.
- Drug may be given with meals to decrease GI adverse effects.
- Store at controlled room temperature (59° to 86° F [15° to 30° C]).

Patient teaching

- Instruct patient to begin treatment as soon as possible after appearance of flu symptoms.
- Inform patient that drug may be taken with or without meals. If nausea or vomiting occurs, he can take drug with food or milk.
- Tell patient that, if a dose is missed, he should take it as soon as possible. However, if next dose is due within 2 hours, tell him to skip the missed dose and take the next dose on schedule.
- Advise patient to complete the full 5 days of treatment, even if symptoms resolve.
- Alert patient that drug isn't a replacement for the annual influenza vaccination. Patients for whom vaccine is indicated should continue to receive the vaccine each fall.

oxaliplatin
Eloxatin

Pregnancy risk category D

Indications & dosages

➲ **First-line treatment of advanced colorectal cancer with 5-fluorouracil/leucovorin (5-FU/LV)**
Adults: On day 1, give 85 mg/m² oxaliplatin I.V. in 250 to 500 ml D_5W and leucovorin 200 mg/m² I.V. in D_5W simultaneously over 120 minutes, in separate bags using a Y-line, followed by 5-FU 400 mg/m² I.V. bolus over 2 to 4 minutes, followed by 600 mg/m² 5-FU I.V. infusion in 500 ml D_5W over 22 hours.

On day 2, give 200 mg/m² leucovorin I.V. infusion over 120 minutes, followed by 400 mg/m² 5-FU I.V. bolus over 2 to 4 minutes, followed by 600 mg/m² 5-FU I.V. infusion in 500 ml D_5W over 22 hours.

Repeat cycle q 2 weeks.

In patients with unresolved and persistent grade 2 neurosensory events, reduce oxaliplatin to 65 mg/m². In those with persistent grade 3 neurosensory events, consider stopping drug. In patients recovering from grade 3 or 4 GI or hematologic events, reduce dose to 65 mg/m² and reduce dose of 5-FU by 20%.

➲ **With 5-fluorouracil (5-FU) and leucovorin for the adjuvant treatment of stage III colon cancer in patients who have had complete resection of the primary tumor**
Adults: On day 1, give oxaliplatin, 85 mg/m² I.V. in 250 to 500 ml D_5W and leucovorin 200 mg/m² I.V. infusion in D_5W, both over 120 minutes at the same time, in separate bags, using a Y-line. Follow with 5-FU 400 mg/m² I.V. bolus over 2 to 4 minutes, then 600 mg/m² 5-FU in 500 ml D_5W as a 22-hour continuous infusion.

On day 2, give leucovorin, 200 mg/m² I.V. infused over 120 minutes followed by 5-FU 400 mg/m² as an I.V. bolus over 2 to 4 minutes, then, 600 mg/m² 5-FU in 500 ml D_5W as a 22-hour infusion.

Repeat cycle q 2 weeks for a total of 6 months. Premedicate with antiemetics, with or without dexamethasone.

For patients with persistent grade 2 neurotoxicity, consider an oxaliplatin dose reduction to 75 mg/m². For patients who recovered from a grade 3/4 GI event or a grade 4 neutropenia or grade 3/4 thrombocytopenia, reduce oxaliplatin to 75 mg/m^2 and 5-FU to a 300-mg/m^2 bolus and 500-mg/m^2 22-hour infusion. Delay dose until neutrophils are 1.5 × 10^9/L or more and platelets are 75 × 10^9/L or more.

Contraindications & cautions

- Contraindicated in patients allergic to drug or other platinum-containing compounds and in pregnant or breast-feeding patients.
- Use cautiously in patients with renal impairment or peripheral sensory neuropathy.

Adverse reactions

CNS: *pain, peripheral neuropathy, fatigue, headache,* dizziness, *insomnia, fever.*
CV: chest pain, ***thromboembolism***, *edema, flushing, peripheral edema.*
EENT: *rhinitis*, pharyngitis, epistaxis, abnormal lacrimation.
GI: *nausea, vomiting, diarrhea, stomatitis, abdominal pain, anorexia, constipation, dyspepsia, taste perversion,* gastroesophageal reflux, flatulence, mucositis.
GU: dysuria, hematuria.
Hematologic: FEBRILE NEUTROPENIA, *anemia,* LEUKOPENIA, THROMBOCYTOPENIA.
Metabolic: hypokalemia, dehydration.
Musculoskeletal: *back pain, arthralgia.*
Respiratory: *dyspnea, cough, upper respiratory tract infection,* hiccups, ***pulmonary toxicity***.
Skin: *injection site reaction,* rash, alopecia.
Other: ***anaphylaxis***, *hand-foot syndrome, allergic reaction,* rigors.

Interactions

Drug-drug. *Nephrotoxic drugs (such as gentamicin):* May decrease elimination of these drugs and increase levels. Monitor patient for signs and symptoms of toxicity.

Nursing considerations

- Drug doesn't require patient prehydration.
- Give antiemetic with or without dexamethasone before drug to reduce nausea.
- Drug clearance is reduced in patients with renal impairment. Dosage adjustment for patients with renal impairment hasn't been established.
- Monitor CBC, platelet count, and liver and kidney function before each chemotherapy cycle.
- Monitor patient for hypersensitivity reactions, which may occur within minutes of administration.
- Monitor patient for injection site reaction; extravasation may occur.
- Monitor patient for neuropathy and pulmonary toxicity. Peripheral neuropathy may be acute or persistent. Acute neuropathy is reversible; it occurs within 2 days of dosing and resolves within 14 days. Persistent peripheral neuropathy occurs more than 14 days after dosing and causes paresthesias, dysesthesias, hypoesthesias, and deficits in proprioception that can interfere with daily activities (such as walking or swallowing).
- Avoid ice and cold exposure during infusion of drug because cold temperatures can worsen acute neurologic symptoms. Cover patient with a blanket during infusion.
- Diarrhea, dehydration, hypokalemia, and fatigue may occur more frequently in elderly patients.

Patient teaching

- Inform patient of potential adverse reactions.
- Tell patient to avoid exposure to cold or cold objects (such as cold drinks or ice cubes), which can bring on or worsen acute symptoms of peripheral neuropathy. Advise patient to have warm drinks, wear warm clothing, and cover any exposed skin (hands, face, and head). Have patient warm the air going into his lungs by wearing a scarf or ski mask. Have him wear gloves when touching cold objects (such as foods in the freezer, outside door handles, or mailbox).
- Tell patient to contact prescriber immediately if he has trouble breathing or experiences signs and symptoms of an allergic reaction, such as rash, hives, swelling of lips or tongue, or sudden cough.
- Tell patient to contact prescriber if fever, signs and symptoms of an infection, persistent vomiting, diarrhea, or signs and symptoms of dehydration (thirst, dry mouth, light-headedness, and decreased urination) occur.

oxazepam

Apo-Oxazepam†, Novoxapam†, Serax

Pregnancy risk category D
Controlled substance schedule IV

Indications & dosages

➲ **Alcohol withdrawal, severe anxiety**
Adults: 15 to 30 mg P.O. t.i.d. or q.i.d.
➲ **Mild to moderate anxiety**
Adults: 10 to 15 mg P.O. t.i.d. or q.i.d.
Elderly patients: Initially, 10 mg t.i.d.; increase to 15 mg t.i.d. to q.i.d.

Contraindications & cautions

- Contraindicated in patients hypersensitive to drug; in pregnant women, especially in the first trimester; and in those with psychoses.
- Use cautiously in elderly patients and in those with history of drug abuse or in whom a decrease in blood pressure might lead to cardiac problems.

Adverse reactions

CNS: *drowsiness*, *lethargy*, dizziness, vertigo, headache, syncope, tremor, slurred speech, changes in EEG patterns.
CV: edema.
GI: nausea.
Hepatic: ***hepatic dysfunction***.
Skin: rash.
Other: altered libido.

Interactions

Drug-drug. *CNS depressants:* May increase CNS depression. Use together cautiously.
Digoxin: May increase digoxin level and risk of toxicity. Monitor patient closely.
Drug-herb. *Kava:* May increase sedation. Discourage use together.
Drug-lifestyle. *Alcohol use:* May cause additive CNS effects. Discourage use together.

Nursing considerations

- Monitor hepatic, renal, and hematopoietic function periodically in patients receiving repeated or prolonged therapy.

!!ALERT Serax tablets may contain tartrazine.
!!ALERT Use of this drug may lead to abuse and addiction. Don't stop drug abruptly because withdrawal symptoms may occur.
!!ALERT Don't confuse oxazepam with oxaprozin.

Patient teaching

- Warn patient to avoid hazardous activities that require alertness or good coordination until effects of drug are known.
- Tell patient to avoid alcohol while taking drug.
- Notify patient that smoking may decrease drug's effectiveness.
- Warn patient not to stop drug abruptly because withdrawal symptoms may occur.
- Warn woman of childbearing age to avoid use during pregnancy.

oxcarbazepine

Trileptal

Pregnancy risk category C

Indications & dosages

➲ **Adjunctive treatment of partial seizures in patients with epilepsy**
Adults: Initially, 300 mg P.O. b.i.d. Increase by a maximum of 600 mg daily (300 mg P.O. b.i.d.) at weekly intervals. Recommended daily dose is 1,200 mg P.O. divided b.i.d.
Children ages 4 to 16: Initially, 8 to 10 mg/kg daily P.O. divided b.i.d., not to exceed 600 mg daily. The target maintenance dose depends on patient's weight and should be divided b.i.d. If patient weighs between 20 and 29 kg (44 and 64 lb), target maintenance dose is 900 mg daily. If patient weighs between 29 and 39 kg (64 and 86 lb), target maintenance dose is 1,200 mg daily. If patient weighs more than 39 kg (86 lb), target maintenance dose is 1,800 mg daily. Target doses should be achieved over 2 weeks.
➲ **To change from multidrug to single-drug treatment of partial seizures in patients with epilepsy**
Adults: Initially, 300 mg P.O. b.i.d., while reducing dose of concomitant anticonvulsant. Increase oxcarbazepine by a maximum of 600 mg daily at weekly intervals over 2 to 4 weeks. Recommended daily dose is 2,400 mg P.O. divided b.i.d. Withdraw other anticonvulsant completely over 3 to 6 weeks.
Children ages 4 to 16: Initially, 8 to 10 mg/kg daily P.O. divided b.i.d., while reducing dose of concomitant anticonvulsant. Increase oxcarbazepine by a maximum of 10 mg/kg daily at weekly intervals. Withdraw other

anticonvulsant completely over 3 to 6 weeks.

➲ **To start single-drug treatment of partial seizures in patients with epilepsy**

Adults: Initially, 300 mg P.O. b.i.d. Increase dosage by 300 mg daily q third day to a daily dose of 1,200 mg divided b.i.d.

Children ages 4 to 16: Initially, 8 to 10 mg/kg daily P.O. divided b.i.d., increasing the dosage by 5 mg/kg daily q third day to the recommended daily dose range shown in the table.

Weight (kg)	Dose (mg/day)
20	600–900
25	900–1,200
30	900–1,200
35	900–1,500
40	900–1,500
45	1,200–1,500
50	1,200–1,800
55	1,200–1,800
60	1,200–2,100
65	1,200–2,100
70	1,500–2,100

If creatinine clearance is less than 30 ml/minute, start therapy at 150 mg P.O. b.i.d. (one-half usual starting dose) and increase slowly to achieve desired response.

Contraindications & cautions

- Contraindicated in patients hypersensitive to drug or its components.

Adverse reactions

CNS: *fatigue*, asthenia, fever, feeling abnormal, *headache*, *dizziness*, *somnolence*, *ataxia*, *abnormal gait*, insomnia, *tremor*, nervousness, agitation, abnormal coordination, speech disorder, confusion, anxiety, amnesia, ***aggravated seizures***, hypesthesia, emotional lability, impaired concentration, *vertigo*.

CV: hypotension, edema, chest pain.

EENT: *nystagmus*, *diplopia*, *abnormal vision*, abnormal accommodation, rhinitis, sinusitis, pharyngitis, epistaxis, ear pain.

GI: *nausea*, *vomiting*, *abdominal pain*, diarrhea, dyspepsia, constipation, gastritis, anorexia, dry mouth, ***rectal hemorrhage***, taste perversion, thirst.

GU: UTI, urinary frequency, vaginitis.

Metabolic: hyponatremia, weight increase.

Musculoskeletal: muscular weakness, back pain.

Respiratory: *upper respiratory tract infection*, coughing, bronchitis, chest infection.

Skin: acne, hot flushes, purpura, rash, bruising, increased sweating.

Other: toothache, allergic reaction, lymphadenopathy, infection.

Interactions

Drug-drug. *Carbamazepine, valproic acid, verapamil:* May decrease level of active metabolite of oxcarbazepine. Monitor patient and level closely.

Felodipine: May decrease felodipine level. Monitor patient closely.

Hormonal contraceptives: May decrease levels of ethinyl estradiol and levonorgestrel, reducing hormonal contraceptive effectiveness. Caution women of childbearing age to use alternative forms of contraception.

Phenobarbital: May decrease level of active metabolite of oxcarbazepine; may increase phenobarbital level. Monitor patient closely.

Phenytoin: May decrease level of active metabolite of oxcarbazepine; may increase phenytoin level in adults receiving high doses of oxcarbazepine. Monitor phenytoin level closely when starting therapy in these patients.

Drug-lifestyle. *Alcohol use:* May increase CNS depression. Discourage use together.

Nursing considerations

!!ALERT Between 25% and 30% of patients with history of hypersensitivity reaction to carbamazepine may develop hypersensitivities to oxcarbazepine. Ask patient about carbamazepine hypersensitivity and stop drug immediately if signs or symptoms of hypersensitivity occur.

- Shake oral suspension well. Suspension can be mixed with water or swallowed directly from syringe.
- Oral suspension and tablets may be interchanged at equal doses.

!!ALERT Withdraw drug gradually to minimize potential for increased seizure frequency.

- Watch for signs and symptoms of hyponatremia, including nausea, malaise, headache, lethargy, confusion, and decreased sensation.

• Monitor sodium level in patients receiving oxcarbazepine for maintenance treatment, especially patients receiving other therapies that may decrease sodium levels.
• Oxcarbazepine use has been linked to several nervous system–related adverse reactions, including psychomotor slowing, difficulty with concentration, speech or language problems, somnolence, fatigue, and coordination abnormalities, such as ataxia and gait disturbances.

Patient teaching

• Drug may be taken with or without food.
• Tell patient to contact prescriber before interrupting or stopping drug.
• Advise patient to report signs and symptoms of low sodium in the blood, such as nausea, malaise, headache, lethargy, and confusion.
!!ALERT Multiorgan hypersensitivity reactions may occur. Tell patient to report fever and swollen lymph nodes to his prescriber.
!!ALERT Serious skin reactions, including Stevens-Johnson syndrome and toxic epidermal necrosis, can occur. Advise patient to immediately report skin rashes to his prescriber.
• Caution patient to avoid driving and other potentially hazardous activities that require mental alertness until effects of drug are known.
• Instruct woman using oral contraceptives to use alternative form of contraception while taking drug.
• Tell patient to avoid alcohol while taking drug.
• Advise patient to inform prescriber if he has ever experienced hypersensitivity reaction to carbamazepine.

oxybutynin chloride

Ditropan, Ditropan XL, Oxytrol

Pregnancy risk category B

Indications & dosages

➲ Uninhibited or reflex neurogenic bladder
Adults: 5 mg P.O. b.i.d. to t.i.d., to maximum of 5 mg q.i.d.
Children age 5 and older: 5 mg P.O. b.i.d., to maximum of 5 mg t.i.d.

➲ Overactive bladder
Adults: Initially, 5 mg P.O. Ditropan XL once daily. Dosage adjustments may be made weekly in 5-mg increments, p.r.n., to maximum of 30 mg P.O. daily. Or, apply one patch twice weekly to dry, intact skin on the abdomen, hip, or buttock.

Contraindications & cautions

• Contraindicated in patients hypersensitive to drug or its components and in those with myasthenia gravis, GI obstruction, untreated angle-closure glaucoma, megacolon, adynamic ileus, severe colitis, ulcerative colitis with megacolon, urine or gastric retention, or obstructive uropathy.
• Contraindicated in elderly or debilitated patients with intestinal atony and in hemorrhaging patients with unstable CV status.
• Use cautiously in elderly, pregnant, or breast-feeding patients and in those with autonomic neuropathy, reflux esophagitis, or hepatic or renal disease.
• Use extended-release form cautiously in patients with bladder outflow obstruction, gastric obstruction, ulcerative colitis, intestinal atony, myasthenia gravis, or gastroesophageal reflux and in those taking drugs that worsen esophagitis (bisphosphonates).

Adverse reactions

CNS: dizziness, insomnia, restlessness, hallucinations, asthenia, fever.
CV: *palpitations, tachycardia,* vasodilation.
EENT: mydriasis, cycloplegia, decreased lacrimation, amblyopia.
GI: nausea, vomiting, *dry mouth, constipation,* decreased GI motility.
GU: impotence, *urinary hesitancy, urine retention.*
Skin: rash, decreased diaphoresis.
Other: suppression of lactation.
Transdermal patch
CNS: fatigue, somnolence, headache.
CV: flushing.
EENT: abnormal vision.
GI: *dry mouth,* diarrhea, abdominal pain, nausea, flatulence.
GU: dysuria.
Musculoskeletal: back pain.
Skin: *pruritus,* erythema, vesicles, macules, rash, burning at injection site.

Interactions

Drug-drug. *Anticholinergics:* May increase anticholinergic effects. Use together cautiously.
Atenolol, digoxin: May increase levels of these drugs. Monitor drug levels closely.
CNS depressants: May increase CNS effects. Use together cautiously.
Haloperidol: May decrease haloperidol level. Monitor drug level closely.
Drug-lifestyle. *Alcohol use:* May increase CNS effects. Discourage use together.
Exercise, hot weather: May cause heatstroke. Advise patient to use with caution in hot weather.

Nursing considerations

- Before giving drug, get confirmation of neurogenic bladder by cystometry and rule out partial intestinal obstruction in patients with diarrhea, especially those with colostomy or ileostomy.
- If patient has UTI, treat him with antibiotics.
- Drug may aggravate symptoms of hyperthyroidism, coronary artery disease, heart failure, arrhythmias, tachycardia, hypertension, or prostatic hyperplasia.
- Obtain periodic cystometry as directed to evaluate response to therapy.

!!ALERT Don't confuse Ditropan with diazepam or Dithranol.

Patient teaching

- Warn patient to avoid hazardous activities, such as operating machinery or driving, until CNS effects of drug are known.
- Caution patient that using drug during very hot weather may cause fever or heatstroke because it suppresses sweating.
- Tell patient to swallow Ditropan XL whole and not to chew or crush it.
- Instruct patient to measure syrup with a teaspoon.
- Advise patient to store drug in tightly closed container at 59° to 86° F (15° to 30° C).
- Instruct patient using transdermal patch to change patch twice a week and to choose a new application site with each new patch to avoid the same site within 7 days. Warn patient to only wear one patch at a time. Tell patient to dispose of old patches carefully in the trash in a manner that prevents accidental application or ingestion by children, pets, and others.
- Advise patient to avoid alcohol while taking drug.
- Tell patient that drug may cause dry mouth.

oxycodone hydrochloride

Endocodone, OxyContin, Oxydose, OxyIR, Roxicodone, Roxicodone Intensol, Supeudol†

oxycodone pectinate

Pregnancy risk category B
Controlled substance schedule II

Indications & dosages

➲ Moderate to severe pain
Adults: 5 mg P.O. q 6 hours. Or, one suppository P.R. three to four times daily, p.r.n. Patients not currently receiving opiates, who need a continuous, around-the-clock analgesic for an extended period of time, give 10 mg controlled-release tablets P.O. q 12 hours. May increase dose q 1 to 2 days p.r.n. The 80-mg formulation is for opioid-tolerant patients only.

Contraindications & cautions

- Contraindicated in patients hypersensitive to drug.
- Contraindicated in those suspected of having paralytic ileus.
- Use with caution in elderly and debilitated patients and in those with head injury, increased intracranial pressure, seizures, asthma, COPD, prostatic hyperplasia, severe hepatic or renal disease, acute abdominal conditions, urethral stricture, hypothyroidism, Addison's disease, and arrhythmias.

Adverse reactions

CNS: sedation, somnolence, clouded sensorium, euphoria, dizziness, light-headedness, physical dependence.
CV: hypotension, ***bradycardia***.
GI: *nausea, vomiting*, constipation, ileus.
GU: urine retention.
Respiratory: ***respiratory depression***.
Skin: diaphoresis, pruritus.

Interactions

Drug-drug. *Anticoagulants:* Oxycodone hydrochloride products containing aspirin may increase anticoagulant effect. Monitor clotting times. Use together cautiously.
CNS depressants, general anesthetics, hypnotics, MAO inhibitors, other opioid analgesics, sedatives, tranquilizers, tricyclic antidepressants: May cause additive effects. Use together with caution. Reduce oxycodone dose and monitor patient response.
Drug-lifestyle. *Alcohol use:* May cause additive effects. Discourage use together.

Nursing considerations

- Reassess patient's level of pain at least 15 and 30 minutes after administration.
- For full analgesic effect, give drug before patient has intense pain.
- To minimize GI upset, give drug after meals or with milk.
- Single-drug oxycodone solution or tablets are especially useful for patients who shouldn't take aspirin or acetaminophen.
- Monitor circulatory and respiratory status. Withhold dose and notify prescriber if respirations are shallow or if respiratory rate falls below 12 breaths/minute.
- Monitor patient's bladder and bowel patterns. Patient may need a laxative because drug has a constipating effect.
- Reserve the 80-mg controlled-release tablets for opioid-tolerant patients who are taking daily doses of 160 mg or more.
- Patients taking around-the-clock controlled-release formulations may need to have immediate-release medication available for pain exacerbation or to prevent incident pain.
- For patients who are taking more than 60 mg daily, stop dosing gradually to prevent withdrawal symptoms.
- OxyContin isn't intended for as-needed use or for immediate postoperative pain. Drug is indicated only for postoperative use if patient was receiving it before surgery or if pain is expected to persist for an extended time.

!!ALERT OxyContin is potentially addictive and abused as much as morphine. Chewing, crushing, snorting, or injecting it can lead to overdose and death.

Patient teaching

- Instruct patient to take drug before pain is intense.
- Tell patient to take drug with milk or after eating.
- Tell patient to swallow extended-release tablets whole.
- Caution ambulatory patient about getting out of bed or walking. Warn outpatient to avoid driving and other hazardous activities that require mental alertness until drug's CNS effects are known.
- Advise patient to avoid alcohol use during therapy.
- Tell patient not to stop drug abruptly.

oxymorphone hydrochloride

Numorphan

Pregnancy risk category C; D if used for prolonged periods or high doses at term
Controlled substance schedule II

Indications & dosages

➲ Moderate to severe pain
Adults: 1 to 1.5 mg I.M. or S.C. q 4 to 6 hours, p.r.n. Or, 0.5 mg I.V. q 4 to 6 hours, p.r.n. Or, 5 mg P.R. q 4 to 6 hours, p.r.n.
➲ Analgesia during labor
Adults: 0.5 to 1 mg I.M.

Contraindications & cautions

- Contraindicated in patients hypersensitive to drug and in those with acute asthma attacks, severe respiratory depression, upper airway obstruction, or paralytic ileus.
- Contraindicated for use in treating pulmonary edema caused by a respiratory irritant.
- Use with caution in elderly or debilitated patients and in those with head injury, increased intracranial pressure, seizures, asthma, COPD, acute abdominal conditions, prostatic hyperplasia, severe hepatic or renal disease, urethral stricture, respiratory depression, hypothyroidism, Addison's disease, and arrhythmias.

Adverse reactions

CNS: *sedation, somnolence, clouded sensorium, euphoria,* dysphoria, dizziness, ***seizures,*** physical dependence, lightheadedness, headache, hallucinations, restlessness.

CV: *hypotension*, ***bradycardia***.
EENT: miosis, diplopia, blurred vision.
GI: *nausea, vomiting, constipation*, ileus.
GU: *urine retention*.
Respiratory: ***respiratory depression***.
Skin: pruritus.

Interactions

Drug-drug. *Anticholinergics:* May increase risk of urinary retention or severe constipation, leading to paralytic ileus. Monitor patient for abdominal pain or distention.
CNS depressants, general anesthetics, MAO inhibitors, phenothiazines, sedative hypnotics, tricyclic antidepressants: May cause additive effects. Use together with caution.
Drug-lifestyle. *Alcohol use:* May cause additive effects. Discourage use together.

Nursing considerations

- Keep opioid antagonist (naloxone) and resuscitation equipment available.
- Use of this drug may worsen gallbladder pain.
- Drug isn't for mild pain. For better effect, give drug before patient has intense pain.
- Monitor CV and respiratory status. Withhold dose and notify prescriber if respirations decrease or rate is below 12 breaths/minute.
- Monitor bladder and bowel function. Patient may need a laxative.

!!ALERT Don't confuse oxymorphone with oxymetholone or oxycodone, and don't confuse Numorphan with nalbuphine.

Patient teaching

- Instruct patient to ask for drug before pain is intense.
- When drug is used after surgery, encourage patient to turn, cough, and deep-breathe and to use incentive spirometer to avoid lung problems.
- Caution ambulatory patient about getting out of bed or walking. Warn outpatient to avoid driving and other hazardous activities that require mental alertness until drug's CNS effects are known.
- Instruct patient to store suppositories in refrigerator.
- Advise patient to avoid alcohol during therapy.

oxytocin, synthetic injection
Pitocin

Pregnancy risk category NR

Indications & dosages

➲ To induce or stimulate labor
Adults: Initially, 10 units in 1,000 ml of D_5W injection, lactated Ringer's, or normal saline solution I.V. infused at 1 to 2 milliunits/minute. Increase rate by 1 to 2 milliunits/minute at 15- to 30-minute intervals until normal contraction pattern is established. Decrease rate when labor is firmly established. Maximum dose is 20 milliunits/minute.
➲ To reduce postpartum bleeding after expulsion of placenta
Adults: 10 to 40 units in 1,000 ml of D_5W injection, lactated Ringer's, or normal saline solution I.V. infused at rate needed to control bleeding, which is usually 20 to 40 milliunits/minute. Also, 10 units may be given I.M. after delivery of placenta.
➲ Incomplete or inevitable abortion
Adults: 10 units I.V. in 500 ml of normal saline solution, lactated Ringer's, or dextrose 5% in normal saline solution. Infuse at 10 to 20 milliunits (20 to 40 drops)/minute.

Contraindications & cautions

- Contraindicated in patients hypersensitive to drug.
- Contraindicated when vaginal delivery isn't advised (placenta previa, vasa previa, invasive cervical carcinoma, genital herpes), when cephalopelvic disproportion is present, or when delivery requires conversion, as in transverse lie.
- Contraindicated in fetal distress when delivery isn't imminent, in prematurity, in other obstetric emergencies, and in patients with severe toxemia or hypertonic uterine patterns.
- Use cautiously during first and second stages of labor because cervical laceration, uterine rupture, and maternal and fetal death have been reported.
- Use cautiously, if at all, in patients with invasive cervical cancer and in those with previous cervical or uterine surgery (including cesarean section), grand multiparity, uterine sepsis, traumatic delivery, or overdistended uterus.

Adverse reactions

Maternal

CNS: ***subarachnoid hemorrhage, seizures, coma.***

CV: hypertension, increased heart rate, systemic venous return, and cardiac output, ***arrhythmias.***

GI: nausea, vomiting.

GU: tetanic uterine contractions, ***abruptio placentae,*** impaired uterine blood flow, pelvic hematoma, increased uterine motility, ***uterine rupture, postpartum hemorrhage.***

Hematologic: ***afibrinogenemia possibly related to postpartum bleeding.***

Other: hypersensitivity reactions, ***anaphylaxis, death from oxytocin-induced water intoxication.***

Fetal

CNS: ***infant brain damage.***

CV: ***bradycardia,*** PVCs, ***arrhythmias.***

EENT: neonatal retinal hemorrhage.

Hepatic: neonatal jaundice.

Respiratory: ***anoxia, asphyxia.***

Other: ***low Apgar scores at 5 minutes.***

Interactions

Drug-drug. *Cyclopropane anesthetics:* May cause less pronounced bradycardia and hypotension. Use together cautiously.

Thiopental anesthetics: May delay induction. Use together cautiously.

Vasoconstrictors: May cause severe hypertension if oxytocin is given within 3 to 4 hours of vasoconstrictor in patient receiving caudal block anesthetic. Avoid using together.

Nursing considerations

- Drug isn't recommended for routine I.M. use, but 10 units may be given I.M. after delivery of placenta to control postpartum uterine bleeding.
- Never give oxytocin simultaneously by more than one route.
- Drug is used to induce or reinforce labor only when pelvis is known to be adequate, when vaginal delivery is indicated, when fetal maturity is assured, and when fetal position is favorable. Use drug only in hospital where critical care facilities and prescriber are immediately available.
- Monitor fluid intake and output. Antidiuretic effect may lead to fluid overload, seizures, and coma from water intoxication.
- Monitor and record uterine contractions, heart rate, blood pressure, intrauterine pressure, fetal heart rate, and character of blood loss every 15 minutes.
- Have 20% magnesium sulfate solution available to relax the myometrium.
- If contractions occur less than 2 minutes apart, exceed 50 mm, or last 90 seconds or longer, stop infusion, turn patient on her side, and notify prescriber.
- Drug doesn't cause fetal abnormalities when used as indicated.

!!ALERT Don't confuse Pitocin with Pitressin.

Patient teaching

- Explain use and administration of drug to patient and family.
- Instruct patient to report adverse reactions promptly.

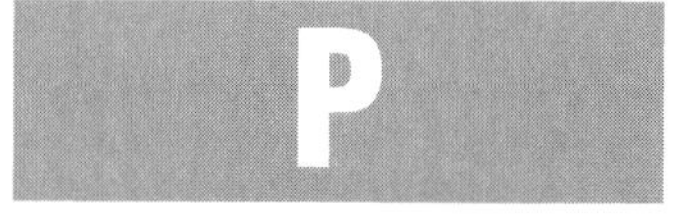

paclitaxel
Onxol, Taxol

Pregnancy risk category D

Indications & dosages

➲ Second-line treatment of AIDS related Kaposi's sarcoma (Taxol)

Adults: 135 mg/m² I.V. over 3 hours q 3 weeks, or 100 mg/m² I.V. over 3 hours q 2 weeks.

Don't give drug if baseline or subsequent neutrophil counts are less than 1,000 cells/mm³. Reduce subsequent doses of Taxol by 20% for patients who experience severe neutropenia (neutrophil count 500 cells/mm³ for 1 week or longer). Patient also may need reduction in dexamethasone premedication dose (10 mg P.O. instead of 20 mg P.O.) and start of a hematopoietic growth factor.

➲ First-line and subsequent therapy for advanced ovarian cancer

Adults (previously untreated): 175 mg/m² over 3 hours q 3 weeks, followed by cisplatin 75 mg/m²; or, 135 mg/m² over 24 hours, followed by cisplatin 75 mg/m², q 3 weeks.

Adults (previously treated): 135 or 175 mg/m^2 I.V. over 3 hours q 3 weeks.

➲ **Breast cancer after failure of combination chemotherapy for metastatic disease or relapse within 6 months of adjuvant chemotherapy (previous therapy should have included an anthracycline unless contraindicated); adjuvant therapy for node-positive breast cancer given sequentially to standard doxorubicin-containing combination chemotherapy**

Adults: 175 mg/m^2 I.V. over 3 hours q 3 weeks.

➲ **First treatment of advanced non–small-cell lung cancer for patients who aren't candidates for curative surgery or radiation (Taxol)**

Adults: 135 mg/m^2 I.V. infusion over 24 hours, followed by cisplatin 75 mg/m^2. Repeat cycle q 3 weeks.

Subsequent courses shouldn't be repeated until neutrophil count is at least 1,500 cells/mm^3 and platelet count is at least 100,000 cells/mm^3. Reduce subsequent doses of Taxol by 20% for patients who experience severe neutropenia (neutrophil less than 500 cells/mm^3 for a week or longer) or severe peripheral neuropathy. For patients with hepatic impairment, adjust doses for the first courses of therapy as follows: For 24-hour infusion of Taxol if transaminase levels are $< 2 \times$ ULN and bilirubin levels are ≤ 1.5 mg/dl, give 135 mg/m^2. If transaminase levels are 2 to $< 10 \times$ ULN and bilirubin levels are ≤ 1.5 mg/dl, give 100 mg/m^2. If transaminase levels are $< 10 \times$ ULN and bilirubin levels are 1.6 to 7.5 mg/dl, give 50 mg/m^2. If transaminase levels are $\geq 10 \times$ ULN or bilirubin levels are > 7.5 mg/dl, don't use drug. For 3-hour infusion of Taxol, if transaminase levels are $< 10 \times$ ULN and bilirubin levels are $\leq 1.25 \times$ ULN, give 175 mg/m^2. If transaminase levels are $< 10 \times$ ULN and bilirubin levels are 1.26 to $2 \times$ ULN, give 135 mg/m^2. If transaminase levels are $< 10 \times$ ULN and bilirubin levels are 2.01 to $5 \times$ ULN, give 90 mg/m^2. If transaminase levels are $\geq 10 \times$ ULN or bilirubin levels are $> 5 \times$ ULN, don't use drug. For subsequent courses, base dosage adjustment on individual tolerance.

Contraindications & cautions

- Contraindicated in patients hypersensitive to drug or polyoxyethylated castor oil (a vehicle used in drug solution) and in those with baseline neutrophil counts below 1,500/mm^3 and platelet counts below 100,000 cells/mm^3, or AIDS-related Kaposi's sarcoma with baseline neutrophil counts below 1,000/mm^3.
- Use cautiously in patients with hepatic impairment.

Adverse reactions

CNS: *peripheral neuropathy, asthenia.*
CV: ***bradycardia****, hypotension, abnormal ECG.*
GI: *nausea, vomiting, diarrhea, mucositis.*
Hematologic: NEUTROPENIA, LEUKOPENIA, THROMBOCYTOPENIA, *anemia, bleeding.*
Musculoskeletal: *myalgia, arthralgia.*
Skin: *alopecia, cellulitis and phlebitis at injection site.*
Other: hypersensitivity reactions, ***anaphylaxis***, *infections.*

Interactions

Drug-drug. *Carbamazepine, phenobarbital:* May increase metabolism and may decrease paclitaxel levels. Use together cautiously.
Cisplatin: May cause additive myelosuppressive effects. Give paclitaxel before cisplatin.
Doxorubicin: May increase plasma levels of doxorubicin and its active metabolite, doxorubicinol. Use together cautiously.
Drugs that inhibit cytochrome P-450, such as cyclosporine, dexamethasone, diazepam, etoposide, ketoconazole, quinidine, retinoic acid, teniposide, testosterone, verapamil, vincristine: May increase paclitaxel level. Monitor patient for toxicity.

Nursing considerations

- Some patients experience peripheral neuropathies, which may be cumulative and dose-related. Patients with severe symptoms may need dosage reduction.
- To reduce risk or severity of hypersensitivity, patients must receive pretreatment with corticosteroids, such as dexamethasone, and antihistamines. Both H_1-receptor antagonists, such as diphenhydramine, and H_2-receptor antagonists, such as cimetidine or ranitidine, may be used. Severe hypersensitivity reactions have occurred in as many as 2% of patients.

- Monitor blood counts often during therapy. Bone marrow toxicity is most common and dose-limiting toxicity. Packed RBC or platelet transfusions may be needed in severe cases. Institute bleeding precautions as appropriate.
- Patient may receive injections of RBC colony–stimulating factors to promote RBC production and decrease need for blood transfusions.
- Avoid all I.M. injections when platelet count is below 50,000/mm³.
- If patient develops significant cardiac conduction abnormalities, use appropriate therapy and continuous cardiac monitoring during therapy and subsequent infusions.

!!ALERT Don't confuse paclitaxel with paroxetine; don't confuse Taxol with Paxil or Taxotere.

Patient teaching

- Advise patient to report any pain or burning at site of injection during or after administration.
- Urge patient to watch for fever, sore throat, and fatigue and for easy bruising, nosebleeds, bleeding gums, or tarry stools. Tell patient to take temperature daily.
- Teach patient symptoms of peripheral neuropathy, such as a tingling or burning sensation or numbness in limbs, and advise her to report these symptoms immediately.
- Warn patient that reversible hair loss is common (up to 82% of patients).
- Caution woman of childbearing age to avoid becoming pregnant during therapy. Recommend that she consult prescriber before becoming pregnant.

paclitaxel protein-bound particles
Abraxane

Pregnancy risk category D

Indications & dosages

➲ **Metastatic breast cancer after failure of combination chemotherapy or relapse within 6 months of adjuvant chemotherapy (previous therapy should have included an anthracycline unless clinically contraindicated at the time)**
Adults: 260 mg/m² I.V. over 30 minutes q 3 weeks.

For patients with severe sensory neuropathy or a neutrophil count less than 500/mm³ for a week or longer, reduce dose to 220 mg/m². For recurring severe sensory neuropathy or severe neutropenia, reduce dose to 180 mg/m². For grade 3 (severe) sensory neuropathy, stop drug until condition improves to a grade 1 or 2 (mild to moderate); then restart at a reduced dose for the rest of treatment.

Contraindications & cautions

- Contraindicated in patients with baseline neutrophil counts of under 1,500/mm³.
- Avoid using in patients with baseline neutrophil counts under 1,500/mm³.
- In patients with creatinine level over 2 mg/dl or bilirubin level over 1.5 mg/dl, use hasn't been studied.

Adverse reactions

CNS: *asthenia, sensory neuropathy.*
CV: *abnormal ECG,* ***cardiac arrest, chest pain,*** *edema,* hypertension, hypotension, ***supraventricular tachycardia, thromboembolism, thrombosis.***
EENT: *visual disturbances.*
GI: *diarrhea,* ***intestinal obstruction, ischemic colitis,*** mucositis, *nausea, oral candidiasis,* ***pancreatitis, perforation,*** *vomiting.*
Hematologic: *anemia,* bleeding, **NEUTROPENIA,** ***thrombocytopenia.***
Hepatic: ***hepatic encephalopathy, hepatic necrosis.***
Musculoskeletal: *arthralgia, myalgia.*
Respiratory: ***PE,*** *cough, dyspnea, pneumonia, respiratory tract infection.*
Skin: *alopecia,* injection site reactions.
Other: hypersensitivity reactions, *infections.*

Interactions

Drug-drug. *CYP-450 inhibitors:* May decrease Abraxane metabolism. Use together cautiously.

Nursing considerations

- Give only under supervision of practitioner experienced in using chemotherapy in facility that can manage complications of therapy.

!!ALERT Don't substitute Abraxane for other forms of paclitaxel.

- Because drug contains human albumin, a remote risk exists of transmitting viruses and Creutzfeldt-Jakob disease.

- Assess patient for symptoms of sensory neuropathy and severe neutropenia.
- Monitor liver and kidney function test results.
- Monitor infusion site closely.

Patient teaching

- Warn patient that alopecia commonly occurs but that it's reversible after therapy.
- Teach patient to recognize signs of neuropathy, such as tingling, burning, and numbness in arms and legs.
- Tell patient to report fever or other signs of infection, severe abdominal pain, or severe diarrhea.
- Advise patient to contact prescriber if nausea and vomiting persist or interfere with adequate nutrition. Reassure patient that a drug can be prescribed that may help.
- Explain that many patients experience weakness and fatigue, so it's important to rest. Tiredness, paleness, and shortness of breath may result from low blood counts, and patient may need a transfusion.
- To reduce or prevent mouth sores, remind patient to perform proper oral hygiene.
- Tell women of childbearing age to avoid becoming pregnant or breast-feeding.
- Advise men to avoid fathering children while taking this drug.

palifermin
Kepivance

Pregnancy risk category C

Indications & dosages

➲ **To decrease frequency and duration of severe oral mucositis in patients with hematologic malignancies who are receiving myelotoxic chemotherapy requiring hematopoietic stem cell support**

Adults: 60 mcg/kg/day by I.V. bolus for 3 consecutive days before myelotoxic chemotherapy, with the third dose 24 to 48 hours before myelotoxic chemotherapy starts. Repeat dose for 3 consecutive days after myelotoxic chemotherapy ends, for a total of six doses. Give first dose after myelotoxic therapy endson the same day as, but after, hematopoietic stem cell infusion and at least 4 days after the most recent palifermin dose.

Contraindications & cautions

- Contraindicated in patients hypersensitive to ***Escherichia coli***-derived proteins or to drug or any of its components.
- Use cautiously in patients with nonhematologic malignancies.

Adverse reactions

CNS: *dysesthesia, fever, hyperesthesia, hypoesthesia, pain, paresthesia.*
CV: *edema,* hypertension.
GI: *mouth or tongue thickness or discoloration, taste alteration.*
Musculoskeletal: *arthralgia.*
Skin: *erythema, pruritus, rash.*

Interactions

Drug-drug. *Heparin:* May bind to palifermin and alter dose. Flush I.V. line with normal saline solution before and after giving palifermin.
Myelotoxic chemotherapy: May increase severity and duration of oral mucositis. Don't give palifermin within 24 hours of chemotherapy.

Nursing considerations

!!ALERT To avoid increasing severity and duration of oral mucositis, don't give palifermin within 24 hours of myelotoxic chemotherapy.
- Monitor patient for fever, arthralgia, and adverse mucocutaneous effects.
- Skin-related toxicities are most likely to occur 6 days after the first three consecutive doses.
- Drug may enhance growth of tumor cells.

Patient teaching

- Tell patient to report to prescriber rash, reddening, swelling, or itching of skin; unpleasant sensation around the mouth; tongue discoloration or thickening; altered taste; fever; and joint pain.
- Explain that drug may stimulate growth of other types of cancer cells.
- Urge patient to keep all scheduled appointments for treatment.

palivizumab
Synagis

Pregnancy risk category C

Indications & dosages
➲ **To prevent serious lower respiratory tract disease caused by respiratory syncytial virus (RSV) in children at high risk**
Children: 15 mg/kg I.M. monthly throughout RSV season (November to April in the northern hemisphere). Give first dose before start of RSV season.

Contraindications & cautions
- Contraindicated in children hypersensitive to drug or its components.
- Use cautiously in patients with thrombocytopenia or other coagulation disorders.

Adverse reactions
CNS: nervousness, pain.
EENT: *otitis media, rhinitis,* pharyngitis, sinusitis, conjunctivitis.
GI: diarrhea, vomiting, gastroenteritis, oral candidiasis.
Hematologic: anemia.
Respiratory: *upper respiratory tract infection,* cough, wheeze, bronchiolitis, ***apnea,*** pneumonia, bronchitis, asthma, croup, dyspnea.
Skin: *rash,* fungal dermatitis, eczema, seborrhea.
Other: hernia, ***failure to thrive,*** injection site reaction, viral infection, flu syndrome.

Interactions
None significant.

Nursing considerations
- Patients should receive monthly doses throughout RSV season, even if RSV infection develops. In the northern hemisphere, RSV season typically lasts from November to April.
- To reconstitute, slowly add 1 ml of sterile water for injection into a 100-mg vial or 0.6 ml of sterile water for injection into a 50-mg vial. Gently swirl the vial for 30 seconds to avoid foaming. Don't shake vial. Let reconstituted solution stand at room temperature for 20 minutes until the solution clears. Give within 6 hours of reconstitution.
- Give drug into anterolateral aspect of thigh. Don't use gluteal muscle routinely as an injection site because of risk of damage to sciatic nerve. Give injection volumes over 1 ml as a divided dose.

!! ALERT Rarely, patient may have an anaphylactoid reaction after using this drug. If anaphylaxis or severe allergic reaction occurs, give epinephrine (1:1,000), and provide supportive care as needed. If reaction is mild, use caution when giving again; if severe, stop therapy.

Patient teaching
- Explain to parent or caregiver that drug is used to prevent RSV and not to treat it.
- Advise parent that monthly injections are recommended throughout RSV season (November to April in the northern hemisphere).
- Tell parent to immediately report adverse reactions or any unusual bruising, bleeding, or weakness.

palonosetron hydrochloride
Aloxi

Pregnancy risk category B

Indications & dosages
➲ **To prevent acute nausea and vomiting from moderately or highly emetogenic chemotherapy or delayed nausea and vomiting from moderately emetogenic chemotherapy**
Adults: 0.25 mg given I.V. over 30 seconds, 30 minutes before chemotherapy starts. Drug is given on the first day of each cycle, no more than q 7 days.

Contraindications & cautions
- Contraindicated in patents hypersensitive to palonosetron or its ingredients.
- Use cautiously in patients hypersensitive to other 5-HT_3 antagonists, in those taking drugs that affect cardiac conduction, and in those with cardiac conduction abnormalities, hypokalemia, or hypomagnesemia.
- Safety and efficacy in children haven't been established.

Adverse reactions
CNS: anxiety, dizziness, headache, weakness.

CV: ***bradycardia***, hypotension, ***nonsustained ventricular tachycardia***.
GI: constipation, diarrhea.
Metabolic: *hyperkalemia*.

Interactions

Drug-drug. *Antiarrhythmics or other drugs that prolong the QTc interval, diuretics that induce electrolyte abnormalities, high-dose anthracycline:* May increase risk of prolonged QTc interval. Use together cautiously.

Nursing considerations

- Before giving this drug, check patient's potassium level.
- Consider adding corticosteroids to the antiemetic regimen, particularly for patients receiving highly emetogenic chemotherapy.
- Make sure patient has additional antiemetics to take for breakthrough nausea or vomiting.
- If patient has cardiac conduction abnormalities, check the ECG before giving drug.

Patient teaching

- Advise patient to take a different antiemetic for breakthrough nausea or vomiting.
- Instruct patient to take the breakthrough antiemetic at the first sign of nausea rather than waiting until symptoms are severe.
- Urge patient with a history of cardiac conduction abnormalities to report any changes in medication regimen (such as adding or stopping an antiarrhythmic).

pamidronate disodium
Aredia

Pregnancy risk category D

Indications & dosages

➲ **Moderate to severe hypercalcemia from cancer (with or without bone metastases)**
Adults: Dosage depends on severity of hypercalcemia. Correct calcium level for albumin. Corrected calcium (CCa) level is calculated using this formula:

CCa (mg/dl) = serum calcium (mg/dl) + 0.8 (4 - serum albumin) (g/dl)

Patients with CCa levels of 12 to 13.5 mg/dl may receive 60 to 90 mg by I.V. infusion as a single dose over 2 to 24 hours. Patients with CCa levels greater than 13.5 mg/dl may receive 90 mg by I.V. infusion over 2 to 24 hours. Allow at least 7 days before retreatment to permit full response to first dose.
➲ **Moderate to severe Paget's disease**
Adults: 30 mg I.V. as a 4-hour infusion on 3 consecutive days for total dose of 90 mg. Repeat cycle, p.r.n.
➲ **Osteolytic bone metastases of breast cancer with standard antineoplastic therapy**
Adults: 90 mg I.V. infusion over 2 hours q 3 to 4 weeks.
➲ **Osteolytic bone lesions of multiple myeloma**
Adults: 90 mg I.V. over 4 hours once monthly.

Contraindications & cautions

- Contraindicated in patients hypersensitive to drug or other bisphosphonates, such as etidronate.
- Use with caution, considering risks versus benefits, in patients with renal impairment.

Adverse reactions

CNS: ***seizures***, *fatigue*, somnolence, syncope, fever.
CV: ***atrial fibrillation***, tachycardia, *hypertension, fluid overload*.
GI: *abdominal pain, anorexia, constipation, nausea, vomiting*, ***GI hemorrhage***.
GU: renal dysfunction, ***renal failure***.
Hematologic: ***leukopenia***, ***thrombocytopenia***, *anemia*.
Metabolic: hypophosphatemia, hypokalemia, hypomagnesemia, hypocalcemia.
Musculoskeletal: osteonecrosis of the jaw.
Skin: *infusion-site reaction, pain at infusion site*.

Interactions

None significant.

Nursing considerations

- Assess hydration status before treatment. Use drug only after patient has been vigorously hydrated with normal saline solution. In patients with mild to moderate hypercalcemia, hydration alone may be sufficient.
- Because drug can cause electrolyte disturbances, carefully monitor electrolyte levels, especially calcium, phosphate, and magnesium. Short-term administration of calcium

may be needed in patients with severe hypocalcemia. Also monitor CBC and differential count, creatinine and hemoglobin levels, and hematocrit.

- Carefully monitor patients with anemia, leukopenia, or thrombocytopenia during first 2 weeks of therapy.
- Monitor patient's temperature. Some patients experience an elevation of 1.8° F (1° C) for 24 to 48 hours after therapy.

!!ALERT Because renal dysfunction may lead to renal failure, single doses of pamidronate shouldn't exceed 90 mg.

- Monitor creatinine level before each treatment.
- In patients treated for bone metastases who have renal dysfunction withhold dose until renal function returns to baseline. Treatment of bone metastases in patients with severe renal impairment isn't recommended. For other indications, determine whether the potential benefit outweighs the potential risk.

!!ALERT Patients should have a dental examination with appropriate preventive dentistry before being treated with bisphosphonates, especially those with risk factors including cancer, chemotherapy or corticosteroid therapy, and poor oral hygiene.

- Use cautiously in breast-feeding women; it's unknown if drug appears in breast milk.

Patient teaching

- Explain use and administration of drug to patient and family.
- Instruct patient to report adverse reactions promptly.
- Advise patient to alert her health care provider if she is pregnant or breast-feeding.

pancreatin

Donnazyme, Kutrase, Ku-Zyme, Pancreatin 4X ◇, Pancreatin 8X ◇

Pregnancy risk category C

Indications & dosages

➲ **Exocrine pancreatic secretion insufficiency; digestive aid in diseases related to deficiency of pancreatic enzymes, such as cystic fibrosis**

Adults and children: Dosage varies with condition treated. Usual first dose is 8,000 to 24,000 units of lipase activity P.O. before or with each meal or snack. Total daily dose also may be given in divided doses q 1 to 2 hours throughout.

Contraindications & cautions

- Contraindicated in patients hypersensitive to drug, pork protein, or pork enzymes and in those with acute pancreatitis or acute worsening of chronic pancreatitis.
- Use with caution in pregnant or breast-feeding women.

Adverse reactions

GI: nausea, diarrhea with high doses.
Skin: perianal irritation.
Other: allergic reactions.

Interactions

Drug-drug. *Antacids:* May negate pancreatin's beneficial effect. Avoid using together. *Oral iron supplement:* May reduce oral iron supplement level. Separate doses.

Nursing considerations

- The different available products aren't interchangeable.
- To avoid indigestion, monitor patient's diet to ensure proper balance of fat, protein, and starch. Dosage varies according to degree of maldigestion and malabsorption, amount of fat in diet, and enzyme activity of individual preparations.
- Fewer bowel movements and improved stool consistency indicate effective therapy.
- Drug isn't effective in GI disorders unrelated to pancreatic enzyme deficiency.
- Enteric coating on some products may reduce available enzyme in upper portion of jejunum.

Patient teaching

- Instruct patient to take drug before or with meals and snacks.
- Tell patient not to crush or chew enteric-coated forms. Capsules containing enteric-coated microspheres may be opened and sprinkled on a small quantity of cool, soft food. Stress importance of swallowing immediately, without chewing, and following with a glass of water or juice.
- Warn patient not to inhale powder form or powder from capsules; it may irritate skin or mucous membranes.
- Tell patient to store drug in airtight container at room temperature.

• Instruct patient not to change brands without consulting prescriber.

pancrelipase

Creon 5, Creon 10, Creon 20, Ku-Zyme HP, Lipram 4500, Lipram-CR5, Lipram-CR10, Lipram-CR20, Lipram-PN10, Lipram-PN16, Lipram-PN20, Lipram-UL12, Lipram-UL18, Lipram-UL20, Pancrease, Pancrease MT4, Pancrease MT10, Pancrease MT 16, Pancrease MT 20, Pancrecarb MS4, Pancrecarb MS8, Panokase, Plaretase 8000, Ultrase MT12, Ultrase, Ultrase MT18, Ultrase MT20, Viokase, Viokase 8, Viokase 16, Viokase Powder, Viokase Tablets

Pregnancy risk category C; B for Pancrease and Pancrease MT

Indications & dosages

➲ **Exocrine pancreatic secretion insufficiency; cystic fibrosis in adults and children; steatorrhea and other disorders of fat metabolism caused by insufficient pancreatic enzymes**

Adults and children older than age 12: Adjust dosage to patient's response. Usual first dosage 4,000 to 48,000 units of lipase with each meal.

Children ages 7 to 12: 4,000 to 12,000 units of lipase activity with each meal or snack. More can be taken, if needed.

Children ages 1 to 6: 4,000 to 8,000 units of lipase with each meal and 4,000 units of lipase with each snack.

Children ages 6 months to 11 months: 2,000 units of lipase with each meal.

Contraindications & cautions

• Contraindicated in patients with severe hypersensitivity to pork and in those with acute pancreatitis or acute worsening of chronic pancreatic diseases.

Adverse reactions

GI: *nausea*, cramping, diarrhea with high doses.

Interactions

Drug-drug. *Antacids:* May destroy enteric coating and enhance degradation of pancrelipase. Avoid using together.

Oral iron supplement: May decrease iron response. Monitor patient for decreased effectiveness.

Nursing considerations

!!ALERT Use drug only for confirmed exocrine pancreatic insufficiency. It isn't effective in GI disorders unrelated to enzyme deficiency.

• Lipase activity is greater than with other pancreatic enzymes.

• For infants, mix powder with applesauce and give with meals. Avoid contact with or inhalation of powder because it may be highly irritating. Older children may take capsules with food.

• Monitor patient's stools. Adequate replacement decreases number of bowel movements and improves stool consistency.

• Minimal USP standards dictate that each milligram of pancrelipase contains 24 units lipase, 100 units protease, and 100 units amylase.

• Dosage varies with degree of maldigestion and malabsorption, amount of fat in diet, and enzyme activity of individual preparations.

• Enteric coating on some products may reduce available enzyme in upper portion of jejunum.

Patient teaching

• Instruct patient to take drug before or with meals and snacks.

• Advise patient not to crush or chew enteric-coated forms. Capsules containing enteric-coated microspheres may be opened and sprinkled on a small quantity of cool, soft food. Stress importance of swallowing immediately, without chewing, and following with glass of water or juice.

• Warn patient not to inhale powder form or powder from capsules; it may irritate skin or mucous membranes.

• Tell patient to store drug in airtight container at room temperature.

• Instruct patient not to change brands without consulting prescriber.

pancuronium bromide

Pregnancy risk category C

Indications & dosages

➲ Adjunct to anesthesia to relax skeletal muscle, facilitate intubation, assist with mechanical ventilation
Adults and children age 1 month and older: Initially, 0.04 to 0.1 mg/kg I.V.; then 0.01 mg/kg q 30 to 60 minutes.
Neonates: Individualized.

Contraindications & cautions

- Contraindicated in patients hypersensitive to bromides, those with tachycardia, and those for whom even a minor increase in heart rate is undesirable.
- Use cautiously in elderly or debilitated patients; in patients with renal, hepatic, or pulmonary impairment; and in those with respiratory depression, myasthenia gravis, myasthenic syndrome related to lung cancer, dehydration, thyroid disorders, CV disease, collagen diseases, porphyria, electrolyte disturbances, hyperthermia, and toxemic states. Also, use large doses cautiously in patients undergoing cesarean section.

Adverse reactions

CV: tachycardia, increased blood pressure.
EENT: excessive salivation.
Musculoskeletal: residual muscle weakness.
Respiratory: ***prolonged respiratory insufficiency or apnea.***
Skin: transient rashes.
Other: ***allergic or idiosyncratic hypersensitivity reactions.***

Interactions

Drug-drug. *Aminoglycosides (amikacin, gentamicin, neomycin, streptomycin, tobramycin):* May increase the effects of nondepolarizing muscle relaxant, including prolonged respiratory depression. Use together only when necessary. Dose of nondepolarizing muscle relaxant may need to be reduced.
Azathioprine: May reverse neuromuscular blockade induced by pancuronium. Monitor patient.
Beta blockers, clindamycin, general anesthetics (such as enflurane, halothane, isoflurane), lincomycin, magnesium sulfate, polymyxin antibiotics (colistin, polymyxin B sulfate), quinidine, quinine: May enhance neuromuscular blockade, increasing skeletal muscle relaxation and prolonging effect of pancuronium. Use together cautiously during and after surgery.
Carbamazepine, phenytoin: May decrease effects of pancuronium. May need to increase pancuronium dose.
Lithium, opioid analgesics: May enhance neuromuscular blockade, increasing skeletal muscle relaxation and possibly causing respiratory paralysis. Use cautiously, and reduce dose of pancuronium.
Succinylcholine: May increase intensity and duration of neuromuscular blockade. Allow effects of succinylcholine to subside before giving pancuronium.

Nursing considerations

- Dosage depends on anesthetic used, individual needs, and response. Dosages are representative and must be adjusted.
- Only staff skilled in airway management should use drug.
- Allow succinylcholine effects to subside before giving pancuronium.
- Monitor baseline electrolyte determinations (electrolyte imbalance can potentiate neuromuscular effects) and vital signs, especially respirations and heart rate.
- Measure fluid intake and output; renal dysfunction may prolong duration of action because 25% of drug is excreted unchanged in the urine.
- A nerve stimulator and train-of-four monitoring are recommended to confirm antagonism of neuromuscular blockade and recovery of muscle strength. Make sure there is some evidence of spontaneous recovery before attempting pharmacologic reversal with neostigmine.
- Monitor respirations closely until patient recovers fully from neuromuscular blockade, as indicated by tests of muscle strength (hand grip, head lift, and ability to cough).
- Once spontaneous recovery starts, pancuronium-induced neuromuscular blockade may be reversed with an anticholinesterase (such as neostigmine or edrophonium), which is usually given with an anticholinergic (such as atropine).

- Drug doesn't cause histamine release or hypotension, but it may raise heart rate and blood pressure.
- Give analgesics for pain.

!! ALERT Careful dosage calculation is essential. Always verify dosage with another health care professional.

!! ALERT Don't confuse pancuronium with pipecuronium.

Patient teaching

- Explain all events and procedures to patient because he can still hear.

pantoprazole sodium

Protonix, Protonix I.V.

Pregnancy risk category B

Indications & dosages

➲ **Erosive esophagitis with gastroesophageal reflux disease (GERD)**

Adults: 40 mg P.O. once daily for up to 8 weeks. For patients who haven't healed after 8 weeks of treatment, another 8-week course may be considered.

➲ **Short-term treatment of GERD in patients who can't take delayed-release tablets orally**

Adults: 40 mg I.V. daily for 7 to 10 days.

➲ **Short-term treatment of GERD linked to history of erosive esophagitis**

Adults: 40 mg I.V. once daily for 7 to 10 days. Switch to P.O. form as soon as patient is able to take orally.

➲ **Long-term maintenance of healing erosive esophagitis and reduction in relapse rates of daytime and nighttime heartburn symptoms in patients with GERD**

Adults: 40 mg P.O. once daily.

➲ **Short-term treatment of pathological hypersecretion conditions caused by Zollinger-Ellison syndrome or other neoplastic conditions**

Adults: Individualize dosage. Usual dose is 80 mg I.V. q 12 hours for no more than 6 days. For those needing a higher dose, 80 mg q 8 hours is expected to maintain acid output below 10 mEq/hour. Maximum daily dose is 240 mg/day.

➲ **Long-term treatment of pathological hypersecretory conditions, including with Zollinger-Ellison syndrome**

Adults: Individualize dosage. Usual starting dose is 40 mg P.O. b.i.d. Adjust dose to a maximum of 240 mg/day. Stop treatment with I.V. pantoprazole when P.O. pantoprazole is warranted.

Contraindications & cautions

- Contraindicated in patients hypersensitive to any component of the formulation.
- Safety and efficacy of using the I.V. formulation to start therapy for GERD are unknown.

Adverse reactions

CNS: headache, insomnia, asthenia, migraine, anxiety, dizziness.
CV: chest pain.
EENT: pharyngitis, rhinitis, sinusitis.
GI: diarrhea, flatulence, abdominal pain, eructation, constipation, dyspepsia, gastroenteritis, GI disorder, nausea, vomiting, rectal disorder.
GU: urinary frequency, UTI.
Metabolic: hyperglycemia, hyperlipemia.
Musculoskeletal: back pain, neck pain, arthralgia, hypertonia.
Respiratory: bronchitis, increased cough, dyspnea, upper respiratory tract infection.
Skin: rash.
Other: flulike syndrome, infection, pain.

Interactions

Drug-drug. *Ampicillin esters, iron salts, ketoconazole:* May decrease absorption of these drugs. Monitor patient closely and separate doses.
Drug-herb. *St. John's wort:* May increase risk of sunburn. Advise patient to avoid excessive sunlight exposure.
Drug-lifestyle. *Sunlight:* May increase risk of sunburn. Advise patient to avoid excessive sunlight exposure.

Nursing considerations

- Stop treatment with I.V. pantoprazole when P.O. form is warranted.

!! ALERT Don't confuse Protonix with Prilosec, Prozac, or Prevacid.

- Drug can be given without regard to meals.
- Symptomatic response to therapy doesn't preclude the presence of gastric malignancy.

Patient teaching

- Instruct patient to take exactly as prescribed and at about the same time every day.
- Advise patient that drug can be taken without regard to meals.
- Tell patient to swallow tablet whole and not to crush, split, or chew it.
- Tell patient that antacids don't affect pantoprazole absorption.

paroxetine hydrochloride

Paxil, Paxil CR

Pregnancy risk category C

Indications & dosages

➲ Depression

Adults: Initially, 20 mg P.O. daily, preferably in morning, as indicated. If patient doesn't improve, dosage may be increased by 10 mg daily at intervals of at least 1 week to maximum of 50 mg daily. If using controlled-release formulation, initially 25 mg P.O. daily. Dose may be increased by 12.5 mg daily at weekly intervals, to maximum of 62.5 mg daily.

Elderly patients: Initially, 10 mg P.O. daily, preferably in morning, as indicated. If patient doesn't improve, dose may be increased by 10 mg daily at weekly intervals, to maximum of 40 mg daily. If using controlled-release formulation, start therapy at 12.5 mg P.O. daily. Don't exceed 50 mg daily.

➲ Obsessive-compulsive disorder (OCD)

Adults: Initially, 20 mg P.O. daily, preferably in morning. Dose may be increased by 10 mg daily at weekly intervals. Recommended daily dose is 40 mg. Maximum daily dose is 60 mg.

➲ Panic disorder

Adults: Initially, 10 mg P.O. daily. Dose may be increased by 10 mg at no less than weekly intervals, to maximum of 60 mg daily. Or, 12.5 mg Paxil CR P.O. as a single daily dose, usually in the morning, with or without food; may increase dose at intervals of at least 1 week by 12.5 mg daily, up to a maximum of 75 mg daily.

In elderly or debilitated patients and in those with severe renal or hepatic impairment, the first dose of Paxil CR is 12.5 mg daily; may increase if indicated. Dosage shouldn't exceed 50 mg daily.

➲ Social anxiety disorder

Adults: Initially, 20 mg P.O. daily, preferably in morning. Dosage range is 20 to 60 mg daily. Adjust dosage to maintain patient on lowest effective dose Or, 12.5 mg Paxil CR P.O. as a single daily dose, usually in the morning, with or without food. Increase dosage at weekly intervals in increments of 12.5 mg daily, up to a maximum of 37.5 mg daily.

➲ Generalized anxiety disorder

Adults: 20 mg P.O. daily initially, increasing by 10 mg per day weekly up to 50 mg daily.

For debilitated patients or those with renal or hepatic impairment taking immediate-release form, initially, 10 mg P.O. daily, preferably in morning. If patient doesn't respond after full antidepressant effect has occurred, dosage may be increased by 10 mg per day at weekly intervals, to maximum of 40 mg daily. If using controlled-release formulation, start therapy at 12.5 mg daily. Don't exceed 50 mg daily.

➲ Posttraumatic stress disorder

Adults: Initially, 20 mg P.O. daily. Increase dose by 10 mg daily at intervals of at least 1 week. Maximum daily dose is 50 mg P.O.

➲ Premenstrual dysphoric disorder

Adults: Initially, 12.5 mg Paxil CR P.O. as a single daily dose, usually in the morning, with or without food. Dose changes should occur at intervals of at least a week. Maximum dose is 25 mg P.O. daily. May be given daily or limited to the luteal phase of the menstrual cycle.

➲ Premature ejaculation♦

Adults: 10 to 40 mg P.O. daily. Or, 20 mg P.O. p.r.n. 3 to 4 hours before planned intercourse.

➲ Diabetic neuropathy♦

Adults: 40 mg P.O. daily.

Contraindications & cautions

- Contraindicated in patients hypersensitive to drug, within 14 days of MAO inhibitor therapy, and in those taking thioridazine.
- Contraindicated in children and adolescents under age 18 with major depressive disorder.

- Use cautiously in patients with history of seizure disorders or mania and in those with other severe, systemic illness.
- Use cautiously in patients at risk for volume depletion and monitor them appropriately.
- Use in third trimester of pregnancy may be associated with neonatal complications at birth. Consider the risk versus benefit of treatment during this time.

Adverse reactions

CNS: *somnolence, dizziness, insomnia, tremor, nervousness,* anxiety, paresthesia, confusion, *headache,* agitation, *asthenia,* ***suicidal behavior***.
CV: palpitations, vasodilation, orthostatic hypotension.
EENT: lump or tightness in throat.
GI: *dry mouth, nausea, constipation, diarrhea,* flatulence, vomiting, dyspepsia, dysgeusia, increased or decreased appetite, abdominal pain.
GU: *ejaculatory disturbances, sexual dysfunction,* urinary frequency, other urinary disorders.
Musculoskeletal: myopathy, myalgia, myasthenia.
Skin: rash, pruritus, *diaphoresis.*
Other: yawning, *decreased libido.*

Interactions

Drug-drug. *Cimetidine:* May decrease hepatic metabolism of paroxetine, leading to risk of adverse reactions. Dosage adjustments may be needed.
Digoxin: May decrease digoxin level. Use together cautiously.
MAO inhibitors (phenelzine, selegiline, tranylcypromine): May cause serotonin syndrome. Avoid using within 14 days of MAO inhibitor therapy.
Phenobarbital, phenytoin: May alter pharmacokinetics of both drugs. Dosage adjustments may be needed.
Procyclidine: May increase procyclidine level. Watch for excessive anticholinergic effects.
Sumatriptan: May cause weakness, hyperreflexia, and incoordination. Monitor patient closely.
Theophylline: May decrease theophylline clearance. Monitor theophylline level.
Thioridazine: May prolong QTc interval and increase risk of serious ventricular arrhythmias, such as torsade de pointes, and sudden death. Avoid using together.
Tramadol: May cause serotonin syndrome. Monitor patient if used together.
Tricyclic antidepressants: May inhibit tricyclic antidepressant metabolism. Dose of tricyclic antidepressant may need to be reduced. Monitor patient closely.
Tryptophan: May cause adverse reactions, such as diaphoresis, headache, nausea, and dizziness. Avoid using together.
Warfarin: May cause bleeding. Use together cautiously.
Drug-herb. *St. John's wort:* May increase sedative-hypnotic effects. Discourage use together.
Drug-lifestyle. *Alcohol use:* May alter psychomotor function. Discourage use together.

Nursing considerations

- Patients taking drug may be at increased risk for developing suicidal behavior, but this hasn't been definitively attributed to use of the drug.
- Patients taking Paxil CR for premenstrual dysphoric disorder should be periodically reassessed to determine the need for continued treatment.
- If signs or symptoms of psychosis occur or increase, expect prescriber to reduce dosage. Record mood changes. Monitor patient for suicidal tendencies, and allow only a minimum supply of drug.
- Monitor patient for complaints of sexual dysfunction. In men, they include anorgasmy, erectile difficulties, delayed ejaculation or orgasm, or impotence; in women, they include anorgasmy or difficulty with orgasm.

!!ALERT Don't stop drug abruptly. Withdrawal or discontinuation syndrome may occur if drug is stopped abruptly. Symptoms include headache, myalgia, lethargy, and general flulike symptoms. Taper drug slowly over 1 to 2 weeks.

!!ALERT Don't confuse paroxetine with paclitaxel, or Paxil with Doxil, paclitaxel, Plavix, or Taxol.

Patient teaching

- Tell patient that drug may be taken with or without food, usually in morning.

- Tell patient not to break, crush, or chew controlled-release tablets.
- Warn patient to avoid activities that require alertness and good coordination until effects of drug are known.
- Advise woman of childbearing age to contact prescriber if she becomes pregnant or plans to become pregnant during therapy, or if she's currently breast-feeding.
- Tell patient to avoid alcohol and to consult prescriber before taking other prescription or OTC drugs or herbal medicines.
- Instruct patient not to stop taking medication abruptly.

pegaspargase (PEG-L-asparaginase)

Oncaspar

Pregnancy risk category C

Indications & dosages

➲ Acute lymphoblastic leukemia in patients who need L-asparaginase but have become hypersensitive to native forms of L-asparaginase

Adults and children with body surface area (BSA) of at least 0.6 m^2: 2,500 IU/m^2 I.V. or I.M. q 14 days.

Children with BSA below 0.6 m^2: 82.5 IU/ kg I.V. or I.M. q 14 days.

Contraindications & cautions

- Contraindicated in patients with pancreatitis or history of pancreatitis, in those who have had significant hemorrhagic events related to previous treatment with L-asparaginase, and in those with history of serious allergic reactions to drug, such as generalized urticaria, bronchospasm, laryngeal edema, hypotension, or other unacceptable adverse reactions.
- Use cautiously in patients with liver dysfunction; use only when clearly indicated in pregnant women.

Adverse reactions

CNS: ***seizures***, headache, paresthesia, ***status epilepticus***, somnolence, ***coma***, mental status changes, dizziness, emotional lability, mood changes, parkinsonism, confusion, disorientation, fatigue, malaise.

CV: hypotension, tachycardia, chest pain, subacute bacterial endocarditis, hypertension, peripheral edema.

EENT: epistaxis.

GI: nausea, vomiting, abdominal pain, anorexia, diarrhea, constipation, indigestion, flatulence, mucositis, mouth tenderness, ***pancreatitis***, severe colitis.

GU: increased urinary frequency, hematuria, proteinuria, severe hemorrhagic cystitis, renal dysfunction, ***renal failure***.

Hematologic: ***thrombosis***, ***disseminated intravascular coagulation***, hemolytic anemia, ***leukopenia***, ***pancytopenia***, ***agranulocytosis***, ***thrombocytopenia***, easy bruising, ***hemorrhage***.

Hepatic: jaundice, ascites, hypoalbuminemia, fatty changes in liver, ***liver failure***.

Metabolic: hyperuricemia, hyponatremia, uric acid nephropathy, hypoproteinemia, weight loss, metabolic acidosis, hyperglycemia, ***hypoglycemia***.

Musculoskeletal: arthralgia, myalgia, musculoskeletal pain, joint stiffness, cramps, pain in limbs.

Respiratory: cough, ***bronchospasm***, upper respiratory tract infection.

Skin: urticaria, itching, alopecia, fever blister, purpura, hand whiteness, fungal changes, nail whiteness and ridging, erythema simplex, petechial rash, injection pain or reaction, localized edema, rash, erythema, ecchymoses.

Other: hypersensitivity reactions, night sweats, infection, ***sepsis***, ***septic shock***, ***anaphylaxis***.

Interactions

Drug-drug. *Aspirin, dipyridamole, heparin, NSAIDs, warfarin:* May cause imbalances in coagulation factors, predisposing patient to bleeding or thrombosis. Use together cautiously.

Methotrexate: May interfere with action of methotrexate. Check patient for decreased effectiveness.

Protein-bound drugs: May increase toxicity of other drugs that bind to proteins and may interfere with enzymatic detoxification of other drugs, especially in the liver. Check for toxicity, and use together cautiously.

Nursing considerations

- Use drug as sole induction drug only in patients refractory to other therapy, or when combined regimen using other chemotherapeutic drugs is inappropriate because of toxicity or other specific patient-related factors.

- Take preventive measures (including adequate hydration) before starting treatment. Hyperuricemia may result from rapid lysis of leukemic cells. Allopurinol may be ordered.
- I.M. route is preferred because it has the lowest risk of hepatotoxicity, coagulopathy, and GI and renal disorders.
- When giving I.M., limit volume given at a single injection site to 2 ml. If volume to be given exceeds 2 ml, use multiple injection sites.

!!ALERT Monitor patient closely for hypersensitivity (including life-threatening anaphylaxis), especially those hypersensitive to other forms of L-asparaginase. As a routine precaution, keep patient under observation for 1 hour and have readily available resuscitation equipment and other drugs needed to treat anaphylaxis (such as epinephrine, oxygen, and I.V. corticosteroids). Moderate to life-threatening hypersensitivity requires stopping L-asparaginase.

- To assess effects of therapy, monitor patient's peripheral blood count and bone marrow. A drop in circulating lymphoblasts is often noted after therapy starts, sometimes accompanied by a marked rise in uric acid level.
- Obtain frequent amylase and lipase determinations to detect pancreatitis. Monitor patient's glucose level during therapy to detect hyperglycemia.
- Monitor patient for liver dysfunction when drug is used with hepatotoxic chemotherapeutic drugs.
- Drug may affect several plasma proteins; monitoring of fibrinogen, PT, INR, and PTT may be indicated.

Patient teaching

- Inform patient of risk of hypersensitivity reactions and importance of reporting them immediately.
- Tell patient not to take other drugs, including OTC preparations, until approved by prescriber because risk of bleeding is higher when pegaspargase is given with drugs such as aspirin. Pegaspargase may also increase toxicity of other drugs.
- Urge patient to report signs and symptoms of infection (fever, chills, and malaise); drug may suppress the immune system.
- Caution woman of childbearing age to avoid pregnancy and breast-feeding during therapy.

pegfilgrastim
Neulasta

Pregnancy risk category C

Indications & dosages

➲ **To reduce frequency of infection in patients with nonmyeloid malignancies receiving myelosuppressive anticancer drugs that may cause febrile neutropenia**
Adults: 6 mg S.C. once per chemotherapy cycle. Don't give in period between 14 days before and 24 hours after administration of cytotoxic chemotherapy.

Contraindications & cautions

- Contraindicated in patients hypersensitive to ***Escherichia coli***-derived proteins, filgrastim, or any component of the drug. Don't use for peripheral blood progenitor cell mobilization.
- Use cautiously in patients with sickle cell disease, those receiving chemotherapy causing delayed myelosuppression, or those receiving radiation therapy.
- Infants, children, and adolescents weighing less than 45 kg (99 lb) shouldn't receive the 6-mg single-use syringe dose. Safety and effectiveness in children haven't been established.

Adverse reactions

CNS: *dizziness, headache, fatigue, insomnia, fever.*
GI: *nausea, diarrhea, vomiting, constipation, anorexia, taste perversion, dyspepsia, abdominal pain, stomatitis, mucositis.*
Hematologic: **GRANULOCYTOPENIA, NEUTROPENIC FEVER.**
Musculoskeletal: *skeletal pain, generalized weakness, arthralgia, myalgia, bone pain.*
Respiratory: ***acute respiratory distress syndrome (ARDS).***
Skin: *alopecia.*
Other: *peripheral edema,* **splenic rupture.**

Interactions

Drug-drug. *Lithium:* May increase the release of neutrophils. Monitor neutrophil counts closely.

Nursing considerations

!!ALERT Splenic rupture has occurred rarely with filgrastim use. Evaluate patient who experiences signs or symptoms of left upper abdominal or shoulder pain for an enlarged spleen or splenic rupture.

- Obtain CBC and platelet count before therapy.
- Monitor patient's hemoglobin level, hematocrit, CBC, and platelet count, as well as LDH, alkaline phosphatase, and uric acid levels during therapy.
- Monitor patient for allergic-type reactions, including anaphylaxis, skin rash, and urticaria, which can occur with first or subsequent treatment.
- Evaluate patient with fever, lung infiltrates, or respiratory distress for ARDS. If ARDS develops, notify prescriber.
- Keep patient with sickle cell disease well hydrated, and monitor him for symptoms of sickle cell crisis.
- Pegfilgrastim may act as a growth factor for tumors.

Patient teaching

- Inform patient of the potential side effects of the drug.
- Tell patient to report signs and symptoms of allergic reactions, fever, or breathing problems.

!!ALERT Rarely, splenic rupture may occur. Advise patient to immediately report upper left abdominal or shoulder tip pain.

- Tell patient with sickle cell disease to keep drinking fluids and report signs or symptoms of sickle cell crisis.
- Instruct patient or caregiver how to give drug if it's to be given at home.

---

peginterferon alfa-2a

Pegasys

Pregnancy risk category C

Indications & dosages

➲ **Chronic hepatitis C with compensated hepatic disease in patients not previously treated with interferon alfa; Chronic hepatitis C in patients with clinically stable HIV who have not previously been treated with interferon**

Adults: 180 mcg S.C. in abdomen or thigh, once weekly for 48 weeks.

For patients who experience moderate adverse reactions, decrease dose to 135 mcg S.C. once a week; for severe adverse reactions, decrease to 90 mcg S.C. once a week. For patients who experience hematologic reactions, if the neutrophil count is less than 750 cells/mm^3, reduce dose to 135 mcg S.C. once a week; if the absolute neutrophil count (ANC) is less than 500 cells/mm^3, stop drug until ANC exceeds 1,000 cells/mm^3 and restart at 90 mcg S.C. once a week. If platelet count is less than 50,000 cells/mm^3, reduce dose to 90 mcg S.C. once a week; stop drug if platelet count drops below 25,000 cells/mm^3. In patients with end-stage renal disease requiring hemodialysis, decrease dose to 135 mcg S.C. once a week. In patients with ALT increases above baseline, decrease dose to 90 mcg S.C. once a week.

Contraindications & cautions

- Contraindicated in patients hypersensitive to interferon alfa-2a or any components of formulation.
- Contraindicated in patients with autoimmune hepatitis or decompensated liver disease (with monoinfection or coinfected with HIV) before or during treatment with drug and in neonates and infants.
- Safety and efficacy has not been established in patients who have failed to respond to other alfa interferon treatments, in organ transplant recipients, and in patients who are also infected with hepatitis B.
- Use cautiously in patients with a history of depression.
- Use cautiously in patients with baseline neutrophil counts less than 1,500 cells/mm^3, baseline platelet counts less than 90,000 cells/mm^3, or baseline hemoglobin less than 10 g/dl.
- Use cautiously in patients with creatinine clearance less than 50 ml/minute.
- Use cautiously in patients with cardiac disease or hypertension, thyroid disease, autoimmune disorders, pulmonary disorders, colitis, pancreatitis, and ophthalmologic disorders.

- Use cautiously in elderly patients because they may be at increased risk for adverse reactions.

!!ALERT Drug may cause an abortion in a pregnant woman. Use in pregnant patient only if benefit outweighs risk.

Adverse reactions

CNS: *fatigue*, asthenia, *headache*, *insomnia*, *dizziness*, concentration impairment, memory impairment, *depression*, *irritability*, anxiety.
GI: *nausea*, *diarrhea*, *abdominal pain*, vomiting, dry mouth, *anorexia*.
Hematologic: NEUTROPENIA, ***thrombocytopenia***.
Musculoskeletal: *myalgia*, *arthralgia*, back pain.
Skin: *alopecia*, *pruritus*, increased sweating, dermatitis, rash.
Other: *pain*, *pyrexia*, *rigors*, *injection site reaction*.

Interactions

Drug-drug. *Ribavirin:* May cause additive hematologic toxicity. Monitor hematologic function.
Theophylline, other drugs metabolized by CYP1A2: May increase theophylline level and may interact with other drugs metabolized by this enzyme system. Monitor theophylline level and adjust dosage as needed.

Nursing considerations

- Monitor patient for neuropsychiatric reactions, including depression and suicidal ideation. These symptoms may occur in patients without previous psychiatric illness. If severe depression occurs, stop drug and start psychiatric treatment.
- Obtain CBC before treatment and monitor counts routinely during therapy. Stop drug in patients who develop severe decrease in neutrophil or platelet counts.
- Stop drug if uncontrollable thyroid disease, hyperglycemia, hypoglycemia, or diabetes mellitus occurs during treatment.
- If persistent or unexplained pulmonary infiltrates or pulmonary dysfunction occur, stop drug.
- Stop drug if signs and symptoms of colitis occur, such as abdominal pain, bloody diarrhea, and fever. Symptoms should resolve within 1 to 3 weeks.
- Stop drug if signs and symptoms of pancreatitis occur, including fever, malaise, and abdominal pain.
- Obtain baseline eye examination and periodically monitor eye exams during treatment. Stop drug if new or worsening eye disorders occur.
- Monitor patient with impaired renal function for interferon toxicity.
- Use in women of childbearing potential only when effective contraception is being used.

Patient teaching

- Teach patient proper way to give drug and dispose of needles and syringes.
- Tell patient to immediately report depression or suicidal ideation.
- Tell patient to report signs and symptoms of pancreatitis, colitis, eye disorders, or respiratory disorders.
- Advise patient to avoid driving or operating machinery if he feels dizzy, tired, confused, or sleepy.

pemetrexed
Alimta

Pregnancy risk category D

Indications & dosages

➲ Malignant pleural mesothelioma, with cisplatin, in patients whose disease is unresectable or who aren't candidates for surgery
Adults: 500 mg/m^2 I.V. over 10 minutes on day 1 of each 21-day cycle. Starting 30 minutes after pemetrexed infusion ends, give cisplatin 75 mg/m^2 I.V. over 2 hours.

➲ Locally advanced or metastatic non-small-cell lung cancer after chemotherapy
Adults: 500 mg/m^2 I.V. over 10 minutes on day 1 of each 21-day cycle.

In patients who develop toxic reactions, adjust dosage according to the table.

Toxic reaction	Dosage change
– Grade 3 (severe or undesirable) or grade 4 (life-threatening or disabling) diarrhea – Diarrhea that warrants hospitalization – Any grade 3 toxicity (except mucositis and increased transaminase levels) – Any grade 4 toxicity (except mucositis) – Platelet count ≥ 50,000/mm³ and absolute neutrophil count < 500/mm³	Give 75% of previous pemetrexed and cisplatin doses.
Platelet count < 50,000/mm³	Give 50% of previous pemetrexed and cisplatin doses.
Grade 3 or 4 mucositis	Give 50% of previous pemetrexed dose and 100% of previous cisplatin dose.
Grade 2 (moderate) neurotoxicity	Give 100% of previous pemetrexed dose and 50% of previous cisplatin dose.
– Grade 3 or 4 neurotoxicity – Any grade 3 or 4 toxicity (except increased transaminase levels) present after two dose reductions	Stop therapy.

Contraindications & cautions

- Contraindicated in patients with a history of severe hypersensitivity reaction to pemetrexed or its ingredients. Don't use in patients with creatinine clearance less than 45 ml/minute.

Adverse reactions

CNS: *depression, fatigue, fever, neuropathy.*
CV: cardiac ischemia, *chest pain, edema,* ***emboli***, thrombosis.
EENT: *pharyngitis.*
GI: *anorexia, constipation, diarrhea,* esophagitis, *nausea,* painful difficult swallowing, *stomatitis, vomiting.*
GU: ***renal failure***.
Hematologic: ANEMIA, LEUKOPENIA, NEUTROPENIA, THROMBOCYTOPENIA.
Metabolic: dehydration.
Musculoskeletal: arthralgia, *myalgia.*
Respiratory: *dyspnea.*
Skin: *alopecia, rash.*
Other: allergic reaction, *infection.*

Interactions

Drug-drug. *Ibuprofen:* May decrease pemetrexed clearance in patients with mild to moderate renal insufficiency. Use together cautiously.
Nephrotoxic drugs, probenecid: May delay pemetrexed clearance. Monitor patient.
NSAIDs: May decrease pemetrexed clearance in patients with mild to moderate renal insufficiency. For NSAIDs with short half-lives, avoid use for 2 days before, during, and 2 days after pemetrexed therapy. For NSAIDs with long half-lives, avoid use for 5 days before, during, and 2 days after pemetrexed therapy.

Nursing considerations

- Patient shouldn't start a new cycle of treatment unless ANC is 1,500 cells/mm³ or more, platelet count is 100,000 cells/mm³ or more, and creatinine clearance is 45 ml/minute or more.
- Patients with pleural effusion and ascites may need to have effusion drained before therapy.
- Monitor renal function, CBC, platelet count, hemoglobin level, hematocrit, and liver function test values.
- Assess patient for neurotoxicity, mucositis, and diarrhea. Severe symptoms may warrant dosage adjustment.

!!ALERT To reduce the occurrence and severity of cutaneous reactions, give a corticosteroid, such as dexamethasone 4 mg P.O. b.i.d., the day before, the day of, and the day after giving pemetrexed.
!!ALERT To reduce toxicity, patient should take 350 to 1,000 mcg of folic acid starting 5 days before the first pemetrexed dose and continue it for 21 days after therapy.
!!ALERT Give vitamin B_{12} 1,000 mcg I.M. once during the week before the first dose and every three cycles thereafter. After the first cycle, vitamin injections may be given on the first day of the cycle.

Patient teaching

- Inform patient that he may receive corticosteroids and vitamins before pemetrexed to help minimize its adverse effects.
- Tell patient to avoid NSAIDs for several days before, during, and after treatment.
- Urge patient to report adverse effects, especially fever, sore throat, infection, diarrhea, fatigue, and limb pain.

• It isn't known if drug appears in breast milk. Advise patient to stop breast-feeding during treatment.

penicillin G benzathine (benzathine benzylpenicillin)
Bicillin L-A, Permapen

Pregnancy risk category B

Indications & dosages

➲ **Congenital syphilis**
Children younger than age 2: 50,000 units/kg I.M. as a single dose.

➲ **Group A streptococcal upper respiratory tract infections**
Adults: 1.2 million units I.M. as a single injection.
Children weighing 27 kg (59.5 lb) or more: 900,000 units I.M. as a single injection.
Children weighing less than 27 kg: 300,000 to 600,000 units I.M. as a single injection.

➲ **To prevent poststreptococcal rheumatic fever**
Adults and children: 1.2 million units I.M. once monthly or 600,000 units I.M. q 2 weeks.

➲ **Syphilis of less than 1 year's duration**
Adults: 2.4 million units I.M. as a single dose.
Children: 50,000 units/kg I.M. as a single dose. Don't exceed adult dosage.

➲ **Syphilis of more than 1 year's duration**
Adults: 2.4 million units I.M. weekly for 3 weeks.
Children: 50,000 units/kg I.M. weekly for 3 weeks.

Contraindications & cautions

• Contraindicated in patients hypersensitive to drug or other penicillins.
• Use cautiously in patients allergic to other drugs, especially to cephalosporins, because of possible cross-sensitivity.

Adverse reactions

CNS: neuropathy, ***seizures***, lethargy, hallucinations, anxiety, confusion, agitation, depression, dizziness, fatigue.
GI: nausea, vomiting, enterocolitis, ***pseudomembranous colitis***.
GU: interstitial nephritis, nephropathy.
Hematologic: eosinophilia, hemolytic anemia, ***thrombocytopenia***, ***leukopenia***, anemia, ***agranulocytosis***.
Skin: maculopapular rash, exfoliative dermatitis.
Other: hypersensitivity reactions, ***anaphylaxis***, pain, sterile abscess at injection site.

Interactions

Drug-drug. *Aminoglycosides:* Physical and chemical incompatibility. Give separately.
Colestipol: May decrease penicillin G benzathine level. Give penicillin G benzathine 1 hour before or 4 hours after colestipol.
Hormonal contraceptives: May decrease hormonal contraceptive effectiveness. Advise use of additional form of contraception during penicillin therapy.
Probenecid: May increase penicillin level. Probenecid may be used for this purpose.
Tetracycline: May antagonize penicillin G benzathine effects. Avoid using together.

Nursing considerations

• Before giving drug, ask patient about allergic reactions to penicillin.
!!ALERT Bicillin L-A is the only penicillin G benzathine product indicated for sexually transmitted infections. Don't substitute Bicillin C-R because it may not be effective.
• Obtain specimen for culture and sensitivity tests before giving first dose. Therapy may begin pending results.
• Shake well before injection.
!!ALERT Never give I.V. Inadvertent I.V. use may cause cardiac arrest and death.
• Inject deep into upper outer quadrant of buttocks in adults and in midlateral thigh in infants and small children. Rotate injection sites. Avoid injection into or near major nerves or blood vessels to prevent permanent neurovascular damage.
• Give drug at least 1 hour before a bacteriostatic antibiotic.
• Drug's extremely slow absorption time makes allergic reactions difficult to treat.
• If large doses are given or if therapy is prolonged, bacterial or fungal superinfection may occur, especially in elderly, debilitated, or immunosuppressed patients.
!!ALERT Don't confuse drug with Polycillin, penicillamine, or the various types of penicillin.

Patient teaching

- Tell patient to report adverse reactions promptly.
- Inform patient that fever and increased WBC count are the most common reactions.
- Warn patient that I.M. injection may be painful, but that ice applied to the site may ease discomfort.

penicillin G potassium (benzylpenicillin potassium)

Pfizerpen

Pregnancy risk category B

Indications & dosages

➲ Moderate to severe systemic infection
Adults and children age 12 and older: Highly individualized; 1 to 30 million units I.M. or I.V. daily in divided doses q 2 to 6 hours or via continuous I.V. infusion.
Children younger than age 12: 25,000 to 400,000 units/kg I.M. or I.V. daily in divided doses q 4 to 6 hours.

➲ Anthrax
Adults: 5 to 20 million units I.V. daily in divided doses q 4 to 6 hours, for at least 14 days after symptoms diminish. Or, 80,000 units/kg in the first hour, followed by a maintenance dose of 320,000 units/kg/day. The average adult dosage is 4 million units q 4 hours or 2 million units q 2 hours.
Children: 100,000 to 150,000 units/kg/day I.V. in divided doses q 4 to 6 hours for at least 14 days after symptoms diminish.

If creatinine clearance is 10 to 50 ml/minute, give the usual dose q 8 to 12 hours. If clearance is less than 10 ml/minute, give 50% of usual dose q 8 to 10 hours or the usual dose q 12 to 18 hours. If patient is uremic and creatinine clearance is more than 10 ml/minute, give full loading dose; then give half the loading dose q 4 to 5 hours for additional doses.

Contraindications & cautions

- Contraindicated in patients hypersensitive to drug or other penicillins.
- Use cautiously in patients with other drug allergies, especially to cephalosporins, because of possible cross-sensitivity.

Adverse reactions

CNS: neuropathy, ***seizures***, lethargy, hallucinations, anxiety, confusion, agitation, depression, dizziness, fatigue.
CV: thrombophlebitis.
GI: nausea, vomiting, enterocolitis, ***pseudomembranous colitis***.
GU: interstitial nephritis, nephropathy.
Hematologic: hemolytic anemia, ***leukopenia***, ***thrombocytopenia***, anemia, eosinophilia, ***agranulocytosis***.
Metabolic: ***possible severe potassium poisoning***.
Skin: maculopapular eruptions, exfoliative dermatitis, pain at injection site.
Other: hypersensitivity reactions, ***anaphylaxis***, overgrowth of nonsusceptible organisms.

Interactions

Drug-drug. *Aminoglycosides:* Physically and chemically incompatible. Give separately.
Colestipol: May decrease penicillin G potassium level. Give penicillin G potassium 1 hour before or 4 hours after colestipol.
Hormonal contraceptives: May decrease hormonal contraceptive effectiveness. Advise use of additional form of contraception during penicillin therapy.
Oral anticoagulants: May increase risk of bleeding. Monitor PT and INR.
Potassium-sparing diuretics: May increase risk of hyperkalemia. Avoid using together.
Probenecid: May increase penicillin level. Probenecid may be used for this purpose.

Nursing considerations

- Before giving drug, ask patient about allergic reactions to penicillin.
- Obtain specimen for culture and sensitivity tests before giving first dose. Therapy may begin pending results.
- For I.M. injection, give deep into large muscle; injection may be extremely painful.
- Monitor renal function closely. Patients with poor renal function are predisposed to high blood levels of drug.
- Monitor potassium and sodium levels closely in patients receiving more than 10 million units I.V. daily.
- Observe patient closely. With large doses and prolonged therapy, bacterial or fungal superinfection may occur, especially in eld-

erly, debilitated, or immunosuppressed patients.
!!ALERT Don't confuse drug with Polycillin, penicillamine, or the various types of penicillin.

Patient teaching

- Tell patient to notify prescriber if rash, fever, or chills develop. A rash is the most common allergic reaction.
- Warn patient that I.M. injection may be painful, but that ice applied to the site may help alleviate discomfort.

penicillin G procaine (benzylpenicillin procaine)

Ayercillin†, Wycillin

Pregnancy risk category B

Indications & dosages

➲ **Moderate to severe systemic infection**
Adults: 600,000 to 1.2 million units I.M. daily for a minimum of 10 days.
Children older than age 1 month: 25,000 to 50,000 units/kg I.M. daily in a single dose.
➲ **Anthrax caused by *Bacillus anthracis*, including inhalation anthrax after exposure**
Adults: 1,200,000 units I.M. q 12 hours.
Children: 25,000 units/kg I.M.; not to exceed 1,200,000 units q 12 hours.
➲ **Cutaneous anthrax**
Adults: 600,000 to 1,000,000 units I.M. daily.

Contraindications & cautions

- Contraindicated in patients hypersensitive to drug or other penicillins.
- Use cautiously in patients with other drug allergies, especially to cephalosporins, because of possible cross-sensitivity. Some formulations contain sulfites, which may cause allergic reactions in sensitive people.

Adverse reactions

CNS: ***seizures***, lethargy, hallucinations, anxiety, confusion, agitation, depression, dizziness, fatigue.
GI: nausea, vomiting, enterocolitis, ***pseudomembranous colitis***.
GU: interstitial nephritis, nephropathy.
Hematologic: ***thrombocytopenia***, ***hemolytic anemia***, ***leukopenia***, anemia, eosinophilia, ***agranulocytosis***.
Musculoskeletal: arthralgia.
Other: hypersensitivity reactions, ***anaphylaxis***, overgrowth of nonsusceptible organisms.

Interactions

Drug-drug. *Aminoglycosides:* Physically and chemically incompatible. Give separately.
Colestipol: May decrease penicillin G procaine level. Give penicillin G procaine 1 hour before or 4 hours after colestipol.
Hormonal contraceptives: May decrease hormonal contraceptive effectiveness. Advise use of additional form of contraception during penicillin therapy.
Probenecid: May increase penicillin level. Probenecid may be used for this purpose.

Nursing considerations

- Before giving drug, ask patient about allergic reactions to penicillin.
- Obtain specimen for culture and sensitivity tests before giving first dose. Therapy may begin pending results.
- Give deep I.M. in upper outer quadrant of buttocks in adults; in midlateral thigh in small children. Rotate injection sites. Don't give S.C. Don't massage injection site. Avoid injection near major nerves or blood vessels to prevent permanent neurovascular damage.

!!ALERT Continue postexposure treatment for inhalation anthrax for 60 days. Prescriber should consider the risk-benefit ratio of continuing penicillin longer than 2 weeks, compared with switching to an effective alternate drug.
!!ALERT Never give by I.V. route. Inadvertent I.V. administration has resulted in death from CNS toxicity.

- Allergic reactions are hard to treat because of drug's slow absorption rate.
- Monitor renal and hematopoietic function periodically.
- If large doses are given or if therapy is prolonged, bacterial or fungal superinfection may occur, especially in elderly, debilitated, or immunosuppressed patients.
- Treatment duration depends on site and cause of infection.

!!ALERT Don't confuse drug with Polycillin, penicillamine, or the various types of penicillin.

Patient teaching

- Tell patient to report adverse reactions promptly. A rash is the most common allergic reaction.
- Warn patient that I.M. injection may be painful, but that ice applied to the site may help alleviate discomfort.

penicillin G sodium (benzylpenicillin sodium)

Crystapen†

Pregnancy risk category B

Indications & dosages

➲ Moderate to severe systemic infection

Adults and children age 12 and older: 1.2 to 24 million units daily I.M. or I.V. in divided doses q 4 to 6 hours.

Children younger than age 12: 25,000 to 400,000 units/kg daily I.M. or I.V. in divided doses q 4 to 6 hours.

➲ Neurosyphilis

Adults: 18 to 24 million units I.V. daily in divided doses q 4 hours for 10 to 14 days.

If creatinine clearance is 10 to 50 ml/minute, give the usual dose q 8 to 12 hours. If clearance is less than 10 ml/minute, give 50% of usual dose q 8 to 10 hours or the usual dose q 12 to 18 hours. If patient is uremic and creatinine clearance is more than 10 ml/minute, give full loading dose; then give half the loading dose q 4 to 5 hours for additional doses.

Contraindications & cautions

- Contraindicated in patients hypersensitive to drug or other penicillins and in those on sodium-restricted diets.
- Use cautiously in patients with other drug allergies, especially to cephalosporins, because of possible cross-sensitivity.

Adverse reactions

CNS: neuropathy, ***seizures***, lethargy, hallucinations, anxiety, confusion, agitation, depression, dizziness, fatigue.
CV: ***heart failure***, thrombophlebitis.
GI: nausea, vomiting, enterocolitis, ***pseudomembranous colitis***.
GU: interstitial colitis, nephropathy.
Hematologic: hemolytic anemia, ***leukopenia, thrombocytopenia, agranulocytosis***, anemia, eosinophilia.
Musculoskeletal: arthralgia.
Other: hypersensitivity reactions, ***anaphylaxis***, overgrowth of nonsusceptible organisms, pain at injection site, vein irritation.

Interactions

Drug-drug. *Aminoglycosides:* Physically and chemically incompatible. Give separately.
Colestipol: May decrease penicillin G sodium level. Give penicillin G sodium 1 hour before or 4 hours after colestipol.
Hormonal contraceptives: May decrease hormonal contraceptive effectiveness. Advise use of additional form of contraception during penicillin therapy.
Oral anticoagulants: May increase risk of bleeding. Monitor PT and INR.
Probenecid: May increase penicillin level. Probenecid may be used for this purpose.

Nursing considerations

- Before giving drug, ask patient about allergic reactions to penicillin.
- Obtain specimen for culture and sensitivity tests before giving first dose. Therapy may begin pending results.
- Observe patient closely. With large doses and prolonged therapy, bacterial or fungal superinfection may occur, especially in elderly, debilitated, or immunosuppressed patients.

!!ALERT Don't confuse drug with Polycillin, penicillamine, or the various types of penicillin.

Patient teaching

- Tell patient to report adverse reactions promptly.
- Instruct patient to report discomfort at I.V. site.
- Warn patient receiving I.M. injection that the injection may be painful, but that ice applied to site may help alleviate discomfort.

penicillin V potassium (phenoxymethylpenicillin potassium)

Apo-Pen VK†, Nadopen-V 200†, Nadopen-V 400†, Novo-Pen-VK†, Nu-Pen-VK†, Pen-Vee†, PVF K†, Veetids

Pregnancy risk category B

Indications & dosages

➲ Mild to moderate systemic infections
Adults and children age 12 and older: 125 to 500 mg or P.O. q 6 hours.
Children younger than age 12: 15 to 62.5 mg/kg P.O. daily in divided doses q 6 to 8 hours.

➲ To prevent recurrent rheumatic fever
Adults and children: 250 mg P.O. b.i.d.

➲ Erythema chronica migrans in Lyme disease♦
Adults: 250 to 500 mg P.O. q.i.d. for 10 to 20 days.
Children younger than age 2: 50 mg/kg/day (up to 2 g/day) P.O. in four divided doses for 10 to 20 days.

➲ To prevent inhalation anthrax after possible exposure♦
Adults: 7.5 mg/kg P.O. q.i.d. Continue treatment until exposure is ruled out. If exposure is confirmed, anthrax vaccine may be indicated. Continue treatment for 60 days.
Children younger than age 9: 50 mg/kg P.O. daily given in four divided doses. Continue treatment until exposure is ruled out. If exposure is confirmed, anthrax vaccine may be indicated. Continue treatment for 60 days.

Contraindications & cautions

- Contraindicated in patients hypersensitive to drug or other penicillins.
- Use cautiously in patients with GI disturbances and in those with other drug allergies, especially to cephalosporins, because of possible cross-sensitivity.

Adverse reactions

CNS: neuropathy.
GI: *epigastric distress*, vomiting, diarrhea, *nausea*, black hairy tongue.
GU: nephropathy.
Hematologic: eosinophilia, hemolytic anemia, ***leukopenia, thrombocytopenia***.
Other: hypersensitivity reactions, ***anaphylaxis***, overgrowth of nonsusceptible organisms.

Interactions

Drug-drug. *Hormonal contraceptives:* May decrease hormonal contraceptive effectiveness. Advise use of additional form of contraception during penicillin therapy.
Probenecid: May increase penicillin level. Probenecid may be used for this purpose.

Nursing considerations

- Before giving drug, ask patient about allergic reactions to penicillins.
- Obtain specimen for culture and sensitivity tests before giving first dose. Therapy may begin pending results.
- Periodically assess renal and hematopoietic function in patients receiving long-term therapy.
- If large doses are given or if therapy is prolonged, bacterial or fungal superinfection may occur, especially in elderly, debilitated, or immunosuppressed patients.
- The American Heart Association considers amoxicillin the preferred drug to prevent endocarditis because GI absorption is better and drug levels are sustained longer. Penicillin V is considered an alternative drug.

!!ALERT Don't confuse drug with Polycillin, penicillamine, or the various types of penicillin.

Patient teaching

- Instruct patient to take entire quantity of drug exactly as prescribed, even after he feels better.
- Tell patient to take drug with food if stomach upset occurs.
- Advise patient to notify prescriber if rash, fever, or chills develop. A rash is the most common allergic reaction.

pentamidine isethionate
NebuPent, Pentam 300

Pregnancy risk category C

Indications & dosages

➲ ***Pneumocystis carinii*** **pneumonia**
Adults and children age 4 months and older: 3 to 4 mg/kg I.V. or I.M. once daily for 14 to 21 days.

➲ **To prevent** ***P. carinii*** **pneumonia in high-risk patients**
Adults and children capable of effectively using a nebulizer: 300 mg by inhalation using a Respirgard II nebulizer once q 4 weeks.

➲ **Visceral leishmaniasis caused by** ***Leishmania donovani***♦
Adults and children: 2 to 4 mg/kg I.V. or I.M. once daily or once every other day for up to 15 doses.

➲ **Cutaneous leishmaniasis**♦
Adults and children: 2 mg/kg I.M. every other day for seven doses or 3 mg/kg I.M. every other day for four doses.

Contraindications & cautions

- Contraindicated in patients with history of anaphylactic reaction to drug.
- Use cautiously in patients with hypertension, hypotension, hypoglycemia, hypocalcemia, leukopenia, thrombocytopenia, anemia, diabetes, pancreatitis, Stevens-Johnson syndrome, or hepatic or renal dysfunction.
- Use cautiously in breast-feeding women; it's unknown if drug appears in breast milk.

Adverse reactions

CNS: confusion, hallucinations, *fatigue, dizziness,* headache.
CV: ***severe hypotension, ventricular tachycardia,*** *chest pain,* edema.
EENT: burning in throat (with inhaled form), *pharyngitis.*
GI: *nausea, metallic taste, decreased appetite, vomiting,* diarrhea, abdominal pain, anorexia, ***pancreatitis.***
GU: ***acute renal failure.***
Hematologic: ***leukopenia, thrombocytopenia,*** anemia.
Metabolic: ***hypoglycemia,*** hyperglycemia, hypocalcemia.
Musculoskeletal: myalgia.
Respiratory: *cough,* ***bronchospasm,*** *shortness of breath,* pneumothorax, *congestion.*
Skin: rash, ***Stevens-Johnson syndrome.***
Other: *night sweats, chills, sterile abscess, pain, induration at injection site.*

Interactions

Drug-drug. *Aminoglycosides, amphotericin B, capreomycin, cisplatin, methoxyflurane, polymyxin B, vancomycin:* May increase risk of nephrotoxicity. Monitor renal function test results closely.
Antineoplastics: May cause additive bone marrow suppression. Use together cautiously; monitor hematologic study results.
Drugs that prolong the QT interval (antipsychotics; antiarrhythmics, such as amiodarone, disopyramide, procainamide, quinidine, and sotalol; fluoroquinolones; macrolides; tricyclic antidepressants): May cause additive effect. Use together cautiously; monitor patient for adverse cardiac effects.

Nursing considerations

- Give aerosol form only by Respirgard II nebulizer. Dosage recommendations are based on particle size and delivery rate of this device. To give aerosol, mix contents of one vial in 6 ml sterile water for injection. Don't use normal saline solution. Don't mix with other drugs.
- Don't use low-pressure (less than 20 pounds per square inch [psi]) compressors. The flow rate should be 5 to 7 L/minute from a 40- to 50-psi air or oxygen source.
- For I.M. injection, reconstitute drug with 3 ml sterile water for a solution containing 100 mg/ml; administer deep into muscle. Expect patient to report pain and induration at injection site. Rotate injection sites.

!!ALERT Monitor glucose, calcium, creatinine, and BUN levels daily. After parenteral administration, glucose level may decrease initially; hypoglycemia may be severe in 5% to 10% of patients. After several months of therapy, this may be followed by hyperglycemia and type 1 diabetes mellitus, which may be permanent because of pancreatic cell damage.

- In patients with AIDS, pentamidine may produce less severe adverse reactions than co-trimoxazole.

Patient teaching

- Instruct patient to use the aerosol device until the chamber is empty, which may take up to 45 minutes.
- Warn patient that I.M. injection is painful.
- Instruct patient to complete the full course of pentamidine therapy, even if he's feeling better.

pentazocine hydrochloride
Talwin†

pentazocine hydrochloride and naloxone hydrochloride
Talwin NX

pentazocine lactate
Talwin

Pregnancy risk category C
Controlled substance schedule IV

Indications & dosages

➲ Moderate to severe pain
Adults: 50 to 100 mg P.O. q 3 to 4 hours, p.r.n. Maximum oral dose is 600 mg/day. Or, 30 mg I.M., I.V., or S.C. q 3 to 4 hours, p.r.n. Maximum parenteral dose is 360 mg/day. Single doses above 30 mg I.V. or 60 mg I.M. or S.C. aren't recommended.

➲ Labor
Adults: 30 mg I.M. as a single dose or 20 mg I.V. q 2 to 3 hours when contractions become regular for two to three doses.

Contraindications & cautions

- Contraindicated in patients hypersensitive to drug or its components and in children younger than age 12.
- Use cautiously in patients with hepatic or renal disease, acute MI, head injury, increased intracranial pressure, and respiratory depression.

Adverse reactions

CNS: *sedation*, visual disturbances, hallucinations, drowsiness, *dizziness*, *lightheadedness*, confusion, *euphoria*, headache, psychotomimetic effects.
CV: circulatory depression, ***shock***, hypertension, hypotension.
EENT: dry mouth.
GI: *nausea*, *vomiting*, constipation.
GU: urine retention.
Respiratory: ***respiratory depression***, dyspnea, ***apnea***.
Skin: induration, nodules, sloughing, sclerosis at injection site, diaphoresis, pruritus.
Other: hypersensitivity reactions, ***anaphylaxis***, physical and psychological dependence.

Interactions

Drug-drug. *CNS depressants:* May cause additive effects. Use together cautiously.
Fluoxetine: May cause additive effects resulting in serotonin syndrome. Use together cautiously.
Opioid analgesics: May decrease analgesic effect. Avoid using together.
Drug-lifestyle. *Alcohol use:* May cause additive effects. Discourage use together.
Smoking: May increase requirements for pentazocine. Monitor drug's effectiveness.

Nursing considerations

- Reassess patient's level of pain at least 15 and 30 minutes after parenteral administration and 30 minutes after oral administration.
- Have naloxone readily available. Respiratory depression can be reversed with naloxone.

!!ALERT When giving by S.C. or I.M. injection, rotate injection sites to minimize tissue irritation. If possible, avoid giving by S.C. route.

- Drug has opioid antagonist properties. May cause withdrawal syndrome in opioid-dependent patients.
- Psychological and physical dependence may occur with prolonged use.

Patient teaching

- Instruct patient to ask for drug before pain is intense.
- Caution ambulatory patient about getting out of bed or walking. Warn outpatient to avoid driving and other hazardous activities that require mental alertness until drug's CNS effects are known.
- Advise patient to avoid alcohol during therapy.
- Instruct patient or family to report skin rash, disorientation, or confusion to prescriber.

pentetate calcium trisodium (Ca-DTPA)

pentetate zinc trisodium (Zn-DTPA)

Pregnancy risk category C (Ca-DTPA); B (Zn-DTPA)

Indications & dosages

➲ To increase rate of plutonium, americium, or curium elimination in patients with internal contamination

Adults and children age 12 and older: Initially, 1 g Ca-DTPA by slow I.V. push over 3 to 4 minutes (or diluted in 100 to 250 ml D_5W, Ringer's lactate, or normal saline solution and infused over 30 minutes) within the first 24 hours of exposure. Then, 1 g once daily of Zn-DTPA by slow I.V. push over 3 to 4 minutes (or diluted in 100 to 250 ml D_5W, Ringer's lactate, or normal saline solution and infused over 30 minutes) until radioactive substances are removed.

If patient was exposed by inhalation, solution may be given by nebulized inhalation at a rate of 1:1 with sterile water or saline.

Children younger than age 12: Initially, 14 mg/kg Ca-DTPA (maximum dose, 1 g) by slow I.V. push over 3 to 4 minutes within the first 24 hours of exposure. Then, 14 mg/kg once daily of Zn-DTPA by slow I.V. push over 3 to 4 minutes (maximum dose, 1 g) until radioactive substances are removed.

Contraindications & cautions

- No known contraindications.
- Use cautiously in patients with severe hemochromatosis.
- Use inhalation route cautiously in patients with asthma.

Adverse reactions

CNS: headache, light-headedness.
CV: chest pain.
GI: diarrhea, metallic taste, nausea.
Skin: dermatitis, injection site reactions.
Other: allergic reaction.

Interactions

None reported.

Nursing considerations

- Binding capacity of Ca-DTPA is greatest in first 24 hours after exposure.

!!ALERT If patient needs further therapy after receiving Ca-DTPA, switch to Zn-DTPA to avoid mineral depletion. If Zn-DTPA isn't available, treatment may continue with Ca-DTPA as long as the patient receives supplemental zinc.

- I.V. administration is preferred when the route of contamination is unknown or if contamination occurred by multiple routes.
- If contamination occurred only by inhalation and within 24 hours, drug may be delivered by nebulized inhalation. It should be diluted 1:1 with sterile water or saline solution.
- Before treatment starts, obtain baseline CBC, serum zinc level, BUN level, serum chemistries and electrolytes, urine analysis, and blood and urine radioassays.
- The elimination rate is based on the quantity of radioactivity taken in.
- During treatment, measure the radioactivity of blood, urine, and feces weekly.
- Monitor CBC, BUN level, serum chemistries and electrolytes, and urine analysis regularly during treatment.
- Treatment of pregnant patients should start and continue with Zn-DTPA (if available) unless patient has a high level of internal radioactive contamination. If the level of contamination is high, therapy may start with a single dose of Ca-DTPA and zinc-containing vitamin or minerals supplements.
- Nebulized inhalation isn't indicated for children.

Patient teaching

- Instruct patient to drink plenty of fluids to cause frequent urination.
- Remind patient that drug enhances elimination of radioactivity in urine, which may make urine highly radioactive and dangerous to others.
- Instruct patient to flush the toilet several times after each use and to wash hands thoroughly after urinating.
- If the patient is coughing, tell him to dispose of phlegm carefully and not to swallow it, if possible.
- Tell parents of young children to dispose of dirty diapers properly and to avoid han-

dling urine, feces, or phlegm of children receiving treatment.

- Tell patient it isn't known if drug appears in breast milk, but radiocontaminants do. Patient shouldn't breast-feed during therapy and should take precautions when discarding breast milk.

pentobarbital
Nembutal†*

pentobarbital sodium
Nembutal Sodium*, Nova Rectal†, NovoPentobarb†

Pregnancy risk category D
Controlled substance schedule II; Controlled substance schedule: III for suppositories

Indications & dosages

➲ Sedation
Adults: 20 mg P.O. t.i.d. or q.i.d.
Children: 2 to 6 mg/kg P.O. daily in three divided doses. Maximum daily dose is 100 mg.

➲ Insomnia
Adults: 100 to 200 mg P.O. h.s. Or, 150 to 200 mg deep I.M. Or, 100 mg I.V. initially, with further small doses up to total of 500 mg. Or, 120 or 200 mg P.R.
Children: 2 to 6 mg/kg or 125 mg/m^2 I.M. Maximum dose is 100 mg.
Children ages 12 to 14: 60 or 120 mg P.R.
Children ages 5 to 11: 60 mg P.R.
Children ages 1 to 4: 30 or 60 mg P.R.
Children ages 2 months to 1 year: 30 mg P.R.

➲ Preoperative sedation
Adults: 150 to 200 mg I.M.
Children age 10 and older: 5 mg/kg P.O. or I.M.
Children younger than age 10: 5 mg/kg I.M. or P.R.

Contraindications & cautions

- Contraindicated in patients hypersensitive to barbiturates and in those with porphyria, bronchopneumonia, or other severe pulmonary insufficiency, and in severe liver or renal dysfunction.
- Use cautiously in elderly or debilitated patients and in patients with acute or chronic pain, mental depression, suicidal tendencies, history of drug abuse, or hepatic impairment.

Adverse reactions

CNS: *drowsiness, lethargy, hangover,* paradoxical excitement in elderly patients, somnolence, physical and psychological dependence.
GI: nausea, vomiting.
Hematologic: worsening porphyria.
Respiratory: ***respiratory depression.***
Skin: rash, urticaria, ***Stevens-Johnson syndrome.***
Other: *angioedema.*

Interactions

Drug-drug. *CNS depressants, including opioid analgesics:* May cause excessive CNS and respiratory depression. Use together cautiously.
Corticosteroids, digitoxin, doxycycline, estrogens and hormonal contraceptives, oral anticoagulants, theophylline, verapamil: May enhance metabolism of these drugs. Watch for decreased effect.
Griseofulvin: May decrease absorption of griseofulvin. Monitor effectiveness of griseofulvin.
MAO inhibitors, valproic acid: May inhibit metabolism of barbiturates; may prolong CNS depression. Reduce barbiturate dosage.
Metoprolol, propranolol: May reduce effects of these drugs. May need to increase beta-blocker dose.
Rifampin: May decrease barbiturate level. Watch for decreased effect of pentobarbital.
Drug-lifestyle. *Alcohol use:* May impair coordination, increase CNS effects, and cause death. Strongly discourage alcohol use with these drugs.

Nursing considerations

- Assess mental status before starting therapy and reduce doses in elderly patients; these patients may be more sensitive to drug's adverse CNS effects.

‼ALERT Give I.M. injection deeply with no more than 5 ml of drug at any one site. Superficial injection may cause pain, sterile abscess, and sloughing.

- To ensure accurate dosage, don't divide suppositories.

• Take precautions to prevent hoarding or overdosing by patients who are depressed, suicidal, or drug-dependent or who have a history of drug abuse.
• Watch for signs of barbiturate toxicity: coma, pupillary constriction, cyanosis, clammy skin, and hypotension. Overdose can be fatal.
• Inspect patient's skin. Skin eruptions may precede potentially fatal reactions to barbiturate therapy. Stop drug when skin reactions occur and call prescriber. In some patients, high temperature, stomatitis, headache, or rhinitis may precede skin reactions.
• Drug has no analgesic effect and may cause restlessness or delirium in patients with pain.
• Long-term use isn't recommended; drug loses its effectiveness in promoting sleep after 14 days of continuous use. Long-term high dosage may cause drug dependence, and patient may experience withdrawal symptoms if drug is suddenly stopped. Withdraw barbiturates gradually.
• EEG patterns show a change in low-voltage fast activity; changes persist after stopping therapy.
!!ALERT Don't confuse pentobarbital with phenobarbital.
!!ALERT Nembutal may contain tartrazine.

Patient teaching

• Inform patient that morning hangover is common after hypnotic dose, which suppresses REM sleep. Patient may experience increased dreaming after drug is stopped.
• Caution patient to avoid performing activities that require mental alertness or physical coordination.
• Tell patient to avoid alcohol use while taking drug.
• Instruct patient using hormonal contraceptives to consider alternative birth control methods, because drug may decrease contraceptive's effect.

pergolide mesylate
Permax

Pregnancy risk category B

Indications & dosages

➲ Adjunctive treatment with levodopa and carbidopa to manage signs and symptoms of Parkinson's disease
Adults: Initially, 0.05 mg P.O. daily for first 2 days; then increase by 0.1 to 0.15 mg q third day over 12 days. Increase subsequent dosage by 0.25 mg q third day, if needed, until optimum response is achieved. Maximum dose is 5 mg daily. Drug is usually given in divided doses t.i.d. Gradual reduction in levodopa and carbidopa dosage may be needed during dosage adjustment.

Contraindications & cautions

• Contraindicated in patients hypersensitive to drug or to ergot alkaloids.
• Use cautiously in patients prone to arrhythmias.
• Use cautiously in patients with a history of pleuritis, pleural effusion, pleural fibrosis, pericarditis, pericardial effusion, cardiac valvulopathy, or retroperitoneal fibrosis.
• Because of the possible additive sedative effects, use cautiously in patients taking other CNS depressants with pergolide mesylate.

Adverse reactions

CNS: headache, chills, asthenia, *dyskinesia, dizziness, hallucinations, dystonia, confusion, somnolence*, insomnia, anxiety, depression, tremor, abnormal dreams, personality disorder, psychosis, abnormal gait, akathisia, extrapyramidal syndrome, incoordination, akinesia, hypertonia, neuralgia, speech disorder, syncope, twitching, paresthesia.
CV: *orthostatic hypotension*, vasodilation, palpitations, ***valvulopathy***, ***fibrosis***, hypotension, hypertension, ***arrhythmias***, ***MI***.
EENT: *rhinitis*, epistaxis, abnormal vision, diplopia, eye disorder.
GI: dry mouth, taste perversion, abdominal pain, *nausea, constipation*, diarrhea, dyspepsia, anorexia, vomiting.
GU: urinary frequency, UTI, hematuria.
Metabolic: weight gain.

Musculoskeletal: arthralgia, bursitis, myalgia, chest, neck, and back pain.
Respiratory: dyspnea.
Skin: rash, diaphoresis.
Other: flulike syndrome, infection, facial, peripheral, and generalized edema.

Interactions

Drug-drug. *Dopamine antagonists:* May antagonize effects of pergolide. Avoid using together.

Nursing considerations

!!ALERT Monitor blood pressure. Symptomatic orthostatic or sustained hypotension may occur, especially at start of therapy.

- Periodically evaluate patient for somnolence. If a patient develops significant daytime sleepiness or episodes of falling asleep during activities that require participation (such as conversations and eating), stop drug. If a decision is made to continue drug, advise patient not to drive and to avoid other potentially dangerous activities. Although dose reduction may reduce the degree of somnolence, it may not eliminate abnormal somnolence altogether.
- Patient should be evaluated for underlying valvular disease, including echocardiogram, before beginning therapy with pergolide.
- Therapy should be stopped if patient develops a fibrotic condition or cardiac valvular disease during treatment.

!!ALERT Don't confuse Permax with Permitil.

Patient teaching

- Inform patient about possible adverse reactions, especially hallucinating, being confused, and suddenly falling asleep during daily activities.
- Advise patient that if he has increased somnolence or new episodes of falling asleep during daily activities, he shouldn't drive or participate in potentially dangerous activities until he has notified his prescriber.
- Warn patient to avoid activities that could result in injury from fainting or dizziness upon standing up quickly.
- Remind patient of the need for regular cardiovascular follow-up during the course of the drug therapy.
- Advise patient to take drug with food.

permethrin

Acticin, Elimite, Nix ◇

Pregnancy risk category B

Indications & dosages

➲ **Infestation with *Pediculus humanus capitis* (head louse) and its nits**
Adults and children age 2 and older: Use after hair has been washed with shampoo, rinsed with water, and towel-dried. Apply 25 to 50 ml of liquid to saturate hair and scalp. Allow drug to remain on hair for 10 minutes before rinsing off with water. Usually only one application is needed.
➲ **Infestation with *Sarcoptes scabiei***
Adults and children age 2 months and older: Thoroughly massage into the skin from the head to the soles. Treat infants on hairline, neck, scalp, temple, and forehead. Wash cream off after 8 to 14 hours.

Contraindications & cautions

- Contraindicated in patients hypersensitive to pyrethrins, chrysanthemums, or components of drug.

Adverse reactions

Skin: pruritus, *burning, stinging,* edema, tingling, scalp numbness or discomfort, mild erythema, scalp rash.

Interactions

None significant.

Nursing considerations

- Usually only one application is needed. Combing of nits isn't needed for effectiveness, but drug package supplies a fine-tooth comb for cosmetic use, as desired.
- Re-treat for lice, as prescribed, if lice are observed 7 days after first application.
- Treat sexual contacts simultaneously.

Patient teaching

- Explain that treatment may temporarily worsen signs and symptoms of head lice infestation, such as itching, redness, and swelling.
- Tell patient to disinfect headgear, comb and brush, scarves, coats, and bed linens by machine washing with hot water and machine drying for at least 20 minutes, using hot cycle. Tell him to seal nonwashable

items in plastic bag for 2 weeks or spray with product designed to eliminate lice and their nits.
- Warn patient not to use drug on eyes, eyelashes, eyebrows, nose, mouth, or mucous membranes.
- Tell patient to warn other family members and sexual contacts about infestation.

perphenazine
Apo-Perphenazine†, Trilafon

Pregnancy risk category NR

Indications & dosages

➲ Psychosis in nonhospitalized patients
Adults and children older than age 12: Initially, 4 to 8 mg P.O. t.i.d.; reduce as soon as possible to minimum effective dose.

➲ Psychosis in hospitalized patients
Adults and children older than age 12: Initially, 8 to 16 mg P.O. b.i.d., t.i.d., or q.i.d.; increase to 64 mg daily, p.r.n. Or, 5 to 10 mg I.M. q 6 hours, p.r.n. Maximum dose, 30 mg.

➲ Severe nausea and vomiting
Adults: 8 to 16 mg P.O. daily in divided doses to maximum of 24 mg. Or, 5 to 10 mg I.M., p.r.n. May be given I.V., diluted to 0.5 mg/ml with saline solution. Dose given I.V. shouldn't exceed 5 mg.

Contraindications & cautions

- Contraindicated in patients hypersensitive to drug and in those with CNS depression, blood dyscrasia, bone marrow depression, liver damage, or subcortical damage; also contraindicated in those experiencing coma or receiving large doses of CNS depressants.
- Use cautiously in elderly or debilitated patients and in those taking other CNS depressants or anticholinergics.
- Use cautiously in patients with alcohol withdrawal, psychotic depression, suicidal tendency, severe adverse reactions to other phenothiazines, renal impairment, CV disease, or respiratory disorders.

Adverse reactions

CNS: *extrapyramidal reactions, tardive dyskinesia,* sedation, pseudoparkinsonism, dizziness, ***seizures***, drowsiness, ***neuroleptic malignant syndrome***.
CV: *orthostatic hypotension,* tachycardia, ECG changes.
EENT: ocular changes, *blurred vision,* nasal congestion.
GI: *dry mouth, constipation,* nausea, vomiting, diarrhea.
GU: *urine retention,* dark urine, menstrual irregularities, inhibited ejaculation.
Hematologic: ***leukopenia***, ***agranulocytosis***, eosinophilia, hemolytic anemia, ***thrombocytopenia***.
Hepatic: cholestatic jaundice.
Metabolic: weight gain.
Skin: *mild photosensitivity reactions,* allergic reactions, pain at I.M. injection site, sterile abscess.
Other: gynecomastia.

Interactions

Drug-drug. *Antacids:* May inhibit absorption of oral phenothiazines. Separate antacid and phenothiazine doses by at least 2 hours.
Barbiturates: May decrease phenothiazine effect. Monitor patient.
CNS depressants: May increase CNS depression. Use together cautiously.
Fluoxetine, paroxetine, sertraline, tricyclic antidepressants: May increase phenothiazine level. Monitor patient for increased adverse effects.
Lithium: May increase neurologic adverse effects. Monitor patient closely.
Drug-herb. *St. John's wort:* May cause photosensitivity reactions. Advise patient to avoid excessive sunlight exposure.
Drug-lifestyle. *Alcohol use:* May increase CNS depression, particularly psychomotor skills. Strongly discourage alcohol use.
Sun exposure: May increase risk of photosensitivity reactions. Advise patient to avoid excessive sunlight exposure.

Nursing considerations

- Obtain baseline blood pressure measurements before starting therapy and monitor pressure regularly. Watch for orthostatic hypotension, especially with parenteral administration. Keep patient supine for 1 hour after giving drug; tell him to change positions slowly.
- Protect drug from light. Slight yellowing of injection or concentrate is common and doesn't affect potency. Discard markedly discolored solutions.

- Prevent contact dermatitis by keeping drug away from skin and clothes. Wear gloves when preparing liquid forms.
- Dilute liquid concentrate with fruit juice, milk, carbonated beverage, or semisolid food just before giving. Don't use colas, black coffee, grape juice, apple juice, or tea because turbidity or precipitation may result.
- Give by deep I.M. injection only in upper outer quadrant of buttocks. Massage slowly afterward to prevent sterile abscess. Injection may sting.
- Monitor patient for tardive dyskinesia, which may occur after prolonged use. It may not appear until months or years later and may disappear spontaneously or persist for life, despite ending drug.

!!ALERT Watch for evidence of neuroleptic malignant syndrome (extrapyramidal effects, hyperthermia, autonomic disturbance), which is rare but commonly fatal. It may not be related to length of drug use or type of neuroleptic; more than 60% of affected patients are men.

- Monitor therapy with weekly bilirubin tests during first month, periodic blood tests (CBCs and liver function tests), and ophthalmic tests (long-term use).
- Withhold dose and notify prescriber if jaundice, symptoms of blood dyscrasia (fever, sore throat, infection, cellulitis, weakness), or persistent extrapyramidal reactions (longer than a few hours) develop.
- Don't withdraw drug abruptly unless severe adverse reactions occur.
- After abrupt withdrawal of long-term therapy, gastritis, nausea, vomiting, dizziness, tremor, feeling of warmth or cold, diaphoresis, tachycardia, headache, or insomnia may occur.

Patient teaching

- Tell patient which beverages to use to dilute oral concentrate.
- Warn patient to avoid activities that require alertness or good coordination until effects of drug are known. Drowsiness and dizziness usually subside after a few weeks.
- Tell patient to avoid alcohol while taking drug.
- Advise patient to report signs of urine retention or constipation.
- Tell patient to use sunblock and wear protective clothing to avoid oversensitivity to the sun.
- Advise patient to relieve dry mouth with sugarless gum or hard candy.

phenazopyridine hydrochloride

Azo-Standard ◇, Baridium ◇, Geridium, Phenazo†, Prodium ◇, Pyridiate, Pyridium, Urodine, Urogesic, UTI-Relief

Pregnancy risk category B

Indications & dosages

➲ Pain with urinary tract irritation or infection

Adults: 200 mg P.O. t.i.d. after meals for 2 days.

Children ages 6 to 12: 12 mg/kg P.O. daily in three equally divided doses after meals for 2 days.

Contraindications & cautions

- Contraindicated in patients hypersensitive to drug and in those with glomerulonephritis, severe hepatitis, uremia, renal insufficiency, or pyelonephritis during pregnancy.

Adverse reactions

CNS: headache.
EENT: staining of contact lenses.
GI: nausea, GI disturbances.
Hematologic: hemolytic anemia, methemoglobinemia.
Skin: rash, pruritus.
Other: ***anaphylactoid reactions***.

Interactions

None significant.

Nursing considerations

- When drug is used with an antibacterial, therapy shouldn't extend beyond 2 days.

!!ALERT Don't confuse Pyridium with pyridoxine.

Patient teaching

- Advise patient that taking drug with meals may minimize GI distress.
- Caution patient to stop drug and notify prescriber immediately if skin or sclera becomes yellow-tinged, which may indicate drug accumulation from impaired renal excretion.

- Inform patient that drug colors urine red or orange and may stain fabrics and contact lenses.
- Tell diabetic patient to use Clinitest for accurate urine glucose test results. Also tell patient that drug may interfere with urinary ketone tests (Acetest or Ketostix).
- Advise patient to notify prescriber if urinary tract pain persists. Tell him that drug shouldn't be used for long-term treatment.

phentermine hydrochloride

Adipex-P, Ionamin, Pro-Fast HS, Pro-Fast SA, Pro-Fast SR

Pregnancy risk category NR
Controlled substance schedule IV

Indications & dosages

➲ **Short-term adjunct in exogenous obesity**

Adults: 8 mg P.O. t.i.d. 30 minutes before meals. Or, 15 to 37.5 mg or 15 to 30 mg (as resin complex) P.O. daily as a single dose in the morning. Give Pro-Fast HS and Pro-Fast SR 2 hours after breakfast. Give Adipex-P before breakfast or 1 to 2 hours after breakfast.

Contraindications & cautions

- Contraindicated in patients hypersensitive to sympathomimetic amines, in those with idiosyncratic reactions to them, in agitated patients, and in those with hyperthyroidism, moderate-to-severe hypertension, advanced arteriosclerosis, symptomatic CV disease, or glaucoma.
- Contraindicated within 14 days of MAO inhibitor therapy.
- Use cautiously in patients with mild hypertension.

Adverse reactions

CNS: overstimulation, headache, euphoria, dysphoria, dizziness, *insomnia*.
CV: *palpitations*, *tachycardia*, increased blood pressure.
GI: dry mouth, dysgeusia, constipation, diarrhea, unpleasant taste, other GI disturbances.
GU: impotence.
Skin: urticaria.
Other: altered libido.

Interactions

Drug-drug. *Acetazolamide, antacids, sodium bicarbonate:* May increase renal reabsorption. Monitor patient for enhanced effects.
Ammonium chloride, ascorbic acid: May decrease level and increase renal excretion of phentermine. Monitor patient for decreased phentermine effects.
Insulin, oral antidiabetics: May alter antidiabetic requirements. Monitor glucose level.
MAO inhibitors: May cause severe hypertension or hypertensive crisis. Avoid using within 14 days of MAO inhibitor therapy.
Drug-food. *Caffeine:* May increase CNS stimulation. Discourage use together.

Nursing considerations

- Use drug with a weight-reduction program.
- Monitor patient for tolerance or dependence.

!!ALERT Don't confuse phentermine with phentolamine.

Patient teaching

- Tell patient to take drug at least 10 hours before bedtime to avoid sleep interference.
- Advise patient to avoid products that contain caffeine. Tell him to report evidence of excessive stimulation.
- Warn patient that fatigue may result as drug effects wear off, and that he'll need more rest.
- Warn patient that drug may lose its effectiveness over time.

phenylephrine hydrochloride (nasal)

Alconefrin Nasal Drops 12 ◇, Alconefrin Nasal Drops 25 ◇, Alconefrin Nasal Drops 50 ◇, Doktors ◇, Duration ◇, Little Noses Gentle Formula ◇, Neo-Synephrine ◇, Nostril ◇, Rhinall ◇, Rhinall-10 Children's Flavored Nose Drops ◇, Sinex ◇

Pregnancy risk category C

Indications & dosages

➲ **Nasal congestion**

Adults and children age 12 and older: 2 or 3 drops or 1 to 2 sprays in each nostril q 4

hours, p.r.n. Don't use for longer than 3 to 5 days.
Children ages 6 to 12: 2 or 3 drops or 1 to 2 sprays of 0.25% solution in each nostril q 4 hours, p.r.n.
Children ages 2 to 6: 2 or 3 drops of 0.125% solution q 4 hours, p.r.n.

Contraindications & cautions

- Contraindicated in patients hypersensitive to drug.
- Use cautiously in patients with hyperthyroidism, marked hypertension, type 1 diabetes mellitus, cardiac disease, or advanced arteriosclerotic changes; in children with low body weight; and in elderly patients.

Adverse reactions

CNS: headache, tremor, dizziness, nervousness.
CV: *palpitations, tachycardia,* PVCs, hypertension, pallor.
EENT: transient burning or stinging, dryness of nasal mucosa, rebound nasal congestion.
GI: nausea.

Interactions

None significant.

Nursing considerations

- Monitor patient for systemic adverse effects.
- Don't use in children who are younger than age 2.

Patient teaching

- Teach patient how to use drug. Tell him to hold head upright to minimize swallowing of drug and to sniff spray briskly.
- Caution patient not to share drug because this could spread infection.
- Tell patient not to exceed recommended dosage and to use only when needed.
- Advise patient to contact prescriber if signs and symptoms persist longer than 3 days.
- Inform patient that prolonged use may result in rebound congestion.

phenylephrine hydrochloride (ophthalmic)

AK-Dilate, AK-Nefrin, Ophthalmic ◇, Isopto Frin ◇, Mydfrin, Neo-Synephrine, Phenoptic, Prefrin Liquifilm ◇, Relief ◇

Pregnancy risk category C

Indications & dosages

➲ Mydriasis without cycloplegia
Adults and children: Instill 1 drop of 2.5% or 10% solution before examination. May repeat in 1 hour, p.r.n. May need to apply topical anesthetic before use to prevent stinging and dilution from lacrimation.
➲ Mydriasis and vasoconstriction
Adults and adolescents: 1 drop of 2.5% or 10% solution.
Children: 1 drop of 2.5% solution.
➲ Chronic mydriasis
Adults and adolescents: 1 drop of 2.5% or 10% solution b.i.d. or t.i.d.
Children: Instill 1 drop of 2.5% solution b.i.d. or t.i.d.
➲ Posterior synechia (adhesion of iris)
Adults and children: Instill 1 drop of 2.5% or 10% solution. Don't use 10% concentration in infants.
➲ Minor eye irritations
Adults and children: 1 or 2 drops of the 0.12% solution in affected eye up to q.i.d., p.r.n.

Contraindications & cautions

- Contraindicated in patients hypersensitive to drug, in those with angle-closure glaucoma, and in those who wear soft contact lenses.
- Use cautiously in patients with marked hypertension, cardiac disorders, advanced arteriosclerotic changes, type 1 diabetes, or hyperthyroidism; in children with low body weight; and in elderly patients.

Adverse reactions

CNS: brow ache, headache.
CV: *hypertension,* with 10% solution, tachycardia, palpitations, PVCs, ***MI.***
EENT: transient eye burning or stinging on instillation, blurred vision, increased intraocular pressure, keratitis, lacrimation, reactive hyperemia of eye, allergic conjunctivitis, rebound miosis.

Skin: pallor, dermatitis, diaphoresis.
Other: trembling.

Interactions

Drug-drug. *Atropine (topical), cyclopentolate, homatropine, scopolamine:* May increase pupil dilation. Use together cautiously.
Beta blockers, MAO inhibitors: May cause arrhythmias because of increased pressor effect. Use together cautiously.
Guanethidine: May increase mydriatic and pressor effects of phenylephrine. Use together cautiously.
Levodopa: May reduce mydriatic effect of phenylephrine. Use together cautiously.
Tricyclic antidepressants: May increase cardiac effects of epinephrine. Use together cautiously.
Drug-lifestyle. *Sun exposure:* May cause photophobia. Advise patient to wear sunglasses.

Nursing considerations

- Systemic adverse reactions are least likely with 0.12% and 2.5% solutions and most likely with 10% solution.

!!ALERT Don't confuse Mydfrin with Midrin.

Patient teaching

- Teach patient how to instill drug. Advise him to wash hands before and after instillation and to apply light finger pressure on lacrimal sac for 1 minute after drops are instilled. Warn him not to touch tip of dropper to eye or surrounding tissue.
- Warn patient not to exceed recommended dosage because systemic effects can result. Monitor blood pressure and pulse rate.
- Tell patient not to use brown solution or solution that contains precipitate.
- Warn patient to avoid hazardous activities, such as operating machinery or driving, until temporary blurring subsides.
- Advise patient to contact prescriber if condition persists longer than 12 hours after stopping drug.
- Advise patient to ease photophobia by wearing dark glasses.

phenylephrine hydrochloride (systemic)

Neo-Synephrine

Pregnancy risk category C

Indications & dosages

➲ Hypotensive emergencies during spinal anesthesia
Adults: Initially, 0.2 mg I.V.; don't let subsequent doses exceed the preceding dose by more than 0.2 mg. Maximum single dose is 0.5 mg.

➲ To maintain blood pressure during spinal or inhaled anesthesia
Adults: 2 to 3 mg S.C. or I.M. 3 to 4 minutes before anesthesia.
Children: 0.044 mg to 0.088 mg/kg S.C. or I.M.

➲ To prolong spinal anesthesia
Adults: 2 to 5 mg added to anesthetic solution.

➲ Vasoconstrictor for regional anesthesia
Adults: 1 mg phenylephrine added to each 20 ml local anesthetic.

➲ Mild to moderate hypotension
Adults: 2 to 5 mg S.C. or I.M.; repeat in 1 or 2 hours as needed and tolerated. First dose shouldn't exceed 5 mg. Or, 0.1 to 0.5 mg slow I.V., not to be repeated more often than 10 to 15 minutes.
Children: 0.1 mg/kg or 3 mg/m^2 I.M. or S.C.; repeat in 1 or 2 hours as needed and tolerated.

➲ Severe hypotension and shock (including drug-induced)
Adults: 10 mg in 250 to 500 ml of D_5W or normal saline solution for injection. I.V. infusion started at 100 to 180 mcg/minute; then decrease to maintenance infusion of 40 to 60 mcg/minute when blood pressure stabilizes.

➲ Paroxysmal supraventricular tachycardia
Adults: Initially, 0.5 mg rapid I.V.; increase in increments of 0.1 to 0.2 mg. Use cautiously. Maximum single dose is 1 mg.

Contraindications & cautions

- Contraindicated in patients hypersensitive to drug and in those with severe hypertension or ventricular tachycardia.

• Use with caution in elderly patients and in patients with heart disease, hyperthyroidism, severe atherosclerosis, bradycardia, partial heart block, myocardial disease, or sulfite sensitivity.

Adverse reactions

CNS: *headache*, excitability, restlessness, anxiety, nervousness, dizziness, weakness.
CV: ***bradycardia***, ***arrhythmias***, hypertension.
Respiratory: ***asthmatic episodes***.
Skin: tissue sloughing with extravasation.
Other: tachyphylaxis and decreased organ perfusion with continued use, ***anaphylaxis***.

Interactions

Drug-drug. *Alpha blockers, phenothiazines:* May decrease pressor response. Monitor patient closely.
Beta blockers: May block cardiostimulatory effects. Monitor patient closely.
Guanethidine, oxytocics: May increase pressor response. Monitor patient.
Halogenated hydrocarbon anesthetics, sympathomimetics: May cause serious arrhythmias. Use together with caution.
MAO inhibitors (phenelzine, tranylcypromine): May cause severe headache, hypertension, fever, and hypertensive crisis. Avoid using together.
Tricyclic antidepressants: May potentiate pressor response and cause arrhythmias. Use together cautiously.

Nursing considerations

• Drug causes little or no CNS stimulation.
• Drug may lower intraocular pressure in normal eyes or in open-angle glaucoma. It also may cause false-normal tonometry readings.
• Drug is incompatible with butacaine sulfate, alkalis, ferric salts, and oxidizing drugs.
• Drug used in eyedrops and OTC cold preparations for decongestant effects.

Patient teaching

• Tell patient to report adverse reactions promptly.
• Instruct patient to report discomfort at I.V. insertion site.

phenytoin (diphenylhydantoin)
Dilantin 125, Dilantin Infatabs

phenytoin sodium (prompt)
Dilantin

phenytoin sodium (extended)
Dilantin Kapseals, Phenytek

Pregnancy risk category D

Indications & dosages

➲ To control tonic-clonic (grand mal) and complex partial (temporal lobe) seizures
Adults: Highly individualized. Initially, 100 mg P.O. t.i.d., increasing by 100 mg P.O. q 2 to 4 weeks until desired response is obtained. Usual range is 300 to 600 mg daily. If patient is stabilized with extended-release capsules, once-daily dosing with 300-mg extended-release capsules is possible as an alternative.
Children: 5 mg/kg or 250 mg/m^2 P.O. divided b.i.d. or t.i.d. Usual dose range is 4 to 8 mg/kg daily. Maximum daily dose is 300 mg.
➲ For patient requiring a loading dose
Adults: Initially, 1 g P.O. daily divided into three doses and given at 2-hour intervals. Or, 10 to 15 mg/kg I.V. at a rate not exceeding 50 mg/minute. Normal maintenance dosage is started 24 hours after loading dose.
Children: 500 to 600 mg P.O. in divided doses, followed by maintenance dosage 24 hours after loading dose.
➲ To prevent and treat seizures occurring during neurosurgery
Adults: 100 to 200 mg I.M. q 4 hours during and after surgery.
➲ Status epilepticus
Adults: Loading dose of 10 to 15 mg/kg I.V. (1 to 1.5 g may be needed) at a rate not exceeding 50 mg/minute; then maintenance dosage of 100 mg P.O. or I.V. q 6 to 8 hours.
Children: Loading dose of 15 to 20 mg/kg I.V., at a rate not exceeding 1 to 3 mg/kg/minute; then highly individualized maintenance dosages.
Elderly patients: May need lower dosages.

Contraindications & cautions

• Contraindicated in patients hypersensitive to hydantoin and in those with sinus bra-

dycardia, SA block, second- or third-degree AV block, or Adams-Stokes syndrome.
- Use cautiously in patients with hepatic dysfunction, hypotension, myocardial insufficiency, diabetes, or respiratory depression; in elderly or debilitated patients; and in those receiving other hydantoin derivatives.
- Elderly patients tend to metabolize phenytoin slowly and may need reduced dosages.

Adverse reactions

CNS: *ataxia, slurred speech*, dizziness, insomnia, nervousness, twitching, headache, *mental confusion, decreased coordination.*
CV: periarteritis nodosa.
EENT: *nystagmus, diplopia*, blurred vision.
GI: *gingival hyperplasia, nausea, vomiting*, constipation.
Hematologic: ***thrombocytopenia, leukopenia, agranulocytosis, pancytopenia***, macrocythemia, megaloblastic anemia.
Hepatic: ***toxic hepatitis***.
Metabolic: hyperglycemia.
Musculoskeletal: osteomalacia.
Skin: scarlatiniform or morbilliform rash, bullous or purpuric dermatitis, exfoliative dermatitis, ***Stevens-Johnson syndrome***, lupus erythematosus, ***toxic epidermal necrolysis***, photosensitivity reactions, discoloration of skin if given by I.V. push in back of hand, hypertrichosis, pain, necrosis, inflammation at injection site.
Other: *hirsutism*, lymphadenopathy.

Interactions

Drug-drug. *Amiodarone, antihistamines, chloramphenicol, cimetidine, cycloserine, diazepam, isoniazid, metronidazole, omeprazole, phenylbutazone, salicylates, sulfamethizole, valproate:* May increase phenytoin activity and toxicity. Monitor patient.
Atracurium, cisatracurium, doxacurium, mivacurium, pancuronium, rocuronium, tubocurarine, vecuronium: May decrease the effects of nondepolarizing muscle relaxant. May need to increase the nondepolarizing muscle relaxant dose.
Barbiturates, carbamazepine, dexamethasone, diazoxide, folic acid, rifampin: May decrease phenytoin activity. Monitor phenytoin level.
Carbamazepine, cardiac glycosides, hormonal contraceptives, quinidine, theophylline, valproic acid: May decrease effects of these drugs. Monitor patient.
Disulfiram: May increase toxic effects of phenytoin. Monitor phenytoin level closely and adjust dose as necessary.
Drug-food. *Enteral tube feedings:* May interfere with absorption of oral phenytoin. Stop enteral feedings for 2 hours before and 2 hours after phenytoin administration.
Drug-lifestyle. *Long-term alcohol use:* May decrease phenytoin activity. Strongly discourage patient from heavy alcohol use.

Nursing considerations

- Phenytoin requirements usually increase during pregnancy.
- Use only clear solution for injection. A slight yellow color is acceptable. Don't refrigerate.
- Don't give I.M. unless dosage adjustments are made; drug may precipitate at injection site, cause pain, and be absorbed erratically.
- Divided doses given with or after meals may decrease adverse GI reactions.
- Stop drug if rash appears. If rash is scarlatiniform or morbilliform, resume drug after rash clears. If rash reappears, stop therapy. If rash is exfoliative, purpuric, or bullous, don't resume drug.
- Don't stop drug suddenly because this may worsen seizures. Call prescriber at once if adverse reactions develop.
- Monitor drug level in blood. Therapeutic level is 10 to 20 mcg/ml.
- Allow at least 7 to 10 days to elapse between dosage changes.
- Monitor CBC and calcium level every 6 months, and periodically monitor hepatic function. If megaloblastic anemia is evident, prescriber may order folic acid and vitamin B_{12}.
- If using to treat seizures, take appropriate safety precautions.
- Mononucleosis may decrease phenytoin level. Watch for increased seizures.
- Watch for gingival hyperplasia, especially in children.

!!ALERT Doubling the dose doesn't result in twice initial serum levels but may result in toxic serum levels. Consult pharmacist for specific dosing recommendations.

- If seizure control is established with divided doses, once-a-day dosing may be considered.

!!ALERT Don't confuse phenytoin with mephenytoin or fosphenytoin or Dilantin with Dilaudid.

Patient teaching

- Tell patient to notify prescriber if skin rash develops.
- Advise patient to avoid driving and other potentially hazardous activities that require mental alertness until drug's CNS effects are known.
- Advise patient not to change brands or dosage forms once he's stabilized on therapy.
- Dilantin capsules are the only oral form that can be given once daily. Toxic levels may result if any other brand or form is given once daily. Dilantin tablets and oral suspension should never be taken once daily.
- Tell patient not to use capsules that are discolored.
- Advise patient to avoid alcohol.
- Warn patient and parents not to stop drug abruptly.
- Stress importance of good oral hygiene and regular dental examinations. Surgical removal of excess gum tissue may be needed periodically if dental hygiene is poor.
- Caution patient that drug may color urine pink, red, or reddish brown.

physostigmine salicylate (eserine salicylate)

Antilirium

Pregnancy risk category C

Indications & dosages

➲ To reverse CNS toxicity from clinical or toxic dosages of drugs capable of producing anticholinergic syndrome

Adults: 0.5 to 2 mg I.M. or I.V. or 1 mg/minute I.V. repeated q 20 minutes p.r.n. until patient responds or develops adverse cholinergic effects. Give additional 1 to 4 mg I.M. or I.V. q 30 to 60 minutes if life-threatening problems such as coma, seizures, and arrhythmias recur.

Children: Only for life-threatening situations. Give 0.02 mg/kg I.M. or slow I.V. at 0.5 mg/minute or slower, and repeat q 5 to 10 minutes until patient responds, adverse cholinergic reactions develop, or a total dose of 2 mg has been given.

Contraindications & cautions

- Contraindicated in patients with mechanical obstruction of the intestine or urogenital tract; in patients with asthma, gangrene, diabetes, CV disease, or vagotonia; and in patients receiving choline esters or depolarizing neuromuscular blockers.
- Use cautiously in pregnant patients and patients with epilepsy, parkinsonism, or bradycardia.

Adverse reactions

CNS: ***seizures***, muscle weakness, *restlessness, excitability.*
CV: ***bradycardia***, hypotension, palpitation, irregular pulse.
EENT: miosis, lacrimation.
GI: nausea, vomiting, epigastric pain, *diarrhea, excessive salivation.*
GU: urinary urgency.
Respiratory: ***bronchospasm***, ***bronchial constriction***, dyspnea, ***respiratory paralysis***.
Skin: diaphoresis.

Interactions

Drug-drug. *Anticholinergics, atropine, local and general anesthetics, procainamide, quinidine:* May reverse cholinergic effects. Observe patient for lack of drug effect.
Ganglionic blockers: May decrease blood pressure. Avoid using together.
Neuromuscular blockers (succinylcholine): May increase neuromuscular blockade, respiratory depression. Use together cautiously.
Drug-herb. *Jaborandi tree, pill-bearing spurge:* May have additive effect. Ask patient about use of herbal remedies, and recommend caution.

Nursing considerations

- Use only clear solution. Darkening may indicate loss of potency.

!!ALERT Watch closely for adverse reactions, particularly CNS disturbances. Raise side rails of bed if patient becomes restless or hallucinates. Adverse reactions may indicate drug toxicity.

- Effectiveness is typically immediate and dramatic but may be transient. Patient may need repeated dosages.

Patient teaching

- Inform patient of need for drug, explain its use and adverse reactions, and answer any questions or concerns.
- Tell patient to report adverse reactions promptly.
- Instruct patient to report discomfort at I.V. site.

pilocarpine hydrochloride
Salagen

Pregnancy risk category C

Indications & dosages

➲ Xerostomia from salivary gland hypofunction caused by radiotherapy for cancer of head and neck
Adults: 5 mg P.O. t.i.d.; may increase to 10 mg P.O. t.i.d., p.r.n.

➲ Dry mouth in patients with Sjögren's syndrome
Adults: 5 mg P.O. q.i.d.

Contraindications & cautions

- Contraindicated in patients hypersensitive to pilocarpine, in breast-feeding patients, in those with uncontrolled asthma, and in those for whom miosis is undesirable, as in acute iritis or angle-closure glaucoma.
- Use cautiously in patients with CV disease, controlled asthma, chronic bronchitis, COPD, cholelithiasis, biliary tract disease, nephrolithiasis, or cognitive or psychiatric disturbances.
- Safety and efficacy of drug in children haven't been established.

Adverse reactions

CNS: *dizziness*, *headache*, tremor, *asthenia*.
CV: hypertension, tachycardia, *flushing*, edema.
EENT: *rhinitis*, lacrimation, amblyopia, pharyngitis, voice alteration, conjunctivitis, epistaxis, *sinusitis*, *abnormal vision*.
GI: *nausea*, dyspepsia, diarrhea, abdominal pain, vomiting, dysphagia, taste perversion.
GU: *urinary frequency*.
Musculoskeletal: myalgia.
Skin: rash, pruritus, *sweating*.
Other: *chills*.

Interactions

Drug-drug. *Beta blockers:* May increase risk of conduction disturbances. Use together cautiously.
Drugs with anticholinergic effects: May antagonize anticholinergic effects. Use together cautiously.
Drugs with parasympathomimetic effects: May result in additive pharmacologic effects. Monitor patient closely.
Drug-food. *High-fat meals:* May reduce drug absorption. Discourage patient from eating high-fat meals.

Nursing considerations

- Examine patient's fundus carefully before beginning therapy because retinal detachment may occur in patients with retinal disease.
- Monitor patient for signs and symptoms of toxicity: headache, visual disturbance, lacrimation, sweating, respiratory distress, GI spasm, nausea, vomiting, diarrhea, AV block, tachycardia, bradycardia, hypotension, hypertension, shock, mental confusion, arrhythmia, and tremors. Immediately notify prescriber of suspected toxicity.

Patient teaching

- Warn patient that driving ability may be impaired, especially at night, by drug-induced visual disturbances.
- Advise patient to drink plenty of fluids to prevent dehydration.
- Tell elderly patient with Sjögren's syndrome that he may be especially prone to urinary frequency, diarrhea, and dizziness.
- Advise patient not to take drug with a high-fat meal.

pilocarpine hydrochloride
Adsorbocarpine, Akarpine, Isopto Carpine, Miocarpine†, Pilocar, Pilopine HS, Pilostat

pilocarpine nitrate
Pilagan Liquifilm

Pregnancy risk category C

Indications & dosages

➲ Primary open-angle glaucoma
Adults and children: Instill 1 or 2 drops up to q.i.d. or apply 1-cm ribbon of 4% gel h.s.

➲ **Emergency treatment of acute angle-closure glaucoma**
Adults and children: Instill 1 drop of 2% solution q 5 to 10 minutes for three to six doses; then 1 drop q 1 to 3 hours until pressure is controlled.
➲ **Mydriasis caused by mydriatic or cycloplegic drugs**
Adults and children: 1 drop of 1% solution.

Contraindications & cautions

- Contraindicated in patients hypersensitive to drug and in conditions in which cholinergic effects, such as constriction, are undesirable (acute iritis, some forms of secondary glaucoma, pupillary block glaucoma, or acute inflammatory disease of the anterior chamber).
- Use cautiously in patients with acute cardiac failure, bronchial asthma, peptic ulcer, hyperthyroidism, GI spasm, urinary tract obstruction, and Parkinson's disease.

Adverse reactions

CV: hypertension, tachycardia.
EENT: periorbital or supraorbital headache, *myopia*, ciliary spasm, *blurred vision*, conjunctival irritation, transient stinging and burning, keratitis, lens opacity, retinal detachment, lacrimation, changes in visual field, *brow pain*, salivation.
GI: nausea, vomiting, diarrhea.
Respiratory: bronchiolar spasm, ***pulmonary edema***.
Other: diaphoresis.

Interactions

Drug-drug. *Carbachol, echothiophate:* May cause additive effects. Avoid using together.
Cyclopentolate, ophthalmic belladonna alkaloids such as atropine, scopolamine: May decrease pilocarpine antiglaucoma effectiveness and block mydriatic effects of these drugs. Avoid using together.
Phenylephrine: May decrease dilation by phenylephrine. Avoid using together.

Nursing considerations

- Monitor vital signs.

!!ALERT Patients with hazel or brown irises may need stronger solutions or more frequent instillation because eye pigment may absorb drug.

Patient teaching

- Instruct patient to apply gel at bedtime because it will blur vision. Warn him to avoid hazardous activities, such as operating machinery or driving, until temporary blurring subsides.
- Teach patient how to instill drug. Advise him to wash hands before and after instillation and to apply light finger pressure on lacrimal sac for 1 minute after drops are instilled. Warn patient not to touch applicator tip to eye or surrounding tissue.
- Warn patient that transient brow pain and nearsightedness are common at first but usually disappear in 10 to 14 days.
- Advise patient to wear or carry medical identification at all times during therapy.

pimecrolimus
Elidel

Pregnancy risk category C

Indications & dosages

➲ **Short- and intermittent long-term treatment of mild to moderate atopic dermatitis in nonimmunocompromised patients in whom the use of other conventional therapies is deemed inadvisable, or in patients with inadequate response to or intolerance of conventional therapies**
Adults and children age 2 and older: Apply a thin layer to the affected skin b.i.d. and rub in gently and completely.

Contraindications & cautions

- Contraindicated in patients hypersensitive to drug or its components, in patients with Netherton's syndrome, and in immunocompromised patients.
- Contraindicated in patients with active cutaneous viral infections or infected atopic dermatitis.
- Use cautiously in patients with varicella zoster virus infection, herpes simplex virus infection, or eczema herpeticum.
- Safety of use in pregnant women hasn't been established.

Adverse reactions

CNS: *headache, fever.*
EENT: *nasopharyngitis*, otitis media, sinusitis, pharyngitis, tonsillitis, eye infection, nasal congestion, rhinorrhea, sinus conges-

tion, rhinitis, epistaxis, conjunctivitis, earache.
GI: gastroenteritis, abdominal pain, vomiting, diarrhea, nausea, constipation, loose stools.
GU: dysmenorrhea.
Musculoskeletal: back pain, arthralgias.
Respiratory: *upper respiratory tract infections*, pneumonia, *bronchitis*, *cough*, asthma, wheezing, dyspnea.
Skin: skin infections, impetigo, folliculitis, molluscum contagiosum, herpes simplex, varicella, papilloma, *application site reaction*, (burning, irritation, erythema, pruritus), urticaria, acne.
Other: *influenza*, flulike illness, hypersensitivity, toothache, bacterial infection, staphylococcal infection, viral infection.

Interactions

Drug-drug. *Cytochrome P-450 inhibitors (such as erythromycin, itraconazole, ketoconazole, fluconazole, calcium channel blockers):* May affect metabolism of pimecrolimus. Use together cautiously.
Drug-lifestyle. *Natural or artificial sunlight exposure:* May worsen atopic dermatitis. Avoid or minimize exposure.

Nursing considerations

!!ALERT Use drug only after other therapies have failed because of the risk of cancer.
- Drug may be used on all skin surfaces, including the head, neck, and intertriginous areas.
- Clear infections at treatment sites before using.
- If symptoms persist longer than 6 weeks, reevaluate the patient.
- Don't use with occlusive dressing.
- May cause local symptoms such as skin burning. Most local reactions start within 1 to 5 days after treatment, are mild to moderately severe, and last no longer than 5 days.
- Monitor patient for lymphadenopathy. If lymphadenopathy occurs and its cause is unknown, or if the patient develops acute infectious mononucleosis, consider stopping drug.
- Drug use may cause papillomas or warts. Consider stopping drug if papillomas worsen or don't respond to conventional treatment.
- It's unknown if drug appears in breast milk. Serious adverse reactions may occur in breast-feeding infants exposed to drug. Patient should either stop breast-feeding or stop treatment.

Patient teaching

- Inform patient that this medication is for external use only and that he should use it as directed.
- Tell patient to report adverse reactions.
- Tell patient not to use with an occlusive dressing.
- Instruct patient to wash hands after application if hands aren't treated.
- Tell patient to stop therapy after signs and symptoms have resolved. If symptoms persist longer than 6 weeks, tell him to contact his prescriber.
- Tell patient to resume treatment at first signs of recurrence.
- Stress that patient should minimize or avoid exposure to natural or artificial sunlight (including tanning beds and UVA-UVB treatment) while using this drug.
- Tell patient to expect application site reactions but to notify his prescriber if reaction is severe or persists for longer than 1 week.

pioglitazone hydrochloride
Actos

Pregnancy risk category C

Indications & dosages

➲ **Adjunct to diet and exercise to improve glycemic control in patients with type 2 (non–insulin-dependent) diabetes; when diet, exercise, and a sulfonylurea, metformin, or insulin fail to yield adequate glycemic control**
Adults: Initially, 15 or 30 mg P.O. once daily. For patients who respond inadequately to first dosage, it may be increased incrementally; maximum daily dose is 45 mg. If used in combination therapy, maximum daily dose shouldn't exceed 30 mg.

Contraindications & cautions

- Contraindicated in patients hypersensitive to drug or its components and in those with type 1 (insulin-dependent) diabetes, clinical evidence of active liver disease, ALT level greater than $2\frac{1}{2}$ times the upper limit of normal, or New York Heart Association (NYHA) Class III or IV heart failure.

- Contraindicated in patients with diabetic ketoacidosis and in those who experienced jaundice while taking troglitazone.
- Use cautiously in patients with edema or heart failure.

Adverse reactions

CNS: headache.
CV: *edema*, ***heart failure***.
EENT: sinusitis, pharyngitis.
Hematologic: anemia.
Metabolic: ***hypoglycemia with combination therapy***, aggravated diabetes, weight gain.
Musculoskeletal: myalgia.
Respiratory: upper respiratory tract infection.
Other: tooth disorder.

Interactions

Drug-drug. *Ketoconazole:* May inhibit pioglitazone metabolism. Monitor glucose level more frequently.
Hormonal contraceptives: May decrease level of hormonal contraceptives, reducing contraceptive effectiveness. Advise patient taking drug and hormonal contraceptives to consider additional birth control measures.
Drug-herb. *Burdock, dandelion, eucalyptus, marshmallow:* May increase hypoglycemic effects. Discourage use together.
Drug-lifestyle. *Alcohol use:* May alter glycemic control and increase risk of hypoglycemia. Discourage use together.

Nursing considerations

!!ALERT Measure liver enzyme levels at start of therapy, every 2 months for first year of therapy, and periodically thereafter. Obtain liver function test results in patients who develop signs and symptoms of liver dysfunction, such as nausea, vomiting, abdominal pain, fatigue, anorexia, or dark urine. Stop drug if patient develops jaundice or if liver function test results show ALT level greater than 3 times the upper limit of normal.

- Pioglitazone hydrochloride alone or with insulin can cause fluid retention that may lead to or worsen heart failure. Observe patients for these signs or symptoms of heart failure. Stop drug if cardiac status deteriorates. This drug isn't recommended for NYHA Class III or IV cardiac status patients.
- Because ovulation may resume in premenopausal, anovulatory women with insulin resistance, recommend use of additional contraceptive measures.
- Use drug in pregnant patients only if the benefit justifies risk to fetus. Insulin is the preferred antidiabetic for use during pregnancy.
- Monitor patients with heart failure for increased edema.
- Hemoglobin level and hematocrit may drop, usually during first 4 to 12 weeks of therapy.
- Management of type 2 diabetes should include diet control. Because caloric restrictions, weight loss, and exercise help improve insulin sensitivity and help make drug therapy effective, these measures are essential for proper diabetes management.
- Watch for hypoglycemia, especially in patients receiving combination therapy. Dosage adjustments of these drugs may be needed.
- Monitor glucose level regularly, especially during situations of increased stress, such as infection, fever, surgery, and trauma.
- Check glucose level and glycosylated hemoglobin periodically to evaluate therapeutic response to drug.
- Safety and efficacy of drug in children haven't been evaluated.

!!ALERT Don't confuse pioglitazone with rosiglitazone.

Patient teaching

- Instruct patient to adhere to dietary instructions and to have glucose and glycosylated hemoglobin levels tested regularly.
- Teach patient taking pioglitazone with insulin or oral antidiabetics the signs and symptoms of hypoglycemia.
- Advise patient to notify prescriber during periods of stress, such as fever, trauma, infection, or surgery, because dosage may have to be changed.
- Instruct patient how and when to monitor glucose level.
- Notify patient that blood tests of liver function will be performed before therapy starts, every 2 months for the first year, and periodically thereafter.
- Tell patient to report unexplained nausea, vomiting, abdominal pain, fatigue, anorexia,

or dark urine immediately because they may indicate liver problems.
- Warn patient to contact his health care provider if he has signs or symptoms of heart failure (unusually rapid increase in weight or swelling, shortness of breath).
- Advise anovulatory, premenopausal women with insulin resistance that therapy may cause resumption of ovulation; recommend using contraceptive measures.

pirbuterol acetate
Maxair, Maxair Autohaler

Pregnancy risk category C

Indications & dosages
➲ To prevent and reverse bronchospasm; asthma
Adults and children age 12 and older: 1 or 2 inhalations (0.2 to 0.4 mg), repeated q 4 to 6 hours. Don't exceed 12 inhalations daily.

Contraindications & cautions
- Contraindicated in patients hypersensitive to drug.
- Use cautiously in patients unusually responsive to sympathomimetic amines and patients with CV disorders, hyperthyroidism, diabetes, and seizure disorders.

Adverse reactions
CNS: tremor, nervousness, dizziness, insomnia, headache, vertigo.
CV: tachycardia, palpitations, chest tightness.
EENT: dry or irritated throat.
GI: nausea, vomiting, diarrhea, dry mouth.
Respiratory: cough.

Interactions
Drug-drug. *Beta blockers, propranolol:* May decrease bronchodilating effects. Avoid using together.
MAO inhibitors, tricyclic antidepressants: May potentiate action of beta agonist on vascular system. Use together cautiously.

Nursing considerations
- Monitor patient for increased pulse or blood pressure during therapy.
- Stop drug immediately and notify prescriber if paradoxical bronchospasm occurs.
- The likelihood of paradoxical bronchospasm is increased with the first use of a new canister or vial.
- Notify prescriber of decreasing effectiveness of the drug.

Patient teaching
- Teach patient to perform oral inhalation correctly. Give the following instructions for using a metered dose inhaler (MDI):
  - Shake canister.
  - Clear nasal passages and throat.
  - Breathe out, expelling as much air from lungs as possible.
  - Place mouthpiece well into mouth, and inhale deeply as you release dose from inhaler.
  - Hold breath for several seconds, remove mouthpiece, and exhale slowly.
- If more than 1 inhalation is ordered, tell patient to wait at least 2 minutes before repeating procedure.
- Give the following instructions for using Autohaler:
  - Remove mouthpiece cover by pulling down lip on back cover. Inspect mouthpiece for foreign objects. Locate "Up" arrows and air vents.
  - Hold Autohaler upright so that arrows point up; raise lever until it snaps into place.
  - Hold Autohaler around the middle, and shake gently several times.
  - Continue to hold upright, and be careful not to block air vents at bottom. Exhale normally before use.
  - Seal lips around mouthpiece. Inhale deeply through mouthpiece with steady, moderate force to trigger release of the drug. You'll hear a click and feel a soft puff when drug is released. Continue to take a full, deep breath.
  - Take Autohaler away from mouth when done inhaling. Hold breath for 10 seconds; then exhale slowly.
  - Continue to hold Autohaler upright while lowering lever. Lower lever after each puff. If additional puffs are ordered, wait 1 minute before repeating process to obtain the next puff.
- Have patient clean inhaler per manufacturer's instructions.
- If patient also uses a corticosteroid inhaler, tell him to use the bronchodilator first, and then wait about 5 minutes before using the corticosteroid. This allows the bronchodila-

tor to open air passages for maximum effectiveness of the corticosteroid.
- Instruct patient to call prescriber if bronchospasm increases after using drug.
- Advise patient to seek medical attention if a previously effective dosage doesn't control symptoms; this change may signal worsening of disease.

piroxicam
Apo-Piroxicam†, Feldene, Novo-Pirocam†

Pregnancy risk category B; D in 3rd trimester

Indications & dosages
➲ Osteoarthritis, rheumatoid arthritis
Adults: 20 mg P.O. daily. If desired, dose may be divided b.i.d.

Contraindications & cautions
- Contraindicated in patients hypersensitive to drug and in those with bronchospasm or angioedema precipitated by aspirin or NSAIDs.
- Contraindicated in pregnant or breastfeeding patients.
- Use cautiously in elderly patients and in patients with GI disorders, history of renal or peptic ulcer disease, cardiac disease, hypertension, or conditions predisposing to fluid retention.

Adverse reactions
CNS: *headache*, drowsiness, *dizziness*, somnolence, vertigo.
CV: peripheral edema.
EENT: auditory disturbances.
GI: epigastric distress, nausea, vomiting, occult blood loss, peptic ulceration, ***severe GI bleeding***, diarrhea, constipation, abdominal pain, heartburn, dyspepsia, flatulence, anorexia, stomatitis.
GU: ***nephrotoxicity***.
Hematologic: prolonged bleeding time, anemia, ***leukopenia***, ***agranulocytosis***, eosinophilia.
Metabolic: ***hyperkalemia***, ***hypoglycemia in diabetic patients***.
Skin: *pruritus*, *rash*.

Interactions
Drug-drug. *Antihypertensives, diuretics:* May decrease effects of these drugs. Avoid using together.
Aspirin, corticosteroids: May cause GI toxicity; may decrease level of piroxicam. Avoid using together.
Cyclosporine, methotrexate: May increase toxicity. Monitor patient closely.
Lithium: May increase lithium level. Monitor patient for toxicity.
Oral anticoagulants, other highly protein-bound drugs: May be toxic. Monitor patient closely.
Oral antidiabetics: May enhance antidiabetic effects. Monitor patient closely.
Ritonavir: May increase piroxicam level. Monitor patient for signs of toxicity.
Drug-herb. *Dong quai, feverfew, garlic, ginger, horse chestnut, red clover:* May cause bleeding. Discourage use together.
St. John's wort: May cause photosensitivity reaction. Advise patient to avoid excessive sunlight exposure.
White willow: Herb contains components similar to those of aspirin. Discourage use together.
Drug-lifestyle. *Alcohol use:* May cause GI toxicity, may decrease level of piroxicam. Discourage use together.
Sun exposure: May cause photosensitivity reaction. Advise patient to avoid excessive sunlight exposure.

Nursing considerations
- Because NSAIDs impair renal prostaglandin synthesis, they can decrease renal blood flow and lead to reversible renal impairment, especially in elderly patients, in patients taking diuretics, and in patients with renal failure, heart failure, or liver dysfunction. Monitor these patients closely.
- Check renal, hepatic, and auditory function and CBC periodically during prolonged therapy. Stop drug and notify prescriber if abnormalities occur.
- Serious GI toxicity, including peptic ulcers and bleeding, can occur in patient taking NSAIDs, despite lack of symptoms.
- NSAIDs may mask signs and symptoms of infection because of their antipyretic and anti-inflammatory actions.

Patient teaching

- Tell patient to take drug with milk, antacids, or meals if adverse GI reactions occur.
- Inform patient that full therapeutic effects may be delayed for 2 to 4 weeks.
- Teach patient signs and symptoms of GI bleeding, including blood in vomit, urine, or stool; coffee-ground vomit; and black, tarry stool. Tell him to notify prescriber immediately if any of these occurs.
- Warn patient against hazardous activities that require mental alertness until CNS effects are known.
- Because drug causes adverse skin reactions more often than other drugs in its class, advise patient to use a sunblock, wear protective clothing, and avoid prolonged exposure to sunlight. Sensitivity to the sun is the most common reaction.
- Advise patient that use of OTC NSAIDs in combination with piroxicam may increase the risk of GI toxicity.

plasma protein fractions

Plasmanate, Plasma-Plex, Plasmatein, Protenate

Pregnancy risk category C

Indications & dosages

➲ Shock

Adults: Varies with patient's condition and response, but usual dose is 250 to 500 ml I.V. (12.5 to 25 g protein), usually no faster than 10 ml/minute.

Infants and children: 6.6 to 33 ml/kg (0.33 to 1.65 g/kg of protein) I.V., 5 to 10 ml/minute.

➲ Hypoproteinemia

Adults: 1,000 to 1,500 ml I.V. daily. Maximum infusion rate is 5 to 8 ml/minute.

Contraindications & cautions

- Contraindicated in patients with severe anemia or heart failure and in those undergoing cardiac bypass.
- Use cautiously in patients with hepatic or renal failure, low cardiac reserve, or restricted sodium intake.

Adverse reactions

CNS: headache, fever.
CV: hypotension, ***vascular overload***, tachycardia, flushing.
GI: nausea, vomiting, hypersalivation.
Musculoskeletal: back pain.
Respiratory: dyspnea, ***pulmonary edema***.
Skin: rash, erythema.
Other: chills.

Interactions

None significant.

Nursing considerations

- Hypotension risk is greater when infusion rate exceeds 10 ml/minute.
- Monitor blood pressure. Be prepared to slow or stop infusion if hypotension suddenly occurs. Vital signs should return to normal gradually; assess them hourly.
- Watch for signs of vascular overload (heart failure or pulmonary edema).

!! ALERT Watch for hemorrhage or shock after surgery or injury. A rapid increase in blood pressure may cause bleeding from sites that isn't apparent at lower pressures.

- Report decreased urine output.
- Drug contains 130 to 160 mEq of sodium per liter.

Patient teaching

- Explain use and administration of drug to patient and family.
- Tell patient to report adverse reactions promptly.

pneumococcal vaccine, polyvalent

Pneumovax 23

Pregnancy risk category C

Indications & dosages

➲ Pneumococcal immunization

Adults and children age 2 and older: 0.5 ml I.M. or S.C.

Contraindications & cautions

- Contraindicated in patients hypersensitive to drug or its components (phenol) and in those with Hodgkin's disease who have received extensive chemotherapy or nodal irradiation.
- Postpone use in patients with acute respiratory distress syndrome.
- Vaccine isn't recommended for children younger than age 2.

Adverse reactions

CNS: slight fever.
Musculoskeletal: myalgia, arthralgia.
Skin: injection site rash, *injection site soreness,* severe local reaction caused by revaccination within 3 years.
Other: ***anaphylaxis.***

Interactions

Drug-drug. *Immunosuppressants:* May reduce immune response to vaccine. Postpone immunization until 3 months after immunosuppressant therapy is stopped.

Nursing considerations

- Vaccine is recommended for all adults older than age 65.
- Check immunization history to avoid revaccination within 3 years.
- Obtain history of allergies and reaction to immunization. Eggs and egg protein aren't used during the manufacture of vaccine; contains phenol as a preservative.
- Keep epinephrine 1:1,000 available to treat anaphylaxis.
- Inject in deltoid or midlateral thigh. Don't inject I.V. or I.D.
- When splenectomy is being considered, give vaccine at least 2 weeks before procedure to ensure adequate antibody response. Vaccine may be less effective in splenectomized patients.
- Vaccine protects against 23 pneumococcal types, accounting for 90% of pneumococcal disease.
- Vaccine may be given to children age 2 and older to prevent pneumococcal otitis media, although the Centers for Disease Control and Prevention doesn't recommend otitis media as an indication for vaccine.
- Administration with influenza virus vaccine is safe and effective.

Patient teaching

- Warn patient about adverse reactions linked to vaccine.
- Tell patient to treat fever with mild fever-reducing drugs and local site reaction with cold compresses.
- Warn patient with a skin rash related to low levels of platelets from unknown cause that there is a possibility of relapse 2 to 14 days after vaccination.

poliovirus vaccine, inactivated (IPV)

IPOL

Pregnancy risk category C

Indications & dosages

➲ Poliovirus immunization

Adults: 0.5 ml S.C.; give second dose 4 to 8 weeks later. Give third dose 6 to 12 months later.
Children: 0.5 ml S.C. at ages 2 months and 4 months. Give third dose at ages 15 to 18 months. Give a reinforcing dose of 0.5 ml S.C. before entry into school at ages 4 to 6.

Contraindications & cautions

- Contraindicated in patients hypersensitive to neomycin, streptomycin, or polymyxin B and in neonates younger than age 6 weeks.

Adverse reactions

CNS: *fever,* sleepiness.
GI: decreased appetite.
Skin: injection site erythema, induration, *pain.*
Other: crying, hypersensitivity reaction.

Interactions

Drug-drug. *Immune serum globulin, plasma, whole blood:* Antibodies in serum may interfere with immune response. Don't use vaccine within 3 months of transfusion.
Immunosuppressants: May reduce immune response to vaccine. Postpone immunization until immunosuppressant is stopped.

Nursing considerations

- Vaccine isn't effective in modifying or preventing existing or incubating poliomyelitis.
- Obtain history of allergies and reaction to immunization.
- If skin test is needed, give it either before or with vaccine.
- Keep epinephrine 1:1,000 available to treat anaphylaxis.
- Adults at high risk for exposure who have completed a primary course may receive another dose.
- Document manufacturer, lot number, date given, and name, address, and title of person giving vaccine on patient's record or log.

• Vaccine may temporarily decrease response to tuberculin skin test.

Patient teaching

• Inform patient or parents about risks and benefits of vaccine before administration.
• Warn patient or parents about adverse reactions linked to vaccine.

polyethylene glycol
GlycoLax, MiraLax

Pregnancy risk category C

Indications & dosages

➲ **Short-term treatment of occasional constipation**
Adults: 17 g (about 1 heaping tablespoon) powder P.O. daily, dissolved in 8 ounces (240 ml) of water, juice, soda, coffee, or tea.

Contraindications & cautions

• Contraindicated in patients allergic to polyethylene glycol and those with known or suspected bowel obstruction.

Adverse reactions

GI: abdominal bloating, cramping, diarrhea, excess stool frequency, flatulence, nausea.

Interactions

Drug-drug. *Drugs containing polyethylene glycol:* May cause urticaria. Monitor patient.

Nursing considerations

• Before giving polyethylene glycol, rule out bowel obstruction in patients who have nausea, vomiting, abdominal pain, or distension.
• It may take 2 to 4 days before a bowel movement occurs.
• Drug should be taken for 2 weeks or less to avoid the risk of laxative dependence.
• Occasional use as directed doesn't affect absorption or secretion of glucose or electrolytes.
• Prolonged, frequent, or excessive use may cause electrolyte imbalance and laxative dependence.
• Drug may be more likely to cause diarrhea in older patients.

Patient teaching

• Explain that proper eating habits and lifestyle changes may produce more regular bowel movements. Tell patient to eat adequate amounts of dietary fiber, drink ample fluids, and get appropriate exercise.
• If patient uses bottled form of drug, urge him to measure each 17-g dose using the measuring cup provided in the package. If patient uses drug packets, each one contains 17 g.
• Instruct patient to dissolve dose in 8 ounces of water, juice, soda, coffee, or tea.
• Inform patient that it may take 2 to 4 days to produce a bowel movement.
• Warn patient that taking more than the recommended dose can cause dehydration and severe diarrhea.
• Tell patient that drug should be used for 2 weeks or less to avoid the risk of laxative dependence.
• Urge patient to report unusual cramping, bloating, or diarrhea.

polyethylene glycol and electrolyte solution
CoLyte, Go-Evac, GoLYTELY, Miralax, NuLytely, OCL

Pregnancy risk category C

Indications & dosages

➲ **Bowel preparation before GI examination**
Adults: 240 ml P.O. q 10 minutes until 4 L are consumed or until watery stool is clear. Typically, give 4 hours before examination, allowing 3 hours for drinking and 1 hour for bowel evacuation.

Contraindications & cautions

• Contraindicated in patients with GI obstruction or perforation, gastric retention, toxic colitis, or megacolon.

Adverse reactions

EENT: rhinorrhea.
GI: *nausea, bloating, cramps, vomiting, abdominal fullness.*
Skin: urticaria, dermatitis, allergic reaction, anal irritation.

Interactions

Drug-drug. *Oral drugs:* May decrease absorption if given within 1 hour of starting therapy. Give at least 2 to 3 hours before starting therapy.

Nursing considerations

- Use tap water to reconstitute powder. Shake vigorously to dissolve all powder. Refrigerate reconstituted solution, but use within 48 hours.

!!ALERT Don't add flavoring or additional ingredients to the solution or give chilled solution. Hypothermia has been reported after ingesting large amounts of chilled solution

- Give solution early in the morning if patient is scheduled for a mid-morning examination. Oral solution induces diarrhea (onset 30 to 60 minutes) that rapidly cleans the bowel, usually within 4 hours.
- When using to prepare for barium enema, give solution the evening before the examination to avoid interfering with barium coating of the colonic mucosa.
- If given to semiconscious patient or to patient with impaired gag reflex, take care to prevent aspiration.
- No major shifts in fluid or electrolyte balance have been reported.
- Patient preparation for barium enema may be less satisfactory with this solution because it may interfere with the barium coating of the colonic mucosa using the double-contrast technique.

Patient teaching

- Tell patient to fast for 3 to 4 hours before taking the solution, and thereafter to drink only clear fluids until examination is complete.
- Warn patient about adverse reactions.

polysaccharide-iron complex

Ferrex 150 ◇, Hytinic ◇, Niferex ◇ *, Niferex-150 ◇, Nu-Iron ◇ *, Nu-Iron 150 ◇

Pregnancy risk category NR

Indications & dosages

➲ **Iron deficiency**

Adults: 100 to 200 mg (2 to 3 mg/kg) P.O. elemental iron daily in three divided doses.

Children ages 2 to 12: 50 to 100 mg (1 to 1.5 mg/kg) P.O. elemental iron daily in three or four divided doses.

Children ages 6 months to 2 years: 3 to 6 mg/kg P.O. elemental iron daily in three divided doses.

Infants younger than age 6 months: 10 to 25 mg P.O. elemental iron daily in three or four divided doses.

➲ **As a supplement during pregnancy**

Women: 15 to 30 mg elemental iron P.O. daily during last two trimesters.

Contraindications & cautions

- Contraindicated in patients hypersensitive to drug or its ingredients and in those with hemochromatosis or hemosiderosis.

Adverse reactions

GI: *nausea*, epigastric pain, vomiting, *constipation*, *black stools*, diarrhea, anorexia.

Other: temporarily stained teeth from liquid forms.

Interactions

Drug-drug. *Antacids, cholestyramine resin, cimetidine:* May decrease iron absorption. Separate doses by 2 to 4 hours.

Chloramphenicol: May delay response to iron therapy. Monitor patient.

Fluoroquinolones, levodopa, methyldopa, penicillamine, tetracyclines: May decrease GI absorption of these drugs, possibly causing decreased level or effect. Separate doses by 2 to 4 hours.

Levothyroxine sodium: May decrease levothyroxine effect, leading to hypothyroidism. Separate doses by 2 to 4 hours.

Thyroid: May inhibit thyroid hormone absorption. Separate doses by 2 hours.

Vitamin C: May increase iron absorption. Use together for therapeutic effect.

Drug-herb. *Black cohosh, chamomile, feverfew, gossypol, hawthorn, nettle, plantain, St. John's wort:* May decrease iron absorption. Discourage use together.

Oregano: May decrease iron absorption. Tell patient to separate ingestion of oregano from ingestion of food containing iron or iron supplement by at least 2 hours.

Drug-food. *Cereals, cheese, coffee, eggs, milk, tea, whole-grain breads, yogurt:* May decrease iron absorption. Advise patient to separate use by 2 to 4 hours.

Nursing considerations

!!ALERT Oral iron may turn stools black. Although this unabsorbed iron is harmless, it may mask melena.

- Monitor hemoglobin level, hematocrit, and reticulocyte count.
- Although nausea, constipation, black stools, and epigastric pain are common adverse reactions to iron therapy, few, if any, occur with polysaccharide iron complex.
- Iron overload may decrease uptake of technetium-99m and thus interfere with skeletal imaging.

Patient teaching

- Tell patient to take tablets with juice (preferably orange juice) or water, but not with milk or antacids.

!!ALERT Inform parents that as few as 3 tablets can cause serious iron poisoning in children.

- Caution patient not to substitute one iron salt for another because the amounts of elemental iron vary.

potassium acetate

Pregnancy risk category C

Indications & dosages

➲ Hypokalemia

Adults: No more than 20 mEq/hour in concentration of 40 mEq/L or less. Total 24-hour dose shouldn't exceed 150 mEq (3 mEq/kg in children).

➲ To prevent hypokalemia

Adults: Dosage is individualized to patient's needs, not to exceed 150 mEq daily. Give as an additive to I.V. infusions. Usual dose is 20 mEq/L infused at no more than 20 mEq/hour.

Children: Individualized dose not to exceed 3 mEq/kg daily. Give as an additive to I.V. infusions.

Contraindications & cautions

- Contraindicated in patients with severe renal impairment with oliguria, anuria, or azotemia.
- Contraindicated in those with untreated Addison's disease, acute dehydration, heat cramps, hyperkalemia, hyperkalemic form of familial periodic paralysis, or conditions linked to extensive tissue breakdown.
- Use cautiously in patients with cardiac disease or renal impairment.

Adverse reactions

CNS: paresthesia of limbs, listlessness, mental confusion, weakness or heaviness of legs, flaccid paralysis, pain, fever.
CV: hypotension, ***arrhythmias***, ***heart block***, ECG changes, ***cardiac arrest***.
GI: nausea, vomiting, abdominal pain, diarrhea.
Metabolic: ***hyperkalemia***.
Respiratory: ***respiratory paralysis***.
Skin: redness at infusion site.

Interactions

Drug-drug. *ACE inhibitors, digoxin, potassium-sparing diuretics:* May increase risk of hyperkalemia. Use together with caution.

Nursing considerations

- During therapy, monitor ECG, renal function, fluid intake and output, and potassium, creatinine, and BUN levels. Never give potassium postoperatively until urine flow is established.
- Many adverse reactions may reflect hyperkalemia.

!!ALERT Potassium preparations aren't interchangeable; verify preparation before use.

Patient teaching

- Explain use and administration to patient and family.
- Tell patient to report adverse effects, especially pain at insertion site.

potassium bicarbonate

K+Care ET, K-Lyte

Pregnancy risk category C

Indications & dosages

➲ To prevent hypokalemia

Adults and children: Initially, 25 mEq P.O. daily, in divided doses. Adjust dosage, p.r.n.

➲ Hypokalemia

Adults and children: 50 to 100 mEq P.O. divided into two to four daily doses. Use I.V. potassium chloride when oral replacement isn't feasible. Don't exceed 150 mEq P.O. daily in adults and 3 mEq/kg daily P.O. in children.

Contraindications & cautions

- Contraindicated in patients with severe renal impairment with oliguria, anuria, or azotemia; untreated Addison's disease; or acute dehydration, heat cramps, hyperkalemia, hyperkalemic form of familial periodic paralysis, or other conditions linked to extensive tissue breakdown.
- Use cautiously in patients with cardiac disease or renal impairment.

Adverse reactions

CNS: paresthesia of limbs, listlessness, confusion, weakness or heaviness of legs, flaccid paralysis.
CV: ***arrhythmias***, ECG changes, hypotension, ***heart block, cardiac arrest.***
GI: *nausea, vomiting, abdominal pain,* diarrhea.

Interactions

Drug-drug. *ACE inhibitors, digoxin, potassium-sparing diuretics:* May cause hyperkalemia. Use with extreme caution.

Nursing considerations

- Dissolve potassium bicarbonate tablets completely in 4 to 8 ounces of cold water.
- Ask patient's flavor preference: lime, fruit punch, citrus, or orange.
- Don't give potassium supplements postoperatively until urine flow has been established.

!!ALERT Potassium preparations aren't interchangeable; verify preparation before use. Never switch potassium products without prescriber's order. Potassium chloride can't be given instead of potassium bicarbonate.

- Monitor fluid intake and output and BUN, potassium, and creatinine levels.

Patient teaching

- Tell patient to take drug with meals and sip slowly over 5 to 10 minutes.
- Tell patient to report adverse effects.
- Warn patient not to use salt substitutes at the same time, except with prescriber's permission.

potassium chloride

Apo-K*, Cena-K, Gen-K, K+8, K-10*, K+10, Kaochlor, Kaochlor S-F, Kaon-Cl, Kaon Cl-10, Kaon-Cl 20%, Kay Ciel, K+ Care, K-Dur 10, K-Dur 20, K-Lease, K-Lor, Klor-Con, Klor-Con 8, Klor-Con 10, Klor-Con/25, Klorvess, Klotrix, K-Lyte/Cl, K-Norm, K-Tab, K-vescent Potassium Chloride, Micro-K Extencaps, Micro-K 10 Extencaps, Micro-K LS, Potasalan, Rum-K, Slow-K, Ten-K

Pregnancy risk category C

Indications & dosages

➲ To prevent hypokalemia
Adults and children: Initially, 20 mEq of potassium supplement P.O. daily, in divided doses. Adjust dosage, p.r.n., based on potassium levels.

➲ Hypokalemia
Adults and children: 40 to 100 mEq P.O. in two to four divided doses daily. Maximum dose of diluted I.V. potassium chloride is 40 mEq/L at 10 mEq/hour. Don't exceed 150 mEq daily in adults and 3 mEq/kg daily in children. Further doses are based on potassium levels and blood pH. Give I.V. potassium replacement only with monitoring of ECG and potassium level.

➲ Severe hypokalemia
Adults and children: Dilute potassium chloride in a suitable I.V. solution of less than 80 mEq/L, and give at no more than 40 mEq/hour.

Further doses are based on potassium level. Don't exceed 150 mEq I.V. daily in adults and 3 mEq/kg I.V. daily or 40 mEq/m^2 daily in children. Give I.V. potassium replacement only with monitoring of ECG and potassium level.

➲ Acute MI♦
Adults: For high dose, 80 mEq/L at 1.5 ml/kg/hour for 24 hours with an I.V. infusion of 25% dextrose and 50 units/L regular insulin. For low dose, 40 mEq/L at 1 ml/kg/hour for 24 hours, with an I.V. infusion of 10% dextrose and 20 units/L regular insulin.

Contraindications & cautions

- Contraindicated in patients with severe renal impairment with oliguria, anuria, or az-

otemia; with untreated Addison's disease; or with acute dehydration, heat cramps, hyperkalemia, hyperkalemic form of familial periodic paralysis, or other conditions linked to extensive tissue breakdown.
- Use cautiously in patients with cardiac disease or renal impairment.

Adverse reactions

CNS: paresthesia of limbs, listlessness, confusion, weakness or heaviness of limbs, flaccid paralysis.
CV: ***arrhythmias*, *heart block*, *cardiac arrest***, ECG changes, hypotension, *postinfusion phlebitis*.
GI: nausea, vomiting, abdominal pain, diarrhea.
Metabolic: ***hyperkalemia***.
Respiratory: ***respiratory paralysis***.

Interactions

Drug-drug. *ACE inhibitors, digoxin, potassium-sparing diuretics:* May cause hyperkalemia. Use together with extreme caution.

Nursing considerations

!!ALERT Potassium preparations aren't interchangeable; verify preparation before use. Never switch products without prescriber's order.
- Make sure powders are completely dissolved before giving.
- Enteric-coated tablets aren't recommended because of increased risk of GI bleeding and small-bowel ulcerations.
- Tablets in wax matrix sometimes lodge in the esophagus and cause ulceration in cardiac patients with esophageal compression from an enlarged left atrium. Use liquid form in such patients and in those with esophageal stasis or obstruction.
- Drug is commonly used orally with potassium-wasting diuretics to maintain potassium levels.
- Sugar-free liquid is available (Kaochlor S-F 10%); use if tablet or capsule passage is likely to be delayed, as in GI obstruction. Have patient sip slowly to minimize GI irritation.
- Don't crush sustained-release potassium products.
- Monitor ECG and electrolyte levels during therapy.
- Monitor renal function. Don't give potassium during immediate postoperative period until urine flow is established.
- Many adverse reactions may reflect hyperkalemia.

Patient teaching

- Teach patient how to prepare (powders) and give drug form prescribed. Tell patient to take with or after meals with full glass of water or fruit juice to lessen GI distress.
- Teach patient signs and symptoms of hyperkalemia, and tell patient to notify prescriber if they occur.
- Tell patient to report discomfort at I.V. insertion site.
- Warn patient not to use salt substitutes concurrently, except with prescriber's permission.

!!ALERT Patient shouldn't be concerned if controlled-release tablets in a wax matrix appear in stool. The potassium has already been absorbed.

potassium gluconate
Kaon, Kaylixir*, K-G Elixir*

Pregnancy risk category C

Indications & dosages

➲ To prevent hypokalemia
Adults and children: Initially, 20 mEq of potassium supplement P.O. daily, in divided doses. Adjust dosage, p.r.n., based on potassium level.

➲ Hypokalemia
Adults and children: 40 to 100 mEq P.O. divided into two to four daily doses. Use I.V. potassium chloride when oral replacement isn't feasible. Don't exceed 150 mEq P.O. daily in adults and 3 mEq/kg daily P.O. in children.

Contraindications & cautions

- Contraindicated in patients with severe renal impairment with oliguria, anuria, or azotemia; untreated Addison's disease; or acute dehydration, heat cramps, hyperkalemia, hyperkalemic form of familial periodic paralysis, or other conditions linked to extensive tissue breakdown.
- Use cautiously in patients with cardiac disease or renal impairment.

Adverse reactions

CNS: paresthesia of limbs, listlessness, confusion, weakness or heaviness of legs, flaccid paralysis.
CV: ***arrhythmias***, ECG changes.
GI: *nausea, vomiting, abdominal pain*, diarrhea.

Interactions

Drug-drug. *ACE inhibitors, digoxin, potassium-sparing diuretics:* May cause hyperkalemia. Use with caution.

Nursing considerations

!!ALERT Give oral potassium supplements with caution because different forms deliver varying amounts of potassium. Never switch products without prescriber's order.
- Don't give potassium supplements postoperatively until urine flow has been established.
- Monitor ECG, fluid intake and output, and BUN, potassium, and creatinine levels.

Patient teaching

- Advise patient to sip liquid potassium slowly to minimize GI irritation. Also tell him to take drug with meals, with a full glass of water or fruit juice.
- Warn patient not to use potassium gluconate with a salt substitute, except with prescriber's permission.
- Teach patient signs and symptoms of hyperkalemia, and tell patient to notify prescriber if they occur.

potassium iodide

Pima, saturated solution (SSKI), strong iodine solution (Lugol's solution), Thyro-Block

Pregnancy risk category D

Indications & dosages

➲ To prepare for thyroidectomy
Adults and children: 3 to 5 drops strong iodine solution P.O. t.i.d.; or 1 to 5 drops SSKI in water P.O. t.i.d. after meals for 10 days before surgery.
➲ Thyrotoxic crisis
Adults and children: 500 mg P.O. q 4 hours (about 10 drops of SSKI); or 1 ml of strong iodine solution t.i.d. Give at least 1 hour after the first dose of propylthiouracil or methimazole.
➲ Radiation protectant for thyroid gland
Adults: 130 mg P.O. daily for 10 days after radiation exposure. Start no later than 3 or 4 hours after acute exposure. Or, 3 ml Pima P.O. once daily 24 hours before and for 10 days after exposure.
Children ages 3 to 18: 65 mg P.O. daily for 10 days after exposure. Start no later than 3 or 4 hours after acute exposure.
Children ages 1 to 18: 2 ml Pima P.O. once daily 24 hours before and for 10 days after exposure.
Infants and children up to age 1 year: 1 ml Pima P.O. once daily 24 hours before and for 10 days after exposure.

Contraindications & cautions

- Contraindicated in patients with tuberculosis, acute bronchitis, iodide hypersensitivity, or hyperkalemia. Some formulations contain sulfites, which may cause allergic reactions in hypersensitive patients.
- Use cautiously in patients with hypocomplementemic vasculitis, goiter, or autoimmune thyroid disease.

Adverse reactions

CNS: fever.
EENT: periorbital edema.
GI: diarrhea, inflammation of salivary glands, burning mouth and throat, sore teeth and gums, *metallic taste.*
Metabolic: ***potassium toxicity***.
Skin: acneiform rash.
Other: hypersensitivity reactions.

Interactions

Drug-drug. *ACE inhibitors, potassium sparing diuretics:* May cause hyperkalemia. Avoid using together.
Antithyroid drugs: May increase hypothyroid or goitrogenic effects. Monitor patient closely.
Lithium carbonate: May cause hypothyroidism. Use together cautiously.
Drug-food. *Iodized salt, shellfish:* May alter drug's effectiveness. Urge caution.

Nursing considerations

- Expect to give with other antithyroid drugs.

- For thyrotoxicosis, first iodine dose is given at least 1 hour after first dose of propylthiouracil and methimazole.
- Dilute oral solution in water, milk, or fruit juice, and give after meals to prevent gastric irritation, hydrate patient, and mask salty taste.
- Give iodides through straw to avoid tooth discoloration.

!!ALERT Earliest signs of delayed hypersensitivity reactions caused by iodides are irritation and swollen eyelids.

- Monitor patient for iodism, which can cause metallic taste, burning in mouth and throat, sore teeth and gums, increased salivation, coryza, sneezing, eye irritation with swelling of eyelids, severe headache, productive cough, GI irritation, diarrhea, rash, or soreness of the pharynx, larynx, and tonsils.
- Store in light-resistant container.

Patient teaching

- Show patient how to mask salty taste of oral solution. Tell him to take all forms of drug after meals.

!!ALERT Warn patient that sudden withdrawal may precipitate thyroid crisis.

!!ALERT Teach patient signs and symptoms of potassium toxicity, including confusion, irregular heartbeat, numbness, tingling, pain or weakness of hands or feet, and tiredness.

- Tell patient to ask prescriber about using iodized salt and eating shellfish. These foods contain iodine and may alter drug's effectiveness.
- Tell patient not to increase the amount of potassium through diet.
- Tell patient to stop drug and notify prescriber if epigastric pain, rash, metallic taste, nausea, or vomiting occurs.

pramipexole dihydrochloride
Mirapex

Pregnancy risk category C

Indications & dosages

➲ Signs and symptoms of idiopathic Parkinson's disease

Adults: Initially, 0.375 mg P.O. daily in three divided doses. Adjust doses slowly (not more often than q 5 to 7 days) over several weeks until desired therapeutic effect is achieved. Maintenance dosage is 1.5 to 4.5 mg daily in three divided doses.

For patients with creatinine clearance over 60 ml/minute, first dosage is 0.125 mg P.O. t.i.d., up to 1.5 mg t.i.d. For those with clearance of 35 to 59 ml/minute, first dosage is 1.25 mg P.O. b.i.d., up to 1.5 mg b.i.d. For those with clearance of 15 to 34 ml/minute, first dosage is 0.125 mg P.O. daily, up to 1.5 mg daily.

Contraindications & cautions

- Contraindicated in patients hypersensitive to drug or its components.
- Use cautiously in renally impaired patients.
- Use cautiously in breast-feeding women. It's unknown if drug appears in breast milk.

Adverse reactions

CNS: drowsiness, akathisia, amnesia, *asthenia, confusion,* delusions, *dizziness, dream abnormalities, dyskinesia,* dystonia, *extrapyramidal syndrome,* gait abnormalities, *hallucinations,* hypoesthesia, hypertonia, *insomnia,* myoclonus, paranoid reaction, malaise, *somnolence,* sleep disorders, thought abnormalities, fever.

CV: chest pain, peripheral edema, *orthostatic hypotension.*

EENT: accommodation abnormalities, diplopia, rhinitis, vision abnormalities.

GI: dry mouth, anorexia, *constipation,* dysphagia, *nausea.*

GU: impotence, urinary frequency, UTI, urinary incontinence.

Metabolic: weight loss.

Musculoskeletal: arthritis, bursitis, myasthenia, twitching.

Respiratory: dyspnea, pneumonia.

Skin: skin disorders.

Other: decreased libido, *accidental injury,* general edema.

Interactions

Drug-drug. *Cimetidine, diltiazem, quinidine, quinine, ranitidine, triamterene, verapamil:* May decrease pramipexole clearance. Adjust dosage as needed.

Dopamine antagonists: May reduce pramipexole effectiveness. Monitor patient closely.

Nursing considerations

- If drug must be stopped, withdraw over 1 week.

• Drug may cause orthostatic hypotension, especially during dosage increases. Monitor patient carefully.
• Adjust dosage gradually to achieve maximum therapeutic effect, balanced against the main adverse effects of dyskinesia, hallucinations, somnolence, and dry mouth.

Patient teaching

• Instruct patient not to rise rapidly after sitting or lying down because of risk of dizziness.
• Caution patient to avoid hazardous activities until CNS response to drug is known.
• Tell patient to use caution before taking drug with other CNS depressants.
• Tell patient (especially elderly patient) that hallucinations may occur.
• Advise patient to take drug with food if nausea develops.
• Tell woman to notify prescriber if she is breast-feeding or intends to do so.
• Advise patient that it may take 4 weeks for effects of drug to be noticed because of slow adjustment schedule.

pramlintide acetate
Symlin

Pregnancy risk category C

Indications & dosages

➲ **Adjunct to insulin in patients with type 1 diabetes who haven't achieved the desired glucose control**
Adults: Initially, 15 mcg S.C. before meals of more than 250 calories or 30 g of carbohydrates. Reduce preprandial rapid-acting or short-acting insulin dose, including fixed-mix insulin such as 70/30, by 50%. Increase pramlintide dose by 15-mcg increments q 3 days if no nausea occurs to a maintenance dose of 30 to 60 mcg. Adjust insulin dose as needed.
➲ **Adjunct to insulin in patients with type 2 diabetes who haven't achieved the desired glucose control, with or without a sulfonylurea or metformin**
Adults: Initially, 60 mcg S.C. immediately before major meals. Reduce preprandial rapid-acting or short-acting insulin dose, including fixed-mix insulin, by 50%. Increase pramlintide dose to 120 mcg if no significant nausea occurs for 3 to 7 days. Adjust insulin dose as needed.

Contraindications & cautions

• Contraindicated in patients hypersensitive to drug or its components, including metacresol, and in patients with gastroparesis or hypoglycemia unawareness.
• Don't use in patients noncompliant with current insulin and glucose monitoring regimen, patients with a glycosylated hemoglobin (HbA1c) level greater than 9%, patients with severe hypoglycemia during the previous 6 months, and patients who take drugs that stimulate GI motility.
• Use cautiously in pregnant or breast-feeding women and in elderly patients.

Adverse reactions

CNS: dizziness, fatigue, *headache.*
EENT: pharyngitis.
GI: abdominal pain, *anorexia, nausea, vomiting.*
Metabolic: ***hypoglycemia.***
Musculoskeletal: arthralgia.
Respiratory: cough.
Skin: injection site reaction.
Other: allergic reaction, *accidental injury.*

Interactions

Drug-drug. *ACE inhibitors, disopyramide, fibrates, fluoxetine, MAO inhibitors, oral antidiabetics, pentoxifylline, propoxyphene, salicylates, sulfonamide antibiotics:* May increase risk of hypoglycemia. Monitor glucose level closely.
Alpha glucosidase inhibitors (such as acarbose), anticholinergics (such as atropine, tricyclic antidepressants, benztropine): May alter GI motility. Avoid using together.
Beta blockers, clonidine, guanethidine, reserpine: May mask signs of hypoglycemia. Monitor glucose level closely.
Oral drugs dependent on rapid onset of action (such as analgesics): May delay absorption because of slowed gastric emptying. If rapid effect is needed, give oral drug 1 hour before or 2 hours after pramlintide.

Nursing considerations

• Before starting drug, review patient's HbA1c level, recent blood glucose monitoring data, history of insulin-induced hypoglycemia, current insulin regimen, and body weight.

• To give drug, use a U-100 insulin syringe, preferably a 0.3-ml size.
• Give each dose S.C. into abdomen or thigh. Rotate injection sites, and use site separate from insulin site used at same time.
!!ALERT Drug may increase the risk of insulin-induced severe hypoglycemia, particularly in patients with type 1 diabetes.
• The risk of severe, drug-related hypoglycemia is highest within the first 3 hours after an injection.
• Symptoms of hypoglycemia may be masked in patients with a long history of diabetes, diabetic nerve disease, or intensified diabetes control.
• Monitor patient for severe nausea and vomiting. Reduce dose if needed.
• Don't mix drug with any type of insulin; give drug as separate injection.
• If patient has persistent nausea or recurrent, unexplained hypoglycemia that requires medical assistance, stop drug .
• If patient doesn't comply with glucose monitoring or drug dosage adjustments, stop drug.
• Use during pregnancy only if potential maternal benefit justifies fetal risk.
• It's unknown whether drug appears in breast milk. Use only if benefit to mother outweighs risk to infant.
• Drug seems to have similar effects on elderly and younger adults, but some older adults may be more sensitive to it.

Patient teaching

• Teach patient how to take drug exactly as prescribed, at mealtimes. Explain that it doesn't replace daily insulin but may lower the amount of insulin needed, especially before meals.
• Explain that a meal is considered more than 250 calories or 30 g of carbohydrates.
• Caution patient not to mix drug with insulin; instruct him to give the injections at separate sites.
• Instruct patient not to change doses of pramlintide or insulin without consulting prescriber.
• Tell patient to refrain from driving, operating heavy machinery, or performing other risky activities where he could hurt himself or others, until it's known how drug affects his glucose level.
• Caution patient about possibility of severe hypoglycemia, particularly within 3 hours after injection.
• Teach patient and family members the signs and symptoms of hypoglycemia, including hunger, headache, sweating, tremor, irritability, and difficulty concentrating.
• Instruct patient and family members what to do if patient develops hypoglycemia.
• Tell patient to report to prescriber severe nausea and vomiting.
• Advise women of child-bearing age to tell the prescriber if they are, could be, or are planning to become pregnant.
• Teach patient how to handle unusual situations, such as illness or stress, low or forgotten insulin dose, accidental use of too much insulin or pramlintide, not enough food, or missed meals.
• Tell patient to refrigerate unopened and opened vials. Contents of open vials should be used within 28 days and unopened vials before expiration date.

pravastatin sodium (eptastatin)
Pravachol

Pregnancy risk category X

Indications & dosages

➲ Primary and secondary prevention of coronary events; hyperlipidemia
Adults: Initially, 40 mg P.O. once daily at the same time each day, with or without food. Adjust dosage q 4 weeks, based on patient tolerance and response; maximum daily dose is 80 mg.
➲ Heterozygous familial hypercholesterolemia
Adolescents ages 14 to 18: 40 mg P.O. once daily.
Children ages 8 to 13: 20 mg P.O. once daily.

In patients with renal or hepatic dysfunction, start with 10 mg P.O. daily. In patients taking immunosuppressants, begin with 10 mg P.O. at bedtime and adjust to higher dosages with caution. Most patients treated with the combination of immunosuppressants and pravastatin receive up to 20 mg pravastatin daily.

Contraindications & cautions

• Contraindicated in patients hypersensitive to drug and in those with active liver dis-

ease or conditions that cause unexplained, persistent elevations of transaminase levels.
- Contraindicated in pregnant and breast-feeding women and in women of childbearing age.
- Safety and efficacy in children younger than age 8 haven't been established.
- Use cautiously in patients who consume large quantities of alcohol or have history of liver disease.

Adverse reactions

CNS: headache, dizziness, fatigue.
CV: chest pain.
EENT: rhinitis.
GI: vomiting, diarrhea, heartburn, abdominal pain, constipation, flatulence, *nausea*.
GU: ***renal failure caused by myoglobinuria***, urinary abnormality.
Musculoskeletal: myositis, myopathy, *localized muscle pain*, myalgia, ***rhabdomyolysis***.
Respiratory: cough, common cold.
Skin: rash.
Other: flulike symptoms, influenza.

Interactions

Drug-drug. *Cholestyramine, colestipol:* May decrease pravastatin level. Give pravastatin 1 hour before or 4 hours after these drugs.
Erythromycin, fibric acid derivatives (such as clofibrate, gemfibrozil), immunosuppressants (such as cyclosporine), high dosages (1 g or more daily) of niacin (nicotinic acid): May cause rhabdomyolysis. Avoid using together; if unavoidable, monitor patient closely.
Fluconazole, itraconazole, ketoconazole: May increase pravastatin level and adverse effects. Avoid using together; if unavoidable, reduce dose of pravastatin.
Gemfibrozil: May decrease protein-binding and urinary clearance of pravastatin. Avoid using together.
Hepatotoxic drugs: May increase risk of hepatotoxicity. Avoid using together.
Drug-herb. *Eucalyptus, jin bu huan, kava:* May increase the risk of hepatotoxicity. Discourage use together.
Red yeast rice: May increase risk of adverse reactions because herb contains compounds similar to those of statin drugs. Discourage use together.
Drug-lifestyle. *Alcohol use:* May increase risk of hepatotoxicity. Discourage use together.

Nursing considerations

- Use only after diet and other nondrug therapies prove ineffective. Patients should follow a standard low-cholesterol diet during therapy.
- Use in children with heterozygous familial hypercholesterolemia if LDL cholesterol level is at least 190 mg/dl or if LDL cholesterol is at least 160 mg/dl and patient has either a positive family history of premature CV disease or two or more other CV disease risk factors.
- Obtain liver function test results at start of therapy and then periodically. A liver biopsy may be performed if elevated liver enzyme levels persist.

!!ALERT Don't confuse Pravachol with Prevacid or propranolol.

Patient teaching

- Tell patient to take the prescribed dose in the evening, preferably at bedtime.
- Advise patient who is also taking a bile-acid resin such as cholestyramine to take pravastatin at least 1 hour before or 4 hours after taking resin.
- Tell patient to notify prescriber of adverse reactions, particularly muscle aches and pains.
- Teach patient about proper dietary management of cholesterol and triglycerides. When appropriate, recommend weight control, exercise, and smoking cessation programs.
- Inform patient that it will take up to 4 weeks to achieve full therapeutic effect.

!!ALERT Tell woman of childbearing age to stop drug and notify prescriber immediately if she is or may be pregnant or if she's breast-feeding.

prazosin hydrochloride
Minipress

Pregnancy risk category C

Indications & dosages

➲ Mild to moderate hypertension, alone or with a diuretic or other antihypertensive

Adults: Test dose is 1 mg P.O. h.s. to prevent first-dose syncope (severe syncope with loss of consciousness). First dosage is 1 mg P.O. b.i.d. or t.i.d. Dosage may be increased slowly. Maximum daily dose is 20 mg. Maintenance dosage is 6 to 15 mg daily in three divided doses. Some patients need larger dosages (up to 40 mg daily).

If other antihypertensives or diuretics are added to therapy, decrease prazosin dosage to 1 to 2 mg t.i.d. and readjust to maintenance dosage.

➲ Benign prostatic hyperplasia♦

Adults: 2 mg P.O. b.i.d. Dose range is 1 to 9 mg P.O. daily.

Contraindications & cautions

- Contraindicated in patients hypersensitive to drug or other alpha blockers.
- Use cautiously in patients receiving other antihypertensives.

Adverse reactions

CNS: *dizziness*, headache, drowsiness, nervousness, paresthesia, weakness, *first-dose syncope*, depression, fever.
CV: orthostatic hypotension, palpitations, edema.
EENT: blurred vision, tinnitus, conjunctivitis, epistaxis, nasal congestion.
GI: vomiting, diarrhea, abdominal cramps, nausea.
GU: priapism, impotence, urinary frequency, incontinence.
Musculoskeletal: arthralgia, myalgia.
Respiratory: dyspnea.
Skin: pruritus.

Interactions

Drug-drug. *Acebutolol, atenolol, betaxolol, carteolol, esmolol, metoprolol, nadolol, pindolol, propranolol, sotalol, timolol:* May increase the risk of orthostatic hypotension in the early phases of use together. Help patient stand slowly until effects are known.
Diuretics: May increase frequency of syncope with loss of consciousness. Advise patient to sit or lie down if dizziness occurs.
Verapamil: May increase prazosin level. Monitor patient closely.
Drug-herb. *Butcher's broom:* May reduce effect. Discourage use together.
Ma huang: May decrease antihypertensive effects. Discourage use together.

Nursing considerations

- Monitor patient's blood pressure and pulse rate frequently.
- Elderly patients may be more sensitive to drug's hypotensive effects.
- Compliance might be improved with twice-daily dosing. Discuss this dosing change with prescriber if compliance problems are suspected.
- Drug alters results of screening tests for pheochromocytoma and causes increases in levels of the urinary metabolite of norepinephrine and vanillylmandelic acid; it may cause positive antinuclear antibody titer.

!!ALERT If first dose is more than 1 mg, first-dose syncope may occur.

Patient teaching

- Warn patient that dizziness may occur with first dose. If he experiences dizziness, tell him to sit or lie down. Reassure him that this effect disappears with continued dosing.
- Caution patient to avoid driving or performing hazardous tasks for the first 24 hours after starting this drug or increasing the dose.
- Tell patient not to suddenly stop taking drug, but to notify prescriber if unpleasant adverse reactions occur.
- Advise patient to minimize low blood pressure and dizziness upon standing by rising slowly and avoiding sudden position changes. Dry mouth can be relieved by chewing gum or sucking on hard candy or ice chips.

prednisolone
Delta-Cortef, Prelone

prednisolone acetate
Key-Pred 25, Key-Pred 50, Predalone 50, Predcor-50

prednisolone sodium phosphate
Hydeltrasol, Key-Pred-SP, Orapred, Pediapred, Prelone

prednisolone tebutate
Prednisol TBA, Nor-Pred TBA, Predate TBA, Predcor-TBA

Pregnancy risk category C

Indications & dosages

Severe inflammation, immunosuppression

prednisolone

Adults: 2.5 to 15 mg P.O. b.i.d., t.i.d., or q.i.d.

Children: Initially, 0.14 to 2 mg/kg/day P.O. or 4 to 60 mg/m^2/day in four divided doses.

prednisolone acetate

Adults: 2 to 30 mg I.M. q 12 hours.

Children: 0.04 to 0.25 mg/kg or 1.5 to 7.5 mg/m^2 I.M. once daily or b.i.d.

prednisolone sodium phosphate

Adults: 4 to 60 mg I.M., I.V., or P.O. daily.

Children: Initially, 0.14 to 2 mg/kg/day or 4 to 60 mg/m^2/day in three or four divided doses I.M., I.V., or P.O.

prednisolone tebutate

Adults: 4 to 40 mg into joints and lesions, p.r.n.

Uncontrolled asthma in those taking inhaled corticosteroids and long-acting bronchodilators

Children: 1 to 2 mg/kg/day prednisolone sodium phosphate P.O. in single or divided doses. Continue short course (or "burst" therapy) until child achieves a peak expiratory flow rate of 80% of his or her personal best, or until symptoms resolve. This usually requires 3 to 10 days of treatment but can take longer. Tapering the dose after improvement doesn't necessarily prevent relapse.

Acute exacerbations of multiple sclerosis

Adults and children: 200 mg/day prednisolone sodium phosphate P.O. as single or divided dose for 7 days; then 80 mg every other day for 1 month.

Nephrotic syndrome

Children: 60 mg/m^2/day prednisolone sodium phosphate P.O. in three divided doses for 4 weeks, followed by 4 weeks of single-dose alternate-day therapy at 40 mg/m^2/day.

Contraindications & cautions

- Contraindicated in patients hypersensitive to drug or its ingredients, in those with systemic fungal infections, and in those receiving immunosuppressive doses together with live-virus vaccines.
- Use with caution in patients with recent MI.
- Use cautiously in patients with GI ulcer, renal disease, hypertension, osteoporosis, diabetes mellitus, hypothyroidism, cirrhosis, active hepatitis, lactation, diverticulitis, nonspecific ulcerative colitis, recent intestinal anastomoses, thromboembolic disorders, seizures, myasthenia gravis, heart failure, tuberculosis, ocular herpes simplex, emotional instability, and psychotic tendencies.

Adverse reactions

CNS: *euphoria, insomnia,* psychotic behavior, ***pseudotumor cerebri***, vertigo, headache, paresthesia, ***seizures***.

CV: ***heart failure***, hypertension, edema, ***arrhythmias***, thrombophlebitis, ***thromboembolism***.

EENT: cataracts, glaucoma.

GI: *peptic ulceration*, GI irritation, increased appetite, ***pancreatitis***, nausea, vomiting.

GU: menstrual irregularities, increased urine calcium levels.

Metabolic: hypokalemia, hyperglycemia, carbohydrate intolerance, hypercholesterolemia, hypocalcemia.

Musculoskeletal: growth suppression in children, muscle weakness, osteoporosis.

Skin: hirsutism, delayed wound healing, acne, various skin eruptions.

Other: susceptibility to infections, cushingoid state, ***acute adrenal insufficiency***, af-

ter increased stress or abrupt withdrawal after long-term therapy.
After abrupt withdrawal: rebound inflammation; fatigue; weakness; arthralgia; fever; dizziness; lethargy; depression; fainting; orthostatic hypotension; dyspnea; anorexia, hypoglycemia. After prolonged use, sudden withdrawal may be fatal.

Interactions

Drug-drug. *Aspirin, indomethacin, other NSAIDs:* May increase risk of GI distress and bleeding. Use together cautiously.
Barbiturates, carbamazepine, fosphenytoin, phenytoin, rifampin: May decrease corticosteroid effect. Increase corticosteroid dosage.
Cyclosporine: May increase toxicity. Monitor patient closely.
Oral anticoagulants: May alter dosage requirements. Monitor PT and INR closely.
Potassium-depleting drugs such as thiazide diuretics: May enhance potassium-wasting effects of prednisolone. Monitor potassium level.
Salicylates: May decrease salicylate level. Monitor patient for lack of salicylate effectiveness.
Skin-test antigens: May decrease response. Postpone skin testing until therapy is completed.
Toxoids, vaccines: May decrease antibody response and may increase risk of neurologic complications. Avoid using together.
Drug-herb. *Echinacea:* May increase immune-stimulating effects. Discourage use together.
Ginseng: May increase immune-modulating response. Discourage use together.

Nursing considerations

- Determine whether patient is sensitive to other corticosteroids.
- Always adjust to lowest effective dose.
- Prednisolone salts (sodium phosphate and tebutate) are less often used parenterally than other corticosteroids that have more potent anti-inflammatory action.
- Drug may be used for alternate-day therapy.
- Most adverse reactions to corticosteroids are dose- or duration-dependent.
- Give oral dose with food, when possible, to reduce GI irritation. Patient may need medication to prevent GI irritation.
- Give I.M. injection deeply into gluteal muscle. Rotate injection sites to prevent muscle atrophy. Avoid S.C. injection because atrophy and sterile abscesses may occur.

!!ALERT Prednisolone acetate and tebutate aren't for I.V. use.

- Monitor patient's weight, blood pressure, and electrolyte level.
- Monitor patient for cushingoid effects, including moon face, buffalo hump, central obesity, thinning hair, hypertension, and increased susceptibility to infection.
- Watch for depression or psychotic episodes, especially during high-dose therapy.
- Diabetic patient may need increased insulin; monitor glucose level.
- Unless contraindicated, give low-sodium diet that's high in potassium and protein. Give potassium supplements as needed.
- Drug may mask or worsen infections, including latent amebiasis.
- Elderly patients may be more susceptible to osteoporosis with long-term use.
- Gradually reduce dosage after long-term therapy.

!!ALERT Don't confuse prednisolone with prednisone.

Patient teaching

- Tell patient not to stop drug abruptly or without prescriber's consent.
- Instruct patient to take oral form of drug with food or milk.
- Teach patient signs and symptoms of early adrenal insufficiency: fatigue, muscle weakness, joint pain, fever, anorexia, nausea, shortness of breath, dizziness, and fainting.
- Instruct patient to carry or wear medical identification indicating his need for supplemental systemic glucocorticoids during stress. It should include prescriber's name, and name and dosage of drug.
- Warn patient on long-term therapy about cushingoid effects (moon face, buffalo hump) and the need to notify prescriber about sudden weight gain or swelling.
- Tell patient to report slow healing.
- Advise patient receiving long-term therapy to consider exercise or physical therapy. Also, tell him to ask prescriber about vitamin D or calcium supplement.

- Instruct patient to avoid exposure to infections and to notify prescriber if exposure occurs.
- Tell patient to avoid immunizations while taking drug.
- Tell patient to store Orapred in the refrigerator between 36° to 46° F (2° to 8° C).

prednisolone acetate (suspension)

Econopred Ophthalmic, Econopred Plus Ophthalmic, Pred Forte, Pred Mild Ophthalmic

prednisolone sodium phosphate (solution)

AK-Pred, Inflamase Forte, Inflamase Mild

Pregnancy risk category C

Indications & dosages

➲ Inflammation of palpebral and bulbar conjunctiva, cornea, and anterior segment of globe

Adults and children: Instill 1 or 2 drops into eye. In severe conditions, may be used hourly, tapering to end as inflammation subsides. In mild or moderate inflammation or when a favorable response is attained in severe conditions, dosage may be reduced to 1 or 2 drops q 3 to 12 hours.

Contraindications & cautions

- Contraindicated in patients with acute, untreated, purulent ocular infections; acute superficial herpes simplex (dendritic keratitis); vaccinia, varicella, or other viral or fungal eye diseases; or ocular tuberculosis.
- Use cautiously in patients with corneal abrasions that may be contaminated (especially with herpes).

Adverse reactions

EENT: increased intraocular pressure, thinning of cornea, interference with corneal wound healing, increased susceptibility to viral or fungal corneal infection, corneal ulceration, discharge, discomfort, foreign body sensation, glaucoma worsening, cataracts, visual acuity and visual field defects, optic nerve damage with excessive or long-term use.

Other: systemic effects, adrenal suppression with excessive or long-term use.

Interactions

None significant.

Nursing considerations

- Shake suspension and check dosage before giving to ensure correct strength. Store in tightly covered container.

!!ALERT Don't confuse prednisolone with prednisone.

Patient teaching

- Teach patient how to instill drops. Advise him to wash hands before and after instillation, and warn him not to touch tip of dropper to eye or surrounding area.
- Advise patient to apply light finger pressure on lacrimal sac for 1 minute after instillation.
- Tell patient on long-term therapy to have intraocular pressure tested frequently.
- Tell patient not to share drug, washcloths, or towels with family members and to notify prescriber if anyone develops same signs or symptoms.
- Stress importance of compliance with recommended therapy.
- Tell patient to notify prescriber if improvement doesn't occur within several days or if pain, itching, or swelling of eye occurs.
- Warn patient not to use leftover drug for new eye inflammation because serious problems may occur.

prednisone

Apo-Prednisone†, Deltasone, Liquid Pred*, Meticorten, Orasone, Panasol-S, Prednicen-M, Prednisone Intensol*, Sterapred, Winpred†

Pregnancy risk category C

Indications & dosages

➲ Severe inflammation, immunosuppression

Adults: 5 to 60 mg P.O. daily in single dose or as two to four divided doses. Maintenance dose given once daily or every other day. Dosage must be individualized.

Children: 0.14 to 2 mg/kg or 4 to 60 mg/m² daily P.O. in four divided doses.

➲ **Acute exacerbations of multiple sclerosis**
Adults: 200 mg P.O. daily for 7 days; then 80 mg P.O. every other day for 1 month.

Contraindications & cautions

- Contraindicated in patients hypersensitive to drug or its ingredients, in those with systemic fungal infections, and in those receiving immunosuppressive doses together with live virus vaccines.
- Use cautiously in patients with recent MI, GI ulcer, renal disease, hypertension, osteoporosis, diabetes mellitus, hypothyroidism, cirrhosis, active hepatitis, lactation, diverticulitis, nonspecific ulcerative colitis, recent intestinal anastomoses, thromboembolic disorders, seizures, myasthenia gravis, heart failure, tuberculosis, ocular herpes simplex, emotional instability, and psychotic tendencies.

Adverse reactions

CNS: *euphoria*, *insomnia*, psychotic behavior, ***pseudotumor cerebri***, vertigo, headache, paresthesia, ***seizures***.
CV: ***heart failure***, hypertension, edema, ***arrhythmias***, thrombophlebitis, ***thromboembolism***.
EENT: cataracts, glaucoma.
GI: *peptic ulceration*, GI irritation, increased appetite, ***pancreatitis***, nausea, vomiting.
GU: menstrual irregularities, increased urine calcium level.
Metabolic: hypokalemia, hyperglycemia, carbohydrate intolerance, hypercholesterolemia, hypocalcemia.
Musculoskeletal: growth suppression in children, muscle weakness, osteoporosis.
Skin: hirsutism, delayed wound healing, acne, various skin eruptions.
Other: cushingoid state, susceptibility to infections, ***acute adrenal insufficiency***, after increased stress or abrupt withdrawal after long-term therapy.
After abrupt withdrawal: rebound inflammation; fatigue; weakness; arthralgia; fever; dizziness; lethargy; depression; fainting; orthostatic hypotension; dyspnea; anorexia, hypoglycemia. After prolonged use, sudden withdrawal may be fatal.

Interactions

Drug-drug. *Aspirin, indomethacin, other NSAIDs:* May increase risk of GI distress and bleeding. Use together cautiously.
Barbiturates, carbamazepine, fosphenytoin, phenytoin, rifampin: May decrease corticosteroid effect. Increase corticosteroid dosage.
Cyclosporine: May increase toxicity. Monitor patient closely.
Oral anticoagulants: May alter dosage requirements. Monitor PT and INR closely.
Potassium-depleting drugs such as thiazide diuretics: May enhance potassium-wasting effects of prednisone. Monitor potassium level.
Salicylates: May decrease salicylate level. Monitor patient for lack of salicylate effectiveness.
Skin-test antigens: May decrease response. Postpone skin testing until therapy is completed.
Toxoids, vaccines: May decrease antibody response and may increase risk of neurologic complications. Avoid using together.
Drug-herb. *Echinacea:* May increase immune-stimulating effects. Discourage use together.
Ginseng: May increase immune-modulating response. Discourage use together.

Nursing considerations

- Determine whether patient is sensitive to other corticosteroids.
- Drug may be used for alternate-day therapy.
- Always adjust to lowest effective dose.
- Most adverse reactions to corticosteroids are dose- or duration-dependent.
- For better results and less toxicity, give a once-daily dose in the morning.
- Unless contraindicated, give oral dose with food when possible to reduce GI irritation. Patient may need medication to prevent GI irritation.
- The oral solution may be diluted in juice or other flavored diluent or semi-solid food (such as applesauce) before using.
- Monitor patient's blood pressure, sleep patterns, and potassium level.
- Weigh patient daily; report sudden weight gain to prescriber.
- Monitor patient for cushingoid effects, including moon face, buffalo hump, central

obesity, thinning hair, hypertension, and increased susceptibility to infection.

- Watch for depression or psychotic episodes, especially during high-dose therapy.
- Diabetic patient may need increased insulin; monitor glucose level.
- Elderly patients may be more susceptible to osteoporosis with long-term use.
- Drug may mask or worsen infections, including latent amebiasis.
- Unless contraindicated, give low-sodium diet that's high in potassium and protein. Give potassium supplements, as needed.
- Gradually reduce dosage after long-term therapy.

!! ALERT Don't confuse prednisone with prednisolone, primidone, or prednimustine.

Patient teaching

- Tell patient not to stop drug abruptly or without prescriber's consent.
- Instruct patient to take drug with food or milk.
- Teach patient signs and symptoms of early adrenal insufficiency: fatigue, muscle weakness, joint pain, fever, anorexia, nausea, shortness of breath, dizziness, and fainting.
- Instruct patient to carry or wear medical identification indicating his need for supplemental systemic glucocorticoids during stress. It should include prescriber's name and name and dosage of drug.
- Warn patient on long-term therapy about cushingoid effects (moon face, buffalo hump) and the need to notify prescriber about sudden weight gain or swelling.
- Advise patient receiving long-term therapy to consider exercise or physical therapy. Also, tell patient to ask prescriber about vitamin D or calcium supplement.
- Tell patient to report slow healing.
- Advise patient receiving long-term therapy to have periodic eye examinations.
- Instruct patient to avoid exposure to infections and to contact prescriber if exposure occurs.

primaquine phosphate

Pregnancy risk category NR

Indications & dosages

➲ **Relapsing *Plasmodium vivax* malaria, eliminating symptoms and infection completely; to prevent relapse**

Adults: 15 mg base P.O. daily for 14 days. Begin therapy during the last 2 weeks of, or after, a course of suppression with chloroquine or comparable drug.

Children: 0.3 mg/kg/day base P.O. for 14 days. Maximum 15 mg base/dose. Begin therapy during the last 2 weeks of, or after, a course of suppression with chloroquine or comparable drug.

Contraindications & cautions

- Contraindicated in patients with systemic diseases in which agranulocytosis may develop, such as lupus erythematosus or rheumatoid arthritis, and in those taking a bone marrow suppressant, quinacrine, or potentially hemolytic drug.
- Use cautiously in patients with previous idiosyncratic reaction involving hemolytic anemia, methemoglobinemia, or leukopenia; in those with a family or personal history of favism; and in those with erythrocytic nicotinamide-adenine-dinucleotide (NADH) methemoglobin reductase deficiency or G6PD.

Adverse reactions

GI: nausea, vomiting, epigastric distress, abdominal cramps.

Hematologic: ***hemolytic anemia***, methemoglobinemia, ***leukopenia***.

Interactions

Drug-drug. *Aluminum salts, magnesium:* Decreases GI absorption. Separate dose times.

Nursing considerations

!! ALERT Drug dosage may be discussed in "mg" or "mg base;" be aware of the difference.

- Give drug with meals.
- Drug is used along with a fast-acting antimalarial such as chloroquine to reduce possibility of drug-resistant strains.

• Obtain frequent blood studies and urinalysis in light-skinned patients taking more than 30 mg base daily, dark-skinned patients taking more than 15 mg base daily, and patients with severe anemia or suspected sensitivity.
• Monitor patient for markedly darkened urine and for suddenly reduced hemoglobin level or erythrocyte or leukocyte count, which suggest impending hemolytic reactions. Stop drug immediately and notify prescriber.
• Safe use during pregnancy hasn't been established.

Patient teaching

• Instruct patient to take drug with meals to minimize stomach upset. If nausea, vomiting, or stomach pain persists, tell patient to notify prescriber.
• Tell patient to report to prescriber chills, fever, chest pain, and bluish skin discoloration; these signs and symptoms may suggest a hemolytic reaction.
• Tell patient to stop drug and notify prescriber immediately if urine darkens markedly.
• Stress importance of completing full course of therapy.

primidone

Apo-Primidone†, Mysoline, PMS Primidone†, Sertan†

Pregnancy risk category NR

Indications & dosages

➲ **Tonic-clonic, complex partial, and simple partial seizures**
Adults and children age 8 and older: Initially, 100 to 125 mg P.O. h.s. on days 1 to 3; then 100 to 125 mg P.O. b.i.d. on days 4 to 6; then 100 to 125 mg P.O. t.i.d. on days 7 to 9, followed by maintenance dose of 250 mg P.O. t.i.d. Maintenance dose may be increased to 250 mg q.i.d., if needed. Dosage may be increased to maximum of 2 g daily in divided doses.
Children younger than age 8: Initially, 50 mg P.O. h.s. for 3 days; then 50 mg P.O. b.i.d. for days 4 to 6; then 100 mg P.O. b.i.d. for days 7 to 9, followed by maintenance dose of 125 to 250 mg P.O. t.i.d. or 10 to 25 mg/kg daily in divided doses.

➲ **Essential tremor♦**
Adults: 750 mg P.O. daily.

Contraindications & cautions

• Contraindicated in patients hypersensitive to phenobarbital and in those with porphyria.

Adverse reactions

CNS: *drowsiness, ataxia,* emotional disturbances, vertigo, hyperirritability, fatigue, paranoid symptoms.
EENT: *diplopia,* nystagmus.
GI: anorexia, *nausea, vomiting.*
GU: impotence, polyuria.
Hematologic: megaloblastic anemia, ***thrombocytopenia.***
Skin: morbilliform rash.

Interactions

Drug-drug. *Acetazolamide, succinimide:* May decrease primidone level. Monitor level.
Carbamazepine: May increase carbamazepine level and decrease primidone and phenobarbital levels. Watch for toxicity.
CNS depressants: May cause additive CNS depression. Avoid using together.
Isoniazid: May increase primidone level. Monitor level.
Metoprolol, propranolol: May reduce effects of these drugs. Consider increasing beta-blocker dose.
Phenytoin: May stimulate conversion of primidone to phenobarbital. Watch for increased phenobarbital effect.
Drug-lifestyle. *Alcohol use:* May impair coordination, increase CNS effects, and cause death. Strongly discourage alcohol use with this drug.

Nursing considerations

• Don't withdraw drug suddenly because seizures may worsen. Notify prescriber immediately if adverse reactions develop.
• Therapeutic level of primidone is 5 to 12 mcg/ml. Therapeutic level of phenobarbital is 15 to 40 mcg/ml.
• Monitor CBC and routine blood chemistry every 6 months.
• Brand interchange isn't recommended because of documented bioequivalence problems for primidone products marketed by different manufacturers.

!!ALERT Don't confuse primidone with prednisone or Prinivil.

Patient teaching

- Advise patient to avoid driving and other potentially hazardous activities that require mental alertness until drug's CNS effects are known.
- Warn patient and parents not to stop drug therapy suddenly.
- Tell patient that full therapeutic response may take 2 weeks or longer.
- Advise woman of childbearing age to discuss drug therapy with prescriber if she's considering pregnancy.
- Caution woman of childbearing age that breast-feeding is contraindicated while taking this drug.

probenecid
Benuryl†

Pregnancy risk category B

Indications & dosages

➲ Adjunct to penicillin therapy
Adults and children weighing more than 50 kg (110 lb): 500 mg P.O. q.i.d.
Children ages 2 to 14 or weighing 50 kg or less: Initially, 25 mg/kg P.O.; then 40 mg/kg/day in divided doses q.i.d.

➲ Gonorrhea
Adults: Give 3.5 g ampicillin or 3 g amoxicillin P.O. along with 1 g probenecid P.O. Or, 1 g probenecid P.O. 30 minutes before 4.8 million units of aqueous penicillin G procaine I.M., injected at two different sites.

➲ Hyperuricemia of gout, gouty arthritis
Adults: 250 mg P.O. b.i.d. for first week; then 500 mg b.i.d., to maximum of 2 to 3 g daily. Review maintenance dose q 6 months and reduce by increments of 500 mg, if indicated.

Contraindications & cautions

- Contraindicated in patients hypersensitive to drug and in those with uric acid kidney stones or blood dyscrasias; also contraindicated in patients with an acute gout attack and in children younger than age 2.
- Use cautiously in patients with peptic ulcer or renal impairment.
- Use cautiously in patients with sulfa allergy because probenecid is a sulfonamide derivative.

Adverse reactions

CNS: fever, *headache*, dizziness.
CV: flushing.
GI: anorexia, nausea, vomiting, sore gums.
GU: urinary frequency, renal colic, nephrotic syndrome, costovertebral pain.
Hematologic: ***hemolytic anemia***, anemia, ***aplastic anemia***.
Hepatic: ***hepatic necrosis***.
Skin: dermatitis, pruritus.
Other: worsening of gout; hypersensitivity reactions, including; ***anaphylaxis***.

Interactions

Drug-drug. *Acyclovir, cephalosporins, clofibrate, dapsone, ketamine, lorazepam, meclofenamate, penicillin, rifampin, sulfonamides, thiopental:* May increase levels of these drugs. Use together cautiously.
Allopurinol: May increase uric acid–lowering effects. May be used to therapeutic advantage.
Methotrexate: May impair excretion of methotrexate, causing increased level, effects, and toxicity of methotrexate. Monitor methotrexate level closely and adjust dosage accordingly.
Nitrofurantoin: May increase toxicity and reduce effectiveness of nitrofurantoin. Reduce probenecid dose.
NSAIDs: May increase NSAID toxicity. Avoid using together.
Salicylates: May inhibit uricosuric effect of probenecid, causing urate retention. Avoid using together.
Sulfonylureas: May increase hypoglycemic effect. Monitor glucose level closely. Dosage may need to be adjusted.
Zidovudine: May increase zidovudine level and toxicity symptoms. Monitor patient.
Drug-lifestyle. *Alcohol use:* May increase urate level. Discourage use together.

Nursing considerations

- To minimize GI distress, give drug with milk, food, or antacids. Continued disturbances might indicate need to reduce dosage.
- Force fluids to maintain minimum daily output of 2 to 3 L. Alkalinize urine with sodium bicarbonate or potassium citrate.

These measures prevent hematuria, renal colic, urate stone development, and costovertebral pain.
- Don't start treating gout until acute attack subsides. Drug has no analgesic or anti-inflammatory effects and is of no value during acute gout attacks.
- Monitor BUN and renal function test results periodically in long-term therapy.
- Drug is suitable for long-term use; no cumulative effects or tolerance have been reported.
- Drug is ineffective in patients with glomerular filtration rate below 30 ml/minute.
- Drug may increase frequency, severity, and length of acute gout attacks during first 6 to 12 months of therapy. Colchicine or another anti-inflammatory may be used preventively during first 3 to 6 months.

!!ALERT Don't confuse probenecid with Procanbid.

Patient teaching

- Instruct patient with gout to take drug regularly to prevent recurrence.
- Tell patient to visit prescriber regularly so that uric acid can be monitored and dosage adjusted, if needed. Lifelong therapy may be needed in patients with hyperuricemia.
- Advise patient with gout to avoid all drugs that contain aspirin, which may precipitate gout. Acetaminophen may be used for pain.
- Instruct patient to drink at least 6 to 8 glasses of water per day.
- Urge patient with gout to avoid alcohol; it increases urate level.
- Tell patient with gout to limit intake of foods high in purine, such as anchovies, liver, sardines, kidneys, sweetbreads, peas, and lentils. Also tell him to identify and avoid other foods that may trigger gout attacks.
- Because drug may be prescribed with an antibiotic, instruct patient to take all medicine as prescribed.

procainamide hydrochloride

Procanbid, Pronestyl, Pronestyl Filmlok, Pronestyl-SR Filmlok

Pregnancy risk category C

Indications & dosages

➲ Symptomatic PVCs; life-threatening ventricular tachycardia

Adults: 100 mg q 5 minutes by slow I.V. push, no faster than 25 to 50 mg/minute, until arrhythmias disappear, adverse effects develop, or 500 mg has been given. Usual effective loading dose is 500 to 600 mg. Alternatively, give a loading dose of 500 to 600 mg I.V. infusion over 25 to 30 minutes. Maximum total dose is 1 g. When arrhythmias disappear, give continuous infusion of 2 to 6 mg/minute. If arrhythmias recur, repeat bolus as above and increase infusion rate.

For I.M. administration, give 50 mg/kg divided q 3 to 6 hours; if arrhythmias occur during surgery, give 100 to 500 mg I.M.

For oral therapy, start at 50 mg/kg/day of P.O. of conventional tablets or capsules in divided doses q 3 hours until therapeutic level is reached. For maintenance, substitute extended-release form to deliver the total daily dose divided q 6 hours or extended-release form (Procanbid) at a dose of 50 mg/kg P.O. in two divided doses q 12 hours.

Children♦: Dosage not established. Recommendations include 2 to 5 mg/kg I.V., not exceeding 100 mg, repeated p.r.n. at 5- to 10-minute intervals, not exceeding 15 mg/kg in 24 hours or 500 mg in 30 minutes. Or, 15 mg/kg infused over 30 to 60 minutes; then maintenance infusion of 0.02 to 0.08 mg/kg/minute.

➲ To convert atrial fibrillation or paroxysmal atrial tachycardia♦

Adults: 1.25 g P.O. of conventional tablets or capsules. If arrhythmias persist after 1 hour, give additional 750 mg. If no change occurs, give 500 mg to 1 g P.O. q 2 hours until arrhythmias disappear or adverse effects occur. Maintenance dose is 1 g extended-release q 6 hours.

Children: 15 to 50 mg/kg/day P.O. divided q 3 to 6 hours. Maximum dose 4 g daily. Or, 20 to 30 mg/kg/day I.M. Or, loading dose of 3 to 6 mg/kg I.V. over 5 minutes, up to

100 mg/dose; then maintenance dose 20 to 80 mcg/kg/minute as continuous I.V. infusion. Maximum daily dose is 2 g.

➲ **To maintain normal sinus rhythm after conversion of atrial flutter**♦

Adults: 0.5 to 1 g P.O. of conventional tablets or capsules q 4 to 6 hours.

➲ **Malignant hyperthermia**♦

Adults: 200 to 900 mg I.V., followed by maintenance infusion.

For patients with renal or hepatic dysfunction, decrease dose or increase dosing interval, as needed.

Contraindications & cautions

- Contraindicated in patients hypersensitive to procaine and related drugs.
- Contraindicated in those with complete, second-, or third-degree heart block in the absence of an artificial pacemaker. Also contraindicated in those with myasthenia gravis, systemic lupus erythematosus, or atypical ventricular tachycardia (torsades de pointes).
- Use with extreme caution in patients with ventricular tachycardia during coronary occlusion.
- Use cautiously in patients with heart failure or other conduction disturbances, such as bundle-branch heart block, sinus bradycardia, or digitalis intoxication; in those with hepatic or renal insufficiency; and in those with blood dyscrasias or bone marrow suppression.

Adverse reactions

CNS: *fever*, hallucinations, psychosis, giddiness, confusion, ***seizures***, depression, dizziness.

CV: hypotension, ***bradycardia***, ***AV block***, ***ventricular fibrillation***, ***ventricular asystole***.

GI: abdominal pain, nausea, vomiting, anorexia, diarrhea, bitter taste.

Skin: *maculopapular rash*, *urticaria*, *pruritus*, *flushing*, *angioneurotic edema*.

Other: *lupus-like syndrome*.

Interactions

Drug-drug. *Amiodarone:* May increase procainamide level and toxicity; additive effects on QTc interval and QRS complex. Avoid using together.

Anticholinergics: May increase antivagal effects. Monitor patient closely.

Anticholinesterases: May decrease effect of anticholinesterases. Anticholinesterase dosage may need to be increased.

Beta blockers, ranitidine, trimethoprim: May increase procainamide level. Watch for toxicity.

Cimetidine: May increase procainamide level. Avoid this combination if possible. Monitor procainamide level closely and adjust the dosage as necessary.

Neuromuscular blockers: May increase skeletal muscle relaxant effect. Monitor patient closely.

Drug-herb. *Jimsonweed:* May adversely affect CV function. Discourage use together.

Licorice: May have additive effect and prolong QTc interval. Urge caution.

Drug-lifestyle. *Alcohol use:* May reduce drug level. Discourage use together.

Nursing considerations

- Monitor level of procainamide and its active metabolite NAPA. To suppress ventricular arrhythmias, therapeutic levels of procainamide are 4 to 8 mcg/ml; therapeutic levels of NAPA are 10 to 30 mcg/ml.
- Monitor QTc interval closely. Dosage reduction may be needed if QTc interval is prolonged more than 50% from baseline.
- Hypokalemia predisposes patient to arrhythmias. Monitor electrolytes, especially potassium level.
- Elderly patients may be more likely to develop hypotension. Monitor blood pressure carefully.
- Monitor CBC frequently during first 3 months of therapy.
- Positive ANA titer is common in about 60% of patients who don't have symptoms of lupuslike syndrome. This response seems to be related to prolonged use, not dosage. May progress to systemic lupus erythematosus if drug isn't stopped.

!!ALERT Don't crush the extended-release tablets.

- The Filmlok formulation may contain tartrazine.

!!ALERT Don't confuse Procanbid with probenecid.

Patient teaching

- Stress importance of taking drug exactly as prescribed. This may require use of an alarm clock for nighttime doses.

- Instruct patient to report fever, rash, muscle pain, diarrhea, bleeding, bruises, or pleuritic chest pain.
- Tell patient not to crush or break extended-release tablets.
- Reassure patient who is taking extended-release form that a wax-matrix "ghost" from the tablet may be passed in stools. Drug is completely absorbed before this occurs.

prochlorperazine
Compazine, Compro, PMS Prochlorperazine†, Stemetil†

prochlorperazine edisylate
Compazine, Compazine Syrup

prochlorperazine maleate
Compazine, Compazine Spansule, PMS Prochlorperazine†, Stemetil†

Pregnancy risk category C

Indications & dosages

➲ To control preoperative nausea
Adults: 5 to 10 mg I.M. 1 to 2 hours before induction of anesthesia; repeat once in 30 minutes, if needed. Or, 5 to 10 mg I.V. 15 to 30 minutes before induction of anesthesia; repeat once, if needed.

➲ Severe nausea and vomiting
Adults: 5 to 10 mg P.O., t.i.d. or q.i.d.; 15 mg sustained-release form P.O. on rising; 10 mg sustained-release form P.O. q 12 hours; 25 mg P.R., b.i.d.; or 5 to 10 mg I.M., repeated q 3 to 4 hours, p.r.n. Maximum I.M. dose is 40 mg daily. Or, 2.5 to 10 mg I.V. at no more than 5 mg/minute.
Children weighing 18 to 39 kg (39 to 86 lb): 2.5 mg P.O. or P.R., t.i.d.; or 5 mg P.O. or P.R., b.i.d. Maximum, 15 mg daily. Or, 0.132 mg/kg by deep I.M. injection. Control is usually achieved with one dose.
Children weighing 14 to 17 kg (30 to 38 lb): 2.5 mg P.O. or P.R., b.i.d. or t.i.d. Maximum, 10 mg daily. Or, 0.132 mg/kg by deep I.M. injection. Control is usually achieved with one dose.
Children weighing 9 to 13 kg (20 to 29 lb): 2.5 mg P.O. or P.R. once daily or b.i.d. Maximum, 7.5 mg daily. Or, 0.132 mg/kg by deep I.M. injection. Control is usually achieved with one dose.

➲ To manage symptoms of psychotic disorders
Adults and children age 12 and older: 5 to 10 mg P.O., t.i.d. or q.i.d.
Children ages 2 to 12: 2.5 mg P.O. or P.R., b.i.d. or t.i.d. Don't exceed 10 mg on day 1. Increase dosage gradually to maximum, if needed. In children ages 2 to 5, maximum is 20 mg daily. In children ages 6 to 12, maximum is 25 mg daily.

➲ To manage symptoms of severe psychosis
Adults and children age 12 and older: 10 to 20 mg I.M., repeated in 1 to 4 hours, if needed. Rarely, patients may receive 10 to 20 mg q 4 to 6 hours. Start oral therapy after symptoms are controlled.
Children ages 2 to 12: 0.13 mg/kg I.M.

➲ Nonpsychotic anxiety
Adults: 5 to 10 mg P.O., t.i.d. or q.i.d. Or, 15 mg extended-release capsule once daily. Or, 10 mg extended-release capsule q 12 hours. Don't exceed 20 mg daily, and don't give for longer than 12 weeks.

Contraindications & cautions

- Contraindicated in patients hypersensitive to phenothiazines and in patients with CNS depression, including those in a coma.
- Contraindicated during pediatric surgery, when using spinal or epidural anesthetic or adrenergic blockers, and in children younger than age 2.
- Use cautiously in patients with impaired CV function, glaucoma, seizure disorders, and Parkinson's disease; in those who have been exposed to extreme heat; and in children with acute illness.

Adverse reactions

CNS: *extrapyramidal reactions,* sedation, pseudoparkinsonism, EEG changes, dizziness.
CV: *orthostatic hypotension,* tachycardia, ECG changes.
EENT: *ocular changes, blurred vision.*
GI: *dry mouth, constipation,* increased appetite.
GU: *urine retention,* dark urine, menstrual irregularities, inhibited ejaculation.
Hematologic: ***transient leukopenia, agranulocytosis.***
Hepatic: cholestatic jaundice.
Metabolic: weight gain.

Skin: *mild photosensitivity*, allergic reactions, exfoliative dermatitis.
Other: gynecomastia, hyperprolactinemia.

Interactions

Drug-drug. *Antacids:* May inhibit absorption of oral phenothiazines. Separate antacid and phenothiazine doses by at least 2 hours.
Anticholinergics, including antidepressants and antiparkinsonians: May increase anticholinergic activity and may aggravate parkinsonian symptoms. Use together cautiously.
Barbiturates: May decrease phenothiazine effect. Monitor patient for decreased antiemetic effect.
Drug-herb. *Dong quai, St. John's wort:* May increase risk of photosensitivity. Advise patient to avoid excessive sun exposure.
Kava: May increase risk of dystonic reactions. Discourage use together.
Drug-lifestyle. *Alcohol use:* May increase CNS depression, particularly psychomotor skills. Strongly discourage use together.

Nursing considerations

- Dilute oral solution with tomato juice, fruit juice, milk, coffee, carbonated beverage, tea, water, or soup. Or, mix with pudding.
- Watch for orthostatic hypotension, especially when giving drug I.V.
- For I.M. use, inject deeply into upper outer quadrant of gluteal region.
- Don't give by S.C. route or mix in syringe with another drug.
- To prevent contact dermatitis, avoid getting concentrate or injection solution on hands or clothing.
- Monitor CBC and liver function studies during long-term therapy.

!!ALERT Use drug only when vomiting can't be controlled by other measures or when only a few doses are needed. If more than four doses are needed in 24 hours, notify prescriber.

- Store in light-resistant container. Slight yellowing doesn't affect potency; discard extremely discolored solutions.

Patient teaching

- Teach patient what to use to dilute oral solution.
- Advise patient to wear protective clothing when exposed to sunlight.
- Tell patient to call prescriber if more than four doses are needed within 24 hours.

promethazine hydrochloride
Phenadoz, Phenergan*

promethazine theoclate‡

Pregnancy risk category C

Indications & dosages

➲ Motion sickness
Adults: 25 mg P.O. or P.R. taken 30 minutes to 1 hour before departure. May repeat dose 8 to 12 hours later, if needed.
Children older than age 2: 12.5 to 25 mg P.O. or P.R. 30 minutes to 1 hour before departure. May repeat dose 8 to 12 hours later, if needed.

➲ Nausea and vomiting
Adults: 12.5 to 25 mg P.O., I.M., or P.R. q 4 to 6 hours, p.r.n.
Children older than age 2: 12.5 to 25 mg P.O. or P.R. q 4 to 6 hours, p.r.n. Or, 6.25 to 12.5 mg I.M. q 4 to 6 hours, p.r.n.

➲ Rhinitis, allergy symptoms
Adults: 12.5 mg P.O. or P.R. q.i.d.; or 25 mg P.O. or P.R. h.s.
Children older than age 2: 6.25 to 12.5 mg P.O. or P.R. t.i.d., or 25 mg P.O. or P.R. h.s.

➲ Nighttime sedation
Adults: 25 to 50 mg P.O., P.R., I.V., or I.M. h.s.
Children older than age 2: 12.5 to 25 mg P.O., I.M., or P.R. h.s.

➲ Adjunct to analgesics for routine preoperative or postoperative sedation
Adults: 25 to 50 mg I.M. or I.V., or 25 to 50 mg P.O. or P.R.
Children older than age 2: 0.5 to 1.1 mg/kg P.O., P.R., or I.M.

Contraindications & cautions

- Contraindicated in patients hypersensitive to drug, those who have experienced adverse reactions to phenothiazines, breast-feeding women, children younger than age 2, and acutely ill or dehydrated children.
- Use cautiously in patients with asthma or pulmonary, hepatic, or CV disease and in those with intestinal obstruction, prostatic hyperplasia, bladder-neck obstruction, angle-closure glaucoma, seizure disorders,

coma, CNS depression, and stenosing or peptic ulcerations.

Adverse reactions

CNS: *sedation*, confusion, sleepiness, dizziness, disorientation, extrapyramidal symptoms, *drowsiness*.
CV: hypotension, hypertension.
EENT: blurred vision.
GI: nausea, vomiting, *dry mouth*.
GU: urine retention.
Hematologic: ***leukopenia, agranulocytosis, thrombocytopenia***.
Metabolic: hyperglycemia.
Skin: photosensitivity, rash.

Interactions

Drug-drug. *Anticholinergics, phenothiazines, tricyclic antidepressants:* May increase anticholinergic effects. Avoid using together.
CNS depressants: May increase sedation. Use together cautiously.
Epinephrine: May block or reverse effects of epinephrine. Use other pressor drugs instead.
Levodopa: May decrease antiparkinsonian action of levodopa. Avoid using together.
Lithium: May reduce GI absorption or enhance renal elimination of lithium. Avoid using together.
MAO inhibitors: May increase extrapyramidal effects. Avoid using together.
Drug-herb. *Yohimbe:* May increase risk of yohimbe toxicity. Ask patient about use of herbal remedies, and recommend caution.
Drug-lifestyle. *Alcohol use:* May increase sedation. Discourage use together.
Sun exposure: May cause photosensitivity reactions. Advise patient to avoid extensive sunlight exposure and to use sunblock.

Nursing considerations

- Monitor patient for neuroleptic malignant syndrome: altered mental status, autonomic instability, muscle rigidity, and hyperpyrexia.
- Stop drug 4 days before diagnostic skin testing because antihistamines can prevent, reduce, or mask positive skin test response.
- Pronounced sedative effect limits use in many ambulatory patients.
- Promethazine is used as an adjunct to analgesics (usually to increase sedation); it has no analgesic activity.
- Reduce GI distress by giving drug with food or milk.
- I.M. injection is the preferred parenteral route of administration. Inject deep I.M. into large muscle mass. Rotate injection sites.

!!ALERT Don't give by S.C. route.

- Drug may be mixed with meperidine in same syringe.
- In patients scheduled for a myelogram, stop drug 48 hours before procedure. Don't resume drug until 24 hours after procedure because of the risk of seizures.

!!ALERT Don't confuse promethazine with promazine.

Patient teaching

- Tell patient to take oral form with food or milk.
- When treating motion sickness, tell patient to take first dose 30 to 60 minutes before travel; dose may be repeated in 8 to 12 hours if necessary. On succeeding days of travel, patient should take dose upon arising and with evening meal.
- Warn patient to avoid alcohol and hazardous activities that require alertness until CNS effects of drug are known.
- Inform patient that sugarless gum, hard candy, or ice chips may relieve dry mouth.
- Warn patient about possible photosensitivity reactions. Advise use of a sunblock.

propafenone hydrochloride

Rythmol, Rythmol SR

Pregnancy risk category C

Indications & dosages

➲ **To suppress life-threatening ventricular arrhythmias such as sustained ventricular tachycardia (SVT); to prevent life-threatening paroxysmal SVT and paroxysmal atrial fibrillation or flutter**
Adults: Initially, 150 mg immediate-release tablet P.O. q 8 hours. May increase dosage q 3 or 4 days to 225 mg q 8 hours. If needed, increase dosage to 300 mg q 8 hours. Maximum daily dose, 900 mg.
➲ **To prolong time until recurrence of symptomatic atrial fibrillation**
Adults: Initially, 225 mg extended-release capsule P.O. q 12 hours. May increase dose after 5 days to 325 mg P.O. q 12 hours. May increase dose to 425 mg q 12 hours.

For patients with hepatic impairment, reduce initial dose of immediate-release tablets by 70% to 80%.

Contraindications & cautions

- Contraindicated in patients hypersensitive to drug and in those with severe or uncontrolled heart failure; cardiogenic shock; SA, AV, or intraventricular disorders of impulse conduction without a pacemaker; bradycardia; marked hypotension; bronchospastic disorders; or electrolyte imbalances.
- Use cautiously in patients with a history of heart failure because drug may weaken the contraction of the heart.
- Use cautiously in patients taking other cardiac depressants and in those with hepatic or renal impairment.
- Avoid using in patients with myasthenia gravis.

Adverse reactions

CNS: anxiety, ataxia, *dizziness*, drowsiness, fatigue, headache, insomnia, syncope, tremor, weakness.
CV: atrial fibrillation; ***bradycardia***; bundle-branch block; ***heart failure***; angina; chest pain; edema; first-degree AV block; hypotension; increased QRS complex; intraventricular conduction delay; palpitations; ***arrhythmias, ventricular tachycardia, PVCs, ventricular fibrillation***.
EENT: blurred vision.
GI: abdominal pain or cramps, constipation; diarrhea; dyspepsia; anorexia; flatulence; *nausea*; *vomiting*; dry mouth; unusual taste.
Musculoskeletal: arthralgia.
Respiratory: dyspnea.
Skin: rash, diaphoresis.

Interactions

Drug-drug. *Antiarrhythmics:* May increase risk of prolonged QTc interval. Monitor patient closely.
Beta blockers (metoprolol, propranolol): May decrease metabolism of these drugs. Adjust dosage of beta blocker as needed.
Cyclosporine, digoxin: May increase levels of these drugs, causing toxicity. Monitor patient closely.
Desipramine: May decrease desipramine metabolism. Monitor patient closely.
Lidocaine: May decrease lidocaine metabolism. Monitor patient for increased CNS adverse effects and lidocaine toxicity.
Local anesthetics: May increase risk of CNS toxicity. Monitor patient closely.
Mexiletine: May decrease mexiletine metabolism, increasing level and adverse reactions. Monitor mexiletine level and patient closely.
Phenobarbital, rifampin: May increase propafenone clearance. Watch for decreased antiarrhythmic effect.
Quinidine: May decrease propafenone metabolism; may be useful in certain patients refractory to propafenone and quinidine monotherapy. Monitor patient closely.
Ritonavir: May increase propafenone level, causing life-threatening arrhythmias. Avoid using together.
Theophylline: May decrease theophylline metabolism. Monitor theophylline level and ECG closely.
Warfarin: May increase warfarin level. Monitor PT and INR closely, and adjust warfarin dose as needed.

Nursing considerations

- To minimize adverse GI reactions, give drug with food.

!!ALERT Perform continuous cardiac monitoring at start of therapy and during dosage adjustments. If PR interval or QRS complex increases by more than 25%, reduce dosage.

- If using with digoxin, frequently monitor ECG and digoxin level.
- Pacing and sensing thresholds of artificial pacemakers may change; monitor pacemaker function.
- Agranulocytosis may develop during the first 2 to 3 months of therapy. If patient has an unexplained fever, monitor leukocyte count.

Patient teaching

- Stress importance of taking drug exactly as prescribed.
- Tell patient not to double dose if he misses one, but to take the next dose at the usual time.
- Tell patient to report adverse reactions promptly, including fever, sore throat, chills, and other signs and symptoms of infection.
- Instruct patient to notify prescriber if prolonged diarrhea, sweating, vomiting, or loss of appetite or thirst occurs; these may cause an electrolyte imbalance.

• Tell patient not to crush, chew, or open the extended-release capsules.

propofol
Diprivan

Pregnancy risk category B

Indications & dosages

➲ To induce anesthesia
Adults younger than age 55 classified as American Society of Anesthesiologists (ASA) Physical Status (PS) category I or II: 2 to 2.5 mg/kg. Give in 40-mg boluses q 10 seconds until desired response is achieved.
Children ages 3 to 16 classified as ASA I or II: 2.5 to 3.5 mg/kg over 20 to 30 seconds.

In geriatric, debilitated, hypovolemic, or ASA PS III or IV patients, give half the usual induction dose, in 20-mg boluses, q 10 seconds. For cardiac anesthesia, give 20 mg (0.5 to 1.5 mg/kg) q 10 seconds until desired response is achieved. For neurosurgical patients, give 20 mg (1 to 2 mg/kg) q 10 seconds until desired response is achieved.

➲ To maintain anesthesia
Healthy adults younger than age 55: 0.1 to 0.2 mg/kg/minute (6 to 12 mg/kg/hour). Or, give in 20- to 50-mg intermittent boluses, p.r.n.
Healthy children ages 2 months to 16 years: 125 to 300 mcg/kg/minute (7.5 to 18 mg/kg/hour).

In geriatric, debilitated, hypovolemic, or ASA PS III or IV patients, give half the usual maintenance dose (0.05 to 0.1 mg/kg/minute or 3 to 6 mg/kg/hour). For cardiac anesthesia with secondary opioid, 100 to 150 mcg/kg/minute; low dose with primary opioid, 50 to 100 mcg/kg/minute. For neurosurgical patients, 100 to 200 mcg/kg/minute (6 to 12 mg/kg/hour).

➲ Monitored anesthesia care
Healthy adults younger than age 55: Initially, 100 to 150 mcg/kg/minute (6 to 9 mg/kg/hour) for 3 to 5 minutes or a slow injection of 0.5 mg/kg over 3 to 5 minutes. For maintenance dose, give infusion of 25 to 75 mcg/kg/minute (1.5 to 4.5 mg/kg/hour), or incremental 10- or 20-mg boluses.

In geriatric, debilitated, or ASA PS III or IV patients, give 80% of usual adult maintenance dose. Don't use rapid bolus.

➲ To sedate intubated intensive care unit (ICU) patients
Adults: Initially, 5 mcg/kg/minute (0.3 mg/kg/hour) for 5 minutes. Increments of 5 to 10 mcg/kg/minute (0.3 to 0.6 mg/kg/hour) over 5 to 10 minutes may be used until desired sedation is achieved. Maintenance rate, 5 to 50 mcg/kg/minute (0.3 to 3 mg/kg/hour).

Contraindications & cautions

• Contraindicated in patients hypersensitive to drug or its components (including egg lecithin, soybean oil, and glycerol), in pregnant women (because it may cause fetal depression), and in those unable to undergo general anesthesia or sedation.
• Use cautiously in patients who are hemodynamically unstable or who have seizures, disorders of lipid metabolism, or increased intracranial pressure.
• Because drug appears in breast milk, avoid using in breast-feeding patients.

Adverse reactions

CNS: involuntary movement.
CV: ***bradycardia***, *hypotension*, hypertension, decreased cardiac output.
Metabolic: hyperlipemia.
Respiratory: APNEA, respiratory acidosis.
Skin: rash.
Other: *burning or stinging at injection site.*

Interactions

Drug-drug. *Inhaled anesthetics (such as enflurane, halothane, isoflurane), opioids (alfentanil, fentanyl, meperidine, morphine), sedatives (such as barbiturates, benzodiazepines, chloral hydrate, droperidol):* May increase anesthetic and sedative effects and further decrease blood pressure and cardiac output. Monitor patient closely.
Drug-herb. *St. John's wort:* May prolong anesthetic effects. Advise patient to stop using herb 5 days before surgery.

Nursing considerations

• Urine may turn green if drug is used for prolonged sedation in ICU.
• Titrate drug daily to maintain minimum effective level.
• For general anesthesia or monitored anesthesia care sedation, trained staff not involved in the surgical or diagnostic procedure should give drug. For ICU sedation,

persons skilled in managing critically ill patients and trained in cardiopulmonary resuscitation and airway management should give drug.

- Continuously monitor vital signs.
- Monitor patient at risk for hyperlipidemia for elevated triglyceride levels.
- Drug contains 0.1 g of fat (1.1 kcal)/ml. Reduce other lipid products if given together.
- Drug contains ethylenediaminetetraacetic acid, a strong metal chelator. Consider supplemental zinc during prolonged therapy.
- When giving drug in the ICU, assess patient's CNS function daily to determine minimum dose needed.
- Stop drug gradually to prevent abrupt awakening and increased agitation.

!!ALERT Don't confuse Diprivan with Dipivefrin.

Patient teaching

- Advise patient that performance of activities requiring mental alertness may be impaired for some time after drug use.

propoxyphene hydrochloride (dextropropoxyphene hydrochloride)

Darvon, Darvon Pulvules, 642†,

propoxyphene napsylate (dextropropoxyphene napsylate)

Darvon N

Pregnancy risk category C
Controlled substance schedule IV

Indications & dosages

➲ Mild to moderate pain

Adults: 65 mg propoxyphene hydrochloride P.O. q 4 hours, p.r.n. Maximum daily dose is 390 mg. Or, 100 mg propoxyphene napsylate P.O. q 4 hours, p.r.n. Maximum daily dose is 600 mg.

For patients with hepatic or renal dysfunction, reduce dosage. Consider increasing dosing interval in elderly patients.

Contraindications & cautions

- Contraindicated in patients hypersensitive to drug.
- Contraindicated in suicidal or addiction-prone patients.
- Use cautiously in patients with hepatic or renal disease, emotional instability, or history of drug or alcohol abuse.

Adverse reactions

CNS: *dizziness*, headache, *sedation*, euphoria, light-headedness, weakness, hallucinations, psychological and physical dependence.

GI: *nausea, vomiting*, constipation, abdominal pain.

Respiratory: ***respiratory depression***.

Interactions

Drug-drug. *Carbamazepine:* May increase carbamazepine level. Monitor patient closely.

CNS depressants: May cause additive effects. Use together cautiously.

Tricyclic antidepressants (such as doxepin): Inhibits antidepressant metabolism. Monitor patient for toxicity.

Warfarin: May increase anticoagulant effect. Monitor PT and INR.

Drug-lifestyle. *Alcohol use:* May cause additive effects. Discourage use together.

Smoking: May increase metabolism of propoxyphene. Monitor patient closely.

Nursing considerations

- Reassess patient's pain level at least 30 minutes after giving drug.
- Propoxyphene hydrochloride 65 mg equals propoxyphene napsylate 100 mg.
- Drug is considered a mild opioid analgesic, but pain relief is equivalent to that provided by aspirin. Drug is used with aspirin or acetaminophen to maximize analgesia. Patient may become tolerant and physically dependent on drug.
- Smokers may need increased dosage because smoking may induce liver enzymes responsible for the metabolism of the drug, decreasing its efficacy.

Patient teaching

- Advise patient to take drug with food or milk to minimize GI upset.
- Warn patient not to exceed recommended dosage. Respiratory depression, low blood pressure, profound sedation, coma and death may result if used in excessive doses or with other CNS depressants. Advise pa-

tient to avoid alcohol or other CNS-type drugs when taking propoxyphene.

- Caution ambulatory patient about getting out of bed or walking. Warn outpatient to avoid driving and other hazardous activities that require mental alertness until drug's CNS effects are known.

propranolol hydrochloride

Apo-Propranolol†, Inderal, Inderal LA, InnoPran XL, Novopranol†, pms Propranolol†

Pregnancy risk category C

Indications & dosages

➲ Angina pectoris
Adults: Total daily doses of 80 to 320 mg P.O. when given b.i.d., t.i.d., or q.i.d. Or, one 80-mg extended-release capsule daily. Dosage increased at 3- to 7-day intervals.

➲ To decrease risk of death after MI
Adults: 180 to 240 mg P.O. daily in divided doses beginning 5 to 21 days after MI has occurred. Usually given t.i.d. or q.i.d.

➲ Supraventricular, ventricular, and atrial arrhythmias; tachyarrhythmias caused by excessive catecholamine action during anesthesia, hyperthyroidism, or pheochromocytoma
Adults: 1 to 3 mg by slow I.V. push, not to exceed 1 mg/minute. After 3 mg have been given, another dose may be given in 2 minutes; subsequent doses, no sooner than q 4 hours. Usual maintenance dose is 10 to 30 mg P.O. t.i.d. or q.i.d.

➲ Hypertension
Adults: Initially, 80 mg P.O. daily in two divided doses or extended-release form once daily. Increase at 3- to 7-day intervals to maximum daily dose of 640 mg. Usual maintenance dose is 120 to 240 mg daily or 120 to 160 mg daily as extended-release. For InnoPran XL, dose is 80 mg P.O. once daily h.s. Give consistently with or without food. Adjust to maximum of 120 mg daily if needed. Full effects are seen in about 2 to 3 weeks.
Children: 0.5 mg/kg (conventional tablets) P.O. b.i.d. Increase q 3 to 5 days to a maximum dose of 16 mg/kg daily. Usual dose is 2 to 4 mg/kg daily in two equally divided doses.

➲ To prevent frequent, severe, uncontrollable, or disabling migraine or vascular headache
Adults: Initially, 80 mg P.O. daily in divided doses or 1 extended-release capsule daily. Usual maintenance dose is 160 to 240 mg daily, t.i.d. or q.i.d.

➲ Essential tremor
Adults: 40 mg (tablets or oral solution) P.O. b.i.d. Usual maintenance dose is 120 to 320 mg daily in three divided doses.

➲ Hypertrophic subaortic stenosis
Adults: 20 to 40 mg P.O. t.i.d. or q.i.d.; or 80 to 160 mg extended-release capsules once daily.

➲ Adjunct therapy in pheochromocytoma
Adults: 60 mg P.O. daily in divided doses with an alpha blocker 3 days before surgery.

Contraindications & cautions

- Contraindicated in patients with bronchial asthma, sinus bradycardia and heart block greater than first-degree, cardiogenic shock, and overt and decompensated heart failure (unless failure is secondary to a tachyarrhythmia that can be treated with propranolol).
- Use cautiously in patients with hepatic or renal impairment, nonallergic bronchospastic diseases, or hepatic disease and in those taking other antihypertensives.
- Because drug blocks some symptoms of hypoglycemia, use cautiously in patients who have diabetes mellitus.
- Use cautiously in patients with thyrotoxicosis because drug may mask some signs and symptoms of that disorder.
- Elderly patients may experience enhanced adverse reactions and may need dosage adjustment.

Adverse reactions

CNS: *fatigue, lethargy,* fever, vivid dreams, hallucinations, mental depression, lightheadedness, dizziness, insomnia.
CV: ***bradycardia****, hypotension,* ***heart failure****,* intermittent claudication, ***intensification of AV block****.*
GI: abdominal cramping, constipation, diarrhea, nausea, vomiting.
Hematologic: ***agranulocytosis****.*
Respiratory: ***bronchospasm****.*
Skin: rash.

Interactions

Drug-drug. *Aminophylline:* May antagonize beta-blocking effects of propranolol. Use together cautiously.
Cardiac glycosides: May reduce the positive inotrope effect of the glycoside. Monitor patient for clinical effect.
Cimetidine: May inhibit metabolism of propranolol. Watch for increased beta-blocking effect.
Diltiazem, verapamil: May cause hypotension, bradycardia, and increased depressant effect on myocardium. Use together cautiously.
Epinephrine: May cause severe vasoconstriction. Monitor blood pressure and observe patient carefully.
Glucagon, isoproterenol: May antagonize propranolol effect. May be used therapeutically and in emergencies.
Haloperidol: May cause cardiac arrest. Avoid using together.
Insulin, oral antidiabetics: May alter requirements for these drugs in previously stabilized diabetics. Monitor patient for hypoglycemia.
Phenothiazines, reserpine: May cause additive effect. Use together cautiously.
Drug-herb. *Betel palm:* May decrease temperature-elevating effects and enhanced CNS effects. Discourage use together.
Ma huang: May decrease antihypertensive effects. Discourage use together.
Drug-lifestyle. *Cocaine use:* May increase angina-inducing potential of cocaine. Inform patient of this interaction.

Nursing considerations

- Always check patient's apical pulse before giving drug. If extremes in pulse rates occur, withhold drug and notify prescriber immediately.
- Give drug consistently with meals. Food may increase absorption of propranolol.
- Drug masks common signs and symptoms of shock and hypoglycemia.

!!ALERT Don't stop drug before surgery for pheochromocytoma. Before any surgical procedure, tell anesthesiologist that patient is receiving propranolol.

- Compliance may be improved by giving drug twice daily or as extended-release capsules. Check with prescriber.

!!ALERT Don't confuse propranolol with Pravachol. Don't confuse Inderal with Inderide, Isordil, Adderall, or Imuran.

Patient teaching

- Caution patient to continue taking this drug as prescribed, even when he's feeling well.
- Instruct patient to take drug with food.

!!ALERT Tell patient not to stop drug suddenly because this can worsen chest pain and trigger a heart attack.

propylthiouracil (PTU)

Propyl-Thyracil†

Pregnancy risk category D

Indications & dosages

➲ Hyperthyroidism

Adults: 300 to 450 mg P.O. daily in divided doses. Patients with severe hyperthyroidism or very large goiters may need initial doses of 600 to 1,200 mg daily. Continue until patient is euthyroid; then start maintenance dose of 100 mg to 150 mg P.O. daily.
Children older than age 10: Initially, 150 to 300 mg P.O. daily in divided doses. Continue until patient is euthyroid. Individualize maintenance dose.
Children ages 6 to 10: Initially, 50 to 150 mg P.O. daily in divided doses q 8 hours. Continue until patient is euthyroid. Individualize maintenance dose.
Neonates: 5 to 10 mg/kg P.O. daily in divided doses t.i.d.

➲ Thyrotoxic crisis

Adults: 200 mg P.O. q 4 to 6 hours on first day; once symptoms are fully controlled, gradually reduce dosage to usual maintenance levels.

Contraindications & cautions

- Contraindicated in patients hypersensitive to drug and in breast-feeding women.
- Use cautiously in pregnant patients.

Adverse reactions

CNS: headache, drowsiness, vertigo, paresthesia, neuritis, neuropathies, CNS stimulation, depression, fever.
CV: vasculitis.
EENT: visual disturbances, loss of taste.

GI: diarrhea, *nausea*, *vomiting*, epigastric distress, salivary gland enlargement.
GU: nephritis.
Hematologic: ***agranulocytosis***, ***leukopenia***, ***thrombocytopenia***, ***aplastic anemia***.
Hepatic: jaundice, ***hepatotoxicity***.
Metabolic: dose-related hypothyroidism.
Musculoskeletal: arthralgia, myalgia.
Skin: rash, urticaria, skin discoloration, pruritus, erythema nodosum, exfoliative dermatitis, lupuslike syndrome.
Other: lymphadenopathy.

Interactions

Drug-drug. *Aminophylline, oxtriphylline, theophylline:* May decrease clearance of these drugs. Dosage may need to be adjusted.
Anticoagulants: May increase anticoagulant effects. Monitor PT and INR.
Cardiac glycosides: May increase glycoside level. Dosage may need to be reduced.
Potassium iodide: May decrease response to drug. Dosage of antithyroid drug may need to be increased.
Drug-food. *Iodized salt, shellfish:* May alter drug's effectiveness. Urge caution.

Nursing considerations

- Pregnant women may need less drug as pregnancy progresses. Monitor thyroid function studies closely. Thyroid hormone may be added to regimen. Drug may be stopped during last few weeks of pregnancy.

!!ALERT Patients older than age 40 may have an increased risk of agranulocytosis.

- Give drug with meals to reduce adverse GI reactions.
- Watch for hypothyroidism (mental depression; cold intolerance; hard, nonpitting edema); adjust dosage.
- Monitor CBC periodically to detect impending leukopenia, thrombocytopenia, and agranulocytosis.

!!ALERT Stop drug and notify prescriber if severe rash develops or cervical lymph nodes enlarge.

- Store drug in light-resistant container.

Patient teaching

- Instruct patient to take drug with meals.
- Warn patient to report fever, sore throat, mouth sores, and skin eruptions.
- Tell patient to report unusual bleeding or bruising.
- Tell patient to ask prescriber about using iodized salt and eating shellfish. These foods contain iodine and may alter effectiveness of drug.
- Teach patient to watch for signs and symptoms of hypothyroidism (unexplained weight gain, fatigue, cold intolerance) and to notify prescriber if they occur.

protamine sulfate

Pregnancy risk category C

Indications & dosages

➲ Heparin overdose
Adults: Base dosage on venous blood coagulation studies, usually 1 mg for each 90 to 115 units of heparin. Give by slow I.V. injection over 10 minutes in doses not to exceed 50 mg.

Contraindications & cautions

- Contraindicated in patients hypersensitive to drug.

Adverse reactions

CNS: lassitude.
CV: hypotension, ***bradycardia***, ***circulatory collapse***, transient flushing.
GI: nausea, vomiting.
Respiratory: dyspnea, pulmonary edema, ***acute pulmonary hypertension***.
Other: feeling of warmth, ***anaphylaxis***, ***anaphylactoid reactions***.

Interactions

None significant.

Nursing considerations

- Base postoperative dose on coagulation studies, and repeat activated PTT time 15 minutes after administration.
- Calculate dosage carefully. One milligram of protamine neutralizes 90 to 115 units of heparin, depending on salt (heparin calcium or heparin sodium) and source of heparin (beef or pork).
- Risk of hypersensitivity reaction increases in patients hypersensitive to fish, in vasectomized or infertile men, and in patients taking protamine-insulin products.
- Monitor patient continually.
- Watch for spontaneous bleeding (heparin rebound), especially in dialysis patients and

in those who have undergone cardiac surgery.
- Protamine may act as an anticoagulant in very high doses.

!!ALERT Don't confuse protamine with Protopam or protropin.

Patient teaching
- Explain use and administration of drug to patient and family.
- Tell patient to report adverse effects.

pseudoephedrine hydrochloride
Cenafed ◇, Decofed ◇, Dimetapp, Genaphed ◇, PediaCare Infants' Decongestant Drops ◇, Sudafed ◇, Triaminic

pseudoephedrine sulfate
Drixoral Non-Drowsy Formula ◇

Pregnancy risk category C

Indications & dosages
➲ To decongest nose and eustachian tube

Adults and children older than age 12: 60 mg P.O. q 4 to 6 hours; or 120 mg P.O. extended-release tablet q 12 hours; or 240 mg P.O. extended-release tablet once daily. Maximum dosage is 240 mg daily.

Children ages 6 to 12: 30 mg P.O. q 4 to 6 hours. Maximum dosage is 120 mg daily.

Children ages 2 to 5: 15 mg P.O. q 4 to 6 hours. Maximum dosage is 60 mg daily, or 4 mg/kg or 125 mg/m^2 P.O. divided q.i.d.

Contraindications & cautions
- Contraindicated in patients with severe hypertension or severe coronary artery disease, in those receiving MAO inhibitors, and in breast-feeding women. Extended-release forms are contraindicated in children younger than age 12.
- Use cautiously in patients with hypertension, cardiac disease, diabetes, glaucoma, hyperthyroidism, and prostatic hyperplasia.

Adverse reactions
CNS: *anxiety*, transient stimulation, tremor, dizziness, headache, insomnia, *nervousness*.
CV: ***arrhythmias***, *palpitations*, tachycardia, ***CV collapse***.
GI: anorexia, nausea, vomiting, dry mouth.
GU: difficulty urinating.
Respiratory: respiratory difficulties.
Skin: pallor.

Interactions
Drug-drug. *Antihypertensives:* May inhibit hypotensive effect. Monitor blood pressure closely.

MAO inhibitors (phenelzine, tranylcypromine): May cause severe headache, hypertension, fever, and hypertensive crisis. Avoid using together.

Methyldopa: May increase pressor response. Monitor patient closely.

Nursing considerations
- Elderly patients are more sensitive to drug's effects. Extended-release tablets shouldn't be given to elderly patients until safety with short-acting preparations has been established.

Patient teaching
- Tell patient not to crush or break extended-release forms.
- Warn against using OTC products containing other sympathomimetics.
- Instruct patient not to take drug within 2 hours of bedtime because it can cause insomnia.
- Tell patient to stop drug and notify prescriber if he becomes unusually restless.

psyllium
Fiberall ◇, Genfiber ◇, Hydrocil Instant ◇, Konsyl ◇, Konsyl-D ◇, Metamucil ◇, Metamucil Effervescent Sugar Free ◇, Metamucil Sugar Free ◇, Modane Bulk ◇, Mylanta Natural Fiber Supplement ◇, Perdiem Fiber ◇, Prodiem Plain† ◇, Reguloid Natural ◇, Serutan ◇, Syllact ◇

Pregnancy risk category B

Indications & dosages
➲ Constipation, bowel management

Adults: 1 or 2 rounded tsp P.O. in full glass of liquid once daily, b.i.d., or t.i.d., followed by second glass of liquid. Or, 1 packet dissolved in water once daily, b.i.d., or t.i.d. Up to 30 g daily.

Children older than age 6: ½ rounded tsp P.O. in a full glass of liquid one to three times daily.

Contraindications & cautions

- Contraindicated in patients hypersensitive to drug and in those with intestinal obstruction, intestinal ulceration, disabling adhesions, difficulty swallowing, or signs or symptoms of appendicitis, such as abdominal pain, nausea, or vomiting.

Adverse reactions

GI: nausea; vomiting; diarrhea with excessive use; esophageal, gastric, small intestine, and rectal obstruction when drug is taken in dry form; abdominal cramps, especially in severe constipation.

Interactions

None significant.

Nursing considerations

- Before giving drug for constipation, determine whether patient has adequate fluid intake, exercise, and diet.
- Mix with at least 8 ounces (240 ml) of cold, pleasant-tasting liquid such as orange juice to mask grittiness, and stir only a few seconds. Have patient drink mixture immediately so it doesn't congeal. Follow with additional glass of liquid.
- For dosages in children younger than age 6, consult prescriber.
- Drug may reduce appetite if taken before meals.
- Drug isn't absorbed systemically and is nontoxic. It's especially useful in debilitated patients and in those with postpartum constipation, irritable bowel syndrome, or diverticular disease. It's also used to treat chronic laxative abuse and with other laxatives to empty colon before barium enema examinations.
- Patients with phenylketonuria should avoid psyllium products, which contain phenylalanine (aspartame).

Patient teaching

- Teach patient how to properly mix drug. Tell him to take drug with plenty of water (at least 8 ounces). Advise patient that inhaling powder may cause allergic reactions.
- Advise patient to seek medical attention if he experiences vomiting, chest pain, or difficulty breathing or swallowing after taking medication.
- Tell patient that laxative effect usually occurs in 12 to 24 hours, but may be delayed 3 days.
- Advise diabetic patient to check label and use a brand of psyllium that doesn't contain sugar.
- Teach patient about dietary sources of bulk, including bran and other cereals, fresh fruit, and vegetables.

pyrazinamide

Tebrazid†

Pregnancy risk category C

Indications & dosages

➲ Active tuberculosis (TB), combined with other antituberculotics

Adults and children: 15 to 30 mg/kg P.O. once daily. Maximum daily dose is 2 g. Or, when compliance is a problem, adults may receive an intermittent regimen of 50 to 70 mg/kg based on lean body mass (up to 3 g) P.O. twice weekly. Children may receive an intermittent regimen of 50 mg/kg (up to 2 g) P.O. twice weekly.

Contraindications & cautions

- Contraindicated in patients hypersensitive to drug and in those with severe hepatic disease or acute gout.
- Use cautiously in patients with diabetes mellitus, renal failure, or gout.

Adverse reactions

CNS: malaise, fever.
GI: anorexia, nausea, vomiting.
GU: dysuria, interstitial nephritis.
Hematologic: sideroblastic anemia, ***thrombocytopenia***.
Hepatic: ***hepatotoxicity***, ***hepatitis***.
Metabolic: hyperuricemia.
Musculoskeletal: *arthralgia*, *myalgia*.
Skin: rash, urticaria, pruritus, photosensitivity.
Other: gout, porphyria.

Interactions

None significant.

Nursing considerations

- Always give pyrazinamide with other antituberculotics to prevent the development of resistant organisms.

• Drug is given for the first 2 months of a 6-month or longer treatment regimen for drug-susceptible patients. Patients with HIV infection may need longer courses of therapy.
• Doses greater than 35 mg/kg may damage the liver.
• Obtain baseline uric acid level and liver function test results before treatment.
• Monitor hematopoietic study and liver function test results, as well as uric acid level; assess patient for jaundice and liver tenderness or enlargement before and frequently during therapy.
!!ALERT Immediately report signs and symptoms of gout and liver impairment, such as anorexia, fatigue, malaise, jaundice, dark urine, and liver tenderness.
• When used with surgical management of TB, start pyrazinamide 1 to 2 weeks before surgery and continue for 4 to 6 weeks after surgery.

Patient teaching
• Inform patient that he must take drug with other antituberculotics.
• Tell patient to report adverse reactions promptly, especially fever, malaise, appetite loss, nausea, vomiting, dark urine, yellow skin or eye discoloration, and pain or swelling of the joints.
• Stress importance of compliance with drug therapy. If daily therapy poses a problem, tell patient to ask prescriber about twice-weekly dosing.

pyrethrins
A-200, Barc ◇, Blue, End Lice, Pronto, Pyrinyl ◇, R & C, RID ◇, Tegrin-LT, Tisit ◇, Triple X

Pregnancy risk category C

Indications & dosages
➲ **Infestations of head, body, and pubic (crab) lice and their eggs**
Adults and children: Apply to hair, scalp, or other infested areas until entirely wet. Allow to remain for 10 minutes but no longer. Wash thoroughly with warm water and soap or shampoo. Remove dead lice and eggs with fine-tooth comb. Repeat treatment, if needed, in 7 to 10 days to kill newly hatched lice; don't use more than two applications within 24 hours.

Contraindications & cautions
• Contraindicated in patients hypersensitive to drug, ragweed, or chrysanthemums.
• Use cautiously in infants and small children.

Adverse reactions
Skin: *irritation with repeated use.*

Interactions
None significant.

Nursing considerations
• Apply topical corticosteroids or give oral antihistamines, as prescribed, if dermatitis develops from scratching.
• Discard container by wrapping in several layers of newspaper.
• Inspect all family members daily for at least 2 weeks for infestation.
• Drug isn't effective against scabies.
• Treat sexual contacts simultaneously.

Patient teaching
• Instruct patient not to apply to open areas, acutely inflamed skin, eyebrows, eyelashes, face, eyes, mucous membranes, or urethral opening. If accidental contact with eyes occurs, advise patient to flush with water and notify prescriber.
• Warn patient not to swallow or inhale vapors from the drug.
• Tell patient to stop using drug, wash it off skin, and notify prescriber immediately if skin irritation develops. All preparations contain petroleum distillates.
• Instruct patient to change and sterilize all clothing and bed linens after drug is washed off body. Tell him to disinfect washable items by machine washing in hot water and drying on hot cycle for at least 20 minutes. Other items can be dry-cleaned and sealed in plastic bags for 2 weeks, or treated with products made for this purpose.
• Teach patient to remove dead parasites with a fine-tooth comb.
• Urge patient to warn other family members and sexual contacts about infestation.

pyridostigmine bromide
Mestinon*, Mestinon-SR†, Mestinon Timespans, Regonol

Pregnancy risk category NR

Indications & dosages
➲ Antidote for nondepolarizing neuromuscular blockers
Adults: 10 to 20 mg I.V., preceded by atropine sulfate 0.6 to 1.2 mg I.V.
➲ Myasthenia gravis
Adults: 60 to 120 mg P.O. q 3 or 4 hours. Usual dosage is 600 mg daily but dosages up to 1,500 mg daily may be needed. For I.M. or I.V. use, give 1/30 of oral dose. Dosage must be adjusted for each patient, based on response and tolerance. Or, 180 to 540 mg extended-release tablets P.O. b.i.d., with at least 6 hours between doses.
Children: 7 mg/kg or 200 mg/m^2 daily in five or six divided doses.
➲ Pre-exposure prophylaxis against the deadly effects of nerve agent soman
Adults in military combat: 30 mg P.O. q 8 hours starting at least several hours before soman exposure.

Smaller doses may be required in patients with renal disease. Adjust dosage to achieve desired effect.

Contraindications & cautions
- Contraindicated in patients hypersensitive to anticholinesterases or bromides and in those with mechanical obstruction of the intestinal or urinary tract.
- Use cautiously in patients with bronchial asthma, bradycardia, arrhythmias, epilepsy, recent coronary occlusion, vagotonia, hyperthyroidism, or peptic ulcer.
- Use cautiously in pregnant women.
- Use cautiously in breast-feeding women; drug is excreted in breast milk.

Adverse reactions
CNS: headache with high doses, weakness, syncope.
CV: ***bradycardia***, hypotension, ***cardiac arrest***, thrombophlebitis.
EENT: miosis.
GI: abdominal cramps, *nausea*, *vomiting*, diarrhea, excessive salivation, increased peristalsis.
Musculoskeletal: muscle cramps, muscle fasciculations.
Respiratory: ***bronchospasm***, ***bronchoconstriction***, increased bronchial secretions.
Skin: rash, diaphoresis.

Interactions
Drug-drug. *Aminoglycosides:* May prolong or enhance muscle weakness. Use together cautiously.
Anticholinergics, atropine, corticosteroids, general or local anesthetics, magnesium, procainamide, quinidine: May antagonize cholinergic effects. Observe patient for lack of drug effect.
Ganglionic blockers: May increase risk of hypotension. Monitor patient closely.

Nursing considerations
!!ALERT If taken immediately before or during soman exposure, drug may be ineffective against soman and may worsen soman's effects. At the first sign of soman poisoning, stop pyridostigmine and immediately begin treatment with atropine and pralidoxime.
- Stop all other cholinergics before giving this drug.
- Don't crush extended-release tablets.
- When using sweet syrup for patients who have trouble swallowing, give over ice chips if patient can't tolerate flavor.
- Monitor and document patient's response after each dose. Optimum dosage is difficult to judge.

!!ALERT In the United States, Regonol contains benzyl ethanol preservative, which may cause toxicity in neonates if given in high doses. The Canadian formulation of this drug doesn't contain benzyl ethanol.
- If appropriate, obtain order for hospitalized patient to have bedside supply of tablets. Many patients with long-standing disease insist on self-administration.

!!ALERT Don't confuse Mestinon with Mesantoin or Metatensin.

Patient teaching
- When giving drug for myasthenia gravis, stress importance of taking it exactly as prescribed, on time, in evenly spaced doses. If using extended-release tablets, explain that patient must take tablets at same time each day, at least 6 hours apart.

- Advise patient not to crush or chew extended-release tablets.
- Explain that patient may have to take drug for life.
- Advise patient to wear or carry medical identification that identifies his myasthenia gravis.
- Stress importance to military personnel of taking nerve agent antidotes atropine and pralidoxime rather than pyridostigmine bromide at first sign of nerve agent poisoning.

pyridoxine hydrochloride (vitamin B_6)

Nestrex ◊, Rodex

Pregnancy risk category A; C if dose exceeds RDA

Indications & dosages

➲ RDA
Adults ages 19 to 50: 1.3 mg.
Men age 51 and older: 1.7 mg.
Women age 51 and older: 1.5 mg.
Boys ages 14 to 19: 1.3 mg.
Girls ages 14 to 19: 1.2 mg.
Children ages 9 to 13: 1 mg.
Children ages 4 to 8: 0.6 mg.
Children ages 1 to 3: 0.5 mg.
Infants ages 6 months to 1 year: 0.3 mg.
Neonates and infants younger than age 6 months: 0.1 mg.
Pregnant women: 2.2 mg.
Breast-feeding women: 2.1 mg.

➲ Dietary vitamin B_6 deficiency
Adults: 2.5 to 10 mg P.O., I.V., or I.M. daily for 3 weeks; then 2 to 5 mg daily as supplement to proper diet.

➲ Seizures related to vitamin B_6 deficiency or dependency
Adults and children: 100 mg I.V. or I.M. in single dose.

➲ Vitamin B_6–responsive anemias or dependency syndrome (inborn errors of metabolism)
Adults: Up to 500 mg P.O., I.V., or I.M. daily until symptoms subside; then same dosage daily for life.

➲ To prevent vitamin B_6 deficiency during drug therapy with isoniazid or penicillamine
Adults: 10 to 50 mg P.O. daily.

➲ To prevent seizures during cycloserine therapy
Adults: 100 to 300 mg P.O. daily.

➲ Antidote for isoniazid poisoning
Adults: 4 g I.V.; then 1 g I.M. q 30 minutes until amount of pyridoxine given equals amount of isoniazid ingested.

Contraindications & cautions

- Contraindicated in patients hypersensitive to drug.
- Don't use drug in patients with heart disease.

Adverse reactions

CNS: paresthesia, unsteady gait, numbness, somnolence, ***seizures***, headache.
Skin: photoallergic reaction.

Interactions

Drug-drug. *Levodopa:* May decrease effectiveness of levodopa. Avoid using together. Pyridoxine has little to no effect on the combination drug levodopa and carbidopa.
Phenobarbital, phenytoin: May decrease anticonvulsant level, increasing risk of seizures. Avoid using together.
Drug-lifestyle. *Alcohol use:* May cause delirium and lactic acidosis. Discourage use together.

Nursing considerations

- When used to treat isoniazid toxicity, expect to also give anticonvulsants.
- If sodium bicarbonate is needed to control acidosis in isoniazid toxicity, don't mix in same syringe with pyridoxine.
- Patients taking high doses (2 to 6 g daily) may have difficulty walking because of diminished proprioceptive and sensory function.
- Carefully monitor patient's diet. Excessive protein intake increases daily pyridoxine requirements.
- Long-term use of large doses may cause neurotoxicity.

!!ALERT Don't confuse pyridoxine with pralidoxime or Pyridium.

Patient teaching

- Stress importance of compliance and of good nutrition if drug is prescribed for maintenance therapy to prevent recurrence of deficiency. Explain that pyridoxine with isoniazid has a specific therapeutic purpose and isn't just a vitamin.

- Advise patient taking levodopa alone to avoid multivitamins containing pyridoxine because of decreased levodopa effect.
- Warn patient that there may be burning at the injection site.

pyrimethamine
Daraprim

pyrimethamine with sulfadoxine
Fansidar

Pregnancy risk category C

Indications & dosages

➲ To prevent and control transmission of malaria

pyrimethamine

Adults and children age 10 and older: 25 mg P.O. weekly for 6 to 10 weeks or longer after leaving malaria-endemic areas.

Children ages 4 to 10: 12.5 mg P.O. weekly continued for 6 to 10 weeks or longer after leaving malaria-endemic areas.

Children younger than age 4: 6.25 mg P.O. weekly continued for 6 to 10 weeks or longer after leaving malaria-endemic areas.

pyrimethamine with sulfadoxine

Adults and children age 14 and older: 1 tablet weekly or 2 tablets q 2 weeks during exposure and for 4 to 6 weeks after exposure.

Children ages 9 to 14: ¾ tablet weekly, or 1½ tablets q 2 weeks during exposure and for 4 to 6 weeks after exposure.

Children ages 4 to 8: ½ tablet weekly or 1 tablet q 2 weeks during exposure and for 4 to 6 weeks after exposure.

Children younger than age 4: ¼ tablet weekly, or ½ tablet q 2 weeks during exposure and for 4 to 6 weeks after exposure.

➲ Acute attacks of malaria

pyrimethamine

Adults: 50 mg P.O. daily for 2 days; then 25 mg once weekly for at least 10 weeks.

Children ages 4 to 10: 25 mg P.O. once daily for 2 days; then 12.5 mg once weekly for at least 10 weeks.

pyrimethamine with sulfadoxine

Adults and children age 14 and older: 3 tablets as a single dose, given on the last day of quinine therapy.

Children ages 9 to 14: 2 tablets as a single dose, given on the last day of quinine therapy.

Children ages 4 to 8: 1 tablet as a single dose, given on the last day of quinine therapy.

Children ages 1 to 3: ½ tablet as a single dose, given on the last day of quinine therapy.

Children ages 2 to 11 months: ¼ tablet as a single dose, given on the last day of quinine therapy.

➲ Toxoplasmosis

pyrimethamine

Adults: Initially, 50 to 75 mg P.O. with 1 to 4 g sulfadiazine; continue for 1 to 3 weeks. After 3 weeks, reduce dosage by half and continue for 4 to 5 weeks.

Children: Initially, 1 mg/kg/day P.O. in two equally divided doses for 2 to 4 days; then 0.5 mg/kg daily for 4 weeks, along with 100 mg sulfadiazine/kg P.O. daily, divided q 6 hours. Don't exceed 100 mg.

➲ Primary prevention of toxoplasmosis in patients with HIV infection♦

Adults and adolescents: 50 mg P.O., once weekly, with leucovorin 25 mg P.O. once weekly and dapsone 50 mg P.O. daily; or 75 mg pyrimethamine with leucovorin 25 mg and dapsone 200 mg P.O., all once weekly.

➲ Secondary prevention of toxoplasmosis in patients with HIV infection♦

Adults and adolescents: 25 to 50 mg P.O., once daily, with leucovorin 10 to 25 mg P.O. once daily and either sulfadiazine 0.5 to 1 g P.O. q.i.d. or clindamycin 300 to 450 mg q 6 to 8 hours.

Contraindications & cautions

- Pyrimethamine is contraindicated in patients hypersensitive to drug and in those with megaloblastic anemia from folic acid deficiency. Pyrimethamine with sulfadoxine is contraindicated in patients with porphyria.
- Repeated use of pyrimethamine with sulfadoxine is contraindicated in patients with severe renal insufficiency, marked parenchymal damage to the liver, blood dyscrasias, hypersensitivity to pyrimethamine or sulfonamides, or documented megaloblastic anemia from folic acid deficiency.

• Contraindicated in infants younger than age 2 months and in pregnant (at term) and breast-feeding women.
• Use cautiously after treatment with chloroquine and in patients with impaired hepatic or renal function, severe allergy or bronchial asthma, G6PD deficiency, or seizure disorders (smaller doses may be needed).

Adverse reactions

CNS: headache, peripheral neuritis, mental depression, ***seizures***, ataxia, hallucinations, fatigue.
CV: ***arrhythmias***, allergic myocarditis.
EENT: scleral irritation, periorbital edema.
GI: anorexia, vomiting, atrophic glossitis.
Hematologic: ***agranulocytosis***, ***aplastic anemia***, megaloblastic anemia, ***leukopenia***, ***thrombocytopenia***, ***pancytopenia***.
Skin: ***Stevens-Johnson syndrome***, generalized skin eruptions, urticaria, pruritus, photosensitivity.

Interactions

Drug-drug. *Co-trimoxazole, methotrexate, sulfonamides:* May increase risk of bone marrow suppression. Avoid using together.
Lorazepam: May increase risk of hepatotoxicity. Avoid using together.
PABA: May decrease antitoxoplasmic effects. May need to adjust dosage.

Nursing considerations

• Pyrimethamine alone isn't recommended for treatment of malaria in nonimmune patients. Use drug with faster-acting antimalarials, such as chloroquine, for 2 days to start transmission control and suppressive cure.
• Obtain twice-weekly blood counts, including platelets, for the patient with toxoplasmosis because usual dosages approach toxic levels. If signs of folic acid or folinic acid deficiency develop, expect to reduce dosage or stop drug while patient receives parenteral folinic acid (leucovorin) until blood counts return to normal.
• Adverse drug reactions related to sulfadiazine are similar to those related to sulfonamides.
• When used to treat toxoplasmosis in patients with AIDS, therapy may be lifelong.
• Use pyrimethamine with sulfadoxine only in areas where chloroquine-resistant malaria is prevalent and only if the traveler plans to stay longer than 3 weeks.

Patient teaching

• Instruct patient to take drug with meals.
• Inform patient with toxoplasmosis of importance of frequent laboratory studies and compliance with therapy. Tell patient he may need long-term therapy.
• Warn patient taking pyrimethamine with sulfadoxine to stop drug and notify prescriber at first sign of rash, sore throat, or glossitis.
• Tell patient to take first preventive dose 1 to 2 days before traveling.

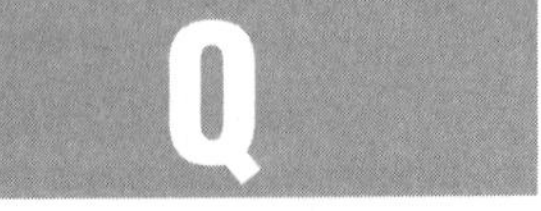

quetiapine fumarate
Seroquel

Pregnancy risk category C

Indications & dosages

➲ To manage signs and symptoms of psychotic disorders
Adults: Initially, 25 mg P.O. b.i.d., with increases in increments of 25 to 50 mg b.i.d. or t.i.d. on days 2 and 3, as tolerated. Target range is 300 to 400 mg daily divided into two or three doses by day 4. Further dosage adjustments, if indicated, should occur at intervals of not less than 2 days. Dosage can be increased or decreased by 25 to 50 mg b.i.d. Antipsychotic effect generally occurs at 150 to 750 mg daily. Safety of dosages over 800 mg daily hasn't been evaluated.
Elderly patients: Give lower dosages, adjust more slowly, and monitor patient carefully in first dosing period.
➲ Monotherapy and adjunct therapy with lithium or divalproex for the short-term treatment of acute manic episodes associated with bipolar I disorder
Adults: Initially, 50 mg P.O. b.i.d. Increase dosage in increments of 100 mg daily in two divided doses up to 200 mg P.O. b.i.d. on day 4. May increase dosage in increments no greater than 200 mg daily up to 800 mg

daily by day 6. Usual dose is 400 to 800 mg daily.

Elderly patients: Give lower dosages, adjust more slowly, and monitor patient carefully in first dosing period.

For debilitated patients and those with hypotension, consider lower dosages and slower adjustment. In patients with hepatic impairment, initial dose is 25 mg daily. Increase daily in increments of 25 to 50 mg daily to an effective dose

Contraindications & cautions

- Contraindicated in patients hypersensitive to drug or its ingredients.
- Use cautiously in patients with CV disease, cerebrovascular disease, conditions that predispose to hypotension, a history of seizures or conditions that lower the seizure threshold, and conditions in which core body temperature may be elevated.
- Use cautiously in patients at risk for aspiration pneumonia.

Adverse reactions

CNS: *dizziness, headache, somnolence,* hypertonia, dysarthria, asthenia, ***neuroleptic malignant syndrome, seizures.***
CV: orthostatic hypotension, tachycardia, palpitations, peripheral edema.
EENT: ear pain, pharyngitis, rhinitis.
GI: dry mouth, dyspepsia, abdominal pain, constipation, anorexia.
Hematologic: ***leukopenia.***
Metabolic: *weight gain,* hyperglycemia.
Musculoskeletal: back pain.
Respiratory: increased cough, dyspnea.
Skin: rash, diaphoresis.
Other: flulike syndrome.

Interactions

Drug-drug. *Antihypertensives:* May increase effects of antihypertensives. Monitor blood pressure.
Carbamazepine, glucocorticoids, phenobarbital, phenytoin, rifampin, thioridazine: May increase quetiapine clearance. May need to adjust quetiapine dosage.
CNS depressants: May increase CNS effects. Use together cautiously.
Dopamine agonists, levodopa: May antagonize the effects of these drugs. Monitor patient.
Erythromycin, fluconazole, itraconazole, ketoconazole: May decrease quetiapine clearance. Use together cautiously.
Lorazepam: May decrease lorazepam clearance. Monitor patient for increased CNS effects.
Drug-lifestyle. *Alcohol use:* May increase CNS effects. Discourage use together.

Nursing considerations

- Dispense lowest appropriate quantity of drug to reduce risk of overdose.

!!ALERT Watch for evidence of neuroleptic malignant syndrome (extrapyramidal effects, hyperthermia, autonomic disturbance), which is rare but commonly fatal. It may not be related to length of drug use or type of neuroleptic; more than 60% of affected patients are men.

- Monitor patient for tardive dyskinesia, which may occur after prolonged use. It may not appear until months or years later and may disappear spontaneously or persist for life, despite ending drug.
- Hyperglycemia may occur in patients taking drug. Monitor patients with diabetes regularly.
- Monitor patient for weight gain.
- Drug use may cause cataract formation. Obtain baseline ophthalmologic examination and reassess every 6 months.

Patient teaching

- Advise patient about risk of dizziness upon standing up quickly. The risk is greatest during the 3- to 5-day period of first dosage adjustment, when resuming treatment, and when increasing dosages.
- Tell patient to avoid becoming overheated or dehydrated.
- Warn patient to avoid activities that require mental alertness until effects of drug are known, especially during first dosage adjustment or dosage increases.
- Remind patient to have an eye examination at start of therapy and every 6 months during therapy to check for cataracts.
- Tell patient to notify prescriber about other prescription or over-the-counter drugs he's taking or plans to take.
- Tell woman of childbearing age to notify prescriber about planned, suspected, or known pregnancy.
- Advise her not to breast-feed during therapy.

• Advise patient to avoid alcohol while taking drug.
• Tell patient to take drug with or without food.

quinapril hydrochloride
Accupril

Pregnancy risk category C; D in 2nd and 3rd trimesters

Indications & dosages

➲ Hypertension
Adults: Initially, 10 to 20 mg P.O. daily. Dosage may be adjusted based on patient response at intervals of about 2 weeks. Most patients are controlled at 20, 40, or 80 mg daily as a single dose or in two divided doses. If patient is taking a diuretic, start therapy with 5 mg daily.
Elderly patients: For patients older than age 65, start therapy at 10 mg P.O. daily.

For adults with creatinine clearance over 60 ml/minute, initially, 10 mg maximum daily; for clearance 30 to 60 ml/minute, 5 mg; for clearance 10 to 30 ml/minute, 2.5 mg.

➲ Heart failure
Adults: If patient is taking a diuretic, give 5 mg P.O. b.i.d. initially. If patient isn't taking a diuretic, give 10 to 20 mg P.O. b.i.d. Dosage may be increased at weekly intervals. Usual effective dose is 20 to 40 mg daily in two equally divided doses.

For patients with creatinine clearance over 30 ml/minute, first dose is 5 mg daily; if clearance is 10 to 30 ml/minute, 2.5 mg.

Contraindications & cautions

• Contraindicated in patients hypersensitive to ACE inhibitors and in those with a history of angioedema related to treatment with an ACE inhibitor.
• Use cautiously in patients with impaired renal function.

Adverse reactions

CNS: somnolence, vertigo, nervousness, headache, dizziness, fatigue, depression.
CV: palpitations, tachycardia, angina pectoris, ***hypertensive crisis***, orthostatic hypotension, rhythm disturbances.
GI: dry mouth, abdominal pain, constipation, vomiting, nausea, ***hemorrhage***, diarrhea.
Metabolic: *hyperkalemia*.
Respiratory: dry, persistent, tickling, nonproductive cough.
Skin: pruritus, photosensitivity reactions, diaphoresis.

Interactions

Drug-drug. *Diuretics, other antihypertensives:* May cause excessive hypotension. Stop diuretic or reduce dose of quinapril, as needed.
Lithium: May increase lithium level and lithium toxicity. Monitor lithium level.
NSAIDs: May decrease antihypertensive effects. Monitor blood pressure.
Potassium-sparing diuretics, potassium supplements: May cause hyperkalemia. Monitor patient closely.
Tetracycline: May decrease absorption if taken with quinapril. Avoid using together.
Drug-herb. *Capsaicin:* May cause cough. Discourage use together.
Ma huang: May decrease antihypertensive effects. Discourage use together.
Drug-food. *Salt substitutes containing potassium:* May cause hyperkalemia. Discourage use together.

Nursing considerations

• Assess renal and hepatic function before and periodically throughout therapy.
• Monitor blood pressure for effectiveness of therapy.
• Monitor potassium level. Risk factors for the development of hyperkalemia include renal insufficiency, diabetes, and concomitant use of drugs that raise potassium level.
• Although ACE inhibitors reduce blood pressure in all races, they reduce it less in blacks taking the ACE inhibitor alone. Black patients should take drug with a thiazide diuretic for a more favorable response.
• ACE inhibitors appear to increase risk of angioedema in black patients.
• Other ACE inhibitors have caused agranulocytosis and neutropenia. Monitor CBC with differential counts before therapy and periodically thereafter.

Patient teaching

• Advise patient to report signs of infection, such as fever and sore throat.

!!ALERT Facial and throat swelling (including swelling of the larynx) may occur, especially after first dose. Advise patient to report signs or symptoms of breathing difficulty or swelling of face, eyes, lips, or tongue.

- Light-headedness can occur, especially during first few days of therapy. Tell patient to rise slowly to minimize effect and to report signs and symptoms to prescriber. If he faints, patient should stop taking drug and call prescriber immediately.
- Inform patient that inadequate fluid intake, vomiting, diarrhea, and excessive perspiration can lead to light-headedness and fainting. Tell him to use caution in hot weather and during exercise.
- Tell patient to avoid salt substitutes. These products may contain potassium, which can cause high potassium level in patients taking quinapril.
- Advise woman of childbearing age to notify prescriber if pregnancy occurs. Drug will need to be stopped.

quinidine gluconate

Quinaglute Dura-Tabs, Quinate†

quinidine sulfate

Apo-Quinidine†, Novoquinidin†, Quinidex Extentabs

Pregnancy risk category C

Indications & dosages

➲ Atrial flutter or fibrillation

Adults: 300 to 400 mg quinidine sulfate or equivalent base P.O. q 6 hours. Or, 200 mg P.O. q 2 to 3 hours for five to eight doses, increased daily until sinus rhythm is restored or toxic effects develop. Maximum, 3 to 4 g daily.

Children♦: 30 mg/kg or 900 mg/m^2 P.O. (sulfate) or I.M or I.V. (gluconate) daily in five divided doses.

➲ Paroxysmal supraventricular tachycardia

Adults: 400 to 600 mg P.O. gluconate q 2 to 3 hours until toxic adverse reactions develop or arrhythmia subsides.

Children♦: 30 mg/kg or 900 mg/m^2 P.O. (sulfate) or I.M or I.V. (gluconate) daily in five divided doses.

➲ Premature atrial and ventricular contractions, paroxysmal AV junctional rhythm, paroxysmal atrial tachycardia, paroxysmal ventricular tachycardia, maintenance after cardioversion of atrial fibrillation or flutter

Adults: Test dose is 200 mg P.O. or I.M. Quinidine sulfate or equivalent base 200 to 400 mg P.O. q 4 to 6 hours or 600 mg quinidine sulfate extended-release q 8 to 12 hours; or quinidine gluconate 800 mg (10 ml of commercially available solution) added to 40 ml of D_5W, infused I.V. at 0.25 mg/kg/minute.

Children♦: 30 mg/kg or 900 mg/m^2 P.O. (sulfate) or I.M or I.V. (gluconate) daily in five divided doses.

➲ Severe *Plasmodium falciparum* malaria

Adults: 10 mg/kg gluconate I.V. diluted in 250 ml normal saline solution and infused over 1 to 2 hours; then continuous infusion of 0.02 mg/kg/minute for 72 hours or until parasitemia is reduced to less than 1% or oral therapy can be started.

Children♦: 10 mg/kg gluconate I.V. over 1 to 2 hours; then continuous infusion of 0.02 mg/kg/minute.

Reduce dosage in patients with hepatic impairment or heart failure.

Contraindications & cautions

- Contraindicated in patients with idiosyncrasy or hypersensitivity to quinidine or related cinchona derivatives.
- Contraindicated in those with myasthenia gravis, intraventricular conduction defects, digitalis toxicity when AV conduction is grossly impaired, abnormal rhythms caused by escape mechanisms, and history of prolonged QT interval syndrome.
- Contraindicated in patients who developed thrombocytopenia after exposure to quinidine or quinine.
- Use cautiously in patients with asthma, muscle weakness, or infection accompanied by fever because hypersensitivity reactions to drug may be masked.
- Use cautiously in patients with hepatic or renal impairment because systemic accumulation may occur.

Adverse reactions

CNS: *vertigo, fever, headache,* ataxia, *light-headedness,* confusion, depression, dementia.

CV: ***PVCs, ventricular tachycardia, atypical ventricular tachycardia***, hypotension, ***complete AV block***, *tachycardia*, ***aggravated heart failure***, *ECG changes*.
EENT: *tinnitus*, blurred vision, diplopia, photophobia.
GI: *diarrhea, nausea, vomiting*, anorexia, excessive salivation, abdominal pain.
Hematologic: hemolytic anemia, ***thrombocytopenia, agranulocytosis***.
Hepatic: ***hepatotoxicity***.
Respiratory: ***acute asthmatic attack, respiratory arrest***.
Skin: rash, petechial hemorrhage of buccal mucosa, pruritus, urticaria, photosensitivity.
Other: ***angioedema***, *cinchonism*, lupus erythematosus.

Interactions

Drug-drug. *Acetazolamide, antacids, sodium bicarbonate, thiazide diuretics:* May increase quinidine level. Monitor patient for increased effect.
Amiodarone: May increase quinidine level, producing life-threatening cardiac arrhythmias. Monitor quinidine level closely if use together can't be avoided. Adjust quinidine as needed.
Barbiturates, phenytoin, rifampin: May decrease quinidine level. Monitor patient for decreased effect.
Cimetidine: May increase quinidine level. Monitor patient for increased arrhythmias.
Digoxin: May increase digoxin level after starting quinidine therapy. Monitor digoxin level.
Drugs that prolong the QT interval (antipsychotics, clarithromycin, disopyramide, erythromycin, fluoroquinolones, procainamide, tricyclic antidepressants, sotalol): May have additive effect with quinidine and cause life-threatening cardiac arrhythmias. Avoid use together when possible.
Fluvoxamine, nefazodone, tricyclic antidepressants: May increase antidepressant level, thus increasing its effect. Monitor patient for adverse reactions.
Neuromuscular blockers: May potentiate effects of these drugs. Avoid use of quinidine immediately after surgery.
Nifedipine: May decrease quinidine level. May need to adjust dosage.
Other antiarrhythmics (such as lidocaine, procainamide, propranolol): May increase risk of toxicity. Use together cautiously.
Verapamil: May decrease quinidine clearance and cause hypotension, bradycardia, AV block, or pulmonary edema. Monitor blood pressure and heart rate.
Warfarin: May increase anticoagulant effect. Monitor patient closely.
Drug-herb. *Jimsonweed:* May adversely affect CV function. Discourage use together.
Licorice: May have additive effect and prolong QT interval. Urge caution.
Drug-food. *Grapefruit:* May delay absorption and onset of action of drug. Discourage use together.

Nursing considerations

- Check apical pulse rate and blood pressure before therapy. If extremes in pulse rate are detected, withhold drug and notify prescriber at once.

!!ALERT For atrial fibrillation or flutter, give quinidine only after AV node has been blocked with a beta blocker, digoxin, or a calcium channel blocker to avoid increasing AV conduction.

- Anticoagulant therapy is commonly advised before quinidine therapy in long-standing atrial fibrillation because restoration of normal sinus rhythm may result in thromboembolism caused by dislodgment of thrombi from atrial wall.
- Monitor patient for atypical ventricular tachycardia such as torsades de pointes and ECG changes, particularly widening of QRS complex, widened QT and PR intervals.

!!ALERT When changing route of administration or oral salt form, prescriber should alter dosage to compensate for variations in quinidine base content.

- Never use discolored (brownish) quinidine solution.
- Quinidine gluconate I.M. is no longer recommended for arrhythmias because of erratic absorption.

!!ALERT Hospitalize patients with severe malaria in an intensive care setting, with continuous monitoring. Decrease infusion rate if quinidine level exceeds 6 mcg/ml, uncorrected QT interval exceeds 0.6 second, or QRS complex widening exceeds 25% of baseline.

- Monitor liver function test results during first 4 to 8 weeks of therapy.

• Monitor quinidine level. Therapeutic levels for antiarrhythmic effects are 4 to 8 mcg/ml.
• Monitor patient response carefully. If adverse GI reactions occur, especially diarrhea, notify prescriber. Check quinidine level, which is increasingly toxic when greater than 10 mcg/ml. GI symptoms may be decreased by giving drug with meals or aluminum hydroxide antacids.
• Store drug away from heat and direct light.
!!ALERT Don't crush the extended-release formulation.
!!ALERT Don't confuse quinidine with quinine or clonidine.

Patient teaching

• Stress importance of taking drug exactly as prescribed and taking it with food if adverse GI reactions occur.
• Instruct patient not to crush or chew extended-release tablets.
• Tell patient to avoid grapefruit juice because it may delay drug absorption and inhibit drug metabolism.
• Advise patient to report persistent or serious adverse reactions promptly, especially signs and symptoms of quinidine toxicity (ringing in the ears, visual disturbances, dizziness, headache, nausea).

quinupristin and dalfopristin
Synercid

Pregnancy risk category B

Indications & dosages

➲ **Serious or life-threatening infections with vancomycin-resistant *Enterococcus faecium* bacteremia**
Adults and adolescents age 16 and older: 7.5 mg/kg I.V. over 1 hour q 8 hours. Length of treatment depends on site and severity of infection.
➲ **Complicated skin and skin-structure infections caused by methicillin-susceptible *Staphylococcus aureus* or *Streptococcus pyogenes***
Adults and adolescents age 16 and older: 7.5 mg/kg I.V. over 1 hour q 12 hours for at least 7 days.

Contraindications & cautions

• Contraindicated in patients hypersensitive to drug or other streptogramin antibiotics.

Adverse reactions

CNS: headache.
CV: thrombophlebitis.
GI: nausea, diarrhea, vomiting.
Musculoskeletal: arthralgia, myalgia.
Skin: rash, pruritus, *inflammation, pain, edema at infusion site, infusion site reaction.*

Interactions

Drug-drug. *Cyclosporine:* May lower metabolism; may increase drug level. Monitor cyclosporine level.
Drugs metabolized by CYP3A4, such as carbamazepine, delavirdine, diazepam, diltiazem, disopyramide, docetaxel, indinavir, lidocaine, lovastatin, methylprednisolone, midazolam, nevirapine, nifedipine, paclitaxel, ritonavir, tacrolimus, verapamil, vinblastine: May increase levels of these drugs, which could increase both their therapeutic effects and adverse reactions. Use together cautiously.
Drugs metabolized by CYP3A4 that may prolong the QTc interval, such as quinidine: May decrease metabolism of these drugs, prolonging QTc interval. Avoid using together.

Nursing considerations

• Drug isn't active against *Enterococcus faecalis*. Appropriate blood cultures are needed to avoid misidentifying *E. faecalis* as *E. faecium*.
• Because drug may cause mild to life-threatening pseudomembranous colitis, consider this diagnosis in patient who develops diarrhea during or after therapy.
• Adverse reactions, such as arthralgia and myalgia, may be reduced by decreasing dosage interval to every 12 hours.
• Because overgrowth of nonsusceptible organisms may occur, monitor patient closely for signs and symptoms of superinfection.
• Monitor liver function test results during therapy.

Patient teaching

• Advise patient to immediately report irritation at I.V. site, pain in joints or muscles, and diarrhea.

• Tell patient about importance of reporting persistent or worsening signs and symptoms of infection, such as pain or redness.

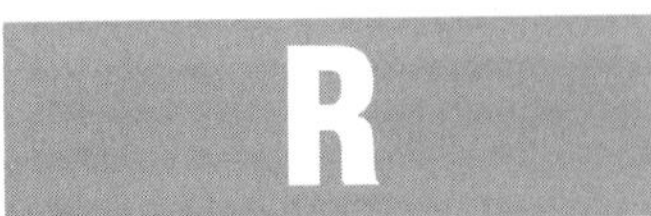

rabeprazole sodium
Aciphex

Pregnancy risk category B

Indications & dosages

➲ Healing of erosive or ulcerative gastroesophageal reflux disease (GERD)
Adults: 20 mg P.O. daily for 4 to 8 weeks. Additional 8-week course may be considered, if needed.

➲ Maintenance of healing of erosive or ulcerative GERD
Adults: 20 mg P.O. daily.

➲ Healing of duodenal ulcers
Adults: 20 mg P.O. daily after morning meal for up to 4 weeks.

➲ Pathologic hypersecretory conditions, including Zollinger-Ellison syndrome
Adults: 60 mg P.O. daily; may be increased, p.r.n., to 100 mg P.O. daily or 60 mg P.O. b.i.d.

➲ Symptomatic GERD, including daytime and nighttime heartburn
Adults: 20 mg P.O. daily for 4 weeks. Additional 4-week course may be considered, if needed.

➲ *Helicobacter pylori* eradication, to reduce the risk of duodenal ulcer recurrence
Adults: 20 mg P.O. b.i.d., combined with amoxicillin 1,000 mg P.O. b.i.d. and clarithromycin 500 mg P.O. b.i.d., for 7 days.

Contraindications & cautions

• Contraindicated in patients hypersensitive to drug, other benzimidazoles (lansoprazole, omeprazole), or components of these formulations.
• In ***H. pylori*** eradication, clarithromycin is contraindicated in pregnant patients, patients hypersensitive to macrolides, and those taking pimozide; amoxicillin is contraindicated in patients hypersensitive to penicillin.
• Use cautiously in patients with severe hepatic impairment.

Adverse reactions

CNS: headache.

Interactions

Drug-drug. *Clarithromycin:* May increase rabeprazole level. Monitor patient closely.
Cyclosporine: May inhibit cyclosporine metabolism. Use together cautiously.
Digoxin, ketoconazole, other gastric pH-dependent drugs: May decrease or increase drug absorption at increased pH values. Monitor patient closely.
Warfarin: May inhibit warfarin metabolism. Monitor PT and INR.

Nursing considerations

• Consider additional courses of therapy if duodenal ulcer or GERD isn't healed after first course of therapy.
• If *H. pylori* eradication is unsuccessful, do susceptibility testing. If patient is resistant to clarithromycin or susceptibility testing isn't possible, expect to start therapy using a different antimicrobial.
!! ALERT Amoxicillin may trigger anaphylaxis in patients with a history of penicillin hypersensitivity.
• Symptomatic response to therapy doesn't preclude presence of gastric malignancy.
!! ALERT Patients treated for *H. pylori* eradication have developed pseudomembranous colitis with nearly all antibacterial agents, including clarithromycin and amoxicillin. Monitor patient closely.

Patient teaching

• Explain importance of taking drug exactly as prescribed.
• Advise patient to swallow delayed-release tablets whole and not to crush, chew, or split it.
• Inform patient that drug may be taken without regard to meals.

rabies immune globulin, human
Hyperab, Imogam Rabies-HT

Pregnancy risk category C

Indications & dosages
➲ Rabies exposure
Adults and children: 20 IU/kg I.M. at time of first dose of rabies vaccine. Half of dose is used to infiltrate wound area; remainder is given I.M. in a different site.

Contraindications & cautions
- No known contraindications.
- Use with caution in patients hypersensitive to thimerosal or history of systemic allergic reactions to human immunoglobulin preparations; also use cautiously in those with immunoglobulin A deficiency.

Adverse reactions
CNS: slight fever.
GU: ***nephrotic syndrome***.
Skin: *rash*, pain, redness, and induration at injection site.
Other: ***anaphylaxis***, ***angioedema***.

Interactions
Drug-drug. *Live-virus vaccines (measles, mumps, polio, or rubella):* May interfere with response to vaccine. Postpone immunization, if possible.

Nursing considerations
- Obtain history of animal bites, allergies, and reactions to immunizations. Have epinephrine 1:1,000 ready to treat anaphylaxis.
- Ask patient when last tetanus immunization was received; many prescribers order a booster at this time.
- Use only with rabies vaccine and immediate local treatment of wound. Don't give rabies vaccine and rabies immune globulin in same syringe or at same site. Give as soon as possible after exposure or through day 7. After day 8, antibody response to culture vaccine has occurred.
- Don't give live-virus vaccines within 3 months of rabies immune globulin.
- Don't give more than 5 ml I.M. at one injection site; divide I.M. doses over 5 ml; give at different sites.
- Give large volumes (5 ml) in adults only. Use upper outer quadrant of gluteal area.

!!ALERT This immune serum provides passive immunity. Don't confuse with rabies vaccine, a suspension of killed microorganisms that confers active immunity. The two drugs are often used together prophylactically after exposure to rabid animals.
- Clean wound thoroughly with soap and water; this is the best prophylaxis against rabies.

Patient teaching
- Inform patient that local reactions may occur at injection site. Instruct him to notify prescriber promptly if reactions persist or become severe.
- Tell patient that a tetanus shot also may be needed.
- Instruct patient in wound care.

rabies vaccine, adsorbed

Pregnancy risk category C

Indications & dosages
➲ Preexposure preventive rabies immunization for persons in high-risk groups
Adults and children: 1 ml I.M. at 0, 7, and 21 or 28 days for total of three injections. Check patients at increased risk for rabies q 6 months and give booster vaccination, 1 ml I.M, p.r.n., to maintain adequate serum titer.
➲ To prevent postexposure rabies
Adults and children not previously vaccinated against rabies: 20-IU/kg doses of human rabies immune globulin (HRIG) I.M. and five 1-ml injections of rabies vaccine, adsorbed I.M. on days 0, 3, 7, 14, and 28.
Adults and children previously vaccinated against rabies: Two 1-ml injections of rabies vaccine, adsorbed I.M. on days 0 and 3. Don't give HRIG.

Contraindications & cautions
- Contraindicated in patients who have experienced life-threatening allergic reactions to previous injections of vaccine or to components of vaccine, including thimerosal.
- Use cautiously in patients hypersensitive to monkey-derived proteins, in those with history of non–life-threatening allergic reactions to previous injections of vaccine, and in children.

Adverse reactions

CNS: *headache, dizziness, slight fever, fatigue.*
GI: *abdominal pain, nausea.*
Musculoskeletal: *myalgia*, aching of injected muscle.
Skin: *transient pain, erythema, swelling, itching*, mild inflammatory reaction at injection site.
Other: reaction resembling serum sickness, ***anaphylaxis***.

Interactions

Drug-drug. *Antimalarials, corticosteroids, immunosuppressants:* May decrease response to rabies vaccine. Avoid using together.

Nursing considerations

- Keep epinephrine 1:1,000 available to treat anaphylaxis.
- Give as I.M. injection into deltoid region in adults and older children. For younger children, the mid-anterolateral aspect of the thigh also is acceptable. Don't use I.D. route. Avoid injecting vaccine near a peripheral nerve or into adipose or S.C. tissue.
- Vaccine is normally a light pink color because of presence of phenol red in suspension.

!!ALERT If patient experiences serious adverse reaction to vaccine, report reaction promptly to local public health officials.
!!ALERT Don't confuse vaccine with rabies immune globulin. Both drugs may be given in some situations.

Patient teaching

- Inform patient about adverse reactions linked to vaccine and importance of reporting serious adverse reactions.
- Warn patient not to perform hazardous activities if dizziness occurs.
- Advise proper fever-reducing drug dose for fever.
- Teach proper wound care and signs and symptoms of infection.

rabies vaccine, human diploid cell (HDCV)

Imovax Rabies, Imovax Rabies I.D. Vaccine

Pregnancy risk category C

Indications & dosages

➲ Postexposure antirabies immunization
Adults and children: Five 1-ml doses of HDCV I.M. Give first dose as soon as possible after exposure; give additional doses on days 3, 7, 14, and 28 after first dose. If no antibody response occurs after this primary series, booster dose is recommended.
➲ Preexposure preventive immunization for persons in high-risk groups
Adults and children: Three 1-ml injections I.M. Give first dose on day 0 (first day of therapy), second dose on day 7, and third dose on day 21 or 28. Or, 0.1 ml I.D. on same dosage schedule.

Contraindications & cautions

- No contraindications reported for persons after exposure. An acute febrile illness contraindicates use of vaccine for persons previously exposed.
- Use cautiously in hypersensitive patients.

Adverse reactions

CNS: *headache, fever*, dizziness, *fatigue.*
GI: *nausea*, abdominal pain, diarrhea.
Musculoskeletal: muscle aches.
Skin: *injection site pain, erythema, swelling, itching.*
Other: ***anaphylaxis***, *serum sickness.*

Interactions

Drug-drug. *Antimalarials, corticosteroids, immunosuppressants:* May decrease response to rabies vaccine. Avoid using together.

Nursing considerations

- Keep epinephrine 1:1,000 available to treat anaphylaxis.
- Use vaccine immediately after reconstitution.

!!ALERT Don't use I.D. route for postexposure rabies vaccination.

- Alternative regimen of 0.1-ml doses given via the intradermal route is only for preexposure prophylaxis.

• Stop corticosteroid therapy during immunizing period unless therapy is essential for treatment of other conditions.
• Some patients who receive booster doses experience serum sickness-like hypersensitivity. These reactions usually respond to antihistamines.
• Report all serious reactions to the State Department of Health.
!!ALERT Don't confuse vaccine with rabies immune globulin. Both drugs may be given in some situations.

Patient teaching

• Inform patient about adverse reactions linked to vaccine. Tell patient to report persistent or severe reactions.
• Stress importance of receiving booster, if appropriate for patient.
• Tell patient to treat mild reaction with appropriate doses of anti-inflammatory or fever-reducing drug.

raloxifene hydrochloride
Evista

Pregnancy risk category X

Indications & dosages

➲ To prevent or treat osteoporosis in postmenopausal women
Adults: 60 mg P.O. once daily.

Contraindications & cautions

• Contraindicated in women hypersensitive to drug or its components; in those with past or current venous thromboembolic events, including deep vein thrombosis, pulmonary embolism, and retinal vein thrombosis; in women who are pregnant, planning to get pregnant, or breast-feeding; and in children.
• Use cautiously in patients with severe hepatic impairment.
• Safety and efficacy of drug haven't been evaluated in men.

Adverse reactions

CNS: depression, insomnia, fever, migraine.
CV: chest pain.
EENT: *sinusitis*, pharyngitis, laryngitis.
GI: nausea, dyspepsia, vomiting, flatulence, gastroenteritis, abdominal pain.
GU: vaginitis, UTI, cystitis, leukorrhea, endometrial disorder, vaginal bleeding.
Metabolic: weight gain.
Musculoskeletal: *arthralgia*, myalgia, arthritis, leg cramps.
Respiratory: increased cough, pneumonia.
Skin: rash, diaphoresis.
Other: breast pain, *infection*, *flulike syndrome*, *hot flashes*, peripheral edema.

Interactions

Drug-drug. *Cholestyramine:* May cause significant reduction in absorption of raloxifene. Avoid using together.
Highly protein-bound drugs (such as clofibrate, diazepam, diazoxide, ibuprofen, indomethacin, naproxen): May interfere with binding sites. Use together cautiously.
Warfarin: May cause a decrease in PT. Monitor PT and INR closely.

Nursing considerations

• Watch for signs of blood clots. Greatest risk of thromboembolic events occurs during first 4 months of treatment.
• Stop drug at least 72 hours before prolonged immobilization and resume only after patient is fully mobilized.
• Report unexplained uterine bleeding; drug isn't known to cause endometrial proliferation.
• Watch for breast abnormalities; drug isn't known to cause an increased risk of breast cancer.
• Effect on bone mineral density beyond 2 years of drug treatment isn't known.
• Use with hormone replacement therapy or systemic estrogen hasn't been evaluated and isn't recommended.

Patient teaching

• Advise patient to avoid long periods of restricted movement (such as during traveling) because of increased risk of venous thromboembolic events.
• Inform patient that hot flashes or flushing may occur and that drug doesn't aid in reducing them.
• Instruct patient to practice other bone loss–prevention measures, including taking supplemental calcium and vitamin D if dietary intake is inadequate, performing weight-bearing exercises, and stopping alcohol consumption and smoking.

- Tell patient that drug may be taken without regard to food.
- Advise patient to report unexplained uterine bleeding or breast abnormalities during therapy.
- Explain adverse reactions and instruct patient to read patient package insert before starting therapy and each time prescription is renewed.

ramipril
Altace

Pregnancy risk category C; D in 2nd and 3rd trimesters

Indications & dosages

➲ Hypertension
Adults: Initially, 2.5 mg P.O. once daily for patients not taking a diuretic, and 1.25 mg P.O. once daily for patients taking a diuretic. Increase dosage, p.r.n., based on patient response. Maintenance dose is 2.5 to 20 mg daily as a single dose or in divided doses.

For patients with creatinine clearance less than 40 ml/minute, give 1.25 mg P.O. daily. Adjust dosage gradually based on response. Maximum daily dose is 5 mg.

➲ Heart failure after an MI
Adults: Initially, 2.5 mg P.O. b.i.d. If hypotension occurs; decrease dosage to 1.25 mg P.O. b.i.d. Adjust as tolerated to target dosage of 5 mg P.O. twice daily.

For patients with creatinine clearance less than 40 ml/minute, give 1.25 mg P.O. daily. Adjust dosage gradually based on response. Maximum dosage is 2.5 mg b.i.d.

➲ To reduce risk of MI, CVA, and death from CV causes
Adults age 55 and older: 2.5 mg P.O. once daily for 1 week, then 5 mg P.O. once daily for 3 weeks. Increase as tolerated to a maintenance dose of 10 mg P.O. once daily.

In patients who are hypertensive or who have recently had an MI, daily dose may be divided.

Contraindications & cautions

- Contraindicated in patients hypersensitive to ACE inhibitors and in those with a history of angioedema related to treatment with an ACE inhibitor.
- Use cautiously in patients with renal impairment.

Adverse reactions

CNS: headache, dizziness, fatigue, asthenia, malaise, light-headedness, anxiety, amnesia, depression, insomnia, nervousness, neuralgia, neuropathy, paresthesia, somnolence, tremor, vertigo, syncope.
CV: ***heart failure***, *hypotension*, postural hypotension, angina pectoris, chest pain, palpitations, ***MI***, edema.
EENT: epistaxis, tinnitus.
GI: nausea, vomiting, abdominal pain, anorexia, constipation, diarrhea, dyspepsia, dry mouth, gastroenteritis.
GU: impotence.
Metabolic: hyperglycemia, ***hyperkalemia***, weight gain.
Musculoskeletal: arthralgia, arthritis, myalgia.
Respiratory: dyspnea; dry, persistent, tickling, nonproductive cough.
Skin: rash, dermatitis, pruritus, photosensitivity reactions, increased diaphoresis.
Other: hypersensitivity reactions.

Interactions

Drug-drug. *Diuretics:* May cause excessive hypotension, especially at start of therapy. Stop diuretic at least 3 days before therapy begins, increase sodium intake, or reduce starting dose of ramipril.
Insulin, oral antidiabetics: May cause hypoglycemia, especially at start of ramipril therapy. Monitor glucose level closely.
Lithium: May increase lithium level. Use together cautiously and monitor lithium level.
Nesiritide: May increase hypotensive effects. Monitor blood pressure.
NSAIDs: May decrease antihypertensive effects. Monitor blood pressure.
Potassium-sparing diuretics, potassium supplements: May cause hyperkalemia; ramipril attenuates potassium loss. Monitor potassium level closely.
Drug-herb. *Capsaicin:* May cause cough. Discourage use together.
Ma huang: May decrease antihypertensive effects. Discourage use together.
Drug-food. *Salt substitutes containing potassium:* May cause hyperkalemia; ramipril attenuates potassium loss. Discourage use of salt substitutes during therapy.

Nursing considerations

- Monitor blood pressure regularly for drug effectiveness.
- Closely assess renal function in patients during first few weeks of therapy. Regular assessment of renal function is advisable. Patients with severe heart failure whose renal function depends on the renin-angiotensin-aldosterone system have experienced acute renal failure during ACE inhibitor therapy. Hypertensive patients with renal artery stenosis also may show signs of worsening renal function during first few days of therapy.
- Although ACE inhibitors reduce blood pressure in all races, they reduce it less in blacks taking the ACE inhibitor alone. Black patients should take drug with a thiazide diuretic for a more favorable response.
- ACE inhibitors appear to increase risk of angioedema in black patients.
- Monitor CBC with differential counts before therapy and periodically thereafter.
- Drug may reduce hemoglobin and WBC, RBC, and platelet counts, especially in patients with impaired renal function or collagen vascular diseases (systemic lupus erythematosus or scleroderma).
- Monitor potassium level. Risk factors for the development of hyperkalemia include renal insufficiency, diabetes, and concomitant use of drugs that raise potassium level.

Patient teaching

- Tell patient to notify prescriber if any adverse reactions occur. Dosage adjustment or discontinuation of drug may be needed.

!!ALERT Rarely, swelling of the face and throat (including swelling of the larynx) may occur, especially after first dose. Advise patient to report signs or symptoms of breathing difficulty or swelling of face, eyes, lips, or tongue.

- Inform patient that light-headedness can occur, especially during the first few days of therapy. Tell him to rise slowly to minimize this effect and to report signs and symptoms to prescriber. If he faints, patient should stop taking drug and call prescriber immediately.
- Tell patient that if he has difficulty swallowing capsules, he can open drug and sprinkle contents on a small amount of applesauce.
- Advise patient to report signs and symptoms of infection, such as fever and sore throat.
- Tell patient to avoid salt substitutes. These products may contain potassium, which can cause high potassium level in patients taking ramipril.
- Tell woman of childbearing age to notify prescriber if pregnancy occurs. Drug will need to be stopped.

ranitidine hydrochloride

Apo-Ranitidine†, Zantac*, Zantac-C†, Zantac 75 ◇, Zantac 150, Zantac EFFERdose Tablets, Zantac 150 GELdose, Zantac 300, Zantac 300 GELdose

Pregnancy risk category B

Indications & dosages

➲ Duodenal and gastric ulcer (short-term treatment); pathologic hypersecretory conditions, such as Zollinger-Ellison syndrome

Adults: 150 mg P.O. b.i.d. or 300 mg daily h.s. Or, 50 mg I.V. or I.M. q 6 to 8 hours. For Zollinger-Ellison syndrome, up to 6 g P.O. daily has been used for severe disease.
Children ages 1 month to 16 years: For duodenal and gastric ulcers only, 2 to 4 mg/kg P.O. b.i.d., up to 300 mg/day.

➲ Maintenance therapy for duodenal or gastric ulcer

Adults: 150 mg P.O. h.s.
Children ages 1 month to 16 years: 2 to 4 mg/kg P.O. daily, up to 150 mg daily.

➲ Gastroesophageal reflux disease

Adults: 150 mg P.O. b.i.d.
Children ages 1 month to 16 years: 5 to 10 mg/kg P.O. daily given as two divided doses.

➲ Erosive esophagitis

Adults: 150 mg P.O. q.i.d. Maintenance dosage is 150 mg P.O. b.i.d.
Children ages 1 month to 16 years: 5 to 10 mg/kg P.O. daily given as two divided doses.

➲ Heartburn

Adults and children age 12 and older: 75 mg of Zantac 75 P.O. as symptoms occur, up to 150 mg daily, not to exceed 2 weeks of continuous treatment.

For patients with creatinine clearance below 50 ml/minute, 150 mg P.O. q 24 hours or 50 mg I.V. q 18 to 24 hours.

Contraindications & cautions

- Contraindicated in patients hypersensitive to drug and those with acute porphyria.
- Use cautiously in patients with hepatic dysfunction. Adjust dosage in patients with impaired renal function.

Adverse reactions

CNS: vertigo, malaise, headache.
EENT: blurred vision.
Hepatic: jaundice.
Other: burning and itching at injection site, ***anaphylaxis***, ***angioedema***.

Interactions

Drug-drug. *Antacids:* May interfere with ranitidine absorption. Stagger doses, if possible.
Diazepam: May decrease absorption of diazepam. Monitor patient closely.
Glipizide: May increase hypoglycemic effect. Adjust glipizide dosage, as directed.
Procainamide: May decrease renal clearance of procainamide. Monitor patient closely for toxicity.
Warfarin: May interfere with warfarin clearance. Monitor patient closely.

Nursing considerations

- Assess patient for abdominal pain. Note presence of blood in emesis, stool, or gastric aspirate.
- Ranitidine may be added to total parenteral nutrition solutions.

!!ALERT Don't confuse ranitidine with rimantadine; don't confuse Zantac with Xanax or Zyrtec.

Patient teaching

- Instruct patient on proper use of OTC preparation, as indicated.
- Remind patient to take once-daily prescription drug at bedtime for best results.
- Instruct patient to take without regard to meals because absorption isn't affected by food.
- Tell patient taking 150 mg EFFERdose to dissolve drug in 6 to 8 ounces of water before taking.
- Tell parent to dissolve 25 mg EFFERdose tablet in at least 5 ml of water and give with a dosing cup, medicine dropper, or oral syringe.
- Urge patient to avoid cigarette smoking because this may increase gastric acid secretion and worsen disease.
- Advise patient to report abdominal pain and blood in stool or emesis.
- Warn patients with phenylketonuria that EFFERdose granules and tablets contain aspartame.

repaglinide

Prandin

Pregnancy risk category C

Indications & dosages

➲ **Adjunct to diet and exercise to lower glucose level in patients with type 2 diabetes whose hyperglycemia can't be controlled by diet and exercise alone; adjunct to diet, exercise, and metformin; adjunct to diet, exercise, and pioglitazone hydrochloride or rosiglitazone maleate**

Adults: For patients not previously treated or whose HbA_{1c} is below 8%, starting dose is 0.5 mg P.O. taken about 15 minutes before each meal; time may vary from immediately before to as long as 30 minutes before meal. For patients previously treated with glucose-lowering drugs and whose HbA_{1c} is 8% or more, first dose is 1 to 2 mg P.O. with each meal. Recommended dosage range is 0.5 to 4 mg with meals b.i.d., t.i.d., or q.i.d. Maximum daily dose is 16 mg.

Determine dosage by glucose response. May double dosage up to 4 mg with each meal until satisfactory glucose response is achieved. At least 1 week should elapse between dosage adjustments to assess response to each dose.

Metformin may be added if repaglinide monotherapy is inadequate; no repaglinide dosage adjustment is necessary.

In patients with severe renal impairment, starting dose is 0.5 mg P.O. with meals.

Contraindications & cautions

- Contraindicated in patients hypersensitive to drug or its inactive ingredients and in those with type 1 (insulin-dependent) diabetes or diabetic ketoacidosis.

• Use cautiously in patients with hepatic insufficiency in whom reduced metabolism could cause hypoglycemia and elevated blood level of repaglinide.
• Use cautiously in elderly, debilitated, or malnourished patients and in those with adrenal or pituitary insufficiency because these patients are more susceptible to hypoglycemic effect of glucose-lowering drugs.

Adverse reactions

CNS: *headache*, paresthesia.
CV: angina.
EENT: rhinitis, sinusitis.
GI: constipation, diarrhea, dyspepsia, nausea, vomiting.
GU: UTI.
Metabolic: **HYPOGLYCEMIA**, hyperglycemia.
Musculoskeletal: arthralgia, back pain.
Respiratory: bronchitis, *upper respiratory tract infection.*
Other: tooth disorder.

Interactions

Drug-drug. *Barbiturates, carbamazepine, rifampin:* May increase repaglinide metabolism. Monitor glucose level.
Beta blockers, chloramphenicol, coumarins, MAO inhibitors, NSAIDs, other drugs that are highly protein-bound, probenecid, salicylates, sulfonamides: May increase hypoglycemic action of repaglinide. Monitor glucose level.
Calcium channel blockers, corticosteroids, estrogens, fosphenytoin, hormonal contraceptives, isoniazid, nicotinic acid, hormonal contraceptives, phenothiazines, phenytoin, sympathomimetics, thiazides and other diuretics, thyroid products: May produce hyperglycemia, resulting in a loss of glycemic control. Monitor glucose level.
Clarithromycin: May increase repaglinide levels. Adjust repaglinide dosage.
Erythromycin, itraconazole, ketoconazole, miconazole, similar inhibitors of CYP 3A4: May inhibit repaglinide metabolism. Monitor glucose level.
Gemfibrozil: May increase repaglinide levels. Patients taking repaglinide shouldn't start taking gemfibrozil; patients taking gemfibrozil shouldn't start taking repaglinide. If already taking both, monitor glucose levels and adjust repaglinide dosage. Patients shouldn't take repaglinide, gemfibrozil, and itraconazole together due to synergistic metabolic inhibition.
Drug-herb. *Burdock, dandelion, eucalyptus, marshmallow:* May increase hypoglycemic effects. Discourage use together.
Drug-food. *Grapefruit juice:* May inhibit metabolism of repaglinide. Discourage use together.
Drug-lifestyle. *Alcohol use:* May alter glycemic control, most commonly causing hypoglycemia. Discourage use together.

Nursing considerations

• Increase dosage carefully in patients with impaired renal function or renal failure requiring dialysis.
• Adjust dosage by glucose level response. May double dosage up to 4 mg with each meal until satisfactory glucose level is achieved. At least 1 week should elapse between dosage adjustments to assess response.
• Metformin may be added if repaglinide monotherapy is inadequate.
• Administration of oral antidiabetics may cause increased CV mortality compared with diet alone or diet plus insulin treatment. This association may also apply to repaglinide.
• Loss of glycemic control can occur during stress, such as fever, trauma, infection, or surgery. Stop drug and give insulin.
• Hypoglycemia may be difficult to recognize in elderly patients and in patients taking beta blockers.
• When switching to another oral hypoglycemic, begin new drug on day after last dose of repaglinide.

Patient teaching

• Stress importance of diet and exercise with drug therapy.
• Discuss symptoms of low glucose level with patient and family.
• Tell patient to monitor glucose level periodically to determine minimum effective dose.
• Encourage patient to keep regular appointments and have his HbA_{1c} level checked every 3 months to determine long-term glucose control.
• Tell patient to take drug before meals, usually 15 minutes before start of meal; however, time can vary from immediately pre-

ceding meal to up to 30 minutes before meal.
- Tell patient that, if a meal is skipped or added, he should skip dose or add an extra dose of drug for that meal, respectively.
- Instruct patient to monitor glucose level carefully and tell him what to do when he's ill, undergoing surgery, or under added stress.
- Advise woman planning pregnancy to first consult prescriber. Insulin may be needed during pregnancy and breast-feeding.
- Teach patient to carry candy or other simple sugars to treat mild hypoglycemia episodes. Patient experiencing severe episode may need hospital treatment.
- Advise patient to avoid alcohol, which lowers glucose level.

respiratory syncytial virus immune globulin intravenous, human (RSV-IGIV)
RespiGam

Pregnancy risk category C

Indications & dosages

➲ To prevent serious lower respiratory tract infections from RSV in children with bronchopulmonary dysplasia (BPD) or history of premature birth (35 weeks' gestation or less)
Premature infants and children younger than age 2: Single infusion monthly. Give 1.5 ml/kg/hour I.V. for 15 minutes; then, if condition allows higher rate, increase to 3.6 ml/kg/hour until infusion ends. Maximum recommended total dose per monthly infusion is 750 mg/kg.

Contraindications & cautions

- Contraindicated in patients severely hypersensitive to drug or other human immunoglobulin and selective immunoglobulin A deficiency.
- Children with fluid overload shouldn't receive drug.

Adverse reactions

CNS: fever, dizziness, anxiety.
CV: tachycardia, hypertension, palpitations, chest tightness, flushing.
GI: vomiting, diarrhea, gastroenteritis, abdominal cramps.
Metabolic: fluid overload.
Musculoskeletal: myalgia, arthralgia.
Respiratory: respiratory distress, wheezing, crackles, hypoxia, tachypnea, dyspnea.
Skin: rash, pruritus, inflammation at injection site.
Other: overdose effect, hypersensitivity reactions (including *anaphylaxis*) , ***angioneurotic edema***.

Interactions

Drug-drug. *Live-virus vaccines (such as mumps, rubella, and especially measles):* May interfere with response. If such vaccines are given during or within 10 months after RSV-IGIV, reimmunization is recommended, if appropriate.

Nursing considerations

- Give first dose before RSV season (November to April) begins; give subsequent doses monthly throughout RSV season to maintain protection. Children with RSV should continue to receive monthly doses for duration of RSV season.
- Watch patient closely for signs and symptoms of fluid overload. Children with BPD may be more prone to this condition. Report increases in heart rate, respiratory rate, retractions, or crackles. Keep available a loop diuretic, such as furosemide or bumetanide.

Patient teaching

- Explain to parents importance of child receiving drug monthly throughout RSV season, even if he is already infected.
- Teach parents how drug is given and which adverse reactions are related to administration. Tell parents to report all adverse reactions promptly.

reteplase, recombinant
Retavase

Pregnancy risk category C

Indications & dosages

➲ To manage acute MI
Adults: Double-bolus injection of 10 + 10 units. Give each bolus I.V. over 2 minutes. If complications, such as serious bleeding or an anaphylactoid reaction, don't oc-

cur after first bolus, give second bolus 30 minutes after start of first one.

Contraindications & cautions

• Contraindicated in patients with active internal bleeding, known bleeding diathesis, history of CVA, recent intracranial or intraspinal surgery or trauma, severe uncontrolled hypertension, intracranial neoplasm, arteriovenous malformation, or aneurysm.
• Use cautiously in patients with previous puncture of noncompressible vessels; in those with recent (within 10 days) major surgery, obstetric delivery, organ biopsy, GI or GU bleeding, or trauma; in those with cerebrovascular disease, systolic blood pressure 180 mm Hg or higher or diastolic pressure 110 mm Hg or higher, and conditions that may lead to left heart thrombus, including mitral stenosis, acute pericarditis, subacute bacterial endocarditis, and hemostatic defects.
• Use cautiously in those with diabetic hemorrhagic retinopathy, septic thrombophlebitis, and other conditions in which bleeding would be difficult to manage.
• Use cautiously in patients age 75 and older and in breast-feeding women.

Adverse reactions

CNS: ***intracranial hemorrhage***.
CV: ***arrhythmias***, ***cholesterol embolization***, ***hemorrhage***.
GI: ***hemorrhage***.
GU: hematuria.
Hematologic: ***bleeding tendency***, anemia.
Other: bleeding at puncture sites, ***hypersensitivity reaction***.

Interactions

Drug-drug. *Heparin, oral anticoagulants, platelet inhibitors (abciximab, aspirin, dipyridamole, eptifibatide, tirofiban):* May increase risk of bleeding. Use together cautiously.

Nursing considerations

• Drug remains active in vitro and can lead to degradation of fibrinogen in sample, changing coagulation study results. Collect blood samples with phenylalanyl-L-prolyl-L-arginine chloromethylketone at 2-micromolar concentrations.
• Drug may be given to menstruating women.
• Carefully monitor ECG during treatment. Coronary thrombolysis may cause arrhythmias linked with reperfusion. Be prepared to treat bradycardia or ventricular irritability.
• Closely monitor patient for bleeding. Avoid I.M. injections, invasive procedures, and nonessential handling of patient. Bleeding is the most common adverse reaction and may occur internally or at external puncture sites. If local measures don't control serious bleeding, stop anticoagulant and notify prescriber. Withhold second bolus of reteplase.
• Use drug in pregnancy only if benefit to mother justifies risk to fetus.
• Safety and efficacy of drug in children haven't been established.
• Potency is expressed in units specific to reteplase and isn't comparable with other thrombolytic drugs.
• Avoid use of noncompressible pressure sites during therapy. If an arterial puncture is needed, use an arm vessel that can be compressed manually. Apply pressure for at least 30 minutes; then apply a pressure dressing. Check site frequently.

Patient teaching

• Explain use and administration of drug to patient and family.
• Tell patient to report adverse reactions immediately.

Rh_0 (D) immune globulin, human

BayRho-D Full Dose, BayRho-D Mini-Dose, MICRhoGAM, RhoGAM

Rh_0(D) immune globulin intravenous, human

Pregnancy risk category C

Indications & dosages

➲ **Rh exposure after abortion, miscarriage, ectopic pregnancy, or childbirth**
Rh_0(D) immune globulin, human
Adults: Transfusion unit or blood bank determines fetal packed RBC volume entering patient's blood; one vial is given I.M. if fetal packed RBC volume is less than 15 ml. More than one vial I.M. may be needed if severe fetomaternal hemorrhage occurs;

must be given within 72 hours after delivery or miscarriage.

➲ To prevent Rh antibody formation after abortion or miscarriage

Adults: Consult transfusion unit or blood bank. One microdose vial I.M. will suppress immune reaction to 2.5 ml Rh_0(D)-positive RBCs. Ideally, give within 3 hours, but may be given up to 72 hours after abortion or miscarriage.

➲ Rh exposure after abortion, amniocentesis after 34 weeks' gestation, or other manipulations past 34 weeks' gestation with increased risk of Rh isoimmunization

Rho(D) immune globulin I.V., human

Adults: 120 mcg I.V. or I.M.; must be given within 72 hours after delivery, miscarriage, or manipulation.

➲ Pregnancy

Adults: 300 mcg I.V. or I.M. at 28 weeks' gestation. If given early in pregnancy, give additional doses at 12-week intervals to maintain adequate levels of passively acquired anti-Rh antibodies. Then, within 72 hours of delivery, give 120 mcg I.M. or I.V. If 72 hours have elapsed, give drug as soon as possible, up to 28 days.

➲ Transfusion accidents

Adults: 600 mcg I.V. q 8 hours or 1,200 mcg I.M. q 12 hours until total dose given. Total dose depends on volume of packed RBCs or whole blood infused. Consult blood bank or transfusion unit at once; must be given within 72 hours.

➲ Idiopathic thrombocytopenic purpura in Rh_0(D) antigen-positive adults

Adults: Initially, 50 mcg/kg I.V. as single dose or divided into two doses on separate days. If hemoglobin is less than 10 g/dl, reduce first dose to 25 to 40 mcg/kg. Then, give 25 to 60 mcg/kg I.V. p.r.n. to elevate platelet counts with specific individually determined dosage.

Contraindications & cautions

- Contraindicated in Rh_0(D)-positive or D^u-positive patients and in those previously immunized to Rh_0(D) blood factor. Contraindicated in patients with anaphylactic or severe systemic reaction to human globulin.
- Use extreme caution when giving drug to patients with immunoglobulin A deficiency.

Adverse reactions

CNS: slight fever.
Skin: discomfort at injection site.
Other: ***anaphylaxis***.

Interactions

Drug-drug. *Live-virus vaccines:* May interfere with response. Postpone immunization for 3 months, if possible.

Nursing considerations

- Patients with immunoglobulin A deficiency may develop immunoglobulin A antibodies and have anaphylactic reaction; prescriber must weigh benefits of treatment against risk of hypersensitivity reactions before giving.
- Obtain history of allergies and reactions to immunizations. Keep epinephrine 1:1,000 ready to treat anaphylaxis.

!!ALERT Immediately after delivery, send a sample of neonate's cord blood to laboratory for typing and crossmatching. Confirm if mother is Rh_0(D)-negative and D^u-negative. Give drug to mother only if infant is Rh_0(D)- or D^u-positive. Administration must occur within 72 hours of delivery.

- This immune serum provides passive immunity to patient exposed to Rh_0(D)-positive fetal blood during pregnancy and prevents formation of maternal antibodies (active immunity), which would endanger future Rh_0(D)-positive pregnancies.
- Postpone vaccination with live-virus vaccines for 3 months after administration of Rh_0(D) immune globulin.
- Minidose preparations are recommended for patient undergoing abortion or miscarriage up to 12 weeks' gestation unless she is Rh_0(D)-positive or D^u-positive or has Rh antibodies, or unless the father or fetus is Rh-negative.

Patient teaching

- Explain how drug protects future Rh_0(D)-positive fetuses if used because of pregnancy, or explain other use, if indicated.
- Warn patient about adverse reactions related to drug.
- Reassure patient receiving this drug that there's no risk of HIV transmission.

ribavirin
Virazole

Pregnancy risk category X

Indications & dosages

➲ **Hospitalized infants and young children infected by respiratory syncytial virus (RSV)**
Infants and young children: Solution in concentration of 20 mg/ml delivered via the Viratek Small Particle Aerosol Generator (SPAG-2) and mechanical ventilator or oxygen hood, face mask, or oxygen tent at a rate of about 12.5 L of mist/minute. Treatment is given for 12 to 18 hours/day for at least 3 days, and no longer than 7 days.

Contraindications & cautions

- Contraindicated in patients hypersensitive to drug. Although drug is used in children, manufacturer states that it's contraindicated in women who are or may become pregnant during treatment.

Adverse reactions

CV: ***cardiac arrest***, hypotension, ***bradycardia***.
EENT: conjunctivitis, rash or erythema of eyelids.
Hematologic: anemia, reticulocytosis.
Respiratory: ***bronchospasm***, pulmonary edema, worsening respiratory state, ***apnea***, bacterial pneumonia, pneumothorax.

Interactions

None significant.

Nursing considerations

- Give ribavirin aerosol by the Viratek SPAG-2 only. Don't use any other aerosol-generating device.
- Use sterile USP water for injection, not bacteriostatic water. Water used to reconstitute this drug must not contain any antimicrobial product.
- Discard solutions placed in the SPAG-2 unit at least every 24 hours before adding newly reconstituted solution.

!!ALERT The most frequent adverse effects reported in health care personnel exposed to aerosolized ribavirin include eye irritation and headache. Advise pregnant personnel of these effects.

!!ALERT Monitor ventilator function frequently. Ribavirin may precipitate in ventilator apparatus, causing equipment malfunction with serious consequences.

- Store reconstituted solutions at room temperature for 24 hours.
- Ribavirin aerosol is indicated only for severe lower respiratory tract infection caused by RSV. Although treatment may begin while awaiting diagnostic test results, existence of RSV infection must be documented eventually.
- Most infants and children with RSV infection don't require treatment with antivirals because the disease is commonly mild and self-limiting. Premature infants or those with cardiopulmonary disease experience RSV in its severest form and benefit most from treatment with ribavirin aerosol.

Patient teaching

- Inform parents of need for drug, and answer any questions.
- Encourage parents to immediately report any subtle change in child.

rifabutin
Mycobutin

Pregnancy risk category B

Indications & dosages

➲ **To prevent disseminated *Mycobacterium avium* complex in patients with advanced HIV infection**
Adults: 300 mg P.O. daily as a single dose or divided b.i.d.

Contraindications & cautions

- Contraindicated in patients hypersensitive to drug or other rifamycin derivatives, such as rifampin, and in patients with active tuberculosis, because single-drug therapy with rifabutin increases risk of inducing bacterial resistance to both rifabutin and rifampin.
- Use cautiously in patients with neutropenia and thrombocytopenia.

Adverse reactions

CNS: headache, fever.
EENT: uveitis.

GI: dyspepsia, eructation, flatulence, diarrhea, nausea, vomiting, abdominal pain, anorexia, taste perversion.
GU: discolored urine.
Hematologic: ***neutropenia***, ***leukopenia***, ***thrombocytopenia***, eosinophilia.
Musculoskeletal: myalgia.
Skin: *rash*.

Interactions

Drug-drug. *Azole antifungals, benzodiazepines, beta blockers, buspirone, corticosteroids, cyclosporine, delavirdine, doxycycline, hydantoins, indinavir, losartan, macrolides, methadone, morphine, nelfinavir, quinidine, quinine, theophylline, tricyclic antidepressants, zolpidem:* May decrease effectiveness of these drugs. Monitor patient for drug effects.
Hormonal contraceptives: May decrease contraceptive effectiveness. Tell patient to use alternate form of birth control.
Indinavir: May increase rifabutin level. Decrease rifabutin dosage by 50%.
Warfarin: May decrease effectiveness of warfarin. May require higher dosages of anticoagulants. Monitor PT and INR.
Drug-food. *High-fat foods:* May reduce rate but not extent of absorption. Discourage use together.

Nursing considerations

- In patients with neutropenia or thrombocytopenia, obtain baseline hematologic studies and repeat periodically.
- Mix drug with soft foods such as applesauce for patients who have difficulty swallowing.
- Dosage may be divided and taken twice daily to decrease GI adverse effects. Drug also may be taken with food to avoid GI upset.

!!ALERT Don't confuse rifabutin with rifampin or rifapentine.

Patient teaching

- Instruct patient to take drug for as long as prescribed, exactly as directed, even after feeling better.
- Tell patient that drug or its metabolites may cause brownish orange staining of urine, feces, sputum, saliva, tears, and skin. Tell him to avoid wearing soft contact lenses because they may be permanently stained.
- Instruct patient to report sensitivity to light, excessive tears, or eye pain immediately; drug rarely may cause eye inflammation.
- Advise patient to report tingling and joint stiffness, swelling, or tenderness.

rifampin (rifampicin)

Rifadin, Rimactane, Rofact†

Pregnancy risk category C

Indications & dosages

➲ **Pulmonary tuberculosis, with other antituberculotics**
Adults: 10 mg/kg P.O. or I.V. daily in single dose. Give oral doses 1 hour before or 2 hours after meals. Maximum daily dose is 600 mg.
Children age 5 and older: 10 to 20 mg/kg P.O. or I.V. daily in single dose. Give oral doses 1 hour before or 2 hours after meals. Maximum daily dose is 600 mg. Give with other antituberculotics.
➲ **Meningococcal carriers**
Adults: 600 mg P.O. or I.V. q 12 hours for 2 days; or 600 mg P.O. or I.V. once daily for 4 days.
Children ages 1 month to 12 years: 10 mg/kg P.O. or I.V. q 12 hours for 2 days, not to exceed 600 mg/day; or 20 mg/kg once daily for 4 days.
Neonates: 5 mg/kg P.O. or I.V. q 12 hours for 2 days.
➲ ***Mycobacterium avium*** **complex♦**
Adults: 600 mg P.O. or I.V. daily as part of a multiple-drug regimen.

Contraindications & cautions

- Contraindicated in patients hypersensitive to rifampin or related drugs.
- Use cautiously in patients with liver disease.

Adverse reactions

CNS: headache, fatigue, drowsiness, behavioral changes, dizziness, mental confusion, generalized numbness, ataxia.
CV: ***shock***.
EENT: visual disturbances, exudative conjunctivitis.
GI: epigastric distress, anorexia, nausea, vomiting, abdominal pain, diarrhea, flatu-

lence, sore mouth and tongue, ***pseudomembranous colitis, pancreatitis***.
GU: hemoglobinuria, hematuria, ***acute renal failure***, menstrual disturbances.
Hematologic: eosinophilia, ***thrombocytopenia, transient leukopenia***, hemolytic anemia.
Hepatic: ***hepatotoxicity***.
Metabolic: hyperuricemia.
Musculoskeletal: osteomalacia.
Respiratory: shortness of breath, wheezing.
Skin: pruritus, urticaria, rash.
Other: flulike syndrome, discoloration of body fluids, porphyria exacerbation.

Interactions

Drug-drug. *Acetaminophen, amiodarone, analgesics, anticonvulsants, barbiturates, beta blockers, cardiac glycosides, chloramphenicol, clofibrate, corticosteroids, cyclosporine, dapsone, delavirdine, diazepam, digoxin, disopyramide, doxycycline, enalapril, fluoroquinolones, hormonal contraceptives, hydantoins, losartan, methadone, mexiletine, midazolam, nifedipine, opioids, ondansetron, progestins, propafenone, quinidine, sulfonylureas, tacrolimus, theophylline, tocainide, triazolam, tricyclic antidepressants, verapamil, zidovudine, zolpidem:* May decrease effectiveness of these drugs. Monitor patient for clinical effects.
Anticoagulants: May increase requirements for anticoagulant. Monitor PT and INR closely and adjust dosage of anticoagulant as needed.
Halothane: May increase risk of hepatotoxicity. Monitor liver function test results.
Isoniazid: May increase risk of hepatotoxicity. Monitor liver function test results.
Ketoconazole, para-aminosalicylate sodium: May interfere with absorption of rifampin. Separate doses by 8 to 12 hours.
Macrolide antibiotics, protease inhibitors: Rifampin metabolism may be inhibited, whereas other drug metabolism may be increased. Monitor patient for clinical effects and adverse effects.
Probenecid: May increase rifampin levels. Use together cautiously.
Drug-lifestyle. *Alcohol use:* May increase risk of hepatotoxicity. Discourage use together.

Nursing considerations

- Give drug with at least one other antituberculotic.
- Give P.O. doses 1 hour before or 2 hours after meals for optimal absorption; if GI irritation occurs, may give with meals.
- Monitor hepatic function, hematopoietic studies, and uric acid levels. Drug's systemic effects may cause asymptomatic elevation of liver function test results and uric acid level.
- Watch for and report to prescriber signs and symptoms of hepatic impairment.
- Drug may cause hemorrhage in neonates of rifampin-treated mothers.

!!ALERT Don't confuse rifampin with rifabutin or rifapentine.

Patient teaching

- Instruct patient who develops drug-induced GI upset to take drug with meals.
- Warn patient that he may feel drowsy and that urine, feces, saliva, sweat, sputum, and tears may turn red-orange. Use of drug may permanently stain soft contact lenses.
- Advise a woman using hormonal contraceptive to consider an alternative form of birth control.
- Advise patient to contact prescriber if he experiences fever, loss of appetite, malaise, nausea, vomiting, dark urine, or yellow discoloration of the eyes or skin.
- Advise patient to avoid alcohol during drug therapy.

rifapentine
Priftin

Pregnancy risk category C

Indications & dosages

➲ Pulmonary tuberculosis (TB), with at least one other antituberculotic to which the isolate is susceptible
Adults: During intensive phase of short-course therapy, 600 mg P.O. twice weekly for 2 months, with an interval between doses of at least 3 days (72 hours). During continuation phase of short-course therapy, 600 mg P.O. once weekly for 4 months, combined with isoniazid or another drug to which the isolate is susceptible.

Contraindications & cautions

- Contraindicated in patients hypersensitive to rifamycins (rifapentine, rifampin, or rifabutin).
- Use drug cautiously and with frequent monitoring in patients with liver disease.

Adverse reactions

CNS: headache, dizziness, pain.
CV: hypertension.
GI: anorexia, nausea, vomiting, dyspepsia, diarrhea.
GU: pyuria, proteinuria, hematuria, urinary casts.
Hematologic: ***neutropenia***, lymphopenia, anemia, ***leukopenia***, thrombocytosis.
Metabolic: *hyperuricemia.*
Musculoskeletal: arthralgia.
Respiratory: hemoptysis.
Skin: rash, pruritus, acne, maculopapular rash.

Interactions

Drug-drug. *Antiarrhythmics (disopyramide, mexiletine, quinidine, tocainide), antibiotics (chloramphenicol, clarithromycin, dapsone, doxycycline, fluoroquinolones), anticonvulsants (phenytoin), antifungals (fluconazole, itraconazole, ketoconazole), barbiturates, benzodiazepines (diazepam), beta blockers, calcium channel blockers (diltiazem, nifedipine, verapamil), cardiac glycosides, clofibrate, corticosteroids, haloperidol, HIV protease inhibitors (indinavir, nelfinavir, ritonavir, saquinavir), hormonal contraceptives, immunosuppressants (cyclosporine, tacrolimus), levothyroxine, opioid analgesics (methadone), oral anticoagulants (warfarin), oral hypoglycemics (sulfonylureas), progestins, quinine, reverse transcriptase inhibitors (delavirdine, zidovudine), sildenafil, theophylline, tricyclic antidepressants (amitriptyline, nortriptyline):* May decrease activity of these drugs because of cytochrome P-450 enzyme metabolism. May need to adjust dosage.

Nursing considerations

- Rifamycin antibiotics may cause hepatotoxicity. Obtain baseline liver function test results before therapy starts.
- Give drug with pyridoxine (vitamin B_6) in malnourished patients; in those predisposed to neuropathy, such as alcoholics and diabetics; and in adolescents.

!!ALERT Give drug with appropriate daily companion drugs. Compliance with all drug regimens, especially with daily companion drugs on the days when rifapentine isn't given, is crucial for early sputum conversion and protection from relapse of TB.

- If used during the last 2 weeks of pregnancy, drug may lead to postnatal hemorrhage in mother or infant. Monitor clotting parameters closely if drug is used at that time.

!!ALERT Don't confuse rifapentine with rifabutin or rifampin.

Patient teaching

- Stress importance of strict compliance with this drug regimen and that of daily companion drugs, as well as needed follow-up visits and laboratory tests.
- Advise a woman to use nonhormonal birth control methods.
- Tell patient to take drug with food if nausea, vomiting, or GI upset occurs.
- Instruct patient to report to prescriber fever, appetite loss, malaise, nausea, vomiting, darkened urine, yellowish skin and eyes, joint pain or swelling, or excessive loose stools or diarrhea.
- Instruct patient to protect pills from excessive heat.
- Tell patient that rifapentine can turn body fluids red-orange and permanently stain contact lenses.

rifaximin
Xifaxan

Pregnancy risk category C

Indications & dosages

➲ Traveler's diarrhea from noninvasive strains of *Escherichia coli*
Adults and children age 12 and older: 200 mg P.O. t.i.d. for 3 days.

Contraindications & cautions

- Contraindicated in patients hypersensitive to rifaximin or any rifamycin antibacterial.

Adverse reactions

CNS: fever, headache.
GI: abdominal pain, constipation, defecation urgency, flatulence, nausea, rectal tenesmus, vomiting.

Interactions
None significant

Nursing considerations
- Don't use drug in patients whose illness may be caused by *Campylobacter jejuni, Shigella,* or *Salmonella.*

!!ALERT Don't use drug in patients with blood in the stool, diarrhea with fever, or diarrhea from pathogens other than *E. coli.*
- Stop drug if diarrhea worsens or lasts longer than 24 to 48 hours. The patient may need a different antibiotic.
- Patients who have diarrhea after antibiotic therapy may have pseudomembranous colitis, which may range from mild to life-threatening.
- Monitor patient for overgrowth of nonsusceptible organisms.

Patient teaching
- Explain that drug may be taken with or without food.
- Tell patient to take all of the prescribed drug, even if he feels better before the drug is finished.
- Advise patient to notify his prescriber if diarrhea worsens or lasts longer than 1 or 2 days after starting treatment. A different treatment may be needed.
- Tell patient to call the prescriber if he develops a fever or has blood in his stool.
- Explain that this drug is only for treating diarrhea caused by contaminated foods or beverages while traveling and not for any other type of infection.
- Caution patient not to share this drug with others.

riluzole
Rilutek

Pregnancy risk category C

Indications & dosages
➲ Amyotrophic lateral sclerosis

Adults: 50 mg P.O. q 12 hours, taken on empty stomach 1 hour before or 2 hours after a meal.

Contraindications & cautions
- Contraindicated in patients with history of severe hypersensitivity to drug or its components.
- Use cautiously in patients with hepatic or renal dysfunction, in elderly patients, and in women and Japanese patients (who may have lower metabolic capacity to eliminate drug than men and white patients, respectively).

Adverse reactions
CNS: headache, aggravation reaction, *asthenia,* hypertonia, depression, dizziness, insomnia, malaise, somnolence, vertigo, circumoral paresthesia.
CV: hypertension, tachycardia, palpitations, orthostatic hypotension.
EENT: rhinitis, sinusitis.
GI: abdominal pain, *nausea,* vomiting, dyspepsia, anorexia, diarrhea, flatulence, stomatitis, dry mouth, oral candidiasis.
GU: UTI, dysuria.
Metabolic: weight loss.
Musculoskeletal: back pain, arthralgia.
Respiratory: *decreased lung function,* increased cough.
Skin: pruritus, eczema, alopecia, exfoliative dermatitis.
Other: phlebitis, peripheral edema, tooth disorder.

Interactions
Drug-drug. *Allopurinol, methyldopa, sulfasalazine:* May increase risk of hepatotoxicity. Monitor liver function closely.
Cytochrome P-450 inducers (omeprazole, rifampin): May increase riluzole elimination. Monitor for lack of effect.
Cytochrome P-450 inhibitors (amitriptyline, caffeine, phenacetin, quinolones, theophylline): May decrease riluzole elimination. Watch for adverse effects.
Drug-food. *Any food:* May decrease drug bioavailability. Advise patient to take drug 1 hour before or 2 hours after meals.
Charcoal-broiled foods: May increase elimination of drug. Discourage use together.
Drug-lifestyle. *Alcohol use:* May increase risk of hepatotoxicity. Discourage excessive use.
Smoking: May increase riluzole elimination. Discourage patient from smoking.

Nursing considerations
- Elevations in baseline liver function studies (especially bilirubin) preclude drug use. Perform liver function studies periodically during therapy. In many patients, drug may

increase aminotransferase level; if level exceeds five times upper limit of normal or if clinical jaundice develops, notify prescriber.
- Give drug at least 1 hour before or 2 hours after meals to avoid decreased bioavailability.

Patient teaching
- Tell patient to take drug at same time each day. If a dose is missed, tell him to take next tablet when planned.
- Instruct patient to take drug on an empty stomach to facilitate full dose absorption.
- Instruct patient to report fever to prescriber, who may order a WBC count.
- Warn patient to avoid hazardous activities until CNS effects of drug are known and to limit alcohol use during therapy.
- Tell patient to store drug at room temperature, protect from bright light, and keep out of children's reach.

risedronate sodium
Actonel

Pregnancy risk category C

Indications & dosages
➲ To prevent and treat postmenopausal osteoporosis
Adults: 5-mg tablet P.O. once daily, or 35-mg tablet once weekly.
➲ Glucocorticoid-induced osteoporosis in patients taking 7.5 mg or more of prednisone or equivalent glucocorticoid daily
Adults: 5 mg P.O. daily.
➲ Paget's disease
Adults: 30 mg P.O. daily for 2 months. If relapse occurs or alkaline phosphatase level doesn't normalize, may repeat treatment course 2 months or more after completing first treatment course.

Don't use if creatinine clearance is less than 30 ml/minute.

Contraindications & cautions
- Contraindicated in patients hypersensitive to any component of the product, in hypocalcemic patients, in patients with creatinine clearance less than 30 ml/minute, and in those who can't stand or sit upright for 30 minutes after administration.
- Use cautiously in patients with upper GI disorders such as dysphagia, esophagitis, and esophageal or gastric ulcers.

Adverse reactions
CNS: asthenia, *headache*, depression, dizziness, insomnia, anxiety, neuralgia, vertigo, hypertonia, paresthesia, *pain*.
CV: *hypertension*, CV disorder, angina pectoris, chest pain, peripheral edema.
EENT: pharyngitis, rhinitis, sinusitis, cataract, conjunctivitis, otitis media, amblyopia, tinnitus.
GI: *nausea, diarrhea, abdominal pain*, flatulence, gastritis, rectal disorder, constipation.
GU: *UTI*, cystitis.
Hematologic: ecchymosis, anemia.
Musculoskeletal: *arthralgia*, neck pain, *back pain*, myalgia, bone pain, leg cramps, bursitis, tendon disorder.
Respiratory: dyspnea, pneumonia, bronchitis.
Skin: *rash*, pruritus, skin carcinoma.
Other: *infection*, tooth disorder.

Interactions
Drug-drug. *Calcium supplements, antacids that contain calcium, magnesium, or aluminum:* May interfere with risedronate absorption. Advise patient to separate dosing times.
Drug-food. *Any food:* May interfere with absorption of drug. Advise patient to take drug at least 30 minutes before first food or drink of the day (other than water).

Nursing considerations
- Risk factors for the development of osteoporosis include family history, previous fracture, smoking, a decrease in bone mineral density below the premenopausal mean, a thin body frame, White or Asian race, and early menopause.

!!ALERT Give drug with 6 to 8 ounces of water at least 30 minutes before patient's first food or drink of the day, to facilitate delivery to the stomach. Don't allow patient to lie down for 30 minutes after taking drug.
- Consider weight-bearing exercise along with cessation of smoking and alcohol consumption, as appropriate.

!!ALERT Bisphosphonates have been linked to such GI disorders as dysphagia, esophagitis, and esophageal or gastric ulcers. Mon-

itor patient for symptoms of esophageal disease (such as dysphagia, retrosternal pain, or severe persistent or worsening heartburn).
- Patients should receive supplemental calcium and vitamin D if dietary intake is inadequate. Because calcium supplements and drugs containing calcium, aluminum, or magnesium may interfere with risedronate absorption, separate dosing times.
- Store drug at 68° to 77° F (20° to 25° C).
- Bisphosphonates can interfere with bone-imaging agents.

Patient teaching

- Explain that risedronate is used to replace bone lost because of certain disease processes.
- Caution patient about the importance of adhering to special dosing instructions.
- Tell patient to take drug at least 30 minutes before the first food or drink of the day other than water. Urge patient to take the drug with 6 to 8 ounces of water while sitting or standing. Warn patient against lying down for 30 minutes after taking risedronate.
- Tell patient not to chew or suck the tablet because doing so may irritate his mouth.
- Advise patient to contact prescriber immediately if he develops symptoms of esophageal disease (such as difficulty or pain when swallowing, retrosternal pain, or severe heartburn).
- Advise patient to take calcium and vitamin D if dietary intake is inadequate, but to take them at a different time than risedronate.
- Advise patient to stop smoking and drinking alcohol, as appropriate. Also, advise patient to perform weight-bearing exercise.
- Tell patient to store drug in a cool, dry place, at room temperature, and away from children.
- Urge patient to read the Patient Information Guide before starting therapy.
- Tell patient if he misses a dose of the 35-mg tablet, he should take 1 tablet on the morning after he remembers and return to taking 1 tablet once a week, as originally scheduled on his chosen day. Patient shouldn't take 2 tablets on the same day.

risperidone

Risperdal, Risperdal Consta, Risperdal M-Tab

Pregnancy risk category C

Indications & dosages

➲ Short-term (6 to 8 weeks) treatment of schizophrenia

Adults: Initially, 1 mg P.O. b.i.d. Increase by 1 mg b.i.d. on days 2 and 3 of treatment to a target dose of 3 mg b.i.d. Or, 1 mg P.O. on day 1, increase to 2 mg once daily on day 2, and 4 mg once daily on day 3. Wait at least 1 week before adjusting dosage further. Adjust doses by 1 to 2 mg. Maximum, 8 mg daily.

➲ To delay relapse in schizophrenia therapy lasting 1 to 2 years

Adults: Initially, 1 mg P.O. on day 1, increase to 2 mg once daily on day 2, and 4 mg once daily on day 3. Dosage range is 2 to 8 mg daily.

➲ Monotherapy or combination therapy with lithium or valproate for 3-week treatment of acute manic or mixed episodes from bipolar I disorder

Adults: 2 to 3 mg P.O. once daily. Adjust dose by 1 mg daily. Dosage range is 1 to 6 mg daily.

In elderly or debilitated patients, hypotensive patients, or those with severe renal or hepatic impairment, start with 0.5 mg P.O. b.i.d. Increase dosage by 0.5 mg b.i.d. Increase in dosages above 1.5 mg b.i.d. should occur at least 1 week apart. Subsequent switches to once-daily dosing may be made after patient is on a twice-daily regimen for 2 to 3 days at the target dose.

➲ 12-week therapy for schizophrenia

Adults: Establish tolerability to oral risperidone before giving I.M. formulation. Give 25 mg deep I.M. gluteal injection q 2 weeks; alternating injections between the two buttocks. Adjust dose no sooner than q 4 weeks. Maximum, 50 mg I.M. q 2 weeks. Continue oral antipsychotic for 3 weeks after first I.M. injection. Then stop oral therapy.

Contraindications & cautions

- Contraindicated in patients hypersensitive to drug and in breast-feeding women.

- Use cautiously in patients with prolonged QT interval, CV disease, cerebrovascular disease, dehydration, hypovolemia, history of seizures, or conditions that could affect metabolism or hemodynamic responses.
- Use cautiously in patients exposed to extreme heat.
- Use caution in patients at risk for aspiration pneumonia.
- Use I.M. injection cautiously in those with hepatic or renal impairment.

Adverse reactions

CNS: ***neuroleptic malignant syndrome***, somnolence, *extrapyramidal reactions, headache, insomnia, agitation, anxiety*, tardive dyskinesia, aggressiveness, dizziness, ***suicide attempt***, fever, ***TIA or stroke in elderly patients with dementia***, hallucination, abnormal thinking and dreaming, akathisia, *parkinsonism*, tremor, *pain*, hypoesthesia, fatigue, depression, nervousness (I.M.).
CV: tachycardia, chest pain, orthostatic hypotension, ***prolonged QT interval***, peripheral edema, syncope, hypertension (I.M.).
EENT: *rhinitis*, sinusitis, pharyngitis, abnormal vision, ear disorder (I.M.).
GI: *constipation, nausea, vomiting, dyspepsia, abdominal pain, anorexia*, dry mouth, increased saliva, diarrhea (I.M.).
Hematologic: anemia.
Metabolic: *weight gain*, ***hyperglycemia***, weight decrease (I.M.).
Musculoskeletal: arthralgia, back pain, leg pain, myalgia (I.M.).
Respiratory: coughing, upper respiratory infection.
Skin: rash, dry skin, photosensitivity, acne, injection site pain (I.M.).
Other: tooth disorder, toothache.

Interactions

Drug-drug. *Antihypertensives:* May enhance hypotensive effects. Monitor blood pressure.
Carbamazepine: May increase risperidone clearance and decreases effectiveness. Monitor patient closely.
Clozapine: May decrease risperidone clearance, increasing toxicity. Monitor patient closely.
CNS depressants: May cause additive CNS depression. Use together cautiously.
Dopamine agonists, levodopa: May antagonize effects of these drugs. Use together cautiously and monitor patient.
Drug-lifestyle. *Alcohol use:* May cause additive CNS depression. Discourage use together.
Sun exposure: May increase risk of photosensitivity reactions. Advise patient to avoid excessive sunlight exposure.

Nursing considerations

!! ALERT Obtain baseline blood pressure measurements before starting therapy, and monitor pressure regularly. Watch for orthostatic hypotension, especially during first dosage adjustment.
- Cerebrovascular adverse events (stroke, TIA), including fatalities, may occur in elderly patients with dementia. Risperidone isn't safe or effective in these patients.
- Monitor patient for tardive dyskinesia, which may occur after prolonged use. It may not appear until months or years later and may disappear spontaneously or persist for life, despite ending drug.
- Monitor patient for weight gain.
- Potentially severe or fatal hyperglycemia may occur in patients taking atypical antipsychotics. Monitor patients with diabetes regularly.
- The effectiveness of risperidone for use longer than 3 weeks to treat an acute episode and for prophylactic use in mania isn't known. If using drug for extended time, periodically reevaluate its risks and benefits.
- Give oral antipsychotic for the first 3 weeks of I.M. injection therapy because injection's effects take a long time. Then stop oral therapy.
- To reconstitute I.M. injection, inject premeasured diluent into vial and shake vigorously for at least 10 seconds. Suspension appears uniform, thick, and milky; particles are visible, but no dry particles remain. Drug should be used immediately, but may be refrigerated up to 6 hours of reconstitution. If more than 2 minutes pass before injection, shake vigorously again. See manufacturer's package insert for more detailed instructions.
- Refrigerate I.M. injection kit and protect it from light. Drug can be stored at temperature less than 77°F (25° C) for no more than 7 days before administration.
- Dosages above 6 mg daily may be no more effective than lower doses and may cause more extrapyramidal reactions. Safety of

dosages above 16 mg daily hasn't been evaluated.

!!ALERT Watch for evidence of neuroleptic malignant syndrome (extrapyramidal effects, hyperthermia, autonomic disturbance), which is rare but commonly fatal. It may not be related to length of drug use or type of neuroleptic; more than 60% of patients are men.

- Phenylalanine contents of orally disintegrating tablets are as follows: 0.5-mg tablet contains 0.14 mg phenylalanine; 1-mg tablet contains 0.28 mg phenylalanine; 2-mg tablet contains 0.56 mg phenylalanine.

!!ALERT Don't confuse risperidone with reserpine.

Patient teaching

- Warn patient to avoid activities that require alertness until effects of drug are known.
- Warn patient to rise slowly, avoid hot showers, and use other cautions when starting therapy, to avoid fainting.
- Advise patient to use caution in hot weather to prevent heatstroke.
- Tell patient to take drug with or without food.
- Instruct patient to release the orally disintegrating tablets from their blister pack just before taking them.
- Advise patient to open the pack and dissolve orally disintegrating tablet on tongue; tell him not to split or chew tablet.
- Tell patient to use sunblock and wear protective clothing outdoors.
- Tell patient to notify prescriber if she becomes pregnant, intends to become pregnant during therapy, or becomes pregnant within 12 weeks after the last I.M. injection.
- Warn patient not to breast-feed an infant during treatment and for at least 12 weeks after the last I.M. injection.

ritonavir
Norvir

Pregnancy risk category B

Indications & dosages

➲ HIV infection, with other antiretrovirals, when antiretroviral therapy is warranted

Adults: 600 mg P.O. b.i.d with meals. To reduce adverse GI effects, begin with 300 mg P.O. b.i.d. and increase by 100 mg b.i.d. at 2- to 3-day intervals.

Children age 2 and older: 400 mg/m^2 P.O. b.i.d.; don't exceed 600 mg P.O. b.i.d. Initially, may start with 250 mg/m^2 b.i.d. and increase by 50 mg/m^2 P.O. q 12 hours at 2- to 3-day intervals. If children can't reach b.i.d. doses of 400 mg/m^2 because of adverse effects, consider alternative therapy.

Contraindications & cautions

- Contraindicated in patients hypersensitive to drug or its components.
- Drug also contraindicated with concomitant alfuzosin, amiodarone, bepridil, flecainide, propafenone, quinidine, ergot derivatives, pimozide, lovastatin, simvastatin, midazolam, and triazolam.
- Use cautiously in patients with hepatic insufficiency.
- Safety and effectiveness in children younger than age 12 haven't been established.
- It's unknown if ritonavir appears in breast milk. Use cautiously in breast-feeding women.

Adverse reactions

CNS: *asthenia*, fever, headache, malaise, circumoral paresthesia, dizziness, insomnia, paresthesia, peripheral paresthesia, somnolence, thinking abnormality, ***generalized tonic-clonic seizure***, depression, anxiety, pain, malaise, confusion.

CV: vasodilation, syncope.

EENT: pharyngitis.

GI: abdominal pain, anorexia, constipation, *diarrhea, nausea, vomiting*, dyspepsia, flatulence, *taste perversion*, ***pancreatitis***, ***pseudomembranous colitis***.

Hematologic: ***leukopenia***, ***thrombocytopenia***.

Hepatic: ***hepatitis***.
Metabolic: ***diabetes mellitus***, weight loss.
Musculoskeletal: myalgia, arthralgia.
Skin: rash, sweating.
Other: fat redistribution or accumulation, ***hypersensitivity reactions***.

Interactions

Drug-drug. *Alfuzosin, amiodarone, bepridil, ergot derivatives, flecainide, midazolam, pimozide, propafenone, quinidine, triazolam:* May cause serious and life-threatening adverse reactions. Use together is contraindicated.
Atovaquone, divalproex, lamotrigine, phenytoin, warfarin: May decrease levels of these drugs. Use together cautiously and monitor drug levels closely.
Beta blockers, disopyramide, fluoxetine, mexiletine, nefazodone: May increase levels of these drugs, causing cardiac and neurologic events. Use together with caution.
Bupropion, carbamazepine, calcium channel blockers, clonazepam, clorazepate, cyclosporine, dexamethasone, diazepam, dronabinol, estazolam, ethosuximide, flurazepam, lidocaine, methamphetamine, metoprolol, perphenazine, prednisone, propoxyphene, quinine, risperidone, SSRIs, tacrolimus, tricyclic antidepressants, thioridazine, timolol, tramadol, zolpidem: May increase levels of these drugs. Use cautiously together and consider decreasing the dosage of these drugs by almost 50%.
Clarithromycin: May increase clarithromycin level. If creatinine clearance is 30 to 60 ml/minute, reduce clarithromycin dose by 50%. If creatinine clearance is less than 30 ml/minute, reduce clarithromycin dose by 75%.
Didanosine: May decrease didanosine absorption. Separate doses by 2½ hours.
Disulfiram, metronidazole: May increase risk of disulfiram-like reactions because ritonavir formulations contain alcohol. Monitor patient.
Ethinyl estradiol: May decrease ethinyl estradiol level. Use an alternative or additional method of birth control.
Fluticasone: May significantly increase fluticasone exposure, significantly decreasing cortisol concentrations and causing systemic corticosteroid effects (including Cushing syndrome). Don't use together, if possible.
HMG-CoA reductase inhibitors: May cause large increase in statin levels, resulting in myopathy. Avoid use with lovastatin and simvastatin. Use cautiously with atorvastatin. Consider using fluvastatin or pravastatin.
Indinavir: May increase indinavir levels. Use together cautiously.
Meperidine: May decrease levels of meperidine and its metabolite. Dosage adjustment not recommended because of CNS effects. Use cautiously together.
Methadone: May decrease methadone levels. Consider increasing methadone dosage.
Rifabutin: May increase rifabutin levels. Monitor patient and reduce rifabutin daily dosage by at least 75% of usual dose.
Rifampin: May decrease ritonavir levels. Consider using rifabutin.
Saquinavir: May increase saquinavir plasma levels. Adjust dose by taking saquinavir 400 mg b.i.d. and ritonavir 400 mg b.i.d.
Sildenafil: May increase levels of sildenafil. Use together cautiously. Tell patient not to exceed 25 mg of sildenafil in a 48-hour period.
Theophylline: May decrease theophylline levels. Increase dose based on blood levels.
Trazodone: May increase trazodone level causing nausea, dizziness, hypotension and syncope. Avoid use together. If unavoidable, use cautiously and lower trazodone dose.
Drug-herb. *St. John's wort:* May substantially reduce ritonavir levels. Discourage use together.
Drug-food. *Any food:* May increase absorption. Advise patient to take drug with food.
Drug-lifestyle. *Smoking:* May decrease serum levels of ritonavir. Discourage smoking.

Nursing considerations

- Patients beginning combination regimens with ritonavir and nucleosides may improve GI tolerance by starting ritonavir alone and then adding nucleosides before completing 2 weeks of ritonavir.

!!ALERT Don't confuse Norvir with Norvasc.

Patient teaching

- Inform patient that drug doesn't cure HIV infection. He may continue to develop opportunistic infections and other complications of HIV infection. Drug hasn't been shown to reduce the risk of transmitting HIV to others through sexual contact or blood contamination.

- Caution patient to take drug as prescribed and not to adjust dosage or stop therapy without first consulting prescriber.
- Tell patient that taste of ritonavir oral solution may be improved by mixing it with chocolate milk, Ensure, or Advera within 1 hour of the scheduled dose.
- Instruct patient to take drug with a meal to improve absorption.
- Tell patient that if a dose is missed, he should take the next dose as soon as possible. If a dose is skipped, he shouldn't double the next dose.
- Advise patients taking sildenafil to promptly report hypotension, visual changes, and priapism to their prescriber. Caution against exceeding 25 mg of sildenafil in a 48-hour period.
- Advise patient to report use of other drugs, including OTC drugs; ritonavir interacts with many drugs.
- Advise woman not to breast-feed to prevent transmission of infection.

rituximab
Rituxan

Pregnancy risk category C

Indications & dosages

➲ **Relapsed or refractory low-grade or follicular, CD20-positive, B-cell non-Hodgkin's malignant lymphoma**

Adults: Initially, 375 mg/m^2 I.V. infusion at rate of 50 mg/hour once weekly for four or eight doses. If no hypersensitivity or infusion-related events occur, increase rate by 50 mg/hour q 30 minutes, to maximum of 400 mg/hour. Start subsequent infusions at 100 mg/hour and increase by 100 mg/hour q 30 minutes, to maximum of 400 mg/hour as tolerated.

Retreatment for patients with progressive disease, 375 mg/m^2 I.V. infusion once weekly for four doses.

Contraindications & cautions

- Contraindicated in patients with type I hypersensitivity or anaphylactic reactions to murine proteins or components of rituximab.

Adverse reactions

CNS: dizziness, *asthenia, headache,* fatigue, paresthesia, malaise, agitation, insomnia, hypesthesia, hypertonia, nervousness, *fever,* pain, vertigo, somnolence.
CV: *hypotension,* ***arrhythmias,*** hypertension, peripheral edema, chest pain, tachycardia, ***bradycardia,*** flushing, edema.
EENT: sore throat, rhinitis, sinusitis, lacrimation disorder, conjunctivitis.
GI: *nausea,* vomiting, abdominal pain or enlargement, diarrhea, dyspepsia, anorexia, taste perversion.
GU: ***acute renal failure.***
Hematologic: **LEUKOPENIA,** ***thrombocytopenia, neutropenia,*** anemia.
Metabolic: hyperglycemia, hypocalcemia, weight decrease.
Musculoskeletal: myalgia, back pain, arthritis.
Respiratory: ***bronchospasm,*** dyspnea, cough increase, bronchitis.
Skin: *pruritus, rash,* urticaria, *severe mucocutaneous reactions,* pain at injection site.
Other: **ANGIOEDEMA,** *chills, rigors,* tumor pain, tumor lysis syndrome, infection.

Interactions

Drug-drug. *Cisplatin:* Use together may result in renal toxicity. Monitor renal function tests if used together.

Nursing considerations

- Monitor patient closely for signs and symptoms of hypersensitivity. Have drugs, such as epinephrine, antihistamines, and corticosteroids, available to immediately treat such a reaction. Premedicate with acetaminophen and diphenhydramine before each infusion.
- Severe mucocutaneous reactions (including toxic epidermal necrolysis, Stevens-Johnson syndrome, paraneoplastic pemphigus, and lichenoid or vesiculobullous dermatitis) have occurred in patients receiving rituximab ranging from 1 to 13 weeks after administration. Avoid further infusions and promptly start treatment of the skin reaction.
- Infusion-related reactions are most severe with the first infusion. Subsequent infusions are generally well tolerated.
- Obtain CBC at regular intervals and more frequently in patients who develop cytopenias.

• Protect vials from direct sunlight.

Patient teaching

• Tell patient to report symptoms of hypersensitivity, such as itching, rash, chills, or rigor, during and after infusion.
• Urge patient to watch for fever, sore throat, fatigue and for easy bruising, nosebleeds, bleeding gums, or tarry stools. Tell him to take temperature daily.
• Advise breast-feeding women to stop breast-feeding until drug levels are undetectable.

rivastigmine tartrate
Exelon

Pregnancy risk category B

Indications & dosages

➲ Symptomatic treatment of patients with mild to moderate Alzheimer's disease
Adults: Initially, 1.5 mg P.O. b.i.d. with food. If tolerated, may increase to 3 mg b.i.d. after 2 weeks. After 2 weeks at this dose, may increase to 4.5 mg b.i.d. and 6 mg b.i.d., as tolerated. Effective dosage range is 6 to 12 mg daily; maximum, 12 mg daily.

Contraindications & cautions

• Contraindicated in patients hypersensitive to drug, other carbamate derivatives, or other components of the drug.

Adverse reactions

CNS: syncope, fatigue, asthenia, malaise, *dizziness*, *headache*, somnolence, tremor, insomnia, confusion, depression, anxiety, hallucinations, aggressive reaction, vertigo, agitation, nervousness, delusion, paranoid reaction.
CV: hypertension, chest pain, peripheral edema.
EENT: rhinitis, pharyngitis.
GI: *nausea*, *vomiting*, *diarrhea*, *anorexia*, *abdominal pain*, dyspepsia, constipation, flatulence, eructation.
GU: UTI, urinary incontinence.
Metabolic: weight loss.
Musculoskeletal: back pain, arthralgia, bone fracture.
Respiratory: upper respiratory tract infection, cough, bronchitis.
Skin: increased sweating, rash.
Other: *accidental trauma*, flulike symptoms, pain.

Interactions

Drug-drug. *Bethanechol, succinylcholine, other neuromuscular blocking drugs or cholinergic antagonists:* May have synergistic effect. Monitor patient closely.
Drug-lifestyle. *Smoking:* May increase rivastigmine clearance. Discourage smoking.

Nursing considerations

• Expect significant GI adverse effects (such as nausea, vomiting, anorexia, and weight loss). These effects are less common during maintenance doses.
• Monitor patient for evidence of active or occult GI bleeding.
• Dramatic memory improvement is unlikely. As disease progresses, the benefits of rivastigmine may decline.
• Monitor patient for severe nausea, vomiting, and diarrhea, which may lead to dehydration and weight loss.
• Carefully monitor patient with a history of GI bleeding, NSAID use, arrhythmias, seizures, or pulmonary conditions for adverse effects.

Patient teaching

• Tell caregiver to give rivastigmine with food in the morning and evening.
• Advise patient that memory improvement may be subtle and that drug more likely slows future memory loss.
• Tell patient to report nausea, vomiting, or diarrhea.
• Tell patient to consult prescriber before using OTC medications.

ropinirole hydrochloride
Requip

Pregnancy risk category C

Indications & dosages

➲ Idiopathic Parkinson's disease
Adults: Initially, 0.25 mg P.O., t.i.d. Increase dose by 0.25 mg t.i.d. at weekly intervals for 4 weeks. After week 4, dosage may be increased by 1.5 mg daily divided t.i.d. at weekly intervals, up to 9 mg daily divided t.i.d.; then dosage may be increased by up

to 3 mg daily divided t.i.d.; at weekly intervals, up to 24 mg daily divided t.i.d.
Elderly patients: Adjust dosages individually, according to patient response; clearance is reduced in these patients.

➲ **Moderate to severe restless leg syndrome**

Adults: Initially, 0.25 mg P.O. 1 to 3 hours before bedtime. May increase dose as needed and tolerated after 2 days to 0.5 mg, then to 1 mg by the end of the first week. May further increase dose as needed and tolerated as follows: week 2, give 1 mg once daily. Week 3, give 1.5 mg once daily. Week 4, give 2 mg once daily. Week 5, give 2.5 mg once daily. Week 6, give 3 mg once daily. And week 7, give 4 mg once daily. All doses should be taken 1 to 2 hours before bedtime.

Contraindications & cautions

- Contraindicated in patients hypersensitive to drug.
- Use cautiously in patients with severe hepatic or renal impairment.

Adverse reactions

Early Parkinson's disease (without levodopa)

CNS: hallucinations, *dizziness*, aggravated Parkinson's disease, *somnolence*, headache, confusion, hyperkinesia, hypoesthesia, vertigo, amnesia, impaired concentration, *syncope*, *fatigue*, malaise, asthenia.
CV: orthostatic hypotension, orthostatic symptoms, hypertension, edema, chest pain, extrasystoles, atrial fibrillation, palpitations, tachycardia, flushing.
EENT: pharyngitis, abnormal vision, eye abnormality, xerophthalmia, rhinitis, sinusitis.
GI: dry mouth, *nausea*, *vomiting*, *dyspepsia*, flatulence, abdominal pain, anorexia, constipation.
GU: UTI, impotence.
Respiratory: bronchitis, dyspnea, yawning.
Other: *viral infection*, pain, increased sweating, peripheral ischemia.

Advanced Parkinson's disease (with levodopa)

CNS: *dizziness*, aggravated parkinsonism, *somnolence*, *headache*, insomnia, *hallucinations*, abnormal dreaming, confusion, tremor, anxiety, nervousness, amnesia, paresis, paresthesia, syncope.
CV: hypotension.
EENT: diplopia.
GI: *nausea*, abdominal pain, dry mouth, vomiting, constipation, diarrhea, dysphagia, flatulence, increased saliva.
GU: UTI, pyuria, urinary incontinence.
Hematologic: anemia.
Metabolic: weight decrease, suppressed prolactin.
Musculoskeletal: arthralgia, arthritis, *dyskinesia*, hypokinesia.
Respiratory: upper respiratory tract infection, dyspnea.
Skin: increased sweating.
Other: injury, *falls*, viral infection, pain.

Restless leg syndrome

CNS: vertigo, *fatigue*, *somnolence*, *dizziness*, paresthesia.
CV: peripheral edema.
EENT: *nasopharyngitis*, nasal congestion.
GI: *nausea*, *vomiting*, diarrhea, dyspepsia, dry mouth.
Musculoskeletal: arthralgia, muscle cramps, extremity pain.
Respiratory: cough.
Skin: increased sweating.
Other: influenza.

Interactions

Drug-drug. *Cimetidine, ciprofloxacin, fluvoxamine, inhibitors or substrates of CYP1A2, ritonavir:* May alter ropinirole clearance. Adjust ropinirole dose if other drugs are started or stopped during treatment.
CNS depressants: May increase CNS effects. Use together cautiously.
Dopamine antagonists (neuroleptics) or metoclopramide: May decrease ropinirole effects. Avoid using together.
Estrogens: May decrease ropinirole clearance. Adjust ropinirole dosage if estrogen therapy is started or stopped during treatment.
Drug-lifestyle. *Alcohol use:* May increase sedative effect. Advise patient to use cautiously.
Smoking: May increase ropinirole clearance. Discourage use together.

Nursing considerations

!!ALERT Monitor patient carefully for orthostatic hypotension, especially during dosage increases.

• Drug may potentiate the dopaminergic adverse effects of levodopa and may cause or worsen dyskinesia. Dosage may be decreased.
• Although not reported with ropinirole, other adverse reactions reported with dopaminergic therapy include hyperpyrexia, fibrotic complications, and confusion, which may occur with rapid dosage reduction or withdrawal of medication.
• Patient may have syncope, with or without bradycardia. Monitor patient carefully, especially for 4 weeks after start of therapy and with dosage increases.
• When used for Parkinson's disease, withdraw drug gradually over 7 days.
• When used for restless leg syndrome, no dose taper is needed when stopping therapy.

Patient teaching

• Advise patient to take drug with food if nausea occurs.
• Inform patient (especially elderly patient) that hallucinations can occur.
• Instruct patient not to rise rapidly after sitting or lying down because of risk of dizziness, which may occur more frequently early in therapy or when dosage increases.
• Sleepiness can occur early in therapy. Warn patient to minimize hazardous activities until CNS effects of drug are known.
• Advise patient to avoid alcohol.
• Tell woman to notify prescriber about planned, suspected, or known pregnancy; also tell her to inform prescriber if she's breast-feeding.

rosiglitazone maleate

Avandia

Pregnancy risk category C

Indications & dosages

➲ **Adjunct to diet and exercise (as monotherapy) to improve glycemic control in patients with type 2 diabetes, or (as combination therapy) with sulfonylurea or metformin, or insulin when diet, exercise, and a single agent don't result in adequate glycemic control**

Adults: Initially, 4 mg P.O. daily in the morning or in divided doses b.i.d. in the morning and evening. Dosage may be increased to 8 mg P.O. daily or in divided doses b.i.d. if fasting glucose level doesn't improve after 12 weeks of treatment.

For patients stabilized on insulin, continue the insulin dose when rosiglitazone therapy starts. Don't give doses of rosiglitazone greater than 4 mg daily with insulin. Decrease insulin dose by 10% to 25% if patient reports hypoglycemia or if fasting glucose level falls to below 100 mg/dl. Individualize further adjustments based on glucose-lowering response.

Contraindications & cautions

• Contraindicated in patients hypersensitive to drug or its components and in those with New York Heart Association Class III or IV cardiac status unless expected benefits outweigh risks.
• Contraindicated in patients with active liver disease, increased baseline liver enzyme levels (ALT level greater than 2½ times upper limit of normal), type 1 (insulin-dependent) diabetes, or diabetic ketoacidosis and in those who experienced jaundice while taking troglitazone.
• Because metformin is contraindicated in patients with renal impairment, combination therapy with rosiglitazone is also contraindicated in patients with renal impairment. Rosiglitazone can be used as monotherapy in patients with renal impairment.
• Use cautiously in patients with edema or heart failure.

Adverse reactions

CNS: headache, fatigue.
CV: edema.
EENT: sinusitis.
GI: diarrhea.
Hematologic: anemia.
Metabolic: hyperglycemia.
Musculoskeletal: back pain.
Respiratory: upper respiratory tract infection.
Other: accidental injury.

Interactions

None significant.

Nursing considerations

• Before starting drug therapy, treat patient for other causes of poor glycemic control, such as infection.

!!ALERT Check liver enzyme levels before therapy starts. Don't use drug in patients with increased baseline liver enzyme levels. In patients with normal baseline liver enzyme levels, monitor these levels every 2 months for first 12 months and periodically thereafter. If ALT level is elevated during treatment, recheck levels as soon as possible. Stop drug if levels remain elevated.

- Rosiglitazone alone or in combination with insulin can cause fluid retention that may lead to or worsen heart failure. Observe patients for these signs or symptoms of heart failure. Stop drug if any deterioration in cardiac status occurs. This drug is not recommended for NYHA Class III or IV cardiac status patients.
- Because ovulation may resume in premenopausal, anovulatory women with insulin resistance, recommend use of contraceptives.
- Management of type 2 diabetes should include diet control. Because caloric restriction, weight loss, and exercise help improve insulin sensitivity and improve effectiveness of drug therapy, these measures are essential to proper diabetes treatment.
- Check glucose and glycosylated hemoglobin levels periodically to monitor therapeutic response to drug.
- Monitor patient with heart failure for increased edema.
- Hemoglobin level and hematocrit may drop during therapy, usually during first 4 to 8 weeks. Increases in total cholesterol, low-density lipoprotein, and high-density lipoprotein levels and decreases in free fatty acid level also may occur.
- For patients inadequately controlled with a maximum dose of a sulfonylurea or metformin, add rosiglitazone to, rather than substitute it for, a sulfonylurea or metformin.

!!ALERT Don't confuse rosiglitazone with pioglitazone.

Patient teaching

- Advise patient that drug can be taken with or without food.
- Notify patient that blood will be tested to check liver function before therapy starts, every 2 months for first 12 months, and then periodically thereafter.
- Tell patient to immediately notify prescriber about unexplained signs and symptoms, such as nausea, vomiting, abdominal pain, fatigue, anorexia, or dark urine; these may indicate liver problems.
- Warn patient to contact his health care provider about signs or symptoms of heart failure (unusually rapid increase in weight or swelling, shortness of breath).
- Recommend use of contraceptives to premenopausal, anovulatory women with insulin resistance because ovulation may resume with therapy.
- Advise patient that management of diabetes should include diet control. Because caloric restriction, weight loss, and exercise help improve insulin sensitivity and improve effectiveness of drug therapy, these measures are essential to proper diabetes treatment.
- Instruct patient to monitor glucose level carefully and tell him what to do when he's ill, undergoing surgery, or under added stress.

rosiglitazone maleate and metformin hydrochloride
Avandamet

Pregnancy risk category C

Indications & dosages

➲ **Adjunct to diet and exercise in patients with type 2 diabetes already treated with rosiglitazone and metformin or in patients who are inadequately controlled on metformin or rosiglitazone alone**

Adults: Dosage is based on patient's current doses of rosiglitazone or metformin (or both), individualized on the basis of efficacy and tolerability, and given in two divided doses with meals.

For patients inadequately controlled on metformin alone, give 2 mg rosiglitazone P.O. b.i.d., plus the dose of metformin already being taken (500 mg or 1,000 mg P.O. b.i.d.). Dosage increases may occur after 8 to 12 weeks.

For patients inadequately controlled on rosiglitazone alone, give 500 mg metformin P.O. b.i.d., plus the dose of rosiglitazone already being taken (2 mg or 4 mg P.O. b.i.d.). Dosage increases may occur after 1 to 2 weeks.

The total daily dose of Avandamet may be increased in increments of 4 mg rosigli-

tazone or 500 mg metformin, or both, up to the maximum daily dose of 8 mg/2,000 mg in two divided doses.
Elderly patients: Initial and maintenance doses should be conservative because kidney function may be reduced in this population. Don't give maximum dose.

For malnourished and debilitated patients, don't give maximum dose.

Contraindications & cautions

- Contraindicated in patients hypersensitive to rosiglitazone or metformin and in those with renal disease or renal dysfunction (abnormal creatinine clearance, or creatinine level 1.5 mg/dl or greater in men or 1.4 mg/dl or greater in women); heart failure requiring drug therapy; type 1 diabetes; acute or chronic metabolic acidosis, including diabetic ketoacidosis, with or without coma; clinical evidence of active liver disease or increased transaminase level (ALT more than 2.5 times the upper limit of normal).
- Contraindicated in pregnant and breast-feeding patients.
- Contraindicated if combined with insulin.
- Use cautiously in patients with edema or at high risk for heart failure.

Adverse reactions

CNS: headache, fatigue.
CV: edema.
EENT: sinusitis.
GI: *diarrhea.*
Hematologic: anemia.
Metabolic: hyperglycemia, ***hypoglycemia***.
Musculoskeletal: back pain, arthralgia.
Respiratory: *upper respiratory tract infection.*
Other: accidental injury, viral infection.

Interactions

Drug-drug. *Calcium channel blocking drugs, corticosteroids, estrogens, hormonal contraceptives, isoniazid, nicotinic acid, phenytoin, phenothiazines, sympathomimetics, thiazides, thyroid products:* May affect glycemic control. Monitor glucose level; may need to adjust dosage.
Cationic drugs (amiloride, digoxin, morphine, procainamide, quinidine, quinine, ranitidine, triamterene, trimethoprim, vancomycin): May decrease metformin excretion. Monitor glucose level; may need to adjust cationic drugs or metformin.
Furosemide: May increase metformin level and decrease furosemide level. Monitor patient closely.
Nifedipine: May increase absorption of metformin. Monitor patient closely.
Drug-herb. *Guar gum:* May decrease hypoglycemic effect. Monitor glucose level.
Drug-lifestyle. *Alcohol use:* May increase effect of metformin on lactate metabolism and increase risk of lactic acidosis. Discourage use together.

Nursing considerations

- Because aging often causes reduced renal function, use drug with caution in elderly patients. Make dose selection carefully and monitor renal function regularly. Don't give elderly patients the maximum daily dose. Don't start treatment in patients older than age 80 unless renal function is normal.
- In patients undergoing radiologic studies involving contrast media containing iodine, stop drug before or during the procedure and withhold for 48 hours after the procedure. Resume treatment only after renal function has been reevaluated and documented to be normal.
- Stop drug temporarily in patients having surgery. Don't restart until oral intake has resumed and renal function is normal.
- Monitor transaminase level at baseline, every 2 months for the first 12 months, and periodically thereafter. If ALT level increases to more than 3 times the upper limit of normal, recheck liver enzymes as soon as possible. If ALT remains more than 3 times the upper limit of normal, stop drug.
- Monitor CBC and vitamin B_{12} level.
- Watch for signs and symptoms of heart failure and hepatic dysfunction. Stop drug use if jaundice occurs.
- Monitor renal function at baseline and at least annually during therapy.
- Monitor glycosylated hemoglobin level every 3 months.
- Stop drug if shock, acute heart failure, acute MI, or other conditions linked to hypoxemia occur.

Patient teaching

- Stress the importance of dietary instructions, weight loss, and a regular exercise program.

- Tell patient to immediately report unexplained hyperventilation, myalgia, malaise, or unusual somnolence.
- Instruct patient to report a rapid increase in weight, swelling, shortness of breath, or other symptoms of heart failure.
- Tell patient to report unexplained nausea, vomiting, abdominal pain, fatigue, anorexia, or dark urine.
- Explain that it may take 1 to 2 weeks for drug to take effect and up to 2 to 3 months for the full effect to occur.
- Stress the importance of avoiding excessive alcohol intake.
- Discuss the possible need for contraception with premenopausal women as ovulation may resume.
- Advise patient to take the medication in divided doses with meals to reduce GI side effects.

rosuvastatin calcium

Crestor

Pregnancy risk category X

Indications & dosages

➲ **Adjunct to diet to reduce LDL cholesterol, total cholesterol, apolipoprotein B, non-HDL cholesterol, and triglyceride (TG) levels and to increase HDL cholesterol level in patients with primary hypercholesterolemia (heterozygous familial and nonfamilial) and mixed dyslipidemia (Fredrickson types IIa and IIb); adjunct to diet to treat elevated TG level (Fredrickson type IV)**

Adults: Initially, 10 mg P.O. once daily; 5 mg P.O. once daily in patients needing less-aggressive LDL cholesterol level reduction or those predisposed to myopathy. For aggressive lipid lowering, initially, 20 mg P.O. once daily. Increase p.r.n. to maximum of 40 mg P.O. daily. Dosage may be increased every 2 to 4 weeks, based on lipid levels.

➲ **Adjunct to lipid-lowering therapies; to reduce LDL cholesterol, apolipoprotein B, and total cholesterol levels in homozygous familial hypercholesterolemia**

Adults: Initially, 20 mg P.O. once daily. Maximum, 40 mg once daily.

If creatinine clearance is less than 30 ml/minute, initially, 5 mg once daily; don't exceed 10 mg once daily. For patient's requiring less aggressive treatment, those at risk for myopathy, Asian patients, and patients also taking cyclosporine, initial dose is 5 mg.

Contraindications & cautions

- Contraindicated in patients hypersensitive to rosuvastatin or its components, pregnant patients, patients with active liver disease, and those with unexplained persistently increased transaminases.
- Use cautiously in patients who drink substantial amounts of alcohol or have a history of liver disease and in those at increased risk for myopathies, such as those with renal impairment, advanced age, or hypothyroidism.
- Use cautiously in Asian patients since they have a greater risk of elevated drug levels.

Adverse reactions

CNS: anxiety, asthenia, depression, dizziness, headache, insomnia, neuralgia, paresthesia, vertigo.
CV: angina pectoris, chest pain, hypertension, palpitations, peripheral edema, vasodilation.
EENT: pharyngitis, rhinitis, sinusitis.
GI: abdominal pain, constipation, diarrhea, dyspepsia, flatulence, gastritis, gastroenteritis, nausea, periodontal abscess, vomiting.
GU: UTI.
Hematologic: anemia, ecchymosis.
Metabolic: diabetes mellitus.
Musculoskeletal: arthralgia, arthritis, back pain, hypertonia, myalgia, neck pain, pain, pathological fracture, pelvic pain.
Respiratory: asthma, bronchitis, dyspnea, increased cough, pneumonia.
Skin: pruritus, rash.
Other: accidental injury, flulike syndrome, infection.

Interactions

Drug-drug. *Antacids:* May decrease rosuvastatin level. Give antacids at least 2 hours after rosuvastatin.
Cimetidine, ketoconazole, spironolactone: May decrease level or effect of endogenous steroid hormones. Use together cautiously.
Cyclosporine: May increase rosuvastatin level and risk of myopathy or rhabdomyolysis. Don't exceed 5 mg of rosuvastatin daily. Watch for evidence of toxicity.
Gemfibrozil: May increase rosuvastatin level and risk of myopathy or rhabdomyolysis.

Don't exceed 10 mg of rosuvastatin once daily. Watch for evidence of toxicity.
Hormonal contraceptives: May increase ethinyl estradiol and norgestrel levels. Watch for adverse effects.
Warfarin: May increase INR and risk of bleeding. Monitor INR, and watch for evidence of increased bleeding.
Drug-lifestyle. *Alcohol use:* May increase risk of hepatotoxicity. Discourage use together.

Nursing considerations

- Before therapy starts, assess patient for underlying causes of hypercholesterolemia, including poorly controlled diabetes, hypothyroidism, nephrotic syndrome, dyslipoproteinemias, obstructive liver disease, drug interaction, and alcoholism.
- Before therapy starts, advise patient to control hypercholesterolemia with diet, exercise, and weight reduction.
- Test liver function before therapy starts, 12 weeks afterward, 12 weeks after any increase in dosage, and twice a year routinely. If AST or ALT level persists at more than three times the upper limit of normal, decrease dose or stop drug.

!!ALERT Rarely, rhabdomyolysis with acute renal failure has developed in patients taking drugs in this class, including rosuvastatin.

- Patients who are 65 or older, have hypothyroidism, or have renal insufficiency may be at a greater risk for developing myopathy while receiving a statin.
- Notify prescriber if CK level becomes markedly elevated or myopathy is suspected, or if routine urinalysis shows persistent proteinuria and patient is taking 40 mg daily.
- Withhold drug temporarily if patient becomes predisposed to myopathy or rhabdomyolysis because of sepsis, hypotension, major surgery, trauma, uncontrolled seizures, or severe metabolic, endocrine, or electrolyte disorders.

Patient teaching

- Instruct patient to take drug exactly as prescribed.
- Teach patient about diet, exercise, and weight control.
- Tell patient to immediately report unexplained muscle pain, tenderness, or weakness, especially if accompanied by malaise or fever.
- Instruct patient to take rosuvastatin at least 2 hours before taking antacids containing aluminum or magnesium.

rubella and mumps virus vaccine, live

Biavax II

Pregnancy risk category C

Indications & dosages

➲ **Rubella and mumps immunization**
Adults and children age 1 and older: 0.5 ml S.C.

Contraindications & cautions

- Contraindicated in immunosuppressed patients; in those with cancer, blood dyscrasia, gamma globulin disorders, fever, active untreated tuberculosis, or history of anaphylaxis or anaphylactoid reactions to neomycin or eggs; in those receiving corticosteroid (except those receiving corticosteroids as replacement therapy) or radiation therapy; and in pregnant women.
- Postpone vaccination in patients with acute illness and after giving immune serum globulin, blood, or plasma.
- Allow an interval of at least 3 weeks between BCG and rubella vaccines.

Adverse reactions

CNS: fever, polyneuritis.
GI: diarrhea.
Musculoskeletal: *arthritis, arthralgia.*
Skin: rash, pain, erythema, and induration at injection site, ***thrombocytopenic purpura***, urticaria.
Other: ***anaphylaxis***, lymphadenopathy.

Interactions

Drug-drug. *Immune serum globulin, plasma, whole blood:* Antibodies in serum may interfere with immune response. Don't give vaccine for at least 3 months after use of these products.
Immunosuppressants: May reduce immune response to vaccine. Postpone immunization until immunosuppressant is stopped.

Nursing considerations

- Obtain history of allergies, especially anaphylactic reaction to antibiotics, and reaction to immunization.
- Keep epinephrine 1:1,000 available to treat anaphylaxis.
- If skin test is needed, give it either before or with vaccine.
- Use only diluent supplied. Discard vaccine 8 hours after reconstituting.
- Inject into outer upper arm. Don't inject I.V.
- Document drug manufacturer, lot number, date, and name, address, and title of person giving dose on patient record or log.
- Consider patients born before 1956 to have acquired natural immunity.

Patient teaching

- Inform patient about adverse reactions linked to vaccine.
- Stress importance of avoiding pregnancy for 3 months after vaccination. Provide contraception information, if needed.
- Inform women and girls older than age 12 about risk of self-limited joint pain or arthritis 2 to 4 weeks after vaccination.

rubella virus vaccine, live attenuated (RA 27/3)

Meruvax II

Pregnancy risk category C

Indications & dosages

➲ Rubella immunization

Adults and children age 1 and older: 0.5 ml or 1,000 units S.C.

Contraindications & cautions

- Contraindicated in immunosuppressed patients; in patients with cancer, blood dyscrasia, gamma globulin disorders, fever, or active untreated tuberculosis; in patients hypersensitive to neomycin; in patients receiving corticosteroids (except those receiving corticosteroids as replacement therapy) or radiation therapy; in pregnant women; and in those with AIDS or symptomatic HIV infection.
- Postpone immunization in patients with acute illness and after administration of human immune serum globulin, blood, or plasma.
- Allow at least 3 weeks between BCG and rubella vaccinations.

Adverse reactions

CNS: fever, headache, malaise, polyneuritis.
EENT: sore throat.
Musculoskeletal: arthralgia, arthritis.
Skin: rash, pain, erythema, and induration at injection site, ***thrombocytopenic purpura***, urticaria.
Other: ***anaphylaxis***, lymphadenopathy.

Interactions

Drug-drug. *Immune serum globulin, plasma, whole blood:* Antibodies in serum may interfere with immune response. Don't give vaccine for at least 3 months after use of these products.
Immunosuppressants, interferon: May reduce immune response to vaccine. Postpone vaccine until immunosuppressant is stopped.

Nursing considerations

- Obtain history of allergies and reaction to immunization.
- Keep epinephrine 1:1,000 available to treat anaphylaxis.
- If skin test is needed, give it either before or with vaccine.
- Use only diluent supplied. Discard vaccine 8 hours after reconstituting. Protect from light.
- Inject into outer upper arm. Don't inject vaccine I.V.
- Document drug manufacturer, lot number, date, and name, address, and title of person giving dose on patient record or log.

Patient teaching

- Inform patient about adverse reactions linked to vaccine.
- Stress importance of avoiding pregnancy for 3 months after vaccination. Provide contraception information, if needed.
- Tell patient to use correct dose of fever-reducing drug for treating fever.

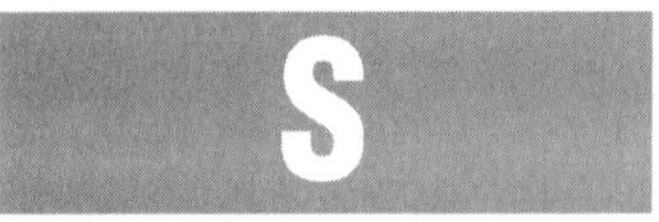

salmeterol xinafoate

Serevent Diskus

Pregnancy risk category C

Indications & dosages

➲ **Long-term maintenance of asthma; to prevent bronchospasm in patients with nocturnal asthma or reversible obstructive airway disease who need regular treatment with short-acting beta agonists**
Adults and children age 4 and older: 1 inhalation (50 mcg) q 12 hours, morning and evening.

➲ **To prevent exercise-induced bronchospasm**
Adults and children age 4 and older: 1 inhalation (50 mcg) at least 30 minutes before exercise. Additional doses shouldn't be taken for at least 12 hours.

➲ **COPD or emphysema**
Adults: 1 inhalation (50 mcg) b.i.d. in the morning and evening, about 12 hours apart.

Contraindications & cautions

- Contraindicated in patients hypersensitive to drug or its ingredients.
- Use cautiously in patients unusually responsive to sympathomimetics and those with coronary insufficiency, arrhythmias, hypertension, other CV disorders, thyrotoxicosis, or seizure disorders.

Adverse reactions

CNS: headache, sinus headache, tremor, nervousness, giddiness, dizziness.
CV: tachycardia, palpitations, ***ventricular arrhythmias***.
EENT: *nasopharyngitis*, pharyngitis, nasal cavity or sinus disorder.
GI: nausea, vomiting, diarrhea, heartburn.
Musculoskeletal: joint and back pain, myalgia.
Respiratory: cough, lower respiratory tract infection, *upper respiratory tract infection*, ***bronchospasm***.
Other: hypersensitivity reactions.

Interactions

Drug-drug. *Beta agonists, other methylxanthines, theophylline:* May cause adverse cardiac effects with excessive use. Monitor patient.
MAO inhibitors: May cause risk of severe adverse CV effects. Avoid use within 14 days of MAO inhibitor therapy.
Tricyclic antidepressants: May cause risk of moderate to severe adverse CV effects. Use together with caution.

Nursing considerations

- Drug isn't indicated for acute bronchospasm.

!!ALERT Monitor patient for rash and urticaria, which may signal a hypersensitivity reaction.

!!ALERT Don't confuse Serevent with Serentil.

Patient teaching

- Remind patient to take drug at about 12-hour intervals for optimum effect and to take drug even when feeling better.
- If patient is taking drug to prevent exercise-induced bronchospasm, tell him to take it 30 to 60 minutes before exercise.

!!ALERT Tell patient that although drug is a beta agonist, it shouldn't be used to treat acute bronchospasm. He must be given a short-acting beta agonist, such as albuterol, to treat worsening symptoms.

!!ALERT Rare serious asthma episodes or asthma-related deaths may occur in patients using salmeterol. Blacks may be at greater risk.

- Tell patient to contact prescriber if the short-acting agonist no longer provides sufficient relief or if he needs more than 4 inhalations daily. This may be a sign that the asthma symptoms are worsening. Tell him not to increase the dosage of salmeterol.
- If patient takes an inhaled corticosteroid, he should continue to use it regularly. Warn patient not to take other drugs without prescriber's consent.
- If patient takes the inhalation powder (in a multidose inhaler), instruct him not to exhale into the device. He should activate and use it only in a level, horizontal position.
- Tell patient not to use the dry-powder multidose inhaler with a spacer.

• Instruct patient never to wash the mouthpiece or any part of the the dry-powder multidose inhaler; it must be kept dry.

saquinavir
Fortovase

saquinavir mesylate
Invirase

Pregnancy risk category B

Indications & dosages

➲ Adjunct treatment of advanced HIV infection in selected patients

Adults: Invirase 1,000 mg (five 200-mg capsules) P.O. b.i.d. given with ritonavir 100 mg P.O. b.i.d; or Fortovase 1,200 mg P.O. t.i.d. Alternatively, 1,000 mg (Fortovase) P.O. b.i.d. given with ritonavir 100 mg P.O. b.i.d. Either formulation is to be taken within 2 hours after a full meal.

Contraindications & cautions

• Contraindicated in patients hypersensitive to drug or its components.
• Safety of drug hasn't been established in pregnant or breast-feeding women or in children younger than age 16. Use cautiously in these patients.

Adverse reactions

CNS: paresthesia, headache, dizziness, asthenia, numbness, depression, insomnia, anxiety.
CV: chest pain.
GI: *diarrhea*, ulcerated buccal mucosa, abdominal pain, *nausea*, dyspepsia, ***pancreatitis***, flatulence, vomiting, altered taste, constipation.
Hematologic: ***pancytopenia***, ***thrombocytopenia***.
Musculoskeletal: musculoskeletal pain.
Respiratory: bronchitis, cough.
Skin: rash.

Interactions

Drug-drug. *Amprenavir:* May decrease amprenavir level. Use together cautiously.
Carbamazepine, phenobarbital, phenytoin: May decrease saquinavir level. Avoid using together.
Delavirdine: May increase saquinavir level. Use cautiously and monitor hepatic enzymes. Decrease dose when used together.
Dexamethasone: May decrease saquinavir level. Avoid using together.
Efavirenz: May decrease levels of both drugs. Avoid using together.
HMG-CoA reductase inhibitors: May increase levels of these drugs, which increases risk of myopathy, including rhabdomyolysis. Avoid using together.
Indinavir, lopinavir and ritonavir combination, nelfinavir, ritonavir: May increase saquinavir level. Use together cautiously.
Ketoconazole: May increase saquinavir level. Don't adjust dosage.
Macrolide antibiotics, such as clarithromycin: May increase levels of both drugs. Use together cautiously.
Nevirapine: May decrease saquinavir level. Monitor patient.
Rifabutin, rifampin: May decrease saquinavir level. Use with rifabutin cautiously. Don't use with rifampin.
Sildenafil: May increase peak level and exposure of sildenafil to the body. Reduce first dose of sildenafil to 25 mg when giving with saquinavir.
Drug-herb. *Garlic supplements:* May decrease saquinavir level by about 50%. Discourage use together.
St. John's wort: May substantially reduce drug level, which could cause loss of therapeutic effects. Discourage use together.
Drug-food. *Any food:* May increase drug absorption. Advise patient to take drug with food.
Grapefruit juice: May increase drug level. Take with liquid other than grapefruit juice.

Nursing considerations

!!ALERT Don't confuse the two forms of this drug because dosages are different.
• Evaluate CBC, platelets, electrolytes, uric acid, liver enzymes, and bilirubin before therapy begins and at appropriate intervals throughout therapy.
• If serious toxicity occurs during treatment, stop drug until cause is identified or toxicity resolves. Drug may be resumed with no dosage modifications.
• Monitor patient's hydration if adverse GI reactions occur.

• Monitor patient for adverse reactions to adjunct therapy (zidovudine or zalcitabine).

Patient teaching

• Advise patient to take drug with food or within 2 hours of a full meal to increase drug absorption.
• Inform patient that drug is usually given with other AIDS-related antivirals.
• Instruct patient to avoid missing any doses, to decrease the risk of developing HIV resistance.
• Inform patient to change from Invirase to Fortovase capsules only under prescriber's supervision.
• Inform patient that drug doesn't cure HIV infection, that opportunistic infections and other complications of HIV infection may continue to occur, and that transmission of HIV to others through sexual contact or blood contamination is still possible.
• Advise patient taking sildenafil about an increased risk of sildenafil-related adverse events, including low blood pressure, visual changes, and painful erections. Tell him to promptly report any symptoms to his prescriber. Tell patient not to exceed 25 mg of sildenafil in a 48-hour period.
• Tell patient to store Fortovase capsules in the refrigerator; Invirase capsules can be kept at room temperature.

sargramostim (GM-CSF; granulocyte macrophage-colony stimulating factor)

Leukine

Pregnancy risk category C

Indications & dosages

➲ Accelerate hematopoietic reconstitution after autologous bone marrow transplantation in patients with malignant lymphoma or acute lymphoblastic leukemia or during autologous bone marrow transplantation in patients with Hodgkin's disease

Adults: 250 mcg/m^2 daily for 21 consecutive days given as 2-hour I.V. infusion beginning 2 to 4 hours after bone marrow transplantation.

➲ Bone marrow transplantation failure or engraftment delay

Adults: 250 mcg/m^2 daily for 14 days as 2-hour I.V. infusion. Dose may be repeated after 7 days of no therapy. If engraftment still hasn't occurred, a third course of 500 mcg/m^2 daily I.V. for 14 days may be attempted after another therapy-free 7 days.

Stimulation of marrow precursors may result in rapid rise of WBC count. If blast cells appear or increase to 10% or more of WBC count or if the underlying disease progresses, stop therapy. If absolute neutrophil count is above 20,000/mm^3 or if platelet count is above 50,000/mm^3, temporarily stop drug or reduce dose by 50%.

Contraindications & cautions

• Contraindicated in patients hypersensitive to drug or its components or to yeast-derived products and in those with excessive leukemic myeloid blasts in bone marrow or peripheral blood.
• Use cautiously in patients with cardiac disease, hypoxia, fluid retention, pulmonary infiltrates, heart failure, or impaired renal or hepatic function because these conditions may be worsened.

Adverse reactions

CNS: *malaise, fever, CNS disorders, asthenia.*
CV: *blood dyscrasias, edema,* ***supraventricular arrhythmias***, pericardial effusion.
GI: *nausea, vomiting, diarrhea, anorexia,* ***hemorrhage***, *GI disorders, stomatitis.*
GU: *urinary tract disorder,* abnormal kidney function.
Hepatic: *liver damage.*
Respiratory: *dyspnea, lung disorders,* pleural effusion.
Skin: *alopecia, rash.*
Other: *mucous membrane disorder, peripheral edema,* SEPSIS.

Interactions

Drug-drug. *Corticosteroids, lithium:* May increase myeloproliferative effects of sargramostim. Use cautiously together.

Nursing considerations

• Anticipate reducing dose by 50% or temporarily stopping drug if severe adverse reactions occur; notify prescriber. Therapy may be resumed when reactions abate.

Transient rash and local reactions at injection site may occur.
- Don't give within 24 hours of last dose of chemotherapy or within 12 hours of last dose of radiotherapy because rapidly dividing progenitor cells may be sensitive to these cytotoxic therapies and drug would be ineffective.
- Monitor CBC with differential, including examination for presence of blast cells, biweekly.
- Drug accelerates myeloid recovery in patients receiving bone marrow that is either unpurged or purged by anti-B cell monoclonal antibodies more than in those who receive bone marrow that is chemically purged.
- Drug may produce a limited response in transplant patients who have received extensive radiotherapy or who have received other myelotoxic drugs.
- Drug can act as a growth factor for any tumor type, particularly myeloid malignant disease.

Patient teaching

- Review administration schedule with patient and caregivers, and address their concerns.
- Urge patient to report adverse reactions promptly.

scopolamine (hyoscine)
Transderm-Scop

scopolamine butylbromide (hyoscine butylbromide)
Buscopan†

scopolamine hydrobromide (systemic) (hyoscine hydrobromide)
Scopolamine Hydrobromide Injection

Pregnancy risk category C

Indications & dosages

➲ Spastic states
Adults: 10 to 20 mg P.O. t.i.d. or q.i.d. or 10 mg P.R. t.i.d. or q.i.d. Adjust dosage, p.r.n. Or, 10 to 20 mg butylbromide S.C., I.M., or I.V., t.i.d. or q.i.d.

➲ Delirium, preanesthetic sedation, and obstetric amnesia with analgesics
Adults: 0.3 to 0.65 mg I.M., S.C., or I.V. Dilute solution with sterile water for injection before giving I.V.
Children: 0.006 mg/kg I.M., S.C., or I.V. Maximum dose, 0.3 mg. Dilute solution with sterile water for injection before giving I.V.

➲ To prevent nausea and vomiting from motion sickness
Adults: One Transderm-Scop, formulated to deliver 1 mg scopolamine over 3 days, applied to the skin behind the ear at least 4 hours before antiemetic is needed. Or, 300 to 600 mcg hydrobromide S.C., I.M., or I.V.
Children: 6 mcg/kg or 200 mcg/m^2 hydrobromide S.C., I.M., or I.V.

Contraindications & cautions

- Contraindicated in patients with angle-closure glaucoma, obstructive uropathy, obstructive disease of the GI tract, asthma, chronic pulmonary disease, myasthenia gravis, paralytic ileus, intestinal atony, unstable CV status in acute hemorrhage, tachycardia from cardiac insufficiency, or toxic megacolon.
- Use cautiously in patients with autonomic neuropathy, hyperthyroidism, coronary artery disease, arrhythmias, heart failure, hypertension, hiatal hernia with reflux esophagitis, hepatic or renal disease, known or suspected GI infection, or ulcerative colitis.
- Use cautiously in children younger than age 6.
- Use cautiously in patients in hot or humid environments; drug can cause heatstroke.

Adverse reactions

CNS: disorientation, restlessness, irritability, dizziness, drowsiness, headache, confusion, hallucinations, delirium, impaired memory.
CV: palpitations, tachycardia, ***paradoxical bradycardia***, flushing.
EENT: dilated pupils, blurred vision, photophobia, increased intraocular pressure, difficulty swallowing.
GI: *constipation, dry mouth, nausea, vomiting, epigastric distress.*

GU: urinary hesitancy, urine retention.
Respiratory: bronchial plugging, depressed respirations.
Skin: rash, dryness, contact dermatitis with transdermal patch.

Interactions

Drug-drug. *Amantadine, antihistamines, antiparkinsonians, disopyramide, glutethimide, meperidine, phenothiazines, procainamide, quinidine, tricyclic antidepressants:* May increase risk of adverse CNS reactions. Avoid using together.
Antacids: May decrease oral absorption of anticholinergics. Separate doses by 2 or 3 hours.
CNS depressants: May increase risk of CNS depression. Monitor patient closely.
Digoxin: May increase digoxin level. Monitor patient for digoxin toxicity.
Ketoconazole: May interfere with ketoconazole absorption. Separate doses by 2 or 3 hours.
Drug-herb. *Jaborandi tree:* May decrease drug effects. Discourage use together.
Pill-bearing spurge: May decrease drug effects. Inform patient of this interaction.
Squaw vine: May decrease metabolic breakdown. Discourage use together.
Drug-lifestyle. *Alcohol use:* May increase risk of CNS depression. Discourage use together.

Nursing considerations

- Raise side rails as a precaution because some patients become temporarily excited or disoriented and some develop amnesia or become drowsy. Reorient patient, as needed.
- Tolerance may develop when therapy is prolonged.
- Atropine-like toxicity may cause dose-related adverse reactions. Individual tolerance varies greatly.

!! ALERT Overdose may cause curarelike effects, such as respiratory paralysis. Keep emergency equipment available.

Patient teaching

- Advise patient to apply patch the night before a planned trip. Transdermal method releases a controlled therapeutic amount of scopolamine. Transderm-Scop is effective if applied 2 or 3 hours before experiencing motion but is more effective if applied 12 hours before.
- Instruct patient to wash and dry hands thoroughly before and after applying the transdermal patch (on dry skin behind the ear) and before touching the eye, because pupil may dilate. Tell patient to discard patch after removing it and to wash application site thoroughly.
- Tell patient that if patch becomes displaced, he should remove it and apply another patch on a fresh skin site behind the ear.
- Alert patient to possible withdrawal signs or symptoms (nausea, vomiting, headache, dizziness) when transdermal system is used for longer than 72 hours.
- Advise patient that eyes may be more sensitive to light while wearing patch.
- Warn patient to avoid activities that require alertness until CNS effects of drug are known.
- Instruct patient to ask pharmacist for brochure that comes with the transdermal product.
- Urge patient to report urinary hesitancy or urine retention.

scopolamine hydrobromide (ophthalmic)

Isopto Hyoscine

Pregnancy risk category NR

Indications & dosages

➲ Cycloplegic refraction
Adults: Instill 1 or 2 drops of 0.25% solution 1 hour before refraction.
Children: Instill 1 drop of 0.25% solution b.i.d. for 2 days before refraction.
➲ Iritis, uveitis
Adults: Instill 1 or 2 drops of 0.25% solution once daily to q.i.d.
Children: Instill 1 drop of 0.25% solution once daily to q.i.d.

Contraindications & cautions

- Contraindicated in patients hypersensitive to drug and in those with shallow anterior chamber, angle-closure glaucoma, or adhesions between the iris and lens.
- Contraindicated in children with previous severe systemic reaction to atropine.

• Use cautiously in patients with cardiac disease and in infants, small children, and elderly patients.

Adverse reactions

CNS: acute psychotic reactions, confusion, delirium, somnolence, headache, hallucinations.
CV: tachycardia, edema.
EENT: ocular congestion with prolonged use, conjunctivitis, *blurred vision*, eye dryness, increased intraocular pressure, *photophobia*, transient stinging and burning.
GI: dry mouth.
Skin: dryness, contact dermatitis.

Interactions

Drug-lifestyle. *Sun exposure:* May cause photophobia. Advise patient to wear sunglasses.

Nursing considerations

• Observe patients closely for adverse CNS effects such as disorientation and delirium.
• Drug may be used in patients sensitive to atropine because it's faster acting and has a shorter duration of action and fewer adverse reactions.

Patient teaching

• Teach patient how to instill drug. Advise him to wash hands before and after instillation and to apply light finger pressure on lacrimal sac for 1 minute after drops are instilled. Warn him to avoid touching tip of dropper to eye or surrounding tissue.
• Warn patient to avoid hazardous activities, such as operating machinery or driving, until temporary blurring subsides.
• Advise patient to ease sun sensitivity by wearing dark glasses.
• Instruct patient to wear or carry medical identification at all times during therapy.

secobarbital sodium
Seconal Sodium

Pregnancy risk category D
Controlled substance schedule II

Indications & dosages

➲ Preoperative sedation
Adults: 200 to 300 mg P.O. 1 to 2 hours before surgery.
Children: 2 to 6 mg/kg P.O. 1 to 2 hours before surgery. Maximum single dose is 100 mg P.O.
➲ Insomnia
Adults: 100 mg P.O. h.s.

In debilitated, elderly, and patients with renal or hepatic impairment, consider reducing dose.

Contraindications & cautions

• Contraindicated in patients hypersensitive to barbiturates and in those with marked liver or renal impairment, respiratory disease in which dyspnea or obstruction is evident, or porphyria.
• Use cautiously in elderly or debilitated patients and in patients with acute or chronic pain, depression, suicidal tendencies, history of drug abuse, or hepatic or renal impairment.

Adverse reactions

CNS: *drowsiness, lethargy, hangover*, paradoxical anxiety, somnolence.
GI: nausea, vomiting.
Hematologic: worsening of porphyria.
Respiratory: ***respiratory depression***.
Skin: rash, urticaria, ***Stevens-Johnson syndrome***, tissue reactions.
Other: ***angioedema***, physical and psychological dependence.

Interactions

Drug-drug. *Chloramphenicol, MAO inhibitors, valproic acid:* May inhibit metabolism of barbiturates; may cause prolonged CNS depression. Reduce barbiturate dosage.
CNS depressants, including opioid analgesics: May cause excessive CNS and respiratory depression. Use together cautiously.
Corticosteroids, digitoxin, doxycycline, estrogens and hormonal contraceptives, oral anticoagulants, theophylline, tricyclic antidepressants, verapamil: May enhance metabolism of these drugs. Watch for decreased effect.
Griseofulvin: May decrease absorption of griseofulvin. Monitor effectiveness of griseofulvin.
Metoprolol, propranolol: May reduce the effects of these drugs. May need to increase beta-blocker dose.
Rifampin: May decrease barbiturate level. Watch for decreased effect.

Drug-lifestyle. *Alcohol use:* May impair coordination, increase CNS effects, and cause death. Strongly discourage alcohol use with these drugs.

Nursing considerations

- Assess mental status before starting therapy and reduce doses in elderly patients; these patients may be more sensitive to drug's adverse CNS effects. Also watch for paradoxical excitement in this population.
- Take precautions to prevent hoarding or overdosing by patients who are depressed, suicidal, or drug-dependent or who have history of drug abuse.
- Watch for signs of barbiturate toxicity: coma, pupillary constriction, cyanosis, clammy skin, and hypotension. Overdose can be fatal.
- Inspect patient's skin. Skin eruptions may precede potentially fatal reactions to barbiturate therapy. Stop drug when skin reactions occur and notify prescriber. In some patients, high temperature, stomatitis, headache, or rhinitis may precede skin reactions.
- Long-term use isn't recommended; drug loses its effect of promoting sleep after 14 days of continued use.
- Drug changes EEG patterns, altering low-voltage fast activity; changes persist for a time after stopping therapy.

Patient teaching

- Tell patient that morning hangover is common after hypnotic dose, which suppresses REM sleep. Patient may experience increased dreaming after drug is stopped.
- Advise patient to avoid alcohol use while taking drug.
- Caution patient to avoid performing activities that require mental alertness or physical coordination.
- Tell patient using hormonal contraceptives to consider a different birth control method.

selegiline hydrochloride (L-deprenyl hydrochloride)

Carbex, Eldepryl

Pregnancy risk category C

Indications & dosages

➲ Adjunctive treatment with levodopa and carbidopa in managing signs and symptoms of Parkinson's disease
Adults: 10 mg P.O. daily, 5 mg at breakfast and 5 mg at lunch. After 2 or 3 days, gradual decrease of levodopa and carbidopa dosage may be needed.

Contraindications & cautions

- Contraindicated in patients hypersensitive to drug and in those receiving meperidine.

Adverse reactions

CNS: *dizziness*, increased tremor, chorea, loss of balance, restlessness, increased bradykinesia, facial grimacing, stiff neck, dyskinesia, involuntary movements, twitching, increased apraxia, behavioral changes, fatigue, headache, confusion, hallucinations, vivid dreams, anxiety, insomnia, lethargy, malaise, syncope.
CV: orthostatic hypotension, hypertension, hypotension, ***arrhythmias***, palpitations, new or increased angina, tachycardia, peripheral edema.
EENT: blepharospasm.
GI: dry mouth, *nausea*, vomiting, constipation, abdominal pain, anorexia or poor appetite, dysphagia, diarrhea, heartburn.
GU: slow urination, transient nocturia, prostatic hyperplasia, urinary hesitancy, urinary frequency, urine retention, sexual dysfunction.
Metabolic: weight loss.
Skin: rash, hair loss, diaphoresis.

Interactions

Drug-drug. *Citalopram, fluoxetine, fluvoxamine, nefazodone, paroxetine, sertraline, venlafaxine:* May cause serotonin syndrome (CNS irritability, shivering, and altered consciousness). Separate dosages by at least 2 weeks.
MAO inhibitors: May cause hypertensive crisis. Avoid using together.

Meperidine: May cause stupor, muscle rigidity, severe agitation, and fever. Avoid using together.
Sympathomimetics: May cause increased pressor response, particularly in patients who have taken an overdose of selegiline. Use together cautiously.
Tricyclic antidepressants: May cause mental status change. Avoid using together.
Drug-herb. *Cacao:* May cause vasopressor effects. Discourage use together.
Ginseng: May cause headache, tremors, or mania. Discourage use together.
Drug-food. *Foods high in tyramine:* May cause hypertensive crisis. Monitor blood pressure.

Nursing considerations

!!ALERT Some patients experience increased adverse reactions to levodopa when it's used with selegiline and need a 10% to 30% reduction of levodopa and carbidopa dosage.
!!ALERT Don't confuse selegiline with Stelazine or Eldepryl with enalapril.
!!ALERT Severe adverse reactions may occur if used with antidepressants.

Patient teaching

- Warn patient to move cautiously at start of therapy because he may become dizzy.
- Advise patient not to take more than 10 mg daily. A larger amount may increase adverse reactions.

sertaconazole nitrate
Ertaczo

Pregnancy risk category C

Indications & dosages

Interdigital tinea pedis caused by *Trichophyton rubrum, Trichophyton mentagrophytes,* or *Epidermophyton floccosum* in immunocompetent patients
Adults and children age 12 and older: Apply cream twice daily to affected areas between toes and healthy surrounding areas for 4 weeks.

Contraindications & cautions

- Contraindicated in patients hypersensitive to drug, its components, or other imidazoles.
- Use cautiously in pregnant or breast-feeding women.

Adverse reactions

Skin: application site reaction, contact dermatitis, dryness, burning, tenderness.

Interactions

None known.

Nursing considerations

- Before treatment starts, diagnosis should be confirmed by direct microscopic examination of infected tissue in potassium hydroxide solution or by culture on an appropriate medium.
- Drug is for use only on skin and not for ophthalmic, oral, or intravaginal use.
- If condition hasn't improved after 2 weeks, review diagnosis.
- Stop drug if skin irritation or sensitivity develops.

Patient teaching

- Warn patient to stop using drug if he develops increased irritation, redness, itching, burning, blistering, swelling, or oozing at the site of application.
- Caution patient that drug is for external use on skin only. Discourage contact with eyes, nose, mouth, and other mucous membranes.
- If cream is to be applied after bathing, tell patient to dry affected area thoroughly before application.
- Tell patient to wash hands after applying cream.
- Urge patient to use drug for full duration of treatment, even if symptoms have improved.
- Instruct patient to notify prescriber if condition worsens or fails to improve.
- Caution patient to avoid occlusive coverings unless directed by prescriber.
- Teach patient proper foot hygiene.

sertraline hydrochloride
Zoloft

Pregnancy risk category C

Indications & dosages

➲ Depression
Adults: 50 mg P.O. daily. Adjust dosage as needed and tolerated; dosages range from 50 to 200 mg daily.

➲ Obsessive-compulsive disorder
Adults: 50 mg P.O. once daily. If patient doesn't improve, increase dosage, up to 200 mg daily.
Children ages 6 to 17: Initially, 25 mg P.O. daily in children ages 6 to 12, or 50 mg P.O. daily in children ages 13 to 17. May increase dosage, p.r.n., up to 200 mg daily at intervals of no less than 1 week.

➲ Panic disorder
Adults: Initially, 25 mg P.O. daily. After 1 week, increase dose to 50 mg P.O. daily. If patient doesn't improve, dose may be increased to maximum of 200 mg daily.

➲ Posttraumatic stress disorder
Adults: Initially, 25 mg P.O. once daily. Increase dosage to 50 mg P.O. once daily after 1 week. Dosage may be increased at weekly intervals to a maximum of 200 mg daily. Maintain patient on lowest effective dose.

➲ Premenstrual dysphoric disorder
Adults: Initially, 50 mg daily P.O. either continuously or only during the luteal phase of the menstrual cycle. If patient doesn't respond, dose may be increased 50 mg per menstrual cycle, up to 150 mg daily for use throughout the menstrual cycle or 100 mg daily for luteal-phase doses. If a 100-mg daily dose has been established with luteal-phase dosing, use a 50-mg daily adjustment for 3 days at the beginning of each luteal phase.

➲ Social anxiety disorder
Adults: Initially, 25 mg P.O. once daily. Increase dosage to 50 mg P.O. once daily after 1 week of therapy. Usual dosage range is 50 to 200 mg daily. Adjust to the lowest effective dosage and periodically reassess patient to determine the need for long-term treatment.

➲ Premature ejaculation♦
Adults: 25 to 50 mg P.O. daily or p.r.n.

For patients with hepatic disease, use lower or less-frequent doses.

Contraindications & cautions

- Contraindicated in patients with a hypersensitivity to drug or its components. Contraindicated in patients taking pimozide or MAO inhibitors or within 14 days of MAO inhibitor therapy.
- Use cautiously in patients at risk for suicide and in those with seizure disorders, major affective disorder, or diseases or conditions that affect metabolism or hemodynamic responses.
- Use in third trimester of pregnancy may cause neonatal complications at birth. Consider the risk versus benefit of treatment during this time.

Adverse reactions

CNS: *headache*, ***suicidal behavior***, *tremor*, *dizziness*, *insomnia*, *somnolence*, paresthesia, hypesthesia, *fatigue*, nervousness, anxiety, agitation, hypertonia, twitching, confusion.
CV: palpitations, chest pain, hot flashes.
GI: *dry mouth*, *nausea*, *diarrhea*, *loose stools*, *dyspepsia*, vomiting, constipation, thirst, flatulence, anorexia, abdominal pain, increased appetite.
GU: *male sexual dysfunction.*
Musculoskeletal: myalgia.
Skin: rash, pruritus, diaphoresis.

Interactions

Drug-drug. *Benzodiazepines, tolbutamide:* May decrease clearance of these drugs. Significance unknown; monitor patient for increased drug effects.
Cimetidine: May decrease clearance of sertraline. Monitor patient closely.
Disulfiram: Oral concentrate contains alcohol, which may react with drug. Avoid using together.
MAO inhibitors (phenelzine, selegiline, tranylcypromine): May cause serotonin syndrome. Avoid using within 14 days of MAO inhibitor therapy.
Pimozide: May increase pimozide level. Avoid using together.
Warfarin, other highly protein-bound drugs: May increase level of sertraline or other highly protein-bound drug. May increase PT or INR may increase by 8%. Monitor patient closely.

Drug-herb. *St. John's wort:* May cause additive effects and serotonin syndrome. Discourage use together.

Nursing considerations

- Give sertraline once daily, either in morning or evening, with or without food.
- Make dosage adjustments at intervals of no less than 1 week.
- Record mood changes. Monitor patient for suicidal tendencies and allow only a minimum supply of drug.
- Don't use the oral concentrate dropper, which is made of rubber, in a patient with latex allergy.

Patient teaching

- Advise patient to use caution when performing hazardous tasks that require alertness.
- Tell patient to avoid alcohol and to consult prescriber before taking OTC drugs.
- Advise patient to mix the oral concentrate with 4 ounces (½ cup) of water, ginger ale, lemon or lime soda, lemonade, or orange juice only, and to take the dose right away.
- Instruct patient to avoid stopping the medication abruptly.

sibutramine hydrochloride monohydrate

Meridia

Pregnancy risk category C
Controlled substance schedule IV

Indications & dosages

➲ To manage obesity

Adults: 10 mg P.O. given once daily with or without food. May increase to 15 mg P.O. daily after 4 weeks if weight loss is inadequate. Patients who don't tolerate 10 mg daily may receive 5 mg P.O. daily. Don't exceed 15 mg daily.

Contraindications & cautions

- Contraindicated in patients hypersensitive to drug or its active ingredients, in those taking MAO inhibitors or other centrally acting appetite suppressants, and in those with anorexia nervosa.
- Contraindicated in patients with severe renal or hepatic dysfunction, history of hypertension, coronary artery disease, heart failure, arrhythmias, or CVA.
- Contraindicated in elderly patients.
- Use cautiously in patients with history of seizures or angle-closure glaucoma.

Adverse reactions

CNS: *headache, insomnia,* dizziness, nervousness, anxiety, depression, paresthesia, somnolence, CNS stimulation, emotional lability, asthenia, migraine.
CV: tachycardia, vasodilation, hypertension, palpitations, chest pain.
EENT: *rhinitis, pharyngitis,* sinusitis, ear disorder, ear pain.
GI: thirst, *anorexia, constipation,* increased appetite, nausea, dyspepsia, gastritis, vomiting, *dry mouth,* taste perversion, abdominal pain, rectal disorder.
GU: dysmenorrhea, UTI, vaginal candidiasis, metrorrhagia.
Musculoskeletal: arthralgia, myalgia, tenosynovitis, joint disorder, neck or back pain.
Respiratory: increased cough, laryngitis.
Skin: rash, sweating, acne.
Other: herpes simplex, flulike syndrome, accidental injury, allergic reaction, generalized edema.

Interactions

Drug-drug. *CNS depressants:* May enhance CNS depression. Use together cautiously.
Dextromethorphan, dihydroergotamine, fentanyl, fluoxetine, fluvoxamine, lithium, MAO inhibitors, meperidine, paroxetine, pentazocine, sertraline, sumatriptan, tryptophan, venlafaxine: May cause hyperthermia, tachycardia, and loss of consciousness. Avoid using together.
Ephedrine, pseudoephedrine: May increase blood pressure or heart rate. Use together cautiously.
Drug-lifestyle. *Alcohol use:* May enhance CNS depression. Discourage use together.

Nursing considerations

- Rule out organic causes of obesity before starting therapy.
- Measure blood pressure and pulse before starting therapy, with dosage changes, and at regular intervals during therapy.
- Use drug in obese patients with a body mass index of 30 kg/m² or more (27 kg/m² or more if patient has other risk factors,

such as hypertension, diabetes, or dyslipidemia).
- Avoid using within 2 weeks of MAO inhibitor.

Patient teaching

- Advise patient to report rash, hives, or other allergic reactions immediately.
- Instruct patient to notify prescriber before taking other prescription or OTC drugs.
- Advise patient to have blood pressure and pulse monitored at regular intervals. Stress importance of regular follow-up visits with prescriber.
- Advise patient to follow a reduced calorie diet.
- Tell patient that weight loss can cause gallstones. Teach signs and symptoms, and tell patient to notify prescriber promptly if they occur.

sildenafil citrate
Viagra

Pregnancy risk category B

Indications & dosages

➲ Erectile dysfunction

Adults younger than age 65: 50 mg P.O., p.r.n., about 1 hour before sexual activity. Dosage range is 25 to 100 mg based on effectiveness and tolerance. Maximum is one dose daily.

Elderly patients (age 65 and older): 25 mg P.O., p.r.n., about 1 hour before sexual activity. Dosage may be adjusted based on patient response. Maximum is one dose daily.

For adults with hepatic or severe renal impairment, 25 mg P.O. about 1 hour before sexual activity. Dosage may be adjusted based on patient response. Maximum is one dose daily.

Contraindications & cautions

- Contraindicated in patients hypersensitive to drug or its components and in those taking organic nitrates.
- Use cautiously in patients age 65 and older; in patients with hepatic or severe renal impairment, retinitis pigmentosa, bleeding disorders, or active peptic ulcer disease; in those who have suffered an MI, a CVA, or life-threatening arrhythmia within last 6 months; in those with history of cardiac failure, coronary artery disease, uncontrolled high or low blood pressure, or anatomic deformation of the penis (such as angulation, cavernosal fibrosis, or Peyronie's disease); and in those with conditions that may predispose them to priapism (such as sickle cell anemia, multiple myeloma, or leukemia).

Adverse reactions

CNS: anxiety, *headache*, dizziness, ***seizures***, somnolence, vertigo.
CV: ***MI, sudden cardiac death, ventricular arrhythmias, cerebrovascular hemorrhage, transient ischemic attack***, hypotension, flushing.
EENT: diplopia, temporary vision loss, ocular redness or bloodshot appearance, increased intraocular pressure, retinal vascular disease, retinal bleeding, vitreous detachment or traction, paramacular edema, photophobia, altered color perception, blurred vision, burning, swelling, pressure, nasal congestion.
GI: *dyspepsia*, diarrhea.
GU: hematuria, prolonged erection, priapism, UTI.
Musculoskeletal: arthralgia, back pain.
Respiratory: respiratory tract infection.
Skin: rash.
Other: flulike syndrome.

Interactions

Drug-drug. *Beta blockers, loop and potassium-sparing diuretics:* May increase sildenafil metabolite level. Monitor patient.
Cytochrome P-450 inducers, rifampin: May reduce sildenafil level. Monitor effect.
Delavirdine, protease inhibitors: May increase sildenafil level, increasing risk of adverse events, including hypotension, visual changes, and priapism. Reduce initial sildenafil dose to 25 mg.
Hepatic isoenzyme inhibitors (such as cimetidine, erythromycin, itraconazole, ketoconazole): May reduce sildenafil clearance. Avoid using together.
Isosorbide, nitroglycerin: May cause severe hypotension. Use of nitrates in any form with sildenafil is contraindicated.
Drug-food. *High-fat meal:* May reduce absorption rate and peak level of drug. Advise patient to take drug on empty stomach.

Grapefruit: May increase drug level, while delaying absorption. Advise patient to avoid using together.

Nursing considerations

!!ALERT Drug increases risk of cardiac events. Systemic vasodilatory properties cause transient decreases in supine blood pressure and cardiac output (about 2 hours after ingestion). Patients with underlying CV disease are at increased risk for cardiac effects related to sexual activity.

!!ALERT Serious CV events, including MI, sudden cardiac death, ventricular arrhythmias, cerebrovascular hemorrhage, transient ischemic attack, and hypertension, have been reported with drug use. Most, but not all, of these incidents involved CV risk factors. Many events occurred during or shortly after sexual activity; a few occurred shortly after drug use without sexual activity; and others occurred hours to days after drug use and sexual activity.

- Drug isn't indicated for use in newborns, children, or women.

Patient teaching

- Advise patient that drug shouldn't be used with nitrates under any circumstances.
- Advise patient of potential cardiac risk of sexual activity, especially in presence of CV risk factors. Instruct patient to notify prescriber and refrain from further activity if such symptoms as chest pain, dizziness, or nausea occur when starting sexual activity.
- Warn patient that erections lasting longer than 4 hours and priapism (painful erections lasting longer than 6 hours) can occur, and tell him to seek immediate medical attention. Penile tissue damage and permanent loss of potency may result if priapism isn't treated immediately.
- Inform patient that drug doesn't protect against sexually transmitted diseases; advise patient to use protective measures such as condoms.
- Tell patient receiving HIV medications that he's at increased risk for sildenafil adverse events, including low blood pressure, visual changes, and priapism, and that he should promptly report such symptoms to his prescriber. Tell him not to exceed 25 mg of sildenafil in 48 hours.
- Instruct patient to take drug 30 minutes to 4 hours before sexual activity; maximum benefit can be expected less than 2 hours after ingestion.
- Advise patient that drug is most rapidly absorbed if taken on an empty stomach.
- Inform patient that impairment of color discrimination (blue, green) may occur and to avoid hazardous activities that rely on color discrimination.
- Instruct patient to notify prescriber of visual changes.
- Advise patient that drug is effective only in presence of sexual stimulation.
- Caution patient to take drug only as prescribed.

sildenafil citrate
Revatio

Pregnancy risk category B

Indications & dosages

➲ **To improve exercise ability in patients with World Health Organization group I pulmonary arterial hypertension**
Adults: 20 mg P.O. t.i.d., 4 to 6 hours apart.

Contraindications & cautions

- Contraindicated in patients hypersensitive to drug or its components and in those taking organic nitrates.
- Don't use in patients with pulmonary veno-occlusive disease.
- Use cautiously in patients with resting hypotension, severe left ventricular outflow obstruction, autonomic dysfunction, and volume depletion.
- Use cautiously in elderly patients; in patients with hepatic or severe renal impairment, retinitis pigmentosa, bleeding disorders, or active peptic ulcer disease; in those who have suffered an MI, stroke, or life-threatening arrhythmia in last 6 months; in those with history of coronary artery disease causing unstable angina, uncontrolled high or low blood pressure, or deformation of the penis; in those with conditions that may cause priapism (such as sickle cell anemia, multiple myeloma, or leukemia); and in those taking bosentan.

Adverse reactions

CNS: fever, *headache*, dizziness.
CV: hypotension, *flushing*.

EENT: epistaxis; rhinitis; sinusitis; photophobia; impaired color discrimination; blurred vision; burning.
GI: *dyspepsia*, diarrhea, gastritis.
Musculoskeletal: myalgia.
Skin: erythema.

Interactions

Drug-drug. *Alpha blockers:* May cause symptomatic hypotension. Use together cautiously.
Amlodipine: May further reduce blood pressure. Monitor blood pressure closely.
Bosentan: May decrease sildenafil level. Monitor patient.
Cytochrome P-450 inducers, rifampin: May reduce sildenafil level. Monitor effect.
Hepatic isoenzyme inhibitors (such as cimetidine, erythromycin, itraconazole, ketoconazole): May increase sildenafil level. Avoid using together.
Isosorbide, nitroglycerin: May cause severe hypotension. Use of nitrates in any form is contraindicated during therapy.
Protease inhibitors (ritonavir): May significantly increase sildenafil level. Don't use together.
Vitamin K antagonists: May increase risk of bleeding (primarily epistaxis). Monitor patient.
Drug-food. *Grapefruit:* May increase drug level, while delaying absorption. Advise patient to avoid using together.

Nursing considerations

- The serious CV events linked to this drug's use in erectile dysfunction mainly involve patients with underlying CV disease who are at increased risk for cardiac effects related to sexual activity.
- Patients with pulmonary arterial hypertension caused by connective tissue disease are more prone to epistaxis during therapy than those with primary pulmonary hypertension.

!!ALERT Don't substitute Viagra for Revatio because there isn't an equivalent dose.

- It's unknown if drug appears in breast milk. Use cautiously in breast-feeding women.
- Safety and efficacy in children haven't been established.

Patient teaching

- Warn patient that drug should never be used with nitrates.
- Advise patient to rise slowly from lying down.
- Inform patient that drug can be taken with or without food.
- Warn patient that discrimination between colors, such as blue and green, may become impaired during therapy; warn him to avoid hazardous activities that rely on color discrimination.
- Instruct patient to notify prescriber of visual changes, dizziness, or fainting.
- Caution patient to take drug only as prescribed.

silver sulfadiazine

Flamazine†, Silvadene, SSD, SSD AF, Thermazene

Pregnancy risk category B

Indications & dosages

➲ To prevent or treat wound infection in second- and third-degree burns
Adults: Apply ¼ -inch ribbon of cream to clean, debrided wound daily or b.i.d.

Contraindications & cautions

- Contraindicated in patients hypersensitive to drug and in those with G6PD deficiency.
- Contraindicated in pregnant women at or near term and in premature or full-term neonates during first 2 months after birth. Drug may increase possibility of kernicterus.

!!ALERT Use cautiously in patients hypersensitive to sulfonamides.

Adverse reactions

Hematologic: ***leukopenia***.
Metabolic: altered serum osmolality.
Skin: pain, burning, rash, pruritus, skin necrosis, ***erythema multiforme***, skin discoloration.

Interactions

Drug-drug. *Topical proteolytic enzymes:* May inactivate enzymes. Avoid using together.
Drug-lifestyle. *Sun exposure:* May cause photosensitivity. Advise patient to avoid excessive sun exposure.

Nursing considerations

- Use sterile application technique to prevent wound contamination.
- Use drug only on affected areas. Keep these areas medicated at all times.
- Bathe patient daily, if possible.
- Inspect patient's skin daily, and note any changes. Notify prescriber if burning or excessive pain develops.
- Monitor sulfadiazine levels and renal function, and check urine for sulfa crystals in patients with extensive burns.
- Tell prescriber if hepatic or renal dysfunction occurs; drug may need to be stopped.
- Leukopenia usually resolves without intervention and doesn't always require stopping drug.
- Absorption of propylene glycol (contained in the cream) can interfere with serum osmolality.
- Discard darkened cream because drug is ineffective.

Patient teaching

- Instruct patient to promptly report adverse reactions, especially burning or excessive pain with application.
- Inform patient of need for frequent blood and urine tests to watch for adverse effects.
- Tell patient that he may develop sensitivity to the sun.
- Tell patient to continue treatment until satisfactory healing occurs or until site is ready for grafting.

simvastatin (synvinolin)

Zocor

Pregnancy risk category X

Indications & dosages

➲ To reduce risk of death from CV disease and CV events in patients at high-risk for coronary events

Adults: Initially, 20 mg P.O. daily in evening. Adjust dosage every 4 weeks based on patient tolerance and response. Maximum, 80 mg daily.

➲ To reduce total and LDL cholesterol levels in patients with homozygous familial hypercholesterolemia

Adults: 40 mg daily in evening; or, 80 mg daily in three divided doses of 20 mg in morning, 20 mg in afternoon, and 40 mg in evening.

➲ Heterozygous familial hypercholesterolemia

Children ages 10 to 17: 10 mg P.O. once daily in the evening. Maximum, 40 mg daily.

For patients taking cyclosporine, begin with 5 mg P.O. simvastatin daily; don't exceed 10 mg P.O. simvastatin daily. In patients taking fibrates or niacin, maximum is 10 mg P.O. simvastatin daily. In patients taking amiodarone or verapamil, maximum is 20 mg P.O. simvastatin daily. In patients with severe renal insufficiency, start with 5 mg P.O. daily.

Contraindications & cautions

- Contraindicated in patients hypersensitive to drug and in those with active liver disease or conditions that cause unexplained persistent elevations of transaminase levels.
- Contraindicated in pregnant and breast-feeding women and in women of childbearing age.
- Use cautiously in patients who consume substantial quantities of alcohol or have a history of liver disease.

Adverse reactions

CNS: headache, asthenia.
GI: abdominal pain, constipation, diarrhea, dyspepsia, flatulence, *nausea, vomiting.*
Respiratory: upper respiratory tract infection.

Interactions

Drug-drug. *Amiodarone, verapamil:* May increase risk of myopathy and rhabdomyolysis. Don't exceed 20 mg simvastatin daily.
Clarithromycin, erythromycin, HIV protease inhibitors, nefazodone: May increase risk of myopathy and rhabdomyolysis. Avoid using together, or suspend therapy during treatment with clarithromycin or erythromycin.
Cyclosporine, fibrates, niacin: May increase risk of myopathy and rhabdomyolysis. Avoid using together; if unavoidable, monitor patient closely and don't exceed 10 mg simvastatin daily.
Digoxin: May slightly increase digoxin level. Closely monitor digoxin levels at the start of simvastatin therapy.

Fluconazole, itraconazole, ketoconazole: May increase simvastatin level and adverse effects. Avoid using together, or, if combination can't be avoided, reduce dose of simvastatin.
Hepatotoxic drugs: May increase risk for hepatotoxicity. Avoid using together.
Warfarin: May slightly enhance anticoagulant effect. Monitor PT and INR when therapy starts or dose is adjusted.
Drug-herb. *Eucalyptus, jin bu huan, kava:* May increase risk of hepatotoxicity. Discourage use together.
Red yeast rice: May increase risk of adverse events or toxicity because it contains similar components to those of statin drugs. Discourage use together.
Drug-food. *Grapefruit juice:* May increase drug levels, increasing risk of adverse effects including myopathy and rhabdomyolysis. Discourage use together.
Drug-lifestyle. *Alcohol use:* May increase risk of hepatotoxicity. Discourage use together.

Nursing considerations

- Use drug only after diet and other nondrug therapies prove ineffective. Patient should follow a standard low-cholesterol diet during therapy.
- Obtain liver function test results at start of therapy and then periodically. A liver biopsy may be performed if enzyme elevations persist.
- Simvastatin 40 mg daily significantly reduces risk of death from coronary heart disease, nonfatal MIs, CVA, and revascularization procedures.

!!ALERT Don't confuse Zocor with Cozaar.

Patient teaching

- Instruct patient to take drug with the evening meal because taking this enhances absorption and increases cholesterol biosynthesis.
- Teach patient about proper dietary management of cholesterol and triglycerides. When appropriate, recommend weight control, exercise, and smoking cessation programs.
- Tell patient to inform prescriber if adverse reactions occur, particularly muscle aches and pains.

!!ALERT Tell woman to stop drug and notify prescriber immediately if she is or may be pregnant or if she's breast-feeding.

sirolimus
Rapamune

Pregnancy risk category C

Indications & dosages

➲ To prevent organ rejection in patients receiving renal transplants with cyclosporine and corticosteroids
Adults and adolescents: Initially, 6 mg P.O. as one-time dose as soon as possible after transplantation; then maintenance dose of 2 mg P.O. once daily.
Children age 13 and older weighing less than 40 kg (88 lb): First dose is 3 mg/m^2 P.O. as one-time dose after transplantation; then 1 mg/m^2 P.O. once daily.

For patients with mild to moderate hepatic impairment, reduce maintenance dose by about one-third. It isn't necessary to reduce loading dose. Two to 4 months after transplantation in patients with low-to-moderate risk of graft rejection, taper off cyclosporine over 4 to 8 weeks. During the taper, adjust sirolimus dose q 1 to 2 weeks to obtain blood levels between 12 and 24 ng/ml. Base dosage adjustments on clinical status, tissue biopsies, and laboratory findings.

Maximum daily dose shouldn't exceed 40 mg. If a daily dose exceeds 40 mg due to a loading dose, give the loading dose over 2 days. Monitor trough concentrations at least 3 to 4 days after a loading dose.

Contraindications & cautions

- Contraindicated in patients hypersensitive to active drug, its derivatives, or components of product.
- Use cautiously in patients with hyperlipidemia and impaired liver or renal function.
- Safety and effectiveness of sirolimus as immunosuppressive therapy haven't been established in liver or lung transplant patients and such use isn't recommended.

Adverse reactions

CNS: *headache, insomnia, tremor, anxiety, depression, asthenia,* malaise, *fever,* syncope, confusion, dizziness, emotional labil-

ity, hypertonia, hypesthesia, hypotonia, neuropathy, paresthesia, somnolence.
CV: *hypertension*, ***heart failure***, ***atrial fibrillation***, tachycardia, hypotension, *chest pain*, *edema*, ***hemorrhage***, palpitations, peripheral vascular disorder, thrombophlebitis, thrombosis, vasodilatation, *peripheral edema*.
EENT: facial edema, *pharyngitis*, epistaxis, rhinitis, sinusitis, abnormal vision, cataract, conjunctivitis, deafness, ear pain, otitis media, tinnitus.
GI: *diarrhea*, *nausea*, *vomiting*, *constipation*, *abdominal pain*, *dyspepsia*, hernia, enlarged abdomen, ascites, peritonitis, anorexia, dysphagia, eructation, esophagitis, flatulence, gastritis, gastroenteritis, gingivitis, gum hyperplasia, ileus, mouth ulceration, oral candidiasis, stomatitis.
GU: dysuria, hematuria, albuminuria, ***kidney tubular necrosis***, *UTI*, pelvic pain, glycosuria, bladder pain, hydronephrosis, impotence, kidney pain, nocturia, oliguria, pyuria, scrotal edema, testis disorder, ***toxic nephropathy***, urinary frequency, urinary incontinence, urine retention.
Hematologic: *anemia*, **THROMBOCYTOPENIA**, ***leukopenia***, ***thrombotic thrombocytopenia purpura***, ecchymosis, leukocytosis, polycythemia.
Hepatic: ***hepatotoxicity***, ***hepatic artery thrombosis***.
Metabolic: *hypercholesteremia*, *hyperlipidemia*, *hypokalemia*, *weight gain*, *hypophosphatemia*, *hyperkalemia*, hypervolemia, Cushing's syndrome, diabetes mellitus, acidosis, dehydration, hypercalcemia, hyperglycemia, hyperphosphatemia, hypocalcemia, ***hypoglycemia***, hypomagnesemia, hyponatremia, weight loss.
Musculoskeletal: *back pain*, *arthralgia*, myalgia, arthrosis, bone necrosis, leg cramps, osteoporosis, tetany.
Respiratory: *dyspnea*, *cough*, *atelectasis*, *upper respiratory tract infection*, asthma, bronchitis, hypoxia, lung edema, pleural effusion, pneumonia, ***interstitial lung disease***.
Skin: *rash*, *acne*, hirsutism, fungal dermatitis, pruritus, skin hypertrophy, skin ulcer, sweating.
Other: *pain*, abscess, cellulitis, chills, flu syndrome, infection, ***sepsis***, lymphadenopathy, lymphocele, abnormal healing, including fascial dehiscence and anastomotic disruption (wound, vascular, airway, ureteral, biliary).

Interactions

Drug-drug. *Aminoglycosides, amphotericin B, other nephrotoxic drugs:* May increase risk of nephrotoxicity. Use with caution.
Bromocriptine, cimetidine, clarithromycin, clotrimazole, danazol, erythromycin, fluconazole, indinavir, itraconazole, metoclopramide, nicardipine, ritonavir, verapamil, other drugs that inhibit CYP3A4: May increase blood levels of sirolimus. Monitor sirolimus levels closely.
Carbamazepine, phenobarbital, phenytoin, rifabutin, rifapentine, other drugs that induce CYP3A4: May decrease blood levels of sirolimus. Monitor patient closely.
Cyclosporine: May inhibit sirolimus metabolism. Sirolimus levels decrease when cyclosporine is stopped. Carefully increase sirolimus dose during cyclosporine taper to eventually be about fourfold higher.
Diltiazem: May increase sirolimus levels. Monitor sirolimus level, as needed.
HMG-CoA reductase inhibitors or fibrates: May increase risk of rhabdomyolysis with the combination of sirolimus and cyclosporine. Monitor patient closely.
Ketoconazole: May increase rate and extent of sirolimus absorption. Avoid using together.
Live-virus vaccines (BCG; measles, mumps, rubella; yellow fever; varicella; TY21a typhoid): May reduce vaccine effectiveness. Avoid using together.
Rifampin: May decrease sirolimus level. Alternative therapy to rifampin may be prescribed.
Drug-food. *Grapefruit juice:* May decrease metabolism of sirolimus. Discourage use together.
Drug-lifestyle. *Sun exposure:* May increase risk of skin cancer. Tell patient to take precautions.

Nursing considerations

!!ALERT Use of sirolimus plus tacrolimus or cyclosporine was linked to an increase in hepatic artery thrombosis, leading to an excessive rate of death and graft loss in a liver transplant study. Most cases occurred within 30 days after transplant, and many of these patients had evidence of infection at or near the time of death.

- Only those experienced in immunosuppressive therapy and management of renal transplant patients should prescribe drug.
- Cases of bronchial anastomotic dehiscence, some fatal, have been reported in lung transplant recipients treated with sirolimus in combination with tacrolimus and corticosteroids.
- Use drug in regimen with cyclosporine and corticosteroids; have patient take drug 4 hours after cyclosporine dose.
- Cyclosporine withdrawal in patients with high-risk of graft rejection isn't recommended. This includes patients with Banff grade III acute rejection or vascular rejection before cyclosporine withdrawal, those who are dialysis-dependent, those with serum creatinine level greater than 4.5 mg/dl, black patients, patients with retransplants or multiorgan transplants, and patients with high panel of reactive antibodies.
- Patient should take drug consistently either with or without food.
- Dilute oral solution before use. After dilution, use immediately and discard oral solution syringe.
- When diluting oral solution, empty correct amount into glass or plastic (not Styrofoam) container holding at least 1/4 cup (60 ml) of either water or orange juice. Don't use grapefruit juice or any other liquid. Stir vigorously and have patient drink immediately. Refill container with at least 1/2 cup (120 ml) of water or orange juice, stir again, and have patient drink all contents.
- After transplantation, give antimicrobial prophylaxis for *Pneumocystis carinii* for 1 year and for cytomegalovirus for 3 months.

!!ALERT Patients taking drug are more susceptible to infection and lymphoma.

- Monitor renal function tests, because use with cyclosporine may cause creatinine level to increase. Adjustment of immunosuppressive regimen may be needed.
- Monitor cholesterol and triglyceride levels. Treatment with lipid-lowering drugs during therapy isn't uncommon. If hyperlipidemia is detected, additional interventions, such as diet and exercise, should begin.
- Check for rhabdomyolysis.
- Monitor drug levels in patients age 13 and older who weigh less than 40 kg (88 lb), patients with hepatic impairment, those also receiving drugs that induce or inhibit CYP3A4, and patients in whom cyclosporine dosing is markedly reduced or stopped.
- A slight haze may develop during refrigeration. This doesn't affect potency of drug. If haze develops, bring to room temperature and shake until haze disappears.
- Store away from light, and refrigerate at 36° to 46° F (2° to 8° C). After opening bottle, use contents within 1 month. If needed, store bottles and pouches at room temperature (up to 77° F [25° C]) for several days. Drug may be kept in oral syringe for 24 hours at room temperature.

Patient teaching

- Tell patient how to properly store, dilute, and give drug.
- Advise woman of childbearing age about risks during pregnancy. Tell her to use effective contraception before and during therapy, and for 12 weeks after stopping therapy.
- Tell patient to take drug consistently with or without food to minimize absorption variability.
- Tell patient to take drug 4 hours after cyclosporine to avoid drug interactions.
- Advise patient to wash area with soap and water if drug solution touches skin or mucous membranes.

smallpox vaccine, dried
Dryvax

Pregnancy risk category C

Indications & dosages

➲ Active immunization to prevent smallpox disease

Adults and children: One drop of vaccine deposited over the deltoid or triceps muscle, followed by a multiple-puncture technique into the superficial layers of skin (two or three needle punctures for primary vaccination and 15 for revaccination).

Contraindications & cautions

Nonemergency situations

- Contraindicated in patients allergic to any component of the vaccine, including polymyxin B sulfate, dihydrostreptomycin sulfate, chlortetracycline hydrochloride, and neomycin sulfate; in infants younger than age 12 months.

• Contraindicated in patients or household contacts of patients with eczema, past history of eczema, or other exfoliative skin conditions; congenital or acquired immune system deficiencies, including HIV, leukemia, lymphomas, malignancy, organ transplantation, stem cell transplantation, agammaglobulinemia, and other malignant neoplasms affecting the bone marrow or lymphatic systems; of those receiving systemic corticosteroids, immunosuppressive drugs, or radiation; of women who are or may be pregnant, breast-feeding women, and elderly people.
• Contraindicated in patients with heart disease (such as cardiomyopathy, heart failure, previous MI, history of angina, or evidence of coronary artery disease).
• Contraindicated in those who have three or more of these risk factors: hypertension, hypercholesterolemia, diabetes mellitus or hyperglycemia, smoking, or a first-degree relative with a heart condition before age 50.

Emergency situations

• For patients at high risk of exposure to smallpox, no contraindications exist for vaccination.

Adverse reactions

CNS: *fever.*
Skin: rash.
Other: accidental spread to another part of the body or to another person.

Interactions

None reported.

Nursing considerations

• Don't give I.M., I.V., or S.C.
!!ALERT The vial stopper contains latex, which may cause hypersensitivity in patients with latex allergy.
• Give vaccination in the deltoid or posterior aspect of the arm over the triceps muscle.
!!ALERT Rapidly make punctures into skin, and allow 15 to 20 seconds for blood to appear. After vaccination, blot off any vaccine remaining on skin at vaccination site with clean, dry gauze or cotton.
• Burn, boil, or autoclave all items that come in contact with the vaccine before their disposal.
• Inspect the site 6 to 8 days after vaccination to determine whether a major or equivocal reaction has occurred.
• Contact transmission of the virus can occur until the scab separates from the skin lesion, usually 14 to 21 days after vaccination.
• Accidental inoculation of other sites is a common complication of the vaccine. The face, eyelid, nose, mouth, genitalia, and rectum are most frequently involved. Autoinoculation of the eye may cause blindness.
• Recently vaccinated health care workers should avoid contact with patients until the scab has separated from the skin at the vaccination site. If continued contact is essential and unavoidable, cover the vaccination site and maintain good hand-washing technique.
• Cardiac complications such as myopericarditis have occurred within 2 weeks of patients being vaccinated.
• The Centers for Disease Control and Prevention (CDC) can help diagnose and manage patients with suspected complications.
• Contact the Advisory Committee on Immunization Practices (ACIP), the Armed Forces, and the CDC for the most updated information and recommendations for use of the smallpox vaccine.

Patient teaching

• Tell patient that although he should keep the vaccination site dry, he can still bathe the rest of the body.
• Advise patient that smallpox may be spread to another part of the body or to another person until the scab separates from the skin lesion (14 to 21 days after vaccination). Hand washing is essential for preventing inadvertent contact transmission of the virus.
• Tell patient to leave vaccination site uncovered or to cover it with a porous bandage, such as gauze, until the scab has separated and the underlying skin has healed. He shouldn't routinely use an occlusive bandage.
• Warn patient not to use salves or ointments on vaccination site.
• Instruct patient to seek immediate medical attention if he has chest pain, dyspnea, or other symptoms of cardiac disease in the first 2 weeks after vaccination.

• Instruct patient to place contaminated bandages in sealed plastic bags before trash disposal.

sodium bicarbonate

Arm & Hammer Baking Soda ◇, Bell/ans ◇, Neut, Soda Mint ◇ ♦

Pregnancy risk category C

Indications & dosages

➲ Metabolic acidosis

Adults and children: Dosage depends on blood carbon dioxide content, pH, and patient's condition; usually, 2 to 5 mEq/kg I.V. infused over 4- to 8-hour period.

➲ Systemic or urinary alkalinization

Adults: Initially, 4 g P.O.; then 1 to 2 g q 6 hours.

Children: 84 to 840 mg/kg P.O. daily.

➲ Antacid

Adults: 300 mg to 2 g P.O. up to q.i.d. taken with glass of water.

➲ Cardiac arrest

Adults: 1 mEq/kg I.V. of 7.5% or 8.4% solution; then 0.5 mEq/kg I.V. q 10 minutes, depending on arterial blood gas (ABG) level. Base further dosages on results of ABG analysis. If ABG level is unavailable, use 0.5 mEq/kg I.V. q 10 minutes until spontaneous circulation returns.

Infants and children: 1 mEq/kg (1 ml/kg of 8.4% solution) I.V. slowly followed by 1 mEq/kg q 10 minutes of arrest. Don't give more than 8 mEq/kg I.V. total; a 4.2% solution may be preferred.

Contraindications & cautions

• Contraindicated in patients with metabolic or respiratory alkalosis and in those with hypocalcemia in which alkalosis may produce tetany, hypertension, seizures, or heart failure.

• Contraindicated in patients losing chloride because of vomiting or continuous GI suction and in those receiving diuretics that produce hypochloremic alkalosis. Oral sodium bicarbonate is contraindicated for acute ingestion of strong mineral acids.

• Use with caution in patients with renal insufficiency, heart failure, or other edematous or sodium-retaining condition.

Adverse reactions

CNS: tetany.
CV: edema.
GI: gastric distention, belching, flatulence.
Metabolic: hypokalemia, ***metabolic alkalosis***, hypernatremia, hyperosmolarity with overdose.
Skin: pain and irritation at injection site.

Interactions

Drug-drug. *Anorexiants, flecainide, mecamylamine, methenamine, quinidine, sympathomimetics:* May decrease renal clearance of these drugs and increase risk of toxicity. Monitor patient closely for toxicity.

Chlorpropamide, lithium, methotrexate, salicylates, tetracycline: May increase urine alkalinization, increase renal clearance of these drugs, and decrease their effect. Monitor patient closely for drug's effect.

Enteric-coated drugs: May be released prematurely in stomach. Avoid using together.

Ketoconazole: May decrease ketoconazole absorption. Separate dosage times.

Nursing considerations

• To avoid risk of alkalosis, obtain blood pH, partial pressure of arterial oxygen, partial pressure of arterial carbon dioxide, and electrolyte levels. Tell prescriber laboratory results.

Patient teaching

• Tell patient not to take drug with milk because doing so may cause high levels of calcium in the blood, abnormally high alkalinity in tissues and fluids, or kidney stones.

sodium chloride

Pregnancy risk category C

Indications & dosages

➲ Fluid and electrolyte replacement in hyponatremia caused by electrolyte loss or in severe salt depletion

Adults: Dosage is individualized. Use 3% or 5% solution only with frequent electrolyte level determination and only slow I.V. For 0.45% solution, 3% to 8% of body weight, according to deficiencies, over 18 to 24 hours. For 0.9% solution, 2% to 6% of body weight, according to deficiencies, over 18 to 24 hours.

➲ **Heat cramp caused by excessive perspiration**
Adults: 1 g P.O. with each glass of water.

Contraindications & cautions

- Contraindicated in patients with conditions in which sodium and chloride administration is detrimental.
- Sodium chloride 3% and 5% injections contraindicated in patients with increased, normal, or only slightly decreased electrolyte levels.
- Use cautiously in elderly or postoperative patients and in patients with heart failure, circulatory insufficiency, renal dysfunction, or hypoproteinemia.

Adverse reactions

CV: ***aggravation of heart failure***, thrombophlebitis, edema when given too rapidly or in excess.
Metabolic: hypernatremia, aggravation of existing metabolic acidosis with excessive infusion.
Respiratory: ***pulmonary edema***.
Skin: local tenderness, tissue necrosis at injection site.
Other: abscess.

Interactions

None significant.

Nursing considerations

- Monitor electrolyte levels.

Patient teaching

- Explain use and administration of drug to patient and family.
- Tell patient to report adverse reactions promptly.

sodium chloride, hypertonic
Adsorbonac, AK-NaCl, Muro 128, Muroptic-5

Pregnancy risk category NR

Indications & dosages

➲ **To temporarily relieve corneal edema**
Adults and children: Apply 1 or 2 drops of solution or 1/4 inch (6 mm) of ointment q 3 to 4 hours.

Contraindications & cautions

- Contraindicated in patients hypersensitive to drug or its components.

Adverse reactions

EENT: slight eye stinging.
Other: hypersensitivity reactions.

Interactions

None significant.

Nursing considerations

- Drug is for ophthalmic use only. Don't inject or give orally.
- Check expiration date before use.

Patient teaching

- Teach patient how to instill drug. Advise him to wash hands before and after instillation and to apply light finger pressure on lacrimal sac for 1 minute after drops are instilled. Warn patient not to touch dropper to eye or surrounding tissue.
- Tell patient to prevent caking on dropper bottle tip by putting a few drops of sterile irrigation solution inside bottle cap.
- Warn patient that ointment may cause blurred vision.
- If patient experiences severe headache, pain, rapid change in vision, acute redness of eyes, sudden appearance of floating spots, pain on exposure to light, or double vision, tell him to stop drug and notify prescriber.
- Advise patient to store drug in tightly closed container.

sodium ferric gluconate complex
Ferrlecit

Pregnancy risk category B

Indications & dosages

➲ **Iron deficiency anemia in patients receiving long-term hemodialysis and supplemental erythropoietin**
Adults: Before starting therapeutic doses, give test dose of 2 ml sodium ferric gluconate complex (25 mg elemental iron) I.V. over 1 hour. If patient tolerates test dose, give therapeutic dose of 10 ml (125 mg elemental iron) I.V. over 1 hour. Most patients need minimum cumulative dose of 1 g elemental iron given at more than eight se-

quential dialysis treatments to achieve a favorable hemoglobin or hematocrit response.

Contraindications & cautions

- Contraindicated in patients hypersensitive to drug or its components (such as benzyl alcohol) and in those with iron overload or anemias not related to iron deficiency.
- Use cautiously in elderly patients.

Adverse reactions

CNS: asthenia, headache, fatigue, malaise, *dizziness*, paresthesia, agitation, insomnia, somnolence, syncope, pain, chills, fever.
CV: *hypotension*, *hypertension*, tachycardia, ***bradycardia***, angina, chest pain, ***MI***, edema, flushing.
EENT: conjunctivitis, abnormal vision, rhinitis.
GI: *nausea, vomiting, diarrhea*, rectal disorder, dyspepsia, eructation, flatulence, melena, abdominal pain.
GU: urinary tract infection.
Hematologic: anemia.
Metabolic: ***hyperkalemia***, ***hypoglycemia***, hypokalemia, hypervolemia.
Musculoskeletal: myalgia, arthralgia, back pain, arm pain, *cramps*.
Respiratory: *dyspnea*, coughing, upper respiratory tract infection, pneumonia, pulmonary edema.
Skin: pruritus, increased sweating, rash, *injection site reaction*.
Other: infection, rigors, flu syndrome, ***sepsis***, ***carcinoma***, hypersensitivity reactions, lymphadenopathy.

Interactions

None significant.

Nursing considerations

!!ALERT Dosage is expressed in milligrams of elemental iron.

- Drug shouldn't be given to patients with iron overload, which often occurs in hemoglobinopathies and other refractory anemias.

!!ALERT Potentially life-threatening hypersensitivity reactions (with CV collapse, cardiac arrest, bronchospasm, oral or pharyngeal edema, dyspnea, angioedema, urticaria, or pruritus sometimes linked to pain and muscle spasm of chest or back) may occur during infusion. Have adequate supportive measures readily available. Monitor patient closely during infusion.

- Monitor ferritin, iron saturation, and hemoglobin levels and hematocrit.
- Some adverse reactions in hemodialysis patients may be related to dialysis itself or to chronic renal failure.
- Check with patient about other potential sources of iron, such as OTC iron preparations and iron-containing multiple vitamins with minerals.

Patient teaching

- Urge patient to notify prescriber immediately if abdominal pain, diarrhea, vomiting, drowsiness, or rapid breathing occurs. These symptoms may indicate iron poisoning.

sodium lactate

Pregnancy risk category NR

Indications & dosages

To alkalinize urine
Adults: 30 ml/kg (1/6 M solution) I.V. daily, in divided doses.

Metabolic acidosis
Adults: Dosage of 1/6 M solution depends on degree of bicarbonate deficit. A suggested formula follows:

$$(60 - \text{plasma } CO_2) \times (0.8 \times \text{body weight in pounds}) = \text{Dose in ml}$$

Contraindications & cautions

- Contraindicated in patients with hypernatremia, severe acidosis, lactic acidosis, or conditions in which sodium administration is detrimental, such as heart failure or during corticosteroid administration.
- Use cautiously in patients with metabolic or respiratory alkalosis, severe hepatic or renal disease, heart failure, shock, hypoxia, or beriberi.

Adverse reactions

CNS: fever.
CV: thrombophlebitis at injection site.
Metabolic: ***metabolic alkalosis***, hypernatremia, hyperosmolarity with overdose.
Other: infection.

Interactions
None significant.

Nursing considerations
- Monitor electrolyte levels to avoid alkalosis.

Patient teaching
- Explain use and administration of drug to patient and family.
- Tell patient to report adverse reactions to prescriber.

sodium phosphate monohydrate and sodium phosphate dibasic anhydrous
Visicol

Pregnancy risk category C

Indications & dosages
➲ To cleanse the bowel before colonoscopy

Adults: 40 tablets taken in the following manner: The evening before the procedure, 3 tablets P.O. with at least 8 ounces of clear liquid q 15 minutes, for a total of 20 tablets. The last dose will be only 2 tablets. The day of the procedure, 3 tablets P.O. with at least 8 ounces of clear liquid q 15 minutes, for a total of 20 tablets, starting 3 to 5 hours before the procedure. The last dose will be only 2 tablets.

Contraindications & cautions
- Contraindicated in patients hypersensitive to sodium phosphate or any of its ingredients. Avoid giving drug to patients with heart failure, ascites, unstable angina, gastric retention, ileus, acute intestinal obstruction, pseudo-obstruction, severe chronic constipation, bowel perforation, acute colitis, toxic megacolon, or hypomotility syndrome (hypothyroidism, scleroderma).
- Use cautiously in patients with a history of electrolyte abnormalities, current electrolyte abnormalities, or impaired renal function. Also use cautiously in patients who take drugs that can induce electrolyte abnormalities or prolong the QT interval.
- Use cautiously in elderly patients because they may be more sensitive to drug effects.

Adverse reactions
CNS: headache, dizziness.
GI: nausea, vomiting, abdominal bloating, abdominal pain.

Interactions
Drug-drug. *Any drugs:* Reduces absorption of these drugs. Separate doses.

Nursing considerations
- Correct electrolyte imbalances before giving drug.
- As with other sodium phosphate cathartic preparations, this drug may induce colonic mucosal ulceration.
- Monitor patient for signs of dehydration.
- Don't repeat administration within 7 days.
- No enema or laxative is needed in addition to drug. Patients shouldn't take any additional purgatives, particularly those that contain sodium phosphate.

!!ALERT Administration of other sodium phosphate products has caused death from significant fluid shifts, electrolyte abnormalities, and cardiac arrhythmias. Patients with electrolyte disturbances have an increased risk of prolonged QT interval. Use drug cautiously in patients who are taking other drugs known to prolong the QT interval.

Patient teaching
- Urge patient to drink at least 8 ounces of clear liquid with each dose. Inadequate fluid intake may lead to excessive fluid loss and hypovolemia.
- Tell patient to drink only clear liquids for at least 12 hours before starting the purgative regimen.
- Caution patient against taking an additional enema or laxative, particularly one that contains sodium phosphate.
- Tell patient that undigested or partially digested Visicol tablets and other drugs may appear in the stool.

sodium phosphates

Fleet Enema ◇, Fleet Phospho-soda ◇

Pregnancy risk category NR

Indications & dosages

➲ Constipation

Adults and children age 12 and older: 20 to 45 ml solution mixed with 120 ml cold water P.O. Or, 60 to 150 ml as an enema.
Children ages 10 to 11: 10 to 20 ml solution mixed with 120 ml cold water P.O.
Children ages 5 to 9: 5 to 10 ml solution mixed with 120 ml cold water P.O. Or, 30 to 60 ml as an enema.
Children ages 2 to 5: 60 ml P.R. as an enema.

Contraindications & cautions

- Contraindicated in patients on sodium-restricted diets and in patients with intestinal obstruction, intestinal perforation, edema, heart failure, megacolon, impaired renal function, or signs and symptoms of appendicitis or acute surgical abdomen, such as abdominal pain, nausea, or vomiting.
- Use cautiously in patients with large hemorrhoids or anal excoriations.

Adverse reactions

GI: *abdominal cramping.*
Metabolic: fluid and electrolyte disturbances, such as hypernatremia and hyperphosphatemia, with daily use.
Other: laxative dependence with long-term or excessive use.

Interactions

None significant.

Nursing considerations

- Before giving drug for constipation, determine whether patient has adequate fluid intake, exercise, and diet.

!!ALERT Up to 10% of sodium content of drug may be absorbed.

!!ALERT Severe electrolyte imbalances may occur if recommended dosage is exceeded.

Patient teaching

- Teach patient about dietary sources of bulk, including bran and other cereals, fresh fruit, and vegetables.
- Warn patient about adverse reactions, and stress importance of using drug only for short-term therapy.

sodium polystyrene sulfonate

Kayexalate, Kionex, SPS

Pregnancy risk category C

Indications & dosages

➲ Hyperkalemia

Adults: 15 g P.O. daily to q.i.d. in water or sorbitol (3 to 4 ml/g of resin). Or, mix powder with appropriate medium—aqueous suspension or diet appropriate for renal failure—and instill through a nasogastric tube. Or, 30 to 50 g/dl of sorbitol q 6 hours as warm emulsion deep into sigmoid colon (20 cm).
Children: 1 g/kg of body weight/dose P.O. q 6 hours, p.r.n.

Contraindications & cautions

- Contraindicated in patients hypersensitive to drug and in those with hypokalemia.
- Use cautiously in patients with severe heart failure, severe hypertension, or marked edema. Drug provides 100 mg of sodium per gram.

Adverse reactions

GI: *constipation*, fecal impaction, anorexia, gastric irritation, nausea, vomiting, *diarrhea with sorbitol emulsions.*
Metabolic: hypokalemia, hypocalcemia, hypomagnesemia, sodium retention.

Interactions

Drug-drug. *Antacids and laxatives (nonabsorbable cation-donating types, including magnesium hydroxide):* May cause systemic alkalosis and reduce potassium exchange capability. Avoid using together.

Nursing considerations

- Don't heat resin; this impairs drug's effect. Mix resin only with water or sorbitol for P.O. administration. Never mix with orange juice (high potassium content) to disguise taste.
- Chill oral suspension for greater palatability.

- Oral administration is preferred because drug should remain in intestine for at least 30 minutes.
- If sorbitol is given, mix with resin suspension.
- Consider giving in solid form. Resin cookie and candy recipes are available; ask pharmacist or dietitian to supply.
- Premixed forms (SPS and others) are available. If preparing manually, mix polystyrene resin only with water or sorbitol for rectal use. Don't use mineral oil for P.R. administration to prevent impaction; ion exchange needs aqueous medium. Sorbitol content prevents impaction.
- Prepare P.R. dose at room temperature. Stir emulsion gently during administration.
- Use #28 French rubber tube for rectal dose; insert 20 cm into sigmoid colon. Tape tube in place. Or, consider an indwelling urinary catheter with a 30-ml balloon inflated distal to anal sphincter to aid in retention. This is especially helpful for patients with poor sphincter control. Use gravity flow. Drain returns constantly through Y-tube connection. Place patient in knee-chest position or with hips on pillow for a while if back leakage occurs.
- After P.R. administration, flush tubing with 50 to 100 ml of non-sodium fluid to ensure delivery of all drug. Flush rectum to remove resin.
- Prevent fecal impaction in elderly patients by giving resin P.R. Give cleansing enema before P.R. administration. Have patient retain enema for 6 to 10 hours if possible, but 30 to 60 minutes is acceptable.
- Watch for constipation with oral or nasogastric administration. Give 10 to 20 ml of 70% sorbitol syrup every 2 hours, as needed, to produce one or two watery stools daily.
- Monitor potassium level at least once daily. Treatment may result in potassium deficiency and is usually stopped when potassium is reduced to 4 or 5 mEq/L.
- Watch for signs of hypokalemia: irritability, confusion, arrhythmias, ECG changes, severe muscle weakness or even paralysis, and digitalis toxicity in digitalized patients.
- When hyperkalemia is severe, polystyrene resin alone isn't adequate for lowering potassium. Dextrose 50% with regular insulin I.V. push may also be given.
- Watch for symptoms of other electrolyte deficiencies (magnesium, calcium) because drug is nonselective. Monitor calcium level in patients receiving sodium polystyrene therapy for more than 3 days. Supplementary calcium may be needed.
- Watch for sodium overload. Drug contains about 100 mg sodium per gram. About one-third of resin's sodium is retained.

Patient teaching

- Explain use and administration of drug to patient.
- Advise patient to report adverse reactions promptly.
- Teach patient about low-potassium diet.

solifenacin succinate

VESIcare

Pregnancy risk category C

Indications & dosages

➲ **Overactive bladder with urinary urgency, frequency, and urge incontinence.** *Adults:* 5 mg P.O. once daily. May increase to 10 mg once daily if 5-mg dose is well tolerated.

If creatinine clearance is less than 30 ml/minute or the patient has moderate liver impairment (Child-Pugh score B), maintain the dose at 5 mg.

Contraindications & cautions

- Contraindicated in patients hypersensitive to drug or its components and in patients with urine or gastric retention or uncontrolled narrow-angle glaucoma. Don't use in patients with severe hepatic impairment.
- Use cautiously in patients with a history of prolonged QT interval, those being treated for narrow-angle glaucoma, and those with bladder outflow obstruction, decreased GI motility, renal insufficiency, or moderate liver impairment.

Adverse reactions

CNS: depression, dizziness, fatigue.
CV: hypertension, leg swelling.
EENT: blurred vision, dry eyes, pharyngitis.
GI: *constipation, dry mouth,* dyspepsia, nausea, upper abdominal pain, vomiting.
GU: urinary retention, UTI.

Respiratory: cough.
Other: influenza.

Interactions

Drug-drug. *Drugs that prolong the QT interval:* May increase the risk of serious cardiac arrhythmias. Monitor patient and ECG closely.
Potent CYP3A4 inhibitors (such as ketoconazole): May increase solifenacin levels. Don't exceed solifenacin dose of 5 mg daily when used together.

Nursing considerations

- Assess bladder function, and monitor drug effects.
- If patient has bladder outlet obstruction, watch for urine retention.
- Monitor patient for decreased gastric motility and constipation.
- Safety and effectiveness are similar in older and younger adults, but blood levels and half-life may increased in the elderly.

Patient teaching

- Explain that drug may cause blurred vision. Tell patient to use caution when performing hazardous activities or tasks that require clear vision until effects of the drug are known.
- Discourage use of other drugs that may cause dry mouth, constipation, urine retention, or blurred vision.
- Urge patient to notify prescriber about abdominal pain or constipation that lasts 3 days or longer.
- Tell patient that drug decreases the ability to sweat normally, and advise cautious use in hot environments or during strenuous activity.
- Tell patient to swallow tablet whole with liquid.
- Inform patient that drug may be taken with or without food.

somatrem
Protropin

Pregnancy risk category C

Indications & dosages

➲ **Long-term treatment of children who have growth failure because of lack of adequate endogenous growth hormone (GH) secretion**
Children (prepubertal): Highly individualized; up to 0.1 mg/kg S.C. (preferred) or I.M. three times weekly. Don't exceed 0.3 mg/kg per week.

Contraindications & cautions

- Contraindicated in patients hypersensitive to benzyl alcohol and in those with epiphyseal closure or active neoplasia.
- Use cautiously in patients with hypothyroidism and in those whose GH deficiency is caused by an intracranial lesion.

Adverse reactions

Metabolic: hypothyroidism, hyperglycemia.
Other: *antibodies to GH.*

Interactions

Drug-drug. *Glucocorticoids:* May inhibit growth-promoting action of somatrem. Adjust glucocorticoid dosage as needed.

Nursing considerations

- Check product's expiration date.
- To prepare solution, inject supplied bacteriostatic water for injection into vial containing drug. Then swirl vial gently until contents are completely dissolved. Don't shake vial.
- After reconstitution, make sure solution is clear. Don't inject solution if it's cloudy or contains particles.
- If prepared for other than neonatal use, store reconstituted drug in refrigerator; use within 14 days.

!! ALERT Toxicity in neonates may occur from exposure to benzyl alcohol used as a preservative. When you give this drug to neonates, reconstitute immediately before use with sterile water for injection (without bacteriostat). Use vial once; then discard.

- Patients will need regular checkups, including height measurement and blood and radiologic studies.
- Observe patient for evidence of glucose intolerance and hyperglycemia.
- Watch for slipped capital femoral epiphysis or progression of scoliosis in patients with rapid growth.
- Monitor periodic thyroid function tests for hypothyroidism; condition may need treatment with a thyroid hormone.

• Do funduscopic examination of patient for intracranial hypertension at start of therapy and periodically thereafter.
!!ALERT Don't confuse somatrem with somatropin, Serostim, or sumatriptan.

Patient teaching

• Reassure patient and caregivers that somatrem is pure and safe. Drug replaces pituitary-derived human GH, which was removed from the market in 1985 because of its link with the rare but fatal Creutzfeldt-Jakob disease.
• Review evidence of hypothyroidism and hyperglycemia. Instruct patient and parents to report such evidence promptly.
• Instruct patient to report to prescriber headache, weakness, localized muscle pain, swelling, and limb, hip, or knee pain.

somatropin

Genotropin, Genotropin MiniQuick, Humatrope, Norditropin, Nutropin, Nutropin AQ, Saizen, Serostim

Pregnancy risk category C; B (Serostim)

Indications & dosages

➲ Long-term treatment of growth failure in children with inadequate secretion of endogenous growth hormone (GH)
Children: 0.18 mg/kg Humatrope I.M. or S.C. weekly, divided equally and given on 3 alternate days, six times weekly or once daily. Or, 0.3 mg/kg Nutropin or Nutropin AQ S.C. weekly in daily divided doses. Or, 0.06 mg/kg Saizen I.M. or S.C. three times weekly. Or, 0.024 to 0.034 mg/kg Norditropin S.C. six to seven times weekly. Or, 0.16 to 0.24 mg/kg Genotropin S.C. weekly, divided into five to seven doses.
➲ Growth failure from chronic renal insufficiency up to time of renal transplantation
Children: Up to 0.35 mg/kg weekly Nutropin or Nutropin AQ S.C. divided into daily doses.
➲ Long-term treatment of short stature caused by Turner's syndrome
Children: Up to 0.375 mg/kg/week Humatrope, Nutropin, or Nutropin AQ S.C. divided into equal doses given three to seven times weekly.
➲ Long-term treatment of growth failure in children with Prader-Willi syndrome diagnosed by genetic testing
Children: 0.24 mg/kg Genotropin S.C. weekly, divided into six to seven doses.
➲ Replacement of endogenous GH in adult patients with GH deficiency
Adults: Initially, not more than 0.006 mg/kg Genotropin, Humatrope, Nutropin, or Nutropin AQ S.C. daily. May be increased to maximum of 0.0125 mg/kg Humatrope daily.

Nutropin or Nutropin AQ dosages may be increased to maximum of 0.025 mg/kg daily in patients younger than age 35 or 0.0125 mg/kg daily in patients older than age 35. Or, starting dosages not exceeding 0.04 mg/kg Genotropin S.C. weekly, divided into six to seven doses, may be increased at 4- to 8-week intervals to a maximum dose of 0.08 mg/kg S.C. weekly, divided into six to seven doses.
➲ Replacement of endogenous GH in adult patients with GH deficiency (Saizen)
Adults: Initially, not more than 0.005 mg/kg daily. May increase after 4 weeks to a maximum dose of 0.01 mg/kg daily based on patient tolerance and clinical response.
➲ AIDS wasting or cachexia
Adults and children weighing more than 55 kg (121 lb): 6 mg Serostim S.C. h.s.
Adults and children weighing 45 to 55 kg (99 to 121 lb): 5 mg Serostim S.C. h.s.
Adults and children weighing 35 to 45 kg (77 to 99 lb): 4 mg Serostim S.C. h.s.
Adults and children weighing less than 35 kg: 0.1 mg/kg/day Serostim S.C. h.s.
➲ Long-term treatment of growth failure in children born small for gestational age (SGA) who don't achieve catch-up growth by age 2
Children: 0.48 mg/kg Genotropin S.C. weekly, divided into five to seven doses.
➲ Idiopathic short stature
Children: Up to 0.37 mg/kg Humatrope S.C. weekly, divided into six to seven equal doses.

Contraindications & cautions

• Contraindicated in patients with closed epiphyses or an active underlying intracranial lesion. Humatrope shouldn't be reconstituted with supplied diluent for patients hypersensitive to either Metacresol or glycerin. Genotropin is also contraindicated in

patients with Prader-Willi syndrome who are severely obese or have severe respiratory impairment.
- Use cautiously in children with hypothyroidism and in those whose GH deficiency is caused by an intracranial lesion.

Adverse reactions

CNS: headache, weakness.
CV: mild, transient edema.
Hematologic: ***leukemia***.
Metabolic: mild hyperglycemia, hypothyroidism.
Musculoskeletal: localized muscle pain.
Skin: injection site pain.
Other: antibodies to GH.

Interactions

Drug-drug. *Corticotropin, corticosteroids:* Long-term use may inhibit growth response to GH. Monitor patient for lack of effect.

Nursing considerations

- Frequently examine children with hypothyroidism and those whose GH deficiency is caused by an intracranial lesion for progression or recurrence of underlying disease.
- To prepare solution, inject supplied diluent into vial containing drug by aiming stream of liquid against wall of glass vial. Then swirl vial gently until contents are completely dissolved. Don't shake vial.
- After reconstitution, make sure solution is clear. Don't inject solution if it's cloudy or contains particles.
- Patients on dialysis need changes in drug administration schedule as follows: For hemodialysis, give drug before bedtime or 3 to 4 hours after dialysis. For long-term cycling peritoneal dialysis, give drug in the morning after completion of dialysis. For long-term ambulatory peritoneal dialysis, give drug in the evening at the time of the overnight exchange.
- Store reconstituted drug in refrigerator; use within 14 days.
- If patient develops sensitivity to diluent, reconstitute drug with sterile water for injection. When drug is reconstituted in this manner, use only one reconstituted dose per vial, refrigerate solution if it isn't used immediately after reconstitution, use reconstituted dose within 24 hours, and discard unused portion.

!!ALERT Fatalities have occurred in patients with Prader-Willi syndrome who are morbidly obese and in those with a history of respiratory impairment, sleep apnea, or unidentified respiratory infection. Evaluate patients with Prader-Willi syndrome for sleep apnea and upper airway obstruction before starting treatment. Interrupt treatment if signs of upper airway obstruction occur.
- Monitor patient with Prader-Willi syndrome for signs of respiratory infection.
- Monitor child's height regularly. Regular checkups, including monitoring of blood and radiologic studies, also are needed.
- Monitor patient's glucose level regularly because GH may induce a state of insulin resistance.
- Excessive glucocorticoid therapy inhibits somatropin's growth-promoting effect. Patients with coexisting corticotropin deficiency should have their glucocorticoid replacement dosage carefully adjusted to avoid growth inhibition.
- Watch for slipped capital femoral epiphysis or progression of scoliosis in patients with rapid growth.
- Monitor results of periodic thyroid function tests for hypothyroidism; condition may need thyroid hormone treatment. Laboratory measurements of thyroid hormone may change.
- Do funduscopic examination of patient for intracranial hypertension when therapy starts and periodically during therapy.

!!ALERT Don't confuse somatropin with somatrem or sumatriptan.
- To be treated with Saizen for GH replacement, an adult must have GH deficiency alone or together with multiple hormone deficiencies, as a result of pituitary or hypothalamic disease, surgery, radiation, or trauma; or he must have been GH deficient as a child and be confirmed as GH deficient as an adult before Saizen treatment starts.

Patient teaching

- Inform parents that child with endocrine disorders (including GH deficiency) may have an increased risk of slipped capital epiphyses. Tell parents to notify prescriber if they notice their child limping.
- Instruct patients with diabetes to monitor glucose level closely and report changes to prescriber.
- Stress importance of close follow-up care.

sotalol hydrochloride
Betapace, Betapace AF

Pregnancy risk category B

Indications & dosages

➲ Documented, life-threatening ventricular arrhythmias
Adults: Initially, 80 mg Betapace P.O. b.i.d. Increase dosage q 3 days as needed and tolerated. Most patients respond to 160 to 320 mg/day, although some patients with refractory arrhythmias need up to 640 mg/day.

If creatinine clearance is 30 to 60 ml/minute, increase dosage interval to q 24 hours; if clearance is 10 to 30 ml/minute, increase interval to q 36 to 48 hours; and if clearance is less than 10 ml/minute, individualize dosage.

➲ To maintain normal sinus rhythm or to delay recurrence of atrial fibrillation or atrial flutter in patients with symptomatic atrial fibrillation or flutter who are currently in sinus rhythm
Adults: 80 mg Betapace AF P.O. b.i.d. Increase dosage p.r.n. to 120 mg P.O. b.i.d. after 3 days if the QTc interval is less than 500 msec. Maximum dose is 160 mg P.O. b.i.d.

If creatinine clearance is 40 to 60 ml/minute, increase dosage interval to q 24 hours.

Contraindications & cautions

- Contraindicated in patients hypersensitive to drug.
- Contraindicated in those with severe sinus node dysfunction, sinus bradycardia, second- and third-degree AV block unless patient has a pacemaker, congenital or acquired long QT-interval syndrome, cardiogenic shock, uncontrolled heart failure, and bronchial asthma.
- Use cautiously in patients with renal impairment or diabetes mellitus (beta blockers may mask signs and symptoms of hypoglycemia).

Adverse reactions

CNS: *asthenia, headache, dizziness, weakness, fatigue,* sleep problems, *lightheadedness.*
CV: ***bradycardia, arrhythmias, heart failure, AV block, proarrhythmic events (including polymorphic ventricular tachycardia, PVCs, ventricular fibrillation),*** edema, *palpitations, chest pain,* ECG abnormalities, hypotension.
GI: *nausea, vomiting,* diarrhea, dyspepsia.
Metabolic: hyperglycemia.
Respiratory: *dyspnea,* ***bronchospasm.***

Interactions

Drug-drug. *Antiarrhythmics:* May increase drug effects. Avoid using together.
Antihypertensives, catecholamine-depleting drugs (such as guanethidine, reserpine): May increase hypotensive effects. Monitor blood pressure closely.
Calcium channel blockers: May increase myocardial depression. Avoid using together.
Clonidine: May enhance rebound effect after withdrawal of clonidine. Stop sotalol several days before withdrawing clonidine.
General anesthetics: May increase myocardial depression. Monitor patient closely.
Insulin, oral antidiabetics: May cause hyperglycemia and may mask signs and symptoms of hypoglycemia. Adjust dosage accordingly.
Prazosin: May increase the risk of orthostatic hypotension. Assist patient to stand slowly until effects are known.
Drug-food. *Any food:* May decrease absorption by 20%. Advise patient to take on empty stomach.

Nursing considerations

- Because proarrhythmic events may occur at start of therapy and during dosage adjustments, hospitalize patient for a minimum of 3 days. Facilities and personnel should be available for cardiac rhythm monitoring and interpretation of ECG.
- Assess patient for new or worsened symptoms of heart failure.
- Although patients receiving I.V. lidocaine may start sotalol therapy without ill effect, withdraw other antiarrhythmics before therapy begins. Sotalol therapy typically is delayed until two or three half-lives of the withdrawn drug have elapsed. After withdrawing amiodarone, give sotalol only after QT interval normalizes.
- Adjust dosage slowly, allowing 3 days between dosage increments for adequate mon-

itoring of QT intervals and for drug levels to reach a steady-state level.

!!ALERT Don't substitute Betapace for Betapace AF.

- Monitor electrolytes regularly, especially if patient is receiving diuretics. Electrolyte imbalances, such as hypokalemia or hypomagnesemia, may enhance QT-interval prolongation and increase the risk of serious arrhythmias such as torsades de pointes.

!!ALERT Don't confuse sotalol with Stadol.

Patient teaching

- Explain to patient that he will need to be hospitalized for initiation of drug therapy.
- Stress need to take drug as prescribed, even when he is feeling well. Caution patient against stopping drug suddenly.
- Caution patient against using nonprescription drugs and decongestants while taking drug.
- Because food and antacids can interfere with absorption, tell patient to take drug on an empty stomach, 1 hour before or 2 hours after meals or antacids.

spironolactone

Aldactone, Novospiroton†

Pregnancy risk category D

Indications & dosages

➲ Edema

Adults: 25 to 200 mg P.O. daily or in two to four divided doses.

Children: 3.3 mg/kg P.O. daily or in divided doses.

➲ Hypertension

Adults: 50 to 100 mg P.O. daily or in divided doses.

Children: 1 to 2 mg/kg P.O. b.i.d.

➲ Diuretic-induced hypokalemia

Adults: 25 to 100 mg P.O. daily.

➲ To detect primary hyperaldosteronism

Adults: 400 mg P.O. daily for 4 days (short test) or 3 to 4 weeks (long test). If hypokalemia and hypertension are corrected, a presumptive diagnosis of primary hyperaldosteronism is made.

➲ To manage primary hyperaldosteronism

Adults: 100 to 400 mg P.O. daily. Use lowest effective dose.

➲ Heart failure, as adjunct to ACE inhibitor or loop diuretic, with or without cardiac glycoside) ♦

Adults: 12.5 to 25 mg P.O. daily. May increase to 50 mg daily after 8 weeks.

➲ Hirsutism in women ♦

Adults: 50 to 200 mg P.O. daily. Or, 50 mg P.O. b.i.d. days 4 to 21 of menstrual cycle.

➲ Premenstrual syndrome ♦

Adults: 25 mg P.O. q.i.d. starting on day 14 of the menstrual cycle.

➲ Acne vulgaris ♦

Adults: 100 mg P.O. daily.

➲ Familial male precocious puberty ♦

Boys: 2 mg/kg spironolactone P.O. daily with 20 to 40 mg/kg testolactone P.O. daily for at least 6 months.

Contraindications & cautions

- Contraindicated in patients hypersensitive to drug.
- Contraindicated in those with anuria, acute or progressive renal insufficiency, or hyperkalemia.
- Use cautiously in patients with fluid or electrolyte imbalances, impaired renal function, or hepatic disease.
- Use with extreme caution in pregnant women.

Adverse reactions

CNS: headache, drowsiness, lethargy, confusion, ataxia.

GI: diarrhea, gastric bleeding, ulceration, cramping, gastritis, vomiting.

GU: inability to maintain erection, menstrual disturbances.

Hematologic: ***agranulocytosis***.

Metabolic: hyponatremia, ***hyperkalemia***, dehydration, mild acidosis.

Skin: urticaria, hirsutism, maculopapular eruptions.

Other: gynecomastia, breast soreness, drug fever, ***anaphylaxis***.

Interactions

Drug-drug. *ACE inhibitors, indomethacin, other potassium-sparing diuretics, potassium supplements:* May increase risk of hyperkalemia. Use together cautiously, especially in patients with renal impairment.

Anticoagulants: May decrease anticoagulant effects. Monitor PT and INR.

Aspirin: May block diuretic effect of spironolactone. Watch for diminished spironolactone response.
Digoxin: May alter digoxin clearance, increasing risk of digoxin toxicity. Monitor digoxin level.
Drug-herb. *Licorice:* May block ulcer-healing and aldosterone-like effects of licorice; increases risk of hypokalemia. Discourage use together.
Drug-food. *Potassium-containing salt substitutes, potassium-rich foods (such as citrus fruits, tomatoes):* May increase risk of hyperkalemia. Urge caution.

Nursing considerations

- To enhance absorption, give drug with meals.
- Protect drug from light.
- Monitor electrolyte levels, fluid intake and output, weight, and blood pressure.
- Monitor elderly patients closely, who are more susceptible to excessive diuresis.
- Inform laboratory that patient is taking spironolactone because drug may interfere with tests that measure digoxin level.
- Drug is less potent than thiazide and loop diuretics and is useful as an adjunct to other diuretic therapy. Diuretic effect is delayed 2 to 3 days when used alone.
- Maximum antihypertensive response may be delayed for up to 2 weeks.
- Watch for hyperchloremic metabolic acidosis, which may occur during therapy, especially in patients with hepatic cirrhosis.
- Breast cancer has been reported in some patients taking spironolactone, although a causal relationship hasn't been established.

!!ALERT Don't confuse Aldactone with Aldactazide.

Patient teaching

- Instruct patient to take drug in morning to prevent need to urinate at night. If second dose is needed, tell him to take it with food in early afternoon.

!!ALERT To prevent serious hyperkalemia, warn patient to avoid excessive ingestion of potassium-rich foods (such as citrus fruits, tomatoes, bananas, dates, and apricots), potassium-containing salt substitutes, and potassium supplements.

- Caution patient not to perform hazardous activities if adverse CNS reactions occur.
- Advise men about possible breast tenderness or breast enlargement.

stavudine (2, 3 didehydro-3-deoxythymidine, d4T)
Zerit, Zerit XR

Pregnancy risk category C

Indications & dosages

➲ HIV-infection, with other antiretrovirals

Adults weighing 60 kg (132 lb) or more: 40 mg P.O. regular-release q 12 hours or 100 mg P.O. extended-release once daily.
Adults weighing 30 kg (66 lb) to 60 kg: 30 mg P.O. regular-release q 12 hours or 75 mg P.O. extended-release once daily.
Children weighing 60 kg or more: 40 mg P.O. regular-release q 12 hours.
Children weighing 30 kg to 60 kg: 30 mg P.O. regular-release q 12 hours.
Children 14 days or older weighing less than 30 kg: 1 mg/kg P.O. regular-release q 12 hours.
Newborns 0 to 13 days old: 0.5 mg/kg P.O. regular-release q 12 hours.

For patients experiencing peripheral neuropathy, withdraw temporarily; then resume therapy at 50% recommended dose. Consider stopping therapy if neuropathy recurs. For patients with creatinine clearance 26 to 50 ml/minute, adjust dosage to 20 mg (if weight exceeds 60 kg) or 15 mg (if weight is less than 60 kg) P.O. q 12 hours; if clearance is 10 to 25 ml/minute, 20 mg (if weight exceeds 60 kg) or 15 mg (if weight is less than 60 kg) P.O. q 24 hours. Don't use extended-release form in patients with creatinine clearance of 50 ml/minute or less.

Contraindications & cautions

- Contraindicated in patients hypersensitive to drug.
- Use cautiously in patients with renal impairment or history of peripheral neuropathy. Adjust dosage for creatinine clearance of less than 50 ml/minute; adjust dosage or stop drug in patients with peripheral neuropathy.
- Use cautiously in pregnant women; fatal lactic acidosis may occur in pregnant women who receive stavudine and didanosine with other antiretrovirals.

• Safety and efficacy of extended-release form in children haven't been established. Don't give extended-release form to children.

Adverse reactions

CNS: peripheral neuropathy, *fever*, headache, malaise, insomnia, anxiety, *asthenia*, depression, nervousness, dizziness.
CV: chest pain.
EENT: conjunctivitis.
GI: *abdominal pain, diarrhea, nausea, vomiting, anorexia*, dyspepsia, constipation, ***pancreatitis***.
Hematologic: ***neutropenia, thrombocytopenia***, anemia.
Hepatic: ***hepatotoxicity, severe hepatomegaly with steatosis***.
Metabolic: weight loss, ***lactic acidosis***.
Musculoskeletal: *arthralgia, myalgia, back pain.*
Respiratory: *dyspnea.*
Skin: *rash, diaphoresis, pruritus*, maculopapular rash.
Other: *chills.*

Interactions

Drug-drug. *Methadone:* May decrease stavudine absorption and level. Separate dosage times and monitor patient for clinical effect if drugs must be used together.
Zidovudine: May inhibit phosphorylation of stavudine. Avoid using together.

Nursing considerations

• Monitor patient for signs and symptoms of pancreatitis, especially if he takes stavudine with didanosine or hydroxyurea. If patient has pancreatitis, reinstate drug cautiously.
• Monitor liver function test results.
!!ALERT Motor weakness, mimicking the clinical presentation of Guillain-Barré syndrome (including respiratory failure) in HIV patients taking stavudine with other antiretrovirals has been reported. Most of the cases were reported in the setting of lactic acidosis. Monitor patient for factors of lactic acidosis, including generalized fatigue, GI problems, tachypnea, or dyspnea. Symptoms may continue or worsen when drug is stopped. Patients with these symptoms should promptly interrupt antiretroviral therapy and rapidly receive a full medical work-up. Consider permanent discontinuation of stavudine.
!!ALERT Peripheral neuropathy appears to be the major dose-limiting adverse effect of stavudine. It may or may not resolve after drug is stopped.
• Monitor CBC results and creatinine.

Patient teaching

• Tell patient that drug may be taken without regard to meals.
• Warn patient not to take other drugs for HIV or AIDS unless prescriber has approved them.
• Inform patient that drug doesn't cure HIV infection, that opportunistic infections and other complications of HIV infection may still occur, and that transmission of HIV to others through sexual contact or blood contamination is still possible.
• Teach patient signs and symptoms of peripheral neuropathy (pain, burning, aching, weakness, or pins and needles in the limbs) and tell him to report these immediately.
• Tell patient to report symptoms of lactic acidosis, including fatigue, GI problems, dyspnea, or tachypnea.
• Tell patient to report symptoms of pancreatitis, including abdominal pain, nausea, vomiting, weight loss, or fatty stools.
• Tell patient to monitor weight patterns and report weight loss or gain.
• Explain to patient who has difficulty swallowing that extended-release capsules can be opened and contents mixed with 2 tablespoons of yogurt or applesauce. Caution patient not to chew or crush the beads while swallowing.

streptokinase
Streptase

Pregnancy risk category C

Indications & dosages

➲ Arteriovenous cannula occlusion
Adults: 250,000 IU in 2 ml I.V. solution by I.V. pump infusion into each occluded limb of the cannula over 25 to 35 minutes. Clamp off cannula for 2 hours. Then aspirate contents of cannula, flush with normal saline solution, and reconnect.
➲ Venous thrombosis, pulmonary embolism, arterial thrombosis, and embolism
Adults: Loading dose is 250,000 IU by I.V. infusion over 30 minutes. Sustaining dose

is 100,000 IU/hour I.V. infusion for 72 hours for deep vein thrombosis and 100,000 IU/hour over 24 to 72 hours by I.V. infusion pump for pulmonary embolism and arterial thrombosis or embolism.

➲ **Lysis of coronary artery thrombi following acute MI**

Adults: 1.5 million IU infused I.V. over 60 minutes.

Contraindications & cautions

- Contraindicated in patients with ulcerative wounds, active internal bleeding, recent CVA, recent trauma with possible internal injuries, visceral or intracranial malignant neoplasms, ulcerative colitis, diverticulitis, severe hypertension, acute or chronic hepatic or renal insufficiency, uncontrolled hypocoagulation, chronic pulmonary disease with cavitation, subacute bacterial endocarditis or rheumatic valvular disease, previous severe allergic reaction to streptokinase, or recent cerebral embolism, thrombosis, or hemorrhage.
- Contraindicated within 10 days after intra-arterial diagnostic procedure or any surgery, including liver or kidney biopsy, lumbar puncture, thoracentesis, paracentesis, or extensive or multiple cutdowns.
- Contraindicated with I.M. injections and other invasive procedures.
- Use cautiously when treating arterial embolism that originates from left side of heart because of danger of cerebral infarction.

Adverse reactions

CNS: polyradiculoneuropathy, headache, *fever.*

CV: ***reperfusion arrhythmias***, *hypotension*, vasculitis, flushing.

EENT: periorbital edema.

GI: nausea.

Hematologic: ***bleeding***, moderately decreased hematocrit.

Respiratory: minor breathing difficulty, ***bronchospasm***, ***pulmonary edema***.

Skin: urticaria, pruritus.

Other: phlebitis at injection site, hypersensitivity reactions, ***anaphylaxis***, delayed hypersensitivity reactions, ***angioedema***.

Interactions

Drug-drug. *Anticoagulants:* May increase risk of bleeding. Monitor patient closely.

Antifibrinolytic drugs (such as aminocaproic acid): May inhibit and reverse streptokinase activity. Avoid using together.

Aspirin, dipyridamole, drugs affecting platelet activity (abciximab, eptifibatide, tirofiban), indomethacin, phenylbutazone: May increase risk of bleeding. Monitor patient closely.

Nursing considerations

- Drug may be given to menstruating women.
- Only prescribers with experience managing thrombotic disease should use streptokinase. Give drug only where clinical and laboratory monitoring can be performed.
- Before using streptokinase to clear an occluded arteriovenous cannula, try flushing with heparinized saline solution.
- Keep aminocaproic acid available to treat bleeding, and corticosteroids to treat allergic reactions.
- Before starting therapy, draw blood for coagulation studies, hematocrit, platelet count, and type and crossmatching. Rate of I.V. infusion depends on thrombin time and streptokinase resistance.
- To check for hypersensitivity reactions, give 100 IU intradermally; a wheal-and-flare response within 20 minutes means patient is probably allergic. Monitor vital signs frequently.
- If patient has had either a recent streptococcal infection or recent treatment with streptokinase, a higher loading dose may be needed. Consider alternative thrombolytics.
- Combined therapy with low-dose aspirin (162.5 mg) or dipyridamole has improved short- and long-term results.
- Monitor patient for excessive bleeding every 15 minutes for first hour, every 30 minutes for second through eighth hours, and then every 4 hours. If bleeding is evident, stop therapy and notify prescriber. Pretreatment with heparin or drugs that affect platelets causes high risk of bleeding but may improve long-term results.
- Monitor pulse, color, and sensation of arms and legs every hour.
- Keep involved limb in straight alignment to prevent bleeding from infusion site.
- Avoid unnecessary handling of patient; pad side rails. Bruising is more likely during therapy.

- Keep a laboratory flow sheet on patient's chart to monitor PTT, PT, thrombin time, hemoglobin level, and hematocrit. Monitor vital signs and neurologic status.
- Avoid I.M. injection. Keep venipuncture sites to a minimum; use pressure dressing on puncture sites for at least 15 minutes.

!!ALERT Watch for signs of hypersensitivity and notify prescriber immediately if any occur. Antihistamines or corticosteroids may be used to treat mild allergic reactions. If a severe reaction occurs, stop infusion immediately and notify prescriber.

- Thrombolytic therapy in patients with acute MI may decrease infarct size, improve ventricular function, and decrease risk of heart failure. For optimal effect, streptokinase must be given within 6 hours after symptoms start.

Patient teaching

- Explain use and administration of drug to patient and family.
- Tell patient to report adverse reactions promptly.

streptomycin sulfate

Pregnancy risk category D

Indications & dosages

➲ Streptococcal endocarditis

Adults: 1 g q 12 hours I.M. for 1 week; then 500 mg I.M. q 12 hours for 1 week, given with penicillin.

In patients older than age 60, give 500 mg I.M. q 12 hours for entire 2 weeks, with penicillin.

➲ Second-line treatment of tuberculosis (TB), given with other antituberculotics

Adults: 15 mg/kg (maximum of 1 g) I.M. daily, continued long enough to prevent relapse. For intermittent use, 25 to 30 mg/kg (maximum of 1.5 g) two to three times weekly.

Children: 20 to 40 mg/kg (maximum of 1 g) I.M. daily. Give with other antituberculotics, except capreomycin; continue until sputum test result becomes negative. For intermittent use, 25 to 30 mg/kg (maximum of 1.5 g) two to three times weekly.

Adults older than 59: 10 mg/kg I.M. daily.

➲ Enterococcal endocarditis

Adults: 1 g I.M. q 12 hours for 2 weeks; then 500 mg I.M. q 12 hours for 4 weeks, given with penicillin.

➲ Tularemia

Adults: 1 to 2 g I.M. daily in divided doses injected deep into upper outer quadrant of buttocks; continued for 7 to 14 days or until patient is afebrile for 5 to 7 days.

Contraindications & cautions

- Contraindicated in patients hypersensitive to drug or other aminoglycosides.
- Use cautiously in elderly patients and in patients with impaired renal function or neuromuscular disorders.

Adverse reactions

CNS: ***neuromuscular blockade***, vertigo, facial paresthesia.
EENT: *ototoxicity*.
GI: vomiting, nausea.
GU: ***nephrotoxicity***, increase in urinary excretion of casts.
Hematologic: eosinophilia, ***leukopenia***, ***thrombocytopenia***, ***hemolytic anemia***.
Respiratory: ***apnea***.
Skin: exfoliative dermatitis.
Other: hypersensitivity reactions, ***anaphylaxis***.

Interactions

Drug-drug. *Acyclovir, amphotericin B, cephalosporins, cidofovir, cisplatin, methoxyflurane, vancomycin, other aminoglycosides:* May increase nephrotoxicity. Monitor renal function test results.
Atracurium, doxacurium, mivacurium, pancuronium, rocuronium, tubocurarine, vecuronium: May increase effects of nondepolarizing muscle relaxants, including prolonged respiratory depression. Use together only when necessary, and expect to reduce dosage of nondepolarizing muscle relaxant.
General anesthetics: May increase neuromuscular blockade. Monitor patient closely.
I.V. loop diuretics (such as furosemide): May increase ototoxicity. Monitor patient's hearing.

Nursing considerations

- Obtain specimen for culture and sensitivity tests before giving first dose, except

when treating TB. Therapy may begin while awaiting results.
- Evaluate patient's hearing before therapy and for 6 months afterward. Notify prescriber if patient has hearing loss, feels fullness in ears, or hears roaring noises.
- To avoid irritation, protect hands when preparing drug.
- When giving I.M., inject deep into upper outer quadrant of buttocks or midlateral thigh. Rotate injection sites.
- In children, give I.M. injection in midlateral thigh, if possible, to minimize possibility of damaging sciatic nerve.
- Obtain blood for peak streptomycin level 1 to 2 hours after I.M. injection; obtain blood for trough level just before next dose. Don't use a heparinized tube; heparin is incompatible with aminoglycosides.
- Drug has been given as I.V. infusion over 30 to 60 minutes without unusual adverse effects in patients unable to tolerate I.M. injections.
- Watch for signs and symptoms of superinfection, such as continued fever, chills, and increased pulse rate.
- Nephrotoxicity occurs less frequently with streptomycin than with other aminoglycosides.
- When drug is used for primary treatment of TB, stop therapy when sputum test result becomes negative.
- Total dose for TB treatment shouldn't exceed 120 g over the course of therapy unless there are no other treatment options.

Patient teaching
- Instruct patient to report adverse reactions promptly.
- Encourage patient to maintain adequate fluid intake.
- Emphasize need for blood tests to monitor streptomycin levels and determine effectiveness of therapy.

succimer
Chemet

Pregnancy risk category C

Indications & dosages
➲ Lead poisoning in children with lead levels greater than 45 mcg/dl
Children: Initially, 10 mg/kg or 350 mg/m^2 q 8 hours for 5 days. Because capsules come only in 100 mg, round dose to nearest 100 mg, as appropriate (see table). Then reduce frequency of administration to q 12 hours for another 2 weeks.

Weight in kg (lb)	Dose (mg)
> 45 (> 100)	500
35–44 (76–100)	400
24–34 (56–75)	300
16–23 (36–55)	200
8–15 (18–35)	100

Contraindications & cautions
- Contraindicated in patients hypersensitive to drug.
- Use cautiously in patients with compromised renal function.

Adverse reactions
CNS: *drowsiness, dizziness, sensorimotor neuropathy, sleepiness, paresthesia, headache.*
CV: ***arrhythmias.***
EENT: plugged ears, cloudy film in eyes, otitis media, watery eyes, sore throat, rhinorrhea, nasal congestion.
GI: *nausea, vomiting, diarrhea, anorexia, abdominal cramps, hemorrhoidal symptoms, metallic taste in mouth, loose stools.*
GU: decreased urination, difficult urination, proteinuria.
Hematologic: increased platelet count, intermittent eosinophilia, ***neutropenia.***
Musculoskeletal: *leg, kneecap, back, stomach, rib, or flank pain.*
Respiratory: cough, head cold.
Skin: papular rash, herpetic rash, mucocutaneous eruptions, pruritus.
Other: *flulike syndrome,* candidiasis.

Interactions
Drug-drug. *Other chelating drugs (such as calcium EDTA):* May cause unknown ad-

verse effects. Separate administration times by 4 weeks.

Nursing considerations

- Measure severity of poisoning by initial lead level and by rate and degree of rebound of lead level. Use severity as a guide for more frequent lead monitoring.
- Monitor patient at least once weekly for rebound lead levels. Elevated levels and associated symptoms may return rapidly after drug is stopped because of redistribution of lead from bone to soft tissues and blood.
- Monitor transaminase levels before and at least weekly during therapy. Transient mild elevations may occur.
- Course of treatment lasts 19 days and may be repeated if indicated by weekly monitoring of lead levels.
- Minimum of 2 weeks between courses is recommended unless high lead levels indicate need for immediate therapy.
- Don't give with other chelating drugs. Patient who has received edetate calcium disodium with or without dimercaprol may use succimer after a 4-week interval.

Patient teaching

- Explain drug use and administration to parents and child. Stress importance of complying with frequent blood tests.
- Tell parents of young child who can't swallow capsules that capsule can be opened and its contents sprinkled on a small amount of soft food. Or, beads from capsule may be poured on a spoon and followed with flavored beverage.
- Tell parents to give child adequate fluids.
- Assist parents with identifying and removing sources of lead in child's environment. Chelation therapy isn't a substitute for preventing further exposure.
- Tell parents to notify prescriber if rash occurs. Tell them allergic or other mucocutaneous reactions may occur each time drug is used.

sucralfate
Carafate

Pregnancy risk category B

Indications & dosages

➲ Short-term (up to 8 weeks) treatment of duodenal ulcer
Adults: 1 g P.O. q.i.d. 1 hour before meals and h.s.

➲ Maintenance therapy for duodenal ulcer
Adults: 1 g P.O. b.i.d.

Contraindications & cautions

- Use cautiously in patients with chronic renal failure.

Adverse reactions

CNS: dizziness, sleepiness, headache, vertigo.
GI: *constipation,* nausea, gastric discomfort, diarrhea, bezoar formation, vomiting, flatulence, dry mouth, indigestion.
Musculoskeletal: back pain.
Skin: rash, pruritus.

Interactions

Drug-drug. *Antacids:* May decrease binding of drug to gastroduodenal mucosa, impairing effectiveness. Separate doses by 30 minutes.
Cimetidine, digoxin, fosphenytoin, ketoconazole, phenytoin, quinidine, ranitidine, tetracycline, theophylline: May decrease absorption. Separate doses by at least 2 hours.
Ciprofloxacin, lomefloxacin, moxifloxacin, norfloxacin, ofloxacin: May decrease absorption of these drugs, reducing antiinfective response. If use together can't be avoided, give at least 6 hours apart.

Nursing considerations

- Reconstitute drug before instillation through a nasogastric tube. Flush tube with water to ensure passage into stomach.
- Drug is minimally absorbed and causes few adverse reactions.
- Monitor patient for severe, persistent constipation.
- Sucralfate is as effective as cimetidine in healing duodenal ulcer.

• Drug contains aluminum but isn't classified as an antacid. Monitor patient with renal insufficiency for aluminum toxicity.

Patient teaching

• Tell patient to take sucralfate on an empty stomach, 1 hour before each meal and h.s.
• Instruct patient to continue prescribed regimen to ensure complete healing. Pain and other ulcer signs and symptoms may subside within first few weeks of therapy.
• Urge patient to avoid cigarette smoking, which may increase gastric acid secretion and worsen disease.
• Antacids may be used while taking sucralfate, but separate antacid and sucralfate doses by 30 minutes.

sulfacetamide sodium 10%

AK-Sulf, Bleph-10, Cetamide, OcuSulf-10, Sodium Sulamyd Ophthalmic, Storz Sulf, Sulf-10 Ophthalmic

sulfacetamide sodium 15%

Isopto-Cetamide Ophthalmic

sulfacetamide sodium 30%

Sodium Sulamyd Ophthalmic

Pregnancy risk category C

Indications & dosages

➲ **Inclusion conjunctivitis, corneal ulcers, chlamydial infection**
Adults and children: 1 or 2 drops of 10% solution into lower conjunctival sac q 2 to 3 hours during day, less often at night. Or, 1 or 2 drops of 15% solution instilled into lower conjunctival sac q 1 to 2 hours initially. Increase interval as condition responds. Or, instill 1 drop of 30% solution into lower conjunctival sac q 2 hours. Apply 0.5 inch of 10% ointment into conjunctival sac t.i.d. to q.i.d. and h.s. Ointment may be used at night along with drops during the day.
➲ **Trachoma**
Adults and children: 2 drops of 30% solution into lower conjunctival sac q 2 hours with systemic sulfonamide or tetracycline.

Contraindications & cautions

• Contraindicated in patients hypersensitive to sulfonamides and children younger than age 2 months.
• Contraindicated in epithelial herpes simplex keratitis, vaccinia, varicella, and many other viral diseases of the cornea and conjunctiva; in mycobacterial or fungal diseases of ocular structures; and after uncomplicated removal of a corneal foreign body (corticosteroid combinations).

Adverse reactions

EENT: slowed corneal wound healing with ointment, pain on instillation of eyedrops, headache or brow pain, photophobia, periorbital edema, eye itching, burning.
Other: overgrowth of nonsusceptible organisms.

Interactions

Drug-drug. *Gentamicin (ophthalmic):* May cause in vitro antagonism. Avoid using together.
Local anesthetics (procaine, tetracaine), PABA derivatives: May decrease sulfacetamide sodium action. Wait 30 minutes to 1 hour after instilling anesthetic or PABA derivative before instilling sulfacetamide.
Silver preparations: May cause precipitate formation. Avoid using together.
Drug-lifestyle. *Sun exposure:* May cause photophobia. Advise patient to avoid excessive sunlight exposure.

Nursing considerations

• Drug is often used with oral tetracycline to treat trachoma and inclusion conjunctivitis.
• Store drug away from heat in tightly closed, light-resistant container.

Patient teaching

• Tell patient to clean excessive discharge from eye area before application.
• Teach patient how to instill drops or apply ointment. Advise him to wash hands before and after applying ointment or solution and not to touch tip of dropper to eye or surrounding tissue.
• Instruct patient to apply light finger pressure on lacrimal sac for 1 minute after drops are instilled.
• Warn patient that eyedrops burn slightly.

- Advise patient to watch for and report signs and symptoms of sensitivity (itching lids, swelling, or constant burning).
- Tell patient to wait at least 5 minutes before instilling other eyedrops.
- Warn patient that solution may stain clothing.
- Tell patient to minimize sensitivity to sunlight by wearing sunglasses and avoiding prolonged exposure to sunlight.
- Advise patient not to use discolored solution.
- Tell patient not to share drug, washcloths, or towels with family members and to notify prescriber if anyone develops same signs or symptoms.
- Stress importance of compliance with recommended therapy.
- Advise patient to alert prescriber if no improvement occurs.

sulfinpyrazone

Antazone†, Anturane, Apo sulfinpyrazone†, Novo-Pyrazone†, Nu-sulfinpyrazone†

Pregnancy risk category NR

Indications & dosages

➲ **Intermittent or chronic gouty arthritis**
Adults: 200 to 400 mg P.O. b.i.d. first week; then 200 mg P.O. b.i.d. Maximum dose is 800 mg daily.

➲ **To decrease the risk of sudden cardiac death 1 to 6 months after an MI♦**
Adults: 300 mg P.O. q.i.d.

Contraindications & cautions

- Contraindicated in patients hypersensitive to pyrazole derivatives (including oxyphenbutazone and phenylbutazone) and in those with blood dyscrasias, active peptic ulcer, or symptoms of GI inflammation or ulceration.
- Use cautiously in patients with healed peptic ulcer and in pregnant women.

Adverse reactions

GI: *nausea, dyspepsia,* epigastric pain, reactivation of peptic ulcerations.
Hematologic: anemia, ***leukopenia, agranulocytosis, thrombocytopenia, aplastic anemia.***
Respiratory: ***bronchoconstriction in patients with aspirin-induced asthma.***
Skin: rash.

Interactions

Drug-drug. *Aspirin, niacin, salicylates:* May inhibit uricosuric effect of sulfinpyrazone. Avoid using together.
Oral anticoagulants: May increase anticoagulant effect and risk of bleeding. Use together cautiously.
Oral antidiabetics: May increase effects of these drugs. Monitor glucose level.
Probenecid: May inhibit renal excretion of sulfinpyrazone. Use together cautiously.
Theophylline, verapamil: May increase clearance of these drugs. Use together cautiously.
Drug-lifestyle. *Alcohol use:* May decrease effectiveness. Discourage use together.

Nursing considerations

- Monitor BUN, CBC, and renal function studies periodically during long-term use.
- Monitor fluid intake and output closely. Therapy, especially at start, may lead to renal colic and formation of uric acid stones until acid levels are normal (about 6 mg/dl).
- Force fluids to maintain minimum daily output of 2 to 3 L. Alkalinize urine with sodium bicarbonate or other drug.
- Drug has no anti-inflammatory or analgesic effects and is of no value during acute gout attacks.
- Drug may increase frequency, severity, and length of acute gout attacks during first 6 to 12 months of therapy. Colchicine or another anti-inflammatory may be used preventively during first 3 to 6 months.
- Lifelong therapy may be needed in patients with hyperuricemia.

!!ALERT Don't confuse Anturane with Accutane, Artane, or Antabuse.

Patient teaching

- Instruct patient and family that drug must be taken regularly, even during acute exacerbations.
- Tell patient to take drug with food, milk, or antacids to reduce GI upset.
- Tell patient to visit prescriber regularly so blood levels can be monitored and dosage adjusted, if needed.
- Warn patient with gout not to take aspirin-containing drugs because these may precipitate gout. Acetaminophen may be used for pain.

• Tell patient with gout to avoid foods high in purine, such as anchovies, liver, sardines, kidneys, sweetbreads, peas, and lentils, and to identify and avoid any other foods that may trigger gout attacks.
• Instruct patient to drink at least 10 to 12 glasses of fluid daily.
• Advise patient to avoid alcohol during therapy.
• Instruct patient to report unusual bleeding, bruising, or flulike symptoms.

sulindac
Apo-Sulin†, Clinoril, Novo-Sundac†

Pregnancy risk category B; D in 3rd trimester

Indications & dosages
➲ Osteoarthritis, rheumatoid arthritis, ankylosing spondylitis
Adults: Initially, 150 mg P.O. b.i.d.; increase to 200 mg b.i.d., p.r.n. Maximum dose is 400 mg daily.
➲ Acute subacromial bursitis or supraspinatus tendinitis, acute gouty arthritis
Adults: 200 mg P.O. b.i.d. for 7 to 14 days. Reduce dosage as symptoms subside. Maximum dose is 400 mg daily.

Contraindications & cautions
• Contraindicated in patients hypersensitive to drug and in those for whom aspirin or NSAIDs precipitate acute asthmatic attacks, urticaria, or rhinitis.
• Don't use drug in pregnant women.
• Use cautiously in patients with a history of ulcers and GI bleeding, renal dysfunction, compromised cardiac function, hypertension, or conditions predisposing to fluid retention.

Adverse reactions
CNS: dizziness, headache, nervousness, psychosis.
CV: hypertension, ***heart failure***, palpitations, edema.
EENT: tinnitus, transient visual disturbances.
GI: *epigastric distress*, peptic ulceration, occult blood loss, nausea, constipation, dyspepsia, flatulence, anorexia, GI bleeding.
GU: interstitial nephritis.
Hematologic: prolonged bleeding time.
Metabolic: ***hyperkalemia***.
Skin: rash, pruritus.
Other: drug fever, ***anaphylaxis***, ***angioedema***, hypersensitivity reactions.

Interactions
Drug-drug. *Anticoagulants:* May cause bleeding. Monitor PT and INR closely.
Aspirin: May decrease sulindac level and increase risk of GI adverse reactions. Avoid using together.
Cyclosporine: May increase nephrotoxicity of cyclosporine. Avoid using together.
Diflunisal, dimethyl sulfoxide: May hinder metabolism of sulindac to its metabolite, reducing its effectiveness. Avoid using together.
Methotrexate: May increase methotrexate toxicity. Avoid using together.
Probenecid: May increase levels of sulindac and its metabolite. Monitor patient for toxicity.
Sulfonamides, sulfonylureas, other highly protein-bound drugs: May cause these drugs to be displaced from protein-binding sites, increasing toxicity. Monitor patient closely.
Drug-herb. *Dong quai, feverfew, garlic, ginger, horse chestnut, red clover:* May cause bleeding, based on the known effects of components. Discourage use together.
White willow: Herb contains components similar to those of aspirin. Discourage use together.
Drug-lifestyle. *Alcohol use:* May increase risk of adverse GI reactions. Discourage use together.

Nursing considerations
• Periodically monitor hepatic and renal function and CBC in patient receiving long-term therapy.
• Serious GI toxicity, including peptic ulcers and bleeding, can occur in patient taking NSAIDs, despite lack of symptoms.
• NSAIDs may mask signs and symptoms of infection.

Patient teaching
• Tell patient to take drug with food, milk, or antacids.
• Teach patient signs and symptoms of GI bleeding, including blood in vomit, urine, or stool; coffee-ground vomit; and black, tarry stool. Tell him to notify prescriber immediately if any of these occurs.

!!ALERT Tell patient to notify prescriber immediately if easy bruising or prolonged bleeding occurs.

- Advise patient to avoid hazardous activities that require mental alertness until CNS effects are known.
- Instruct patient to report edema and have blood pressure checked monthly. Drug causes sodium retention but is thought to have less effect on the kidneys than other NSAIDs.
- Advise patient to notify prescriber and have complete eye examination if visual disturbances occur.
- Advise patient that use of OTC NSAIDs in combination with sulindac may increase the risk of GI toxicity.

sumatriptan succinate
Imitrex

Pregnancy risk category C

Indications & dosages

➲ Acute migraine attacks (with or without aura)

Adults: For injection, 6 mg S.C. Maximum dose is two 6-mg injections in 24 hours, separated by at least 1 hour.

For tablets, 25 to 100 mg P.O., initially. If desired response isn't achieved in 2 hours, may give second dose of 25 to 100 mg. Additional doses may be used in at least 2-hour intervals. Maximum daily dose, 200 mg.

For nasal spray, give 5 mg, 10 mg, or 20 mg once in one nostril; may repeat once after 2 hours, for maximum daily dose of 40 mg. A 10-mg dose may be achieved by giving a 5-mg dose in each nostril.

➲ Cluster headache

Adults: 6 mg S.C. Maximum recommended dose is two 6-mg injections in 24 hours, separated by at least 1 hour.

In patients with hepatic impairment, the maximum single oral dose shouldn't exceed 50 mg.

Contraindications & cautions

- Contraindicated in patients with hypersensitivity to drug or its components; those with history, symptoms, or signs of ischemic cardiac, cerebrovascular (such as CVA or transient ischemic attack), or peripheral vascular syndromes (such as ischemic bowel disease); significant underlying CV diseases, including angina pectoris, MI, and silent myocardial ischemia; uncontrolled hypertension; or severe hepatic impairment.
- Contraindicated within 24 hours of another 5-HT agonist or drug containing ergotamine and within 2 weeks of MAO inhibitor.

Adverse reactions

CNS: *dizziness, vertigo,* drowsiness, headache, anxiety, malaise, fatigue.
CV: ***atrial fibrillation, ventricular fibrillation, ventricular tachycardia, coronary artery vasospasm, transient myocardial ischemia, MI,*** pressure or tightness in chest.
EENT: discomfort of throat, nasal cavity or sinus, mouth, jaw, or tongue, altered vision.
GI: abdominal discomfort, dysphagia, diarrhea, nausea, vomiting, unusual or bad taste (nasal spray).
Musculoskeletal: myalgia, muscle cramps, neck pain.
Respiratory: upper respiratory inflammation and dyspnea (P.O.).
Skin: diaphoresis, flushing, *tingling, injection site reaction,* (S.C.).
Other: *warm or hot sensation, burning sensation,* heaviness, pressure or tightness, tight feeling in head, cold sensation, numbness.

Interactions

Drug-drug. *Ergot and ergot derivatives, other 5-HT_1 agonists:* May prolong vasospastic effects. Don't use within 24 hours of sumatriptan therapy.
MAO inhibitors: May reduce sumatriptan clearance. Avoid using within 2 weeks of MAO inhibitor. Use injection cautiously and decrease sumatriptan dose.
SSRIs: May cause weakness, hyperreflexia, and incoordination. Monitor patient closely if use together can't be avoided.
Drug-herb. *Horehound:* May enhance serotonergic effects. Discourage use together.

Nursing considerations

- Use cautiously in patient who is or may become pregnant.
- Use cautiously in patient with risk factors for coronary artery disease (CAD), such as postmenopausal women, men older than age 40, or patients with hypertension, hy-

percholesterolemia, obesity, diabetes, smoking, or family history of CAD.

!!ALERT When giving drug to patient at risk for CAD, consider giving first dose in presence of other medical personnel. Serious adverse cardiac effects can follow administration of drug, but such events are rare.

- After S.C. injection, most patients experience relief in 1 to 2 hours.
- Redness or pain at injection site should subside within 1 hour after injection.

!!ALERT Don't confuse sumatriptan with somatropin.

Patient teaching

- Inform patient that drug is intended only to treat migraine attacks, not to prevent them or reduce their occurrence.
- If patient is pregnant or may become pregnant, tell her not to use drug but to discuss with prescriber the risks and benefits of using drug during pregnancy.
- Tell patient that drug may be taken any time during a migraine attack, as soon as signs or symptoms appear.
- Review information about drug's injectable form, which is available in a spring-loaded injector system for easier patient use. Make sure patient understands how to load the injector, give the injection, and dispose of used syringes.

!!ALERT Tell patient to tell prescriber immediately about persistent or severe chest pain. Warn him to stop using drug and to call prescriber if he develops pain or tightness in the throat, wheezing, heart throbbing, rash, lumps, hives, or swollen eyelids, face, or lips.

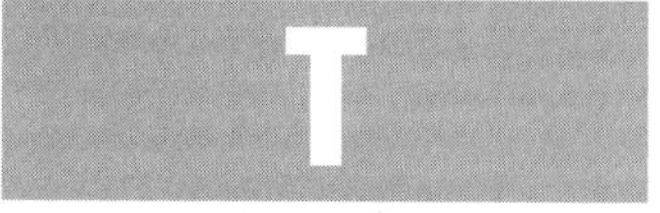

tacrine hydrochloride
Cognex

Pregnancy risk category C

Indications & dosages

➲ Mild to moderate Alzheimer's dementia

Adults: Initially, 10 mg P.O. q.i.d. After 4 weeks, if patient tolerates treatment and has no increase in transaminase levels, increase dosage to 20 mg q.i.d. After an additional 4 weeks, increase to 30 mg q.i.d. If still tolerated, increase dosage to 40 mg q.i.d. after another 4 weeks.

Contraindications & cautions

- Contraindicated in patients hypersensitive to drug or to acridine derivatives.
- Contraindicated in patients for whom tacrine-related jaundice has previously been confirmed, with a total bilirubin level of more than 3 mg/dl.
- Use cautiously in patients with sick sinus syndrome or bradycardia, in patients at risk for peptic ulcers (including those taking NSAIDs or those with history of peptic ulcer), and in those with a history of hepatic disease.
- Use cautiously in patients with renal disease, asthma, prostatic hyperplasia, or other urine outflow impairment.

Adverse reactions

CNS: agitation, ataxia, insomnia, abnormal thinking, somnolence, depression, anxiety, *headache*, fatigue, *dizziness*, confusion.
CV: chest pain.
EENT: rhinitis.
GI: *nausea, vomiting, diarrhea*, dyspepsia, loose stools, changes in stool color, anorexia, abdominal pain, flatulence, constipation.
Hepatic: LIVER TOXICITY .
Metabolic: weight loss.
Musculoskeletal: myalgia.
Respiratory: upper respiratory tract infection, cough.
Skin: rash, jaundice, facial flushing.

Interactions

Drug-drug. *Anticholinergics:* May lessen the effects of tacrine. Avoid using together.
Cholinergics such as bethanechol, anticholinesterases: May have additive effects. Monitor patient for toxicity.
Cimetidine, ciprofloxacin, fluvoxamine, ritonavir: May increase tacrine level. Monitor patient for adverse effects.
Succinylcholine: May enhance neuromuscular blockade and prolong duration of action. Monitor patient closely.
Theophylline: May increase theophylline level and prolong theophylline half-life.

Carefully monitor theophylline level and adjust dosage.

Drug-food. *Any food:* May delay drug absorption. Give drug 1 hour before meals.

Drug-lifestyle. *Smoking:* May decrease drug level. Ask patient about nicotine use, and monitor him closely.

Nursing considerations

- Monitor ALT level weekly during first 18 weeks of therapy. If ALT is modestly elevated (twice the upper limit of normal range) after first 18 weeks, continue weekly monitoring. If no problems are detected, ALT tests may be decreased to once every 3 months. Each time dosage is increased, resume weekly monitoring for at least 6 weeks.
- If drug is stopped for 4 weeks or longer, full dosage adjustment and monitoring schedule must be restarted.

Patient teaching

- Stress that drug doesn't alter the underlying degenerative disease but can stabilize or alleviate symptoms. Effect of therapy depends on regular drug administration.

!!ALERT Remind caregiver that dosage adjustment is an integral part of safe drug use. Abrupt discontinuation or a large reduction in daily dosage (80 mg daily or more) may cause behavioral disturbances and a decline in cognitive function.

- Tell caregiver to give drug between meals whenever possible. If GI upset becomes a problem, drug may be taken with meals, although doing so may reduce plasma levels by 30% to 40%.
- Advise patient and caregiver to immediately report significant adverse reactions or changes in status.

tacrolimus (FK506)

Prograf

Pregnancy risk category C

Indications & dosages

➲ To prevent organ rejection in allogenic liver or kidney transplants

Adults: 0.03 to 0.05 mg/kg daily I.V. as continuous infusion given no sooner than 6 hours after transplantation. Substitute P.O. therapy as soon as possible, with first oral dose given 8 to 12 hours after stopping I.V. infusion. Or, give P.O. dose within 24 hours of transplantation after renal function has recovered. Recommended first P.O. dosage for allogenic liver transplants is 0.1 to 0.15 mg/kg daily P.O. in two divided doses q 12 hours. Recommended first P.O. dosage for allogenic kidney transplants is 0.2 mg/kg daily in two divided doses q 12 hours. Adjust dosages based on clinical response.

Children: Initially, 0.03 to 0.05 mg/kg daily I.V.; then 0.15 to 0.2 mg/kg daily P.O. on schedule similar to that of adults, adjusted p.r.n.

Give lowest recommended P.O. and I.V. dosages to patients with renal or hepatic impairment.

Contraindications & cautions

- Contraindicated in patients hypersensitive to drug.
- I.V. form is contraindicated in patients hypersensitive to castor oil derivatives.

Adverse reactions

CNS: *headache, tremor, insomnia, paresthesia, delirium,* ***coma****, fever, asthenia.*

CV: hypertension, *peripheral edema.*

GI: *diarrhea, nausea, vomiting, constipation, anorexia, abdominal pain, ascites.*

GU: *abnormal renal function, UTI, oliguria.*

Hematologic: *anemia, leukocytosis,* THROMBOCYTOPENIA.

Metabolic: *hyperkalemia, hypokalemia, hyperglycemia, hypomagnesemia.*

Musculoskeletal: *back pain.*

Respiratory: *pleural effusion, atelectasis, dyspnea.*

Skin: *pruritus, burning, rash, photosensitivity,* alopecia.

Other: *pain.*

Interactions

Drug-drug. *Bromocriptine, cimetidine, clarithromycin, clotrimazole, cyclosporine, danazol, diltiazem, erythromycin, fluconazole, itraconazole, ketoconazole, methylprednisolone, metoclopramide, nicardipine, verapamil:* May increase tacrolimus level. Watch for adverse effects.

Carbamazepine, phenobarbital, phenytoin, rifabutin, rifampin: May decrease tacrolimus level. Monitor effectiveness of tacrolimus.

Cyclosporine: May increase risk of excess nephrotoxicity. Avoid using together.
Immunosuppressants (except adrenal corticosteroids): May oversuppress immune system. Monitor patient closely, especially during times of stress.
Inducers of cytochrome P-450 enzyme system: May increase tacrolimus metabolism and decrease blood levels. Dosage adjustment may be needed.
Inhibitors of cytochrome P-450 enzyme system (phenobarbital, phenytoin, rifampin): May decrease tacrolimus metabolism and increase blood level. Dosage adjustment may be needed.
Live-virus vaccines: May interfere with immune response to live-virus vaccines. Postpone routine immunizations.
Nephrotoxic drugs (such as aminoglycosides, amphotericin B, cisplatin, cyclosporine): May cause additive or synergistic effects. Monitor patient closely.
Drug-food. *Any food:* May inhibit drug absorption. Urge patient to take drug on empty stomach.
Grapefruit juice: May increase drug level. Discourage patient from taking together.

Nursing considerations

!!ALERT Because of risk of anaphylaxis, use injection only in patients who can't take oral form.
- Keep epinephrine 1:1,000 and oxygen available to treat anaphylaxis.
- Children with normal renal and hepatic function may need higher dosages than adults.
- Patients with hepatic or renal dysfunction should receive lowest dosage possible.
- Expect to give adrenal corticosteroids with drug.
- Monitor patient for signs and symptoms of neurotoxicity and nephrotoxicity, especially if patient is receiving a high dose or has renal or hepatic dysfunction.
- Monitor patient for signs and symptoms of hyperkalemia, such as palpitations and muscle weakness or cramping. Obtain potassium levels regularly. Avoid potassium-sparing diuretics during drug therapy.
- Monitor patient's glucose level regularly. Also monitor patient for signs and symptoms of hyperglycemia, such as dizziness, confusion, and frequent urination. Treatment of hyperglycemia may be needed. Insulin-dependent posttransplant diabetes may occur; in some cases, it's reversible.
- Patient receiving drug is at increased risk for infections, lymphomas, and other malignant diseases.

Patient teaching

- Advise patient to check with prescriber before taking other drugs during therapy.
- Urge patient to report adverse reactions promptly.
- Tell diabetic patient that glucose levels may increase.

tacrolimus (topical)
Protopic

Pregnancy risk category C

Indications & dosages

➲ **Moderate to severe atopic dermatitis in patients unresponsive to other therapies or unable to use other therapies because of potential risks**
Adults: Thin layer of 0.03% or 0.1% strength applied to affected areas b.i.d. and rubbed in completely. Continue for 1 week after affected area clears.
Children age 2 and older: Thin layer of 0.03% strength applied to affected areas b.i.d. and rubbed in completely. Continue for 1 week after affected area clears.

Contraindications & cautions

- Contraindicated in patients hypersensitive to drug.
- Don't use in patients with Netherton's syndrome or generalized erythroderma.

!!ALERT Use only after other therapies have failed because of the risk of cancer.

Adverse reactions

CNS: *headache*, hyperesthesia, asthenia, insomnia.
CV: peripheral edema.
EENT: *otitis media*, *pharyngitis*, rhinitis, sinusitis, conjunctivitis.
GI: diarrhea, vomiting, nausea, abdominal pain, gastroenteritis, dyspepsia.
GU: dysmenorrhea.
Musculoskeletal: back pain, myalgia.
Respiratory: *increased cough*, *asthma*, pneumonia, bronchitis.

Skin: *burning, pruritus, erythema, infection, herpes simplex,* eczema herpeticum, pustular rash, *folliculitis,* urticaria, maculopapular rash, fungal dermatitis, acne, sunburn, tingling, benign skin neoplasm, vesiculobullous rash, dry skin, varicella zoster, herpes zoster, eczema, exfoliative dermatitis, contact dermatitis.
Other: *flulike symptoms, accidental injury, infection,* facial edema, alcohol intolerance, periodontal abscess, cyst, *allergic reaction, fever,* pain, lymphadenopathy.

Interactions

Drug-drug. *Calcium channel blockers, cimetidine, CYP3A4 inhibitors (erythromycin, itraconazole, ketoconazole, fluconazole):* May interfere with effects of tacrolimus. Use together cautiously.
Drug-lifestyle. *Sun exposure:* May cause phototoxicity. Advise patient to avoid excessive sunlight or artificial ultraviolet light exposure.

Nursing considerations

- Use drug only for short-term or intermittent long-term therapy.
- In patients with infected atopic dermatitis, clear infections at treatment site before using drug.
- Don't use with occlusive dressings.
- Use of this drug may increase the risk of varicella zoster, herpes simplex virus, and eczema herpeticum.
- Consider stopping drug in patients with lymphadenopathy if cause is unknown or acute mononucleosis is diagnosed.
- Monitor all cases of lymphadenopathy until resolution.
- Local adverse effects are most common during the first few days of treatment.
- Use only the 0.03% ointment in children ages 2 to 15.

Patient teaching

- Tell patient to wash hands before and after applying drug and to avoid applying drug to wet skin.
- Urge patient not to use bandages or other occlusive dressings.
- Tell patient not to bathe, shower, or swim immediately after application because doing so could wash the ointment off.
- Tell patient to continue treatment for 1 week after affected area clears.
- Advise patient to avoid or minimize exposure to natural or artificial sunlight.
- Caution patient not to use drug for any disorder other than that for which it was prescribed.
- Encourage patient to report adverse reactions.
- Tell patient to store the ointment at room temperature.

tadalafil
Cialis

Pregnancy risk category B

Indications & dosages

➲ **Erectile dysfunction**
Adults: 10 mg P.O. as a single dose, p.r.n., before sexual activity. Range is 5 to 20 mg, based on effectiveness and tolerance. Maximum is one dose daily.

If creatinine clearance is 31 to 50 ml/minute, starting dosage is 5 mg once daily and maximum is 10 mg once q 48 hours. If clearance is 30 ml/minute or less, maximum is 5 mg once daily. Patients with Child-Pugh category A or B shouldn't exceed 10 mg daily. Patients taking potent Cytochrome P-450 inhibitors (such as erythromycin, itraconazole, ketoconazole, and ritonavir) shouldn't exceed one 10-mg dose q 72 hours.

Contraindications & cautions

- Contraindicated in patients hypersensitive to drug or its components and in those taking nitrates or alpha blockers (other than tamsulosin 0.4 mg once daily).
- Drug isn't recommended for patients with Child-Pugh category C, unstable angina, angina that occurs during sexual intercourse, New York Heart Association class II or greater heart failure within past 6 months, uncontrolled arrhythmias, hypotension (lower than 90/50 mm Hg), uncontrolled hypertension (higher than 170/100 mm Hg), CVA within past 6 months, or an MI within past 90 days.
- Drug isn't recommended for patients whose cardiac status makes sexual activity inadvisable or for those with hereditary degenerative retinal disorders.
- Use cautiously in patients taking potent Cytochrome P-450 inhibitors (such as eryth-

romycin, itraconazole, ketoconazole, and ritonavir) and in patients with bleeding disorders, significant peptic ulceration, or renal or hepatic impairment.
- Use cautiously in patients with conditions predisposing them to priapism (such as sickle cell anemia, multiple myeloma, and leukemia), anatomical penis abnormalities, or left ventricular outflow obstruction.
- Use cautiously in elderly patients, who may be more sensitive to drug effects.

Adverse reactions

CNS: *headache.*
CV: flushing.
EENT: nasal congestion.
GI: *dyspepsia.*
Musculoskeletal: back pain, limb pain, myalgia.

Interactions

Drug-drug. *Alpha blockers (except tamsulosin 0.4 mg daily), nitrates:* May enhance hypotensive effects. Use together is contraindicated.
Potent cytochrome P-450 inhibitors (such as erythromycin, itraconazole, ketoconazole, ritonavir): May increase tadalafil level. Patient shouldn't exceed a 10-mg dose q 72 hours.
Rifampin and other cytochrome P-450 inducers: May decrease tadalafil level. Monitor patient closely.
Drug-food. *Grapefruit:* May increase tadalafil level. Discourage use together.
Drug-lifestyle. *Alcohol use:* May increase risk of headache, dizziness, orthostatic hypotension, and increased heart rate. Discourage use together.

Nursing considerations

!!ALERT Sexual activity may increase cardiac risk. Evaluate patient's cardiac risk before he starts taking drug.
- Before patient starts drug, assess him for underlying causes of erectile dysfunction.
- Transient decreases in supine blood pressure may occur.
- Prolonged erections and priapism may occur.

Patient teaching

- Warn patient that taking drug with nitrates could cause a serious drop in blood pressure, which increases the risk of heart attack or stroke.
- Tell patient to seek immediate medical attention if chest pain develops after taking the drug.
- Tell patient that drug doesn't protect against sexually transmitted diseases and that he should use protective measures.
- Urge patient to seek emergency medical care if his erection lasts more than 4 hours.
- Tell patient to take drug about 60 minutes before anticipated sexual activity. Explain that drug has no effect without sexual stimulation.
- Warn patient not to change dosage unless directed by prescriber.
- Caution patient against drinking large amounts of alcohol while taking drug.

tamoxifen citrate

Nolvadex, Novo-Tamoxifen†, Tamofen†, Tamone†

Pregnancy risk category D

Indications & dosages

➲ **Advanced breast cancer in women and men**
Adults: 20 mg to 40 mg P.O. daily; divide doses greater than 20 mg per day b.i.d.
➲ **Adjunct treatment of breast cancer in women**
Adults: 20 mg to 40 mg P.O. daily for 5 years; divide doses greater than 20 mg per day b.i.d.
➲ **To reduce breast cancer occurrence in high-risk women**
Adults: 20 mg P.O. daily for 5 years.
➲ **Ductal carcinoma in situ (DCIS) after breast surgery and radiation**
Adults: 20 mg P.O. daily for 5 years.
➲ **McCune-Albright syndrome and precocious puberty♦**
Children ages 2 to 10: 20 mg P.O. daily. Treat for up to 12 months.
➲ **To stimulate ovulation♦**
Adults: 5 to 40 mg P.O. b.i.d. for 4 days.
➲ **Mastalgia♦**
Adults: 10 mg P.O. daily for 10 months.

Contraindications & cautions

- Contraindicated in patients hypersensitive to drug. Also contraindicated as therapy to reduce risk of breast cancer in high-risk

women who also need coumarin-type anticoagulant therapy or in women with history of deep vein thrombosis or pulmonary embolism.
- Use cautiously in patients with leukopenia or thrombocytopenia. Monitor CBC closely.

Adverse reactions

CNS: confusion, weakness, sleepiness, headache, ***CVA***.
CV: *fluid retention*, ***thromboembolism***, *hot flashes*.
EENT: corneal changes, cataracts, retinopathy.
GI: *nausea, vomiting, diarrhea*.
GU: *vaginal discharge*, vaginal bleeding, *irregular menses, amenorrhea*, ***endometrial cancer, uterine sarcoma***.
Hematologic: ***leukopenia, thrombocytopenia***.
Hepatic: fatty liver, cholestasis, ***hepatic necrosis***.
Metabolic: *hypercalcemia, weight gain or loss*.
Musculoskeletal: brief worsening of pain from osseous metastases.
Respiratory: ***pulmonary embolism***.
Skin: *skin changes*, rash.
Other: temporary bone or tumor pain, alopecia.

Interactions

Drug-drug. *Antacids:* May affect absorption of enteric-coated tablet. Separate doses by 2 hours.
Bromocriptine: May elevate tamoxifen level. Monitor patient closely.
Coumarin-type anticoagulants: May cause significant increase in anticoagulant effect. Monitor patient, PT, and INR closely.
Cytotoxic drugs: May increase risk of thromboembolic events. Monitor patient.
CYP3A4 inducers (such as rifampin): May increase tamoxifen metabolism and lower drug levels. Monitor patient for clinical effects.

Nursing considerations

- Monitor lipid levels during long-term therapy in patients with hyperlipidemia.
- Monitor calcium level. At start of therapy, drug may compound hypercalcemia related to bone metastases.
- Patient should have baseline and periodic gynecologic examinations because of the small increased risk of endometrial cancer.
- Rule out pregnancy before treatment begins.
- Patient may initially experience worsening symptoms.
- Adverse reactions are usually minor and well tolerated.
- Variations on karyopyknotic index in vaginal smears and various degrees of estrogen effect on Papanicolaou smears may occur in postmenopausal patients.

!!ALERT Women at high risk for breast cancer or who have DCIS taking tamoxifen to reduce risk may experience serious, life-threatening, or fatal endometrial cancer, uterine sarcoma, stroke, and pulmonary embolism. Prescriber should discuss with these patients the benefits of the drug versus the risks of these serious events. The benefits of tamoxifen outweigh its risks in women already diagnosed with breast cancer.

Patient teaching

- For patient taking enteric-coated Nolvadex-D tablets, tell him to swallow them whole without crushing or chewing. Tell him not to take antacids within 2 hours of dose.
- Reassure patient that acute worsening of bone pain during therapy usually indicates drug will produce good response. Recommend analgesics to relieve pain.
- Strongly encourage woman who is taking or has taken tamoxifen to have regular gynecologic examinations because drug may increase risk of uterine cancer.
- Encourage woman to have annual mammograms and breast examinations.
- Advise patient to use barrier form of contraception because short-term therapy induces ovulation in premenopausal patients.
- Instruct patient to report vaginal bleeding or changes in menstrual cycle.
- Caution woman of childbearing age to avoid becoming pregnant during therapy and first 2 months after stopping drug. Recommend that she consult prescriber before becoming pregnant.
- Advise patient that breast cancer risk assessment tools are available and that she should discuss her concerns with her prescriber.
- Tell patient to report symptoms of stroke (headache; vision changes; weakness of

face, arm, or leg, especially on one side of the body; confusion; difficulty speaking or walking).
- Tell patients to report symptoms of pulmonary embolism (chest pain, difficulty breathing, rapid breathing, sweating, or fainting).

tamsulosin hydrochloride
Flomax

Pregnancy risk category B

Indications & dosages
➲ BPH
Adults: 0.4 mg P.O. once daily, given 30 minutes after same meal each day. If no response after 2 to 4 weeks, increase dosage to 0.8 mg P.O. once daily.

Contraindications & cautions
- Contraindicated in patients hypersensitive to drug or its components.

Adverse reactions
CNS: asthenia, *dizziness*, *headache*, insomnia, somnolence, syncope, vertigo.
CV: chest pain, orthostatic hypotension.
EENT: amblyopia, pharyngitis, *rhinitis*, sinusitis.
GI: diarrhea, nausea.
GU: decreased libido, abnormal ejaculation, priapism.
Musculoskeletal: back pain.
Respiratory: increased cough.
Other: *infection*, tooth disorder.

Interactions
Drug-drug. *Alpha blockers:* May interact with tamsulosin. Avoid using together.
Cimetidine: May decrease tamsulosin clearance. Use together cautiously.

Nursing considerations
- Monitor patient for decreases in blood pressure.
- Symptoms of BPH and prostate cancer are similar; rule out prostate cancer before starting therapy.
- If treatment is interrupted for several days or more, restart therapy at 1 capsule daily.

!!ALERT Don't confuse Flomax with Fosamax or Volmax.

Patient teaching
- Instruct patient not to crush, chew, or open capsules.
- Tell patient to rise slowly from chair or bed when starting therapy and to avoid situations in which injury could occur as a result of fainting. Advise him that drug may cause sudden drop in blood pressure, especially after first dose or when changing doses.
- Instruct patient not to drive or perform hazardous tasks for 12 hours after first dose or changes in dose until response can be monitored.
- Tell patient to take drug about 30 minutes after same meal each day.

tegaserod maleate
Zelnorm

Pregnancy risk category B

Indications & dosages
➲ Short-term treatment of women with irritable bowel syndrome, when the primary bowel symptom is constipation
Women: 6 mg P.O. b.i.d. before meals for 4 to 6 weeks. May add another 4- to 6-week course for patients who respond to therapy at 4 to 6 weeks.
➲ Chronic idiopathic constipation
Men and women younger than age 65: 6 mg P.O. b.i.d. before meals.

Contraindications & cautions
- Contraindicated in patients hypersensitive to drug or its components and in those with severe renal impairment, moderate or severe hepatic impairment, a history of bowel obstruction, symptomatic gallbladder disease, suspected sphincter of Oddi dysfunction or abdominal adhesions, or frequently or currently occurring diarrhea.
- Use cautiously in patient who now has or often has diarrhea.

Adverse reactions
CNS: *headache*, dizziness, migraine.
GI: *abdominal pain*, diarrhea, nausea, flatulence.
Musculoskeletal: back pain, leg pain, arthropathy.
Other: accidental injury.

Interactions

Drug-drug. *Digoxin:* May reduce peak level and exposure of digoxin by 15%. No need to adjust digoxin dose.
Drug-food. *Food:* May reduce bioavailability of drug. Advise patient to take drug on an empty stomach.

Nursing considerations

- Stop drug if patient has new or sudden worsening of abdominal pain.
- Diarrhea sometimes develops during therapy, usually in the first week of treatment, and resolves as therapy continues.
- If serious diarrhea with hypovolemia, hypotension, and syncope occurs, stop drug. Don't start in patients with frequent diarrhea.
- Stop drug in patients who develop ischemic colitis or other forms of intestinal ischemia characterized by rectal bleeding, bloody diarrhea, or abdominal pain. Don't restart treatment with tegaserod if ischemic colitis has occurred.

Patient teaching

- Tell patient to take drug on an empty stomach, before a meal.
- Inform patient that diarrhea might develop during therapy.
- Tell patient to stop drug and consult prescriber if he gets severe diarrhea, bloody diarrhea, or diarrhea accompanied by severe cramping, abdominal pain, or dizziness.
- Advise patient not to start therapy if he now has or often has diarrhea.
- Warn patient not to use drug during pregnancy or breast-feeding.

telithromycin

Ketek

Pregnancy risk category C

Indications & dosages

➲ **Acute bacterial worsening of chronic bronchitis caused by *Streptococcus pneumoniae, Haemophilus influenzae,* or *Moraxella catarrhalis*; acute bacterial sinusitis caused by *S. pneumoniae, H. influenzae, M. catarrhalis,* or *Staphylococcus aureus***
Adults: 800 mg P.O. once daily for 5 days.

➲ **Mild to moderate community-acquired pneumonia caused by *S. pneumoniae* (including multi–drug-resistant isolates), *H. influenzae, M. catarrhalis, Chlamydophila pneumoniae,* or *Mycoplasma pneumoniae***
Adults: 800 mg P.O. once daily for 7 to 10 days.

In patients with creatinine clearance less than 30 ml/minute, including those on dialysis, give 600 mg P.O. once daily. On dialysis days, give after session. In patients with hepatic impairment and clearance less than 30 ml/minute, 400 mg once daily.

Contraindications & cautions

- Contraindicated in patients hypersensitive to telithromycin or any macrolide antibiotic. Also contraindicated in patients taking cisapride or pimozide.
- Avoid use in those with congenital prolongation of the QTc interval, those with ongoing proarrhythmic conditions (such as uncorrected hypokalemia, hypomagnesemia, or bradycardia), or those taking class IA antiarrhythmics (such as quinidine or procainamide) or class III antiarrhythmics (such as dofetilide).
- Not recommended for patients with myasthenia gravis, because telithromycin may worsen symptoms and increase the risk of acute respiratory failure.
- Use cautiously in patients with a history of hepatitis or jaundice caused by telithromycin.

Adverse reactions

CNS: dizziness, headache.
EENT: blurred vision, diplopia, difficulty focusing.
GI: *diarrhea,* loose stools, nausea, taste disturbance, vomiting.

Interactions

Drug-drug. *Atorvastatin, lovastatin, simvastatin:* May increase levels of these drugs, increasing the risk of myopathy. Avoid using together.
Benzodiazepines (midazolam): May increase benzodiazepine level. Monitor patient closely and consider adjusting benzodiazepine dosage.
CYP3A4 inhibitors (itraconazole, ketoconazole): May increase telithromycin level. Monitor patient closely.

CYP3A4 inducers (carbamazepine, phenobarbital, phenytoin): May decrease telithromycin level. Avoid using together.
Digoxin: May increase digoxin level. Monitor digoxin level.
Drugs metabolized by the cytochrome P-450 system (carbamazepine, cyclosporine, hexobarbital, phenytoin, sirolimus, tacrolimus): May increase levels of these drugs, increasing or prolonging their effects. Use together cautiously.
Ergot alkaloid derivatives (such as ergotamine): May increase the risk of ergot toxicity, characterized by severe peripheral vasospasm and dysesthesia. Avoid using together.
Metoprolol: May increase metoprolol level. Use together cautiously.
Oral anticoagulants: May increase the effects of anticoagulant. Monitor PT and INR.
Pimozide: May increase pimozide level. Avoid using together.
Rifampin: May significantly decrease telithromycin level. Avoid using together.
Sotalol: May decrease sotalol level. Monitor patient for lack of effect.
Theophylline: May increase theophylline level and cause nausea and vomiting. Separate telithromycin and theophylline doses by 1 hour.

Nursing considerations

- Telithromycin may cause visual disturbances, particularly in women and patients younger than age 40. Adverse visual effects occur most often after the first or second dose, last several hours, and sometimes return with later doses.
- Patients with diarrhea may have pseudomembranous colitis.
- This drug may prolong the QTc interval. Rarely, an irregular heartbeat may cause the patient to faint.
- Use with caution in breast-feeding women.

Patient teaching

- Tell patient to take entire amount of drug exactly as directed, even if he feels better.
- Tell patient that drug can be taken with or without food.
- Explain that this drug may cause visual disturbances. Caution patient to avoid hazardous activities.
- Tell patient to report diarrhea or any episodes of fainting that occur while taking this drug.

telmisartan
Micardis

Pregnancy risk category C; D in 2nd and 3rd trimesters

Indications & dosages

➲ Hypertension (used alone or with other antihypertensives)
Adults: 40 mg P.O. daily. Blood pressure response is dose-related over a range of 20 to 80 mg daily.

Contraindications & cautions

- Contraindicated in patients hypersensitive to drug or its components.
- Use cautiously in patients with biliary obstruction disorders or renal and hepatic insufficiency and in those with an activated renin-angiotensin system, such as volume- or salt-depleted patients (for example, those being treated with high doses of diuretics).
- Drugs such as telmisartan that act on the renin-angiotensin system can cause fetal and neonatal morbidity and death when given to pregnant women. These problems haven't been detected when exposure has been limited to the first trimester. If pregnancy is suspected, notify prescriber because drug should be stopped.

Adverse reactions

CNS: dizziness, pain, fatigue, headache.
CV: chest pain, hypertension, peripheral edema.
EENT: pharyngitis, sinusitis.
GI: abdominal pain, diarrhea, dyspepsia, *nausea.*
GU: UTI.
Musculoskeletal: back pain, myalgia.
Respiratory: cough, upper respiratory tract infection.
Other: flulike symptoms.

Interactions

Drug-drug. *Digoxin:* May increase digoxin level. Monitor digoxin level closely.
Warfarin: May decrease warfarin level. Monitor INR.

Drug-herb. *Ma huang:* May decrease antihypertensive effects. Discourage use together.
Drug-food. *Salt substitutes containing potassium:* May cause hyperkalemia. Discourage use together.

Nursing considerations

- Monitor patient for hypotension after starting drug. Place patient supine if hypotension occurs, and give I.V. normal saline, if needed.
- Most of the antihypertensive effect occurs within 2 weeks. Maximal blood pressure reduction is usually reached after 4 weeks. Diuretic may be added if blood pressure isn't controlled by drug alone.
- For patients whose renal function may depend on the activity of the renin-angiotensin-aldosterone system (such as those with severe heart failure), treatment with ACE inhibitors and angiotensin receptor antagonists has caused oliguria or progressive azotemia and (rarely) acute renal failure or death.
- Drug isn't removed by hemodialysis. Patients undergoing dialysis may develop orthostatic hypotension. Closely monitor blood pressure.

Patient teaching

- Instruct patient to report suspected pregnancy to prescriber immediately.
- Inform woman of childbearing age of the consequences of second and third trimester exposure to drug.
- Advise breast-feeding woman about risk of adverse drug effects in infants and the need to stop either drug or breast-feeding.
- Tell patient that if he feels dizzy or has low blood pressure on standing, he should lie down, rise slowly from a lying to standing position, and climb stairs slowly.
- Tell patient that drug may be taken without regard to meals.
- Tell patient not to remove drug from blister-sealed packet until immediately before use.

temazepam
Restoril

Pregnancy risk category X
Controlled substance schedule IV

Indications & dosages

➲ Insomnia
Adults: 15 to 30 mg P.O. h.s.
Elderly or debilitated patients: 15 mg P.O. h.s. until individualized response is determined.

Contraindications & cautions

- Contraindicated in pregnant patients and those hypersensitive to drug or other benzodiazepines.
- Use cautiously in patients with chronic pulmonary insufficiency, impaired hepatic or renal function, severe or latent mental depression, suicidal tendencies, and history of drug abuse.

Adverse reactions

CNS: drowsiness, dizziness, lethargy, disturbed coordination, daytime sedation, confusion, nightmares, vertigo, euphoria, weakness, headache, fatigue, nervousness, anxiety, depression, minor changes in EEG patterns (usually low-voltage fast activity).
EENT: blurred vision.
GI: diarrhea, nausea, dry mouth.
Other: physical and psychological dependence.

Interactions

Drug-drug. *CNS depressants:* May increase CNS depression. Use together cautiously.
Drug-herb. *Calendula, hops, kava, lemon balm, passion flower, skullcap, valerian:* May enhance sedative effect of drug. Discourage use together.
Drug-lifestyle. *Alcohol use:* May cause additive CNS effects. Discourage use together.

Nursing considerations

- Assess mental status before starting therapy and reduce doses in elderly patients; these patients may be more sensitive to drug's adverse CNS effects.
- Take precautions to prevent hoarding or overdosing by patients who are depressed, suicidal, or drug-dependent or who have history of drug abuse.

!!ALERT Don't confuse Restoril with Vistaril.

Patient teaching

- Tell patient to avoid alcohol during therapy.
- Caution patient to avoid performing activities that require mental alertness or physical coordination.
- Warn patient not to stop drug abruptly if taken for 1 month or longer.
- Tell patient that onset of drug's effects may take as long as 2 to 2¼ hours.

tenecteplase
TNKase

Pregnancy risk category C

Indications & dosages

➲ Reduction of mortality from an acute MI

Adults weighing 90 kg (198 lb) or more: 50 mg (10 ml) by I.V. bolus over 5 seconds.
Adults weighing 80 to 89 kg (176 to 196 lb): 45 mg (9 ml) by I.V. bolus over 5 seconds.
Adults weighing 70 to 79 kg (154 to 174 lb): 40 mg (8 ml) by I.V. bolus over 5 seconds.
Adults weighing 60 to 69 kg (132 to 152 lb): 35 mg (7 ml) by I.V. bolus over 5 seconds.
Adults weighing less than 60 kg (132 lb): 30 mg (6 ml) by I.V. bolus over 5 seconds.
Maximum dose is 50 mg.

Contraindications & cautions

- Contraindicated in patients with active internal bleeding; history of CVA; intracranial or intraspinal surgery or trauma during previous 2 months; intracranial neoplasm, aneurysm, or arteriovenous malformation; severe uncontrolled hypertension; or bleeding diathesis.
- Use cautiously in patients who have had recent major surgery (such as coronary artery bypass graft), organ biopsy, obstetric delivery, or previous puncture of noncompressible vessels.
- Use cautiously in pregnant women, patients age 75 and older, and patients with recent trauma, recent GI or GU bleeding, high risk of left ventricular thrombus, acute pericarditis, systolic blood pressure 180 mm Hg or higher or diastolic pressure 110 mm Hg or higher, severe hepatic dysfunction, hemostatic defects, subacute bacterial endocarditis, septic thrombophlebitis, diabetic hemorrhagic retinopathy, or cerebrovascular disease.

Adverse reactions

CNS: *CVA*, ***intracranial hemorrhage***.
CV: ***arrhythmias***.
EENT: pharyngeal bleeding, epistaxis.
GI: ***GI bleeding***.
GU: hematuria.
Skin: *hematoma*.
Other: bleeding at puncture site, ***hypersensitivity reactions***.

Interactions

Drug-drug. *Anticoagulants (heparin, vitamin K antagonists), drugs that alter platelet function (acetylsalicylic acid, dipyridamole, glycoprotein IIb/IIIa inhibitors):* May increase risk of bleeding when used before, during, or after tenecteplase use. Use together cautiously.

Nursing considerations

- Begin therapy as soon as possible after onset of MI symptoms.
- Minimize arterial and venous punctures during treatment.
- Avoid noncompressible arterial punctures and internal jugular and subclavian venous punctures.
- Give heparin with tenecteplase but not in the same I.V. line.
- Monitor patient for bleeding. If serious bleeding occurs, stop heparin and antiplatelet drugs immediately.

!!ALERT Use exact patient weight for dosage. An overestimation in patient weight can lead to significant increase in bleeding or intracerebral hemorrhage.

- Monitor ECG for reperfusion arrhythmias.
- Cholesterol embolism is rarely related to thrombolytic use, but it may be lethal. Signs and symptoms may include livedo reticularis ("purple toe" syndrome), acute renal failure, gangrenous digits, hypertension, pancreatitis, MI, cerebral infarction, spinal cord infarction, retinal artery occlusion, bowel infarction, and rhabdomyolysis.

Patient teaching

- Advise patient about proper dental care to avoid excessive gum bleeding.
- Tell patient to report any adverse effects or excess bleeding immediately.

• Explain to patient and family about the use of tenecteplase.

teniposide (VM-26)
Vumon

Pregnancy risk category D

Indications & dosages

➲ Refractory childhood acute lymphoblastic leukemia

Children: Optimum dosage hasn't been established. Dosages ranging from 165 to 250 mg/m^2 I.V. once or twice weekly for 4 to 8 weeks have been used. Usually given with other drugs.

Patients with both Down syndrome and leukemia are at higher risk for myelosuppression. Give first course of treatment at half the recommended dosage.

Contraindications & cautions

• Contraindicated in patients hypersensitive to drug or to polyoxyethylated castor oil, an injection vehicle.

Adverse reactions

CNS: fever.

CV: hypotension.

GI: *nausea, vomiting, mucositis, diarrhea.*

Hematologic: MYELOSUPPRESSION, LEUKOPENIA, NEUTROPENIA, THROMBOCYTOPENIA, *anemia.*

Skin: rash, alopecia, *extravasation at injection site.*

Other: *infection*, bleeding, hypersensitivity reactions, ***anaphylaxis***, *phlebitis.*

Interactions

Drug-drug. *Methotrexate:* May increase clearance and intracellular levels of methotrexate. Avoid using together.

Sodium salicylate, sulfamethizole, tolbutamide: May displace teniposide from protein-binding sites and increase toxicity. Avoid using together.

Nursing considerations

• Drug may be prescribed despite patient's history of hypersensitivity because therapeutic benefits outweigh risks. Treat such patients with antihistamines and corticosteroids before infusion begins, and observe continuously for first hour of infusion and at frequent intervals thereafter.

• Obtain baseline blood counts and renal and hepatic function tests.

• Monitor blood pressure before and during therapy. Hypotension can occur from rapid infusion.

• Have on hand diphenhydramine, hydrocortisone, epinephrine, and emergency equipment to establish an airway in case of anaphylaxis. Signs of hypersensitivity include chills, fever, urticaria, tachycardia, bronchospasm, dyspnea, hypotension, and flushing.

• Monitor blood counts and renal and hepatic function tests.

Patient teaching

• Advise patient to report any pain or burning at site of injection during or after administration.

• Tell patient to report signs and symptoms of infection (fever, sore throat, fatigue) and bleeding (easy bruising, nosebleeds, bleeding gums, tarry stools). Tell patient to take temperature daily.

• Caution woman of childbearing age to avoid becoming pregnant during therapy and to consult prescriber before becoming pregnant.

tenofovir disoproxil fumarate
Viread

Pregnancy risk category B

Indications & dosages

➲ HIV-1 infection, with other antiretrovirals

Adults: 300 mg P.O. once daily with a meal. When given with didanosine, give 2 hours before or 1 hour after didanosine.

For patients with creatinine clearance of 30 to 49 ml/minute, 300 mg P.O. q 48 hours. For a clearance of 10 to 29 ml/minute, 300 mg P.O. twice weekly. For patients receiving hemodialysis, 300 mg P.O. q 7 days or after a total of about 12 hours of hemodialysis. Give dose after session. There are no recommendations for patients with a creatinine clearance of less than 10 ml/minute not receiving hemodialysis.

Contraindications & cautions

- Contraindicated in patients hypersensitive to any component of the drug. Don't use in patients with creatinine clearance less than 60 ml/minute.
- Use very cautiously in patients with risk factors for liver disease or with hepatic impairment.
- Because of a high rate of early virologic failure and emergence of resistance, combination therapy with tenofovir, didanosine, and lamivudine isn't recommended as a new treatment regimen for therapy-naïve or experienced patients with HIV infection. Patients on this regimen should be considered for treatment modification.
- Because the effects of tenofovir on pregnant women aren't known, give this drug to pregnant women only if its benefits clearly outweigh the risks.
- It's unknown if tenofovir appears in breast milk. Use cautiously in breast-feeding women.
- Safety and efficacy haven't been studied in children. Don't use drug in children.

Adverse reactions

CNS: asthenia, headache.
GI: abdominal pain, anorexia, diarrhea, flatulence, *nausea*, vomiting.
GU: glycosuria.
Hematologic: ***neutropenia***.
Metabolic: hyperglycemia.

Interactions

Drug-drug. *Atazanavir:* May decrease atazanavir levels, causing resistance. Give both drugs with ritonavir.
Didanosine (buffered formulation): May increase didanosine bioavailability. Monitor patient for didanosine-related adverse effects, such as bone marrow suppression, GI distress, and peripheral neuropathy. Give tenofovir 2 hours before or 1 hour after didanosine.
Drugs that reduce renal function or compete for renal tubular secretion (acyclovir, cidofovir, ganciclovir, valacyclovir, valganciclovir): May increase levels of tenofovir or other renally eliminated drugs. Monitor patient for adverse effects.

Nursing considerations

!!ALERT Antiretrovirals, alone or combined, have been linked to lactic acidosis and severe (including fatal) hepatomegaly with steatosis. These effects may occur without elevated transaminase levels. Risk factors may include long-term antiretroviral use, obesity, and being female. Monitor all patients for hepatotoxicity, including lactic acidosis and hepatomegaly with steatosis.

- Antiretrovirals may cause body fat to accumulate and be redistributed, resulting in central obesity, peripheral wasting, and a buffalo hump. The long-term effects of these changes are unknown. Monitor patient for changes in body fat.
- Tenofovir may be linked to osteomalacia and decreased bone mineral density and increased creatinine and phosphaturia levels. Monitor patient carefully during long-term treatment.
- Drug may lead to decreased HIV-1 RNA level and CD4 + cell counts.
- The effects of tenofovir on the progression of HIV infection are unknown.
- Use tenofovir cautiously in elderly patients because these patients are more likely to have renal impairment and concurrent drug therapy.
- Because of a high rate of early virologic resistance, triple antiretroviral therapy with abacavir, lamivudine, and tenofovir shouldn't be used as new treatment regimen for naive or pretreated patient. Monitor patients currently controlled with this combination and those who use this combination in addition to other antiretrovirals, and consider modification of therapy.

Patient teaching

- Instruct patient to take tenofovir with a meal to enhance bioavailability.
- Inform patient that drug doesn't cure HIV infection, that opportunistic infections and other complications of HIV infection may still occur, and that transmission of HIV to others through sexual contact or blood contamination is still possible.
- If patient takes tenofovir and didanosine (buffered form), instruct him to take tenofovir 2 hours before or 1 hour after didanosine.
- Tell patient to report adverse effects, including nausea, vomiting, diarrhea, flatulence, and headache.

terazosin hydrochloride
Hytrin

Pregnancy risk category C

Indications & dosages
➲ Hypertension
Adults: Initially, 1 mg P.O. h.s. Dosage may be increased gradually based on response. Usual dosage range is 1 to 5 mg daily. Maximum recommended dose is 20 mg daily.
➲ Symptomatic BPH
Adults: Initially, 1 mg P.O. h.s. Dosage may be increased in a stepwise fashion to 2, 5, or 10 mg once daily to achieve optimal response. Most patients need 10 mg daily for optimal response.

Contraindications & cautions
- Contraindicated in patients hypersensitive to drug.

Adverse reactions
CNS: asthenia, *dizziness*, *headache*, nervousness, paresthesia, somnolence.
CV: palpitations, orthostatic hypotension, tachycardia, *peripheral edema*, atrial fibrillation.
EENT: *nasal congestion*, sinusitis, blurred vision.
GI: nausea.
GU: impotence, priapism.
Hematologic: ***thrombocytopenia***.
Musculoskeletal: back pain, muscle pain.
Respiratory: dyspnea.

Interactions
Drug-drug. *Antihypertensives:* May cause excessive hypotension. Use together cautiously.
Drug-herb. *Butcher's broom:* May cause diminished effect of drug. Discourage use together.
Ma-huang: May decrease antihypertensive effects. Discourage use together.

Nursing considerations
- Monitor blood pressure frequently.

!!ALERT If terazosin is stopped for several days, readjust dosage using first dosing regimen (1 mg P.O. h.s.).

Patient teaching
- Tell patient not to stop drug suddenly, but to notify prescriber if adverse reactions occur.
- Warn patient to avoid hazardous activities that require mental alertness, such as driving or operating heavy machinery, for 12 hours after first dose.
- Tell patient that light-headedness can occur, especially during the first few days of therapy. Advise him to rise slowly to minimize this effect and to report signs and symptoms to prescriber.

terbinafine hydrochloride
Lamisil

Pregnancy risk category B

Indications & dosages
➲ Fingernail onychomycosis caused by dermatophytes (tinea unguium)
Adults: 250 mg P.O. once daily for 6 weeks.
➲ Toenail onychomycosis caused by dermatophytes (tinea unguium)
Adults: 250 mg P.O. once daily for 12 weeks.

Contraindications & cautions
- Contraindicated in patients hypersensitive to drug, pregnant or breast-feeding patients, those with liver disease, and those with creatinine clearance less than 50 ml/minute.

Adverse reactions
CNS: *headache*.
EENT: visual disturbances.
GI: taste disturbances, diarrhea, dyspepsia, abdominal pain, nausea, flatulence.
Hematologic: ***neutropenia***.
Hepatic: hepatobiliary dysfunction, including cholestatic jaundice.
Skin: rash, pruritus, urticaria, ***Stevens-Johnson syndrome***, ***toxic epidermal necrolysis***.
Other: hypersensitivity reactions, ***anaphylaxis***.

Interactions
Drug-drug. *Caffeine:* May decrease I.V. caffeine clearance. Use cautiously together.
Cimetidine: May decrease clearance of terbinafine by one-third. Avoid using together.
Cyclosporine: May increase cyclosporine clearance. Monitor cyclosporine level.

Rifampin: May increase terbinafine clearance by 100%. Monitor response to therapy.

Nursing considerations

!!ALERT Rarely, patients with and without liver disease may suffer liver failure, which can lead either to death or to liver transplant.

- Obtain pretreatment transaminase levels for all patients taking terbinafine. Tablets aren't recommended for patients with acute or chronic liver disease.
- Monitor CBC and hepatic enzyme levels in patients receiving drug for longer than 6 weeks. Stop drug if hepatobiliary dysfunction or cholestatic hepatitis develops.

!!ALERT Don't confuse terbinafine with terbutaline or Lamisil with Lamictal.

Patient teaching

- Inform patient that successful treatment may take 10 weeks for toenail infections and 4 weeks for fingernail infections.
- Tell patient to report visual disturbances immediately; changes in the ocular lens and retina may occur. Patient should also immediately report persistent nausea, anorexia, fatigue, vomiting, right upper quadrant pain, jaundice, dark urine, or pale stools.

terbutaline sulfate

Brethine

Pregnancy risk category B

Indications & dosages

➲ **Bronchospasm in patients with reversible obstructive airway disease**

Injection

Adults and children age 12 and older: 0.25 mg S.C. May be repeated in 15 to 30 minutes, p.r.n. Maximum, 0.5 mg in 4 hours.

Tablets

Adults and adolescents older than age 15: 2.5 to 5 mg P.O. t.i.d. in 6-hour intervals during waking hours. Maximum, 15 mg daily.

Children ages 12 to 15: 2.5 mg P.O. t.i.d. in 6-hour intervals during waking hours. Maximum, 7.5 mg daily.

Contraindications & cautions

- Contraindicated in patients hypersensitive to drug or sympathomimetic amines.
- Use cautiously in patient with CV disorders, hyperthyroidism, diabetes, or seizure disorders.

Adverse reactions

CNS: *nervousness, tremor, drowsiness, dizziness, headache,* weakness.
CV: *palpitations,* tachycardia, ***arrhythmias,*** flushing.
GI: *vomiting, nausea,* heartburn.
Metabolic: hypokalemia.
Respiratory: ***paradoxical bronchospasm with prolonged use,*** dyspnea.
Skin: diaphoresis.

Interactions

Drug-drug. *Cardiac glycosides, cyclopropane, halogenated inhaled anesthetics, levodopa:* May increase risk of arrhythmias. Monitor patient closely, and avoid using together with levodopa.
CNS stimulants: May increase CNS stimulation. Avoid using together.
MAO inhibitors: When given with sympathomimetics, may cause severe hypertension (hypertensive crisis). Avoid using together.
Propranolol, other beta blockers: May block bronchodilating effects of terbutaline. Avoid using together.

Nursing considerations

- Give S.C. injections in lateral deltoid area.
- Protect medication from light. Don't use if discolored.
- Terbutaline may reduce the sensitivity of spirometry for the diagnosis of bronchospasm.

!!ALERT Don't confuse terbutaline with tolbutamide or terbinafine.

Patient teaching

- Make sure patient and caregivers understand why patient needs drug.
- Remind patient to separate oral doses by 6-hour intervals.

terconazole

Terazol 3, Terazol 7

Pregnancy risk category C

Indications & dosages

➲ **Vulvovaginal candidiasis**

Adults: 1 applicatorful of cream or 1 suppository inserted into vagina h.s.; 0.4% cream used for 7 consecutive days; 0.8% cream or 80-mg suppository for 3 consecutive days. Repeat course, if needed, after reconfirmation by smear or culture.

Contraindications & cautions

- Contraindicated in patients hypersensitive to drug or its inactive ingredients.

Adverse reactions

CNS: fever, *headache.*
GI: abdominal pain.
GU: dysmenorrhea, genital pain, vulvovaginal burning.
Skin: irritation, *pruritus*, photosensitivity.
Other: chills, body aches.

Interactions

None significant.

Nursing considerations

- Therapeutic effect of drug is unaffected by menstruation or hormonal contraceptive use.

!!ALERT Don't confuse terconazole with tioconazole.

Patient teaching

- Advise patient to continue treatment during menstrual period. However, tell her not to use tampons.
- Instruct patient to insert drug high in vagina (except during pregnancy).
- Tell patient to use drug for full treatment period prescribed. Explain how to prevent reinfection.
- Instruct patient to notify prescriber and stop drug if fever, chills, other flulike signs and symptoms, or sensitivity develops.
- Caution patient to refrain from sexual intercourse during treatment.
- Tell patient that drug base may react with latex, causing decreased effectiveness of condoms and diaphragms (for up to 72 hours after treatment is completed).
- Instruct patient to store drug at room temperature.

teriparatide (rDNA origin)

Forteo

Pregnancy risk category C

Indications & dosages

➲ **Osteoporosis in postmenopausal women at high risk for fracture; primary or hypogonadal osteoporosis in men at high risk for fracture**

Adults: 20 mcg S.C. in thigh or abdominal wall once daily.

Contraindications & cautions

- Contraindicated in patients hypersensitive to teriparatide or its components.
- Contraindicated in patients at increased risk for osteosarcoma, such as those with Paget's disease or unexplained alkaline phosphatase elevations, children, and patients who have had skeletal radiation; in patients with bone metastases, a history of skeletal malignancies, hypercalcemia, or metabolic bone diseases other than osteoporosis; and in patients with hypercalcemia.
- Use cautiously in patients with active or recent urolithiasis or hepatic, renal, or cardiac disease.

Adverse reactions

CNS: asthenia, depression, dizziness, headache, insomnia, syncope, vertigo.
CV: angina pectoris, hypertension, orthostatic hypotension.
EENT: pharyngitis, rhinitis.
GI: constipation, diarrhea, dyspepsia, nausea, tooth disorder, vomiting.
Metabolic: hypercalcemia.
Musculoskeletal: *arthralgia*, leg cramps, neck pain.
Respiratory: dyspnea, increased cough, pneumonia.
Skin: rash, sweating.
Other: *pain.*

Interactions

Drug-drug. *Calcium supplements:* May increase urinary calcium excretion. Dosage may need adjustment.

Digoxin: May predispose hypercalcemic patient to digitalis toxicity. Use together cautiously.

Nursing considerations

!!ALERT Because of the risk of osteosarcoma, give drug only to patients for whom benefits outweigh risk.
- Don't continue therapy for longer than 2 years.
- If patient may have urolithiasis or hypercalciuria, measure urinary calcium excretion before treatment.
- Monitor patient for orthostatic hypotension, which may occur within 4 hours of dosing.
- Monitor calcium level. If persistent hypercalcemia develops, stop drug and evaluate possible cause.

Patient teaching

- Instruct patient on proper use and disposal of prefilled pen.
- Tell patient not to share pen with others.
- Advise patient to sit or lie down if drug causes a fast heartbeat, light-headedness, or dizziness. Tell patient to report persistent or worsening symptoms.
- Urge patient to report persistent symptoms of hypercalcemia, which include nausea, vomiting, constipation, lethargy, and muscle weakness.

testolactone
Teslac

Pregnancy risk category C
Controlled substance schedule III

Indications & dosages

➲ **Advanced premenopausal breast cancer in women whose ovarian function has been terminated; advanced postmenopausal breast cancer**
Adults: 250 mg P.O. q.i.d for at least 3 months unless disease is actively progressing.

Contraindications & cautions

- Contraindicated in patients hypersensitive to drug and in men with breast cancer.

Adverse reactions

CNS: paresthesia, peripheral neuropathy.
CV: increased blood pressure, edema.
GI: nausea, vomiting, diarrhea, anorexia, glossitis.
Skin: alopecia, erythema, nail changes.

Interactions

Drug-drug. *Oral anticoagulants:* May increase anticoagulant effects. Monitor patient, PT, and INR carefully.

Nursing considerations

- Monitor fluid and electrolyte levels, especially calcium level.
- Force fluids to aid calcium excretion and encourage exercise to prevent hypercalcemia. Immobilized patients are susceptible to hypercalcemia.
- While higher-than-recommended doses don't increase likelihood of remission, patients with visceral metastases may benefit from a dosage of 2 g daily.
- Although similar to testosterone, drug has no androgenic effects.

Patient teaching

- Inform patient that therapeutic response isn't immediate; 3 months is an adequate trial for drug.
- Tell patient to notify prescriber if numbness or tingling occurs in fingers, toes, or face.
- Advise patient to use contraception during therapy.

testosterone transdermal system
Androderm, AndroGel, Testoderm, Testoderm TTS, Testoderm w/Adhesive

Pregnancy risk category X
Controlled substance schedule III

Indications & dosages

➲ **Primary or hypogonadotropic hypogonadism in men**
Androderm
Men: One or two patches applied to back, abdomen, arm, or thigh h.s. for total dosage of 5 mg daily.
AndroGel
Men: Initially, 50 mg applied q morning to shoulders, upper arms, or abdomen. Check testosterone level after about 2 weeks. If re-

sponse is inadequate, may increase to 75 mg daily. Subsequently, adjust to 100 mg, if needed. Or, for AndroGel pump, 5 g (4 pump actuations) applied q morning to shoulders, upper arms, or abdomen. Check testosterone level after about 2 weeks. If response is inadequate, may increase to 7.5 g (6 pump actuations) daily or from 7.5 g to 10 g (8 pump actuations) daily.

Testoderm

Men: One 6-mg/day patch applied to scrotal area daily; or 4 mg/day if scrotal area is small. Patch is worn for 22 to 24 hours daily.

Testoderm TTS

Men: One 5-mg/day patch applied to arm, back, or upper buttock.

Contraindications & cautions

- Contraindicated in patients hypersensitive to drug, in women, in men with known or suspected breast or prostate cancer, and in patients with CV, renal, or hepatic disease.
- Use cautiously in elderly men.

Adverse reactions

CNS: ***CVA***, asthenia, depression, headache.
GI: GI bleeding.
GU: prostatitis, prostate abnormalities, UTI.
Hepatic: reversible jaundice, ***cholestatic hepatitis***.
Metabolic: hypernatremia, hyperkalemia, hypercalcemia, hyperphosphatemia, hypercholesterolemia.
Skin: acne irritation, *pruritus*, *blister under system*, allergic contact dermatitis, burning.
Other: gynecomastia, breast tenderness, flu-like syndrome.

Interactions

Drug-drug. *Insulin:* May alter insulin dosage requirements. Monitor glucose level.
Oral anticoagulants: May alter anticoagulant dosage requirements. Monitor PT and INR.

Nursing considerations

- Apply Androderm system or gel to clean, dry skin on back, abdomen, upper arms, or thigh. Apply Testoderm TTS to arm, back, or upper buttock. Rotate application site every 7 days.
- Wear gloves when handling transdermal patches. Fold used patches with adhesive sides together, and discard so they can't be handled.
- Periodically assess liver function test results, lipid profiles, hemoglobin level, hematocrit (with long-term use), and levels of prostatic acid phosphatase and prostate-specific antigen.
- Watch for excessive hormonal effects in male patients.

!!ALERT Don't confuse Testoderm with Estraderm.

!!ALERT Testoderm and Androderm aren't interchangeable.

Patient teaching

- Teach patient how to apply transdermal system. Warn him that adequate serum level won't be attained if Testoderm patch isn't applied to genital skin. Scrotal area may be dry-shaved for best contact. Application sites should be rotated, with 7 days between applications to same site. Avoid bony prominences.
- Tell patient to fully prime the AndroGel pump by depressing the pumping mechanism three times before first use and discard that portion. The gel can be pumped into the palm of the hand then applied to application sites.
- Advise against changing patch brands.
- Tell patient not to apply Androderm or Testoderm TTS to scrotum.
- Tell patient that if the patch falls off, it may be reapplied. If patch falls off and can't be reapplied, and it has been worn at least 12 hours, a new patch may be applied at the next application time.
- Advise patient to wear brief-style underwear to prevent patch from falling off.
- Instruct patient that system must be changed every 24 hours.
- Tell patient to apply gel to clean, dry, intact skin of the shoulders, upper arms, or abdomen only and not to scrotum.
- Tell patient to wash his hands thoroughly with soap and water after applying gel.
- For best results, advise patient to wait to swim or shower for at least 5 hours after applying gel. Showering or swimming 1 hour after gel application, if done infrequently, should have minimal effects on drug absorption.
- Warn diabetic patient that testosterone may decrease glucose level and to be alert for hypoglycemia.
- Tell patient that topical testosterone has caused virilization in women partners, who

should report acne or changes in body hair distribution.

- Advise patient to report persistent erections, nausea, vomiting, changes in skin color, ankle swelling, or sudden weight gain to prescriber.
- Tell patient that Androderm doesn't have to be removed during sexual intercourse or while showering.

testosterone
Striant, Testopel Pellets

testosterone cypionate
Depo-Testosterone

testosterone enanthate
Delatestryl

testosterone propionate
Malogen†

Pregnancy risk category X
Controlled substance schedule III

Indications & dosages

➲ Male hypogonadism

Men: 10 to 25 mg propionate I.M. two to three times weekly; or 50 to 400 mg cypionate or enanthate I.M. q 2 to 4 weeks. Or, 150 to 450 mg (2 to 6 pellets) implanted S.C. q 3 to 6 months. Or, apply 1 buccal system (30 mg) to the gum region just above the incisor tooth on either side of the mouth, b.i.d., morning and evening about 12 hours apart. Alternate sides of the mouth with each application.

➲ Metastatic breast cancer in women 1 to 5 years after menopause

Women: 50 to 100 mg propionate I.M. three times weekly; or 200 to 400 mg cypionate or enanthate I.M. q 2 to 4 weeks.

Contraindications & cautions

- Contraindicated in patients hypersensitive to drug and in those with hypercalcemia or cardiac, hepatic, or renal decompensation.
- Contraindicated in men with breast or prostate cancer and in pregnant or breast-feeding women.
- Use cautiously in elderly patients.

Adverse reactions

CNS: headache, anxiety, depression, paresthesia, sleep apnea.
CV: edema.
GI: nausea; gum or mouth irritation; bitter taste; gum pain, tenderness, or edema; taste perversion (with buccal application).
GU: amenorrhea.
Hematologic: polycythemia, ***suppression of clotting factors***.
Hepatic: reversible jaundice, ***cholestatic hepatitis***.
Metabolic: hypernatremia, hyperkalemia, hypercalcemia, hyperphosphatemia, hypercholesterolemia.
Skin: pain, induration at injection site, local edema, acne.
Other: androgenic effects in women, gynecomastia, hypersensitivity reactions, hypoestrogenic effects in women, excessive hormonal effects in men.

Interactions

Drug-drug. *Corticosteroids:* May increase risk of edema. Use together cautiously, especially in patients with cardiac or hepatic disease.
Hepatotoxic drugs: May increase risk of hepatotoxicity. Monitor liver function closely.
Insulin, oral antidiabetics: May decrease glucose level; may alter dosage requirements. Monitor glucose level in diabetic patients.
Oral anticoagulants: May increase sensitivity; may alter dosage requirements. Monitor PT and INR.
Oxyphenbutazone: May increase oxyphenbutazone level. Monitor patient.

Nursing considerations

- Don't give to woman of childbearing age until pregnancy is ruled out.
- Store I.M. preparations at room temperature. If crystals appear, warm and shake bottle to disperse them.
- Cypionate and enanthate are long-acting solutions.
- Inject deep into upper outer quadrant of gluteal muscle. Rotate injection sites; report soreness at site.
- Unless contraindicated, use with high-calorie, high-protein diet. Give small, frequent meals to help avoid nausea.
- Monitor patient's liver function test results.

- Testosterone may cause abnormal glucose tolerance test results.
- In patients with metastatic breast cancer, hypercalcemia usually indicates progression of bone metastases. Report signs and symptoms of hypercalcemia.
- Report evidence of virilization in women. Androgenic effects include acne, edema, weight gain, increased hair growth, hoarseness, clitoral enlargement, decreased breast size, changes in libido, male-pattern baldness, and oily skin or hair.
- Watch for hypoestrogenic effects in women (flushing; diaphoresis; vaginitis, including itching, drying, and burning; vaginal bleeding; menstrual irregularities).
- Watch for excessive hormonal effects in male patients. If patient is prepubertal, watch for premature epiphyseal closure, acne, priapism, growth of body and facial hair, and phallic enlargement. If he's postpubertal, watch for testicular atrophy, oligospermia, decreased ejaculatory volume, impotence, gynecomastia, and epididymitis.
- Monitor patient's weight and blood pressure routinely.
- Monitor prepubertal boys by X-ray for rate of bone maturation.

!!ALERT Therapeutic response in breast cancer is usually apparent within 3 months. Therapy should be stopped if disease progresses.

- Androgens may alter results of laboratory studies during therapy and for 2 to 3 weeks after therapy ends.

!!ALERT Don't confuse testosterone with testolactone.

!!ALERT Testosterone salts aren't interchangeable.

Patient teaching

- Make sure patient understands importance of using an effective nonhormonal contraceptive during therapy.
- Instruct patient to stop drug immediately and notify prescriber if pregnancy is suspected.
- Review signs and symptoms of virilization with woman, and instruct her to notify prescriber if they occur.
- Advise woman to wear cotton underwear and to wash after intercourse to decrease risk of vaginitis.
- Instruct man to notify prescriber about priapism, reduced ejaculatory volume, or gynecomastia.
- Warn diabetic patient to be alert for hypoglycemia and to notify prescriber if it occurs.
- Instruct boys using testosterone for delayed puberty to have X-rays of hand and wrist obtained every 6 months during treatment.
- Tell patient to report sudden weight gain.
- Warn patient that drug shouldn't be used to enhance athletic performance.
- Instruct patient how to use the buccal system.
- Advise patient to avoid dislodging buccal system and ensure that the system is in place after toothbrushing, use of mouthwash, and eating or drinking.
- Tell patient not to chew or swallow buccal system.

tetanus immune globulin, human
BayTet

Pregnancy risk category C

Indications & dosages

➲ **Postexposure prevention of tetanus after injury, in patients whose immunization is incomplete or unknown**

Adults and children: 250 units deep I.M. injection.

➲ **Tetanus**

Adults and children: Single doses of 3,000 to 6,000 units I.M. have been used. Optimal dosage schedules haven't been established.

Contraindications & cautions

- Contraindicated in patients with thrombocytopenia or other coagulation disorders that would contraindicate I.M. injection unless benefits outweigh risks.
- Use cautiously in patients with history of previous systemic allergic reactions after giving human immunoglobulin preparations and in those allergic to thimerosal.

Adverse reactions

CNS: slight fever.
GU: ***nephrotic syndrome.***
Musculoskeletal: stiffness.
Skin: erythema at injection site.

Other: pain, hypersensitivity reactions, ***anaphylaxis, angioedema.***

Interactions

Drug-drug. *Live-virus vaccines:* May interfere with response. Postpone administration of live-virus vaccines for 3 months after giving tetanus immune globulin.

Nursing considerations

- Obtain history of injury, tetanus immunizations, last tetanus toxoid injection, allergies, and reactions to immunizations. Keep epinephrine 1:1,000 available to treat hypersensitivity reaction.
- Don't give I.V. or I.D. Don't give in gluteal area.
- Tetanus immune globulin is used only if wound is more than 24 hours old or patient has had fewer than two tetanus toxoid injections.
- Thoroughly clean wound and remove all foreign matter.

!!ALERT Don't confuse drug with tetanus toxoid. Tetanus immune globulin isn't a substitute for tetanus toxoid, which should be given at same time to produce active immunization. Don't give at same site as toxoid.

- Antibodies remain at effective levels for about 4 weeks, several times the duration of equine antitetanus antibodies, thereby protecting patients for incubation period of most tetanus cases.
- Don't give live-virus vaccines for 3 months after giving tetanus immune globulin.

!!ALERT Don't confuse Hyper-Tet with HyperHep or Hyperstat.

Patient teaching

- Warn patient about local adverse reactions related to drug.
- Instruct patient to report serious adverse reactions promptly.
- Advise patient to complete full series of tetanus immunizations.
- Instruct patient to take acetaminophen to reduce fever and to apply cool compresses at injection site for comfort.

tetanus toxoid, adsorbed

tetanus toxoid, fluid

Pregnancy risk category C

Indications & dosages

➲ **Primary immunization to prevent tetanus**

Adults and children age 7 and older: 0.5 ml (adsorbed) I.M. 4 to 8 weeks apart for two doses; then give third dose 6 to 12 months after second. Or, 0.5 ml (fluid) I.M. or S.C. 4 to 8 weeks apart for three doses; then give fourth dose of 0.5 ml 6 to 12 months after third dose.

Children ages 6 weeks to 6 years: Although use isn't recommended in children younger than age 7, the following dosage schedule may be used: 0.5 ml (adsorbed) I.M. at ages 2, 4, and 6 months. Give fourth dose at 15 to 18 months. Give fifth dose at ages 4 to 6, just before entry into school, if indicated. Diphtheria and tetanus toxoids and acellular pertussis vaccine adsorbed (DTaP) is recommended for active immunization in children younger than age 7.

➲ **Booster dose to prevent tetanus**

Adults: 0.5 ml I.M. at 10-year intervals.

➲ **Postexposure prevention of tetanus**

Adults: For a clean, minor wound, give emergency booster dose if more than 10 years have elapsed since last dose. For all other wounds, give booster dose if more than 5 years have elapsed since last dose.

Contraindications & cautions

- Contraindicated in immunosuppressed patients, in those with immunoglobulin abnormalities, and in those with severe hypersensitivity or neurologic reactions to toxoid or its ingredients. Contraindicated in patients with thrombocytopenia or other coagulation disorders that would contraindicate I.M. injection unless benefits outweigh risks.
- Use adsorbed form cautiously in infants or children with cerebral damage, neurologic disorders, or history of febrile seizures.
- Postpone vaccination in patients with acute illness and during polio outbreaks, except in emergencies.

Adverse reactions

CNS: slight fever, headache, ***seizures***, malaise, encephalopathy.
CV: tachycardia, hypotension, flushing.
Musculoskeletal: aches, pains.
Skin: erythema, induration, nodule at injection site, urticaria, pruritus.
Other: chills, ***anaphylaxis***.

Interactions

Drug-drug. *Chloramphenicol:* May interfere with response to tetanus toxoid. Monitor patient for effect.
Immunosuppressants, tetanus immune globulin: May reduce immune response to vaccine. Postpone vaccine until 1 month after immunosuppressant is stopped.

Nursing considerations

- Obtain history of allergies and reaction to immunization.
- Determine date of last tetanus immunization.
- Keep epinephrine 1:1,000 available to treat anaphylaxis.
- Adsorbed form produces longer immunity. Fluid form provides quicker booster effect in patients actively immunized previously.
- Document manufacturer, lot number, date, and name, address, and title of person giving dose on patient record or log.

!!ALERT Don't confuse drug with tetanus immune globulin, human. Both drugs may be given in some situations.

Patient teaching

- Advise patient to avoid using hot or cold compresses at injection site; this may increase severity of local reaction.
- Instruct patient to report persistent or severe adverse reactions.
- Advise patient of proper fever-reducing drug dose for fever reaction.
- Tell patient that nodule at injection site may be present for a few weeks.

tetracycline hydrochloride

Achromycin, Apo-Tetra†, Novo-Tetra†, Nu-Tetra†, Sumycin

Pregnancy risk category D

Indications & dosages

➲ Infections caused by susceptible gram-negative and -positive organisms, including *Haemophilus ducreyi, Yersinia pestis, Campylobacter fetus, Rickettsiae* species, *Mycoplasma pneumoniae,* and *Chlamydia trachomatis;* psittacosis; granuloma inguinale
Adults: 1 g to 2 g/day P.O. in two or four equally divided doses depending on the severity of infection.
Children older than age 8: 25 to 50 mg/kg P.O. daily, in divided doses q 6 hours.

➲ Uncomplicated urethral, endocervical, or rectal infections caused by *C. trachomatis*
Adults: 500 mg P.O. q.i.d. for at least 7 days, 10 days for epididymitis, and for at least 14 days for lymphogranuloma venereum.

➲ Brucellosis
Adults: 500 mg P.O. q 6 hours for 3 weeks with 1 g of streptomycin I.M. q 12 hours for first week; once daily for second week.

➲ Gonorrhea in patients allergic to penicillin
Adults: Initially, 1.5 g P.O.; then 500 mg P.O. q 6 hours for total dose of 9 g. For epididymitis, 500 mg P.O. q 6 hours for 7 days.

➲ Syphilis in patients allergic to penicillin
Adults and adolescents: 500 mg P.O. q.i.d. for 2 weeks. If infection has lasted 1 year or longer, treat for 4 weeks.

➲ Acne
Adults and adolescents: Initially, 250 mg P.O. q 6 hours; then 125 to 500 mg daily or every other day.

➲ *Helicobacter pylori* infection
Adults: 500 mg P.O. q 6 hours for 10 to 14 days with other drugs, such as metronidazole, bismuth subsalicylate, amoxicillin, or omeprazole.

➲ Cholera
Adults: 500 mg P.O. q 6 hours for 48 to 72 hours.

➲ **Malaria caused by *Plasmodium falciparum***
Adults: 250 to 500 mg P.O. daily for 7 days with quinine sulfate 650 mg P.O. q 8 hours for 3 to 7 days.
➲ **To prevent infection in rape victims**
Adults: 500 mg P.O. q.i.d. for 7 days.

Contraindications & cautions

- Contraindicated in patients hypersensitive to drug or other tetracyclines.
- Use cautiously in patients with renal or hepatic impairment. Avoid using or use cautiously during last half of pregnancy and in children younger than age 8 because drug may cause permanent discoloration of teeth, enamel defects, and bone growth retardation.

Adverse reactions

CNS: dizziness, headache, ***intracranial hypertension***.
CV: pericarditis.
EENT: sore throat.
GI: anorexia, dysphagia, glossitis, *epigastric distress*, *nausea*, vomiting, *diarrhea*, esophagitis, stomatitis, enterocolitis, oral candidiasis.
GU: inflammatory lesions in anogenital region.
Hematologic: ***neutropenia***, eosinophilia, ***thrombocytopenia***.
Musculoskeletal: *bone growth retardation in children younger than age 8.*
Skin: *candidal superinfection, maculopapular and erythematous rash, urticaria, photosensitivity, increased pigmentation.*
Other: hypersensitivity reactions, permanent discoloration of teeth, enamel defects.

Interactions

Drug-drug. *Antacids (including sodium bicarbonate) and laxatives containing aluminum, magnesium, or calcium; antidiarrheals containing kaolin, pectin, or bismuth subsalicylate:* May decrease antibiotic absorption. Give antibiotic 1 hour before or 2 hours after these drugs.
Digoxin: May increase digoxin absorption. Monitor digoxin levels and monitor patient for signs of toxicity.
Ferrous sulfate and other iron products, zinc: May decrease antibiotic absorption. Give tetracycline 2 hours before or 3 hours after these products.
Hormonal contraceptives: May decrease contraceptive effectiveness and increase risk of breakthrough bleeding. Advise patient to use nonhormonal contraceptive.
Methoxyflurane: May cause severe nephrotoxicity. Avoid using together.
Oral anticoagulants: May increase anticoagulant effects. Monitor PT and INR, and adjust anticoagulant dosage.
Penicillins: May interfere with bactericidal action of penicillins. Avoid using together.
Drug-food. *Dairy products, other foods:* May decrease antibiotic absorption. Give antibiotic 1 hour before or 2 hours after any of these products.
Drug-lifestyle. *Sun exposure:* May cause photosensitivity reactions. Advise patient to avoid excessive sunlight exposure.

Nursing considerations

- Obtain specimen for culture and sensitivity tests before giving first dose. Therapy may begin while awaiting test results.

!!ALERT Check expiration date. Outdated or deteriorated tetracyclines have been linked to reversible nephrotoxicity (Fanconi's syndrome).

- Don't expose drug to light or heat.
- If large doses are given, therapy is prolonged, or patient is at high risk, monitor patient for signs and symptoms of superinfection.
- In patients with renal or hepatic impairment, monitor renal and liver function test results if drug is used.
- Check patient's tongue for signs of candidal infection. Stress good oral hygiene.
- Drug isn't indicated for treatment of neurosyphilis.
- Photosensitivity reactions may occur within a few minutes to several hours after sun exposure. Photosensitivity lasts after therapy ends.

Patient teaching

- Tell patient to take drug exactly as prescribed, even after he feels better, and to take entire amount prescribed.
- Explain that effectiveness is reduced when drug is taken with milk or other dairy products, food, antacids, or iron products. Tell patient to take each dose with a full glass of water on an empty stomach, at least 1 hour before or 2 hours after meals. Also tell him to take it at least 1 hour before bed-

time to prevent esophageal irritation or ulceration.
- Warn patient to avoid direct sunlight and ultraviolet light, wear protective clothing, and use sunscreen.
- Advise patient to promptly report adverse reactions to prescriber.

tetrahydrozoline hydrochloride
Tyzine, Tyzine Pediatric

Pregnancy risk category C

Indications & dosages
➲ Nasal congestion
Adults and children older than age 6: 2 to 4 drops or 3 to 4 sprays of 0.1% solution in each nostril no more than q 3 hours, p.r.n.
Children ages 2 to 6: 2 to 3 drops of 0.05% solution in each nostril no more than q 3 hours, p.r.n.

Contraindications & cautions
- Contraindicated in patients hypersensitive to drug and in children younger than age 2. The 0.1% solution is contraindicated in children younger than age 6.
- Use cautiously in patients with hyperthyroidism, hypertension, or diabetes mellitus.

Adverse reactions
EENT: transient burning or stinging, sneezing, rebound nasal congestion.

Interactions
None significant.

Nursing considerations
- Drug should be used for only 3 to 5 days.
- Overdose in young children may cause oversedation.

Patient teaching
- Teach patient how to use drug. Tell him to hold head upright to minimize swallowing of drug and to sniff spray briskly.
- Caution patient not to share drug because this could spread infection.
- Tell patient not to exceed recommended dosage and to use only as needed for 3 to 5 days.

theophylline

Immediate-release liquids
Accurbron*, Aerolate, Aquaphyllin, Asmalix*, Bronkodyl*, Elixomin*, Elixophyllin*, Lanophyllin*, Slo-Phyllin, Theoclear-80, Theolair Liquid, Theostat 80*

Immediate-release tablets and capsules
Bronkodyl, Elixophyllin, Quibron T Dividose, Slo-Phyllin

Timed-release tablets
Quibron-T/SR, Respbid, Sustaire, Theochron, Theolair-SR, Theo-Sav, Theo-Time, T-Phyl, Uniphyl

Timed-release capsules
Aerolate, Elixophyllin, Slo-bid Gyrocaps, Slo-Phyllin, Theobid Duracaps, Theochron, Theoclear L.A., Theospan-SR, Theo-24, Theovent Long-Acting

Pregnancy risk category C

Indications & dosages
Extended-release preparations shouldn't be used to treat acute bronchospasm.
➲ Oral theophylline for acute bronchospasm in patients not currently receiving theophylline
Adult nonsmokers and children older than age 16: 5 mg/kg P.O., then 3 mg/kg q 6 hours for two doses. Maintenance dosage is 3 mg/kg q 8 hours.
Children ages 9 to 16: 5 mg/kg P.O.; then 3 mg/kg q 4 hours for three dosages. Maintenance dosage is 3 mg/kg q 6 hours.
Children ages 6 months to 9 years: 5 mg/kg P.O.; then 4 mg/kg q 4 hours for three doses. Maintenance dosage is 4 mg/kg q 6 hours.

For otherwise healthy adult smokers, 5 mg/kg P.O.; then 3 mg/kg q 4 hours for three doses. Maintenance dosage is 3 mg/kg q 6 hours. For older adults and patients with cor pulmonale, 5 mg/kg P.O.; then 2 mg/kg q 6 hours for two doses. Maintenance dosage is 2 mg/kg q 8 hours. For adults with heart failure or liver disease, 5 mg/kg P.O.; then 2 mg/kg q 8 hours for two doses.

Maintenance dosage is 1 to 2 mg/kg q 12 hours.

➲ Parenteral theophylline for patients not currently receiving theophylline

Loading dose: 4.7 mg/kg I.V. slowly; then maintenance infusion.

Adult nonsmokers and children older than age 16: 0.55 mg/kg/hour I.V. for 12 hours; then 0.39 mg/kg/hour.

Children ages 9 to 16: 0.79 mg/kg/hour I.V. for 12 hours; then 0.63 mg/kg/hour.

Children ages 6 months to 9 years: 0.95 mg/kg/hour I.V. for 12 hours; then 0.79 mg/kg/hour.

For otherwise healthy adult smokers, 0.79 mg/kg/hour I.V. for 12 hours; then 0.63 mg/kg/hour. For older adults and patients with cor pulmonale, 0.47 mg/kg/hour I.V. for 12 hours; then 0.24 mg/kg/hour. For adults with heart failure or liver disease, 0.39 mg/kg/hour I.V. for 12 hours; then 0.08 to 0.16 mg/kg/hour.

➲ Oral and parenteral theophylline for acute bronchospasm in patients currently receiving theophylline

Adults and children: Ideally, dose is based on current theophylline level. Each 0.5 mg/kg I.V. or P.O. loading dose will increase drug level by 1 mcg/ml. In emergencies, some prescribers recommend a 2.5-mg/kg P.O. dose of rapidly absorbed form if patient develops no obvious signs or symptoms of theophylline toxicity.

➲ Chronic bronchospasm

Adults and children: Initially, 16 mg/kg or 400 mg P.O. daily, whichever is less, given in three or four divided doses at 6- to 8-hour intervals. Or, 12 mg/kg or 400 mg P.O. daily, whichever is less, in an extended-release preparation given in two or three divided doses at 8- or 12-hour intervals. Dosage may be increased, as tolerated, at 2- to 3-day intervals to the following maximums: adults and children older than age 16, 13 mg/kg or 900 mg P.O. daily, whichever is less; children ages 12 to 16, 18 mg/kg P.O. daily; children ages 9 to 12, 20 mg/kg P.O. daily; children younger than age 9, 24 mg/kg P.O. daily.

Contraindications & cautions

- Contraindicated in patients hypersensitive to xanthine compounds (caffeine, theobromine) and in those with active peptic ulcer or poorly controlled seizure disorders.
- Use cautiously in young children, infants, neonates, elderly patients, and those with COPD, cardiac failure, cor pulmonale, renal or hepatic disease, peptic ulceration, hyperthyroidism, diabetes mellitus, glaucoma, severe hypoxemia, hypertension, compromised cardiac or circulatory function, angina, acute MI, or sulfite sensitivity.

Adverse reactions

CNS: *restlessness, dizziness,* headache, *insomnia,* irritability, ***seizures***, muscle twitching.

CV: *palpitations, sinus tachycardia,* extrasystoles, flushing, marked hypotension, ***arrhythmias***.

GI: *nausea, vomiting,* diarrhea, epigastric pain.

Metabolic: urinary catecholamines.

Respiratory: tachypnea, ***respiratory arrest***.

Interactions

Drug-drug. *Adenosine:* May decrease antiarrhythmic effectiveness. Higher doses of adenosine may be needed.

Allopurinol, calcium channel blockers, cimetidine, disulfiram, influenza virus vaccine, interferon, macrolide antibiotics (such as erythromycin), methotrexate, hormonal contraceptives, quinolone antibiotics (such as ciprofloxacin): May decrease hepatic clearance of theophylline; may increase theophylline level. Monitor patient for toxicity.

Barbiturates, nicotine, phenytoin, rifampin: May enhance metabolism and decrease theophylline level. Monitor patient for decreased effect.

Carbamazepine, isoniazid, loop diuretics: May increase or decrease theophylline level. Monitor theophylline level.

Carteolol, pindolol, propranolol, timolol: May act antagonistically, reducing the effects of one or both drugs; may reduce elimination of theophylline. Monitor theophylline level and patient closely.

Ephedrine, other sympathomimetics: May exhibit synergistic toxicity with these drugs, predisposing patient to arrhythmias. Monitor patient closely.

Lithium: May increase lithium excretion. Monitor patient closely.

Drug-herb. *Cacao tree:* May inhibit theophylline metabolism. Discourage use together.

Cayenne: May increase risk of theophylline toxicity. Advise patient to use together cautiously.
Ephedra: May increase risk of adverse reactions. Discourage use together.
Guarana: May cause additive CNS and CV effects. Discourage use together.
Ipriflavone: May increase risk of theophylline toxicity. Advise patient to use together cautiously.
St. John's wort: May decrease theophylline level. Discourage use together.
Drug-food. *Any food:* May cause accelerated release of theophylline from extended-release products. Tell patient to take Theo-24 on an empty stomach.
Caffeine: May decrease hepatic clearance of theophylline; may increase theophylline level. Monitor patient for toxicity.
Drug-lifestyle. *Smoking:* May increase elimination of theophylline, increasing dosage requirements. Monitor theophylline response and level.

Nursing considerations

!!ALERT Don't confuse extended-release forms with regular-release forms.
- Dosage may need to be increased in cigarette smokers and in habitual marijuana smokers because smoking causes drug to be metabolized faster.
- Give drug around the clock, using extended-release product at bedtime.
- Depending on assay used, theophylline levels may be falsely elevated in the presence of furosemide, phenylbutazone, probenecid, theobromine, caffeine, tea, chocolate, cola beverages, and acetaminophen.
- Monitor vital signs; measure and record fluid intake and output. Expect improved quality of pulse and respirations.
- People metabolize xanthines at different rates; dosage is determined by monitoring response, tolerance, pulmonary function, and theophylline level. Theophylline levels range from 10 to 20 mcg/ml; toxicity may occur at levels above 20 mcg/ml.

!!ALERT Evidence of toxicity includes tachycardia, anorexia, nausea, vomiting, diarrhea, restlessness, irritability, and headache. The presence of any of these signs in patients taking theophylline warrants checking theophylline level and adjusting dosage, as indicated.

!!ALERT Don't confuse Theolair with Thyrolar.

Patient teaching

- Supply instructions for home care and dosage schedule.
- Warn patient not to dissolve, crush, or chew extended-release products. Small children unable to swallow these can ingest (without chewing) the contents of capsules sprinkled over soft food.
- Tell patient to relieve GI symptoms by taking oral drug with full glass of water after meals, although food in stomach delays absorption.
- Warn patient to take drug regularly, only as directed. Patients tend to want to take extra "breathing pills."
- Inform elderly patient that dizziness is common at start of therapy.
- Urge patient to tell prescriber about any other medications used. OTC drugs or herbal remedies may contain ephedrine or theophylline salts; excessive CNS stimulation may result.
- If patient smokes, have him inform prescriber if he quits. A dosage reduction may be necessary to prevent toxicity.

thiamine hydrochloride (vitamin B_1)

Pregnancy risk category A; C if dose exceeds RDA

Indications & dosages

➲ RDA
Adult men: 1.2 mg.
Adult women: 1.1 mg.
Boys ages 14 to 18: 1.2 mg.
Girls ages 14 to 18: 1 mg.
Children ages 9 to 13: 0.9 mg.
Children ages 4 to 8: 0.6 mg.
Children ages 1 to 3: 0.5 mg.
Infants ages 6 months to 1 year: 0.3 mg.
Neonates and infants younger than age 6 months: 0.2 mg.
Pregnant women: 1.4 mg.
Breast-feeding women: 1.5 mg.
➲ Beriberi
Adults: Depending on severity, 5 to 30 mg I.M. t.i.d. for 2 weeks; then dietary correction and multivitamin supplement containing 5 to 30 mg thiamine daily for 1 month.

Children: Depending on severity, 10 to 25 mg I.V. or I.M. daily. For noncritically ill children, 10 to 50 mg P.O. daily in divided doses for several weeks with adequate diet.

➲ **Wet beriberi with myocardial failure**

Adults and children: 10 to 30 mg I.V. t.i.d.

➲ **Wernicke's encephalopathy**

Adults: Initially, 100 mg I.V.; then 50 to 100 mg I.V. or I.M. daily until patient is consuming a regular balanced diet.

Contraindications & cautions

- Contraindicated in patients hypersensitive to thiamine products.

Adverse reactions

CNS: restlessness, weakness.
CV: cyanosis, ***CV collapse (with repeated I.V. injections)***.
EENT: tightness of throat.
GI: nausea, ***hemorrhage***.
Respiratory: pulmonary edema.
Skin: feeling of warmth, pruritus, urticaria, diaphoresis.
Other: ***angioedema***, tenderness, induration after I.M. administration.

Interactions

Drug-drug. *Neuromuscular blockers:* May increase effects of these drugs. Monitor patient closely.

Nursing considerations

- Use parenteral route only when use of oral route isn't feasible.
- Thiamine malabsorption is most likely in alcoholism, cirrhosis, and GI disease.
- Thiamine deficiency can occur after about 3 weeks of totally thiamine-free diet.
- Thiamine deficiency usually requires concurrent treatment for multiple deficiencies.
- Dosages over 30 mg t.i.d. may not be fully used. After tissue saturation with thiamine, drug is excreted in urine as pyrimidine.
- In Wernicke's encephalopathy, give thiamine before dextrose because dextrose increases thiamine requirement.

!! ALERT Don't confuse thiamine with Thorazine.

Patient teaching

- Inform breast-feeding woman that if beriberi occurs in infant, both she and her child should be treated with thiamine.
- Stress proper nutritional habits to prevent recurrence of deficiency.
- Instruct patient to protect oral doses from light.

thioridazine hydrochloride

Apo-Thioridazine†, Mellaril*, Mellaril Concentrate, Novo-Ridazine†, PMS Thioridazine†

Pregnancy risk category C

Indications & dosages

➲ **Schizophrenia in patients who don't respond to treatment with other antipsychotic drugs**

Adults: Initially, 50 to 100 mg P.O. t.i.d., increased gradually to 800 mg daily in divided doses, if needed. Dosage varies.

Children: Initially, 0.5 mg/kg daily in divided doses. Increase gradually to optimum therapeutic effect; maximum dose is 3 mg/kg daily.

Contraindications & cautions

- Contraindicated in patients hypersensitive to drug and in those with CNS depression, coma, or severe hypertensive or hypotensive cardiac disease.
- Contraindicated in patients taking fluvoxamine, propranolol, pindolol, fluoxetine, drugs that inhibit the CYP2D6 enzyme, or drugs that prolong the QTc interval.
- Contraindicated in patients with reduced levels of CYP2D6 enzyme, those with congenital long QT interval syndrome, or those with history of cardiac arrhythmias.
- Use cautiously in elderly or debilitated patients and in patients with hepatic disease, CV disease, respiratory disorders, hypocalcemia, seizure disorders, or severe reactions to insulin or electroconvulsive therapy.
- Use cautiously in those exposed to extreme heat or cold (including antipyretic therapy) or organophosphate insecticides.

Adverse reactions

CNS: *tardive dyskinesia*, *sedation*, EEG changes, dizziness, ***neuroleptic malignant syndrome***.
CV: *orthostatic hypotension*, ***prolonged QTc interval, torsades de pointes***, ECG changes, tachycardia.

EENT: *ocular changes, blurred vision*, retinitis pigmentosa.
GI: *dry mouth, constipation*, increased appetite.
GU: *urine retention*, dark urine, menstrual irregularities, inhibited ejaculation.
Hematologic: ***transient leukopenia, agranulocytosis***, hyperprolactinemia.
Hepatic: cholestatic jaundice.
Metabolic: weight gain.
Skin: *mild photosensitivity reactions*, allergic reactions.
Other: gynecomastia, galactorrhea.

Interactions

Drug-drug. *Antacids:* May inhibit absorption of oral phenothiazines. Separate dosages by at least 2 hours.
Barbiturates: May decrease phenothiazine effect. Monitor patient.
Centrally acting antihypertensives: May decrease antihypertensive effect. Monitor blood pressure.
Fluoxetine, fluvoxamine, pindolol, propranolol, other drugs that inhibit CYP2D6 enzyme, drugs that prolong QTc interval (disopyramide, procainamide, quinidine): May inhibit metabolism of thioridazine; may cause arrhythmias resulting from QTc interval prolongation. Avoid using together.
Lithium: May decrease phenothiazine effect and increase neurologic adverse effects. Monitor patient closely.
Other CNS depressants: May increase CNS depression. Use together cautiously.
Drug-herb. *St. John's wort:* May cause photosensitivity reactions. Advise patient to avoid excessive sunlight exposure.
Drug-lifestyle. *Alcohol use:* May increase CNS depression, particularly psychomotor skills. Strongly discourage alcohol use.
Sun exposure: May increase risk of photosensitivity reactions. Advise patient to avoid excessive sunlight exposure.

Nursing considerations

!!ALERT Before starting treatment, obtain baseline ECG and potassium level. Patients with a QTc interval greater than 450 msec shouldn't receive Mellaril. Patients with a QTc interval greater than 500 msec should stop drug.
!!ALERT Drug isn't used in first treatment of schizophrenia.
!!ALERT Different liquid formulations have different concentrations. Check dosage carefully.
- Prevent contact dermatitis by keeping drug away from skin and clothes. Wear gloves when preparing liquid forms.
- Dilute liquid concentrate with water or fruit juice just before giving.
- Shake suspension well before using.
- Monitor patient for tardive dyskinesia, which may occur after prolonged use. It may not appear until months or years later and may disappear spontaneously or persist for life, despite ending drug.

!!ALERT Watch for evidence of neuroleptic malignant syndrome (extrapyramidal effects, hyperthermia, autonomic disturbance), which is rare but commonly fatal. It may not be related to length of drug use or type of neuroleptic; more than 60% of patients are men.
- Monitor periodic blood tests (CBCs and liver function tests), and ophthalmic tests (long-term use).
- Withhold dose and notify prescriber if jaundice, blood dyscrasia (fever, sore throat, infection, cellulitis, weakness), or persistent extrapyramidal reactions develop, especially in children or pregnant women.
- Don't stop drug abruptly unless required by severe adverse reactions.
- After abrupt withdrawal of long-term therapy, gastritis, nausea, vomiting, dizziness, tremor, feeling of warmth or cold, diaphoresis, tachycardia, headache, or insomnia may occur.

!!ALERT Don't confuse thioridazine with Thorazine or Mellaril with Elavil.

Patient teaching

- Tell patient to shake suspension before use.
- Warn patient to avoid activities that require alertness until effects of drug are known.
- Tell patient to watch for dizziness when standing quickly. Advise patient to change positions slowly.
- Instruct patient to report symptoms of dizziness, palpitations, or fainting to prescriber.
- Tell patient to avoid alcohol use.
- Have patient report signs of urine retention, constipation, or blurred vision.
- Tell patient that drug may discolor the urine.

- Advise patient to relieve dry mouth with sugarless gum or hard candy.
- Instruct patient to use sunblock and to wear protective clothing outdoors.

thiotepa (TESPA, triethylenethiophosphoramide, TSPA)

Thioplex

Pregnancy risk category D

Indications & dosages

➲ Breast and ovarian cancers, lymphoma, Hodgkin's disease
Adults and children older than age 12: 0.3 to 0.4 mg/kg I.V. q 1 to 4 weeks or 0.2 mg/kg for 4 to 5 days at intervals of 2 to 4 weeks.

➲ Bladder tumor
Adults and children older than age 12: 30 to 60 mg in 30 to 60 ml of normal saline solution instilled in bladder for 2 hours once weekly for 4 weeks.

➲ Neoplastic effusions
Adults and children older than age 12: 0.6 to 0.8 mg/kg intracavitarily q 1 to 4 weeks.

Contraindications & cautions

- Contraindicated in patients hypersensitive to drug, in breast-feeding patients, and in those with severe bone marrow, hepatic, or renal dysfunction.
- Use in pregnant women only when benefits to mother outweigh risk of teratogenicity.
- Use cautiously in patients with mild bone marrow suppression and renal or hepatic dysfunction.

Adverse reactions

CNS: headache, dizziness, fatigue, weakness, fever.
EENT: blurred vision, conjunctivitis.
GI: *nausea, vomiting,* abdominal pain, anorexia, stomatitis.
GU: amenorrhea, decreased spermatogenesis, dysuria, increased urine levels of uric acid, urine retention, hemorrhagic cystitis (with intravesical administration).
Hematologic: ***leukopenia, thrombocytopenia, neutropenia,*** anemia.
Metabolic: hyperuricemia.
Skin: dermatitis, alopecia, pain at injection site.
Other: hypersensitivity reactions (including, ***anaphylaxis, laryngeal edema,*** urticaria, rash).

Interactions

Drug-drug. *Anticoagulants, aspirin, NSAIDs:* May increase risk of bleeding. Avoid using together.
Myelosuppressives: May increase myelosuppression. Monitor patient.
Neuromuscular blockers: May prolong muscular paralysis. Monitor patient.
Other alkylating drugs, irradiation therapy: May intensify toxicity rather than enhance therapeutic response. Avoid using together.
Pancuronium, succinylcholine: May increase apnea. Avoid using together.

Nursing considerations

- For bladder instillation, dehydrate patient 8 to 10 hours before therapy. Instill drug into bladder by catheter; ask patient to retain solution for 2 hours. Volume may be reduced to 30 ml if discomfort is too great with 60 ml. Reposition patient every 15 minutes for maximum area contact.
- Monitor CBC weekly for at least 3 weeks after last dose.
- Stop drug and notify prescriber if patient's WBC count drops below 3,000/mm^3 or if platelet count falls below 150,000/mm^3. If WBC count falls below 2,000/mm^3 or granulocyte count falls below 1,000/mm^3, follow institutional policy for infection control in immunocompromised patients.
- Monitor uric acid level. To prevent hyperuricemia with resulting uric acid nephropathy, give allopurinol along with adequate hydration.
- Therapeutic effects are commonly accompanied by toxicity.
- To prevent bleeding, avoid all I.M. injections when platelet count is below 50,000/mm^3.
- Anticipate blood transfusions because of cumulative anemia. Patient may need injections of RBC colony-stimulating factor to promote RBC production and decrease need for blood transfusions.

Patient teaching

- Advise patient to watch for signs and symptoms of infection (fever, sore throat, fa-

tigue) and bleeding (easy bruising, nosebleeds, bleeding gums, tarry stools). Tell patient to take temperature daily. Tell patient to report even mild infections.
- Instruct patient to avoid OTC products containing aspirin or NSAIDs.
- Advise woman to stop breast-feeding during therapy because of risk of toxicity to infant.
- Caution woman of childbearing age to consult prescriber before becoming pregnant.

thiothixene
Navane

thiothixene hydrochloride
Navane*

Pregnancy risk category C

Indications & dosages

➲ Mild to moderate psychosis
Adults: Initially, 2 mg P.O. t.i.d. Increased gradually to 15 mg daily, p.r.n.

➲ Severe psychosis
Adults: Initially, 5 mg P.O. b.i.d. Increase gradually to 20 to 30 mg daily, p.r.n. Maximum dose is 60 mg daily.

Contraindications & cautions

- Contraindicated in patients hypersensitive to drug and in those with CNS depression, circulatory collapse, coma, or blood dyscrasia.
- Use with caution in patients with history of seizure disorder and in those undergoing alcohol withdrawal.
- Use cautiously in elderly or debilitated patients and in those with CV disease (may cause sudden drop in blood pressure), hepatic disease, heat exposure, glaucoma, or prostatic hyperplasia.

Adverse reactions

CNS: *extrapyramidal reactions, drowsiness,* restlessness, agitation, insomnia, *tardive dyskinesia,* sedation, EEG changes, pseudoparkinsonism, dizziness, ***neuroleptic malignant syndrome.***
CV: *hypotension,* tachycardia, ECG changes.
EENT: ocular changes, *blurred vision,* nasal congestion.
GI: *dry mouth, constipation.*
GU: *urine retention,* menstrual irregularities, inhibited ejaculation.
Hematologic: ***transient leukopenia,*** leukocytosis, ***agranulocytosis.***
Hepatic: jaundice.
Metabolic: weight gain.
Skin: *mild photosensitivity reactions,* allergic reactions, exfoliative dermatitis.
Other: gynecomastia.

Interactions

Drug-drug. *CNS depressants:* May increase CNS depression. Use together cautiously.
Drug-lifestyle. *Alcohol use:* May increase CNS depression. Discourage use together.
Sun exposure: May increase risk of photosensitivity reactions. Advise patient to avoid excessive sunlight exposure.

Nursing considerations

- Prevent contact dermatitis by keeping drug off skin and clothes. Wear gloves when preparing liquid forms.
- Dilute liquid concentrate with fruit juice, milk, or semisolid food just before giving.
- Slight yellowing of injection or concentrate is common and doesn't affect potency. Discard markedly discolored solutions.
- Monitor patient for tardive dyskinesia, which may occur after prolonged use; it may not appear until months or years later, and may disappear spontaneously or persist for life, despite stopping drug.

!!ALERT Watch for evidence of neuroleptic malignant syndrome (extrapyramidal effects, hyperthermia, autonomic disturbance), which is rare but commonly fatal. It may not be related to length of drug use or type of neuroleptic; more than 60% of patients are men.

- Monitor periodic CBCs, liver function tests, and renal function tests; and ophthalmic tests for long-term use.
- Watch for orthostatic hypotension. Keep patient supine for 1 hour after drug administration, and tell him to change positions slowly.
- Withhold dose and notify prescriber if jaundice, blood dyscrasia (fever, sore throat, infection, cellulitis, weakness), or persistent extrapyramidal reactions develop, especially in pregnant women.
- Don't withdraw drug abruptly unless severe adverse reactions occur.

• After abrupt withdrawal of long-term therapy, gastritis, nausea, vomiting, dizziness, tremor, feeling of warmth or cold, diaphoresis, tachycardia, headache, or insomnia may occur.
‼**ALERT** Don't confuse Navane with Nubain or Norvasc.

Patient teaching

• Warn patient to avoid activities that require alertness until effects of drug are known.
• Tell patient to watch for dizziness upon standing quickly. Advise him to change positions slowly.
• Instruct patient to dilute liquid appropriately.
• Tell patient to avoid alcohol use during therapy.
• Have patient report signs of urine retention, constipation, or blurred vision.
• Instruct patient to use sunblock and to wear protective clothing outdoors.

thyroid, desiccated
Armour Thyroid

Pregnancy risk category A

Indications & dosages

➲ Mild hypothyroidism
Adults: Initially, 60 mg P.O. daily, increased by 60 mg q 30 days until desired response occurs. Usual maintenance dose is 60 to 120 mg daily as single dose.
Elderly patients: Start at lower dose.
➲ Severe hypothyroidism
Adults: Initially, 15 mg P.O. daily; increased by 30 mg daily after 2 weeks, and 2 weeks later increased to 60 mg daily. After 2 months, increased to 120 mg daily if response is still inadequate.
Patients older than age 65: 7.5 to 15 mg daily. May double dose q 6 to 8 weeks until desired result is obtained.
➲ Congenital or severe hypothyroidism in children
Children older than age 12: 1.2 to 1.8 mg/kg daily P.O.
Children ages 6 to 12: 2.4 to 3 mg/kg daily P.O.
Children ages 1 to 5: 3 to 3.6 mg/kg daily P.O.
Children ages 6 months to 1 year: 3.6 to 4.8 mg/kg daily P.O.
Children younger than age 6 months: 4.8 to 6 mg/kg daily P.O.

In patients with long-term disease, other endocrine diseases, severe hypothyroidism, or CV disease, start at lower dose.

Contraindications & cautions

• Contraindicated in patients hypersensitive to drug and in those with acute MI uncomplicated by hypothyroidism, untreated thyrotoxicosis, or uncorrected adrenal insufficiency.
• Use cautiously in elderly patients and in those with angina pectoris, hypertension, other CV disorders, renal insufficiency, or ischemia.
• Use cautiously in patients with myxedema, diabetes mellitus, or diabetes insipidus.

Adverse reactions

CNS: *nervousness*, *insomnia*, tremor, headache.
CV: *tachycardia*, ***arrhythmias***, angina pectoris, ***cardiac decompensation and collapse***.
GI: diarrhea, vomiting.
GU: menstrual irregularities.
Metabolic: weight loss.
Musculoskeletal: accelerated rate of bone maturation in infants and children.
Skin: allergic skin reactions, diaphoresis.
Other: heat intolerance.

Interactions

Drug-drug. *Beta blockers:* May reduce beta-blocker effect. Monitor patient for clinical effect.
Cholestyramine: May impair thyroid absorption. Separate doses by 4 to 5 hours.
Digoxin: May decrease glycoside effect. Monitor patient for clinical effect.
Insulin, oral antidiabetics: May alter glucose level. Monitor glucose level, and adjust dosage as needed.
Oral anticoagulants: May alter PT. Monitor PT and INR, and adjust dosage as needed.
Sympathomimetics, such as epinephrine: May increase risk of coronary insufficiency. Monitor patient closely.
Theophylline: May decrease theophylline clearance in hypothyroidism; clearance may return to normal when euthyroid state is achieved. Monitor theophylline level.

Drug-herb. *Lemon balm:* May have antithyroid effects; may inhibit thyroid-stimulating hormone. Discourage use together.

Nursing considerations

- Check for coronary insufficiency in patients with coronary artery disease.
- Thyroid hormone replacement requirements are about 25% lower in patients older than age 60 than in young adults.
- Dosage may need to be increased in pregnant patients.
- Monitor pulse and blood pressure.
- Reduce dose if angina occurs.
- Long-term therapy causes bone loss in premenopausal and postmenopausal women. Consider a basal bone density measurement, and monitor patient closely for osteoporosis.
- In children, treatment is guided by sleeping pulse rate and basal morning temperature.
- Patient must stop thyroid hormones 7 to 10 days before undergoing ^{131}I studies.

!!ALERT Don't confuse thyroid with Thyrolar.

Patient teaching

- Tell patient to take thyroid hormones at same time each day, preferably before breakfast, to maintain constant hormone levels and help prevent insomnia.
- Tell patient the drug should never be stopped unless directed by prescriber.
- Advise patient who has achieved stable response not to change brands.
- Warn patient (especially elderly patient) to notify prescriber at once about chest pain, palpitations, or other signs of overdose or aggravated CV disease.
- Tell patient to report unusual bleeding and bruising.
- Advise patient not to take OTC or other prescription medications without first consulting his prescriber.
- Advise patient to report pregnancy to prescriber, because dosage may need adjustment.

tiagabine hydrochloride
Gabitril

Pregnancy risk category C

Indications & dosages

➲ Adjunctive treatment of partial seizures

Adults: Initially, 4 mg P.O. once daily. Total daily dose may be increased by 4 to 8 mg at weekly intervals until clinical response or up to 56 mg daily. Give total daily dose in divided doses b.i.d. to q.i.d.

Children ages 12 to 18: Initially, 4 mg P.O. once daily. Total daily dose may be increased by 4 mg at beginning of week 2 and thereafter by 4 to 8 mg per week until clinical response or up to 32 mg daily. Give total daily dose in divided doses b.i.d. to q.i.d.

For patients with hepatic impairment, reduce first and maintenance doses or increase dosing intervals.

Contraindications & cautions

- Contraindicated in patients hypersensitive to drug or its components.

!!ALERT Drug may cause new-onset seizures and status epilepticus in patients without a history of epilepsy. In these patients, stop drug and evaluate for underlying seizure disorder. Drug shouldn't be used for off-label uses.

- Use cautiously in breast-feeding women.

Adverse reactions

CNS: *dizziness, asthenia, somnolence, nervousness*, tremor, difficulty with concentration and attention, insomnia, ataxia, confusion, speech disorder, difficulty with memory, paresthesia, depression, emotional lability, abnormal gait, hostility, language problems, agitation.
CV: vasodilation.
EENT: nystagmus, pharyngitis.
GI: abdominal pain, *nausea*, diarrhea, vomiting, increased appetite, mouth ulceration.
Musculoskeletal: generalized weakness, pain, myasthenia.
Respiratory: increased cough.
Skin: rash, pruritus.

Interactions

Drug-drug. *Carbamazepine, phenobarbital, phenytoin:* May increase tiagabine clearance. Monitor patient closely.
CNS depressants: May enhance CNS effects. Use together cautiously.
Drug-lifestyle. *Alcohol use:* May enhance CNS effects. Discourage use together.

Nursing considerations

- Withdraw drug gradually unless safety concerns require a more rapid withdrawal because sudden withdrawal may cause more frequent seizures.

!!ALERT Use of anticonvulsants, including tiagabine, may cause status epilepticus and sudden unexpected death in patients with epilepsy.
!!ALERT Don't confuse tiagabine with tizanidine; both have 4-mg starting doses.

- Patients who aren't receiving at least one enzyme-inducing anticonvulsant when starting tiagabine may need lower doses or slower dosage adjustment.
- Drug may cause moderately severe to incapacitating generalized weakness, which resolves after dosage is reduced or drug stopped.

Patient teaching

- Advise patient to take drug only as prescribed.
- Tell patient to take drug with food.
- Warn patient that drug may cause dizziness, somnolence, and other signs and symptoms of CNS depression. Advise patient to avoid driving and other potentially hazardous activities that require mental alertness until drug's CNS effects are known.
- Tell woman of childbearing age to call prescriber if she becomes pregnant or plans to become pregnant during therapy.
- Instruct woman of childbearing age to notify prescriber if she's planning to breastfeed because drug may appear in breast milk.

ticarcillin disodium

Ticar

Pregnancy risk category B

Indications & dosages

➲ **Severe systemic infections caused by susceptible strains of gram-positive and especially gram-negative organisms, including *Pseudomonas* and *Proteus species***
Adults and children older than age 1 month: 200 to 300 mg/kg I.V. daily in divided doses q 4 to 6 hours.
➲ **UTIs**
Adults and children weighing at least 40 kg (88 lb): 1 g I.M. or I.V. q 6 hours. For complicated infections, 150 to 200 mg/kg I.V. infusion daily in divided doses q 4 to 6 hours.
Infants and children older than age 1 month, weighing less than 40 kg: 50 to 100 mg/kg I.M. or I.V. daily in divided doses q 6 to 8 hours. For complicated infections, 150 to 200 mg/kg I.V. infusion daily in divided doses q 4 to 6 hours.

If creatinine clearance is 30 to 60 ml/minute, dosage is 2 g I.V. q 4 hours; if clearance is 10 to 29 ml/minute, 2 g I.V. q 8 hours; and if below 10 ml/minute, 2 g I.V. q 12 hours or 1 g I.M. q 6 hours.

Contraindications & cautions

- Contraindicated in patients hypersensitive to drug or other penicillins.
- Use cautiously in patients with other drug allergies, especially to cephalosporins, because of possible cross-sensitivity, and in those with impaired renal function, hemorrhagic conditions, hypokalemia, or sodium restrictions. Drug contains 5.2 to 6.5 mEq sodium/g.

Adverse reactions

CNS: neuromuscular excitability, ***seizures***.
CV: phlebitis, vein irritation.
GI: nausea, diarrhea, vomiting, ***pseudomembranous colitis***.
Hematologic: ***leukopenia***, ***neutropenia***, eosinophilia, ***thrombocytopenia***, hemolytic anemia.
Metabolic: hypokalemia, hypernatremia.
Skin: pain at injection site.
Other: hypersensitivity reactions, ***anaphylaxis***, overgrowth of nonsusceptible organisms.

Interactions

Drug-drug. *Hormonal contraceptives:* May decrease hormonal contraceptive effectiveness. Advise use of additional form of contraception during penicillin therapy.
Lithium: May alter renal elimination of lithium. Monitor lithium level closely.
Oral anticoagulants: May increase risk of bleeding. Monitor PT and INR.
Probenecid: May increase levels of ticarcillin and other penicillins. Probenecid may be used for this purpose.

Nursing considerations

- Before giving drug, ask patient about allergic reactions to penicillin.
- Obtain specimen for culture and sensitivity tests before giving first dose. Therapy may begin pending results.
- Give ticarcillin at least 1 hour before a bacteriostatic antibiotic.
- For I.M. injection, reconstitute drug using sterile water for injection, normal saline solution for injection, or lidocaine 1% (without epinephrine). Use 2 ml diluent for each gram of drug. Use only the 1-g vial for I.M. administration. Give deep into large muscle. Don't exceed 2 g per injection.
- Monitor potassium and sodium levels.
- Check CBC and platelet counts frequently. Drug may cause thrombocytopenia.
- Ticarcillin is typically used with another antibiotic, such as gentamicin.
- If large doses are given or if therapy is prolonged, bacterial or fungal superinfection may occur, especially in elderly, debilitated, or immunosuppressed patients.
- Monitor INR in patients receiving warfarin because drug may prolong PT.
- Give patients receiving hemodialysis a 3-g dose after each dialysis session.

Patient teaching

- Tell patient to report adverse reactions promptly.
- Advise patient to report discomfort at I.V. insertion site.

ticarcillin disodium and clavulanate potassium

Timentin

Pregnancy risk category B

Indications & dosages

➲ **Lower respiratory tract, urinary tract, bone and joint, intra-abdominal, gynecologic, and skin and skin-structure infections and septicemia caused by beta-lactamase–producing strains of bacteria or by ticarcillin-susceptible organisms**
Adults and children weighing more than 60 kg (132 lb): 3 g ticarcillin and 100 mg clavulanic acid, given by I.V. infusion q 4 to 6 hours.
Adults and children ages 3 months to 16 years weighing less than 60 kg: 200 mg ticarcillin/kg I.V. daily in divided doses q 6 hours. For severe infections, 300 mg ticarcillin/kg I.V. daily in divided doses q 4 hours.

If creatinine clearance is 30 to 60 ml/minute, dosage is 2 g I.V. q 4 hours; if clearance is 10 to 29 ml/minute, 2 g I.V. q 8 hours; and if clearance is less than 10 ml/minute, 2 g I.V. q 12 hours. For patients receiving peritoneal dialysis or hemodialysis, give a loading dose of 3.1 g I.V. and then maintenance doses of 3.1 g I.V. q 12 hours for patients receiving peritoneal dialysis or 2 g I.V. q 12 hours for patients receiving hemodialysis. Supplement with 3.1 g after each hemodialysis session.

Contraindications & cautions

- Contraindicated in patients hypersensitive to drug or other penicillins.
- Use cautiously in patients with other drug allergies, especially to cephalosporins because of possible cross-sensitivity, and in those with impaired renal function, hemorrhagic conditions, hypokalemia, or sodium restriction.

Adverse reactions

CNS: neuromuscular excitability, headache, ***seizures***, giddiness.
CV: phlebitis, vein irritation.
EENT: taste and smell disturbances.
GI: nausea, diarrhea, stomatitis, vomiting, epigastric pain, flatulence, ***pseudomembranous colitis***.

Hematologic: ***leukopenia, neutropenia***, eosinophilia, ***thrombocytopenia***, hemolytic anemia, anemia.
Metabolic: hypokalemia, hypernatremia.
Skin: pain at injection site, rash, pruritus, ***Stevens-Johnson syndrome***.
Other: hypersensitivity reactions, ***anaphylaxis***, overgrowth of nonsusceptible organisms.

Interactions

Drug-drug. *Hormonal contraceptives:* May decrease hormonal contraceptive effectiveness. Advise use of additional form of contraception during penicillin therapy.
Oral anticoagulants: May increase risk of bleeding. Monitor PT and INR.
Probenecid: May increase ticarcillin level. Probenecid may be used for this purpose.

Nursing considerations

- Before giving drug, ask patient about allergic reactions to penicillin.
- Obtain specimen for culture and sensitivity tests before giving first dose. Therapy may begin pending results.
- Give drug at least 1 hour before a bacteriostatic antibiotic.
- Check CBC and platelet counts frequently. Drug may cause thrombocytopenia.
- Monitor PT and INR in patients taking oral anticoagulants.
- Monitor potassium and sodium levels.
- If large doses are given or if therapy is prolonged, bacterial or fungal superinfection may occur, especially in elderly, debilitated, or immunosuppressed patients.
- Patients receiving hemodialysis should receive an additional 3.1-g dose after each dialysis session.

Patient teaching

- Tell patient to report adverse reactions promptly.
- Instruct patient to report discomfort at I.V. site.
- Advise patient to limit salt intake during drug therapy because of high sodium content.

ticlopidine hydrochloride
Ticlid

Pregnancy risk category B

Indications & dosages

➲ **To reduce risk of thrombotic CVA in patients who have had a CVA or CVA precursors**
Adults: 250 mg P.O. b.i.d. with meals.
➲ **Adjunct to aspirin to prevent subacute stent thrombosis in patients having coronary stent placement**
Adults: 250 mg P.O. b.i.d., combined with antiplatelet doses of aspirin. Start therapy after stent placement and continue for 30 days.

Contraindications & cautions

- Contraindicated in patients hypersensitive to drug and in those with severe hepatic impairment, hematopoietic disorders, active pathologic bleeding from peptic ulceration, or active intracranial bleeding.
- Use cautiously and with close monitoring of CBC and WBC differentials, watching for signs and symptoms of neutropenia and agranulocytosis.

Adverse reactions

CNS: dizziness, peripheral neuropathy, ***intracranial bleeding***.
CV: vasculitis.
EENT: conjunctival hemorrhage.
GI: *diarrhea*, nausea, dyspepsia, abdominal pain, anorexia, vomiting, flatulence, bleeding.
GU: hematuria, dark urine.
Hematologic: ***neutropenia, pancytopenia, agranulocytosis, immune thrombocytopenia***.
Musculoskeletal: arthropathy, myositis.
Respiratory: *allergic pneumonitis*.
Skin: rash, pruritus, maculopapular rash, urticaria, ***thrombocytopenic purpura***, ecchymoses.
Other: hypersensitivity reactions, postoperative bleeding.

Interactions

Drug-drug. *Antacids:* May decrease ticlopidine level. Separate doses by at least 2 hours.

Aspirin: May increase effect of aspirin on platelets. Use together cautiously.
Cimetidine: May decrease clearance of ticlopidine and increase risk of toxicity. Avoid using together.
Digoxin: May decrease digoxin level. Monitor digoxin level.
Phenytoin: May increase phenytoin level. Monitor patient closely.
Theophylline: May decrease theophylline clearance and risk of toxicity. Monitor patient closely and adjust theophylline dosage.
Drug-herb. *Red clover:* May cause bleeding. Discourage use together.

Nursing considerations

- Because of life-threatening adverse reactions, use drug only in patients who are allergic to, can't tolerate, or have failed aspirin therapy.
- Obtain baseline liver function test results before therapy.
- Determine CBC and WBC differentials at second week of therapy and repeat every 2 weeks until end of third month.
- Monitor liver function test results and repeat if dysfunction is suspected.
- Thrombocytopenia has occurred rarely. Stop drug in patients with platelet count of 80,000/mm^3 or less. If needed, give methylprednisolone 20 mg I.V. to normalize bleeding time within 2 hours.
- When used preoperatively, drug may decrease risk of graft occlusion in patients receiving coronary artery bypass grafts and reduce severity of drop in platelet count in patients receiving extracorporeal hemoperfusion during open heart surgery.

Patient teaching

- Tell patient to take drug with meals.
- Warn patient to avoid aspirin and aspirin-containing products and to check with prescriber or pharmacist before taking OTC drugs.
- Explain that drug will prolong bleeding time and that patient should report unusual or prolonged bleeding. Advise patient to tell dentists and other health care providers that he takes ticlopidine.
- Stress importance of regular blood tests. Because neutropenia can result with increased risk of infection, tell patient to immediately report signs and symptoms of infection, such as fever, chills, or sore throat.
- If drug is being substituted for a fibrinolytic or anticoagulant, tell patient to stop those drugs before starting ticlopidine therapy.
- Advise patient to stop drug 10 to 14 days before undergoing elective surgery.
- Tell patient to immediately report to prescriber yellow skin or sclera, severe or persistent diarrhea, rashes, bleeding under the skin, light-colored stools, or dark urine.

timolol maleate

Betimol, Istalol, Timoptic, Timoptic-XE

Pregnancy risk category C

Indications & dosages

➲ To reduce intraocular pressure (IOP) in ocular hypertension or open-angle glaucoma
Adults: Initially, 1 drop of 0.25% solution in each affected eye b.i.d.; maintenance dosage is 1 drop once daily. If no response, instill 1 drop of 0.5% solution in each affected eye b.i.d. If IOP is controlled, reduce dosage to 1 drop daily. Or, 1 drop of gel in each affected eye once daily. Or, for Istalol, initially 1 drop 0.5% solution in each affected eye once daily in the morning. If response is unsatisfactory, concomitant therapy may be considered.

Contraindications & cautions

- Contraindicated in patients hypersensitive to drug and in those with bronchial asthma, sinus bradycardia, second- or third-degree AV block, cardiac failure, cardiogenic shock, or history of bronchial asthma or severe COPD.
- Use cautiously in patients with nonallergic bronchospasm, chronic bronchitis, emphysema, diabetes mellitus, hyperthyroidism, or cerebrovascular insufficiency.

Adverse reactions

CNS: ***CVA***, depression, fatigue, dizziness, lethargy, hallucinations, confusion, *syncope*.
CV: slight reduction in resting heart rate, ***arrhythmia, cardiac arrest, heart block***, palpitations, *hypotension*, ***bradycardia, heart failure***.

EENT: minor eye irritation, conjunctivitis, blepharitis, keratitis, visual disturbances, diplopia, ptosis, decreased corneal sensitivity with long-term use.
Metabolic: hyperglycemia, hyperuricemia.
Respiratory: ***bronchospasm in patients with history of asthma.***

Interactions

Drug-drug. *Aminophylline, theophylline:* May act antagonistically, reducing effects of one or both drugs; may also reduce elimination of theophylline. Monitor theophylline level and patient closely.
Calcium channel blockers, cardiac glycosides, quinidine: May increase risk of adverse cardiac effects if significant amounts of timolol are systemically absorbed. Use together cautiously.
Cimetidine: May increase beta blocker effects. Consider another H_2 agonist or decrease dose of beta blocker.
Epinephrine: May cause a hypertensive episode, followed by bradycardia. Stop beta blocker 3 days before starting epinephrine. Monitor patient closely.
Insulin: May mask symptoms of hypoglycemia (such as tachycardia) as a result of beta blockade. Use together cautiously in patients with diabetes.
Oral beta blockers: May increase ocular and systemic effects. Use together cautiously.
Prazosin: May increase risk of orthostatic hypotension in early phases of use together. Assist patient to stand slowly until effects are known.
Reserpine, other catecholamine-depleting drugs: May increase hypotensive and bradycardia-induced effects. Avoid using together.
Verapamil: May increase effects of both drugs. Monitor cardiac function closely and decrease dosages as necessary.

Nursing considerations

- Give other ophthalmic drugs at least 10 minutes before giving gel form of drug.
- Monitor diabetic patients carefully. Systemic beta-blocking effects can mask some signs and symptoms of hypoglycemia.
- Some patients may need a few weeks of treatment to stabilize pressure-lowering response. Determine IOP after 4 weeks of treatment.
- Drug can be used safely in patients with glaucoma who wear conventional polymethylmethacrylate (PMMA) hard contact lenses.

!!ALERT Don't confuse timolol with atenolol, or Timoptic with Viroptic.

Patient teaching

- Teach patient how to instill drops. Advise him to wash hands before and after instillation and to apply light finger pressure on lacrimal sac for 1 minute after drops are instilled. Warn patient not to touch tip of dropper to eye or surrounding tissue.
- Instruct patient using gel to invert container and shake once before each use. Also tell him to use other ophthalmic drugs at least 10 minutes before applying gel.
- Tell patient to instill drug without contact lenses in place. Lenses may be reinserted about 15 minutes after drug use.
- Advise patient to monitor pulse rate and report slow rate to prescriber. Drug may be absorbed systemically and produce signs and symptoms of beta blockade.
- Tell patient to report difficulty breathing or chest pain to prescriber.

tinidazole
Tindamax

Pregnancy risk category C

Indications & dosages

➲ Trichomoniasis caused by *Trichomonas vaginalis*
Adults: 2 g P.O. as a single dose taken with food. Sexual partners should be treated at the same time with the same dose.
➲ Giardiasis caused by *Giardia lamblia (G. duodenalis)*
Adults: 2 g P.O. as a single dose taken with food.
Children older than age 3: 50 mg/kg (up to 2 g) as a single dose taken with food.
➲ Intestinal amebiasis caused by *Entamoeba histolytica*
Adults: 2 g P.O. daily for 3 days, taken with food.
Children older than age 3: 50 mg/kg (up to 2 g) P.O. daily for 3 days, taken with food.
➲ Amebic liver abscess (amebiasis)
Adults: 2 g P.O. daily for 3 to 5 days, taken with food.

Children older than age 3: 50 mg/kg (up to 2 g) P.O. daily for 3 to 5 days, taken with food.

For patients receiving hemodialysis, give an additional dose equal to one-half the recommended dose after the hemodialysis session.

Contraindications & cautions

- Contraindicated in patients hypersensitive to tinidazole, its component, or other nitroimidazole derivatives.
- Contraindicated in pregnant women during first trimester of pregnancy.
- Use cautiously in patients with CNS disorders and in those with blood dyscrasias or hepatic dysfunction.

Adverse reactions

CNS: dizziness, fatigue, headache, malaise, peripheral neuropathy, ***seizures***, weakness.
GI: anorexia, constipation, cramps, dyspepsia, metallic taste, nausea, vomiting.

Interactions

Drug-drug. *Cyclosporine, tacrolimus:* May increase cyclosporine or tacrolimus level. Monitor patient closely for toxicity, including headache, nausea, vomiting, nephrotoxicity, and electrolyte abnormalities.
Disulfiram: May increase abdominal cramping, nausea, vomiting, headaches, and flushing. Separate doses by 2 weeks.
Drugs that induce CYP-450, such as fosphenytoin, phenobarbital, phenytoin, and rifampin: May increase tinidazole elimination. Monitor patient.
Drugs that inhibit CYP-450, such as cimetidine and ketoconazole: May prolong tinidazole half-life and decrease clearance. Monitor patient.
Fluorouracil: May decrease fluorouracil clearance, increasing adverse effects without added benefit. Monitor patient for rash, nausea, vomiting, stomatitis, and leukopenia.
Fosphenytoin, phenytoin: May prolong phenytoin half-life and decrease clearance of I.V. drug. Monitor patient for toxicity.
Lithium: May increase lithium level. Monitor patient; monitor lithium and creatinine levels.
Oxytetracycline: May antagonize tinidazole. Assess patient for lack of effect.
Warfarin and other oral anticoagulants: May increase anticoagulant effect. Anticoagulant dosage may need adjustment during and for up to 8 days after tinidazole therapy.
Drug-herb. *St. John's wort:* May increase or decrease tinidazole level. Discourage use together.
Drug-lifestyle. *Use of alcohol and alcohol-containing products:* May increase abdominal cramping, nausea, vomiting, headaches, and flushing. Discourage use together and for 3 days after stopping tinidazole.

Nursing considerations

- Monitor children closely if therapy exceeds 3 days.
- Tablets may be crushed into a fine powder and mixed with artificial cherry syrup for children who can't swallow pills.
- Patient should take drug with food to minimize adverse GI effects.

!!ALERT Stop drug immediately if abnormal neurologic signs occur, such as seizures or numbness of the arms or legs.

- If candidiasis develops during therapy, the patient may need an antifungal.
- Patient shouldn't breast-feed during therapy and for 3 days after the last dose.
- Dose selection for elderly patients should reflect the possibility of decreased liver or kidney function, other medical conditions, and other drugs they may be taking.

Patient teaching

- Tell patient to take drug with food.

!!ALERT Tell patient to report to prescriber seizures and numbness in arms or legs.

- Warn patient not to drink alcohol or use alcohol-containing products while taking tinidazole and for 3 days afterward.
- Advise patient to immediately tell her prescriber if she becomes pregnant.
- Tell patient to stop breast-feeding during therapy and for 3 days after the last dose.
- If patient is being treated for a sexually transmitted disease, explain that sexual partners should be treated at the same time.

tinzaparin sodium
Innohep

Pregnancy risk category B

Indications & dosages

➲ **Symptomatic DVT with or without pulmonary embolism with warfarin sodium**
Adults: 175 anti–factor Xa IU/kg of body weight S.C. once daily for at least 6 days and until patient is adequately anticoagulated with warfarin sodium (INR of at least 2) for 2 consecutive days. Start warfarin sodium therapy when appropriate, usually within 1 to 3 days of tinzaparin initiation. Volume of dose to be given may be calculated as follows:

Patient weight in kg × 0.00875 ml/kg = Volume to be given in ml

Contraindications & cautions

- Contraindicated in patients hypersensitive to tinzaparin sodium or other low-molecular-weight heparins, heparin, sulfites, benzyl alcohol, or pork products. Also contraindicated in patients with active major bleeding and in those with history of heparin-induced thrombocytopenia.
- Use cautiously in patients with increased risk of hemorrhage, such as those with bacterial endocarditis; uncontrolled hypertension; diabetic retinopathy; congenital or acquired bleeding disorders, including hepatic failure and amyloidosis; GI ulceration; or hemorrhagic stroke. Also use cautiously in patients who have recently undergone brain, spinal, or ophthalmologic surgery, and in patients being treated with platelet inhibitors. Elderly patients and patients with renal insufficiency may show reduced elimination of drug. Use drug with care in these patients.
- Use cautiously in breast-feeding women; it's unknown if drug appears in breast milk.

Adverse reactions

CNS: headache, dizziness, insomnia, confusion, ***cerebral or intracranial bleeding***, fever, pain.
CV: ***arrhythmias***, chest pain, hypotension, hypertension, ***MI***, ***thromboembolism***, tachycardia, dependent edema, angina pectoris.
EENT: epistaxis, ocular hemorrhage.
GI: anorectal bleeding, constipation, flatulence, hematemesis, ***GI hemorrhage***, nausea, vomiting, dyspepsia, retroperitoneal or intra-abdominal bleeding, melena.
GU: dysuria, hematuria, UTI, urine retention, ***vaginal hemorrhage***.
Hematologic: ***granulocytopenia***, ***thrombocytopenia***, anemia, ***agranulocytosis***, ***pancytopenia***, ***hemorrhage***.
Musculoskeletal: back pain, hemarthrosis.
Respiratory: pneumonia, respiratory disorder, dyspnea, ***pulmonary embolism***.
Skin: bullous eruption, cellulitis, *injection site hematoma*, pruritus, purpura, rash, skin necrosis, wound hematoma, bullous eruption.
Other: hypersensitivity reaction, ***spinal or epidural hematoma***, infection, impaired healing, ***allergic reaction***, congenital anomaly, ***fetal death***, fetal distress.

Interactions

Drug-drug. *Oral anticoagulants, platelet inhibitors (such as dextran, dipyridamole, NSAIDs, salicylates, sulfinpyrazone), thrombolytics:* May increase risk of bleeding. Use together cautiously. If drugs must be given together, monitor patient.

Nursing considerations

- Drug isn't intended for I.M. or I.V. administration, nor should it be mixed with other injections or infusions.
- Don't interchange drug (unit to unit) with heparin or other low-molecular-weight heparins.
- When giving drug, have patient lie or sit down. Give by deep S.C. injection into abdominal wall. Introduce whole length of needle into skinfold held between thumb and forefinger. Make sure to hold skinfold throughout injection. Rotate injection sites between right and left anterolateral and posterolateral abdominal wall. To minimize bruising, don't rub injection site after administration.
- Use an appropriate calibrated syringe to ensure correct withdrawal of volume of drug from vials.
- Monitor platelet count during therapy. Stop drug if platelet count goes below 100,000/mm^3.

- Periodically monitor CBC count and stool tests for occult blood during treatment.
- Drug may affect PT and INR levels. Patient also receiving warfarin should have blood for PT and INR drawn just before next scheduled dose of tinzaparin.
- Drug contains sodium metabisulfite, which may cause allergic reactions in susceptible people.

!!ALERT When neuraxial anesthesia (epidural or spinal anesthesia) or spinal puncture is used, patient is at risk for developing spinal hematoma, which can result in long-term or permanent paralysis. Watch for signs and symptoms of neurologic impairment. Consider risk versus benefit of neuraxial intervention in patient being treated with low-molecular-weight heparins or heparinoids.

- If patient becomes pregnant while taking drug, warn her of potential hazards to fetus. Cases of gasping syndrome have occurred in premature infants when large amounts of benzyl alcohol have been given.
- Store drug at room temperature.

Patient teaching

- Explain to patient importance of laboratory monitoring to ensure effectiveness of drug while maintaining safety.
- Teach patient warning signs of bleeding and instruct him to report these signs immediately.
- Caution patient to use soft toothbrush and electric razor to prevent cuts and bruises.
- Instruct patient that warfarin therapy will be started when appropriate, within 1 to 3 days of tinzaparin administration. Explain importance of warfarin therapy and monitoring to ensure safety and efficacy.

tiotropium bromide
Spiriva

Pregnancy risk category C

Indications & dosages

➲ Maintenance treatment of bronchospasm in COPD, including chronic bronchitis and emphysema

Adults: 1 capsule (18 mcg) inhaled orally once daily using the HandiHaler inhalation device.

Contraindications & cautions

- Contraindicated in patients hypersensitive to atropine, its derivatives, ipratropium, or any component of the product.
- Use cautiously in women who are pregnant or breast-feeding, patients with creatinine clearance of 50 ml/minute or less, or patients with angle-closure glaucoma, prostatic hyperplasia, or bladder neck obstruction.

Adverse reactions

CNS: depression, paresthesia.

CV: ***angina pectoris***, chest pain, edema.

EENT: cataract, dysphonia, epistaxis, glaucoma, laryngitis, pharyngitis, rhinitis, *sinusitis*.

GI: abdominal pain, constipation, *dry mouth*, dyspepsia, gastroesophageal reflux, stomatitis, vomiting.

GU: UTI.

Metabolic: hypercholesterolemia, hyperglycemia.

Musculoskeletal: arthritis, leg pain, myalgia, skeletal pain.

Respiratory: cough, *upper respiratory tract infection*.

Skin: rash.

Other: *accidental injury*, allergic reaction, candidiasis, flulike syndrome, herpes zoster, infections.

Interactions

Drug-drug. *Anticholinergics:* May increase the risk of adverse reactions. Avoid using together.

Nursing considerations

- Drug is for maintenance treatment of COPD and not for acute bronchospasm.
- Capsules aren't for oral ingestion. Give them only by oral inhalation with the HandiHaler device.
- Watch for evidence of hypersensitivity (especially angioedema) and paradoxical bronchospasm.

Patient teaching

- Inform patient that drug is for maintenance treatment of COPD and not for immediate relief of breathing problems.

!!ALERT Explain that capsules are for inhalation and shouldn't be swallowed

- Provide full instructions for the HandiHaler device.

- Tell patient not to get powder in his eyes.
- Review signs and symptoms of hypersensitivity (especially angioedema) and paradoxical bronchospasm. Tell patient to stop the drug and contact the prescriber if they occur.
- Advise patient to report eye pain, blurred vision, visual halos, colored images, or red eyes immediately.
- Tell patient to keep capsules in sealed blisters and to remove each capsule just before use. Caution against storing capsules in the HandiHaler device.
- Instruct patient to store capsules at 77° F (25° C) and not to expose them to extreme temperatures or moisture.

tirofiban hydrochloride

Aggrastat

Pregnancy risk category B

Indications & dosages

➲ **Acute coronary syndrome, with heparin or aspirin, including patients who are to be managed medically and those undergoing PTCA or atherectomy**

Adults: I.V. loading dose of 0.4 mcg/kg/minute for 30 minutes; then continuous I.V. infusion of 0.1 mcg/kg/minute. Continue infusion through angiography and for 12 to 24 hours after angioplasty or atherectomy.

If creatinine clearance is less than 30 ml/minute, use a loading dose of 0.2 mcg/kg/minute for 30 minutes; then continuous infusion of 0.05 mcg/kg/minute. Continue infusion through angiography and for 12 to 24 hours after angioplasty or atherectomy.

Contraindications & cautions

- Contraindicated in patients hypersensitive to drug or its components.
- Contraindicated in those with active internal bleeding or history of bleeding diathesis within the previous 30 days and in those with history of intracranial hemorrhage, intracranial neoplasm, arteriovenous malformation, aneurysm, thrombocytopenia after previous exposure to tirofiban, CVA within 30 days, or hemorrhagic CVA.
- Contraindicated in those with history, symptoms, or findings suggestive of aortic dissection; severe hypertension (systolic blood pressure higher than 180 mm Hg or diastolic blood pressure higher than 110 mm Hg); acute pericarditis; major surgical procedure or severe physical trauma within previous month; or concomitant use of another parenteral GP IIb/IIIa inhibitor.
- Use cautiously in patients with increased risk of bleeding, including those with hemorrhagic retinopathy or platelet count less than 150,000/mm^3.
- Safety and effectiveness of drug haven't been studied in patients younger than age 18.

Adverse reactions

CNS: dizziness, headache, fever.
CV: ***bradycardia, coronary artery dissection***, edema, vasovagal reaction.
GI: nausea, *occult bleeding*.
Hematologic: *bleeding*, ***thrombocytopenia***.
Musculoskeletal: leg pain.
Skin: sweating.
Other: *bleeding at arterial access site*, pelvic pain.

Interactions

Drug-drug. *Anticoagulants such as warfarin, clopidogrel, dipyridamole, heparin, NSAIDs, thrombolytics, ticlopidine:* May increase risk of bleeding. Monitor patient closely.
Levothyroxine, omeprazole: May increase tirofiban renal clearance. Monitor patient.

Nursing considerations

- Monitor hemoglobin level, hematocrit, and platelet counts before starting therapy, 6 hours after loading dose, and at least daily during therapy. Notify prescriber if thrombocytopenia occurs.
- Give drug with aspirin and heparin.
- Monitor patient for bleeding.

!!ALERT The most common adverse effect is bleeding at the arterial access site for cardiac catheterization.

- The risk of bleeding may be decreased by early sheath removal and by keeping the access site immobile. The sheath may be removed during tirofiban infusion, but only after heparin has been stopped and its effects largely reversed.
- Minimize use of arterial and venous punctures, I.M. injections, urinary catheters, and nasotracheal and nasogastric tubes.

• When obtaining I.V. access, avoid use of noncompressible sites (such as subclavian or jugular veins).
!! **ALERT** Don't confuse Aggrastat with argatroban.

Patient teaching

• Explain that drug is a blood thinner used to prevent chest pain and heart attack.
• Explain that risk of serious bleeding is far outweighed by the benefits of drug.
• Instruct patient to report chest discomfort or other adverse effects immediately.
• Tell patient that frequent blood sampling may be needed to evaluate therapy.

tobramycin
AKTob, Defy, Tobrex

Pregnancy risk category B

Indications & dosages

➲ **External ocular infections by susceptible bacteria**
Adults and children: In mild to moderate infections, instill 1 or 2 drops into affected eye q 4 hours, or apply 1-cm strip of ointment q 8 to 12 hours. In severe infections, instill 2 drops into infected eye q 30 to 60 minutes until condition improves; then reduce frequency. Or, apply 1-cm strip of ointment q 3 to 4 hours until condition improves; then reduce frequency to b.i.d. to t.i.d.

Contraindications & cautions

• Contraindicated in patients hypersensitive to drug or other aminoglycosides.

Adverse reactions

EENT: burning or stinging on instillation, lid itching or swelling, conjunctival erythema, blurred vision with ointment, increased lacrimation.

Interactions

None significant.

Nursing considerations

• When two different ophthalmic solutions are used, allow at least 5 minutes between instillations.
!! **ALERT** Tobramycin ophthalmic solution isn't for injection.
• If topical ocular tobramycin is given with systemic tobramycin, carefully monitor levels.
• Prolonged use may result in overgrowth of nonsusceptible organisms, including fungi.
!! **ALERT** Don't confuse tobramycin with Trobicin, or Tobrex with TobraDex.

Patient teaching

• Tell patient to clean excessive discharge from eye area before application.
• Teach patient how to instill drops or apply ointment. Advise him to wash hands before and after applying and to avoid touching tip of dropper to eye or surrounding tissue.
• Instruct patient to apply light finger pressure on lacrimal sac for 1 minute after drops are instilled.
• Advise patient to watch for itching lids, swelling, or constant burning. Tell him to stop drug and notify prescriber if these signs and symptoms develop.
• Tell patient not to share drug, washcloths, or towels with family members and to notify prescriber if anyone develops same signs or symptoms.
• Stress importance of compliance with recommended therapy.

tobramycin sulfate
Nebcin, TOBI

Pregnancy risk category D

Indications & dosages

➲ **Serious infections caused by sensitive strains of *Escherichia coli, Proteus, Klebsiella, Enterobacter, Serratia, Morganella morganii, Staphylococcus aureus, Citrobacter, Pseudomonas*, or *Providencia***
Adults: 3 mg/kg/day I.M. or I.V. in divided doses. For life-threatening infections, give up to 5 mg/kg/day in divided doses q 6 to 8 hours; reduce to 3 mg/kg daily as soon as clinically indicated.
Children: 6 to 7.5 mg/kg/day I.M. or I.V. in three or four divided doses.
Neonates younger than age 1 week or premature infants: Up to 4 mg/kg/day I.V. or I.M. in two equal doses q 12 hours.

For patients with renal impairment, give loading dose of 1 mg/kg; then give decreased doses at 8-hour intervals or same dose at prolonged intervals. For patients with severe cystic fibrosis, initial dose is 10 mg/kg/day I.V. or I.M. in four divided doses.

➲ **To manage cystic fibrosis patients with *Pseudomonas aeruginosa***

Adults and children age 6 and older: 300 mg via nebulizer q 12 hours for 28 days. Continue cycle of 28 days on drug and 28 days off.

Contraindications & cautions

- Contraindicated in patients hypersensitive to drug or other aminoglycosides.
- Use cautiously in patients with impaired renal function or neuromuscular disorders and in elderly patients.

Adverse reactions

CNS: headache, lethargy, confusion, disorientation, fever, ***seizures***.
EENT: *ototoxicity, hoarseness, pharyngitis*.
GI: vomiting, nausea, diarrhea.
GU: ***nephrotoxicity***, possible increase in urinary excretion of casts.
Hematologic: anemia, eosinophilia, ***leukopenia***, ***thrombocytopenia***, ***agranulocytosis***.
Metabolic: electrolyte imbalances.
Musculoskeletal: muscle twitching.
Respiratory: ***bronchospasm***.
Skin: rash, urticaria, pruritus.

Interactions

Drug-drug. *Acyclovir, amphotericin B, cephalosporins, cidofovir, cisplatin, methoxyflurane, vancomycin, other aminoglycosides:* May increase nephrotoxicity. Monitor renal function test results.
Atracurium, doxacurium, mivacurium, pancuronium, rocuronium, tubocurarine, vecuronium: May increase effects of nondepolarizing muscle relaxants, including prolonged respiratory depression. Use together only when necessary, and expect to reduce dosage of nondepolarizing muscle relaxant.
Dimenhydrinate: May mask symptoms of ototoxicity. Monitor patient's hearing.
General anesthetics: May increase neuromuscular blockade. Monitor patient for increased clinical effects.
I.V. loop diuretics (such as furosemide): May increase ototoxicity. Monitor patient's hearing.
Parenteral penicillins (such as ticarcillin): May inactivate tobramycin in vitro. Don't mix.

Nursing considerations

- Obtain specimen for culture and sensitivity tests before giving first dose. Therapy may begin while awaiting results.
- Weigh patient and review renal function studies before therapy.
- Evaluate patient's hearing before and during therapy. Notify prescriber if patient complains of tinnitus, vertigo, or hearing loss.
- Don't dilute or mix tobramycin sulfate with dornase alpha in the nebulizer.
- Unrefrigerated tobramycin sulfate, which is normally slightly yellow, may darken with age. This change doesn't indicate a change in product quality.
- Avoid exposing tobramycin sulfate ampules to intense light.
- Give nebulizer solution over 10 to 15 minutes using handheld Pari LC Plus reusable nebulizer with DeVilbiss Pulmo-Aide compressor.
- Obtain blood for peak level 1 hour after I.M. injection or ½ hour after infusion stops; draw blood for trough level just before next dose. Don't collect blood in a heparinized tube; heparin is incompatible with aminoglycosides.

!!ALERT Peak blood levels over 12 mcg/ml and trough levels over 2 mcg/ml may increase the risk of toxicity. Reserve higher peak levels for cystic fibrosis patients, who need a greater lung penetration.

- Monitor renal function: urine output, specific gravity, urinalysis, creatinine clearance, and BUN and creatinine levels. Notify prescriber about signs and symptoms of decreasing renal function.
- Watch for signs and symptoms of superinfection, such as continued fever, chills, and increased pulse rate.
- If no response occurs in 3 to 5 days, therapy may be stopped and new specimens obtained for culture and sensitivity testing.

!!ALERT Don't confuse tobramycin with Trobicin.

Patient teaching

- Instruct patient to report adverse reactions promptly.
- Caution patient not to perform hazardous activities if adverse CNS reactions occur.

• Encourage patient to maintain adequate fluid intake.
• Teach patient how to use and maintain nebulizer.
• Tell patient using multiple inhaled therapies to use tobramycin sulfate last.
• Instruct patient not to use tobramycin sulfate if the solution is cloudy or contains particles or if it has been stored at room temperature for longer than 28 days.

tocainide hydrochloride

Tonocard

Pregnancy risk category C

Indications & dosages

➲ **Suppression of symptomatic life-threatening ventricular arrhythmias**
Adults: Initially, 400 mg P.O. q 8 hours. Usual dose is between 1,200 and 1,800 mg daily in three divided doses.
➲ **Myotonic dystrophy**♦
Adults: 800 to 1,200 mg P.O. daily.
➲ **Trigeminal neuralgia**♦
Adults: 20 mg/kg/day P.O. in three divided doses.

For patients with renal or hepatic impairment, a dose less than 1,200 mg daily may be adequate.

Contraindications & cautions

• Contraindicated in patients hypersensitive to lidocaine or other amide-type local anesthetics and in those with second- or third-degree AV block in the absence of an artificial pacemaker.
• Use cautiously in patients with heart failure or diminished cardiac reserve and in those with hepatic or renal impairment. These patients often may be treated effectively with a lower dose.

Adverse reactions

CNS: ataxia, *light-headedness, tremor,* paresthesia, *dizziness, vertigo,* drowsiness, fatigue, confusion, headache.
CV: hypotension, ***new or worsened arrhythmias, heart failure, bradycardia,*** palpitations.
EENT: blurred vision, tinnitus.
GI: *nausea, vomiting,* diarrhea, anorexia.
Hematologic: ***agranulocytosis, bone marrow depression, thrombocytopenia, aplastic anemia, neutropenia.***
Hepatic: ***hepatitis.***
Respiratory: ***pulmonary fibrosis,*** pulmonary edema, interstitial pneumonitis, fibrosing alveolitis.
Skin: rash, diaphoresis.

Interactions

Drug-drug. *Beta blockers:* May decrease myocardial contractility; may increase CNS toxicity. Monitor patient closely.
Cimetidine: May reduce tocainide level. Monitor tocainide effectiveness.
Rifampin: May increase clearance of tocainide. Monitor tocainide effectiveness.

Nursing considerations

• Drug may ease transition from I.V. lidocaine to oral antiarrhythmic. Monitor patient carefully.
• Correct potassium deficits. Drug may be ineffective in patients with hypokalemia.
• Monitor patient for tremor, which may indicate that maximum dosage has been reached.
• Notify prescriber if patient develops signs and symptoms of infection; perform a CBC immediately to rule out agranulocytosis.

Patient teaching

• Instruct patient to immediately report unusual bruising or bleeding or signs or symptoms of infection. Severe blood cell deficiency and bone marrow suppression have been reported in patients taking usual doses of drug, typically within first 12 weeks of therapy.
• Advise patient to report immediately sudden onset of breathing problems, such as coughing, wheezing, or labored breathing after exertion. Drug may cause serious breathing problems.
• Tell elderly patient to take safety precautions to reduce the risk of dizziness and falling.

tolcapone
Tasmar

Pregnancy risk category C

Indications & dosages

➲ **Adjunct to levodopa and carbidopa for treating signs and symptoms of idiopathic Parkinson's disease in patients who have symptom fluctuation or haven't responded to other adjunctive treatment**
Adults: Initially, 100 mg P.O. t.i.d. with levodopa and carbidopa. Recommended daily dosage is 100 mg P.O. t.i.d. Levodopa dosage may need to be reduced by 20% to 30% to minimize risk of dyskinesias. Maximum, 600 mg daily. Stop drug if patient shows no benefit within 3 weeks.

Contraindications & cautions

- Contraindicated in patients hypersensitive to drug or its components and in those with hepatic disease, elevated ALT or AST levels, or history of drug-related confusion and nontraumatic rhabdomyolysis or hyperpyrexia.
- Contraindicated in those who were withdrawn from tolcapone because of drug-induced hepatocellular injury.
- Use cautiously in patients with severe renal impairment and in breast-feeding women.

Adverse reactions

CNS: fever, *dyskinesia, sleep disorder, dystonia, excessive dreaming, somnolence*, dizziness, *confusion, headache, hallucinations*, hyperkinesia, hypertonia, fatigue, falling, syncope, balance loss, depression, tremor, speech disorder, paresthesia, agitation, irritability, mental deficiency, hyperactivity, hypokinesia.
CV: *orthostatic complaints*, chest pain, chest discomfort, palpitations, hypotension.
EENT: pharyngitis, tinnitus, sinus congestion.
GI: *nausea, anorexia, diarrhea*, flatulence, *vomiting*, constipation, abdominal pain, dyspepsia, dry mouth.
GU: UTI, urine discoloration, hematuria, micturition disorder, urinary incontinence, impotence.
Hematologic: bleeding.
Hepatic: ***hepatotoxicity***.
Musculoskeletal: *muscle cramps*, stiffness, arthritis, neck pain.
Respiratory: bronchitis, dyspnea, upper respiratory tract infection.
Skin: increased sweating, rash.
Other: influenza.

Interactions

Drug-drug. *CNS depressants:* May cause additive effects. Monitor patient closely.
Desipramine, SSRIs, tricyclic antidepressants: May increase risk of adverse effects. Use together cautiously.
Nonselective MAO inhibitors (phenelzine, tranylcypromine): May cause hypertensive crisis. Avoid using together.
Warfarin: May cause increased warfarin level. Monitor INR, and adjust warfarin dosage as needed.

Nursing considerations

- Because of risk of liver toxicity, stop treatment if patient shows no benefit within 3 weeks.
- Because of fatal hepatic failure risk, use drug only in patients taking levodopa and carbidopa who don't respond to or who aren't appropriate candidates for other adjunctive therapies.

!!ALERT Make sure patient provides written informed consent before taking drug.

- Monitor liver function test results before starting drug, every 2 weeks for first year of therapy, every 4 weeks for next 6 months, and every 8 weeks thereafter. Stop drug if results are abnormal or if patient appears jaundiced.
- Because drug is highly protein-bound, it isn't significantly removed during dialysis.
- Monitor patient for orthostatic hypotension and syncope.
- Give first dose of the day with first daily dose of levodopa and carbidopa.

Patient teaching

- Advise patient to take drug exactly as prescribed.
- Teach patient to immediately report the signs and symptoms of liver injury (yellow eyes or skin, fatigue, loss of appetite, persistent nausea, itching, dark urine, or right upper abdominal tenderness).
- Warn patient about risk of dizziness upon standing up quickly; tell him to stand up cautiously.

- Advise patient to avoid hazardous activities until CNS effects of drug are known.
- Tell patient that nausea may occur early in therapy.
- Inform patient that diarrhea is common, sometimes occurring 2 to 12 weeks after therapy begins, and usually resolves when therapy stops.
- Advise patient about risk of increased problems making voluntary movements or impaired muscle tone.
- Inform patient that hallucinations may occur.
- Tell woman to notify prescriber about planned, suspected, or known pregnancy.
- Inform patient that drug may be taken without regard to meals.

tolterodine tartrate
Detrol, Detrol LA

Pregnancy risk category C

Indications & dosages

➲ Overactive bladder in patients with symptoms of urinary frequency, urgency, or urge incontinence

Adults: 2-mg tablet P.O. b.i.d. or 4-mg extended-release capsule P.O. daily. Dose may be reduced to 1-mg tablet P.O. b.i.d. or 2-mg extended-release capsule P.O. daily, based on patient response and tolerance.

For patients with significantly reduced hepatic function or those taking a cytochrome P-450 inhibitor, 1-mg tablet P.O. b.i.d. or 2-mg extended-release capsule P.O. daily.

Contraindications & cautions

- Contraindicated in patients hypersensitive to drug or its components and in those with uncontrolled angle-closure glaucoma or urine or gastric retention.
- Use cautiously in patients with significant bladder outflow obstruction, GI obstructive disorders (such as pyloric stenosis), controlled angle-closure glaucoma, and hepatic or renal impairment.

Adverse reactions

CNS: fatigue, paresthesia, vertigo, dizziness, *headache,* nervousness, somnolence.
CV: hypertension, chest pain.
EENT: abnormal vision, xerophthalmia, pharyngitis, rhinitis, sinusitis.
GI: *dry mouth,* abdominal pain, constipation, diarrhea, dyspepsia, flatulence, nausea, vomiting.
GU: dysuria, micturition frequency, urine retention, UTI.
Metabolic: weight gain.
Musculoskeletal: arthralgia, back pain.
Respiratory: bronchitis, coughing, upper respiratory tract infection.
Skin: pruritus, rash, erythema, dry skin.
Other: flulike syndrome, accidental injury, fungal infection, infection.

Interactions

Drug-drug. *Antifungal drugs (itraconazole, ketoconazole, miconazole), cytochrome P-450 inhibitors (such as the macrolide antibiotics clarithromycin and erythromycin):* May increase tolterodine level. Don't give more than 1-mg tablet b.i.d. or 2-mg extended-release capsule daily of tolterodine if used together.

Fluoxetine: May increase tolterodine level. Monitor patient. No dosage adjustment is needed.

Nursing considerations

- Assess baseline bladder function and monitor therapeutic effects.

Patient teaching

- Tell patient that sugarless gum, hard candy, or saliva substitute may help relieve dry mouth.
- Advise patient to avoid driving or other potentially hazardous activities until visual effects of drug are known.
- Advise breast-feeding woman to stop breast-feeding during therapy.
- Instruct patient to immediately report signs of infection, urine retention, or GI problems.
- Tell patient taking extended-release form to swallow capsule whole and take with liquids.

topiramate
Topamax

Pregnancy risk category C

Indications & dosages

➲ Adjunct treatment for partial onset seizures, primary generalized tonic-clonic seizures; Lennox-Gastaut syndrome in children

Adults: Initially, 25 to 50 mg P.O. daily; increase gradually by 25 to 50 mg/week until an effective daily dose is reached. Adjust to recommended daily dose of 200 to 400 mg P.O in two divided doses for adults with partial seizures or 400 mg P.O. in two divided doses for adults with primary generalized tonic-clonic seizures.

Children ages 2 to 16: Initially, 1 to 3 mg/kg daily given h.s. for 1 week. Increase at 1- or 2-week intervals by 1 to 3 mg/kg daily in two divided doses to achieve optimal response Recommended dose is 5 to 9 mg/kg daily given in two divided doses.

➲ To prevent migraine headache

Adults: Initially, 25 mg P.O. daily in the evening for first week. Then, 25 mg P.O. b.i.d. in the morning and evening for the second week. For the third week, 25 mg P.O. in the morning and 50 mg P.O. in the evening. For the fourth week, 50 mg P.O. b.i.d. in the morning and evening.

If creatinine clearance is less than 70 ml/minute, reduce dosage by 50%. For hemodialysis patients, supplemental doses may be needed to avoid rapid drops in drug level during prolonged dialysis treatment.

Contraindications & cautions

- Contraindicated in patients hypersensitive to drug or its components.
- Use with caution in breast-feeding or pregnant women and in those with hepatic impairment.
- Use cautiously with other drugs that predispose patients to heat-related disorders, including other carbonic anhydrase inhibitors and anticholinergics.

Adverse reactions

CNS: fever, abnormal coordination, aggressive reaction, agitation, apathy, asthenia, *ataxia, confusion*, depression, depersonalization, *difficulty with memory, dizziness*, emotional lability, euphoria, ***generalized tonic-clonic seizures***, hallucination, hyperkinesia, hypertonia, hypoesthesia, hypokinesia, insomnia, mood problems, *nervousness, paresthesia*, personality disorder, *psychomotor slowing*, psychosis, *somnolence, speech disorders*, stupor, ***suicide attempts***, *tremor*, vertigo, malaise, *fatigue*, difficulty with concentration, attention, or language.

CV: chest pain, palpitations, vasodilation, edema.

EENT: *abnormal vision*, conjunctivitis, *diplopia*, eye pain, epistaxis, hearing problems, tinnitus, pharyngitis, sinusitis, *nystagmus*.

GI: abdominal pain, *anorexia*, constipation, diarrhea, dry mouth, dyspepsia, flatulence, gastroenteritis, gingivitis, *nausea*, vomiting, taste perversion.

GU: amenorrhea, dysuria, dysmenorrhea, hematuria, impotence, intermenstrual bleeding, menstrual disorder, menorrhagia, urinary frequency, renal calculi, urinary incontinence, UTI, vaginitis, leukorrhea.

Hematologic: anemia, ***leukopenia***.

Metabolic: increased weight, *decreased weight*.

Musculoskeletal: arthralgia, back or leg pain, muscle weakness, myalgia, rigors.

Respiratory: bronchitis, coughing, dyspnea, *upper respiratory tract infection*.

Skin: acne, alopecia, increased sweating, pruritus, rash.

Other: decreased libido, breast pain, body odor, flulike syndrome, hot flashes, lymphadenopathy.

Interactions

Drug-drug. *Carbamazepine:* May decrease topiramate level. Monitor patient.

Carbonic anhydrase inhibitors (acetazolamide, dichlorphenamide): May cause renal calculus formation. Avoid using together.

CNS depressants: May cause CNS depression and other adverse cognitive and neuropsychiatric events. Use together cautiously.

Hormonal contraceptives: May decrease efficacy. Report changes in menstrual patterns. Advise patient to use another contraceptive method.

Phenytoin: May decrease topiramate level and increase phenytoin level. Monitor levels.

Valproic acid: May decrease valproic acid and topiramate level. Monitor patient.
Drug-lifestyle. *Alcohol use:* May cause CNS depression and other adverse cognitive and neuropsychiatric events. Discourage use together.

Nursing considerations

- If needed, withdraw anticonvulsant (including topiramate) gradually to minimize risk of increased seizure activity.
- Monitoring topiramate level isn't necessary.
- Drug may infrequently cause oligohidrosis and hyperthermia, mainly in children. Monitor patient closely, especially in hot weather.
- Topiramate may cause hyperchloremic, non–anion gap metabolic acidosis from renal bicarbonate loss. Factors that may predispose patients to acidosis, such as renal disease, severe respiratory disorders, status epilepticus, diarrhea, surgery, ketogenic diet, or drugs, may add to topiramate's bicarbonate-lowering effects.
- Measure baseline and periodic bicarbonate levels. If metabolic acidosis develops and persists, consider reducing the dose, gradually stopping the drug, or alkali treatment.
- Drug is rapidly cleared by dialysis. A prolonged period of dialysis may cause low drug level and seizures. A supplemental dose may be needed.
- Stop drug if patient experiences acute myopia and secondary angle-closure glaucoma.

!!ALERT Don't confuse Topamax with Toprol-XL.

Patient teaching

- Tell patient to drink plenty of fluids during therapy to minimize risk of forming kidney stones.
- Advise patient not to drive or operate hazardous machinery until CNS effects of drug are known. Drug can cause sleepiness, dizziness, confusion, and concentration problems.
- Tell woman of childbearing age that drug may decrease effectiveness of hormonal contraceptives. Advise woman using hormonal contraceptives to report change in menstrual patterns.
- Tell patient to avoid crushing or breaking tablets because of bitter taste.
- Inform patient that drug can be taken without regard to food.
- Tell patient that capsules may either be swallowed whole or carefully opened and contents sprinkled on a teaspoonful of soft food. Tell patient to swallow immediately without chewing.
- Tell patient to notify prescriber immediately if he experiences changes in vision.

topotecan hydrochloride
Hycamtin

Pregnancy risk category D

Indications & dosages

➲ **Metastatic carcinoma of the ovary after failure of first or subsequent chemotherapy; small-cell lung cancer-sensitive disease after failure of first-line chemotherapy**
Adults: 1.5 mg/m^2 I.V. infusion given over 30 minutes daily for 5 consecutive days, starting on day 1 of a 21-day cycle. Give a minimum of four cycles.

For patients with creatinine clearance of 20 to 39 ml/minute, decrease dosage to 0.75 mg/m^2. If severe neutropenia occurs, decrease dosage by 0.25 mg/m^2 for subsequent courses. Or, if severe neutropenia occurs, give granulocyte colony–stimulating factor after subsequent course (before resorting to dosage reduction) starting from day 6 of course (24 hours after completion of topotecan administration).

Contraindications & cautions

- Contraindicated in patients hypersensitive to drug or its components and in those with severe bone marrow depression.
- Contraindicated in pregnant or breast-feeding women.
- Safety and effectiveness of drug in children haven't been established.

Adverse reactions

CNS: *fatigue, asthenia, headache, fever.*
GI: *nausea, vomiting, diarrhea, constipation, abdominal pain, stomatitis, anorexia.*
Hematologic: NEUTROPENIA, LEUKOPENIA, THROMBOCYTOPENIA, *anemia.*
Hepatic: ***hepatotoxicity.***
Musculoskeletal: *back and skeletal pain.*
Respiratory: *dyspnea, coughing.*

Skin: *alopecia*, rash.
Other: ***sepsis***.

Interactions

Drug-drug. *Cisplatin:* May increase severity of myelosuppression. Use together with extreme caution.
Granulocyte colony–stimulating factor: May prolong duration of neutropenia. If granulocyte colony–stimulating factor is to be used, don't start it until day 6 of the course, 24 hours after completion of topotecan treatment.

Nursing considerations

!!ALERT Before first course of therapy is started, patient must have baseline neutrophil count over 1,500 cells/mm³ and platelet count over 100,000 cells/mm³.
- Prepare drug under vertical laminar flow hood; wear gloves and protective clothing. If drug solution contacts skin, wash immediately and thoroughly with soap and water. If mucous membranes are affected, flush areas thoroughly with water.
- Bone marrow suppression (primarily neutropenia) indicates toxic levels of topotecan. The nadir occurs at about 11 days. Neutropenia isn't cumulative over time.
- Duration of thrombocytopenia is about 5 days, with nadir at 15 days. The nadir for anemia is 15 days. Blood or platelet transfusions may be needed.
- Monitor peripheral blood cell counts frequently. Don't give subsequent courses of topotecan until neutrophil count recovers to more than 1,000 cells/mm³, platelet count recovers to more than 100,000 cells/mm³, and hemoglobin level recovers to more than 9 mg/dl (with transfusion, if needed).
- Patient may receive injections of WBC colony–stimulating factors to promote cell growth and decrease risk for infection.

Patient teaching

- Urge patient to report promptly sore throat, fever, chills, or unusual bleeding or bruising.
- Caution woman of childbearing age to avoid pregnancy or breast-feeding during therapy.
- Teach patient and family about drug's adverse reactions and need for frequent monitoring of blood counts.

toremifene citrate
Fareston

Pregnancy risk category D

Indications & dosages

➲ **Metastatic breast cancer in postmenopausal women with estrogen receptor–positive or estrogen receptor–unknown tumors**
Adults: 60 mg P.O. once daily. Continue until disease progresses.

Contraindications & cautions

- Contraindicated in patients hypersensitive to drug and in those with history of thromboembolic disease.

Adverse reactions

CNS: dizziness, fatigue, depression.
CV: edema, ***thromboembolism***, ***heart failure***, ***MI***, ***pulmonary embolism***, *hot flashes*.
EENT: visual disturbances, glaucoma, dry eyes, *cataracts*.
GI: *nausea*, vomiting.
GU: *vaginal discharge*, vaginal bleeding.
Hepatic: ***hepatotoxicity***.
Metabolic: hypercalcemia.
Skin: *sweating*.

Interactions

Drug-drug. *Calcium-elevating drugs such as hydrochlorothiazide:* May increase risk of hypercalcemia. Monitor calcium level closely.
Coumarin-like anticoagulants such as warfarin: May prolong PT and INR. Monitor PT and INR closely.
CYP3A4 enzyme inducers (such as carbamazepine, phenobarbital, phenytoin): May increase toremifene metabolism rate. Monitor patient closely.
CYP3A4-6 enzyme inhibitors (such as erythromycin, ketoconazole): May increase toremifene metabolism rate. Monitor patient closely.

Nursing considerations

- Obtain periodic CBC, calcium levels, and liver function tests.
- Monitor calcium level closely during first weeks of treatment in patients with bone metastases because of increased risk of hypercalcemia.

Patient teaching

- Instruct patient to take drug exactly as prescribed.
- Advise patient that doses may be taken without regard to meals.
- Warn patient not to stop therapy without consulting prescriber.
- Inform patient about vaginal bleeding and other adverse effects; tell her to notify prescriber if bleeding occurs.
- Warn patient that disease flare-up may occur during first weeks of therapy. Reassure her that this doesn't indicate treatment failure.
- Advise patient to report leg or chest pain, severe headache, visual changes, or shortness of breath.
- Counsel woman of childbearing age about risks of becoming pregnant during therapy.

torsemide
Demadex

Pregnancy risk category B

Indications & dosages

➲ Diuresis in patients with heart failure
Adults: Initially, 10 to 20 mg P.O. or I.V. once daily. If response is inadequate, double dose until desired effect is achieved. Maximum, 200 mg daily.

➲ Diuresis in patients with chronic renal failure
Adults: Initially, 20 mg P.O. or I.V. once daily. If response is inadequate, double dose until response is obtained. Maximum, 200 mg daily.

➲ Diuresis in patients with hepatic cirrhosis
Adults: Initially, 5 to 10 mg P.O. or I.V. once daily with an aldosterone antagonist or a potassium-sparing diuretic. If response is inadequate, double dose until desired effect is achieved. Maximum, 40 mg daily.

➲ Hypertension
Adults: Initially, 5 mg P.O. daily. Increased to 10 mg if needed and tolerated. Add another antihypertensive if response is still inadequate.

Contraindications & cautions

- Contraindicated in patients hypersensitive to drug or other sulfonamide derivatives and in those with anuria.
- Use cautiously in patients with hepatic disease and related cirrhosis and ascites; sudden changes in fluid and electrolyte balance may precipitate hepatic coma in these patients.

Adverse reactions

CNS: asthenia, dizziness, headache, nervousness, insomnia, syncope.
CV: ECG abnormalities, chest pain, edema, orthostatic hypotension.
EENT: rhinitis, sore throat.
GI: *excessive thirst*, diarrhea, constipation, nausea, dyspepsia, ***hemorrhage***.
GU: excessive urination, impotence.
Metabolic: *electrolyte imbalances including hypokalemia and hypomagnesemia*, ***dehydration***, hypochloremic alkalosis, hyperuricemia, hypercholesterolemia.
Musculoskeletal: arthralgia, myalgia.
Respiratory: cough.
Skin: rash.

Interactions

Drug-drug. *Aminoglycoside antibiotics, cisplatin:* May increase ototoxicity. Use together cautiously.
Amphotericin B, corticosteroids, metolazone: May increase risk of hypokalemia. Monitor potassium level.
Antidiabetics: May decrease hypoglycemic effect. Monitor glucose level.
Chlorothiazide, chlorthalidone, hydrochlorothiazide, indapamide, metolazone: May cause excessive diuretic response, resulting in serious electrolyte abnormalities or dehydration. Adjust doses carefully, and monitor patient closely for signs and symptoms of excessive diuretic response.
Cholestyramine: May decrease absorption of torsemide. Separate doses by at least 3 hours.
Digoxin: May decrease torsemide clearance. Use together cautiously.
Indomethacin: May decrease diuretic effect in sodium-restricted patients. Avoid using together.
Lithium: May increase lithium level and cause toxicity. Use together cautiously and monitor lithium level.
NSAIDs: May increase nephrotoxicity of NSAIDs. Use together cautiously.
Probenecid: May decrease diuretic effect. Avoid using together.

Salicylates: May decrease excretion, possibly leading to salicylate toxicity. Avoid using together.
Spironolactone: May decrease renal clearance of spironolactone. Use together cautiously.
Drug-herb. *Dandelion:* May interfere with diuretic activity. Discourage use together.
Licorice: May cause unexpected rapid potassium loss. Discourage use together.

Nursing considerations

- To prevent nocturia, give drug in the morning.
- Monitor fluid intake and output, electrolyte levels, blood pressure, weight, and pulse rate during rapid diuresis and routinely with long-term use. Drug can cause profound diuresis and water and electrolyte depletion.
- Watch for signs of hypokalemia, such as muscle weakness and cramps.
- Consult prescriber and dietitian about providing a high-potassium diet. Foods rich in potassium include citrus fruits, tomatoes, bananas, dates, and apricots.
- Monitor elderly patients, who are especially susceptible to excessive diuresis with potential for circulatory collapse and thromboembolic complications.

!!ALERT Don't confuse torsemide with furosemide.

Patient teaching

- Tell patient to take drug in morning to prevent need to urinate at night.
- Advise patient to change positions slowly to prevent dizziness and to limit alcohol intake and strenuous exercise in hot weather to prevent dizziness.
- Advise patient to immediately report ringing in ears because it may indicate toxicity.
- Tell patient to check with prescriber or pharmacist before taking OTC drugs.

tramadol hydrochloride
Ultram

Pregnancy risk category C

Indications & dosages

➲ Moderate to moderately severe pain
Adults: Initially, 25 mg P.O. in the morning. Adjust by 25 mg q 3 days to 100 mg/day (25 mg q.i.d.). Thereafter, adjust by 50 mg q 3 days to reach 200 mg/day (50 mg q.i.d.). Thereafter, give 50 to 100 mg P.O. q 4 to 6 hours, p.r.n. Maximum, 400 mg daily.
Elderly patients: For patients older than age 75, maximum is 300 mg daily in divided doses.

If creatinine clearance is less than 30 ml/minute, increase dose interval to q 12 hours; maximum is 200 mg daily. For patients with cirrhosis, give 50 mg q 12 hours.

Contraindications & cautions

- Contraindicated in patients hypersensitive to drug or other opioids, in breast-feeding women, and in those with acute intoxication from alcohol, hypnotics, centrally acting analgesics, opioids, or psychotropic drugs. Serious hypersensitivity reactions can occur, usually after the first dose. Patients with history of anaphylactic reaction to codeine and other opioids may be at increased risk.
- Use cautiously in patients at risk for seizures or respiratory depression; in patients with increased intracranial pressure or head injury, acute abdominal conditions, or renal or hepatic impairment; or in patients with physical dependence on opioids.

Adverse reactions

CNS: *dizziness, vertigo, headache, somnolence,* CNS stimulation, asthenia, anxiety, confusion, coordination disturbance, euphoria, nervousness, sleep disorder, ***seizures***, malaise.
CV: vasodilation.
EENT: visual disturbances.
GI: *nausea, constipation, vomiting,* dyspepsia, dry mouth, diarrhea, abdominal pain, anorexia, flatulence.
GU: urine retention, urinary frequency, menopausal symptoms, proteinuria.
Musculoskeletal: hypertonia.
Respiratory: ***respiratory depression***.
Skin: pruritus, diaphoresis, rash.

Interactions

Drug-drug. *Carbamazepine:* May increase tramadol metabolism. Patients receiving long-term carbamazepine therapy up to 800 mg daily may need up to twice the recommended tramadol dose.

CNS depressants: May cause additive effects. Use together cautiously; tramadol dosage may need to be reduced.
Cyclobenzaprine, MAO inhibitors, neuroleptics, other opioids, tricyclic antidepressants: May increase risk of seizures. Monitor patient closely.
Quinidine: May increase level of tramadol. Monitor patient closely.
SSRIs: May increase risk of serotonin syndrome. Use cautiously and monitor patient for adverse effects.

Nursing considerations

- Reassess patient's level of pain at least 30 minutes after administration.
- Monitor CV and respiratory status. Withhold dose and notify prescriber if respirations decrease or rate is below 12 breaths/minute.
- Monitor bowel and bladder function. Anticipate need for laxative.
- For better analgesic effect, give drug before onset of intense pain.
- Monitor patients at risk for seizures. Drug may reduce seizure threshold.
- In the case of an overdose, naloxone may also increase risk of seizures.
- Monitor patient for drug dependence. Drug can produce dependence similar to that of codeine or dextropropoxyphene and thus has potential for abuse.
- Withdrawal symptoms may occur if drug is stopped abruptly. Reduce dosage gradually.

!!ALERT Don't confuse tramadol with trazodone or trandolapril.

Patient teaching

- Tell patient to take drug as prescribed and not to increase dose or dosage interval unless ordered by prescriber.
- Caution ambulatory patient to be careful when rising and walking. Warn outpatient to avoid driving and other potentially hazardous activities that require mental alertness until drug's CNS effects are known.
- Advise patient to check with prescriber before taking OTC drugs because drug interactions can occur.
- Warn patient not to stop the drug abruptly.

trastuzumab
Herceptin

Pregnancy risk category B

Indications & dosages

➲ **Single-drug treatment of metastatic breast cancer in patients whose tumors overexpress the human epidermal growth factor receptor 2 (HER2) protein and who have received one or more chemotherapy regimens for their metastatic disease, or with paclitaxel for metastatic breast cancer in patients whose tumors overexpress the HER2 protein and who haven't received chemotherapy for their metastatic disease**
Adults: First loading dose is 4 mg/kg I.V. over 90 minutes. Maintenance dose is 2 mg/kg I.V. weekly as 30-minute I.V. infusion if first loading dose is well tolerated.

Contraindications & cautions

- Contraindicated in patients hypersensitive to the drug.
- Use cautiously in elderly patients, in patients hypersensitive to drug or its components, and in those with cardiac dysfunction.
- Give drug with extreme caution in patients with pulmonary compromise, symptomatic intrinsic pulmonary disease (such as asthma, COPD), or extensive tumor involvement of the lungs.
- Safety and effectiveness of drug in children haven't been established.

Adverse reactions

CNS: depression, *dizziness*, *insomnia*, neuropathy, paresthesia, peripheral neuritis, *asthenia*, *headache*, *fever*, *pain*.
CV: ***heart failure***, *peripheral edema*, tachycardia, hypotension.
EENT: *rhinitis*, *pharyngitis*, sinusitis.
GI: *anorexia*, *abdominal pain*, *diarrhea*, *nausea*, *vomiting*.
GU: UTI.
Hematologic: ***leukopenia***, anemia.
Musculoskeletal: arthralgia, *back pain*, bone pain.
Respiratory: *dyspnea*, *increased cough*.
Skin: acne, *rash*.

Other: allergic reaction, herpes simplex, *chills, flulike syndrome, infection,* ANAPHYLAXIS.

Interactions

Drug-drug. *Anthracyclines, cyclophosphamide:* May increase cardiotoxicity. Use together very cautiously.

Nursing considerations

- Before beginning therapy, patient should undergo thorough baseline cardiac assessment, including history and physical examination and methods to identify risk of cardiotoxicity.
- Assess patient for signs and symptoms of cardiac dysfunction, especially if he is receiving drug with anthracyclines and cyclophosphamide.
- Check for dyspnea, increased cough, paroxysmal nocturnal dyspnea, peripheral edema, or S_3 gallop. Treatment may be stopped in patients who develop a significant decrease in left ventricular function.
- Monitor patient receiving both drug and chemotherapy closely for cardiac dysfunction or failure, anemia, leukopenia, diarrhea, and infection.
- Use drug only in patients with metastatic breast cancer whose tumors have HER2 protein overexpression.
- Check for first-infusion symptom complex, commonly consisting of chills or fever. Treat with acetaminophen, diphenhydramine, and meperidine (with or without reducing rate of infusion). Other signs or symptoms include nausea, vomiting, pain, rigors, headache, dizziness, dyspnea, hypotension, rash, and asthenia. These symptoms occur infrequently with subsequent infusions.

Patient teaching

- Tell patient about risk of first-dose infusion-related adverse reactions.
- Urge patient to notify prescriber immediately if signs or symptoms of heart problems occur, such as shortness of breath, increased cough, or swelling in arms or legs. Tell patient that these effects can occur after infusion is complete.
- Instruct patient to report adverse effects to prescriber.
- Advise breast-feeding woman to stop breast-feeding during drug therapy and for 6 months after last dose of drug.

travoprost
Travatan

Pregnancy risk category C

Indications & dosages

➲ To reduce intraocular pressure (IOP) in patients with open-angle glaucoma or ocular hypertension who can't tolerate or who respond inadequately to other IOP-lowering drugs
Adults: 1 drop in conjunctival sac of affected eye once daily h.s.

Contraindications & cautions

- Contraindicated in patients hypersensitive to travoprost, benzalkonium chloride, or other drug components; in pregnant women or women trying to become pregnant; and in those with angle-closure, inflammatory, or neovascular glaucoma.
- Use cautiously in patients with renal or hepatic impairment, active intraocular inflammation (iritis, uveitis), or risk factors for macular edema.
- Use cautiously in aphakic patients and pseudophakic patients with a torn posterior lens capsule.

Adverse reactions

CNS: anxiety, depression, headache, pain.
CV: angina pectoris, ***bradycardia***, chest pain, hypertension, hypotension.
EENT: *ocular hyperemia, decreased visual acuity, eye discomfort, foreign body sensation, eye pain, eye pruritus,* conjunctival hyperemia, abnormal vision, blepharitis, blurred vision, cataract, conjunctivitis, eye disorder, iris discoloration, dry eye, keratitis, lid margin crusting, photophobia, subconjunctival hemorrhage, tearing, sinusitis.
GI: dyspepsia, GI disorder.
GU: prostate disorder, urinary incontinence, UTI.
Metabolic: hypercholesterolemia.
Musculoskeletal: arthritis, back pain.
Respiratory: bronchitis.
Other: accidental injury, cold syndrome, infection.

Interactions

Drug-herb. *Areca, jaborandi:* May increase effects. Discourage use together.

Nursing considerations

- Temporary or permanent increased pigmentation of the iris and eyelid may occur as well as increased pigmentation and growth of eyelashes.
- Patient should remove contact lenses before instilling drug and reinsert them 15 minutes after administration.
- If using more than one ophthalmic drug, give the drugs at least 5 minutes apart.
- Store drug between 36° and 77° (2° and 25° C).
- If a pregnant woman or a woman attempting to become pregnant accidentally comes in contact with drug, thoroughly cleanse the exposed area with soap and water immediately.

Patient teaching

- Teach patient how to instill drops, and advise him to wash hands before and after instilling solution. Warn him not to touch tip of dropper to eye or surrounding tissue.
- Advise patient to apply light finger pressure on lacrimal sac for 1 minute after instillation to minimize systemic absorption of drug.
- Tell patient to remove contact lenses before administration and explain that he can reinsert them 15 minutes afterward.
- Tell patient receiving treatment in only one eye about potential for increased iris pigmentation, eyelid darkening, and increased length, thickness, pigmentation, or number of lashes in the treated eye.
- If eye trauma or infection occurs or if eye surgery is needed, advise patient to seek medical advice before continuing to use the multidose container.
- Advise patient to immediately report eye inflammation or lid reactions.
- If patient is using more than one ophthalmic drug, tell him to apply them at least 5 minutes apart.
- Stress importance of compliance with recommended therapy.
- Tell patient to discard container within 6 weeks of removing it from the sealed pouch.
- If a pregnant woman or a woman attempting to become pregnant accidentally comes in contact with drug, tell her to thoroughly cleanse the exposed area with soap and water immediately.

trazodone hydrochloride
Desyrel

Pregnancy risk category C

Indications & dosages

➲ Depression
Adults: Initially, 150 mg P.O. daily in divided doses; then increased by 50 mg daily q 3 to 4 days, p.r.n. Dose ranges from 150 to 400 mg daily. Maximum, 600 mg daily for inpatients and 400 mg daily for outpatients.

Contraindications & cautions

- Contraindicated in patients hypersensitive to drug.
- Use cautiously in patients with cardiac disease or in the initial recovery phase of MI and in patients at risk for suicide.

Adverse reactions

CNS: *drowsiness, dizziness,* nervousness, fatigue, confusion, tremor, weakness, hostility, anger, nightmares, vivid dreams, headache, insomnia, syncope.
CV: orthostatic hypotension, tachycardia, hypertension, shortness of breath, ECG changes.
EENT: blurred vision, tinnitus, nasal congestion.
GI: dry mouth, dysgeusia, constipation, nausea, vomiting, anorexia.
GU: urine retention, priapism possibly leading to impotence, hematuria.
Hematologic: anemia.
Skin: rash, urticaria, diaphoresis.
Other: decreased libido.

Interactions

Drug-drug. *Antihypertensives:* May increase hypotensive effect of trazodone. Antihypertensive dosage may need to be decreased.
Clonidine, CNS depressants: May enhance CNS depression. Avoid using together.
CYP3A4 inducers (carbamazepine): May reduce trazodone level. Monitor patient closely; may need to increase trazodone dose.
CYP3A4 inhibitors (ketoconazole, ritonavir, indinavir): May slow the clearance of trazodone and increase trazodone level. May cause nausea, hypotension, and fainting. Consider decreasing trazodone dose.

Digoxin, phenytoin: May increase levels of these drugs. Watch for toxicity.
MAO inhibitors: Effects unknown. Use together with extreme caution.
Drug-herb. *Ginkgo biloba:* May cause sedation. Discourage use together.
St. John's wort: May cause serotonin syndrome. Discourage use together.
Drug-lifestyle. *Alcohol use:* May enhance CNS depression. Discourage use together.

Nursing considerations

- Give drug after meals or a light snack for optimal absorption and to decrease risk of dizziness.
- Record mood changes. Monitor patient for suicidal tendencies and allow only minimum supply of drug.

!!ALERT Don't confuse trazodone hydrochloride with tramadol hydrochloride.

Patient teaching

!!ALERT Tell patient to report a persistent, painful erection (priapism) right away because he may need immediate intervention.

- Warn patient to avoid activities that require alertness and good coordination until effects of drug are known. Drowsiness and dizziness usually subside after first few weeks.
- Teach caregivers how to recognize signs and symptoms of suicidal tendency or suicidal thoughts.

treprostinil sodium
Remodulin

Pregnancy risk category B

Indications & dosages

➲ To reduce symptoms caused by exercise in patients with New York Heart Association class II to IV pulmonary arterial hypertension
Adults: Initially, 1.25 nanogram/kg/minute by continuous S.C. infusion. If patient doesn't tolerate initial dose, reduce infusion rate to 0.625 nanogram/kg/minute. Increase by 1.25 nanogram/kg/minute each week for the first 4 weeks and then by no more than 2.5 nanogram/kg/minute each week for the remaining duration of infusion. Maximum infusion rate is 40 nanogram/kg/minute.

In patients with mild or moderate hepatic insufficiency, initially, 0.625 nanogram/kg ideal body weight per minute, and increase cautiously.

Contraindications & cautions

- Contraindicated in patients hypersensitive to drug or structurally related compounds.
- Use cautiously in patients with hepatic or renal impairment and in elderly patients.

Adverse reactions

CNS: dizziness, *headache*, fatigue.
CV: *vasodilation*, hypotension, edema, chest pain, right ventricular, ***heart failure***.
GI: *diarrhea, nausea.*
Musculoskeletal: *jaw pain.*
Respiratory: dyspnea.
Skin: *infusion site pain, infusion site reaction, rash*, pruritus, pallor.

Interactions

Drug-drug. *Antihypertensives, diuretics, vasodilators:* May exacerbate reduction in blood pressure. Monitor blood pressure.
Anticoagulants: May increase risk of bleeding. Monitor patient closely for bleeding.

Nursing considerations

- Assess the patient's ability to accept, place, and care for an S.C. catheter and to use an infusion pump.
- Give only by continuous S.C. infusion via a self-inserted S.C. catheter, using an infusion pump designed for S.C. drug delivery. The infusion pump should be small and lightweight; adjustable to approximately 0.002 ml/hour; have occlusion/no delivery, low battery, programming error, and motor malfunction alarms; have delivery accuracy of ± 6% or better; and be positive-pressure driven. The reservoir should be made of polyvinyl chloride, polypropylene, or glass.
- During use, a single reservoir syringe can be given up to 72 hours at 98.6°F (37° C).
- Don't use a single vial longer than 14 days after the initial introduction to the vial.
- Inspect for particulate matter and discoloration before administration.
- Start treatment in setting where adequate monitoring and emergency care are available.
- Increase dose if patient doesn't improve or symptoms worsen, and decrease if drug ef-

fects become excessive or unacceptable infusion site symptoms develop.
- Avoid abrupt withdrawal or sudden large dose reductions because pulmonary arterial hypertension symptoms may worsen.

Patient teaching

- Inform patient that he'll need to continue therapy for prolonged periods, possibly years.
- Tell patient that subsequent disease management may require the initiation of I.V. therapy.
- Inform patient that many side effects may be related to the underlying disease (labored breathing, fatigue, chest pain).
- Tell patient that the most common local reactions are pain, redness, tissue hardening, and rash at the infusion site.

tretinoin (retinoic acid, vitamin A acid)

Avita, Renova, Retin-A, Retin-A Micro, StieVA-A†

Pregnancy risk category C

Indications & dosages

➲ Acne vulgaris

Adults and children: Clean affected area and lightly apply once daily h.s.

➲ Adjunctive use in the mitigation of fine facial wrinkles in patients who use comprehensive skin care and sunlight avoidance programs

Adults: Apply a small, pearl-sized amount (¼ inch or 5 mm in diameter) to cover affected area lightly, once daily in the evening.

Contraindications & cautions

- Contraindicated in patients hypersensitive to drug or its components and in those with sunburn.
- Use cautiously in patients with eczema.

Adverse reactions

Skin: *feeling of warmth, slight stinging, local erythema, peeling,* chapping, swelling, blistering, crusting, temporary hyperpigmentation or hypopigmentation.

Interactions

Drug-drug. *Topical drugs containing benzoyl peroxide, resorcinol, salicylic acid, or sulfur:* May increase risk of skin irritation. Avoid using together.

Topical minoxidil or photosensitizing drugs: May increase risk of skin irritation. Avoid using together.

Drug-lifestyle. *Abrasive cleansers, medicated cosmetics, skin preparations containing alcohol:* May increase risk of skin irritation. Discourage use together.

Sun exposure: May increase photosensitivity reaction. Advise patient to avoid excessive sunlight exposure.

Nursing considerations

- Initially, drug may be applied every 2 to 3 days using a lower concentration to reduce irritation.
- Relapses typically occur within 3 to 6 weeks after therapy is stopped.

!!ALERT Don't confuse tretinoin with trientine.

Patient teaching

- Instruct patient to clean area thoroughly before application and to avoid getting drug in eyes, mouth, or mucous membranes.
- Tell patient to wash hands after application.
- Tell patient to wash face with mild soap no more than b.i.d. or t.i.d. Warn patient against using strong or medicated cosmetics, soaps, or other skin cleansers. Also advise him to avoid topical products containing alcohol, astringents, spices, and lime because they may interfere with drug's actions.
- Tell patient using drug for treatment of fine wrinkles to wait 20 minutes after washing face to apply drug, and to avoid washing face or applying another skin product or cosmetic for 1 hour after application.
- Tell patient that normal use of cosmetics is allowed.
- Advise patient not to stop drug if temporary worsening of inflammatory lesions occurs. If severe local irritation develops, advise patient to stop drug temporarily and notify prescriber. Dosage will be readjusted when application is resumed. Some redness and scaling are normal reactions.
- Warn patient that he may experience increased sensitivity to wind or cold temperatures.
- Instruct patient to minimize exposure to sunlight or ultraviolet rays during treatment.

If he becomes sunburned, he should delay therapy until sunburn subsides. Tell patient who can't avoid exposure to sunlight to use SPF-15 sunblock and to wear protective clothing.
- Warn patient that he may have a temporary increase in lesions, which will improve in 2 to 3 weeks.

triamcinolone acetonide
Nasacort AQ

Pregnancy risk category C

Indications & dosages

➲ Rhinitis, allergic disorders, inflammatory conditions
Adults and children 12 years and older: 2 sprays in each nostril daily; may decrease to 1 spray in each nostril daily for allergic disorders.
Children ages 6 to 11: 1 spray in each nostril daily. Maximum dosage is 2 sprays in each nostril daily.

Contraindications & cautions

- Contraindicated in patients hypersensitive to drug or its components and in those with untreated mucosal infection.
- Use with caution, if at all, in patients with active or quiescent tuberculous infection of respiratory tract and in patients with untreated fungal, bacterial, or systemic viral infection or ocular herpes simplex.
- Use cautiously in patients already receiving systemic corticosteroids because of increased likelihood of hypothalamic-pituitary-adrenal axis suppression.
- Use cautiously in breast-feeding women and in those with recent nasal septal ulcers, nasal surgery, or trauma because drug may inhibit wound healing.

Adverse reactions

CNS: *headache.*
EENT: *nasal irritation,* dry mucous membranes, nasal and sinus congestion, irritation, burning, stinging, throat discomfort, sneezing, epistaxis.

Interactions

None significant.

Nursing considerations

!!ALERT Excessive doses may cause signs and symptoms of hyperadrenocorticism and adrenal axis suppression; stop drug slowly.
!!ALERT Don't confuse triamcinolone with Triaminicin.

Patient teaching

- Urge patient to read patient instruction sheet contained in each package before using drug for first time.
- To instill, instruct patient to shake container before use, blow nose to clear nasal passages, tilt head slightly forward, and insert nozzle into nostril, pointing away from septum. Tell him to hold other nostril closed and inhale gently while spraying. Next, have patient shake container and repeat procedure in other nostril.
- Instruct patient to avoid getting aerosol in eyes. If this occurs, tell him to rinse with copious amounts of cool tap water.
- Stress importance of using drug on a regular schedule because its effectiveness depends on regular use. Warn patient not to exceed prescribed dosage because serious adverse reactions can occur.
- Tell patient to notify prescriber if signs and symptoms don't diminish or if condition worsens in 2 to 3 weeks.
- Warn patient to avoid exposure to chickenpox or measles and, if exposed, to notify prescriber.
- Instruct patient to watch for and report signs and symptoms of nasal infection. Drug may need to be stopped and appropriate local therapy given.

triamcinolone acetonide
Azmacort, Nasacort AQ, Nasacort HFA

Pregnancy risk category C

Indications & dosages

➲ Persistent asthma
Adults and children older than age 12: 2 inhalations t.i.d. to q.i.d. Maximum, 16 inhalations daily. In some patients, maintenance can be achieved when total daily dose is given b.i.d.
Children ages 6 to 12: 1 to 2 inhalations t.i.d. to q.i.d. Maximum, 12 inhalations daily.

➲ **Nasal treatment of symptoms of seasonal and perennial allergic rhinitis**
Adults and children older than age 12: 2 sprays Nasacort HFA in each nostril once daily. May increase to 4 sprays into each nostril once daily. Adjust to minimum effective dosage. Or, 2 sprays Nasacort AQ in each nostril daily; may decrease to 1 spray per nostril daily.
Children ages 6 to 12: Initially, 1 spray Nasacort AQ in each nostril daily. If no response occurs, increase to 2 sprays in each nostril daily. Or, 2 sprays Nasacort HFA into each nostril once daily. Adjust to minimum effective dosage.

Contraindications & cautions

- Contraindicated in patients hypersensitive to drug or its ingredients and in those with status asthmaticus.
- Use with extreme caution, if at all, in patients with tuberculosis of the respiratory tract, ocular herpes simplex, or untreated fungal, bacterial, or systemic viral infections.
- Because of risk of severe adverse effects, don't use in breast-feeding women. It's unknown if drug appears in breast milk.

Adverse reactions

CNS: *headache.*
EENT: dry or irritated nose or throat, hoarseness, *pharyngitis, sneezing,* rhinitis.
GI: oral candidiasis, dry or irritated tongue or mouth.
Metabolic: hypothalamic-pituitary-adrenal function suppression, adrenal insufficiency.
Respiratory: cough, wheezing.
Other: facial edema.

Interactions

None significant.

Nursing considerations

- Unlike other corticosteroids, drug has a spacer built into the drug-delivery device.
- Use cautiously in patients receiving systemic corticosteroids.
- Most adverse reactions to corticosteroids are dose- or duration-dependent.
- Patients who have recently been switched from systemic corticosteroids to oral inhaled corticosteroids may need to resume systemic corticosteroid therapy during periods of stress or severe asthma attacks.
- Taper oral therapy slowly.
- Store drug between 59° and 86° F (15° and 30° C).
- For nasal spray, if symptoms don't improve after 2 to 3 weeks, reevaluate the patient.

!! ALERT Don't confuse triamcinolone with Triaminicin.

Patient teaching

Inhalation aerosol

- Inform patient that inhaled corticosteroids don't relieve emergency asthma attacks.
- Advise patient to warm canister to room temperature before using. Some patients carry canister in a pocket to keep it warm.
- If patient needs a bronchodilator, tell him to use it several minutes before triamcinolone. Tell patient to allow 1 minute to elapse before repeat inhalations and to hold his breath for a few seconds to enhance drug action.
- Teach patient to check mucous membranes frequently for evidence of fungal infection. Advise patient to avoid exposure to chickenpox or measles and to contact provider if exposure occurs.
- Tell patient to prevent oral fungal infections by gargling or rinsing mouth with water after each use of the inhaler. Remind him not to swallow the water.
- Tell patient to keep inhaler clean and unobstructed and to wash it with warm water and dry it thoroughly after use.
- Instruct patient to contact prescriber if response to therapy decreases; dosage may need adjustment. Tell him not to exceed recommended dosage on his own.
- Instruct patient to wear or carry medical identification indicating his need for supplemental systemic glucocorticoids during periods of stress.

Nasal spray

- Advise patient to use at regular intervals for full therapeutic effect.
- Advise patient to clear nasal passages before use.
- Have patient follow manufacturer's recommendations for use and cleaning.

triamcinolone acetonide

Aristocort, Aristocort A, Delta-Tritex, Flutex, Kenalog, Triacet, Triderm

Pregnancy risk category C

Indications & dosages

➲ Inflammation and pruritus from corticosteroid-responsive dermatoses
Adults and children: Clean area; apply aerosol, cream, lotion, or ointment sparingly b.i.d. to q.i.d. Rub in lightly.

➲ Inflammation from oral lesions
Adults and children: Apply paste h.s. and, if needed, b.i.d. or t.i.d., preferably after meals. Apply small amount without rubbing; press to lesion in mouth until thin film develops.

Contraindications & cautions

- Contraindicated in patients hypersensitive to drug or its components.

Adverse reactions

CV: syncope.
GU: glycosuria.
Metabolic: hyperglycemia.
Skin: burning, pruritus, irritation, dryness, erythema, folliculitis, hypertrichosis, hypopigmentation, acneiform eruptions, perioral dermatitis, allergic contact dermatitis, *maceration, secondary infection, atrophy, striae, miliaria with occlusive dressings.*
Other: ***hypothalamic-pituitary-adrenal axis suppression***, Cushing's syndrome.

Interactions

None significant.

Nursing considerations

- Gently wash skin before applying. To avoid skin damage, rub in gently, leaving a thin coat. When treating hairy sites, part hair and apply directly to lesions.
- Don't apply near eyes or in ear canal.
- Stop drug and tell prescriber if skin infection, striae, or atrophy occurs.
- When using aerosol near the face, cover patient's eyes and warn against inhaling spray. Aerosol contains alcohol and may cause irritation or burning when used on open lesions. Don't spray longer than 3 seconds or from closer than 6 inches (15 cm) to avoid freezing tissues.
- If antifungal or antibiotic combined with corticosteroid fails to provide prompt improvement, stop corticosteroid until infection is controlled.
- Systemic absorption is likely with the use of occlusive dressings, prolonged treatment, or extensive body surface treatment. Watch for symptoms, such as hyperglycemia, glycosuria, and hypothalamic-pituitary-adrenal axis suppression.
- Avoid using plastic pants or tight-fitting diapers on treated areas in young children. Children may absorb larger amounts of drug and be more susceptible to systemic toxicity.

!!ALERT Don't confuse triamcinolone with Triaminicin or Triaminicol.

Patient teaching

- Teach patient or family member how to apply drug.
- If an occlusive dressing is ordered, advise patient to leave it in place for no longer than 12 hours each day and not to use the dressing on infected or weeping lesions.
- Tell patient to stop drug and report signs of systemic absorption, skin irritation or ulceration, hypersensitivity, infection, or lack of improvement.

triamterene

Dyrenium

Pregnancy risk category B

Indications & dosages

➲ Edema
Adults: Initially, 100 mg P.O. b.i.d. after meals. Maximum, 300 mg daily.

Contraindications & cautions

- Contraindicated in patients hypersensitive to drug and in those with anuria, severe or progressive renal disease or dysfunction, severe hepatic disease, or hyperkalemia.
- Use cautiously in elderly or debilitated patients and in those with hepatic impairment or diabetes mellitus.

Adverse reactions

CNS: dizziness, weakness, fatigue, headache.
CV: hypotension.
GI: dry mouth, nausea, vomiting, diarrhea.

GU: interstitial nephritis, nephrolithiasis.
Hematologic: megaloblastic anemia related to low folic acid level, ***thrombocytopenia, agranulocytosis***.
Hepatic: jaundice.
Metabolic: azotemia, ***hyperkalemia***, hypokalemia, hyponatremia, hyperglycemia, acidosis.
Musculoskeletal: muscle cramps.
Skin: photosensitivity reactions, rash.
Other: ***anaphylaxis***.

Interactions

Drug-drug. *ACE inhibitors, potassium supplements:* May increase risk of hyperkalemia. If used together, monitor potassium level.
Amantadine: May increase risk of amantadine toxicity. Avoid using together.
Chlorpropamide: May increase risk of hyponatremia. Monitor sodium level.
Cimetidine: May increase bioavailability and decrease renal clearance of triamterene. Monitor potassium level and blood pressure closely.
Lithium: May decrease lithium clearance, increasing risk of lithium toxicity. Monitor lithium level.
NSAIDs: May enhance risk of nephrotoxicity. Use together cautiously.
Quinidine: May interfere with some laboratory tests that measure quinidine level. Inform laboratory that patient is taking triamterene.
Drug-herb. *Licorice:* May increase risk of hypokalemia. Discourage use together.
Drug-food. *Potassium-containing salt substitutes, potassium-rich foods:* May increase risk of hyperkalemia. Urge caution, and monitor potassium level.
Drug-lifestyle. *Sun exposure:* May increase risk for photosensitivity reactions. Advise patient to avoid excessive sunlight exposure.

Nursing considerations

- To minimize nausea, give drug after meals.
- Monitor blood pressure, uric acid, CBC, and glucose, BUN, and electrolyte levels.
- Watch for blood dyscrasia.
- To minimize excessive rebound potassium excretion, withdraw drug gradually.
- Drug is less potent than thiazides and loop diuretics and is useful as an adjunct to other diuretic therapy. It's usually used with potassium-wasting diuretics; full effect is delayed 2 to 3 days when used alone.

!!ALERT Don't confuse triamterene with trimipramine.

Patient teaching

- Tell patient to take drug after meals to minimize nausea.
- If a single daily dose is prescribed, instruct patient to take it in the morning to prevent need to urinate at night.

!!ALERT Warn patient that to prevent serious hyperkalemia, he should avoid excessive ingestion of potassium-rich foods (such as citrus fruits, tomatoes, bananas, dates, and apricots), potassium-containing salt substitutes, and potassium supplements.

- Teach patient to avoid direct sunlight, wear protective clothing, and use sunblock to prevent photosensitivity reactions.
- Tell patient that urine may turn blue.

trifluoperazine hydrochloride

Apo-Trifluoperazine†, Novo-Trifluzine†, PMS Trifluoperazine†

Pregnancy risk category NR

Indications & dosages

➲ Anxiety states
Adults: 1 to 2 mg P.O. b.i.d. Maximum, 6 mg daily. Don't give drug for longer than 12 weeks for anxiety.

➲ Schizophrenia, other psychotic disorders
Adults: In outpatients, 1 to 2 mg P.O. b.i.d. In hospitalized patients, 2 to 5 mg P.O. b.i.d., gradually increased until therapeutic response occurs. Most patients respond to 15 to 20 mg P.O. daily, although some may need 40 mg daily or more. Or, for prompt control of symptoms, 1 to 2 mg deeply I.M. q 4 to 6 hours, p.r.n. More than 6 mg I.M. in 24 hours is rarely needed.
Children ages 6 to 12: For hospitalized or closely supervised patients, 1 mg P.O. daily or b.i.d.; may increase gradually to 15 mg daily, if needed. Or, for prompt control of symptoms, give 1 mg I.M. once or twice daily at least 4 hours apart.

Contraindications & cautions

- Contraindicated in patients hypersensitive to phenothiazines and in those with CNS

depression, coma, bone marrow suppression, or liver damage.
- Use cautiously in elderly or debilitated patients and in patients with CV disease (may decrease blood pressure), seizure disorder, glaucoma, or prostatic hyperplasia; also, use cautiously in those exposed to extreme heat.
- Reserve use in children for those who are hospitalized or under close supervision.

Adverse reactions

CNS: *extrapyramidal reactions, tardive dyskinesia*, pseudoparkinsonism, dizziness, drowsiness, insomnia, fatigue, headache, ***neuroleptic malignant syndrome***.
CV: *orthostatic hypotension*, tachycardia, ECG changes.
EENT: ocular changes, *blurred vision*.
GI: *dry mouth, constipation*, nausea.
GU: *urine retention*, menstrual irregularities, inhibited ejaculation.
Hematologic: ***transient leukopenia, agranulocytosis***.
Hepatic: cholestatic jaundice.
Metabolic: weight gain.
Skin: *photosensitivity reactions*, allergic reactions, pain at I.M. injection site, sterile abscess, rash.
Other: gynecomastia.

Interactions

Drug-drug. *Antacids:* May inhibit absorption of oral phenothiazines. Separate antacid and phenothiazine doses by at least 2 hours.
Barbiturates, lithium: May decrease phenothiazine effect. Monitor patient.
Centrally acting antihypertensives: May decrease antihypertensive effect. Monitor blood pressure.
CNS depressants: May increase CNS depression. Use together cautiously.
Propranolol: May increase propranolol and trifluoperazine levels. Monitor patient.
Warfarin: May decrease effect of oral anticoagulants. Monitor PT and INR.
Drug-herb. *St. John's wort:* May cause photosensitivity reactions. Advise patient to avoid excessive sunlight exposure.
Drug-lifestyle. *Alcohol use:* May increase CNS depression, particularly psychomotor skills. Strongly discourage alcohol use.
Sun exposure: May increase risk of photosensitivity reactions. Advise patient to avoid excessive sunlight exposure.

Nursing considerations

- Wear gloves when preparing liquid forms.
- Protect drug from light. Slight yellowing of injection is common and doesn't affect potency. Discard markedly discolored solutions.
- Give deeply I.M. only in upper outer quadrant of buttocks. Massage slowly afterward to prevent sterile abscess. Injection may sting.
- Watch for orthostatic hypotension, especially with parenteral administration. Keep patient supine for 1 hour after giving drug, and tell him to change positions slowly.
- Monitor patient for tardive dyskinesia, which may occur after prolonged use. It may not appear until months or years later and may disappear spontaneously or persist for life, despite ending drug.

!!ALERT Watch for evidence of neuroleptic malignant syndrome (extrapyramidal effects, hyperthermia, autonomic disturbance), which is rare but commonly fatal. It may not be related to length of drug use or type of neuroleptic; more than 60% of patients are men.

- Monitor periodic CBC and liver function tests, and ophthalmic tests (long-term use).
- Withhold dose and notify prescriber if jaundice, signs and symptoms of blood dyscrasia (fever, sore throat, infection, cellulitis, weakness), or persistent extrapyramidal reactions (longer than a few hours) develop, especially in children or pregnant women.
- Don't withdraw drug abruptly unless severe adverse reactions occur.
- After abrupt withdrawal of long-term therapy, gastritis, nausea, vomiting, dizziness, tremor, feeling of warmth or cold, diaphoresis, tachycardia, headache, insomnia, anorexia, muscle rigidity, altered mental status, or evidence of autonomic instability may occur.

!!ALERT Don't confuse trifluoperazine with triflupromazine.

Patient teaching

- Warn patient to avoid activities that require alertness until effects of drug are known.
- Tell patient to avoid alcohol while taking drug.
- Instruct patient to properly dilute liquid.

- Tell patient to report signs of urine retention or constipation.
- Tell patient to use sunblock and to wear protective clothing outdoors.
- Advise patient to relieve dry mouth with sugarless gum or hard candy.

trihexyphenidyl hydrochloride
Apo-Trihex†, Trihexy-2, Trihexy-5

Pregnancy risk category NR

Indications & dosages
➲ All forms of parkinsonism, including drug-induced parkinsonism; adjunct to levodopa in managing signs and symptoms of parkinsonism
Adults: 1 mg P.O. on day 1, 2 mg on day 2; then increased in 2-mg increments q 3 to 5 days up to total of 6 to 10 mg daily. Usually given t.i.d. with meals; sometimes given q.i.d. (last dose h.s.).

Patients with postencephalitic parkinsonism may need total daily dose of 12 to 15 mg.

Contraindications & cautions
- Contraindicated in patients hypersensitive to drug.
- Use cautiously in patients with glaucoma, cardiac disorders, hepatic disorders, renal disorders, obstructive GI or GU disorders, and prostatic hyperplasia.

Adverse reactions
CNS: nervousness, dizziness, headache, hallucinations, drowsiness, weakness.
CV: tachycardia.
EENT: blurred vision, mydriasis, increased intraocular pressure.
GI: *dry mouth*, constipation, *nausea*, vomiting.
GU: urinary hesitancy, urine retention.

Interactions
Drug-drug. *Amantadine, other anticholinergics:* May cause additive anticholinergic adverse reactions, such as confusion and hallucinations. Reduce trihexyphenidyl dose.
Levodopa: May decrease levodopa bioavailability. May need to reduce doses of both drugs.
Drug-lifestyle. *Alcohol use:* May increase sedative effects. Discourage use together.

Nursing considerations
- Dosage may need to be gradually increased in patients who develop tolerance to drug.
- Monitor patient. Adverse reactions are dose related and transient.
- Elderly patients may be particularly sensitive to the adverse effects of the drug.

Patient teaching
- Tell patient that drug may cause nausea if taken before meals.
- Tell patient to avoid activities that require alertness, until CNS effects of drug are known.
- Advise patient to report signs and symptoms of urinary hesitancy or urine retention.
- Tell patient to relieve dry mouth with cool drinks, ice chips, or sugarless gum or hard candy.
- Advise patient to avoid alcohol while taking drug.
- Advise patient to avoid OTC sleep aids or cold medicines because of possibility of increased anticholinergic effects.

trimethobenzamide hydrochloride
Tebamide, T-Gen, Ticon, Tigan, Triban, Trimazide

Pregnancy risk category C

Indications & dosages
➲ Nausea and vomiting
Adults: 250 to 300 mg P.O. t.i.d. or q.i.d.; or 200 mg I.M. or P.R., t.i.d. or q.i.d.
Children weighing 13 to 40 kg (29 to 88 lb): 100 to 200 mg P.O. or P.R., t.i.d. or q.i.d.
Children weighing less than 13 kg: 100 mg P.R., t.i.d. or q.i.d.

Contraindications & cautions
- Contraindicated in patients hypersensitive to drug. Suppositories contraindicated in patients hypersensitive to benzocaine hydrochloride or similar local anesthetic.
- Use cautiously in children because drug may be linked to Reye's syndrome.

Adverse reactions

CNS: *drowsiness*, dizziness with large doses, headache, disorientation, depression, parkinsonian symptoms, ***coma, seizures***.
CV: hypotension.
EENT: blurred vision.
GI: diarrhea.
Hepatic: jaundice.
Musculoskeletal: muscle cramps.
Other: hypersensitivity reactions.

Interactions

Drug-drug. *CNS depressants:* May cause additive CNS depression. Avoid using together.
Drug-lifestyle. *Alcohol use:* May cause additive CNS depression. Discourage use together.

Nursing considerations

- For I.M. use, inject deep into upper outer quadrant of gluteal region to reduce pain and local irritation.
- Drug may mask signs and symptoms of toxic drug overdose, intestinal obstruction, brain tumor, or other conditions.
- Drug may cause pain, stinging, burning, redness, or swelling at I.M. injection site. Withhold drug if skin hypersensitivity reaction occurs.

!!ALERT Don't confuse Tigan with Ticar.

Patient teaching

- Tell patient to refrigerate suppositories.
- Advise patient of possible drowsiness and dizziness; caution against performing hazardous activities requiring alertness until CNS effects of drug are known.

triptorelin pamoate
Trelstar Depot, Trelstar LA

Pregnancy risk category X

Indications & dosages

➲ Palliative treatment of advanced prostate cancer
Adults: 3.75 mg I.M. Trelstar Depot q 28 days as a single injection or 11.25 mg I.M. Trelstar LA q 84 days as a single injection.

Contraindications & cautions

- Contraindicated in patients hypersensitive to triptorelin, its components, other luteinizing hormone–releasing hormone (LH-RH) agonists, or LH-RH. Contraindicated in women who are or may become pregnant during therapy. Use cautiously in patients with metastatic vertebral lesions or upper or lower urinary tract obstruction during the first few weeks of therapy.
- Patients with renal or hepatic impairment may retain drug longer and have a drug exposure twofold to fourfold higher than those of young healthy men.

Adverse reactions

CNS: headache, dizziness, fatigue, insomnia, emotional lability, pain.
CV: hypertension, edema, *hot flashes*.
GI: diarrhea, vomiting, nausea.
GU: urinary retention, UTI, impotence.
Hematologic: anemia.
Musculoskeletal: *skeletal pain*, leg pain.
Skin: pruritus, injection site pain.
Other: breast pain, gynecomastia.

Interactions

Drug-drug. *Hyperprolactinemic drugs:* May decrease pituitary gonadotropin-releasing hormone (GnRH) receptors. Avoid using together.

Nursing considerations

- Give drug only under the supervision of prescriber.
- Reconstitute only with sterile water. Use no other diluent.
- Change the injection site periodically.
- Monitor testosterone and prostate-specific antigen levels.
- Monitor patients with metastatic vertebral lesions or upper or lower urinary tract obstruction during the first few weeks of therapy.
- Initially, triptorelin causes a transient increase in testosterone level. As a result, signs and symptoms of prostate cancer may worsen during the first few weeks of treatment.
- Patients may experience worsening of symptoms or onset of new symptoms, including bone pain, neuropathy, hematuria, or urethral or bladder outlet obstruction.
- Spinal cord compression may occur, which can cause paralysis, and possibly death. If spinal cord compression or renal impairment develops, give standard treatment. In

extreme cases, consider immediate orchiectomy.
- If patient has a hypersensitivity reaction, stop drug immediately and give supportive and symptomatic care.
- Diagnostic tests of pituitary-gonadal function conducted during and after therapy may be misleading.

Patient teaching

- Inform the patient about adverse reactions.
- Tell patient that symptoms may worsen during the first few weeks of therapy (such as bone pain, nerve inflammation, bloody urine, or obstructed urethral or bladder outlet)
- Inform patient that a blood test will be used to monitor response to therapy.

trospium chloride
Sanctura

Pregnancy risk category C

Indications & dosages

➲ **Overactive bladder with symptoms of urinary urge incontinence, urgency, and frequency**
Adults younger than age 75: 20 mg P.O. b.i.d. taken on an empty stomach or at least 1 hour before a meal.
Adults age 75 and older: Based on patient tolerance, reduce dose to 20 mg once daily.

If patient's creatinine clearance is less than 30 ml/minute, give 20 mg P.O. once daily h.s.

Contraindications & cautions

- Contraindicated in patients hypersensitive to the drug or any of its ingredients and in patients with or at risk for urine retention, gastric retention, or uncontrolled narrow-angle glaucoma.
- Use cautiously in patients with significant bladder outflow obstruction, obstructive GI disorders, ulcerative colitis, intestinal atony, myasthenia gravis, renal insufficiency, moderate or severe hepatic impairment, or controlled narrow-angle glaucoma.

Adverse reactions

CNS: fatigue, headache.
EENT: dry eyes.
GI: abdominal pain, *constipation, dry mouth,* dyspepsia, flatulence.
GU: urine retention.

Interactions

Drug-drug. *Anticholinergics:* May increase dry mouth, constipation, or other adverse effects. Monitor patient.
Digoxin, metformin, morphine, procainamide, pancuronium, tenofovir, vancomycin: May alter elimination of these drugs or trospium, increasing serum levels. Monitor patient closely.
Drug-food. *High fat foods:* May decrease absorption by up to 80%. Give trospium at least 1 hour before meals or on an empty stomach.
Drug-lifestyle. *Alcohol use:* May increase drowsiness. Discourage use together.

Nursing considerations

- Assess patient to determine baseline bladder function, and monitor patient for therapeutic effects.
- If patient has bladder outflow obstruction, watch for evidence of urine retention.
- Monitor patient for decreased gastric motility and constipation.
- Elderly patients typically need a reduced dosage because they have an increased risk of anticholinergic effects.

Patient teaching

- Tell patient to take drug on an empty stomach or at least 1 hour before meals.
- Discourage use of other drugs that may cause dry mouth, constipation, blurred vision, or urine retention.
- Tell patient that alcohol may increase drowsiness and fatigue. Urge him to avoid excessive alcohol consumption while taking trospium.
- Explain that drug may decrease sweating and increase the risk of heatstroke when used in hot environments or during strenuous activities.
- Urge patient to avoid activities that are hazardous or require mental alertness until he knows how the drug affects him.

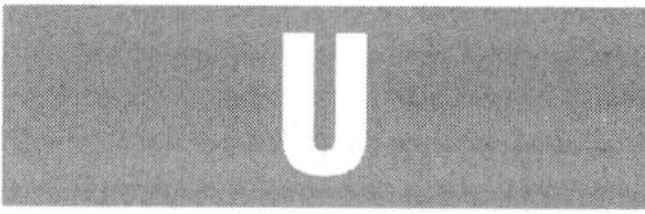

unoprostone isopropyl

Rescula

Pregnancy risk category C

Indications & dosages

➲ **To reduce intraocular pressure (IOP) in patients with open-angle glaucoma or ocular hypertension who can't tolerate or who respond inadequately to other IOP-lowering drugs**

Adults: Instill 1 drop in affected eye b.i.d.

Contraindications & cautions

- Contraindicated in patients hypersensitive to unoprostone isopropyl, benzalkonium chloride, or other components of product.
- Use cautiously in patients with active intraocular inflammation (uveitis) or angle-closure, inflammatory, or neovascular glaucoma.
- Use cautiously in patients with renal or hepatic impairment.

Adverse reactions

CNS: dizziness, headache, insomnia.
CV: hypertension.
EENT: abnormal vision, blepharitis, cataracts, conjunctivitis, corneal lesion, *dry eyes,* eye discharge, *eye burning or stinging, eye itching, eye redness,* eye discomfort, eye irritation, eye hemorrhage, decreased length of eyelashes, *increased length of eyelashes,* eyelid disorder, foreign body sensation, keratitis, lacrimal disorder, pharyngitis, photophobia, rhinitis, sinusitis, vitreous disorder.
Metabolic: diabetes mellitus.
Musculoskeletal: back pain.
Respiratory: bronchitis, increased cough.
Other: accidental injury, ***allergic reaction,*** flulike syndrome, pain.

Interactions

None reported.

Nursing considerations

- Don't give to patient wearing contact lenses because product contains benzalkonium chloride, which may be absorbed by the contact lenses.
- Patient should remove contact lenses before instilling drug and reinsert them 15 minutes after administration.
- Avoid touching tip of dropper to eye to avoid infection.
- Serious eye damage and blindness may result from using contaminated solutions.
- If using more than one ophthalmic drug, give the drugs at least 5 minutes apart.
- Store at 36° to 77° F (2° to 25° C).

Patient teaching

- Instruct patient to report side effects, especially eye inflammation or eyelid reactions.
- Tell patient to remove contact lenses before instilling drops and then wait 15 minutes before reinserting them.
- Instruct patient to avoid touching tip of container to eye because tip could become contaminated, possibly causing an eye infection. Tell him that serious eye damage and blindness may result from using contaminated solutions.
- If eye trauma or infection occurs or if ocular surgery is needed, tell patient to consult prescriber about continued use of multidose container.
- Tell patient that drug can be used with other eye medications but that it's important to separate administration times by 5 minutes.
- Tell patient that drug may permanently change eye color. Change may be gradual, over months to years.
- Warn patient not to use drug if he's allergic to it, to benzalkonium chloride, or to other ingredients in this product.
- Instruct woman to notify prescriber if she's breast-feeding or becomes pregnant while taking drug.

urokinase
Abbokinase

Pregnancy risk category B

Indications & dosages

➲ Lysis of acute massive pulmonary embolism and of pulmonary embolism with unstable hemodynamics

Adults: For I.V. infusion only by constant infusion pump. For priming dose, give 4,400 IU/kg with normal saline solution or D_5 W solution, over 10 minutes, followed by 4,400 IU/kg/hour for 12 hours. Then give continuous I.V. infusion of heparin and oral anticoagulants.

➲ Coronary artery thrombosis♦

Adults: After bolus dose of heparin ranging from 2,500 to 10,000 units, infuse 6,000 IU/minute into occluded artery for up to 2 hours. Average total dose is 500,000 IU. Start drug within 6 hours after symptoms start.

➲ Venous catheter occlusion♦

Adults: Instill 5,000 IU into occluded line.

Contraindications & cautions

- Contraindicated in patients with active internal bleeding, history of CVA, aneurysm, arteriovenous malformation, known bleeding diathesis, recent trauma with possible internal injuries, visceral or intracranial malignancy, ulcerative colitis, diverticulitis, severe hypertension, hemostatic defects including those secondary to severe hepatic or renal insufficiency, uncontrolled hypocoagulation, chronic pulmonary disease with cavitation, subacute bacterial endocarditis or rheumatic valvular disease, and recent cerebral embolism, thrombosis, or hemorrhage
- Contraindicated within 10 days after intra-arterial diagnostic procedure or surgery (liver or kidney biopsy, lumbar puncture, thoracentesis, paracentesis, or extensive or multiple cutdowns) or within 2 months after intracranial or intraspinal surgery.
- Contraindicated during pregnancy and first 10 days postpartum.
- I.M. injections and other invasive procedures are contraindicated during urokinase therapy.

Adverse reactions

CNS: fever.
CV: reperfusion arrhythmias, tachycardia, transient hypotension or hypertension.
GI: nausea, vomiting.
Hematologic: ***bleeding***.
Respiratory: bronchospasm, minor breathing difficulties.
Skin: phlebitis at injection site, rash.
Other: anaphylaxis, chills.

Interactions

Drug-drug. *Anticoagulants, aspirin, dipyridamole, indomethacin, phenylbutazone, other drugs affecting platelet activity:* May increase risk of bleeding. Monitor patient.

Nursing considerations

- Have typed and crossmatched RBCs, whole blood, plasma expanders (other than dextran), and aminocaproic acid available to treat bleeding. Keep corticosteroids, epinephrine, and antihistamines available to treat allergic reactions.
- Drug may be given to menstruating women.
- Only prescribers with extensive experience in thrombotic disease management should use urokinase and only in facilities where clinical and laboratory monitoring can be performed.
- Monitor patient for excessive bleeding every 15 minutes for first hour; every 30 minutes for second through eighth hours; then once every 4 hours. Pretreatment with drugs affecting platelets places patient at high risk of bleeding.
- Monitor pulse, color, and sensation of arms and legs every hour.
- Although risk of hypersensitivity reactions is low, monitor patient.
- Keep a laboratory flow sheet on patient's chart to monitor PTT, PT, thrombin time, hemoglobin level, and hematocrit.
- Monitor vital signs and neurologic status. Don't take blood pressure in legs because doing so could dislodge a clot.
- Keep venipuncture sites to a minimum; use pressure dressing on puncture sites for at least 15 minutes.
- Keep involved limb in straight alignment to prevent bleeding from infusion site.
- Because bruising is more likely during therapy, avoid unnecessary handling of patient, and pad side rails.
- Rare reports of orolingual edema, urticaria, cholesterol embolization, and infusion re-

actions causing hypoxia, cyanosis, acidosis, and back pain have occurred in patients receiving this drug.

Patient teaching

- Explain use and administration of drug to patient and family.
- Instruct patient to report adverse reactions promptly.

ursodiol
Actigall, Urso

Pregnancy risk category B

Indications & dosages

➲ Dissolution of gallstones less than 20 mm in diameter when surgery is prohibited
Adults: 8 to 10 mg/kg P.O. daily in two or three divided doses.
➲ To prevent gallstone formation in obese patients experiencing rapid weight loss
Adults: 300 mg P.O. b.i.d.

Contraindications & cautions

- Contraindicated in patients hypersensitive to ursodiol or other bile acids and in those with chronic hepatic disease, unremitting acute cholecystitis, cholangitis, biliary obstruction, gallstone-induced pancreatitis, or biliary fistula.

Adverse reactions

CNS: *headache*, fatigue, anxiety, depression, *dizziness*, sleep disorders.
EENT: rhinitis.
GI: *nausea, vomiting, dyspepsia*, metallic taste, *abdominal pain*, biliary pain, cholecystitis, *diarrhea, constipation*, stomatitis, flatulence.
GU: *UTI.*
Musculoskeletal: arthralgia, myalgia, *back pain.*
Respiratory: cough.
Skin: pruritus, rash, dry skin, urticaria, hair thinning, diaphoresis.

Interactions

Drug-drug. *Antacids containing aluminum, cholestyramine, colestipol:* May bind ursodiol, preventing its absorption. Avoid using together.
Clofibrate, estrogens, hormonal contraceptives: May increase hepatic cholesterol secretion; may counteract ursodiol effect. Avoid using together.

Nursing considerations

- Drug won't dissolve calcified cholesterol stones, radiolucent bile pigment stones, or radiopaque stones.

!!ALERT Monitor liver function test results, including AST and ALT levels, at the start of therapy and after 1 month, 3 months, and then every 6 months during therapy. Abnormal test results may indicate worsening of the disease. A hepatotoxic metabolite of ursodiol theoretically could form in some patients.

- Therapy usually is long term, taking ultrasound images of the gallbladder every 6 months. If stones don't partially dissolve in 12 months, success is unlikely. Safety of use for longer than 24 months hasn't been established.

Patient teaching

- Advise patient about alternative therapies, including watchful waiting (no intervention) and cholecystectomy, because the relapse rate may be as high as 50% after 5 years.
- Tell patient to report adverse effects.
- Advise patient that dissolution of gallstones requires months of treatment.

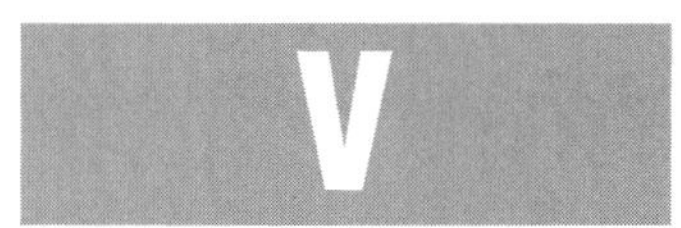

valacyclovir hydrochloride
Valtrex

Pregnancy risk category B

Indications & dosages

➲ Herpes zoster infection (shingles)
Adults: 1 g P.O. t.i.d. for 7 days.

For patients with creatinine clearance of 30 to 49 ml/minute, give 1g P.O. q 12 hours; if clearance is 10 to 29 ml/minute, give 1 g P.O. q 24 hours; if clearance is less than 10 ml/minute, give 500 mg P.O. q 24 hours.
➲ First episode of genital herpes
Adults: 1 g P.O. b.i.d. for 10 days.

For patients with creatinine clearance of 10 to 29 ml/minute, give 1 g P.O. q 24 hours; if clearance is less than 10 ml/minute, give 500 mg P.O. q 24 hours.

➲ **Recurrent genital herpes in immunocompetent patients**

Adults: 500 mg P.O. b.i.d. for 3 days, given at the first sign or symptom of an episode.

For patients with creatinine clearance of 29 ml/minute or less, give 500 mg P.O. q 24 hours.

➲ **Long-term suppression of recurrent genital herpes**

Adults: 1 g P.O. once daily. In patients with a history of nine or fewer recurrences per year, use alternative dose of 500 mg once daily.

For patients with creatinine clearance of 29 ml/minute or less, 500 mg P.O. q 24 hours (q 48 hours if patient has nine or fewer occurrences per year).

➲ **Cold sores (herpes labialis)**

Adults: 2 g P.O. q 12 hours for two doses.

For patients with creatinine clearance of 30 to 49 ml/minute, give 1 g q 12 hours for two doses; if clearance is 10 to 29 ml/minute, give 500 mg q 12 hours for two doses; if clearance is less than 10 ml/minute, give 500 mg as a single dose.

➲ **Long-term suppression of recurrent genital herpes in HIV-infected patients with CD4 cell count of 100 cells/mm^3 or more**

Adults: 500 mg P.O. b.i.d. Safety and efficacy of therapy beyond 6 months hasn't been established.

For patients with creatinine clearance of 29 ml/minute or less, give 500 mg P.O. q 24 hours.

➲ **To reduce transmission of genital herpes in patients with history of nine or fewer occurrences per year**

Adults: 500 mg P.O. daily.

Contraindications & cautions

- Contraindicated in patients hypersensitive to or intolerant of valacyclovir, acyclovir, or components of the formulation.

!!ALERT Valacyclovir isn't recommended for use in patients with HIV infection or in bone marrow or renal transplant recipients because of the occurrence of thrombotic thrombocytopenic purpura and hemolytic uremic syndrome in these patients at doses of 8 g/day.

- Use cautiously in elderly patients, those with renal impairment, and those receiving other nephrotoxic drugs. Monitor renal function test results.
- Consider use of drug during pregnancy only if the benefits outweigh the risks.
- If patient is breast-feeding, drug may need to be stopped.
- Safety and efficacy in prepubertal children haven't been established.

Adverse reactions

CNS: *headache*, dizziness, depression.
GI: *nausea*, vomiting, diarrhea, abdominal pain.
GU: dysmenorrhea.
Musculoskeletal: arthralgia.

Interactions

Drug-drug. *Cimetidine, probenecid:* May reduce rate but not extent of conversion of valacyclovir to acyclovir and may decrease renal clearance of acyclovir, thus increasing acyclovir level. Monitor patient for acyclovir toxicity.

Nursing considerations

!!ALERT Don't confuse valacyclovir (Valtrex) with valganciclovir (Valcyte).

- Although there are no reports of overdose, precipitation of acyclovir in renal tubules may occur when solubility (2.5 mg/ml) is exceeded in the intratubular fluid. With acute renal failure and anuria, the patient may benefit from hemodialysis until renal function is restored.

Patient teaching

- Inform patient that valacyclovir may be taken without regard to meals.
- Teach patient the signs and symptoms of herpes infection (rash, tingling, itching, and pain), and advise him to notify prescriber immediately if they occur. Treatment should begin as soon as possible after symptoms appear, preferably within 48 hours of the onset of zoster rash.
- Tell patient that valacyclovir isn't a cure for herpes but may decrease the length and severity of symptoms.

valdecoxib
Bextra

Pregnancy risk category C; D in 3rd trimester

Indications & dosages

➲ Osteoarthritis, rheumatoid arthritis
Adults: 10 mg P.O. once daily.
➲ Primary dysmenorrhea
Adults: 20 mg P.O. b.i.d., p.r.n.

Contraindications & cautions

- Contraindicated in patients hypersensitive to this drug and in those with sensitivity to aspirin, sulfonamides, or NSAIDs that results in asthma, urticaria, or allergic reactions.
- Contraindicated in patients with advanced renal or hepatic disease.
- Use cautiously in patients with a history of GI bleeding or peptic ulcer disease, in elderly and debilitated patients, and in patients at increased risk of GI bleeding because of smoking, alcoholism, poor general health, or use of corticosteroids, anticoagulants, or long-term NSAIDs.
- Use cautiously in patients with renal impairment, heart failure, hepatic dysfunction, hypertension, and preexisting asthma; in those taking diuretics or ACE inhibitors; and in patients who are dehydrated or have fluid retention.

Adverse reactions

CNS: dizziness, headache, ***cerebrovascular disorder***.
CV: peripheral edema, ***aggravated hypertension***, ***unstable angina***, ***bradycardia***, ***arrhythmia***, ***heart failure***, ***aneurysm***.
EENT: sinusitis.
GI: abdominal fullness, abdominal pain, diarrhea, dyspepsia, flatulence, nausea.
GU: renal impairment.
Hematologic: ***thrombocytopenia***, ***leukopenia***, anemia.
Hepatic: ***hepatitis***.
Metabolic: hyperglycemia, hypercholesterolemia, hyperkalemia, hyperlipidemia, hyperuricemia, hypocalcemia, hypokalemia, increased or decreased weight.
Musculoskeletal: back pain, myalgia.
Respiratory: upper respiratory tract infection, ***bronchospasm***.
Skin: rash.
Other: flulike symptoms, accidental injury.

Interactions

Drug-drug. *ACE inhibitors:* May diminish antihypertensive effect. Monitor blood pressure carefully.
Aspirin: May increase risk of GI ulceration. Use together cautiously.
Dextromethorphan: May increase dextromethorphan level. Monitor patient carefully.
Fluconazole, ketoconazole: May enhance valdecoxib effects. Monitor patient closely.
Furosemide, thiazide diuretics: May reduce natriuretic effect. Monitor patient carefully.
Lithium: May delay lithium clearance. Monitor lithium level.
Warfarin: May increase anticoagulant activity. Monitor INR and PT closely.

Nursing considerations

!!ALERT The manufacturer has suspended production and sales of valdecoxib.
- Rehydrate dehydrated patients before treatment starts.
- Monitor patient carefully for signs and symptoms of GI toxicity, such as bleeding or ulceration.

!!ALERT Drug may cause hypersensitivity reactions, including anaphylaxis, angioedema, and severe skin reactions. Stop therapy at the first sign of these reactions.
- Liver function test values may be elevated, and there may be progression to more serious hepatic abnormalities. Notify prescriber if hepatic disease is suspected or if systemic symptoms such as eosinophilia or rash occur.
- Fluid retention and edema may occur.
- Monitor hemoglobin and hematocrit in patients on long-term therapy; watch for signs and symptoms of anemia.

!!ALERT Don't confuse Bextra with Arixtra.

Patient teaching

- Advise patient to notify his prescriber of signs or symptoms of GI bleeding and ulceration, weight gain, swelling, skin rash, or liver damage (nausea, fatigue, lethargy, yellowed skin or eyes, right upper-quadrant tenderness, flulike symptoms).
- Advise patient to seek emergency attention for trouble breathing, especially if he has a history of aspirin sensitivity.

- Tell patient drug may be taken without regard to meals or antacid administration.
- Advise patient that use of OTC NSAIDs in combination with valdecoxib may increase the risk of GI toxicity.

valganciclovir
Valcyte

Pregnancy risk category C

Indications & dosages

➲ To prevent CMV disease in heart, kidney, and kidney-pancreas transplantation in patients at high risk (donor CMV seropositive or recipient CMV seronegative)
Adults: 900 mg (two 450-mg tablets) P.O. once daily with food starting within 10 days of transplantation until 100 days after transplantation.

➲ Active CMV retinitis in patients with AIDS
Adults: 900 mg (two 450-mg tablets) P.O. b.i.d. with food for 21 days; maintenance dose is 900 mg (two 450-mg tablets) P.O. daily with food.

➲ Inactive CMV retinitis
Adults: 900 mg (two 450-mg tablets) P.O. daily with food.

For patients with creatinine clearance of 40 to 59 ml/minute, induction dosage is 450 mg b.i.d.; maintenance dosage is 450 mg daily. If clearance is 25 to 39 ml/minute, induction dosage is 450 mg daily; maintenance dosage is 450 mg q 2 days. If clearance is 10 to 24 ml/minute, induction dosage is 450 mg q 2 days; maintenance dosage is 450 mg twice weekly.

Contraindications & cautions

- Contraindicated in patients hypersensitive to valganciclovir or ganciclovir. Don't use in patients receiving hemodialysis.
- Drug isn't indicated for use in liver transplant patients.
- The safety and efficacy of drug for the prevention of CMV disease in other solid organ transplant patients, such as lung transplant patients, haven't been established.
- Use cautiously in patients with cytopenias and in those who have received immunosuppressants or radiation.

Adverse reactions

CNS: *headache, insomnia,* peripheral neuropathy, paresthesia, *pyrexia,* ***seizures,*** psychosis, hallucinations, confusion, agitation.
EENT: *retinal detachment.*
GI: *diarrhea, nausea, vomiting, abdominal pain.*
Hematologic: NEUTROPENIA, *anemia,* ***thrombocytopenia, pancytopenia, bone marrow depression, aplastic anemia.***
Other: catheter-related infection, ***sepsis,*** local or systemic infections, hypersensitivity reactions.

Interactions

Drug-drug. *Didanosine:* May increase absorption of didanosine. Monitor patient closely for didanosine toxicity.
Immunosuppressants, zidovudine: May enhance neutropenia, anemia, thrombocytopenia, and bone marrow depression. Monitor CBC results.
Mycophenolate mofetil: May increase levels of both drugs in renally impaired patients. Use together cautiously.
Probenecid: May decrease renal clearance of ganciclovir. Monitor patient for ganciclovir toxicity.
Drug-food. *Any food:* May increase absorption of drug. Give drug with food.

Nursing considerations

- Make sure to adhere to dosing guidelines for valganciclovir because ganciclovir and valganciclovir aren't interchangeable and overdose may occur.
- Clinical toxicities include severe leukopenia, neutropenia, anemia, pancytopenia, bone marrow depression, aplastic anemia, and thrombocytopenia. Don't use if patient's absolute neutrophil count is less than 500 cells/mm^3, platelet count is less than 25,000/mm^3, or hemoglobin level is less than 8 g/dl.
- Monitor CBC, platelet counts, and creatinine level or creatinine clearance values frequently during treatment.
- Cytopenia may occur at any time during treatment and increase with continued use. Cell counts usually recover 3 to 7 days after stopping drug.
- No drug interaction studies have been conducted with valganciclovir; however, because drug is converted to ganciclovir, it can

be assumed that drug interactions would be similar.

- Drug may cause temporary or permanent inhibition of spermatogenesis.

!!ALERT Don't confuse valganciclovir hydrochloride (Valcyte) with valacyclovir (Valtrex).

Patient teaching

- Tell patient to take drug with food.
- Tell patient to follow dosage instructions precisely. Ganciclovir capsules and valganciclovir tablets aren't interchangeable on a one-to-one basis.
- Advise patient that blood tests are needed during treatment. Doses may need to be adjusted based on blood counts.
- Tell woman of childbearing age to use contraception during treatment. Inform man that he should use barrier contraception during and for 90 days after treatment.
- Advise patient that ganciclovir is considered a potential carcinogen.
- Tell patient that CNS effects (seizures, ataxia, dizziness) can occur and to use care in driving or operating machinery.
- Advise patient that this drug isn't a cure for CMV retinitis and that the condition may recur. Tell patient to have ophthalmologic examinations at least every 4 to 6 weeks during treatment.

valproate sodium

Depacon, Depakene

valproic acid

Depakene

divalproex sodium

Depakote, Depakote ER, Depakote Sprinkle, Epival†

Pregnancy risk category D

Indications & dosages

➲ Simple and complex absence seizures, mixed seizure types (including absence seizures)

Adults and children: Initially, 15 mg/kg P.O. or I.V. daily; then increase by 5 to 10 mg/kg daily at weekly intervals up to maximum of 60 mg/kg daily. Don't use Depakote ER in children younger than 10.

➲ Complex partial seizures

Adults and children age 10 and older: 10 to 15 mg/kg Depakote or Depakote ER P.O. or valproate sodium I.V. daily; then increase by 5 to 10 mg/kg daily at weekly intervals, up to 60 mg/kg daily.

➲ Mania

Adults: Initially, 750 mg delayed-release divalproex sodium daily in divided doses. Adjust dosage based on patient's response; maximum dose is 60 mg/kg daily.

➲ To prevent migraine headache

Adults: Initially, 250 mg delayed-release divalproex sodium P.O. b.i.d. Some patients may need up to 1,000 mg daily. Or, 500 mg Depakote ER P.O. daily for 1 week; then 1,000 mg P.O. daily.

For elderly patients, start at lower dosage. Increase dosage more slowly and with regular monitoring of fluid and nutritional intake, and watch for dehydration, somnolence, and other adverse reactions.

Contraindications & cautions

- Contraindicated in patients hypersensitive to drug and in those with hepatic disease or significant hepatic dysfunction, and in patients with a urea cycle disorder (UCD).
- Safety and efficacy of Depakote ER in children younger than age 10 haven't been established.

Adverse reactions

CNS: *insomnia, nervousness, somnolence,* abnormal thinking, amnesia, emotional upset, depression, *tremor,* ataxia, *headache, dizziness, asthenia,* fever.
CV: chest pain, hypertension, hypotension, tachycardia, edema.
EENT: nystagmus, *diplopia, blurred vision,* rhinitis, pharyngitis, tinnitus.
GI: *nausea, vomiting, diarrhea, abdominal pain, dyspepsia,* constipation, increased appetite, *anorexia,* ***pancreatitis.***
Hematologic: petechiae, bruising, ***hemorrhage, bone marrow suppression.***
Hepatic: ***hepatotoxicity.***
Metabolic: weight gain or loss.
Musculoskeletal: back and neck pain.
Respiratory: bronchitis, dyspnea.
Skin: rash, *alopecia,* pruritus, photosensitivity, ***erythema multiforme, Stevens-Johnson syndrome, hypersensitivity reactions,*** *flu syndrome, infection.*

Interactions

Drug-drug. *Aspirin, chlorpromazine, cimetidine, erythromycin, felbamate:* May cause valproic acid toxicity. Use together cautiously and monitor drug level.
Benzodiazepines, other CNS depressants: May cause excessive CNS depression. Avoid using together.
Carbamazepine: May cause carbamazepine CNS toxicity; may decrease valproic acid level. Use together cautiously, if at all.
Lamotrigine: May increase lamotrigine level; may decrease valproate level. Monitor levels closely.
Phenobarbital: May increase phenobarbital level; may increase clearance of valproate. Monitor patient closely.
Phenytoin: May increase or decrease phenytoin level; may decrease valproate level. Monitor patient closely.
Rifampin: May decrease valproate level. Monitor level of valproate.
Warfarin: May displace warfarin from binding sites. Monitor PT and INR.
Zidovudine: May decrease zidovudine clearance. Avoid using together.
Drug-lifestyle. *Alcohol use:* May cause excessive CNS depression. Discourage use together.

Nursing considerations

- Obtain liver function test results, platelet count, and PT and INR before starting therapy, and monitor these values periodically.
- Don't give syrup to patients who need sodium restriction. Check with prescriber.
- Adverse reactions may not be caused by valproic acid alone because it's usually used with other anticonvulsants.
- When converting adults and children age 10 and older with seizures from Depakote to Depakote ER, make sure the extended-release dose is 8% to 20% higher than the regular dose taken previously. See manufacturer's package insert for more details.
- Divalproex sodium has a lower risk of adverse GI reactions.
- Never withdraw drug suddenly because sudden withdrawal may worsen seizures. Call prescriber at once if adverse reactions develop.

!!ALERT Serious or fatal hepatotoxicity may follow nonspecific symptoms, such as malaise, fever, and lethargy. If these symptoms occur during therapy, notify prescriber at once because patient who might be developing hepatic dysfunction must stop taking drug.

- Patients at high risk for hepatotoxicity include those with congenital metabolic disorders, mental retardation, or organic brain disease; those taking multiple anticonvulsants; and children younger than age 2.
- Notify prescriber if tremors occur; a dosage reduction may be needed.
- Monitor drug level. Therapeutic level is 50 to 100 mcg/ml.
- Use caution when converting patients from a brand-name drug to a generic drug because breakthrough seizures are possible.

!!ALERT Sometimes fatal, hyperammonemic encephalopathy may occur when starting valproate therapy in patients with UCD. Evaluate patients with UCD risk factors before starting valproate therapy. Patients who develop symptoms of unexplained hyperammonemic encephalopathy during valproate therapy should stop drug, undergo prompt appropriate treatment, and be evaluated for underlying UCD.

Patient teaching

- Tell patient to take drug with food or milk to reduce adverse GI effects.
- Advise patient not to chew capsules; irritation of mouth and throat may result.
- Tell patient that capsules may be either swallowed whole or carefully opened and contents sprinkled on a teaspoonful of soft food. Tell patient to swallow immediately without chewing.
- Tell patient and parents that syrup shouldn't be mixed with carbonated beverages; mixture may be irritating to mouth and throat.
- Tell patient and parents to keep drug out of children's reach.
- Warn patient and parents not to stop drug therapy abruptly.
- Advise patient to avoid driving and other potentially hazardous activities that require mental alertness until drug's CNS effects are known.
- Instruct patient or parents to call prescriber if malaise, weakness, lethargy, facial swelling, loss of appetite, or vomiting occurs.
- Tell woman to call prescriber if she becomes pregnant or plans to become pregnant during therapy.

valsartan
Diovan

Pregnancy risk category C; D in 2nd and 3rd trimesters

Indications & dosages

➲ Hypertension (used alone or with other antihypertensives)
Adults: Initially, 80 mg P.O. once daily. Expect to see a reduction in blood pressure in 2 to 4 weeks. If additional antihypertensive effect is needed, dose may be increased to 160 or 320 mg daily, or a diuretic may be added. (Addition of a diuretic has a greater effect than dosage increases beyond 80 mg.) Usual dosage range is 80 to 320 mg daily.

➲ New York Heart Association class II to IV heart failure in patients intolerant of ACE inhibitors
Adults: Initially, 40 mg P.O. b.i.d.; increase as tolerated to 80 mg b.i.d. Maximum dose is 160 mg b.i.d.

Contraindications & cautions

- Contraindicated in patients hypersensitive to drug.
- Drug can cause fetal or neonatal morbidity and death if given to a pregnant woman in the second or third trimester. Breast-feeding women shouldn't take drug.
- Safety and effectiveness of drug in children haven't been established. Don't give drug to children.
- Use cautiously in patients with renal or hepatic disease.

Adverse reactions

CNS: *dizziness*, headache, insomnia, fatigue, vertigo.
CV: edema, hypotension, orthostatic hypotension, syncope.
EENT: rhinitis, sinusitis, pharyngitis, blurred vision.
GI: abdominal pain, diarrhea, nausea, dyspepsia.
GU: renal impairment.
Hematologic: ***neutropenia***.
Metabolic: hyperkalemia.
Musculoskeletal: arthralgia, back pain.
Respiratory: upper respiratory tract infection, cough.
Other: viral infection, ***angioedema***.

Interactions

Drug-drug. *Lithium:* May increase lithium level. Monitor lithium level and patient for toxicity.
Potassium-sparing diuretics, potassium supplements, other angiotensin II blockers: May increase potassium level. May also increase creatinine level in heart failure patients. Avoid using together.
Drug-herb. *Ma huang:* May decrease antihypertensive effects. Discourage use together.
Drug-food. *Salt substitutes containing potassium:* May increase potassium level. May also increase creatinine level in heart failure patients. Avoid using together.

Nursing considerations

- Watch for hypotension. Excessive hypotension can occur when drug is given with high doses of diuretics.
- Correct volume and salt depletions before starting drug.

Patient teaching

- Tell woman of childbearing age to notify prescriber if pregnancy occurs. Drug will need to be stopped.
- Advise patient that drug may be taken without regard to food.

vancomycin hydrochloride
Vancocin, Vancoled

Pregnancy risk category C

Indications & dosages

➲ Serious or severe infections when other antibiotics are ineffective or contraindicated, including those caused by methicillin-resistant *Staphylococcus aureus, S. epidermidis,* or diphtheroid organisms
Adults: 1 to 1.5 g I.V. q 12 hours.
Children: 10 mg/kg I.V. q 6 hours.
Neonates and young infants: 15 mg/kg I.V. loading dose; then 10 mg/kg I.V. q 12 hours if child is younger than age 1 week or 10 mg/kg I.V. q 8 hours if age is older than 1 week but younger than 1 month.
Elderly patients: 15 mg/kg I.V. loading dose. Subsequent doses are based on renal function and serum drug levels.

➲ Antibiotic-related pseudomembranous *Clostridium difficile* and *S. enterocolitis*
Adults: 125 to 500 mg P.O. q 6 hours for 7 to 10 days.
Children: 40 mg/kg P.O. daily, in divided doses q 6 hours for 7 to 10 days. Maximum daily dose is 2 g.
➲ Endocarditis prophylaxis for dental procedures
Adults: 1 g I.V. slowly over 1 to 2 hours, completing infusion 30 minutes before procedure.
Children: 20 mg/kg I.V. over 1 to 2 hours, completing infusion 30 minutes before procedure.

In renal insufficiency, adjust dosage based on degree of renal impairment, drug level, severity of infection, and susceptibility of causative organism. Initially, give 15 mg/kg, and adjust subsequent doses, p.r.n. One possible schedule is as follows: If creatinine level is less than 1.5 mg/dl, give 1 g q 12 hours. If creatinine level is 1.5 to 5 mg/dl, give 1 g q 3 to 6 days. If creatinine level is greater than 5 mg/dl, give 1 g q 10 to 14 days. Or, if glomerular filtration rate (GFR) is 10 to 50 ml/minute, give usual dose q 3 to 10 days, and if GFR is less than 10 ml/minute, give usual dose q 10 days.

Contraindications & cautions

- Contraindicated in patients hypersensitive to drug.

Adverse reactions

CNS: fever, pain.
CV: hypotension, thrombophlebitis at injection site.
EENT: tinnitus, ototoxicity.
GI: nausea, ***pseudomembranous colitis***.
GU: ***nephrotoxicity***.
Hematologic: ***neutropenia***, ***leukopenia***, eosinophilia.
Respiratory: wheezing, dyspnea.
Skin: red-man syndrome (with rapid I.V. infusion).
Other: chills, ***anaphylaxis***, superinfection.

Interactions

Drug-drug. *Aminoglycosides, amphotericin B, cisplatin, pentamidine:* May increase risk of nephrotoxicity and ototoxicity. Monitor renal function and hearing function tests.

Nursing considerations

- Use cautiously in patients receiving other neurotoxic, nephrotoxic, or ototoxic drugs; in patients older than age 60; and in those with impaired hepatic or renal function, hearing loss, or allergies to other antibiotics. Patients with renal dysfunction need dosage adjustment. Monitor blood levels to adjust I.V. dosage. Normal therapeutic levels of vancomycin are peak, 30 to 40 mg/L (drawn 1 hour after infusion ends), and trough, 5 to 10 mg/L (drawn just before next dose is given).
- Obtain specimen for culture and sensitivity tests before giving first dose. Because of the emergence of vancomycin-resistant enterococci, reserve use of drug for treatment of serious infections caused by gram-positive bacteria resistant to beta-lactam anti-infectives.
- Obtain hearing evaluation and renal function studies before therapy.
- Monitor patient's fluid balance and watch for oliguria and cloudy urine.
- Monitor patient carefully for red-man syndrome, which can occur if drug is infused too rapidly. Signs and symptoms include maculopapular rash on face, neck, trunk, and limbs and pruritus and hypotension caused by histamine release. If wheezing, urticaria, or pain and muscle spasm of the chest and back occur, stop infusion and notify prescriber.
- Don't give drug I.M.

!! ALERT Oral administration is ineffective for systemic infections, and I.V. administration is ineffective for pseudomembranous (*Clostridium difficile*) diarrhea.

- Oral preparation is stable for 2 weeks if refrigerated.
- Monitor renal function (BUN, creatinine and creatinine clearance levels, urinalysis, and urine output) during therapy.
- Monitor patient for signs and symptoms of superinfection.
- Have patient's hearing evaluated during prolonged therapy.
- When using drug to treat staphylococcal endocarditis, give for at least 4 weeks.

Patient teaching

- Tell patient to take entire amount of drug exactly as directed, even after he feels better.

- Instruct patient receiving drug I.V. to report discomfort at I.V. insertion site.
- Tell patient to report ringing in ears.
- Tell patient to report adverse reactions to prescriber immediately.

vardenafil hydrochloride
Levitra

Pregnancy risk category B

Indications & dosages
➲ Erectile dysfunction
Adults: 10 mg P.O. as a single dose, p.r.n., 1 hour before sexual activity. Dosage range is 5 to 20 mg, based on effectiveness and tolerance. Maximum, one dose daily.
Elderly patients age 65 and older: Initially 5 mg as a single dose, p.r.n., 1 hour before sexual activity.

For patients with Child-Pugh category B, first dose is 5 mg daily, p.r.n. Don't exceed 10 mg daily in patients with hepatic impairment.

Contraindications & cautions
- Contraindicated in patients hypersensitive to drug or its components and in those taking nitrates or alpha blockers.
- Contraindicated in patients with unstable angina, hypotension (systolic less than 90 mm Hg), uncontrolled hypertension (over 170/110 mm Hg), CVA, life-threatening arrhythmia, an MI within past 6 months, severe cardiac failure, Child-Pugh category C, end-stage renal disease requiring dialysis, congenital QTc-interval prolongation, or hereditary degenerative retinal disorders.
- Use cautiously in patients with bleeding disorders or significant peptic ulceration.
- Use cautiously in those with anatomical penis abnormalities or conditions that predispose patient to priapism (such as sickle cell anemia, multiple myeloma, or leukemia).

Adverse reactions
CNS: *headache*, dizziness.
CV: *flushing*.
EENT: rhinitis, sinusitis.
GI: dyspepsia, nausea.
Musculoskeletal: back pain.
Other: flulike syndrome.

Interactions
Drug-drug. *Alpha blockers, nitrates:* May enhance hypotensive effects. Avoid using together.
Antiarrhythmics of class IA (quinidine, procainamide) and class III (amiodarone, sotalol): May prolong QTc interval. Avoid using together.
Erythromycin, indinavir, itraconazole, ketoconazole, ritonavir: May increase vardenafil level. Reduce dose of vardenafil. If taken with ritonavir, reduce and extend dosage interval to once every 72 hours.
Drug-food. *High-fat meals:* May reduce peak level of drug. Discourage use with a high-fat meal.

Nursing considerations
!!ALERT Sexual activity may increase cardiac risk. Evaluate patient's cardiac risk before he starts taking drug.
- Before patient starts drug, assess for underlying causes of erectile dysfunction.
- Transient decreases in supine blood pressure may occur.
- Prolonged erections and priapism may occur.

Patient teaching
- Tell patient that drug doesn't protect against sexually transmitted diseases and that he should use protective measures.
- Advise patient that drug is absorbed most rapidly if taken on an empty stomach.
- Tell patient to notify prescriber about visual changes.
- Urge patient to seek immediate medical care if erection lasts more than 4 hours.
- Tell patient to take drug 60 minutes before anticipated sexual activity. Explain that drug has no effect without sexual stimulation.
- Warn patient not to change dosage unless directed by prescriber.

varicella virus vaccine
Varivax

Pregnancy risk category C

Indications & dosages

➲ **To prevent varicella zoster (chickenpox) infections**
Adults and children age 13 and older: 0.5 ml S.C.; then, second 0.5-ml dose 4 to 8 weeks later.
Children ages 1 to 12: 0.5 ml S.C.

Contraindications & cautions

- Contraindicated in patients hypersensitive to drug; in those with history of anaphylactoid reaction to neomycin; and in those with blood dyscrasia, leukemia, lymphomas, neoplasms affecting bone marrow or lymphatic system, or primary and acquired immunosuppressive states; and in those receiving immunosuppressants.
- Contraindicated in those with active untreated tuberculosis or any febrile illness or infection.
- Contraindicated in pregnant women.

Adverse reactions

CNS: *fever.*
Skin: swelling, redness, pain, rash, varicella-like rash at injection site.
Other: ***anaphylaxis***, herpes zoster, stiffness.

Interactions

Drug-drug. *Blood products, immune globulin:* May inactivate vaccine. Don't give vaccine until at least 5 months after blood or plasma transfusions or administration of immune globulin or varicella zoster immune globulin.
Immunosuppressants: May cause severe reactions to live virus vaccines. Postpone routine vaccination.
Salicylates: May cause Reye's syndrome after natural varicella infection. Avoid using salicylates for 6 weeks after varicella immunization.

Nursing considerations

- To reconstitute vaccine, first withdraw 0.7 ml of diluent into syringe to be used for reconstitution. Inject all diluent in syringe into vial of lyophilized vaccine and gently agitate to mix thoroughly. Give immediately after reconstitution. Discard if not used within 30 minutes.
- Keep epinephrine available to treat anaphylaxis.
- Vaccine has been used safely and effectively with measles, mumps, and rubella vaccine.
- Document manufacturer, lot number, date, and name, address, and title of person giving dose on patient record or log.
- Store vaccine frozen. Store diluent separately at room temperature or refrigerated.

!!ALERT Vaccine contains live, attenuated virus. Vaccinated patients who develop rash may be able to transmit virus.

Patient teaching

- Inform patient or parents about adverse reactions linked to vaccine.
- Caution woman of childbearing age to report suspected pregnancy before administration.
- Instruct patient to avoid salicylates for 6 weeks after vaccination to prevent Reye's syndrome.
- Tell patient to avoid pregnancy for 3 months after vaccination.
- Warn patient to be careful after the injection to avoid close contact with susceptible high-risk people (such as pregnant women or immunocompromised persons).

varicella zoster immune globulin (VZIG)

Pregnancy risk category C

Indications & dosages

➲ **Passive immunization of susceptible immunodeficient patients after exposure to varicella (chickenpox or herpes zoster)**
Adults and children weighing more than 40 kg (88 lb): 625 units I.M.
Children weighing 30 to 40 kg (66 to 88 lb): 500 units I.M.
Children weighing 20 to 30 kg (44 to 66 lb): 375 units I.M.
Children weighing 10 to 20 kg (22 to 44 lb): 250 units I.M.
Children weighing up to 10 kg (22 lb): 125 units I.M.

Contraindications & cautions

- Contraindicated in patients with thrombocytopenia or history of severe reaction to human immune serum globulin or thimerosal; also contraindicated during pregnancy.

Adverse reactions

CNS: headache, malaise.
GI: GI distress.
Respiratory: respiratory distress.
Skin: discomfort at injection site, rash.
Other: ***anaphylaxis***.

Interactions

Drug-drug. *Live-virus vaccines:* May interfere with response. Postpone vaccination for 3 months after administration of VZIG.

Nursing considerations

- Obtain accurate patient history of allergies and reactions to immunizations. Keep epinephrine 1:1,000 ready to treat anaphylaxis.
- For maximum benefit, give as soon as possible after presumed exposure. Drug may be of benefit when given as late as 96 hours after exposure.
- Give only by deep I.M. injection into a large muscle such as gluteal muscle. Never give I.V.
- Don't give in divided doses.
- Although usually restricted to children younger than age 15, VZIG may be given to adolescents and adults, if needed.
- VZIG isn't recommended for patients who aren't immunosuppressed.

!!ALERT VZIG provides passive immunity; don't confuse with varicella vaccine. Don't use these two drugs together.

- Drug isn't commercially distributed and is available only from 20 regional United States distribution centers. These centers will distribute to Canada and overseas. Contact the Massachusetts Public Health Biologic Laboratories or the CDC at (800) 232-2522 for more information.

Patient teaching

- Warn patient about local adverse reactions caused by the drug.
- Instruct patient to report serious adverse reactions to prescriber promptly.
- Suggest use of acetaminophen to reduce fever and cool compresses at injection site for comfort.

vasopressin (ADH)
Pitressin

Pregnancy risk category C

Indications & dosages

➲ Nonnephrogenic, nonpsychogenic diabetes insipidus
Adults: 5 to 10 units I.M. or S.C. b.i.d. to q.i.d., p.r.n. Or, intranasally (aqueous solution used as spray or applied to cotton balls) in individualized dosages, based on response.
Children: 2.5 to 10 units I.M. or S.C. b.i.d. to q.i.d., p.r.n. Or, intranasally (aqueous solution used as spray or applied to cotton balls) in individualized doses.

➲ To prevent and treat abdominal distention
Adults: Initially, 5 units I.M.; give subsequent injections q 3 to 4 hours, increasing to 10 units if needed. Children may receive reduced dosages. Or, for adults, aqueous vasopressin 5 to 15 units S.C. at 2 hours before and again at 30 minutes before abdominal radiography or kidney biopsy.

Contraindications & cautions

- Contraindicated in patients with chronic nephritis and nitrogen retention.
- Use cautiously in children; elderly patients; pregnant women; patients with preoperative or postoperative polyuria; and those with seizure disorders, migraines, asthma, CV disease, heart failure, renal disease, goiter with cardiac complications, arteriosclerosis, or fluid overload.

Adverse reactions

CNS: tremor, headache, vertigo.
CV: vasoconstriction, ***arrhythmias***, ***cardiac arrest***, myocardial ischemia, circumoral pallor, decreased cardiac output, angina in patients with vascular disease.
GI: abdominal cramps, nausea, vomiting, flatulence.
GU: uterine cramps.
Respiratory: ***bronchoconstriction***.
Skin: diaphoresis, cutaneous gangrene, urticaria.
Other: water intoxication, ***hypersensitivity reactions***.

Interactions

Drug-drug. *Carbamazepine, chlorpropamide, clofibrate, fludrocortisone, tricyclic antidepressant:* May increase antidiuretic response. Use together cautiously.
Demeclocycline, heparin, lithium, norepinephrine: May reduce antidiuretic activity. Use together cautiously.
Drug-lifestyle. *Alcohol use:* May reduce antidiuretic activity. Discourage use together.

Nursing considerations

- Monitor patient for hypersensitivity reactions, including urticaria, angioedema, bronchoconstriction, and anaphylaxis.
- Synthetic desmopressin is sometimes preferred because of its longer duration of action and less frequent adverse reactions. Desmopressin also is available commercially as a nasal solution.
- Drug may be used for transient polyuria resulting from ADH deficiency related to neurosurgery or head injury.
- Use minimum effective dose to reduce adverse reactions.
- Give with 1 to 2 glasses of water to reduce adverse reactions and improve therapeutic response.
- Warm the vasopressin vial in your hands, and mix until the hormone is distributed throughout the solution before administration.
- Monitor urine specific gravity and fluid intake and output to aid evaluation of drug effectiveness.
- To prevent possible seizures, coma, and death, observe patient closely for early evidence of water intoxication, including drowsiness, listlessness, headache, confusion, and weight gain.
- Monitor blood pressure of patient taking vasopressin twice daily. Watch for excessively elevated blood pressure or lack of response to drug, which may be indicated by hypotension. Also, monitor weight daily.

!!ALERT Don't confuse vasopressin with desmopressin.

Patient teaching

- Instruct patient to rotate injection sites to prevent tissue damage.
- Tell patient to report adverse reactions to prescriber promptly.
- Tell patient to report drowsiness, listlessness, and headache to prescriber.
- Tell patient to avoid alcohol and OTC medications unless approved by prescriber.
- Tell patient to restrict water intake.

vecuronium bromide

Pregnancy risk category C

Indications & dosages

➲ **Adjunct to general anesthesia to facilitate endotracheal intubation and relax skeletal muscles during surgery or mechanical ventilation**
Adults and children age 10 or older: Initially, 0.08 to 0.1 mg/kg I.V. bolus. Give maintenance doses of 0.01 to 0.015 mg/kg within 25 to 40 minutes of first dose during prolonged surgical procedures. Maintenance doses may be given q 12 to 15 minutes in patients receiving balanced anesthesia.
Children ages 1 to 9: May need a slightly higher first dose and slightly more frequent supplementation than adults. Or, may give continuous I.V. infusion of 1 mcg/kg/minute initially; then 0.8 to 1.2 mcg/kg/minute.
Children ages 7 weeks to 1 year: Doses comparable to those used in adults, possibly with less frequent use of maintenance doses.

Contraindications & cautions

- Contraindicated in patients hypersensitive to drug or to bromides.
- Use cautiously in elderly patients; in patients with altered circulation caused by CV disease or edema; and in those with hepatic disease, severe obesity, bronchogenic carcinoma, electrolyte disturbances, and neuromuscular disease.
- Not recommended for use in infants younger than age 7 weeks.

Adverse reactions

Musculoskeletal: skeletal muscle weakness.
Respiratory: ***prolonged respiratory insufficiency or apnea.***

Interactions

Drug-drug. *Aminoglycosides (amikacin, gentamicin, neomycin, streptomycin, tobramycin):* May increase the effects of nondepolarizing muscle relaxant, including prolonged respiratory depression. Use together

only when necessary. May need to reduce nondepolarizing muscle relaxant dose.
Bacitracin, beta blockers, clindamycin, general anesthetics (enflurane, halothane, isoflurane), magnesium salts, other skeletal muscle relaxants, polymyxin antibiotics (colistin, polymyxin B sulfate), quinidine, quinine, succinylcholine, tetracyclines: May enhance neuromuscular blockade, increasing skeletal muscle relaxation and potentiating effect. Use together cautiously during and after surgery.
Carbamazepine, phenytoin: May decrease effects of vecuronium. May need to increase vecuronium dose.
Opioid analgesics: May enhance neuromuscular blockade, increasing skeletal muscle relaxation and possibly causing respiratory paralysis. Use together cautiously, and reduce vecuronium dose.

Nursing considerations

- Dosage depends on anesthetic used, individual needs, and response. Recommended dosages must be individually adjusted.
- Only staff skilled in airway management should use drug.
- A nerve stimulator and train-of-four monitoring are recommended to confirm antagonism of neuromuscular blockade and recovery of muscle strength. Make sure there is some evidence of spontaneous recovery before attempting pharmacologic reversal with neostigmine.
- Monitor respirations closely until patient recovers fully from neuromuscular blockade, as indicated by tests of muscle strength (hand grip, head lift, and ability to cough).
- Previous use of succinylcholine may enhance the neuromuscular blocking effect and duration of action.
- Vecuronium is well tolerated in patients with renal failure.
- Give analgesics for pain.

!!ALERT Careful dosage calculation is essential. Always verify dosage with another health care professional.

Patient teaching

- Explain all events and procedures to patient because he can still hear.

venlafaxine hydrochloride
Effexor, Effexor XR

Pregnancy risk category C

Indications & dosages

➲ Depression
Adults: Initially, 75 mg P.O. daily in two or three divided doses with food. Increase as tolerated and needed by 75 mg daily q 4 days. For moderately depressed outpatients, usual maximum is 225 mg daily; in certain severely depressed patients, dose may be as high as 375 mg daily. For extended-release capsules, 75 mg P.O. daily in a single dose. For some patients, it may be desirable to start at 37.5 mg P.O. daily for 4 to 7 days before increasing to 75 mg daily. Dosage may be increased by 75 mg daily q 4 days to maximum of 225 mg daily.

➲ Generalized anxiety disorder
Adults: Initially, 75 mg of Effexor XR P.O. daily in a single dose. For some patients, it may be desirable to start at 37.5 mg P.O. daily for 4 to 7 days before increasing to 75 mg daily. Dosage may be increased by 75 mg daily q 4 days to maximum of 225 mg daily.

➲ Social anxiety disorder
Adults: Initially, 75 mg extended-release capsule daily as a single dose. For some patients, it may be desirable to start at 37.5 mg P.O. daily for 4 to 7 days before increasing to 75 mg daily. Increase dosage p.r.n. by 75 mg daily q 4 days. Maximum dosage is 225 mg daily.

For patients with renal impairment, reduce daily amount by 25%. For those undergoing hemodialysis, reduce daily amount by 50% and withhold dose until dialysis is completed. For patients with hepatic impairment, reduce daily amount by 50%.

➲ To prevent major depressive disorder relapse♦
Adults: 100 to 200 mg daily P.O. Effexor or 75 to 225 mg daily P.O. Effexor XR.

Contraindications & cautions

- Contraindicated in patients hypersensitive to drug or within 14 days of MAO inhibitor therapy.
- Use cautiously in patients with renal impairment, diseases or conditions that could affect hemodynamic responses or metabo-

lism, and in those with history of mania or seizures.
- Use in third trimester of pregnancy may be associated with neonatal complications at birth. Consider the risk versus benefit of treatment during this time.

Adverse reactions

CNS: *headache*, ***suicidal behavior***, *somnolence*, *dizziness*, *nervousness*, *insomnia*, anxiety, tremor, abnormal dreams, paresthesia, agitation, *asthenia*.
CV: hypertension, tachycardia, vasodilation.
EENT: blurred vision.
GI: *nausea*, *constipation*, vomiting, *dry mouth*, *anorexia*, diarrhea, dyspepsia, flatulence.
GU: *abnormal ejaculation*, impotence, urinary frequency, impaired urination.
Metabolic: weight loss.
Skin: *diaphoresis*, rash.
Other: yawning, chills, infection.

Interactions

Drug-drug. *MAO inhibitors (phenelzine, selegiline, tranylcypromine):* May cause serotonin syndrome. Avoid using within 14 days of MAO inhibitor therapy.
Drug-herb. *Yohimbe:* May cause additive stimulation. Urge caution.

Nursing considerations

!!ALERT Closely monitor patients being treated for depression for signs and symptoms of clinical worsening and suicidal ideation, especially at the beginning of therapy and dosage adjustments. Symptoms may include agitation, insomnia, anxiety, aggressiveness, or panic attacks.
- Carefully monitor blood pressure. Drug therapy may cause sustained, dose-dependent increases in blood pressure. Greatest increases (averaging about 7 mm Hg above baseline) occur in patients taking 375 mg daily.
- Monitor patient's weight, particularly underweight, depressed patients.

Patient teaching

- If medication is to be stopped, inform patient who has received drug for 6 weeks or longer that drug will be gradually stopped by tapering dosage over a 2-week period as instructed by prescriber. Patient shouldn't abruptly stop taking the drug.

!!ALERT Warn family members to closely monitor patient for signs of worsening condition or suicidal ideation.
- Warn patient to avoid hazardous activities that require alertness and good coordination until effects of drug are known.
- Tell patient to avoid alcohol and to consult prescriber before taking other prescription or OTC drugs.
- Advise woman of childbearing age to contact prescriber if she becomes pregnant or intends to become pregnant during therapy or if she's breast-feeding.

verapamil hydrochloride

Apo-Verap†, Calan, Calan SR, Covera-HS, Isoptin SR, Novo-Veramil†, Nu-Verap†, Verelan, Verelan PM

Pregnancy risk category C

Indications & dosages

➲ **Vasospastic angina (Prinzmetal's or variant angina); classic chronic, stable angina pectoris; chronic atrial fibrillation**
Adults: Starting dose is 80 to 120 mg P.O. t.i.d. Increase dosage at daily or weekly intervals, p.r.n. Some patients may require up to 480 mg daily.
➲ **To prevent paroxysmal supraventricular tachycardia**
Adults: 80 to 120 mg P.O. t.i.d. or q.i.d.
➲ **Supraventricular arrhythmias**
Adults: 0.075 to 0.15 mg/kg (5 to 10 mg) by I.V. push over 2 minutes with ECG and blood pressure monitoring. Repeat dose in 30 minutes if no response occurs.
Children ages 1 to 15: 0.1 to 0.3 mg/kg as I.V. bolus over 2 minutes; not to exceed 5 mg.
Children younger than age 1: 0.1 to 0.2 mg/kg as I.V. bolus over 2 minutes with continuous ECG monitoring. Repeat dose in 30 minutes if no response occurs.
➲ **Digitalized patients with chronic atrial fibrillation or flutter**
Adults: 240 to 320 mg P.O. daily, divided t.i.d. or q.i.d.
➲ **Hypertension**
Adults: 240 mg extended-release tablet P.O. once daily in the morning. If response isn't adequate, give an additional 120 mg in the evening or 240 mg q 12 hours, or an 80-mg immediate-release tablet t.i.d.

Contraindications & cautions

- Contraindicated in patients hypersensitive to drug and in those with severe left ventricular dysfunction, cardiogenic shock, second- or third-degree AV block or sick sinus syndrome except in presence of functioning pacemaker, atrial flutter or fibrillation and accessory bypass tract syndrome, severe heart failure (unless secondary to verapamil therapy), and severe hypotension.
- I.V. verapamil is contraindicated in patients receiving I.V. beta blockers and in those with ventricular tachycardia.
- Use cautiously in elderly patients and in those with increased intracranial pressure or hepatic or renal disease.

Adverse reactions

CNS: dizziness, headache, asthenia.
CV: *transient hypotension*, ***heart failure***, pulmonary edema, ***bradycardia***, ***AV block***, ***ventricular asystole***, ***ventricular fibrillation***, peripheral edema.
GI: *constipation*, nausea.
Skin: rash.

Interactions

Drug-drug. *Acebutolol, atenolol, betaxolol, carteolol, esmolol, metoprolol, nadolol, penbutolol, pindolol, propanolol, timolol:* May increase effects of both drugs. Monitor cardiac function closely and decrease doses as needed.
Antihypertensives, quinidine: May cause hypotension. Monitor blood pressure.
Carbamazepine, cardiac glycosides: May increase levels of these drugs. Monitor patient for toxicity.
Cyclosporine: May increase cyclosporine level. Monitor cyclosporine level.
Disopyramide, flecainide: May cause heart failure. Avoid using together.
Dofetilide: May increase dofetilide level. Avoid using together.
Lithium: May decrease or increase lithium level. Monitor lithium level.
Rifampin: May decrease oral bioavailability of verapamil. Monitor patient for lack of effect.
Drug-herb. *Black catechu:* May cause additive effects. Discourage use together.
Yerba maté: May decrease clearance of yerba maté methylxanthines and cause toxicity. Urge caution.
Drug-food. *Any food:* May increase absorption. Advise patient to take drug with food.
Grapefruit juice: May increase verapamil level . Discourage use together.
Drug-lifestyle. *Alcohol use:* May enhance the effects of alcohol. Discourage use together.

Nursing considerations

- Although drug should be taken with food, taking extended-release tablets with food may decrease rate and extent of absorption but allows smaller fluctuations of peak and trough blood levels.
- Pellet-filled capsules may be given by carefully opening the capsule and sprinkling the pellets on a spoonful of applesauce. This should be swallowed immediately without chewing, followed by a glass of cool water to ensure all pellets are swallowed.
- Patients with severely compromised cardiac function or those receiving beta blockers should receive lower doses of verapamil. Monitor these patients closely.
- If verapamil is being used to terminate supraventricular tachycardia, prescriber may have the patient perform vagal maneuvers after receiving drug.
- Monitor blood pressure at the start of therapy and during dosage adjustments. Assist patient with walking because dizziness may occur.
- Notify prescriber if signs and symptoms of heart failure occur, such as swelling of hands and feet and shortness of breath.
- Monitor liver function test results during prolonged treatment.

!! ALERT Don't confuse Verelan with Vivarin, Voltaren, or Virilon.

Patient teaching

- Instruct patient to take oral form of drug exactly as prescribed.
- Tell patient that long-acting forms shouldn't be crushed or chewed.
- Advise patient to take drug with food.
- Caution patient against abruptly stopping drug.
- If patient continues nitrate therapy during oral verapamil dosage adjustment, urge continued compliance. S.L. nitroglycerin may be taken, as needed, when chest pain is acute.

- Encourage patient to increase fluid and fiber intake to combat constipation. Give a stool softener.
- Advise patient to avoid or severely limit alcohol consumption. Verapamil significantly inhibits alcohol elimination.

vinblastine sulfate (VLB)
Velban

Pregnancy risk category D

Indications & dosages

➲ Breast or testicular cancer, Hodgkin's disease and malignant lymphoma, choriocarcinoma, lymphosarcoma, mycosis fungoides, Kaposi's sarcoma, histiocytosis

Adults: 3.7 mg/m^2 I.V. weekly. May increase to maximum dose of 18.5 mg/m^2 I.V. weekly based on response. Don't repeat dose if WBC count is below 4,000/mm^3. Increase dosage at weekly intervals in increments of 1.8 mg/m^2 until desired therapeutic response is obtained, leukocyte count decreases to 3,000/mm^3, or maximum weekly dose of 18.5 mg/m^2 is reached.
Children: First dose is 2.5 mg/m^2 I.V. weekly. Increase dosage by 1.25 mg/m^2 weekly until WBC count is below 3,000/mm^3 or tumor response is seen. Maximum dose is 12.5 mg/m^2 I.V. weekly.

For patients with direct bilirubin over 3 mg/dl, reduce dose by 50%. For patients with recent exposure to radiation therapy or chemotherapy, single doses usually don't exceed 5.5 mg/m^2. Once a dose is determined to produce a WBC count below 3,000/mm^3, give maintenance doses of one increment less than this amount at weekly intervals.

Contraindications & cautions

- Contraindicated in patients with severe leukopenia or bacterial infection or in patients hypersensitive to the drug.
- Use cautiously in patients with hepatic dysfunction.

Adverse reactions

CNS: depression, *paresthesia, peripheral neuropathy and neuritis, numbness*, headache, ***CVA***.
CV: hypertension, ***MI***.
EENT: pharyngitis.
GI: *nausea, vomiting*, bleeding ulcer, *constipation, ileus, anorexia*, diarrhea, abdominal pain, *stomatitis*.
Hematologic: *anemia*, ***leukopenia, thrombocytopenia***.
Metabolic: hyperuricemia, *weight loss*, SIADH.
Musculoskeletal: *muscle pain and weakness*, jaw pain, *loss of deep tendon reflexes*.
Respiratory: ***acute bronchospasm***, shortness of breath.
Skin: reversible alopecia, vesiculation, *irritation, phlebitis*, cellulitis, and necrosis with extravasation.

Interactions

Drug-drug. *Erythromycin, itraconazole, other drugs that inhibit cytochrome P-450 pathway:* May increase toxicity of vinblastine. Monitor patient closely for toxicity.
Mitomycin: May increase risk of bronchospasm and shortness of breath. Monitor patient's respiratory status.
Ototoxic drugs such as platinum-containing antineoplastics: May cause temporary or permanent hearing impairment. Monitor hearing function.
Phenytoin: May decrease plasma phenytoin level. Monitor phenytoin level closely.

Nursing considerations

- To reduce nausea, give antiemetic before drug.
- Don't give drug into a limb with compromised circulation.

!!ALERT After giving drug, check for development of life-threatening acute bronchospasm. If this occurs, notify prescriber immediately. Reaction is most likely to occur in patients who are also receiving mitomycin.

- Monitor patient for stomatitis. Stop drug if stomatitis occurs and notify prescriber.
- Assess bowel activity. Give laxatives as needed and ordered. Stool softeners may be used prophylactically.
- Dosage shouldn't be repeated more frequently than every 7 days or severe leukopenia will occur. Nadir occurs on days 4 to 10 and lasts another 7 to 14 days.
- Assess patient for numbness and tingling in hands and feet. Assess gait for early evidence of footdrop.
- Drug is less neurotoxic than vincristine.

- Anticipate a decrease in dosage by 50% if bilirubin levels exceed 3 mg/100 ml.
- Stop drugs known to cause urine retention for first few days after vinblastine therapy, particularly in elderly patients.

!!ALERT Don't confuse vinblastine with vincristine, vindesine, or vinorelbine.

Patient teaching

- Tell patient to report evidence of infection (fever, sore throat, fatigue) and bleeding (easy bruising, nosebleeds, bleeding gums, tarry stools). Tell patient to take temperature daily.
- Urge patient to report pain, swelling, burning, or any unusual feeling at injection site during infusion.
- Warn patient that hair loss may occur, but explain that it's usually reversible.
- Caution woman of childbearing age to avoid pregnancy during therapy.
- Tell patient that pain may occur in jaw and in organ containing tumor.

vincristine sulfate (VCR)
Oncovin, Vincasar PFS

Pregnancy risk category D D

Indications & dosages

➲ **Acute lymphoblastic and other leukemias, Hodgkin's disease, malignant lymphoma, neuroblastoma, rhabdomyosarcoma, Wilms' tumor**

Adults: 0.4 to 1.4 mg/m^2 I.V. weekly. Maximum weekly dose is 2 mg.
Children weighing more than 10 kg (22 lb): 1.5 to 2 mg/m^2 I.V. weekly.
Children weighing 10 kg and less or with body surface area less than 1 m^2: Initially, 0.05 mg/kg I.V. weekly.

For patients with direct bilirubin over 3 mg/dl, reduce dose by 50%.

Contraindications & cautions

- Contraindicated in patients hypersensitive to drug and in those with demyelinating form of Charcot-Marie-Tooth syndrome.
- Don't give to patients who are receiving radiation therapy through ports that include the liver.
- Use cautiously in patients with hepatic dysfunction, neuromuscular disease, or infection.

Adverse reactions

CNS: *peripheral neuropathy*, sensory loss, *loss of deep tendon reflexes, paresthesia, wristdrop and footdrop*, ***seizures***, ***coma***, headache, ataxia, cranial nerve palsies, fever.
CV: hypotension, hypertension.
EENT: visual disturbances, blindness, diplopia, optic and extraocular neuropathy, ptosis, hoarseness, vocal cord paralysis, photophobia.
GI: diarrhea, *constipation*, *cramps*, ileus that mimics surgical abdomen, paralytic ileus, *nausea*, *vomiting*, anorexia, dysphagia, ***intestinal necrosis***, *stomatitis*.
GU: urine retention, SIADH, dysuria, polyuria.
Hematologic: anemia, ***leukopenia***, ***thrombocytopenia***.
Metabolic: weight loss, hyponatremia.
Musculoskeletal: *jaw pain, muscle weakness, cramps*.
Respiratory: ***acute bronchospasm***, dyspnea.
Skin: rash, reversible alopecia, severe local reaction following extravasation, *phlebitis*, cellulitis at injection site.

Interactions

Drug-drug. *Asparaginase:* May decrease hepatic clearance of vincristine. Use together also may result in additive neurotoxicity. Monitor patient for toxicity.
Digoxin: May decrease digoxin's effects. Monitor digoxin level.
Mitomycin: May increase frequency of bronchospasm and acute pulmonary reactions. Monitor patient's respiratory status.
Ototoxic drugs: May potentiate loss of hearing. Use together with caution.
Phenytoin: May reduce phenytoin level. Monitor phenytoin level closely.

Nursing considerations

- Don't give 5-mg vial as a single dose. The 5-mg vials are for multiple-dose use.

!!ALERT After giving drug, check for life-threatening acute bronchospasm. If this occurs, notify prescriber immediately. This reaction is most likely to occur in those also receiving mitomycin.

- Check for hyperuricemia, especially in patients with leukemia or lymphoma. Maintain hydration and give allopurinol to prevent uric acid nephropathy. Check for toxicity.

- Monitor fluid intake and output. Fluid restriction may be needed if SIADH develops.
- Because of risk of neurotoxicity, don't give drug more often than once weekly. Children are more resistant to neurotoxicity than adults. Neurotoxicity is dose-related and usually reversible. Some neurotoxicities may be permanent.
- Elderly patients and those with underlying neurologic disease may be more susceptible to neurotoxic effects.
- Check for depression of Achilles tendon reflex, numbness, tingling, footdrop or wristdrop, difficulty in walking, ataxia, and slapping gait. Also check ability to walk on heels. Support patient when walking.
- Monitor bowel function. Give stool softener, laxative, or water before giving dose. Constipation may be an early sign of neurotoxicity.
- All vials (1-mg, 2-mg, 5-mg) contain 1-mg/ml solution; refrigerate them.
- Stop drugs known to cause urine retention, particularly in elderly patients, for first few days after vincristine therapy.

!!ALERT Drug is fatal if given intrathecally; it's for I.V. use only.

!!ALERT Don't confuse vincristine with vinblastine or vindesine.

Patient teaching

- Advise patient to report any pain or burning at site of injection during or after administration.
- Tell patient to report evidence of infection (fever, sore throat, fatigue) and bleeding (easy bruising, nosebleeds, bleeding gums, tarry stools). Tell patient to take temperature daily.
- Warn patient that hair loss may occur, but explain that it's usually reversible.
- Caution woman of childbearing age to avoid becoming pregnant during therapy and to consult prescriber before becoming pregnant.

vinorelbine tartrate
Navelbine

Pregnancy risk category D

Indications & dosages

➲ Alone or as adjunct therapy with cisplatin for first-line treatment of ambulatory patients with nonresectable advanced non–small-cell lung cancer (NSCLC); alone or with cisplatin in stage IV of NSCLC; with cisplatin in stage III of NSCLC

Adults: 30 mg/m^2 I.V. weekly. In combination treatment, same dosage with 120 mg/m^2 of cisplatin given on days 1 and 29, and then q 6 weeks.

If granulocyte count is 1,000 to 1,499 cells/mm^3, give 50% of dose. If less than 1,000 cells/mm^3, dose is withheld. If total bilirubin is 2.1 to 3 mg/dl, reduce dose by 50%; if more than 3 mg/dl, give 25% of dose.

➲ Breast cancer♦

Adults: 20 to 30 mg/m^2 I.V. once weekly.

Contraindications & cautions

- Contraindicated in patients with pretreatment granulocyte counts below 1,000 cells/mm^3 and in patients hypersensitive to the drug.
- Use with caution in patients whose bone marrow may have been compromised by previous exposure to radiation therapy or chemotherapy or whose bone marrow is still recovering from chemotherapy.
- Use with caution in patients with hepatic impairment.
- Safety and effectiveness in children haven't been established.

Adverse reactions

CNS: *peripheral neuropathy, asthenia, fatigue.*
CV: chest pain.
GI: *nausea, vomiting, anorexia, diarrhea, constipation, stomatitis.*
Hematologic: ***bone marrow suppression, agranulocytosis,*** LEUKOPENIA, ***thrombocytopenia,*** *anemia,* ***granulocytopenia.***
Hepatic: hyperbilirubinemia.
Musculoskeletal: myalgia, arthralgia, jaw pain, loss of deep tendon reflexes.
Respiratory: dyspnea, shortness of breath.

Skin: *alopecia*, rash, *injection pain or reaction.*

Interactions

Drug-drug. *Cisplatin:* May increase risk of bone marrow suppression when used with cisplatin. Monitor hematologic status closely.
Cytochrome P-450 inhibitors: May decrease metabolism of vinorelbine. Watch for increased adverse effects.
Mitomycin: May cause pulmonary reactions. Monitor respiratory status closely.

Nursing considerations

- Check patient's granulocyte count before administration; make sure count is 1,000 cells/mm^3 or higher before giving drug. Withhold drug and notify prescriber if count is lower. Granulocyte nadirs occur between days 7 and 10.

!!ALERT Drug is fatal if given intrathecally; it's for I.V. use only.

- Dosage adjustments are made according to hematologic toxicity or hepatic insufficiency, whichever results in the lower dosage. Expect dosage reduction of 50% if granulocyte count falls below 1,500 cells/mm^3 but is greater than 1,000 cells/mm^3. If three consecutive doses are skipped because of agranulocytosis, don't resume vinorelbine therapy.
- Monitor liver enzyme levels in patients with hepatic impairment.
- Patient may receive injections of WBC colony-stimulating factors to promote cell growth and decrease risk of infection.
- Drug may be a contact irritant, and the solution must be handled and given with care. Gloves are recommended. Avoid inhalation of vapors and contact with skin or mucous membranes, especially those of the eyes. In case of contact, wash with generous amounts of water for at least 15 minutes.

!!ALERT Monitor deep tendon reflexes; loss may represent cumulative toxicity.

- Monitor patient closely for hypersensitivity.
- As a guide to the effects of therapy, monitor patient's peripheral blood count and bone marrow.

!!ALERT Don't confuse vinorelbine with vinblastine or vincristine.

Patient teaching

- Advise patient to report any pain or burning at site of injection.
- Instruct patient not to take other drugs, including OTC preparations, until approved by prescriber.
- Tell patient to report evidence of infection (fever, sore throat, fatigue) and bleeding (easy bruising, nosebleeds, bleeding gums, tarry stools). Tell him to take temperature daily.
- Advise patient to report increased shortness of breath, cough, abdominal pain, or constipation.
- Caution woman of childbearing age to avoid becoming pregnant during therapy.

vitamin K analogue

phytonadione (vitamin K_1)

AquaMEPHYTON, Mephyton

Pregnancy risk category C

Indications & dosages

➲ RDA
Men age 19 and older: 120 mcg.
Women age 19 and older, including pregnant and breast-feeding women: 90 mcg.
Children ages 14 to 18: 75 mcg.
Children ages 9 to 13: 60 mcg.
Children ages 4 to 8: 55 mcg.
Children ages 1 to 3: 30 mcg.
Infants ages 7 months to 1 year: 2.5 mcg.
Neonates and infants younger than age 6 months: 2 mcg.

➲ Hypoprothrombinemia caused by vitamin K malabsorption, drug therapy, or excessive vitamin A dosage
Adults: Depending on severity, 2.5 to 10 mg P.O., I.M., or S.C., repeated and increased up to 50 mg, if needed.
Children: 5 to 10 mg P.O. or parenterally.
Infants: 2 mg P.O. or parenterally.

➲ Hypoprothrombinemia caused by effect of oral anticoagulants
Adults: 2.5 to 10 mg P.O., I.M., or S.C. based on PT/INR, repeated if needed within 12 to 48 hours after oral dose or within 6 to 8 hours after parenteral dose. In emergency, 10 to 50 mg slow I.V. at rate not to exceed 1 mg/minute, repeated q 4 hours, p.r.n.

➲ To prevent hemorrhagic disease of newborn
Neonates: 0.5 to 1 mg I.M. within 1 hour after birth.
➲ Hemorrhagic disease of newborn
Neonates: 1 mg S.C. or I.M. Higher doses may be needed if mother has been receiving oral anticoagulants.
➲ To prevent hypoprothrombinemia related to vitamin K deficiency in long-term parenteral nutrition
Adults: 5 to 10 mg P.O. or I.M. weekly.
Children: 2 to 5 mg P.O. or I.M. weekly.
➲ To prevent hypoprothrombinemia in infants receiving less than 0.1 mg/L vitamin K in breast milk or milk substitutes
Infants: 1 mg I.M. monthly.

Contraindications & cautions

- Contraindicated in patients hypersensitive to drug.

Adverse reactions

CNS: dizziness.
CV: flushing, transient hypotension after I.V. administration, rapid and weak pulse.
Skin: diaphoresis, erythema.
Other: ***anaphylaxis or anaphylactoid reactions, usually after excessively rapid I.V. administration***; pain, swelling, and hematoma at injection site.

Interactions

Drug-drug. *Anticoagulants:* May cause temporary resistance to prothrombin-depressing anticoagulants, especially when larger doses of phytonadione are used. Monitor patient closely.
Cholestyramine, mineral oil, orlistat: May inhibit GI absorption of oral vitamin K. Separate doses if possible. If unavoidable, use together cautiously.

Nursing considerations

- Check brand name labels for administration route restrictions.
- For I.M. administration in adults and older children, give in upper outer quadrant of buttocks; for infants, give in anterolateral aspect of thigh or deltoid region. S.C. route is preferred to avoid hematoma formation.
- Allergic reactions may also occur after I.M. or S.C. use.
- Anticipate order for weekly addition of 5 to 10 mg of phytonadione to total parenteral nutrition solutions.
- Monitor PT or INR to determine dosage effectiveness.
- If severe bleeding occurs, don't delay other measures, such as administration of fresh frozen plasma or whole blood.
- Vitamin K doesn't reverse the anticoagulant effects of heparin.

!!ALERT Watch for flushing, weakness, tachycardia, and hypotension; condition may progress to shock.

- Phytonadione therapy for hemorrhagic disease in infants causes fewer adverse reactions than other vitamin K analogues.

Patient teaching

- Explain purpose of drug.
- Tell patient to avoid hazardous activities if dizziness occurs.
- Inform patient that drug is fat soluble; advise her to take drug only as prescribed to avoid accumulation.
- Teach patient that foods that provide vitamin K include cabbage, cauliflower, kale, spinach, fish, liver, eggs, meats, and dairy products.

voriconazole
Vfend

Pregnancy risk category D

Indications & dosages

➲ Esophageal candidiasis
Adults weighing 40 kg (88 lb) or more: 200 mg P.O. q 12 hours. Treat for a minimum of 14 days and for at least 7 days after symptoms resolve.
Adults weighing less than 40 kg: 100 mg P.O. q 12 hours. Treat for a minimum of 14 days and for at least 7 days after symptoms resolve.
➲ Invasive aspergillosis; serious infections caused by *Fusarium* species and *Scedosporium apiospermum* in patients intolerant of or refractory to other therapy
Adults: Initially, 6 mg/kg I.V. q 12 hours for two doses; then maintenance dose of 4 mg/kg I.V. q 12 hours. Switch to P.O. form as tolerated, using the maintenance dosages shown here.

Adults weighing more than 40 kg: 200 mg P.O. q 12 hours. May increase to 300 mg P.O. q 12 hours, if needed.
Adults weighing less than 40 kg: 100 mg P.O. q 12 hours. May increase to 150 mg P.O. q 12 hours, if needed.

➲ **Candidemia in nonneutropenic patients; Candida infections of the kidney, abdomen, bladder wall, or wounds and disseminated skin infections**

Adults: Initially, 6 mg/kg I.V. q 12 hours for two doses, then 4 mg/kg I.V. q 12 hours for maintenance. If patient can't tolerate maintenance dose, decrease to 3 mg/kg. Switch to P.O. form as tolerated. For adults who weigh 40 kg or more, give 200 mg P.O. q 12 hours. May increase to 300 mg P.O. q 12 hours, if needed. For adults who weigh less than 40 kg, give 100 mg P.O. q 12 hours. May increase to 150 mg P.O. q 12 hours, if needed. Patients with candidemia should be treated for at least 14 days after symptoms resolve or after the last positive culture, whichever is longer.

For patients in Child-Pugh classes A or B, decrease the maintenance dosage by 50%. In patients with a creatinine clearance of less than 50 ml/minute, use oral form instead of I.V. form to prevent accumulation of a component of the I.V. mixture.

Contraindications & cautions

- Contraindicated in patients hypersensitive to drug or its components; in those with rare hereditary problems of galactose intolerance, Lapp lactase deficiency, or glucose-galactose malabsorption; and in those taking rifampin, carbamazepine, a long-acting barbiturate, sirolimus, rifabutin, an ergot alkaloid, pimozide, or quinidine.
- Use cautiously in patients hypersensitive to other azoles. Use I.V. form cautiously in patients with creatinine clearance less than 50 ml/minute.

!!ALERT Drug may harm fetus. If drug is used during pregnancy or if the patient becomes pregnant while taking the drug, inform patient of the potential hazard to the fetus.

Adverse reactions

CNS: fever, headache, hallucinations, dizziness.
CV: tachycardia, hypertension, hypotension, vasodilatation.
EENT: *abnormal vision*, photophobia, chromatopsia, dry mouth.
GI: abdominal pain, nausea, vomiting, diarrhea.
Hepatic: cholestatic jaundice.
Metabolic: hypokalemia, hypomagnesemia.
Skin: rash, pruritus.
Other: chills, peripheral edema.

Interactions

Drug-drug. *Benzodiazepines, calcium channel blockers, lovastatin, omeprazole, sulfonylureas, vinca alkaloids:* May increase levels of these drugs. Adjust dosages of these drugs, and monitor patient for adverse reactions.
Carbamazepine, long-acting barbiturates, rifabutin, rifampin: May decrease voriconazole level. Avoid using together.
Coumarin anticoagulants (such as warfarin): May significantly increase PT. Monitor PT and other appropriate anticoagulant test results.
Cyclosporine, tacrolimus: May increase levels of these drugs. Adjust dosages; monitor levels of these drugs.
Efavirenz: May significantly decrease voriconazole levels while significantly increasing efavirenz levels. Avoid use together.
Ergot alkaloids (such as ergotamine), sirolimus: May increase levels of these drugs. Avoid using together.
HIV protease inhibitors (amprenavir, nelfinavir, saquinavir), nonnucleoside reverse transcriptase inhibitors (delavirdine, efavirenz): May increase levels of both drugs. Monitor patient for adverse reactions.
Phenytoin: May decrease voriconazole level and increase phenytoin level. Increase voriconazole maintenance dose; monitor phenytoin level.
Pimozide, quinidine: May increase levels of these drugs, possibly leading to QT interval prolongation and torsades de pointes. Avoid using together.
Drug-lifestyle. *Sun exposure:* May cause photosensitivity. Advise patient to avoid excessive sunlight exposure.

Nursing considerations

- Infusion reactions, including flushing, fever, sweating, tachycardia, chest tightness, dyspnea, faintness, nausea, pruritus, and rash, may occur as soon as infusion is

started. Notify prescriber if reaction occurs. Infusion may need to be stopped.
- Monitor liver function test results at the start of and during therapy. Monitor patients who develop abnormal liver function test results for more severe hepatic injury. Drug may need to be stopped if patient develops signs and symptoms of liver disease.
- Monitor renal function during treatment. Patients with creatinine clearance less than 50 ml/minute may benefit more from oral formulation of drug.
- Visual changes may occur if treatment lasts longer than 28 days.

Patient teaching

- Tell patient to take oral form at least 1 hour before or 1 hour after a meal.
- Tell patient using the oral suspension to only use the dispenser provided with the medication pack.
- Advise patient not to mix oral suspension with other drugs or beverages.
- Tell patient to keep suspension refrigerated and to discard any unused portion after 14 days.
- Advise patient to avoid driving or operating machinery while taking drug, especially at night, because vision changes, including blurring and photophobia, may occur.
- Tell patient to avoid strong, direct sunlight during therapy.
- Advise patient to avoid becoming pregnant during drug therapy because of potential fetal harm.

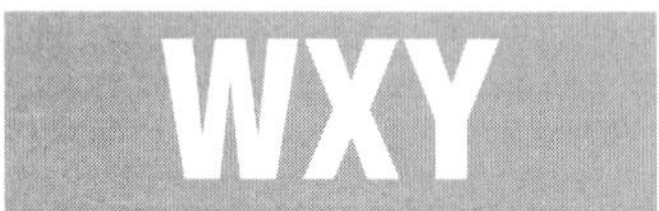

warfarin sodium
Coumadin, Warfilone†

Pregnancy risk category X

Indications & dosages

➲ Pulmonary embolism with DVT, MI, rheumatic heart disease with heart valve damage, prosthetic heart valves, chronic atrial fibrillation

Adults: 2 to 5 mg P.O. daily for 2 to 4 days; then dosage based on daily PT and INR. Usual maintenance dosage is 2 to 10 mg P.O. daily; I.V. dosage is same as that used P.O.

Contraindications & cautions

- Contraindicated in patients hypersensitive to drug and in those with bleeding from the GI, GU, or respiratory tract; aneurysm; cerebrovascular hemorrhage; severe or malignant hypertension; severe renal or hepatic disease; subacute bacterial endocarditis, pericarditis, or pericardial effusion; or blood dyscrasias or hemorrhagic tendencies.
- Contraindicated during pregnancy, threatened abortion, eclampsia, or preeclampsia, and after recent surgery involving large open areas, eye, brain, or spinal cord; recent prostatectomy; major regional lumbar block anesthesia, spinal puncture, or diagnostic or therapeutic invasive procedures.
- Avoid using in patients with a history of warfarin-induced necrosis; in unsupervised patients with senility, alcoholism, or psychosis; or in situations in which there are inadequate laboratory facilities for coagulation testing.
- Use cautiously in patients with diverticulitis, colitis, mild or moderate hypertension, or mild or moderate hepatic or renal disease; with drainage tubes in any orifice; with regional or lumbar block anesthesia; or in conditions that increase risk of hemorrhage.
- Use cautiously in breast-feeding women.

Adverse reactions

CNS: headache, *fever*.
GI: anorexia, nausea, vomiting, cramps, *diarrhea*, mouth ulcerations, sore mouth, melena.
GU: hematuria, excessive menstrual bleeding.
Hematologic: ***hemorrhage***.
Hepatic: ***hepatitis***, jaundice.
Skin: dermatitis, urticaria, necrosis, gangrene, alopecia, *rash*.
Other: enhanced uric acid excretion.

Interactions

Drug-drug. *Acetaminophen:* May increase bleeding with long-term therapy (more than 2 weeks) at high doses (more than 2 g/day) of acetaminophen. Monitor patient very carefully.
Allopurinol, amiodarone, anabolic steroids, antidepressants, antifungals, cephalospor-

ins, chloramphenicol, cimetidine, danazol, diazoxide, diflunisal, disulfiram, erythromycin, ethacrynic acid, fluoroquinolones, glucagon, heparin, influenza virus vaccine, isoniazid, meclofenamate, methimazole, metronidazole, nalidixic acid, neomycin (oral), NSAIDs, omeprazole, pentoxifylline, propafenone, propoxyphene, propylthiouracil, quinidine, sulfinpyrazone, sulfonamides, tamoxifen, tetracyclines, thiazides, thrombolytics, thyroid drugs, vitamin E: May increase PT and INR. Monitor patient carefully for bleeding. Reduce anticoagulant dosage as directed.

Anticonvulsants: May increase levels of phenytoin and phenobarbital. Monitor drug levels closely.

Aspirin, NSAIDs, salicylates: May increase PT and INR; ulcerogenic effects. Avoid using together.

Barbiturates, carbamazepine, corticosteroids, corticotropin, dicloxacillin, ethchlorvynol, griseofulvin, haloperidol, meprobamate, mercaptopurine, nafcillin, oral contraceptives containing estrogen, rifampin, spironolactone, sucralfate, trazodone: May decrease PT and INR with reduced anticoagulant effect. Monitor patient carefully.

Chloral hydrate, hypolipidemics, propylthiouracil: May increase or decrease PT and INR. Avoid using, if possible, and monitor patient carefully.

Cholestyramine: May decrease response when given too closely together. Give 6 hours after oral anticoagulants.

Sulfonylureas (oral antidiabetics): May increase hypoglycemic response. Monitor glucose levels.

Drug-herb. *Angelica:* May significantly prolong PT and INR when *Angelica sinensis* is given with warfarin. Discourage use together.

Anise, arnica flower, asafoetida, bromelain, celery, chamomile, clove, Danshen, devil's claw, dong quai, fenugreek, feverfew, garlic, ginger, ginkgo, ginseng, horse chestnut, licorice, meadowsweet, motherwort, onion, papain, parsley, passion flower, quassia, red clover, reishi mushroom, rue, sweet clover, turmeric, white willow: May increase risk of bleeding. Discourage use together.

Coenzyme Q10, ginseng, St. John's wort: May reduce action of drug. Ask patient about use of herbal remedies, and advise caution.

Green tea: May decrease anticoagulant effect caused by vitamin K content of green tea. Advise patient to minimize variable consumption of green tea and other foods or nutritional supplements containing vitamin K.

Drug-food. *Foods, multivitamins, or enteral products containing vitamin K:* May impair anticoagulation. Tell patient to maintain consistent daily intake of foods containing vitamin K.

Drug-lifestyle. *Alcohol use:* May enhance anticoagulant effects. Tell patient to avoid large amounts of alcohol.

Nursing considerations

- Draw blood to establish baseline coagulation parameters before therapy.
- PT and INR determinations are essential for proper control.
- Give warfarin at same time daily. INR range for chronic atrial fibrillation is usually 2 to 3.
- I.M. administration isn't recommended.
- Regularly inspect patient for bleeding gums, bruises on arms or legs, petechiae, nosebleeds, melena, tarry stools, hematuria, and hematemesis.
- Check for unexpected bleeding in breast-fed infants of women on drug.

!!ALERT Withhold drug and call prescriber at once in the event of fever or rash (signs of severe adverse reactions).

- Half-life of warfarin's anticoagulant effect is 36 to 44 hours. Effect can be neutralized by parenteral or oral vitamin K.
- Elderly patients and patients with renal or hepatic failure are especially sensitive to warfarin effect.

Patient teaching

- Stress importance of complying with prescribed dosage and follow-up appointments. Tell patient to carry a card that identifies his increased risk of bleeding.
- Tell patient and family to watch for signs of bleeding or abnormal bruising and to call prescriber at once if they occur.
- Warn patient to avoid OTC products containing aspirin, other salicylates, or drugs that may interact with warfarin unless ordered by prescriber.
- Tell patient to consult a prescriber before using miconazole vaginal cream or supposi-

tories. Abnormal bleeding and bruising have occurred.
- Instruct woman to notify prescriber if menstruation is heavier than usual; she may need dosage adjustment.
- Tell patient to use electric razor when shaving, and to use a soft toothbrush.
- Tell patient to read food labels. Food, nutritional supplements, and multivitamins that contain vitamin K may impair anticoagulation.
- Tell patient to eat a daily, consistent diet of food and drinks containing vitamin K, because eating varied amounts may alter anticoagulant effects.

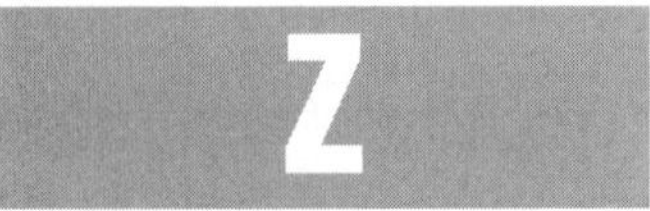

zafirlukast
Accolate

Pregnancy risk category B

Indications & dosages
➲ Prevention and long-term treatment of asthma
Adults and children age 12 and older: 20 mg P.O. b.i.d. taken 1 hour before or 2 hours after meals.
Children ages 5 to 11: 10 mg P.O. b.i.d. taken 1 hour before or 2 hours after meals.

Contraindications & cautions
- Contraindicated in patients hypersensitive to drug.
- Give cautiously to elderly patients and those with hepatic impairment.
- Give to pregnant patients only if clearly needed. Don't use in breast-feeding women.

Adverse reactions
CNS: *headache*, asthenia, dizziness, pain.
GI: nausea, diarrhea, abdominal pain, vomiting, dyspepsia, gastritis.
Musculoskeletal: myalgia, back pain.
Other: infection, accidental injury, fever.

Interactions
Drug-drug. *Aspirin:* May increase zafirlukast level. Monitor patient for adverse effects.
Erythromycin, theophylline: May decrease zafirlukast level. Monitor patient for decreased effectiveness.
Warfarin: May increase PT. Monitor PT and INR, and adjust anticoagulant dosage.
Drug-food. *Food:* May reduce rate and extent of zafirlukast absorption. Give 1 hour before or 2 hours after a meal.

Nursing considerations
!!ALERT Reducing oral corticosteroid dose has been followed in rare cases by eosinophilia, vasculitic rash, worsening pulmonary symptoms, cardiac complications, or neuropathy, sometimes presenting as Churg-Strauss syndrome.
- Drug is not indicated to reverse bronchospasm in acute asthma attacks.

Patient teaching
- Tell patient that drug is used for long-term treatment of asthma and to keep taking it even if symptoms resolve.
- Advise patient to continue taking other antiasthma drugs, as prescribed.
- Instruct patient to take drug 1 hour before or 2 hours after meals.

zalcitabine (ddC, dideoxycytidine)
Hivid

Pregnancy risk category C

Indications & dosages
➲ HIV disease, with other antiretrovirals
Adults and adolescents age 13 and older: 0.75 mg P.O. q 8 hours.

For patients with creatinine clearance of 10 to 40 ml/minute, give 0.75 mg P.O. q 12 hours; if clearance is less than 10 ml/minute, give 0.75 mg P.O. q 24 hours. If patient has moderate discomfort and signs and symptoms of peripheral neuropathy, stop drug temporarily. If symptoms improve after stopping therapy, drug may be reintroduced at 0.375 mg P.O. q 8 hours.

Contraindications & cautions
- Contraindicated in patients hypersensitive to drug or its components.
- Use with extreme caution in patients with peripheral neuropathy.

• Use cautiously in patients with hepatic failure, history of pancreatitis or heart failure, or baseline cardiomyopathy. Monitor liver function test results and pancreatic enzymes.

Adverse reactions

CNS: *peripheral neuropathy, headache, fatigue,* dizziness, *fever,* confusion, ***seizures***, impaired concentration, amnesia, insomnia, mental depression, tremor, hypertonia, anxiety.
CV: cardiomyopathy, ***heart failure***, chest pain.
EENT: pharyngitis, ocular pain, abnormal vision, ototoxicity, nasal discharge.
GI: nausea, vomiting, diarrhea, abdominal pain, anorexia, constipation, stomatitis, esophageal ulcer, glossitis, ***pancreatitis***.
Hematologic: anemia, ***neutropenia, leukopenia, thrombocytopenia***.
Metabolic: ***hypoglycemia***.
Musculoskeletal: myalgia, arthralgia.
Respiratory: cough.
Skin: pruritus; night sweats; *erythematous, maculopapular, or follicular rash*; urticaria.

Interactions

Drug-drug. *Aminoglycosides, amphotericin B, foscarnet, other drugs that may impair renal function:* May increase risk of nephrotoxicity. Monitor renal function.
Antacids containing aluminum or magnesium: May decrease bioavailability of zalcitabine. Separate dosage times.
Chloramphenicol, cisplatin, dapsone, didanosine, disulfiram, ethionamide, glutethimide, gold salts, hydralazine, iodoquinol, isoniazid, metronidazole, nitrofurantoin, other drugs that can cause peripheral neuropathy, phenytoin, ribavirin, stavudine, vincristine: May increase risk of peripheral neuropathy. Avoid using together.
Cimetidine, probenecid: May increase zalcitabine level. Monitor patient closely.
Pentamidine: May increase risk of pancreatitis. Avoid using together.
Drug-food. *Any food:* May decrease rate of absorption. Give drug on an empty stomach.

Nursing considerations

!!ALERT Occasionally fatal cases of lactic acidosis, severe hepatomegaly with steatosis, and hepatic failure have been reported. Monitor patient closely.
• Toxic effects of drug may cause abnormalities in several laboratory tests, including CBC; hemoglobin level; leukocyte, reticulocyte, granulocyte, and platelet counts; and AST, ALT, and alkaline phosphatase levels.
• Don't give drug with food because it decreases the rate and extent of absorption.
• Assess patients for signs and symptoms of peripheral neuropathy, characterized by numbness and burning in the limbs, the drug's major toxic effects. If drug isn't withdrawn, peripheral neuropathy can progress to sharp shooting pain or severe continuous burning pain requiring opioid analgesics. The pain may or may not be reversible.
!!ALERT Don't confuse drug with other antivirals identified by initials.

Patient teaching

• Instruct patient to take drug on an empty stomach.
• Make sure patient understands that the drug doesn't cure HIV infection and that opportunistic infections may occur despite continued use. Review safe sex practices with patient.
• Inform patient that peripheral neuropathy is the major toxic condition associated with drug and that inflammation of the pancreas is the major life-threatening toxic reaction. Review the signs and symptoms of these adverse reactions, and tell patient to call prescriber promptly if any appear.
• Advise patient of childbearing age to use an effective contraceptive while taking drug.

zaleplon
Sonata

Pregnancy risk category C
Controlled substance schedule IV

Indications & dosages

➲ Insomnia
Adults: 10 mg P.O. daily h.s.; may increase to 20 mg, p.r.n. Low-weight adults may respond to 5-mg dose. Limit use to 7 to 10 days. Reevaluate patient if used for more than 2 to 3 weeks.

Elderly patients: initially, 5 mg P.O. daily h.s.; doses of more than 10 mg aren't recommended.

For debilitated patients, initially, 5 mg P.O. daily h.s.; doses of more than 10 mg aren't recommended. For patients with mild to moderate hepatic impairment or those also taking cimetidine, 5 mg P.O. daily h.s.

Contraindications & cautions

- Contraindicated in patients with severe hepatic impairment.
- Use cautiously in elderly, depressed, or debilitated patients, in breast-feeding women, and in patients with compromised respiratory function.

Adverse reactions

CNS: *headache*, amnesia, dizziness, somnolence, depression, hypertonia, nervousness, depersonalization, hallucinations, vertigo, difficulty concentrating, anxiety, paresthesia, hypesthesia, tremor, asthenia, migraine, malaise, fever.
CV: chest pain, peripheral edema.
EENT: abnormal vision, conjunctivitis, eye discomfort, ear discomfort, hyperacusis, epistaxis, smell alteration.
GI: constipation, dry mouth, anorexia, dyspepsia, nausea, abdominal pain, colitis.
GU: dysmenorrhea.
Musculoskeletal: arthritis, myalgia, back pain.
Respiratory: bronchitis.
Skin: pruritus, rash, photosensitivity reactions.

Interactions

Drug-drug. *Carbamazepine, phenobarbital, phenytoin, rifampin, other CYP3A4 inducers:* May reduce zaleplon bioavailability and peak level by 80%. Consider using a different hypnotic.
Cimetidine: May increase zaleplon bioavailability and peak level by 85%. Use an initial zaleplon dose of 5 mg.
CNS depressants (imipramine, thioridazine): May cause additive CNS effects. Use together cautiously.
Drug-food. *High-fat foods, heavy meals:* May prolong absorption, delaying peak zaleplon level by about 2 hours; may delay sleep onset. Advise patient to avoid taking with meals.
Drug-lifestyle. *Alcohol use:* May increase CNS effects. Discourage use together.

Nursing considerations

- Because drug works rapidly, give immediately before bedtime or after patient has gone to bed and has had difficulty falling asleep.
- Closely monitor patients who have compromised respiratory function caused by illness or who are elderly or debilitated because they are more sensitive to respiratory depression.
- Start treatment only after carefully evaluating patient because sleep disturbances may be a symptom of an underlying physical or psychiatric disorder.
- Adverse reactions are usually dose-related. Consult prescriber about dose reduction if adverse reactions occur.

Patient teaching

- Advise patient that drug works rapidly and should only be taken immediately before bedtime or after he has gone to bed and has had trouble falling asleep.
- Advise patient to take drug only if he will be able to sleep for at least 4 undisturbed hours.
- Caution patient that drowsiness, dizziness, light-headedness, and coordination problems occur most often within 1 hour after taking drug.
- Advise patient to avoid performing activities that require mental alertness until CNS adverse reactions are known.
- Advise patient to avoid alcohol use while taking drug and to notify prescriber before taking other prescription or OTC drugs.
- Tell patient not to take drug after a high-fat or heavy meal.
- Advise patient to report sleep problems that continue despite use of drug.
- Notify patient that dependence can occur and that drug is recommended for short-term use only.
- Warn patient not to abruptly stop drug because of the risk of withdrawal symptoms, including unpleasant feelings, stomach and muscle cramps, vomiting, sweating, shakiness, and seizures.
- Notify patient that insomnia may recur for a few nights after stopping drug, but should resolve on its own.

• Warn patient that drug may cause changes in behavior and thinking, including outgoing or aggressive behavior, loss of personal identity, confusion, strange behavior, agitation, hallucinations, worsening of depression, or suicidal thoughts. Tell patient to notify prescriber immediately if these symptoms occur.

zidovudine (azidothymidine, AZT)
Apo-Zidovudine†, Novo-AZT†, Retrovir

Pregnancy risk category C

Indications & dosages

➲ HIV infection, with other antiretrovirals

Adults: 600 mg daily P.O. in divided doses. If patient is unable to tolerate oral zidovudine, give 1 mg/kg I.V. over 1 hour five to six times daily.

Children ages 6 weeks to 12 years: 160 mg/m^2 q 8 hours (480 mg/m^2/day up to a maximum of 200 mg q 8 hours) with other antiretrovirals. Some prescribers recommend 120 mg/m^2 I.V. q 6 hours, or 20 mg/m^2/hour continuous I.V. infusion.

➲ To prevent maternal-fetal transmission of HIV

Pregnant women at more than 14 weeks' gestation: 100 mg P.O. five times daily until the start of labor. Then, 2 mg/kg I.V. over 1 hour followed by a continuous I.V. infusion of 1 mg/kg/hour until the umbilical cord is clamped.

Neonates: 2 mg/kg P.O. q 6 hours starting within 12 hours after birth and continuing until 6 weeks old. Or, give 1.5 mg/kg via I.V. infusion over 30 minutes q 6 hours.

In patients with significant anemia (hemoglobin level less than 7.5 g/dl or more than 25% below baseline) or significant neutropenia (granulocyte count less than 750 cells/mm^3 or more than 50% below baseline), interrupt therapy until evidence proves marrow has recovered. In patients receiving hemodialysis or peritoneal dialysis, give 100 mg P.O. or 1 mg/kg I.V. q 6 to 8 hours. For patients with mild to moderate hepatic dysfunction or liver cirrhosis, daily dose may need to be reduced.

Contraindications & cautions

• Contraindicated in patients hypersensitive to drug.

• Use cautiously and with close monitoring in patients with advanced symptomatic HIV infection and in patients with severe bone marrow depression.

• Use cautiously in patients with hepatomegaly, hepatitis, or other risk factors for liver disease and in those with renal insufficiency. Monitor renal and liver function tests.

Adverse reactions

CNS: *headache*, ***seizures***, paresthesia, *malaise*, insomnia, *asthenia*, *dizziness*, somnolence, *fever*.

GI: nausea, anorexia, abdominal pain, vomiting, constipation, diarrhea, taste perversion, dyspepsia, ***pancreatitis***.

Hematologic: ***severe bone marrow suppression***, anemia, ***agranulocytosis***, ***thrombocytopenia***.

Metabolic: lactic acidosis.

Musculoskeletal: myalgia.

Skin: *rash*, diaphoresis.

Interactions

Drug-drug. *Atovaquone, fluconazole, methadone, probenecid, valproic acid:* May increase bioavailability of zidovudine. May need to adjust dosage.

Doxorubicin, ribavirin, stavudine: May have antagonistic effects. Avoid using together.

Ganciclovir, interferon alfa, other bone marrow suppressive or cytotoxic drugs: May increase hematologic toxicity of zidovudine. Use together cautiously.

Phenytoin: May alter phenytoin level and decrease zidovudine clearance by 30%. Monitor patient closely.

Nursing considerations

!!ALERT Although rare, lactic acidosis without hypoxemia may occur with the use of antiretroviral nucleoside analogues, including zidovudine. Notify prescriber if patient develops unexplained tachypnea, dyspnea, or a decrease in bicarbonate level. Drug therapy may need to be suspended until lactic acidosis is ruled out.

• Monitor blood studies every 2 weeks to detect anemia or agranulocytosis. Patients may need dosage reduction or temporary discontinuation of drug.

• Drug may temporarily decrease morbidity and mortality in certain patients with AIDS.

Patient teaching

• Tell patient to take drug exactly as directed and not to share it with others.
• Instruct patient to take drug on an empty stomach. To avoid esophageal irritation, tell patient to take drug while sitting upright and with adequate fluids.
• Remind patient to comply with the dosage schedule. Suggest ways to avoid missing doses, perhaps by using an alarm clock.
• Advise patient that blood transfusions may be needed during therapy because of zidovudine-related anemia.
• Tell patient that dosages vary among patients and not to change his dosing instructions unless directed to do so by his prescriber.
• Tell patient that his gums may bleed. Recommend good mouth care with a soft toothbrush.
• Warn patient not to take other drugs for AIDS unless prescriber has approved them.
• Advise pregnant, HIV-infected patient that drug therapy only reduces the risk of HIV transmission to her newborn. Long-term risks to infants are unknown.
• Advise patient that monotherapy isn't recommended and to discuss any questions with prescriber.
• Advise health care worker considering zidovudine prophylaxis after occupational exposure (such as needlestick injury) that drug's safety and efficacy haven't been established.
• Tell patient not to keep capsules in the kitchen, bathroom, or other places that may be damp or hot. Heat and moisture may cause the drug to break down and affect the intended results.

ziprasidone
Geodon

Pregnancy risk category C

Indications & dosages

➲ Symptomatic treatment of schizophrenia
Adults: Initially, 20 mg b.i.d. with food. Dosages are highly individualized. Adjust dosage, if necessary, no more frequently than q 2 days; to allow for lowest possible doses, the interval should be several weeks to assess symptom response. Effective dosage range is usually 20 to 80 mg b.i.d. Maximum dosage is 100 mg b.i.d.

➲ Rapid control of acute agitation in schizophrenic patients
Adults: 10 to 20 mg I.M. p.r.n., up to a maximum dosage of 40 mg daily. Doses of 10 mg may be given q 2 hours; doses of 20 mg may be given q 4 hours.

➲ Acute bipolar mania, including manic and mixed episodes, with or without psychotic features
Adults: 40 mg P.O. b.i.d., with food, on day 1. Increase to 60 to 80 mg P.O. b.i.d., with food, on day 2; then adjust dosage based on patient response from 40 to 80 mg b.i.d., with food.

Contraindications & cautions

• Contraindicated in patients hypersensitive to drug and in those with recent MI or uncompensated heart failure.
• Contraindicated in those with history of prolonged QT interval or congenital long QT interval syndrome and in those taking other drugs that prolong QT interval, such as dofetilide, sotalol, quinidine, other class IA and III antiarrhythmics, mesoridazine, thioridazine, chlorpromazine, droperidol, pimozide, sparfloxacin, gatifloxacin, moxifloxacin, halofantrine, mefloquine, pentamidine, arsenic trioxide, levomethadyl acetate, dolasetron mesylate, probucol, and tacrolimus.

P.O.
• Contraindicated in patients with a history of QT interval prolongation or congenital QT syndrome and in those taking other drugs that prolong QT interval.
• Use cautiously in patients with history of seizures, bradycardia, hypokalemia, or hypomagnesemia; in those with acute diarrhea; and in those with conditions that may lower the seizure threshold (such as Alzheimer's dementia).
• Use cautiously in patients at risk for aspiration pneumonia.

I.M.
• Contraindicated in schizophrenic patients already taking P.O. ziprasidone.
• Use cautiously in elderly and renally or hepatically impaired patients.

Adverse reactions

CNS: *somnolence*, akathisia, dizziness, extrapyramidal symptoms, hypertonia, asthenia, dystonia (P.O.), *headache, dizziness*, anxiety, ***suicide attempt***, insomnia, agitation, cogwheel rigidity, paresthesia, personality disorder, psychosis, speech disorder (I.M.).
CV: orthostatic hypotension, ***QT interval prolongation***, tachycardia (P.O.), hypertension, ***bradycardia***, vasodilation (I.M.).
EENT: rhinitis, abnormal vision (P.O.).
GI: *nausea*, constipation, dyspepsia, diarrhea, dry mouth, anorexia, abdominal pain, rectal hemorrhage, vomiting, dyspepsia, tooth disorder (I.M.).
GU: dysmenorrhea, priapism (I.M.).
Metabolic: hyperglycemia.
Musculoskeletal: myalgia (P.O.), back pain (I.M.).
Respiratory: cough (P.O.).
Skin: rash (P.O.), injection site pain, furunculosis, sweating (I.M.).
Other: flulike syndrome (I.M.).

Interactions

Drug-drug. *Antihypertensives:* may enhance hypotensive effects. Monitor blood pressure.
Carbamazepine: May decrease ziprasidone level. May need to increase ziprasidone dose to achieve desired effect.
Drugs that decrease potassium or magnesium, such as diuretics: May increase risk of arrhythmias. Monitor potassium and magnesium levels if using these drugs together.
Drugs that prolong QT interval, such as dofetilide, moxifloxacin, pimozide, quinidine, sotalol, sparfloxacin, thioridazine: May increase risk of arrhythmias. Avoid using together.
Itraconazole, ketoconazole: May increase ziprasidone level. May need to reduce ziprasidone dose to achieve desired effect.

Nursing considerations

!!ALERT Hyperglycemia may occur. Monitor patients with diabetes regularly. Patients with risk factors for diabetes should undergo fasting blood glucose testing at baseline and periodically. Monitor all patients for symptoms of hyperglycemia, including excessive hunger or thirst, frequent urination, and weakness. Hyperglycemia may be reversible when drug is stopped.

P.O.

- Stop drug in patients with a QTc interval more than 500 msec.
- Dizziness, palpitations, or syncope may be symptoms of a life-threatening arrhythmia such as torsades de pointes. Further CV evaluation and monitoring are needed in patients who experience these symptoms.
- Don't give to patients with electrolyte disturbances, such as hypokalemia or hypomagnesemia, because these increase the risk of developing an arrhythmia.
- Patient taking an antipsychotic is at risk for developing life-threatening neuroleptic malignant syndrome (hyperpyrexia, muscle rigidity, altered mental status, and autonomic instability) or tardive dyskinesia. Assess abnormal involuntary movement before starting therapy, at dosage changes, and periodically thereafter, to monitor patient for tardive dyskinesia.
- Monitor patient for abnormal body temperature regulation, especially if patient is exercising strenuously, is exposed to extreme heat, is receiving concomitant anticholinergics, or is subject to dehydration.
- Symptoms may not improve for 4 to 6 weeks.
- Always give drug with food for optimal effect.
- Don't use drug in breast-feeding patients.

I.M.

- To prepare I.M. ziprasidone, add 1.2 ml of sterile water for injection to the vial and shake vigorously until drug is completely dissolved.
- Don't mix injection with other medicinal products or solvents other than sterile water for injection.
- Inspect parenteral drug products for particulate matter and discoloration before administration, whenever possible.
- The effects of giving I.M. ziprasidone for more than three consecutive days are unknown. If long-term therapy of ziprasidone is necessary, switch to P.O. as soon as possible.
- Store injection at controlled room temperature, 59° to 86° F (15° to 30°C) in dry form, and protect from light. After reconstituting the drug, it may be stored away from light for up to 24 hours at 59° to 86° F (15°to 30° C) or up to 7 days refrigerated, 36° to 46° F (2° to 8° C).

Patient teaching

- Tell patient to take drug with food.
- Tell patient to immediately report to prescriber signs or symptoms of dizziness, fainting, irregular heartbeat, or relevant heart problems.
- Advise patient to report any recent episodes of diarrhea, abnormal movements, sudden fever, muscle rigidity, or change in mental status.
- Advise patient that symptoms may not improve for 4 to 6 weeks.

zoledronic acid
Zometa

Pregnancy risk category D

Indications & dosages

➲ Hypercalcemia caused by malignancy
Adults: 4 mg by I.V. infusion over at least 15 minutes. If albumin-corrected calcium level doesn't return to normal, may repeat 4 mg. Let at least 7 days pass before retreatment to allow a full response to the first dose.

For patients in whom drug caused reduced renal function and who must be retreated with the drug, the following applies. For patients with normal baseline creatinine level who experience an increase in creatinine level of 0.5 mg/dl within 2 weeks of the next dose, withhold drug until level is within 10% of baseline value. Likewise, if patient had an abnormal creatinine level before treatment and has an increase of 1 mg/dl within 2 weeks of the next dose, withhold drug until level is within 10% of baseline value.

➲ Multiple myeloma and bone metastases of solid tumors in conjunction with standard antineoplastic therapy; prostate cancer that has progressed after treatment with at least one course of hormonal therapy
Adults: 4 mg I.V. infused over at least 15 minutes q 3 to 4 weeks. Treatment may last 15 months for prostate cancer, 12 months for breast cancer and multiple myeloma, and 9 months for other solid tumors.

For patients with creatinine clearance of 50 to 60 ml/minute, give 3.5 mg. If 40 to 49 ml/minute, give 3.3 mg. If 30 to 39 ml/minute, give 3 mg. For patients with normal baseline creatinine level but an increase of 0.5 mg/dl and in those with abnormal baseline creatinine level who have an increase of 1 mg/dl, withhold drug. Resume treatment only when creatinine level has returned to within 10% of baseline value.

Contraindications & cautions

- Contraindicated in patients hypersensitive to drug, other bisphosphonates, or ingredients in formulation.
- Contraindicated in patients with hypercalcemia of malignancy whose creatinine level is more than 4.5 mg/dl and in patients with bone metastases whose creatinine level is more than 3 mg/dl.
- Contraindicated in breast-feeding women.
- Use cautiously in patients with aspirin-sensitive asthma because other bisphosphonates have been linked to bronchoconstriction in aspirin-sensitive patients with asthma.
- Use cautiously in elderly patients.

Adverse reactions

Hypercalcemia
CNS: headache, somnolence, *anxiety*, confusion, agitation, *insomnia*, *fever*.
CV: hypotension.
GI: *nausea*, *constipation*, *diarrhea*, *abdominal pain*, *vomiting*, anorexia, dysphagia.
GU: ***decreased creatinine level***, *urinary infection*, *candidiasis*.
Hematologic: ANEMIA, ***granulocytopenia***, ***thrombocytopenia***, ***thrombocytopenia***.
Metabolic: *decreased calcium, phosphate, and magnesium levels*, dehydration.
Musculoskeletal: *skeletal pain*, arthralgia.
Respiratory: *dyspnea*, *cough*, pleural effusion.
Other: *progression of cancer*, infection.
Bone metastases
CNS: *headache*, anxiety, *insomnia*, *depression*, *paresthesia*, *hypoesthesia*, *fatigue*, *weakness*, *dizziness*, *fever*.
CV: *hypotension*, *leg edema*.
GI: *nausea*, *constipation*, *diarrhea*, *abdominal pain*, *vomiting*, *anorexia*, *increased appetite*.
GU: ***decreased creatinine level***, *urinary infection*.
Hematologic: *anemia*, ***neutropenia***.
Metabolic: *decreased calcium, phosphate, and magnesium levels*, *dehydration*, *weight decrease*.

Musculoskeletal: *skeletal pain, arthralgia, myalgia, back pain,* osteonecrosis of the jaw.
Respiratory: *dyspnea, cough.*
Skin: alopecia, dermatitis.
Other: PROGRESSION OF CANCER, *rigors,* infection.

Interactions

Drug-drug. *Aminoglycosides, loop diuretics:* May have additive effects that lower calcium level. Use together cautiously, and monitor calcium level.
Thalidomide: May increase risk of renal dysfunction in patients with multiple myeloma. Use together cautiously.

Nursing considerations

- Make sure patient is adequately hydrated before giving drug; urine output should be about 2 L daily.
- Each vial also contains 220 mg mannitol and 24 mg sodium citrate.

!!ALERT Because of the risk of a decline in renal function that could progress to renal failure, single doses shouldn't exceed 4 mg and infusion should last at least 15 minutes.

- No acute overdoses reported, but rapid infusion and high doses may increase risk of renal toxicity. Overdose may cause hypocalcemia, hypophosphatemia, and hypomagnesemia.
- Monitor calcium, phosphate, magnesium, and creatinine levels carefully after giving drug. Correct calcium, phosphorus, and magnesium level reductions by I.V. administration of calcium gluconate, potassium and sodium phosphate, and magnesium sulfate.
- Monitor renal function closely. Drug is excreted mainly through kidneys. The risk of adverse reactions may be greater in patients with impaired renal function; give drug to these patients only if benefits outweigh risks.
- Drug is used cautiously in elderly patients because of the greater likelihood of disease, additional drug therapy, and decreased hepatic, renal, or cardiac function.

!!ALERT Patients should have a dental exam with appropriate preventive dentistry before being treated with bisphosphonates, especially those with risk factors including cancer, receiving chemotherapy or corticosteroids, or those with poor oral hygiene.

- Give patients an oral calcium supplement of 500 mg and a multiple vitamin containing 400 IU of vitamin D daily.

Patient teaching

- Review the use and administration of drug with patient and family.
- Instruct patient to report adverse effects promptly.
- Explain the importance of periodic laboratory tests to monitor therapy and renal function.
- Advise woman to alert prescriber if she is pregnant or breast-feeding.

zolmitriptan
Zomig, Zomig ZMT

Pregnancy risk category C

Indications & dosages

➲ Acute migraine headaches
Adults: Initially, 2.5 mg or less P.O., increased to 5 mg per dosage, p.r.n. Or, disintegrating tablets: initially, 2.5 mg P.O. Don't break tablets in half. Or, 1 spray (5 mg) into nostril. If headache returns after first dose, give a second dose at least 2 hours after the first dose. Maximum dosage is 10 mg in 24 hours.

In patients with hepatic disease, use doses less than 2.5 mg. Don't use orally disintegrating tablets because they shouldn't be broken in half, or nasal spray because 5 mg is the lowest deliverable dose.

Contraindications & cautions

- Contraindicated in patients hypersensitive to drug or its components, pregnant or breast-feeding patients, and those with uncontrolled hypertension, hemiplegic or basilar migraine, ischemic heart disease (angina pectoris, history of MI or documented silent ischemia), symptoms of ischemic heart disease (coronary artery vasospasm, including Prinzmetal's variant angina) or other significant heart disease.
- Contraindicated within 24 hours of other 5-HT_1 agonists or drugs containing ergot or within 2 weeks of stopping MAO inhibitor.
- Use cautiously in patients with liver disease and in those who may be at risk for

coronary artery disease (such as postmenopausal women or men older than age 40) or those with risk factors such as hypertension, hypercholesterolemia, obesity, diabetes, smoking, or family history.

Adverse reactions

CNS: somnolence, vertigo, *dizziness*, hypesthesia, paresthesia, asthenia, pain.
CV: palpitations, ***coronary artery vasospasm, transient myocardial ischemia, MI, ventricular tachycardia, ventricular fibrillation***, pain, tightness, pressure, or heaviness in chest.
EENT: *pain, tightness, or pressure in the neck, throat, or jaw.*
GI: dry mouth, dyspepsia, dysphagia, nausea.
Musculoskeletal: myalgia, myasthenia.
Skin: sweating.
Other: warm or cold sensations.

Interactions

Drug-drug. *Cimetidine:* May double half-life of zolmitriptan. Monitor patient closely.
Ergot-containing drugs, 5-HT$_1$ agonists: May cause additive effects. Avoid using within 24 hours of almotriptan.
Hormonal contraceptives, propranolol: May increase zolmitriptan level. Monitor patient closely.
MAO inhibitors: May increase zolmitriptan level. Avoid using within 2 weeks of MAO inhibitor.
SSRIs: May cause additive serotonin effects, resulting in weakness, hyperreflexia, or incoordination. Monitor patient closely if given together.

Nursing considerations

- Drug isn't intended for preventing migraines or treating hemiplegic or basilar migraines.
- Safety of drug hasn't been established for cluster headaches.

Patient teaching

- Tell patient that drug is intended to relieve, not prevent, signs and symptoms of migraine.
- Advise patient to take drug as prescribed and not to take a second dose unless instructed by prescriber. Tell patient if a second dose is indicated and permitted, he should take it 2 hours after first dose.
- Instruct patient to release the orally disintegrating tablets from the blister pack just before taking; tablet should dissolve on tongue.
- Advise patient not to break the orally disintegrating tablets in half.
- Advise patient to immediately report pain or tightness in the chest or throat, heart throbbing, rash, skin lumps, or swelling of the face, lips, or eyelids.
- Tell patient not to take drug if she is or may become pregnant.

zolpidem tartrate
Ambien

Pregnancy risk category B
Controlled substance schedule IV

Indications & dosages

➲ Short-term management of insomnia
Adults: 10 mg P.O. immediately before h.s.
Elderly patients: 5 mg P.O. immediately before h.s. Maximum daily dose is 10 mg.

For debilitated patients and those with hepatic insufficiency, 5 mg P.O. immediately before h.s. Maximum daily dose is 10 mg.

Contraindications & cautions

- No known contraindications.
- Use cautiously in patients with compromised respiratory status.

Adverse reactions

CNS: daytime drowsiness, lightheadedness, change in dreams, amnesia, dizziness, *headache*, hangover, sleep disorder, nervousness, lethargy, depression.
CV: palpitations.
EENT: sinusitis, pharyngitis.
GI: nausea, vomiting, dry mouth, diarrhea, dyspepsia, constipation, abdominal pain.
Musculoskeletal: myalgia, arthralgia.
Skin: rash.
Other: back or chest pain, flulike syndrome, hypersensitivity reactions.

Interactions

Drug-drug. *CNS depressants:* May cause excessive CNS depression. Use together cautiously.
Rifampin: May decrease effects of zolpidem. Avoid using together, if possible. Consider alternative hypnotic.

Drug-lifestyle. *Alcohol use:* May cause excessive CNS depression. Discourage use together.

Nursing considerations

- Use hypnotics only for short-term management of insomnia, usually 7 to 10 days.
- Use the smallest effective dose in all patients.
- Take precautions to prevent hoarding or overdosing by patients who are depressed, suicidal, or drug-dependent or who have history of drug abuse.

!!ALERT Don't confuse Ambien with Amen.

Patient teaching

- For rapid sleep onset, instruct patient not to take drug with or immediately after meals.
- Instruct patient to take drug immediately before going to bed; onset of action is rapid.
- Tell patient to avoid alcohol use while taking drug.
- Caution patient to avoid performing activities that require mental alertness or physical coordination during therapy.

zonisamide

Zonegran

Pregnancy risk category C

Indications & dosages

➲ **Adjunct therapy for partial seizures in adults with epilepsy**

Adults and children older than age 16: Initially, 100 mg P.O. as a single daily dose for 2 weeks. Then, dosage may be increased to 200 mg daily for at least 2 weeks. Dosage can be increased to 300 mg and 400 mg P.O. daily, with the dose stable for at least 2 weeks to achieve steady state at each level. Doses can be given once or twice daily except for the daily dose of 100 mg at start of therapy. Maximum dose is 600 mg daily.

Contraindications & cautions

- Contraindicated in patients hypersensitive to drug or to sulfonamides.
- Contraindicated in those with glomerular filtration rate less than 50 ml/minute.
- Use cautiously in patients with renal and hepatic dysfunction.
- Use cautiously with other drugs that predispose patients to heat-related disorders, including but not limited to carbonic anhydrase inhibitors and drugs with anticholinergic activity.
- Safety and efficacy in children younger than age 16 haven't been established. Children are at increased risk for oligohidrosis and hyperthermia caused by zonisamide.

Adverse reactions

CNS: *headache, dizziness,* ataxia, nystagmus, paresthesia, confusion, difficulties in concentration or memory, mental slowing, agitation or irritability, depression, insomnia, anxiety, nervousness, schizophrenic or schizophreniform behavior, *somnolence,* fatigue, asthenia, speech disorders, difficulties in verbal expression, hyperesthesia, incoordination, tremor, ***seizures, status epilepticus.***
EENT: taste perversion, diplopia, amblyopia, tinnitus, rhinitis, pharyngitis.
GI: *anorexia,* nausea, vomiting, diarrhea, dyspepsia, constipation, dry mouth, abdominal pain.
GU: kidney stones.
Hematologic: ecchymoses.
Metabolic: weight loss.
Respiratory: cough.
Skin: rash, pruritus.
Other: flulike syndrome, accidental injury.

Interactions

Drug-drug. *Drugs that induce or inhibit CYP3A4:* Changes zonisamide level; phenytoin, carbamazepine, phenobarbital, and valproate increase zonisamide clearance-.Monitor patient closely.

Nursing considerations

!!ALERT Rarely, patients receiving sulfonamides have died because of severe reactions such as Stevens-Johnson syndrome, fulminant hepatic necrosis, aplastic anemia, otherwise unexplained rashes, and agranulocytosis. If signs and symptoms of hypersensitivity or other serious reactions occur, stop drug immediately and notify prescriber.

- If patient develops acute renal failure or a significant sustained increase in creatinine or BUN level, stop drug and notify prescriber.

- Achieving steady-state levels may take 2 weeks.
- Monitor patient for signs and symptoms of hypersensitivity.
- Don't stop drug abruptly because this may cause increased seizures or status epilepticus; reduce dosage or stop drug gradually.
- Increase fluid intake and urine output to help prevent kidney stones, especially in patients with predisposing factors.
- Monitor renal function periodically.

Patient teaching

- Tell patient to take drug with or without food and not to bite or break capsule.
- Advise patient to call prescriber immediately if rash develops or seizures worsen.
- Tell patient to contact prescriber immediately if he develops sudden back or abdominal pain, pain when urinating, bloody or dark urine, fever, sore throat, mouth sores or easy bruising, decreased sweating, fever, depression, or speech or language problems.
- Tell patient to drink 6 to 8 glasses of water a day.
- Caution patient that this drug can cause drowsiness and not to drive or operate dangerous machinery until drug's effects are known.
- Advise patient not to stop taking drug without prescriber's approval.
- Instruct woman of childbearing age to call prescriber if she is pregnant or breastfeeding or plans to become pregnant or breast-feed.
- Advise woman of childbearing age to use contraceptives while taking drug.

Index

B

C

D

E

F

G

H

I

JK

L

M

N

Q

R

S

T

U

V

W

X

YZ